The Child's Foot

MIHRAN O. TACHDJIAN, M.S., M.D.

Professor of Orthopedic Surgery
Northwestern University Medical School
Chicago, Illinois

1985   W.B. SAUNDERS COMPANY
Philadelphia / London / Toronto / Mexico City / Rio de Janeiro / Sydney / Tokyo

W. B. Saunders Company: West Washington Square
Philadelphia, PA 19105

1 St. Anne's Road
Eastbourne, East Sussex BN21 3UN, England

1 Goldthorne Avenue
Toronto, Ontario M8Z 5T9, Canada

Apartado 26370—Cedro 512
Mexico 4, D.F., Mexico

Rua Coronel Cabrita, 8
Sao Cristovao Caixa Postal 21176
Rio de Janeiro, Brazil

9 Waltham Street
Artarmon, N.S.W. 2064, Australia

Ichibancho, Central Bldg., 22-1 Ichibancho
Chiyoda-Ku, Tokyo 102, Japan

Library of Congress Cataloging in Publication Data

Tachdjian, Mihran O.

The child's foot.

1. Foot—Abnormalities. 2. Foot—Diseases. 3. Pediatric orthopedia. I. Title. [DNLM: 1. Foot—Abnormalities. 2. Foot diseases—In infancy and childhood. WE 880 T117c]

RD781.T33	618.92′097585	81-48522
ISBN 0-7216-8734-2		AACR2

The Child's Foot ISBN 0-7216-8734-2

© 1985 by W. B. Saunders Company. Copyright under the Uniform Copyright Convention. Simultaneously published in Canada. All rights reserved. This book is protected by copyright. No part of it may be reproduced, stored in a retrieval system, or transmitted in any form or by any means, electronic, mechanical, photocopying, recording, or otherwise, without written permission from the publisher. Made in the United States of America. Press of W. B. Saunders Company. Library of Congress catalog card number 81-48522.

Last digit is the print number: 9   8   7   6   5   4   3   2   1

Dedicated to Mr. John L. Dusseau, whose intuitive critique, intellectual stimulation, and support have elevated the art of medical writing and publishing.

Preface

The purpose of this book is to provide the reader with a comprehensive presentation of progress made in the orthopedic care of children's foot disorders. It is primarily intended as a guide for the orthopedic resident-in-training, the orthopedic surgeon in practice, and all those who are concerned with the care of the child's foot. It is also hoped that, as a reference work, this book will make available information that will assist the radiologist, the pediatrician, and the general practitioner.

The foot is subject to a wide range of malformations and disease states; its response to them serves as a mirror of the protean affections of the neuromusculoskeletal system. Therefore it is imperative to assess the whole child and not to examine and treat the foot alone. With this objective in mind, Chapter 1 presents details of examination of the foot and of the entire patient. Color drawings of the anatomy of the foot are given to complement descriptions of operative technique. Chapter 2 deals with congenital deformities, and Chapter 3 with neuromuscular affections of the foot. Complex problems of flat foot and pes cavus are presented in Chapters 4 and 5. Chapter 6 discusses the acquired affections of the foot.

Great strides have been made in understanding of the pathogenesis of and in treatment of deformities of the foot. Despite significant progress, however, many controversial issues still remain. For example, on congenital talipes equinovarus, does the primary deformity stem from a defect of the cartilaginous anlage of the talus or from an intrauterine neuromuscular disorder or a contracture of the ligamentous tissues? What is the value of roentgenographic assessment? In nonoperative treatment of clubfoot, should one correct all elements of the contractural deformity simultaneously, or should one correct deformities sequentially? What kind of retentive device should one use? Jones adhesive strapping or cast? How long should one persist in nonoperative treatment? Should one operate in the neonatal period or at two to three months of age, or at six months and older? What are the primary obstacles to anatomic realignment of the talocalcaneonavicular joint? What is the best surgical approach, the transverse Cincinnati incision or posteromedial and lateral incisions?

This author has attempted to present his personal posture and philosophy of care in the various gray areas of management. Basic principles and guidelines of treatment are presented along with indications and prerequisites for and contraindications to operative procedures. Diligent postoperative care is crucial because the result of an operation is often dependent on the adequacy of aftercare.

Many thanks to the W. B. Saunders Company, particularly to Miss Ruth Barker for her editorial assistance and to Mr. Albert Meier for his support and patience in completion of this work. I especially thank Mr. Ernie Beck for his superb medical art work and would like to extend my deep gratitude to Ms. Lynn Ridings for her editorial and secretarial support.

Contents

1
INTRODUCTION 1
  Anatomy and Biomechanics 1
  Development and Ossification of the Foot and Leg 39
  Diagnosis 44
  Growth of the Normal Foot 121
  Normal Variations of the Bones of the Foot and Ankle 123

2
CONGENITAL DEFORMITIES 131
  Postural Deformities of the Foot and Leg 131
  Congenital Talipes Equinovarus 139
  Congenital Convex Pes Valgus 239
  Tarsal Coalition 261
  Congenital Metatarsus Varus 294
  Congenital Metatarsus Primus Varus and Hallux Valgus 308
  Congenital Ball-and-Socket Ankle Joint 312
  Brachymetatarsia (Congenital Short Metatarsal) 314
  Congenital Split or Cleft Foot (Lobster Claw) 317
  Polydactylism 323
  Congenital Hallux Varus 329
  Macrodactylism 333
  Miscellaneous Deformities of Toes 335
  Hammer Toe 350
  Mallet Toe 351

3
NEUROMUSCULAR DISEASES 352
  The Foot and Ankle in Neuromuscular Diseases 352
  Cerebral Palsy 358

Myelomeningocele 418
Diastematomyelia 449
Poliomyelitis 451
Peroneal Muscular Atrophy (Charcot-Marie-Tooth Disease) 496
Friedreich's Ataxia (Hereditary Spinocerebellar Ataxia) 500
Hypertrophic Interstitial Neuritis 503
Progressive Muscular Dystrophy 505
Congenital Absence of Muscles 507
Accessory Muscles 508
Congenital Contracture of Triceps Surae Muscle 508
Achilles Tendinitis 509

4
PES CAVUS AND CLAW TOES 510
Pes Cavus 510
Claw Toes 554

5
FLEXIBLE PES PLANOVALGUS (FLAT FOOT) 556

6
ACQUIRED AFFECTIONS OF BONES, JOINTS, AND SOFT TISSUES 598
Infections and Inflammatory Disorders of the Foot 598
    Pyogenic Osteomyelitis 598
    Tuberculosis of Bones and Joints 604
    Suppurative or Septic Arthritis 605
    Juvenile Rheumatoid Arthritis 608
Circulatory Disturbances 610
    Köhler's Disease of the Tarsal Navicular 610
    Freiberg's Infraction 612
    Miscellaneous Osteochondroses 615
    Osteochondritis Dissecans 616
Affections of the Toes 627
    Hallux Rigidus 627
Tumors of the Foot 635
    Soft-Tissue Tumors 635
    Tumors of Bone 655
Skin and Nail Lesions 658
    Hard Corn (Clavus Durus) 658
    Soft Corn (Clavus Mollis) 658
    Plantar Wart (Verruca Plantaris) 659
    Ingrowing Toenail 660
Fractures and Dislocations 660
    Fractures of the Ankle 660
    Fractures of the Foot 700
    Stress Fractures 703

Index 711

1. Introduction

ANATOMY AND BIOMECHANICS

DEVELOPMENT AND OSSIFICATION OF THE FOOT AND LEG

DIAGNOSIS

GROWTH OF THE NORMAL FOOT

NORMAL VARIATIONS OF THE BONES OF THE FOOT AND ANKLE

ANATOMY AND BIOMECHANICS

The human foot has the dual function of supporting the body in stance and propelling it in gait. It consists of three major parts: (1) the hindfoot, which includes the talus, the calcaneus, and the navicular bone; (2) the midfoot, which contains the cuneiform and the cuboid bones; and (3) the forefoot, which is made up of the metatarsals and the phalanges. Some anatomists include the navicular among the bones of the midfoot.

Descriptions of the normal anatomy of the foot and ankle can be found in any textbook of anatomy. For convenience, however, the principal structures of the foot, ankle, and leg are depicted in Figures 1–1 through 1–37.

Architecturally, the skeletal components of the foot form a longitudinal arch, the function of which is to provide a resilient spring during locomotion. This longitudinal arch, highest medially at the midtarsal joint and shallow laterally, where it is limited by the lateral border of the foot that lies flat on the floor, is maintained by the structure and relationship of the bony parts, by the ligaments, and by the muscle tone of the four long plantar muscles—the posterior tibial, flexor digitorum longus, flexor hallucis longus, and peroneus longus.

Articulating in a complex system of multiplaned synovial joints, the components of the foot form a functional unit capable of the complex motions of flexion, rotation, inversion, eversion, and translation. For description and discussion of the mechanics of the human foot, the reader is referred to the cited literature. [1–37]

Text continued on page 39

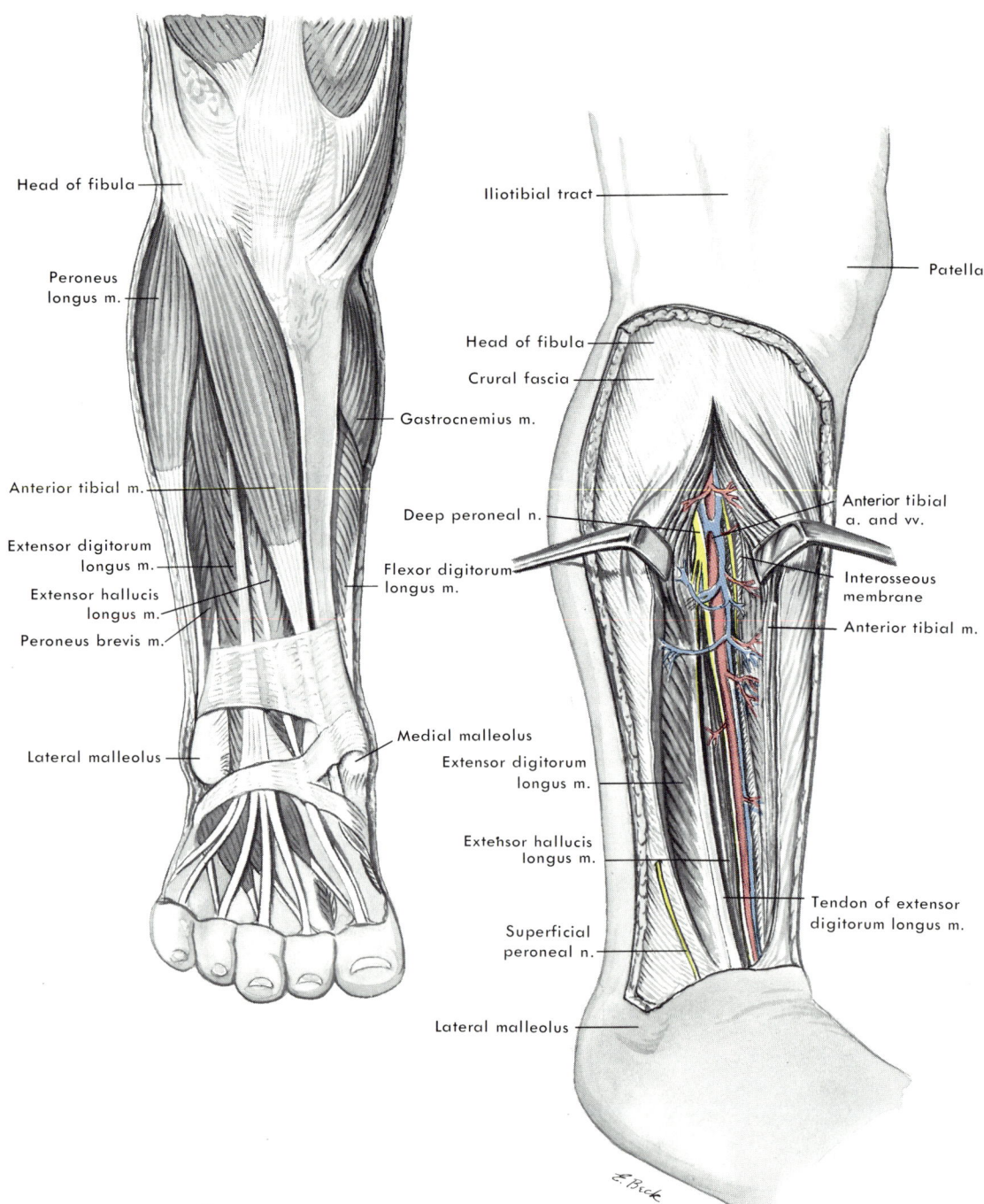

FIGURE 1–1. Muscles and tendons on anterior aspect of right leg and foot.

Dissection of the lateral aspect of the right leg shows the relations of anterior tibial vessels and deep peroneal nerve.

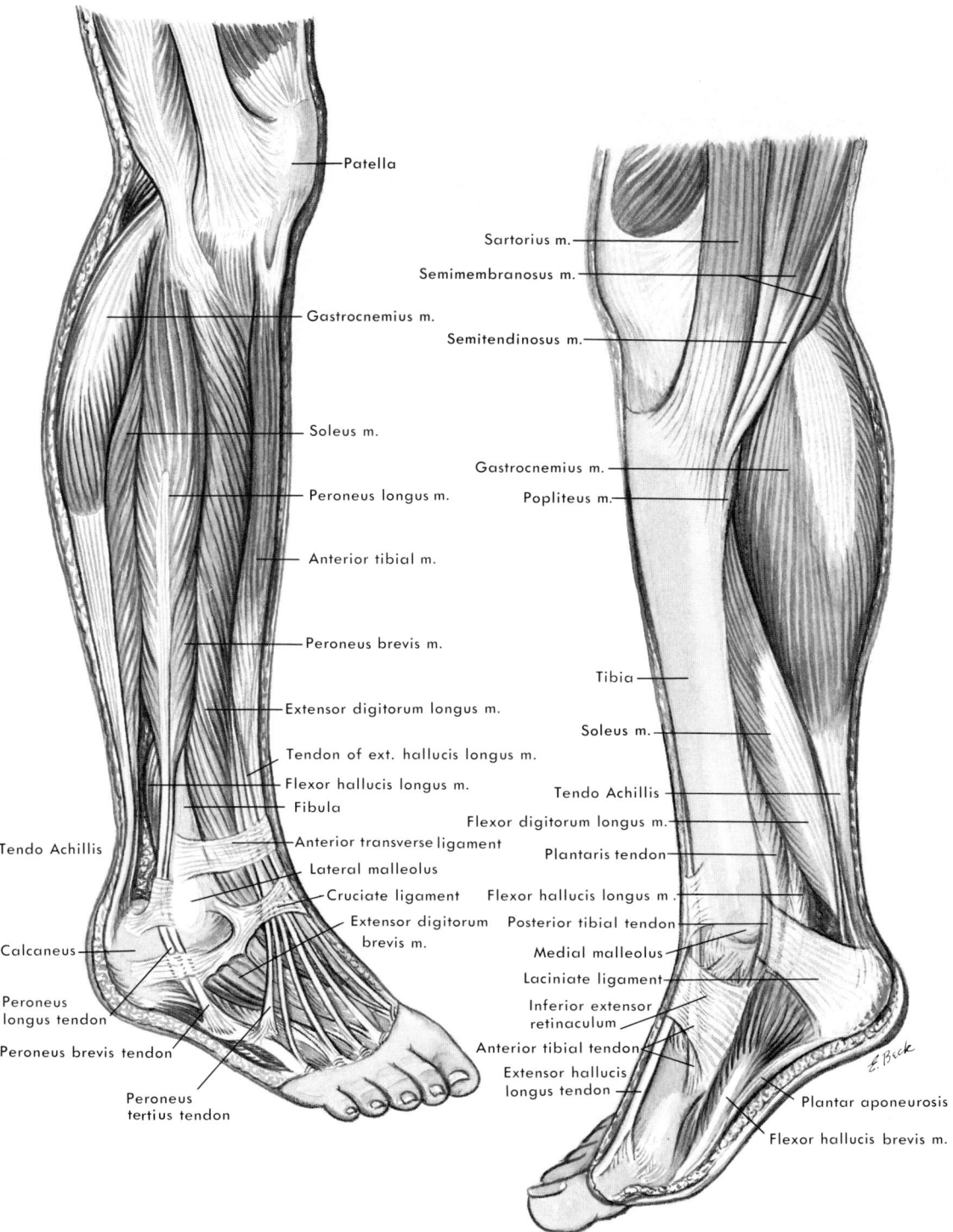

FIGURE 1-2. Muscles of the right leg—lateral and medial aspects.

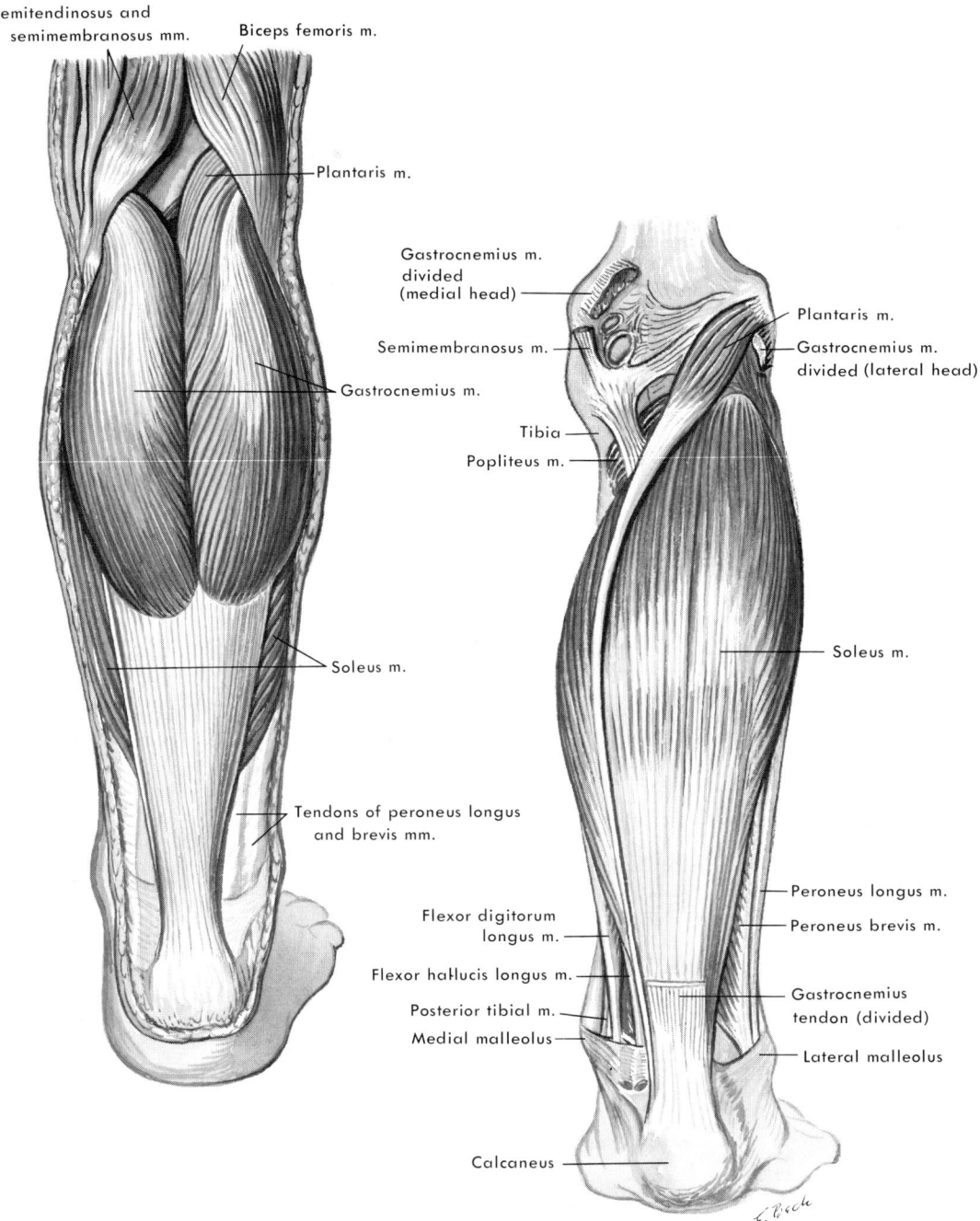

FIGURE 1–3. Muscles of the right calf.
The superficial layer, showing the gastrocnemius muscle and, deep to it, the soleus and plantaris muscles.

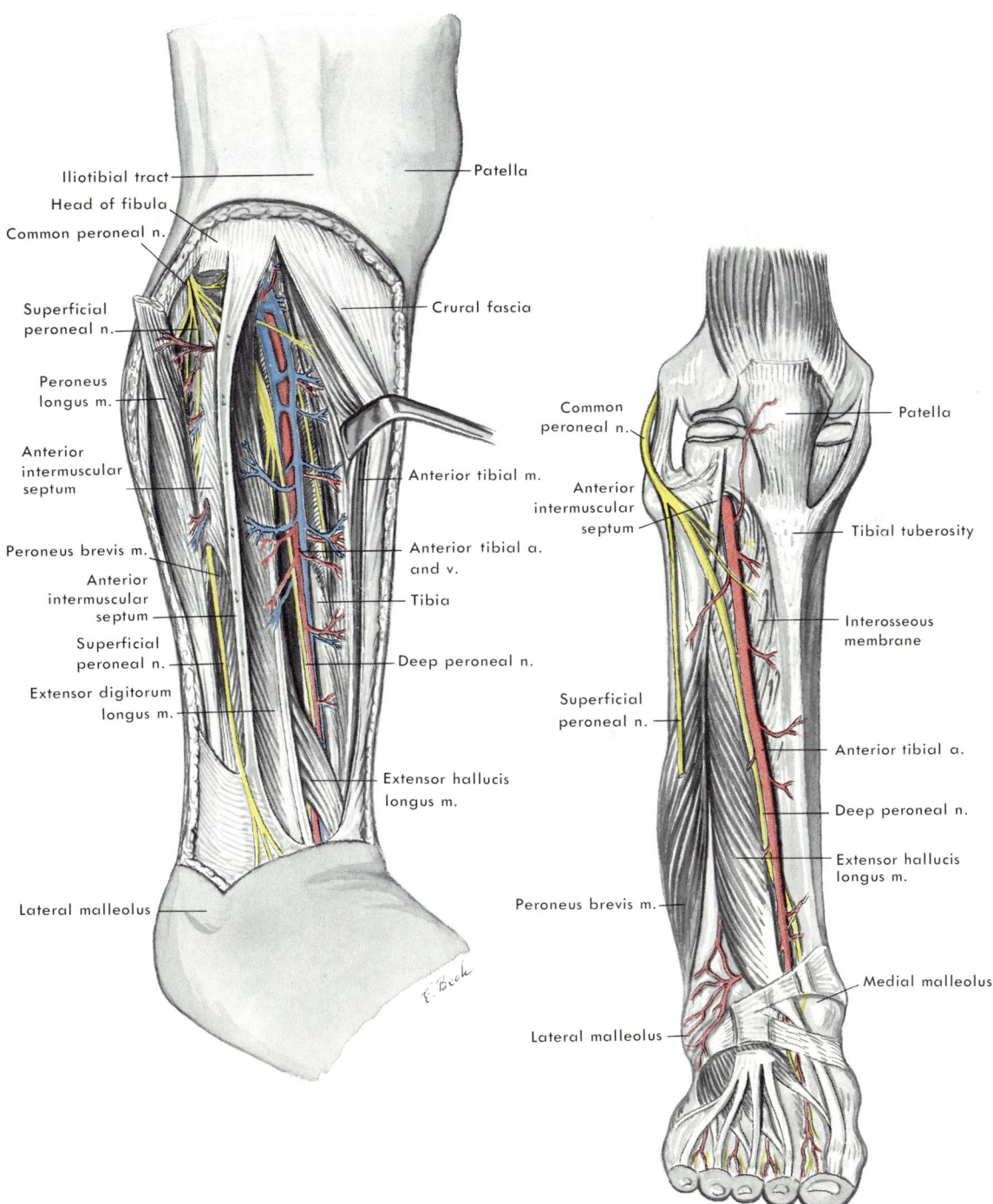

FIGURE 1–4. Dissection of the right leg.

On the lateral aspect the peroneus longus muscle is divided at its origin and retracted posteriorly to show the common peroneal nerve and its subdivision into the superficial and deep peroneal branches; the tibialis anterior is retracted medially to expose the relations of the deep peroneal nerve and the anterior tibial vessels. On the anterior view of the leg, the peroneus longus, anterior tibial, and extensor digitorum longus muscles are excised to demonstrate the course and anatomic relations of the anterior tibial vessels and peroneal nerves.

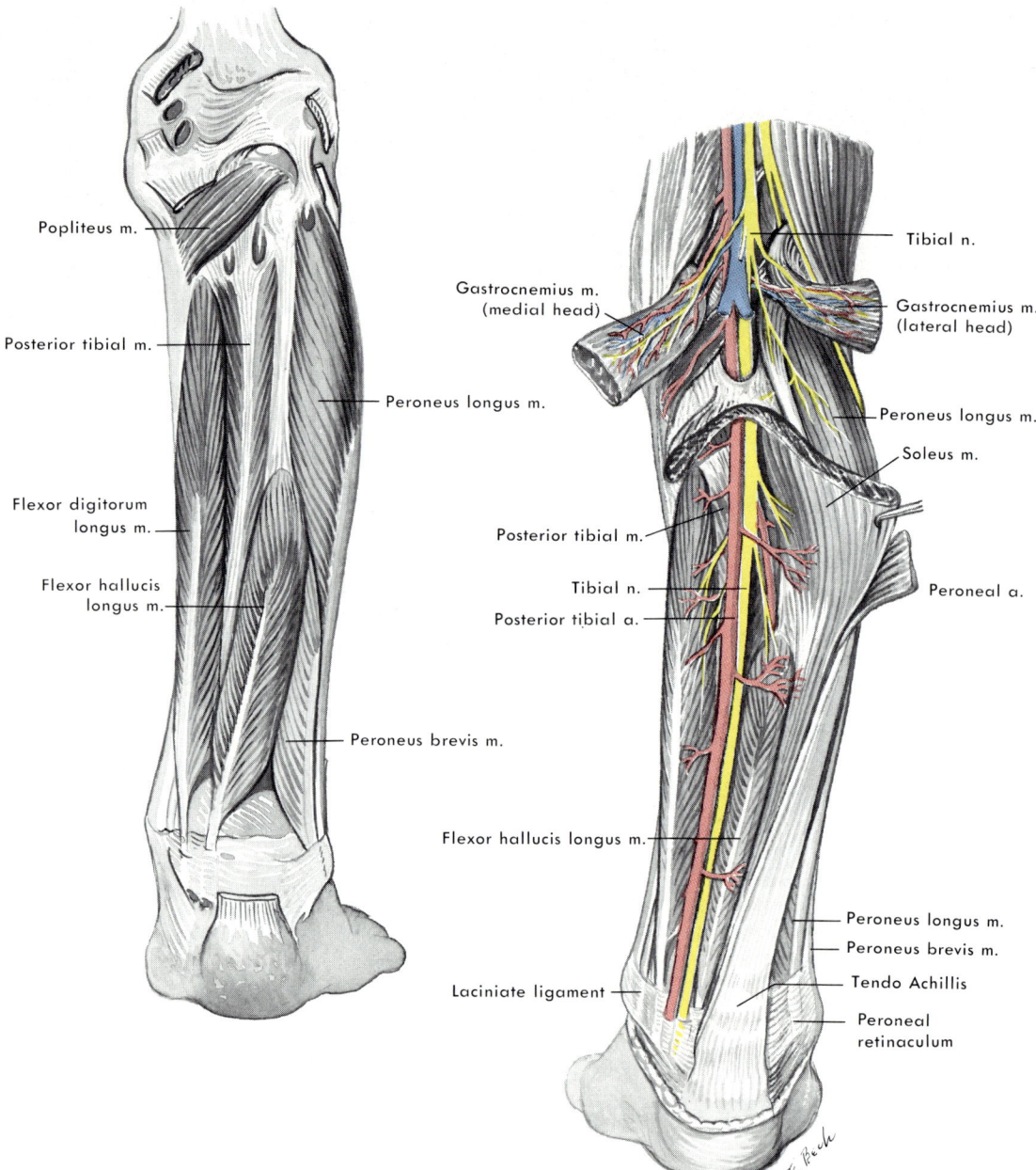

FIGURE 1–5. *Deep posterior crural muscles.*
Dissection of right calf to show tibial nerve and posterior tibial artery.

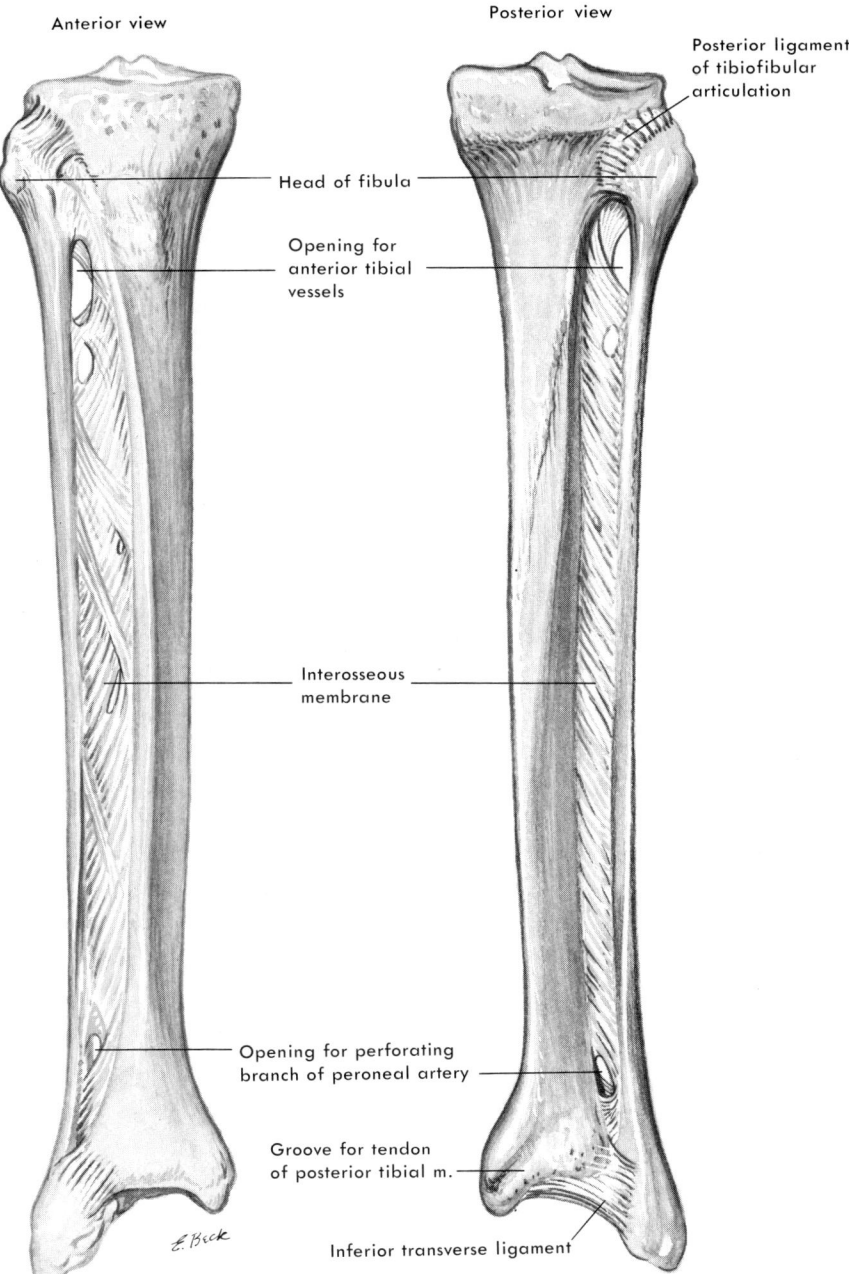

FIGURE 1-6. The crural interosseous membrane—anterior and posterior aspects.

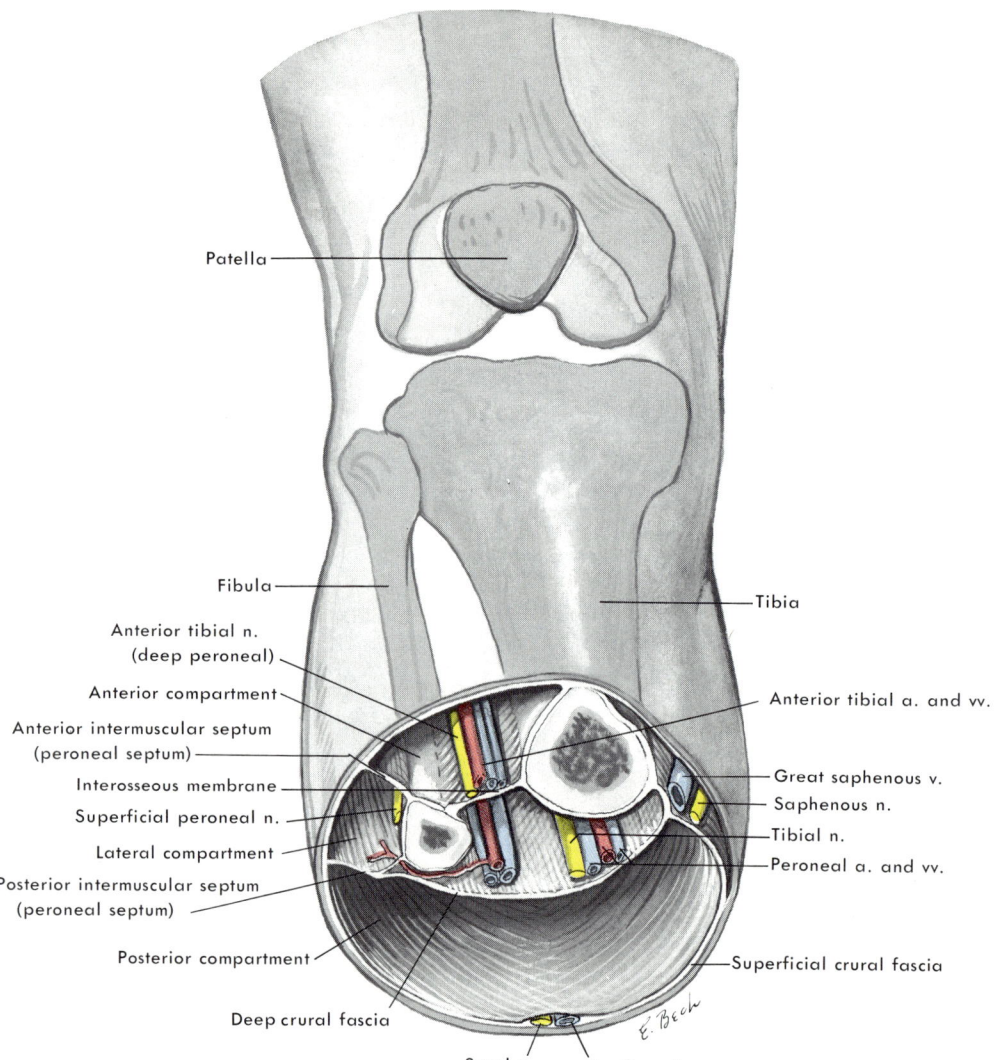

FIGURE 1–7. *Cross section of the leg at the junction of the proximal one third and distal two thirds.* The anterior, lateral, and posterior compartments are shown. Note the relationship of the vessels and nerves.

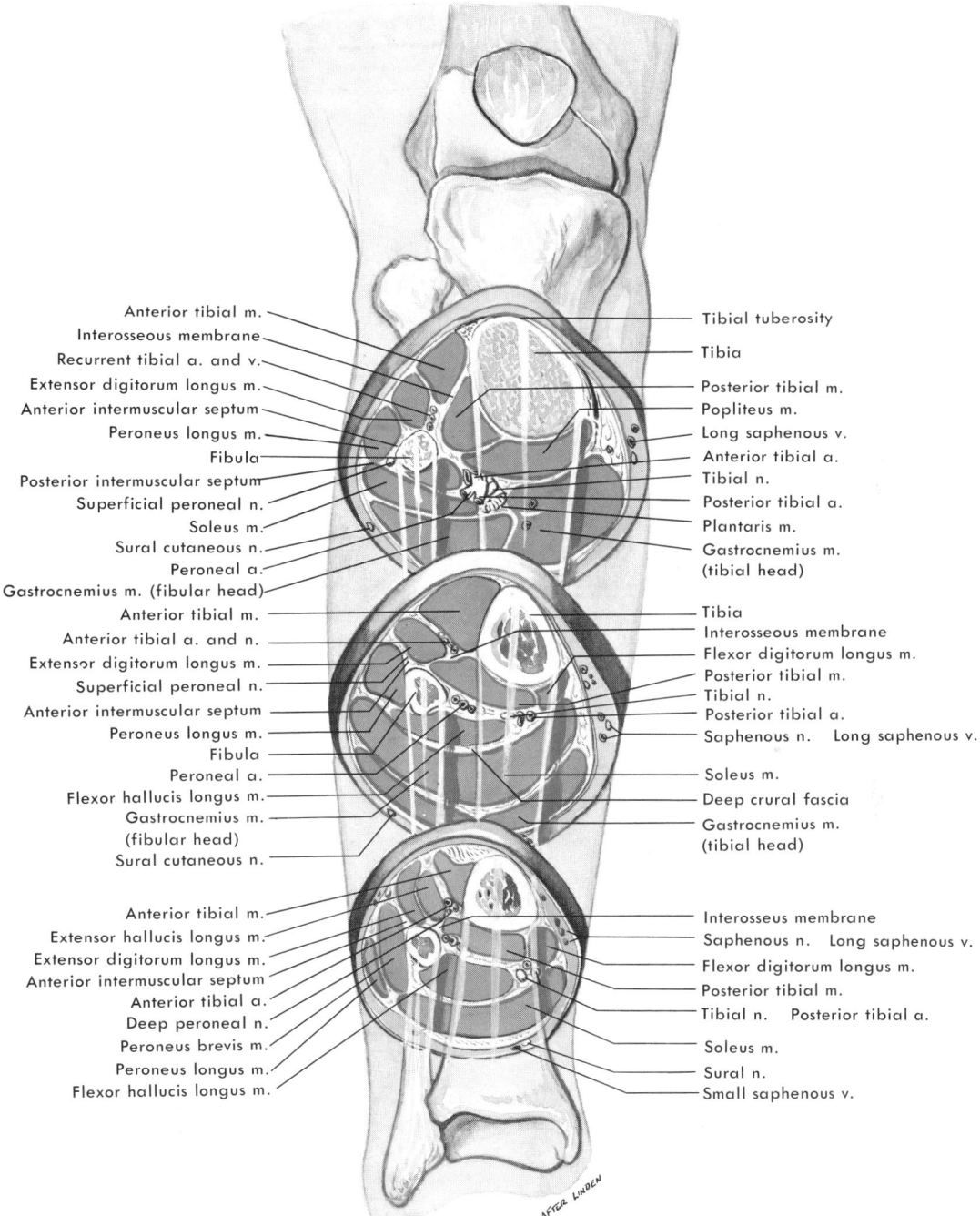

FIGURE 1–8. Cross sections of the right leg at the proximal, middle, and distal thirds.

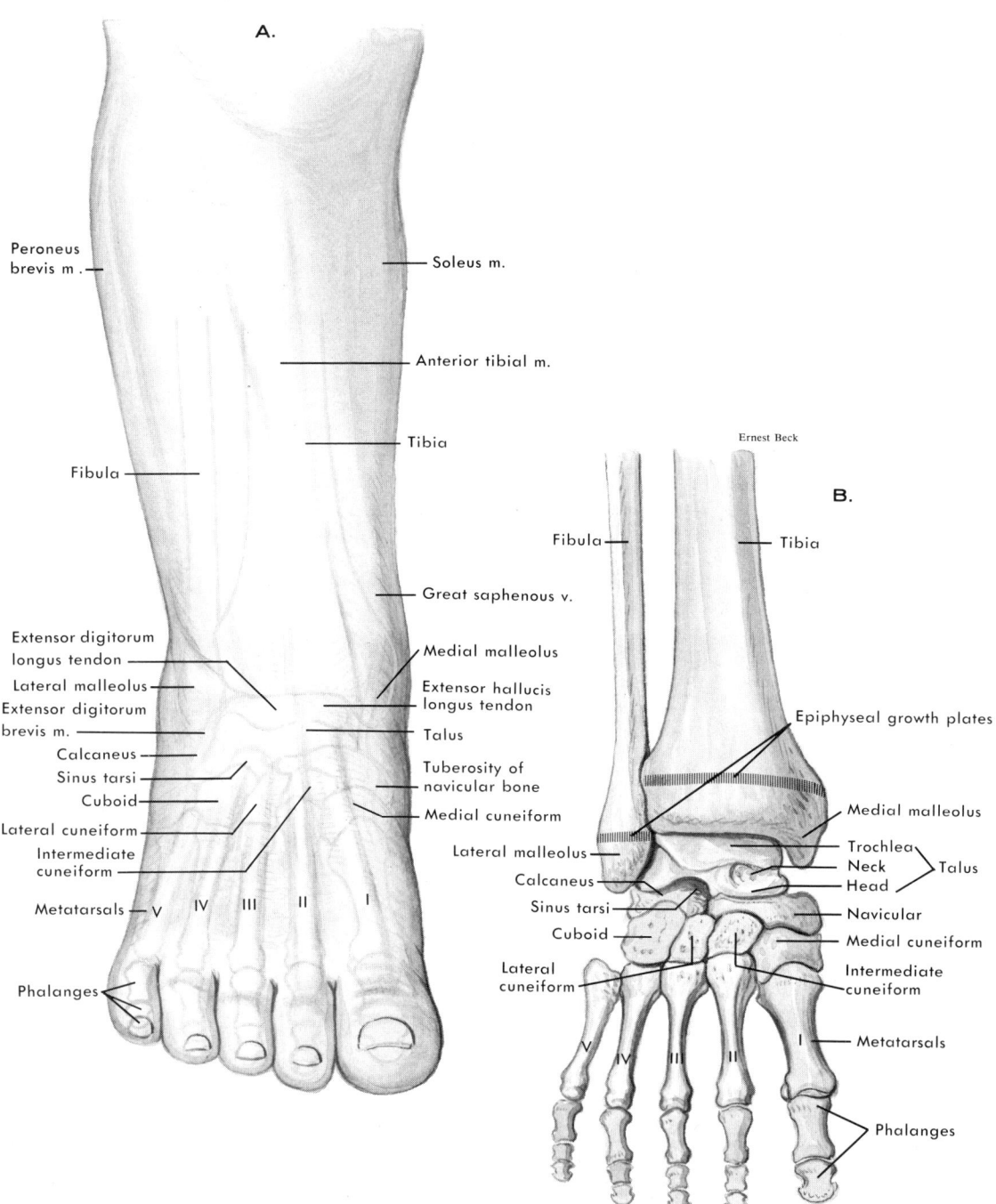

FIGURE 1–9. *The dorsum of the right ankle and foot.*
A. Surface anatomy. **B.** Bony landmarks.

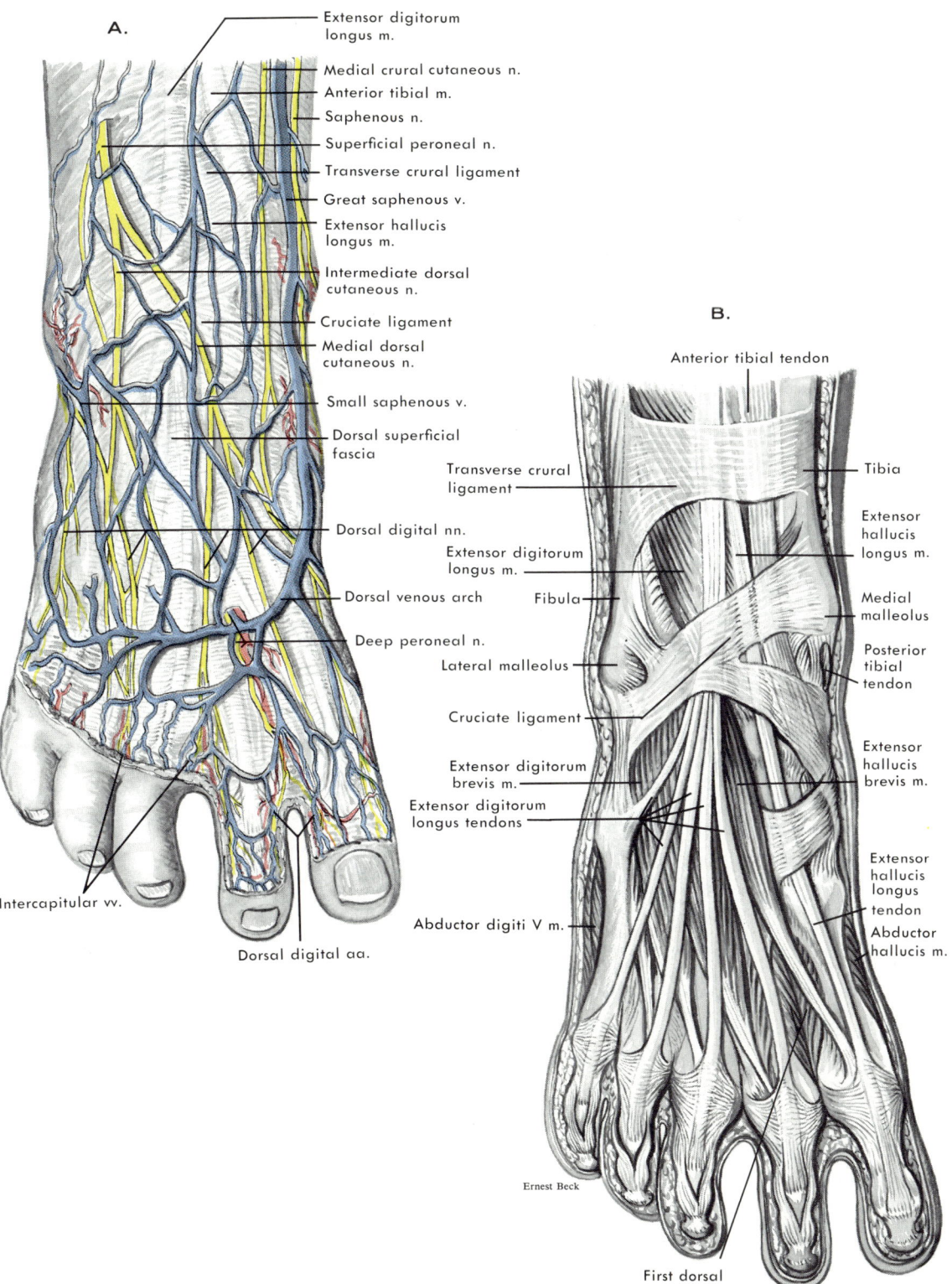

FIGURE 1–10. *The dorsum of the right ankle and foot.*

A. Note the superficial nerves and veins; during surgical exposure one should exercise caution so as not to section them inadvertently. **B.** The long and short extensors of the toes.

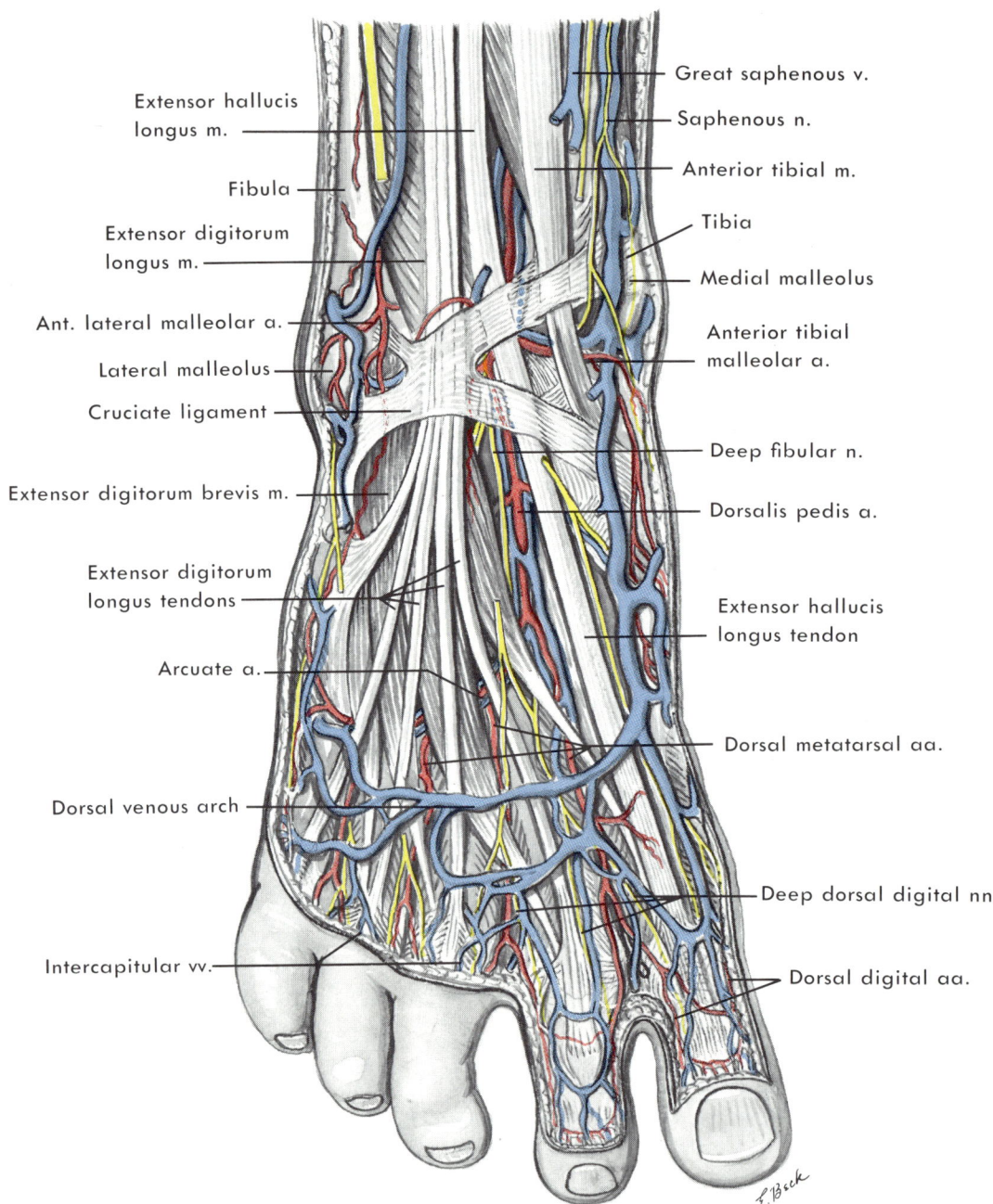

FIGURE 1–11. The dorsum of the right ankle and foot.

The anatomic relations of the superficial vessels and sensory nerves to the extensor tendons and retinacula are shown.

Introduction

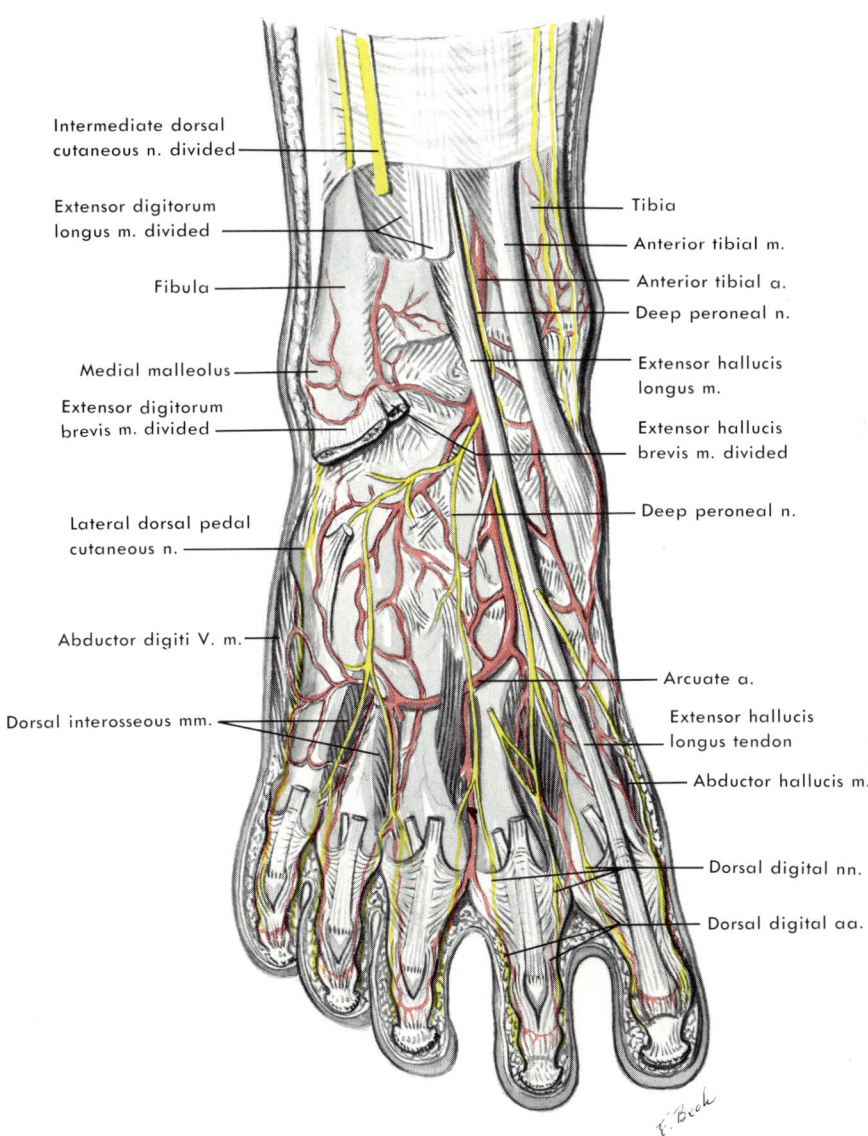

FIGURE 1–12. *Deep vessels and nerves on the dorsal aspect of the right ankle and foot.*

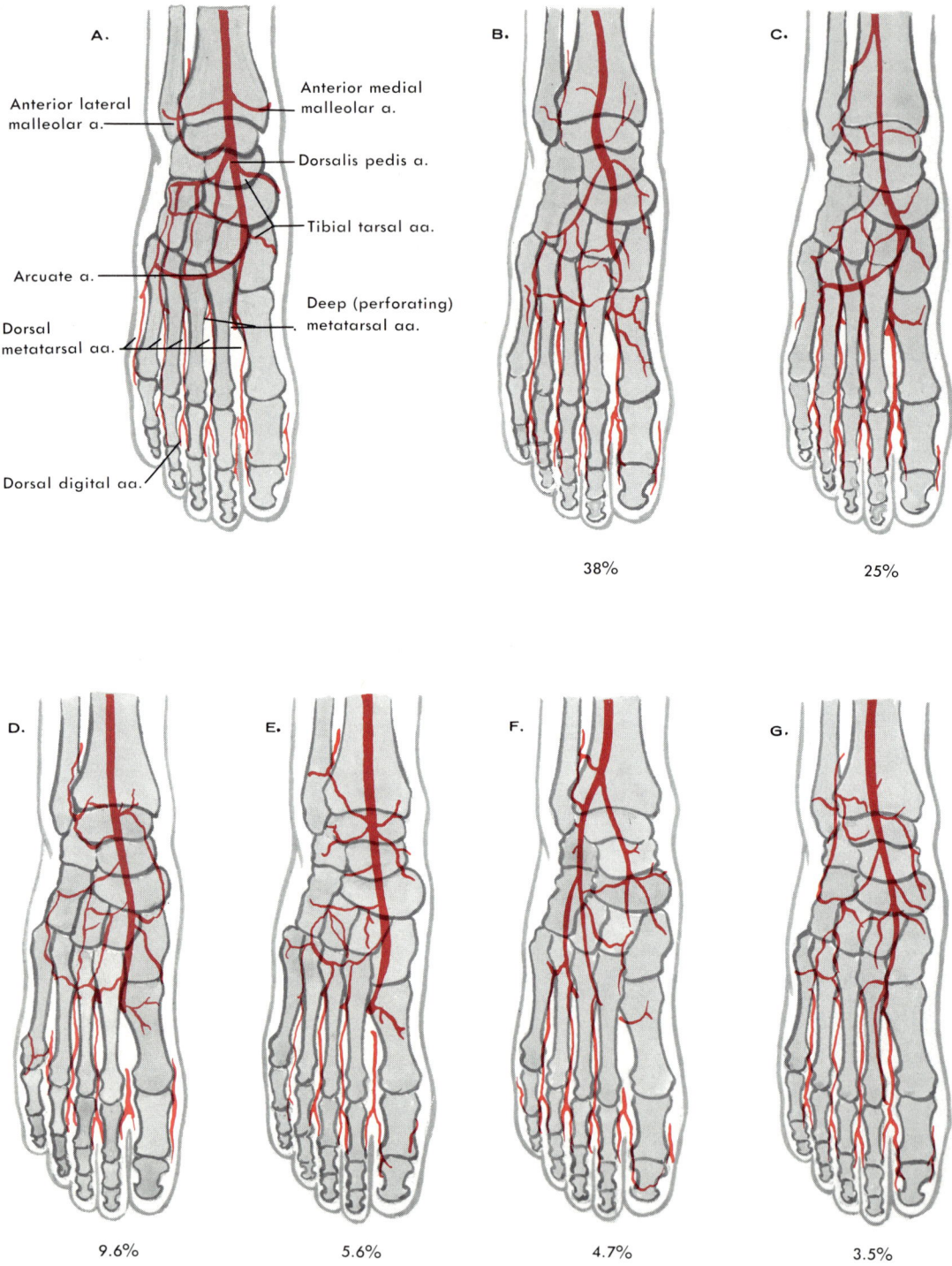

FIGURE 1–13. Variations in origins of metatarsal arteries.

(Adapted from von Lanz, T., and Wachsmuth, W.: Praktische Anatomie. Berlin, Julius Springer, 1938, p. 392.)

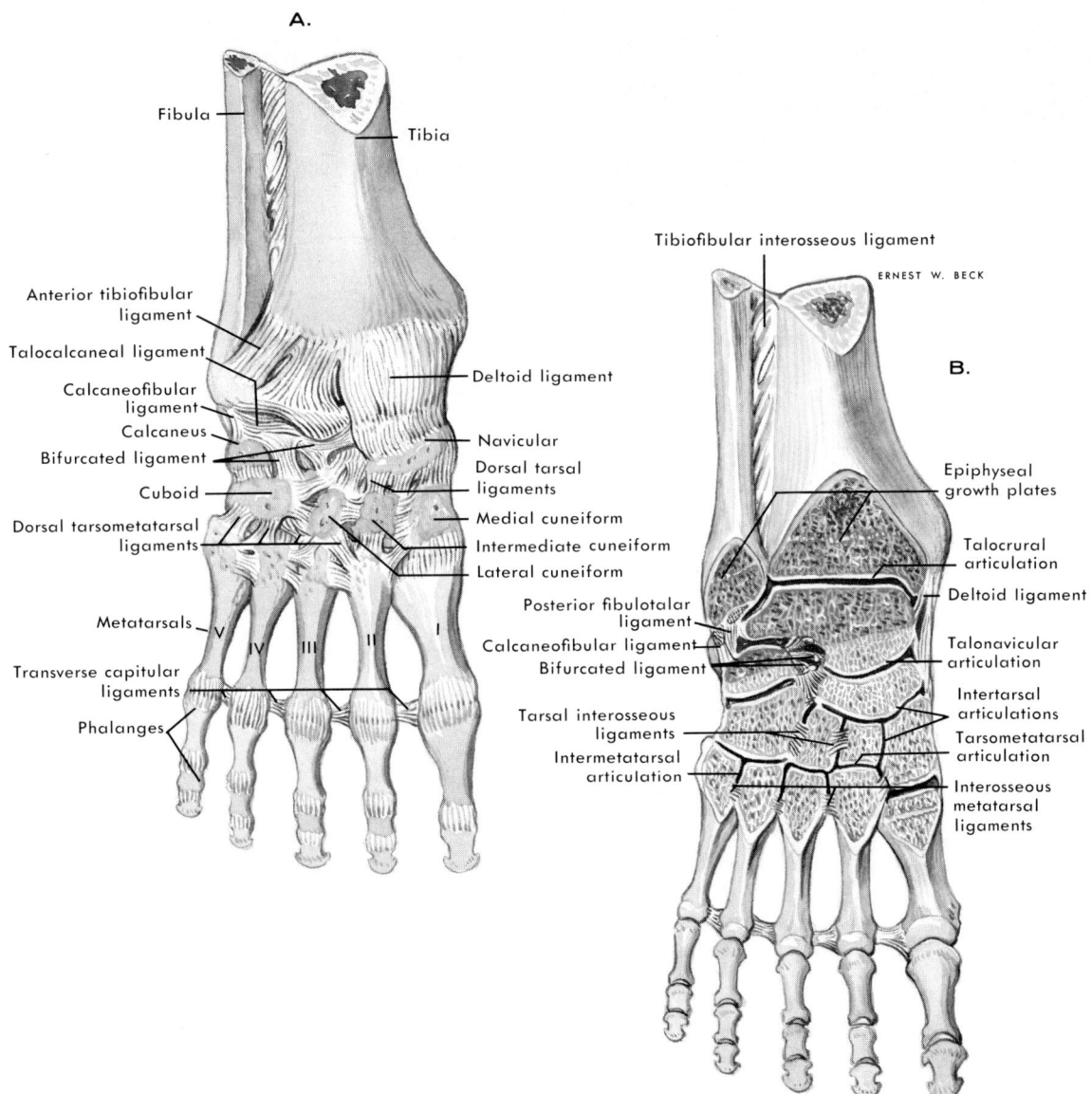

FIGURE 1–14. The dorsum of the right ankle and foot.

Note the ligaments and articulations.

16 *Introduction*

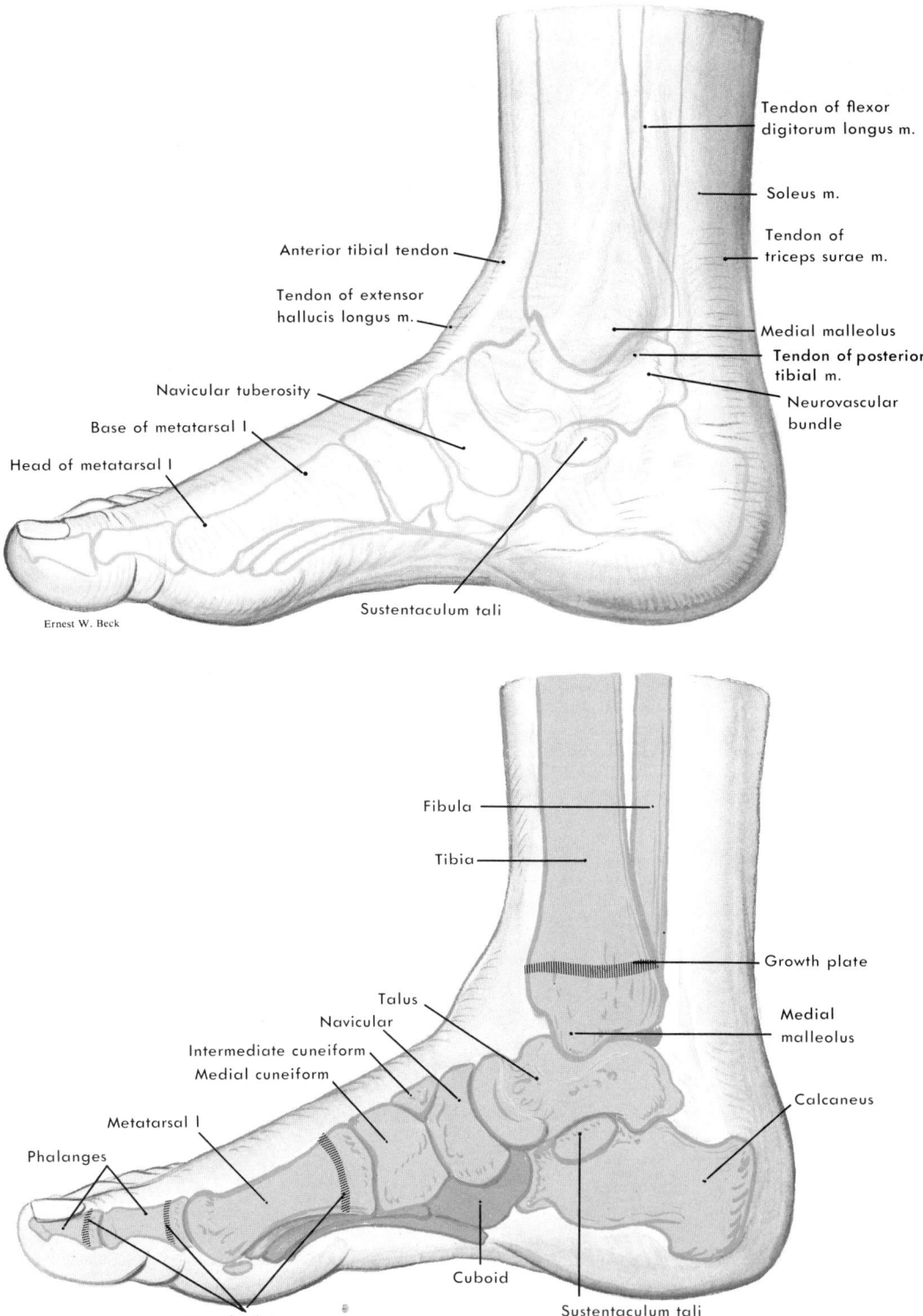

FIGURE 1–15. *Medial aspect of the right ankle and foot.*
Surface anatomy and bony landmarks.

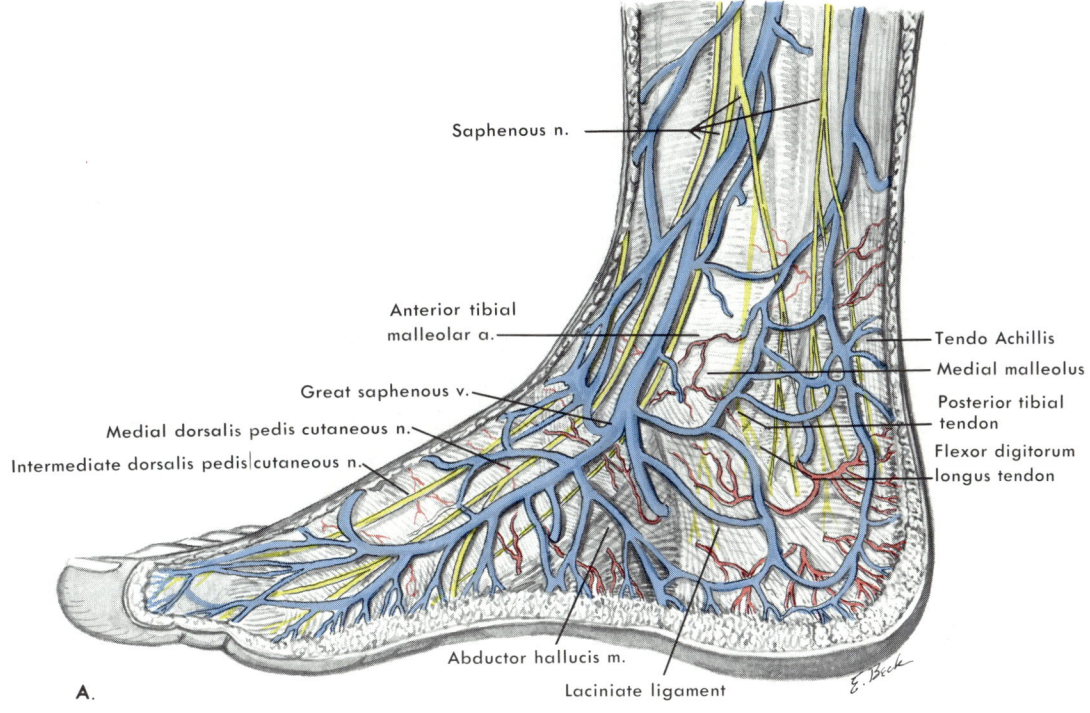

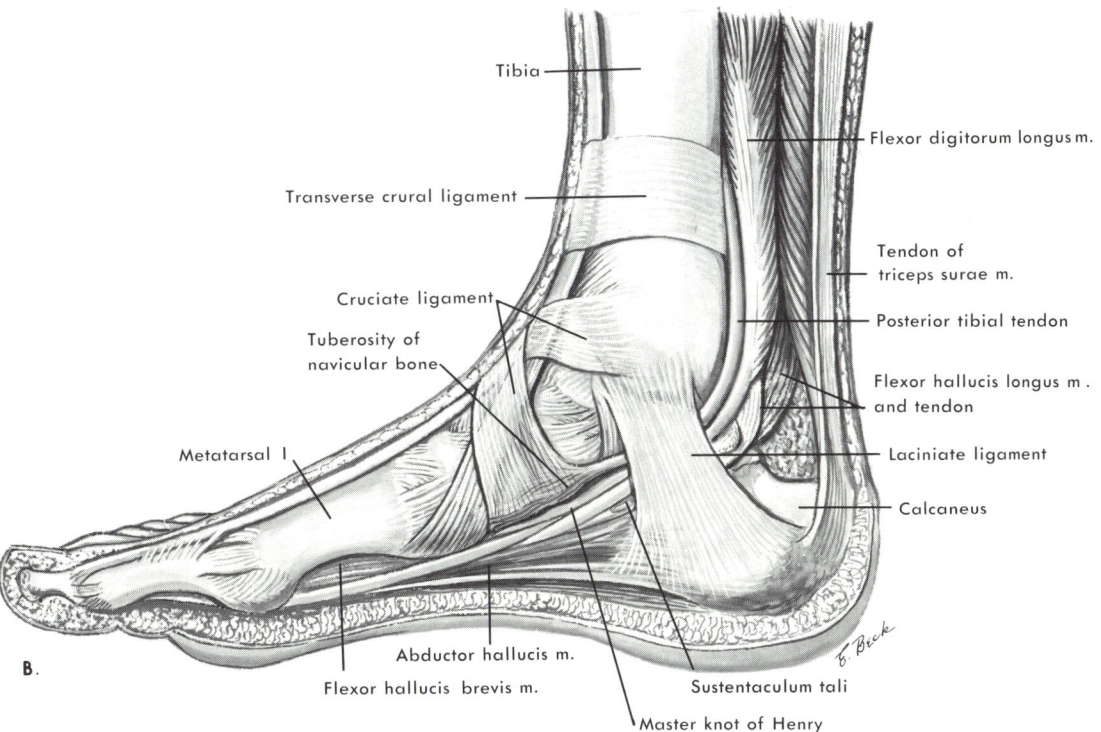

FIGURE 1–16. Medial aspect of the right foot.

A. The superficial veins and sensory nerve. **B.** The anatomic relations of the tendons of the tibialis posterior, flexor digitorum longus, and flexor hallucis longus behind the medial malleolus and as they enter the plantar aspect of the foot deep to the laciniate ligament (or flexor retinaculum). A thick fibrous band (the master knot of Henry) binds the flexor digitorum longus and flexor hallucis longus tendons to the navicular.

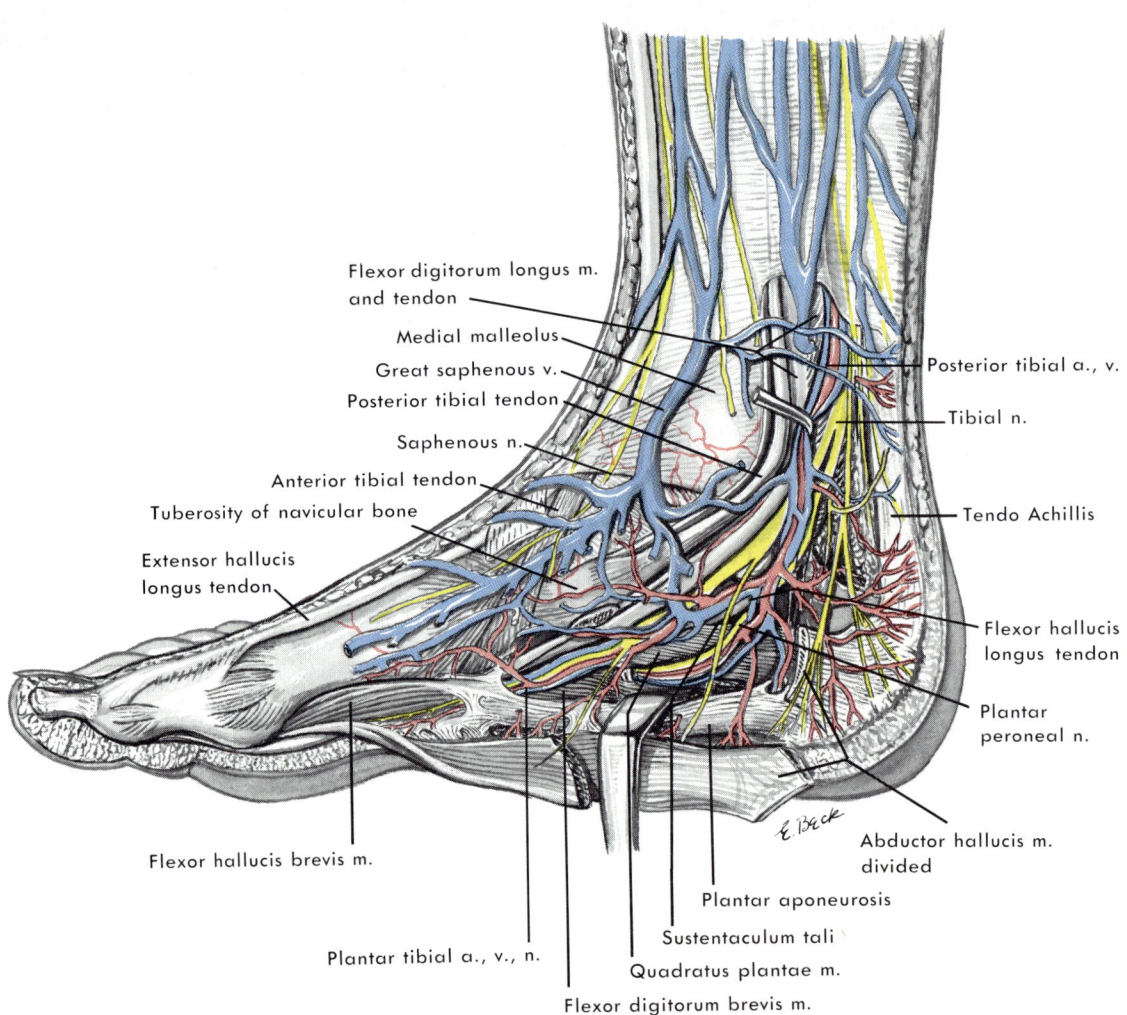

FIGURE 1–17. Medial aspect of the right ankle and foot.

Note the tibial nerve and its branches, the posterior tibial vessels, the saphenous nerve, and the great saphenous vein.

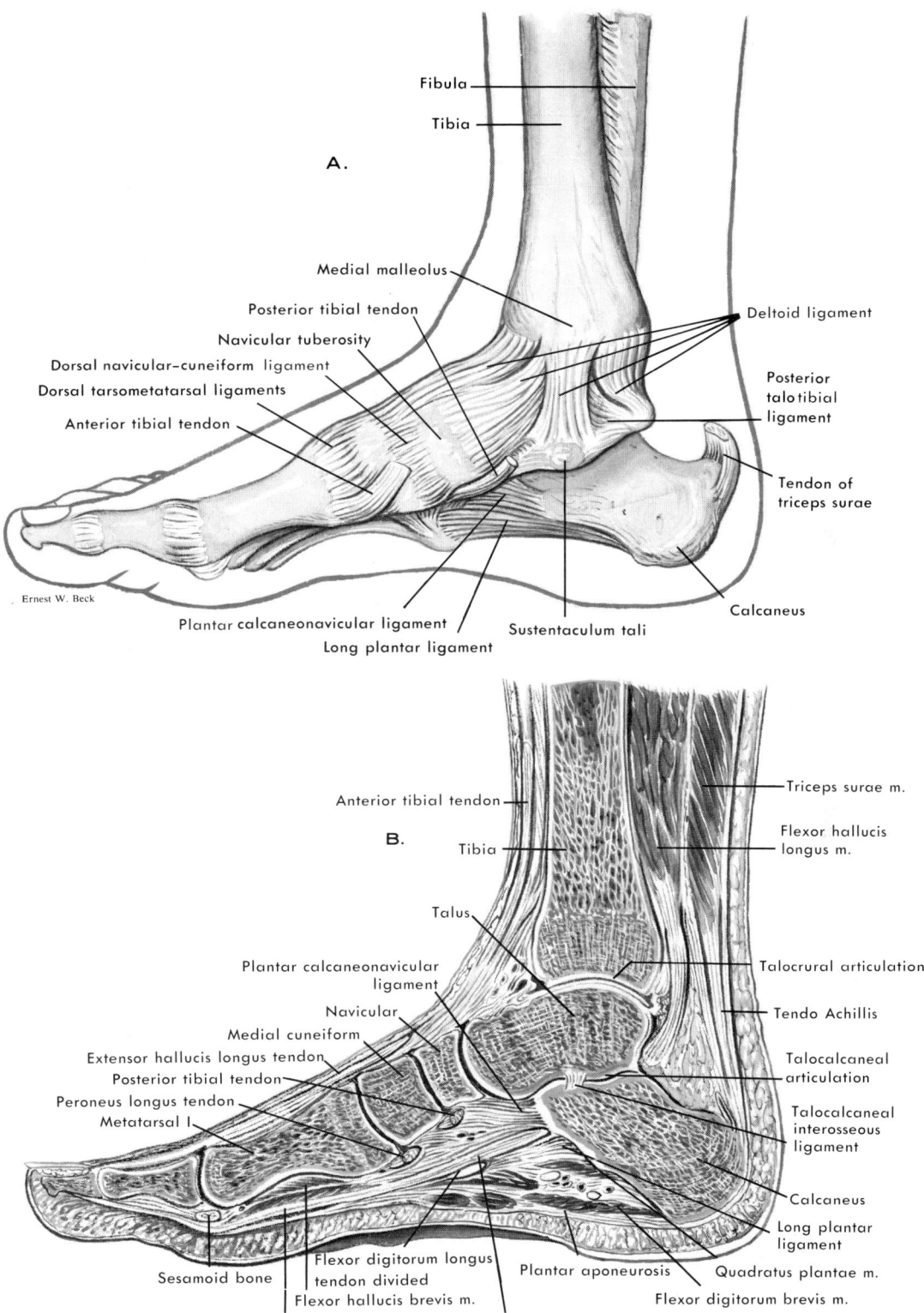

FIGURE 1–18. The ligaments, capsules, and articulations on the medial aspect of the ankle and foot.

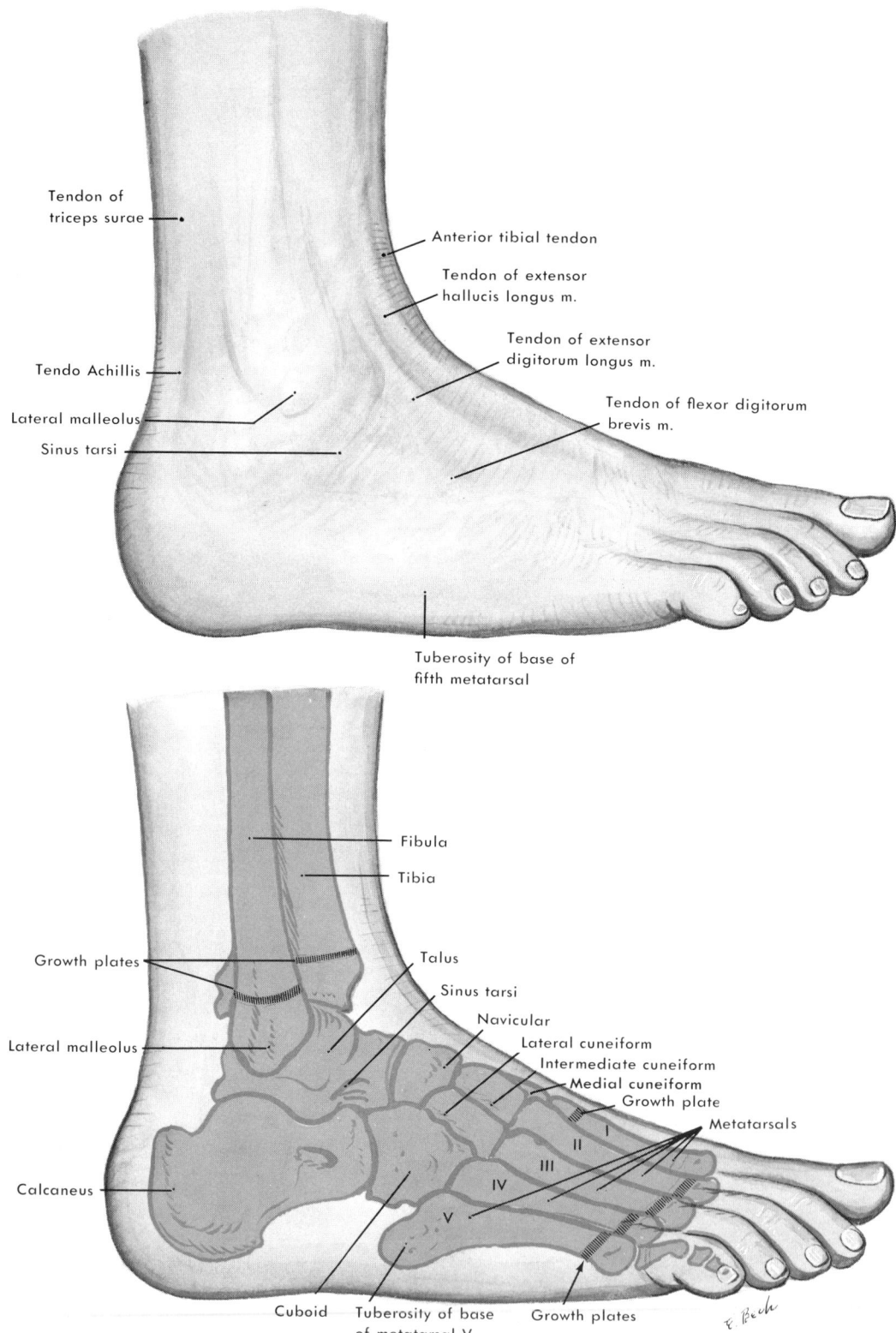

FIGURE 1–19. *The lateral aspect of the right ankle and foot.*
Surface anatomy and anatomic landmarks.

Introduction

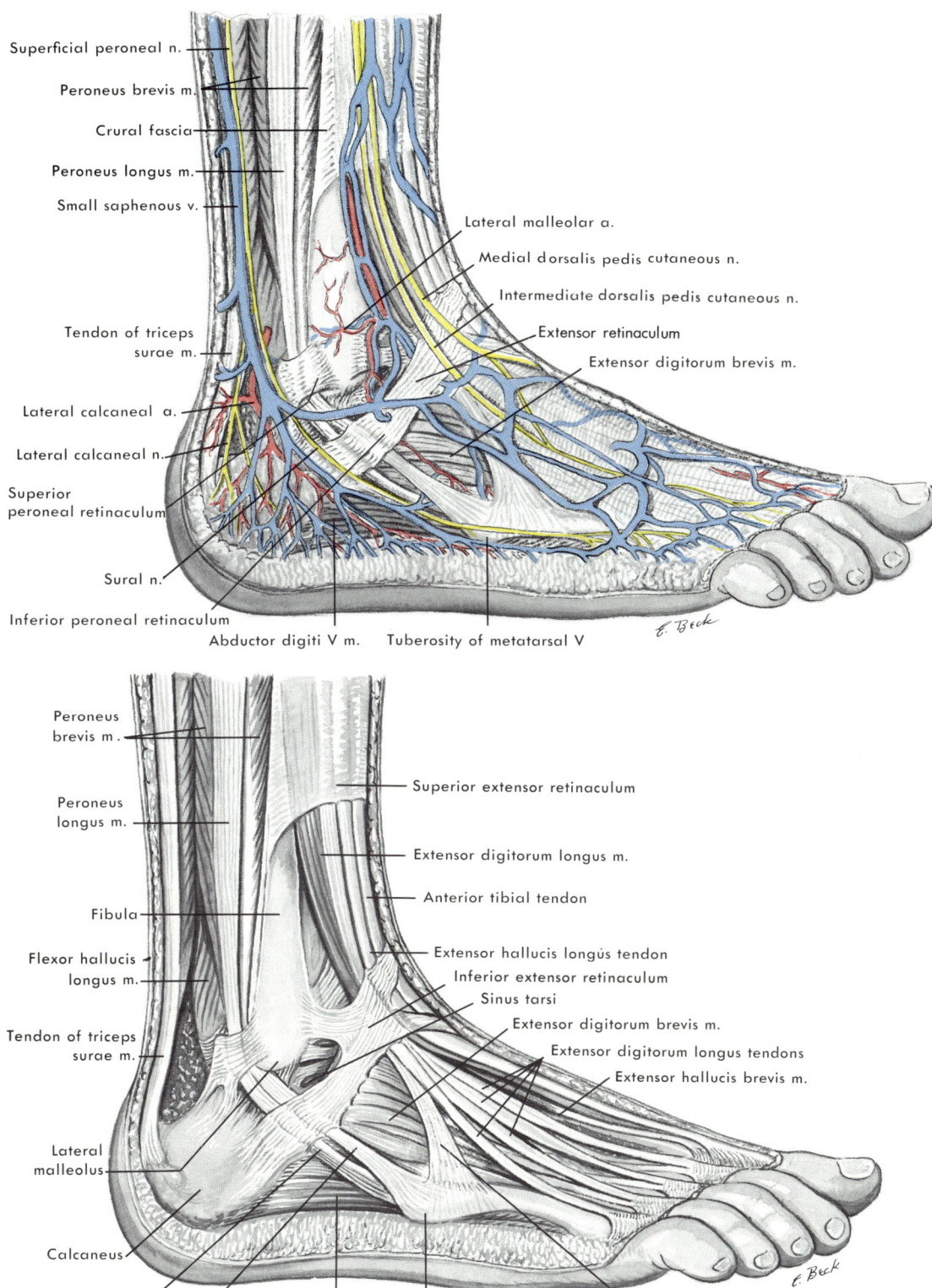

FIGURE 1–20. *Lateral aspect of the right foot.*
Sensory nerves, superficial veins, retinacula and muscles are shown.

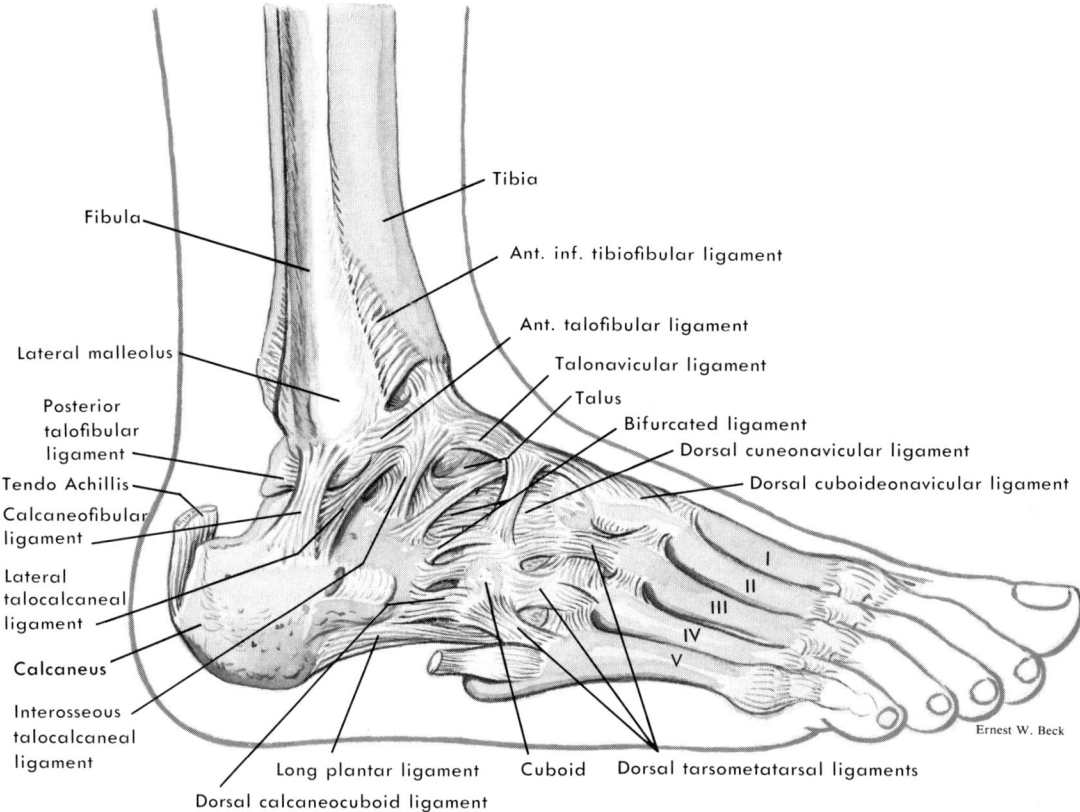

FIGURE 1–21. *The ligaments and capsules on the lateral aspect of the right foot and ankle.*

Introduction

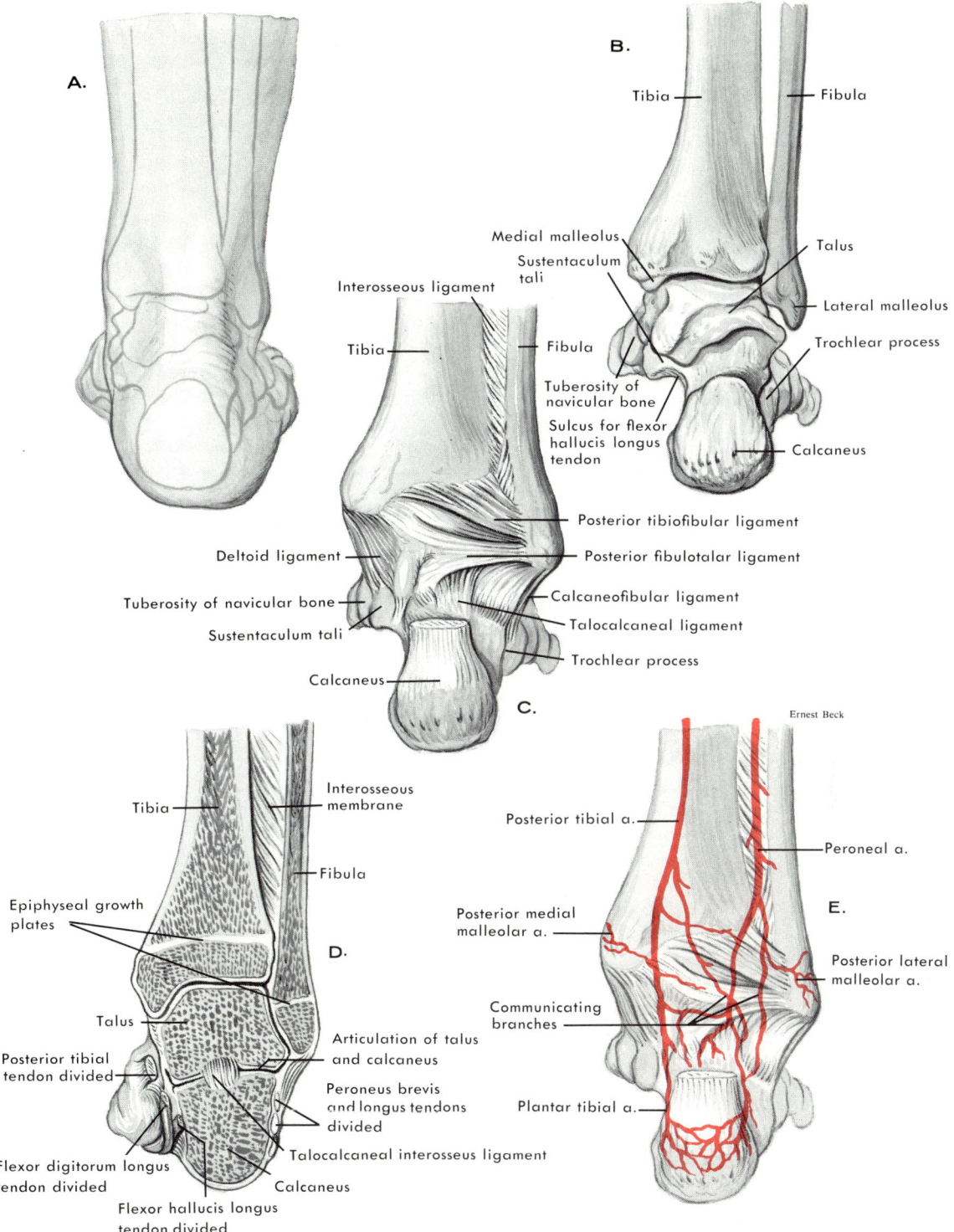

FIGURE 1-22. *The posterior aspect of the right ankle and heel.*

A. Surface anatomy. **B** through **D.** Articulations and ligaments. **E.** Course of the peroneal and posterior tibial arteries.

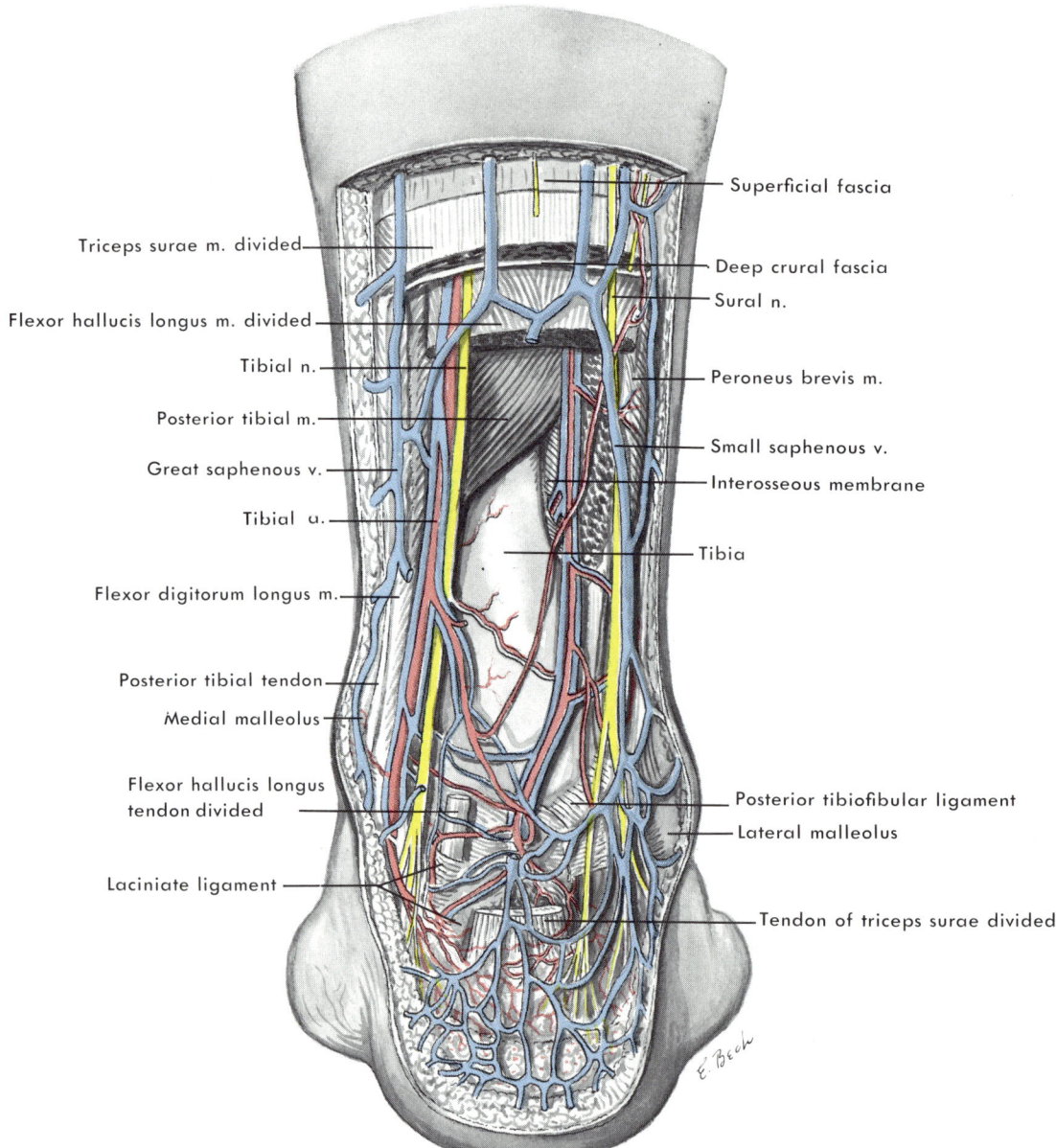

FIGURE 1–23. *Dissection showing the anatomic relations of neurovascular structures on the posterior aspect of the ankle.*

(Redrawn after von Lanz, T., and Wachsmuth, W.: Praktische Anatomie. Berlin, Julius Springer, 1938, p. 332.)

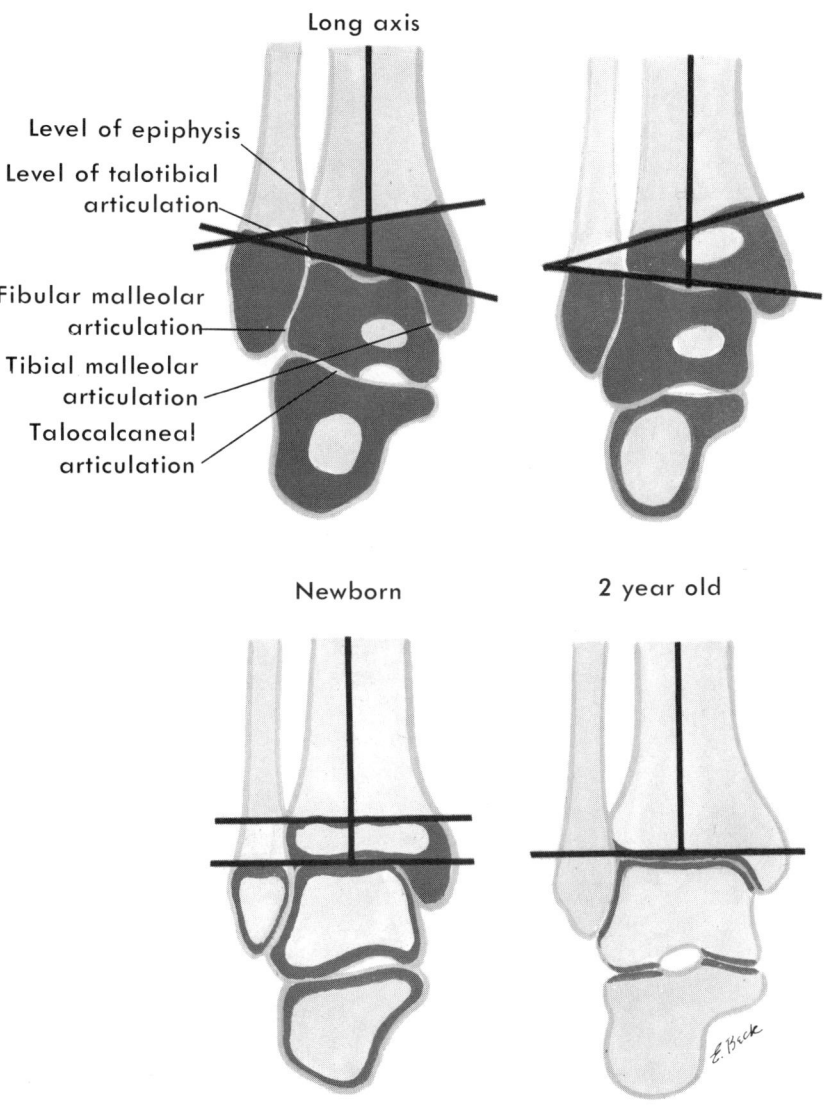

FIGURE 1–24. Obliquity of the ankle mortise in various age groups.

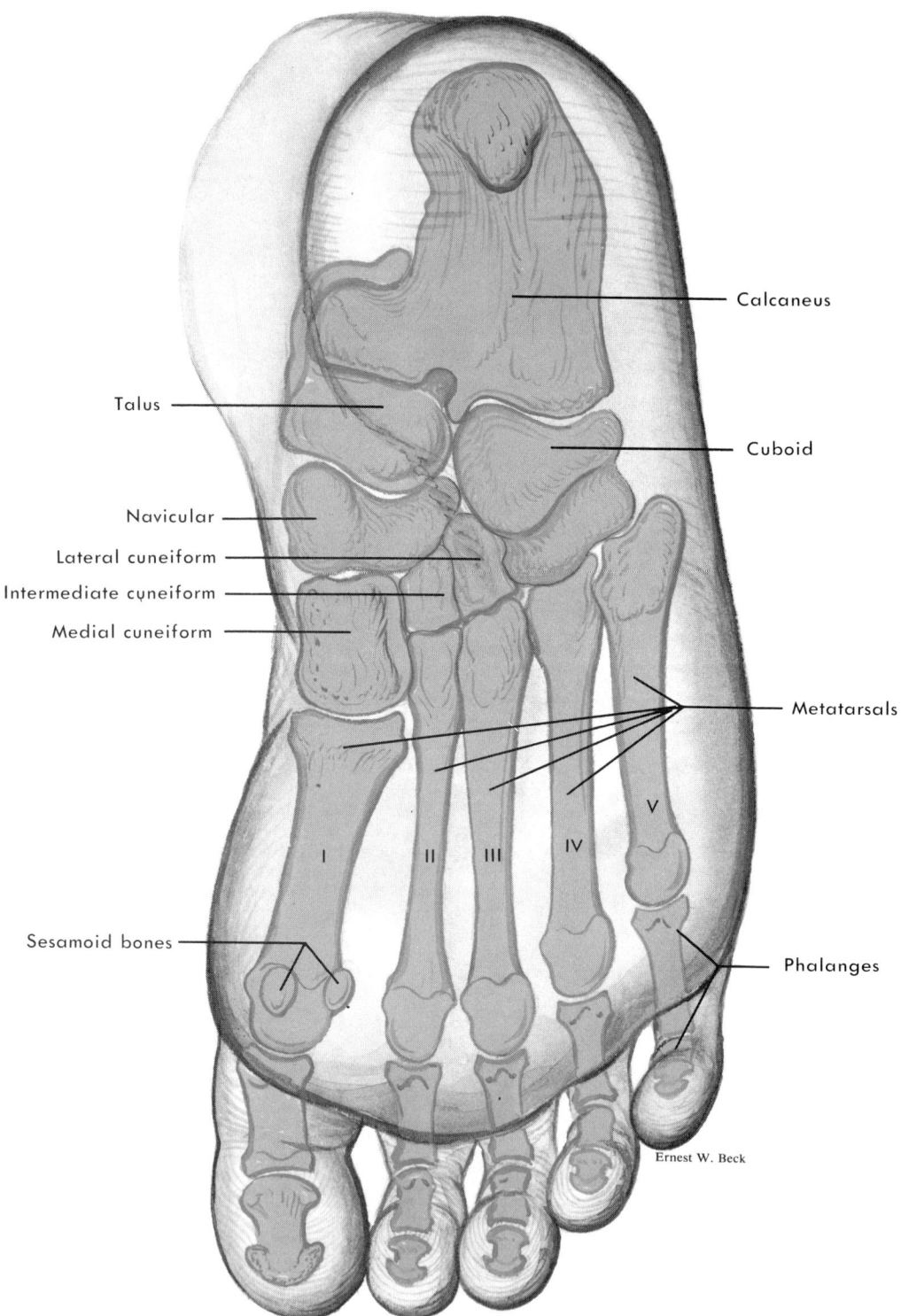

FIGURE 1–25. *Plantar aspect of the right foot: surface anatomy and bony landmarks.*

Introduction

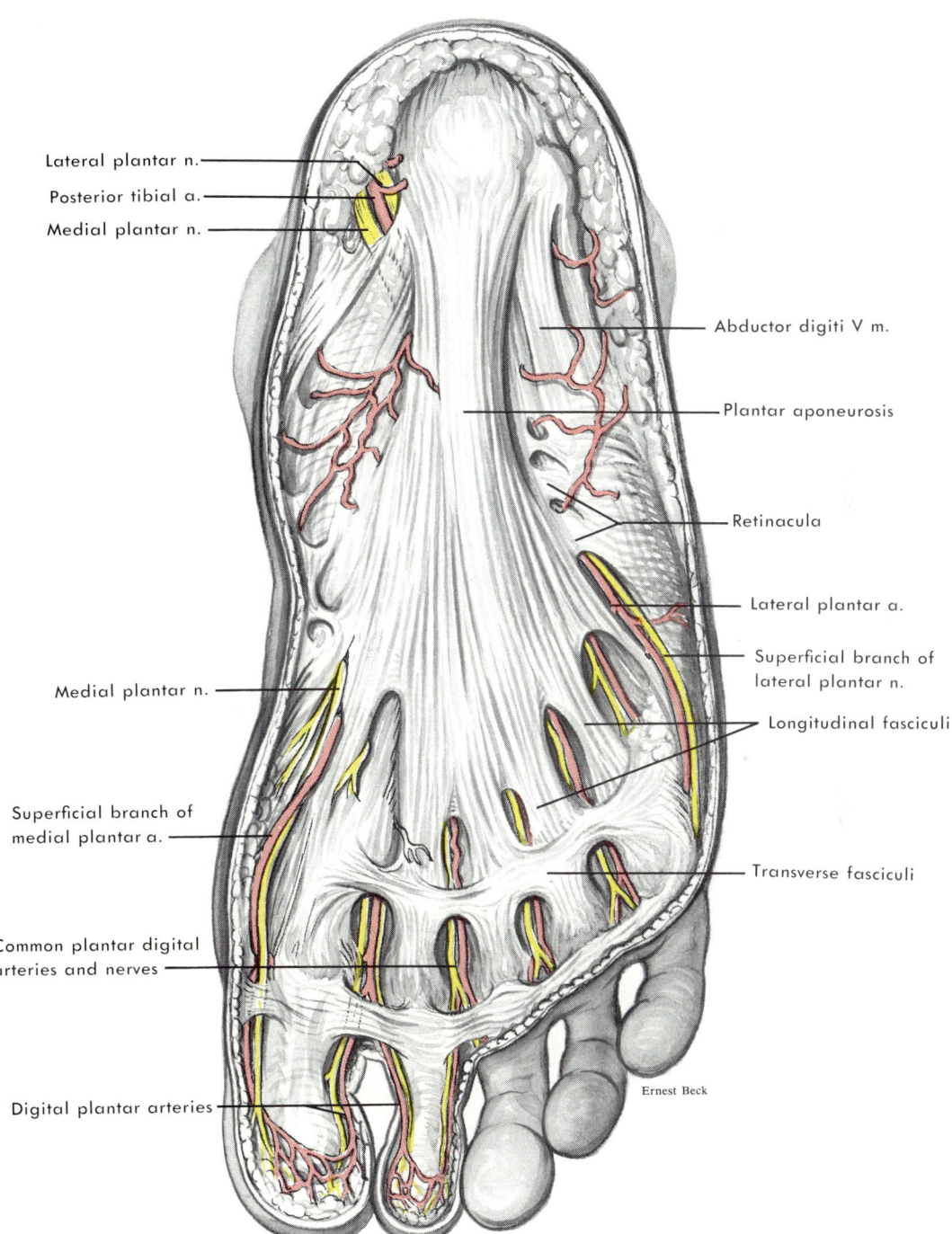

FIGURE 1–26. *Superficial dissection of plantar aspect of right foot.*
Note the plantar fascia, sensory nerves, and superficial vessels.

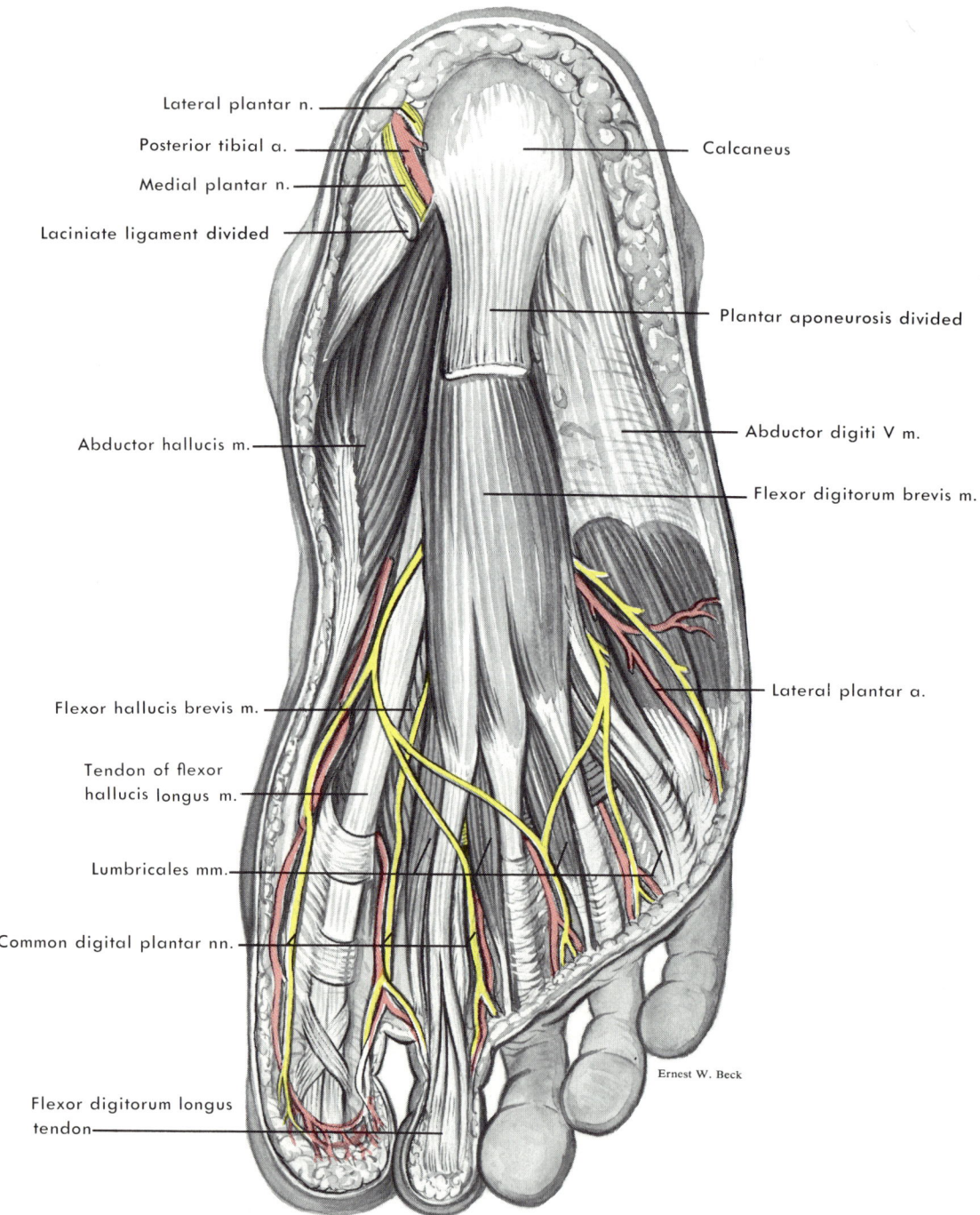

FIGURE 1–27. First layer of plantar muscles of right foot.

Note the relations of the posterior tibial vessels and medial plantar nerve. They are vulnerable to injury during plantar release.

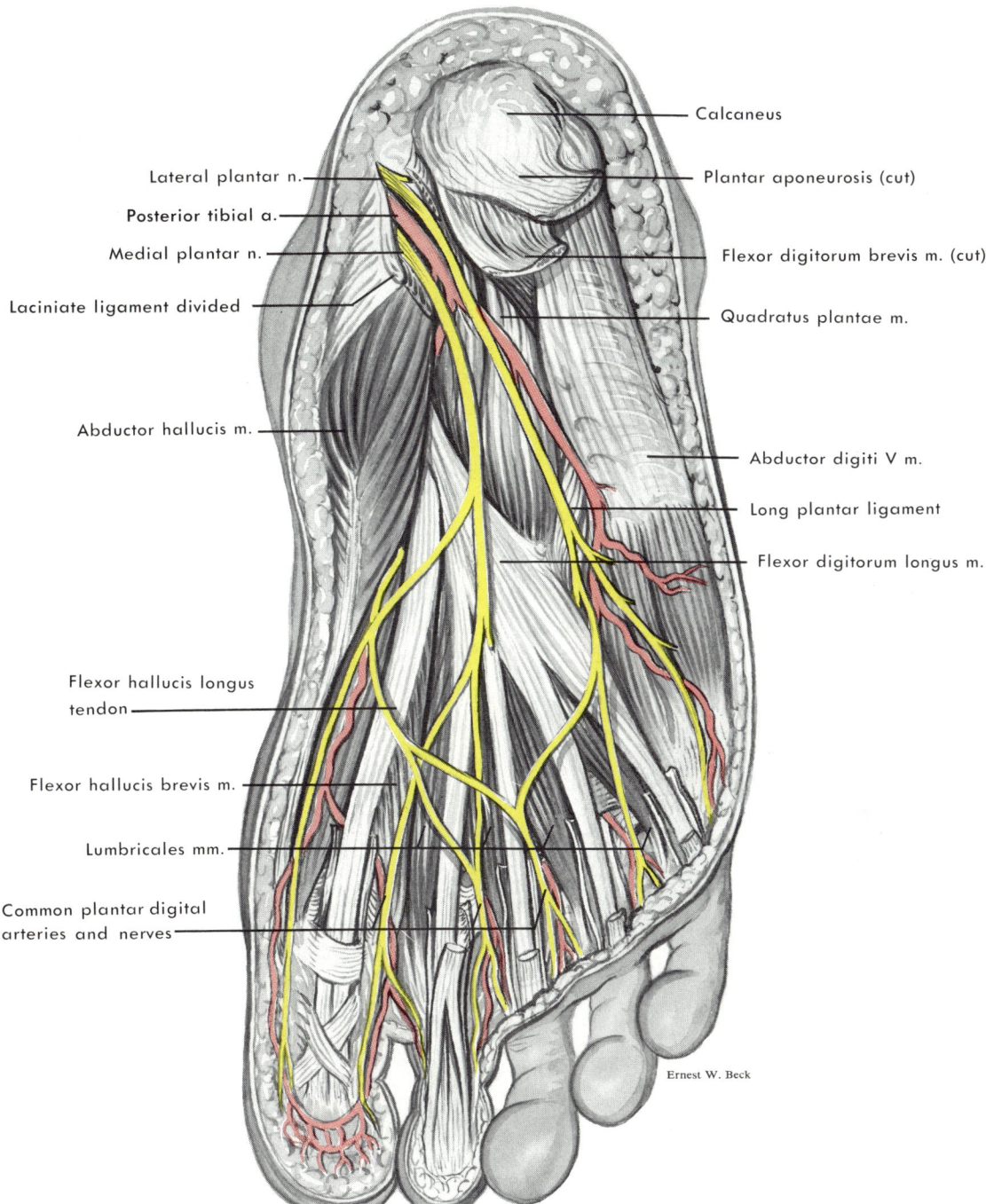

FIGURE 1–28. *Dissection of plantar aspect of right foot.*

The flexor digitorum brevis has been excised to demonstrate the course and anatomic relations of the medial and lateral plantar nerves.

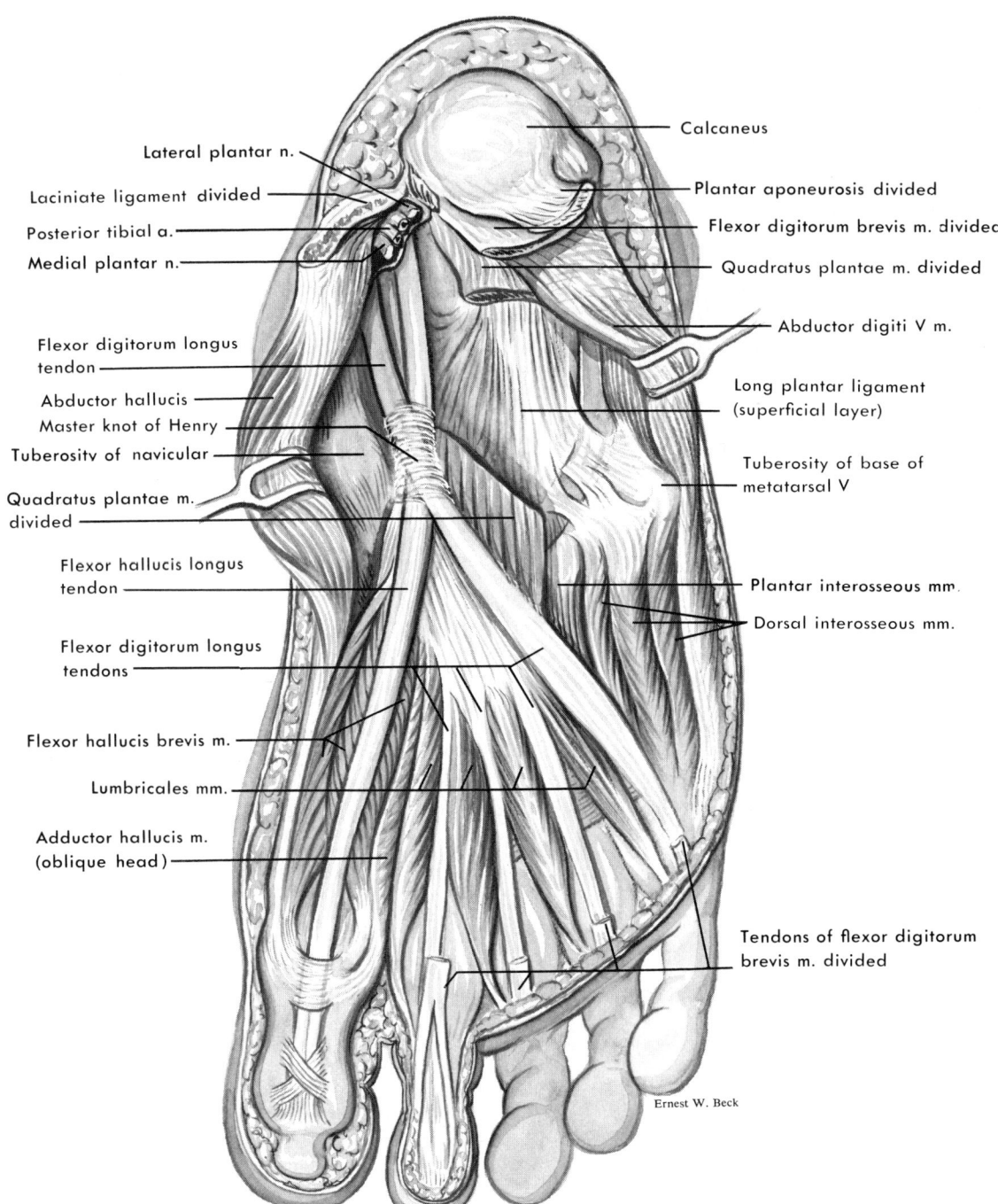

FIGURE 1–29. The second layer of plantar muscles of the right foot.

This layer consists of two long tendons (flexor hallucis longus and flexor digitorum longus) and two short muscles (quadratus plantae and lumbricales) for each digit.

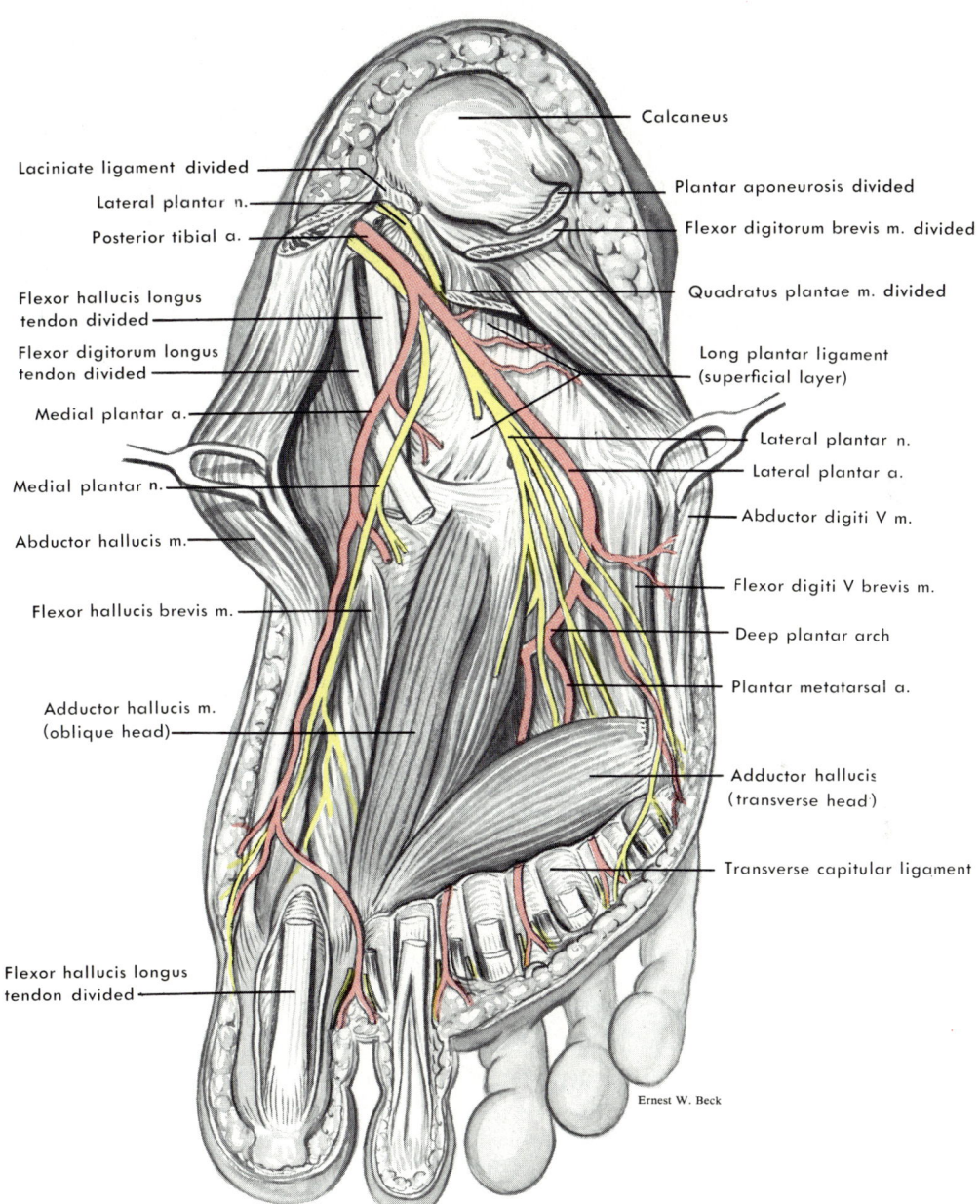

FIGURE 1–30. *The third layer of plantar muscles.*

The third layer comprises the flexor hallucis brevis, adductor hallucis, and flexor digiti quinti brevis. Note the course and relations of the medial plantar artery and nerve, and lateral plantar artery and nerve.

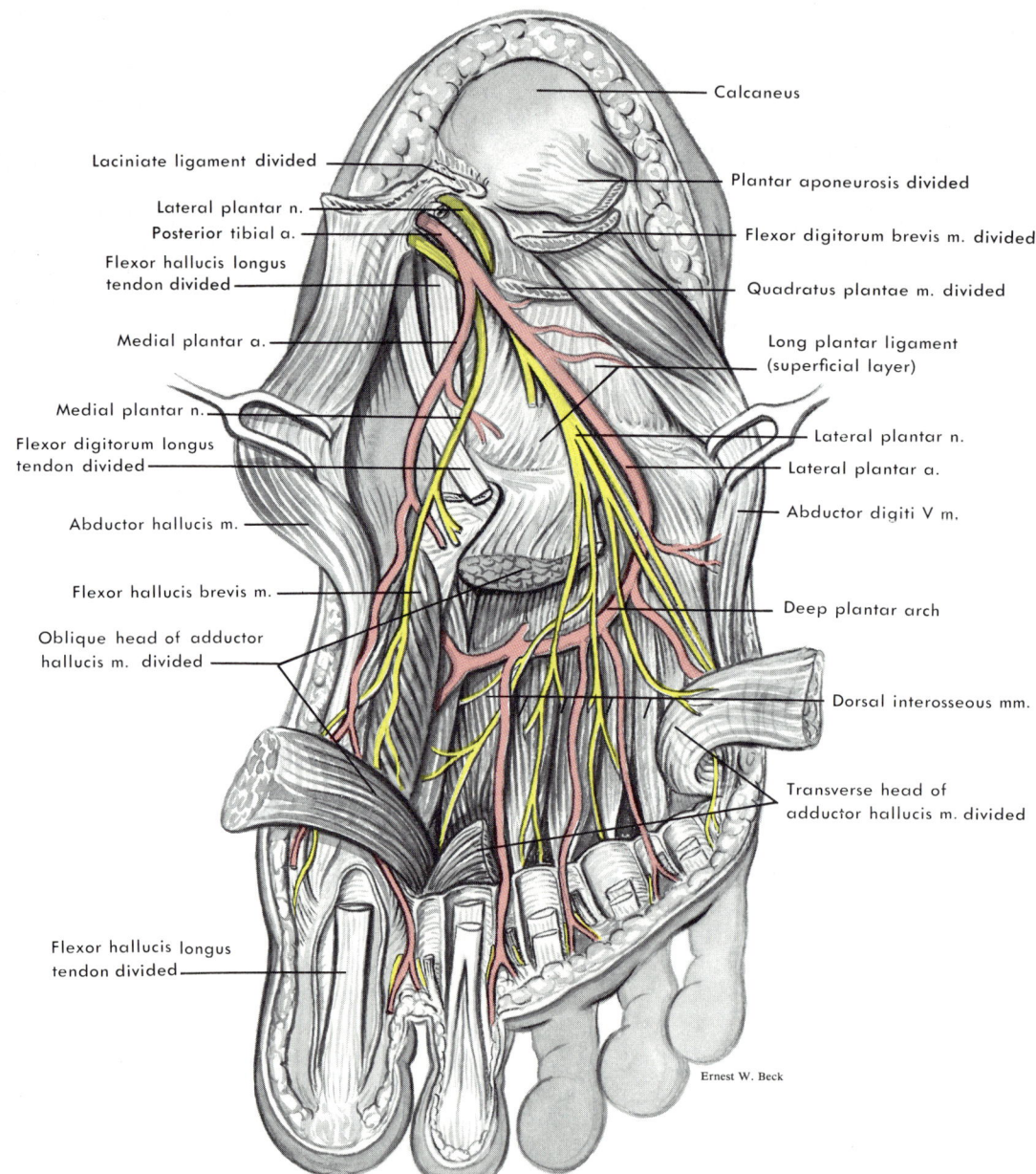

FIGURE 1–31. Deep dissection of the plantar aspect of the right foot.

The formation of the deep plantar arch and its branches is shown. Also note the medial and lateral plantar nerves and their branches.

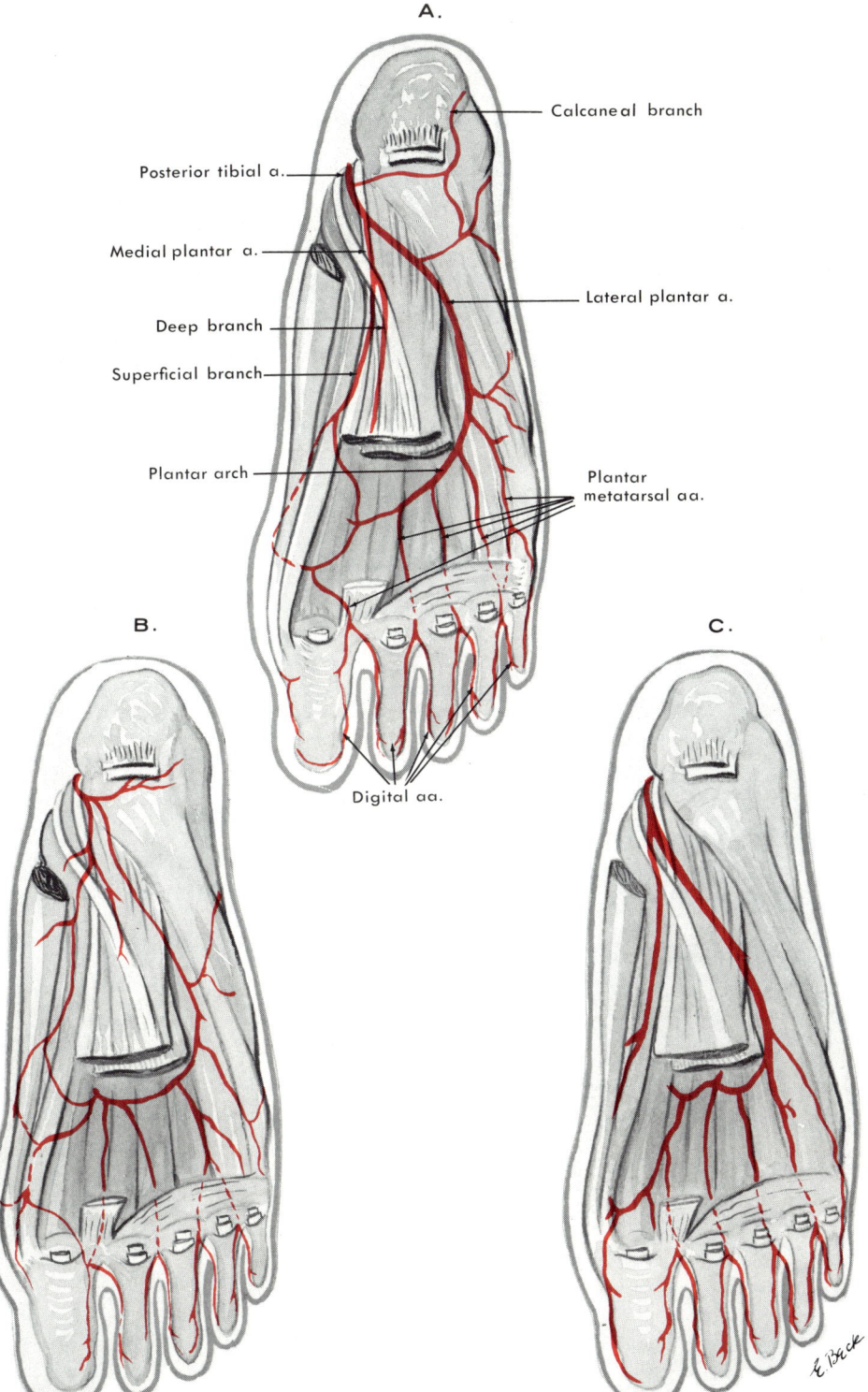

FIGURE 1–32. Variations of blood supply on the plantar aspect of the foot.
(Adapted from von Lanz, T., and Wachsmuth, W.: Praktische Anatomie. Berlin, Julius Springer, 1938, p. 410.)

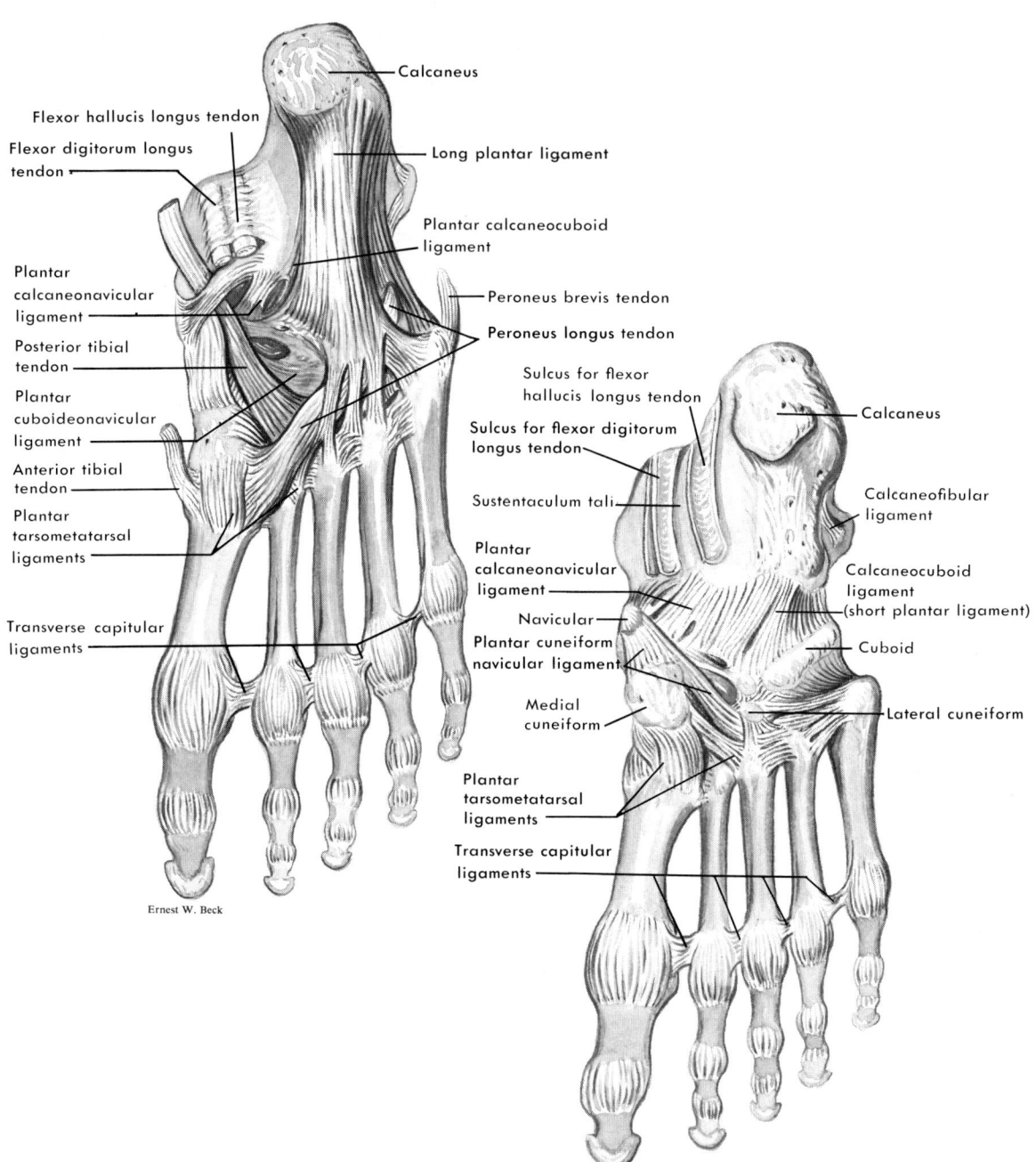

FIGURE 1–33. *The ligaments on the plantar aspect of the right foot.*

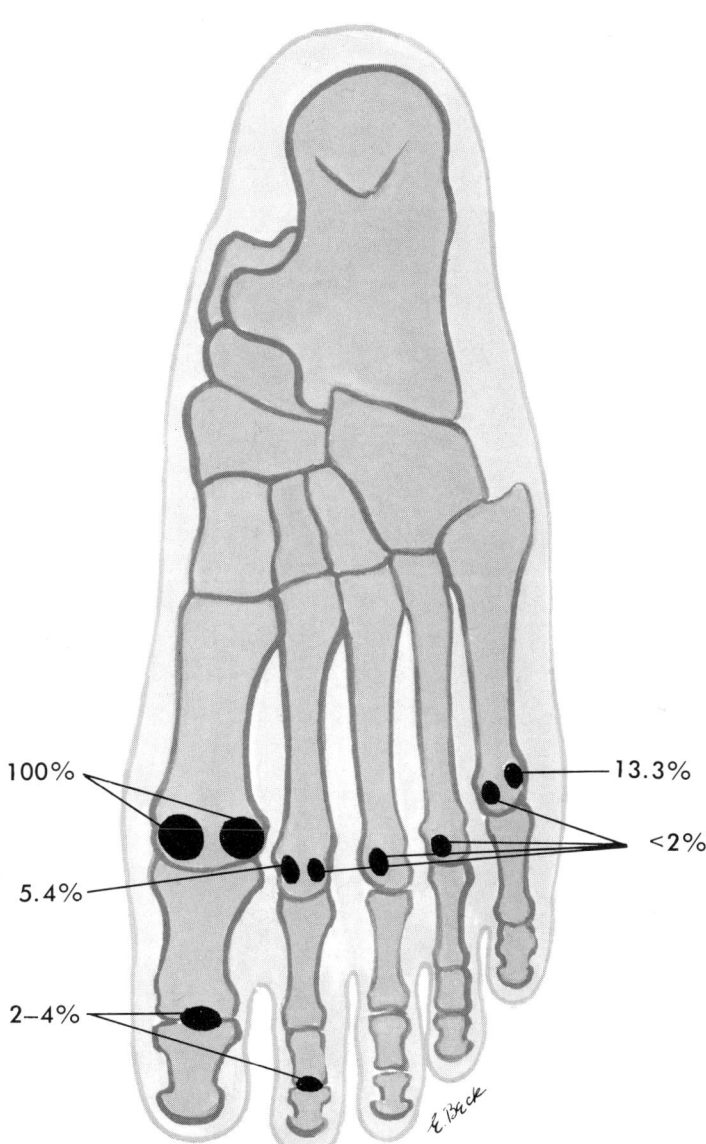

FIGURE 1–34. *The sesamoid bones on the plantar aspect of the right foot.*

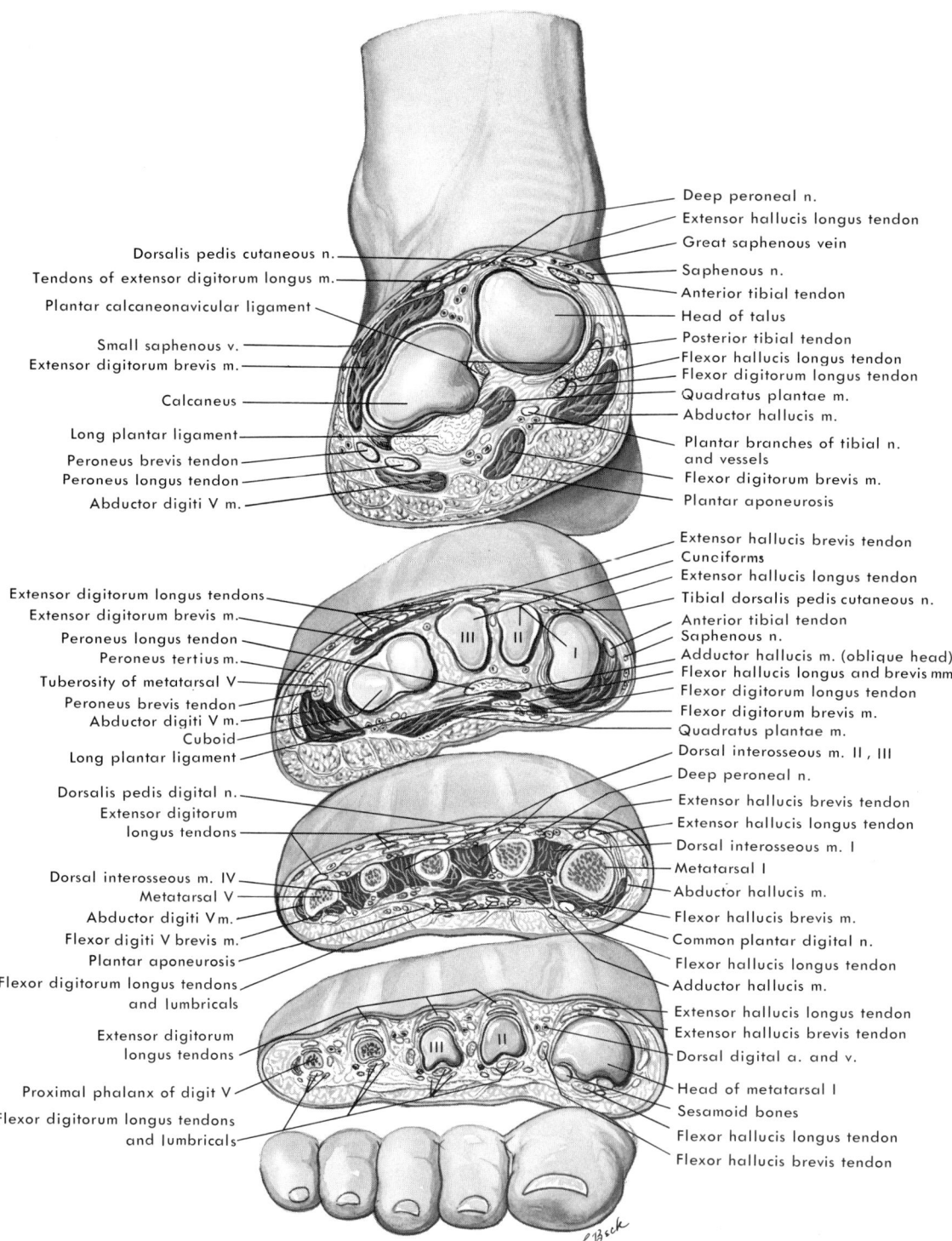

FIGURE 1-35. *Cross sections of the right foot at various levels—at Chopart's joint, at Lisfranc's joint, at the midmetatarsal area, and at the metatarsophalangeal joints.*

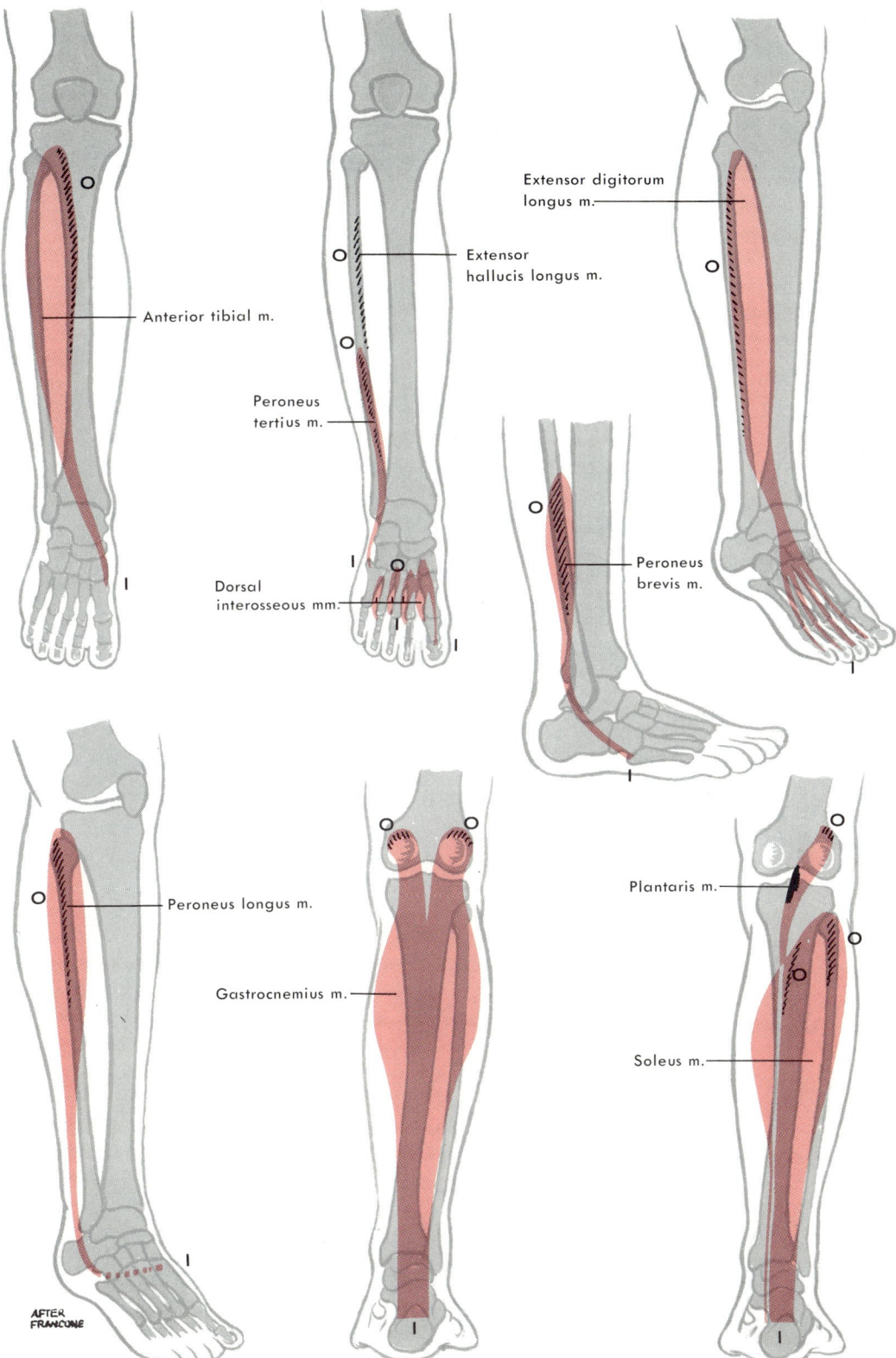

FIGURE 1–36. *The origins and insertions of the anterior, lateral, and posterior crural muscles.*

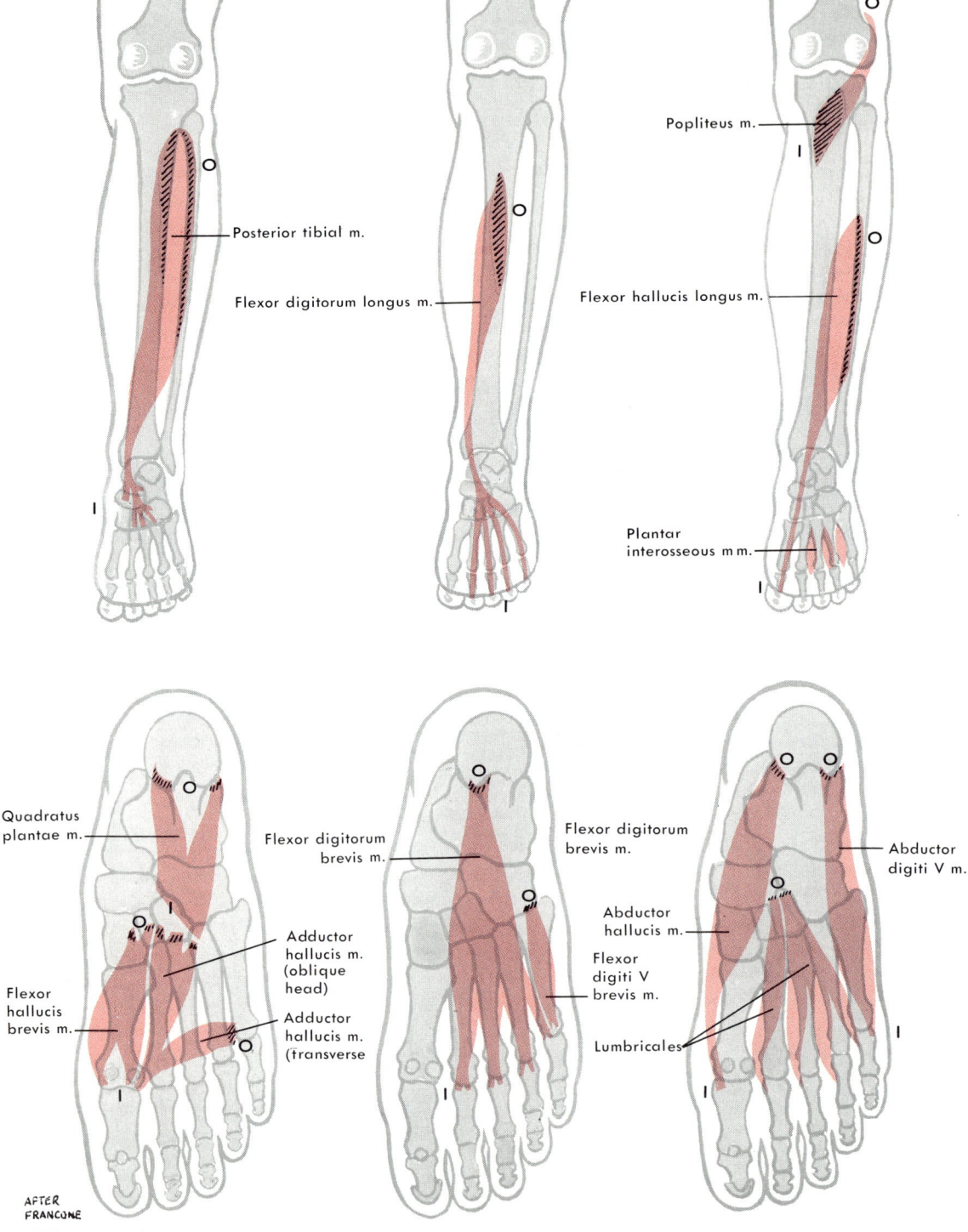

FIGURE 1–37. The origins and insertions of the deep posterior crural muscles, and the muscles on the plantar aspect of the foot.

References (Anatomy and Biomechanics)

1. Barnett, C. H., and Napier, J. R.: The axis of rotation of ankle joint in man. Its importance upon the form of the talus and the mobility of the fibula. J. Anat., 86:1, 1952.
2. Basmajian, J. V.: Electromyography of postural muscle. In Evans, F. G. (ed.): Biomechanical Studies of the Musculoskeletal System. Springfield, Ill., Charles C Thomas, 1961, Chapter 6, pp. 136–160.
3. Basmajian, J. V.: Human locomotion. In Muscles Alive: Their Functions Revealed by Electromyography. 3rd Ed. Baltimore, Williams & Wilkins Co., 1974, Chapter 11, pp. 205–252.
4. Brunnstrom, S.: Ankle and foot. In Clinical Kinesiology. 3rd Ed. Philadelphia, F. A. Davis Co., 1972, Chapter 7, pp. 197–224.
5. Cordier, G.: Etude statigraphique de l'architecture de la voute plantaire. Ann. Anat. Path. (Paris), 16:376, 1939–1940.
6. Elftman, H.: A cinematic study of the distribution of pressure in the human foot. Anat. Rec., 59:481, 1934.
7. Elftman, H.: The function of muscles in locomotion. Amer. J. Physiol., 125:357, 1939.
8. Elftman, H.: The transverse tarsal joint and its control. Clin. Orthop., 16:41, 1960.
9. Elftman, H., and Manter, J. T.: The axes of the human foot. Science, 80:484, 1934.
10. Gardner, G. M., and Murray, M. P.: A method of measuring the duration of foot-floor contact during walking. Phys. Ther., 55:751, 1975.
11. Grundy, M., Tosh, P. A., McLeish, R. D., and Smidt, L.: An investigation of the centers of pressure under the foot while walking. J. Bone Joint Surg., 57-B:98, 1975.
12. Hall, M. C.: The trabecular patterns of the normal foot. Clin. Orthop., 16:15, 1960.
13. Hall, M. C.: The Locomotor System Functional Anatomy. Springfield, Ill., Charles C Thomas, 1965.
14. Hicks, J. H.: Mechanics of the foot. J. Anat., 87:345, 1953.
15. Hiss, J. M.: Foot in motion. In Functional Foot Disorders. Los Angeles, Calif., Univ. Pub. Co., 1937, Chapter II, pp. 35–52.
16. Houtz, S. J., and Walsh, F. P.: Electromyographic analysis of the function of the muscle acting on the ankle during weight-bearing with special reference to the triceps surae. J. Bone Joint Surg., 41-A:1469, 1959.
17. Howorth, B.: Dynamic posture in relation to the foot. Clin. Orthop., 16:74, 1960.
18. Huson, H. H., and Walker, P. S.: Stabilizing mechanisms of the loaded and unloaded knee joint. J. Bone Joint Surg., 58-A:87, 1976.
19. Hutton, W. C., Stott, J. R. R., and Stokes, I. A. F.: The mechanics of the foot. In Klenerman, L. (ed.): The Foot and Its Disorders. Oxford, Blackwell Scientific Publications, Ltd., 1976, Chapter 3, pp. 30–48.
20. Inman, V. T.: The Joints of the Ankle. Baltimore, Williams & Wilkins Co., 1976.
21. Kaplan, E. B.: Some principles of anatomy and kinesiology in stabilization operation of the foot. Clin. Orthop., 34:7, 1964.
22. Klenerman, L.: Functional anatomy. In Klenerman, L. (ed.): The Foot and Its Disorders. Oxford, Blackwell Scientific Publications, Ltd., 1976, pp. 19–29.
23. Lambert, K.: The weight bearing function of the fibula. J. Bone Joint Surg., 53-A:507, 1971.
24. Lapidus, P. W.: Subtalar joint. Its anatomy and mechanics. Bull. Hosp. Joint Dis., 16:179, 1955.
25. Levens, A. S., Inman, V. T., and Blosser, J. A.: Transverse rotation of the segments of the lower extremity in locomotion. J. Bone Joint Surg., 30-A:859, 1948.
26. Mann, R. A.: Biomechanics of the foot. In American Academy of Orthopedic Surgeons: Atlas of Orthotics. Biomechanical Principles and Applications. St. Louis, C. V. Mosby Co., 1975, Chapter 13, pp. 257–266.
27. Mann, R. A., and Inman, V. T.: Phasic activity of intrinsic muscles of the foot. J. Bone Joint Surg., 46-A:469, 1964.
28. Manter, J. T.: Movements of the subtalar and transverse tarsal joints. Anat. Rec., 80:397, 1941.
29. Morris, J. M.: Biomechanics of the foot and ankle. Clin. Orthop., 122:10, 1977.
30. Murray, M. P., Guten, G. N., Baldwin, J. M., and Gardner, G. M.: A comparison of plantar flexion torque with and without the triceps surae. Acta Orthop. Scand., 47:122, 1976.
31. Sammarco, G. J., Burstein, A. H., and Frankel, V. H.: Biomechanics of the ankle: A kinematic study. Proceedings, American Orthopedic Foot Society. Orthop. Clin. N. Amer., 4:75, 1973.
31a. Sarrafian, S.: Anatomy of the Foot and Ankle. Philadelphia, J. B. Lippincott Co., 1983.
32. Scranton, P. E., McMaster, J. H., and Kelly, E.: Dynamic fibular function. A new concept. Clin. Orthop., 118:76, 1976.
33. Weinert, C. R., Jr., McMaster, J. H., and Ferguson, R.: Dynamic function of the human fibula. Amer. J. Anat., 138:145, 1973.
34. Weinert, C. R., Jr., McMaster, J. H., Scranton, P. E., Jr., and Ferguson, R. J.: Human fibular dynamics. In Bateman, J. E. (ed.): Foot Science. Philadelphia, W. B. Saunders Co., 1976, Chapter 1, pp. 1–6.
35. Weseley, M. S., Koval, R., and Kleiger, B.: Roentgen measurement of ankle flexion-extension motion. Clin. Orthop., 65:167, 1969.
36. Wright, D. G., and Rennels, D. C.: A study of the elastic properties of plantar fascia. J. Bone Joint Surg., 46-A:482, 1964.
37. Zitzlsperger, S.: The mechanics of the foot based on the concept of the skeleton as a statically indetermined space framework. Clin. Orthop., 16:47, 1960.

DEVELOPMENT AND OSSIFICATION OF THE FOOT AND LEG

The embryonic period, comprising the first seven postovulatory weeks, is the stage of organogenesis. The lower limb bud first appears in embryos of four postovulatory weeks (3 to 6 mm. crown-rump length) as a minute bud that elongates and develops in a proximal to distal direction. The foot is first seen at four and a half weeks. Soon afterward three or four digital prolongations can be observed.[1-5]

The tarsus is first distinguished as a condensed mesenchyme at five to six weeks (9–14 mm. crown-rump length). A few days later (at 12 to 21 mm.) chondrification begins in the center of each blastemal element. The individual bones of the foot chondrify in a definite sequence, the second to fourth metatarsals first, followed by the cuboid and fifth metatarsal. The navicular bone is the last tarsal element to chondrify. In the digits chondrification proceeds in a proximal to distal direction, with the distal phalanx of the little toe last to chondrify. By the end of the embryonic period the form and arrangement of the bony elements of the foot resemble those of an adult (Fig. 1–38). Although ossification of the foot does not occur during the embryonic period proper, the synovial joints begin to develop as "interzones" between the various elements.

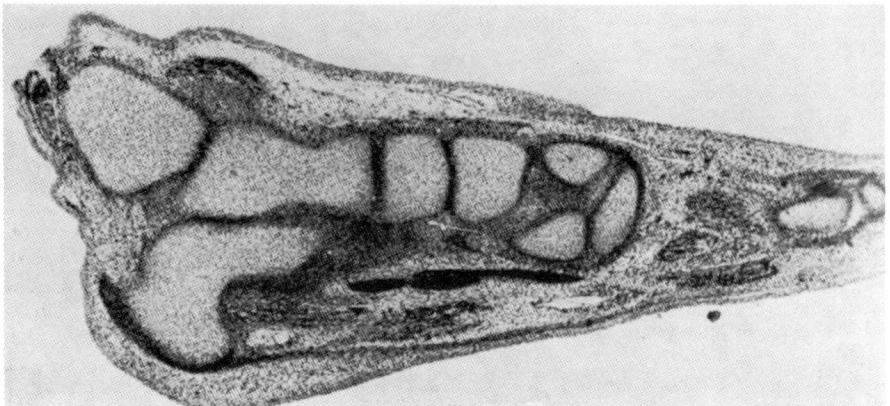

FIGURE 1–38. Sagittal section of the right foot in a 26-mm. crown to rump–length embryo.

The fibula is at the upper left, then the talus, and the calcaneus is at the lower left. × 41. (From Gardner, E., Gray, D. J., and O'Rahilly, R.: The prenatal development of the skeleton and joints of the human foot. J. Bone Joint Surg., 41-A:856, 1959. Reprinted by permission.)

Thus, in considering the pathogenesis of congenital malformations of the feet, it is important to keep in mind that their structure and skeletal components are determined prior to the seventh postovulatory week of intrauterine life. Gardner, Gray, and O'Rahilly noted cartilaginous fusion between the talus and calcaneus in a 28-mm. crown-rump-length embryo, as shown in Figure 1–39; partial fusion between the lateral cuneiform, calcaneus, and cuboid bones in one embryo; and symphalangism of the middle and distal phalanges of the little toe in another embryo. A bipartite medial cuneiform bone was found in both feet of an 18-mm. embryo. Accessory tarsal cartilages were not found in the embryonic foot. The digital sesamoids may chondrify as early as seven weeks, with distribution and frequency very similar to those of the adult.[3]

Vascular invasion of the tarsus, heralding the approach of ossification, first begins in the talus. Vascular channels in the cartilaginous anlage of the talus can be seen at a length of 43 mm. and are constantly present at 78 mm. The vessels in the canals originate principally from the arteries of the sinus tarsi and the tarsal canal; it should be noted that these vessels are the principal source of blood supply to the talus in the adult. The vascular invasion then proceeds in the calcaneus, navicular, cuboid, cuneiforms, metatarsals, and phalanges.

Ossification in the foot first begins in the tips of the distal phalanges and then advances proximally. Soon after, periosteal bone collars are formed around the metatarsal shafts, and later around the proximal and middle phalanges, in that sequential order.

The calcaneus is the first of the tarsal bones to begin ossification; its primary ossific center appears between the fifth and sixth fetal months. Occasionally the body of

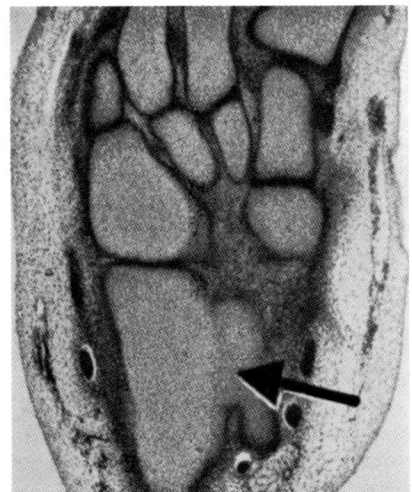

FIGURE 1–39. Horizontal section of the right foot in a 28-mm. embryo.

Note the cartilaginous fusion between the talus (arrow) and the os calcis. × 41. (From Gardner, E., Gray, D. J., and O'Rahilly, R.: The prenatal development of the skeleton and joints of the human foot. J. Bone Joint Surg., 41-A:856, 1959. Reprinted by permission.)

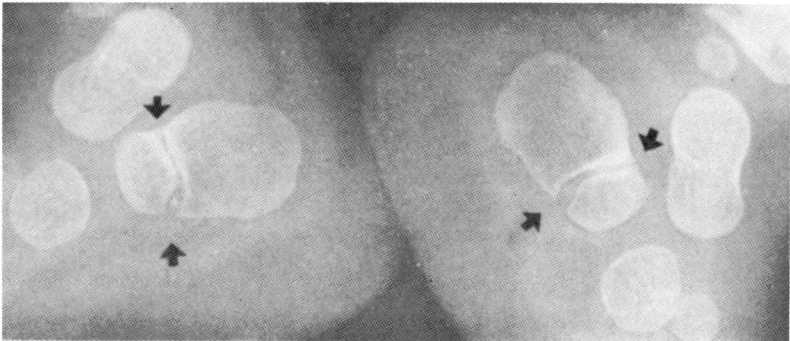

FIGURE 1–40. Two centers of ossification in the body of the calcaneus in a 20-month-old infant.

The cartilaginous line of radiolucency separating the two ossific centers should not be mistaken for a fracture. (From Caffey, J., et al.: Pediatric X-Ray Diagnosis, 7th Ed., Vol. 2, p. 1064. Copyright © 1978, Year Book Medical Publishers, Inc., Chicago. Reprinted by permission.)

the calcaneus appears to have two centers (Fig. 1–40). The apophysis of the os calcis begins to ossify at four to six years of age in girls, and at five to nine years in boys; it fuses with the body of the calcaneus toward 16 years in the female and 20 years in the male. The talus is the second tarsal bone to ossify, usually about the eighth fetal month. Ossification of the cuboid bone takes place at or near birth, but it may be delayed until 21 days of age. In the tarsus, at birth, the primary centers of ossification of the calcaneus, talus, and cuboid bone are usually present. The average age for ossification of the lateral cuneiform bone is 4 to 20 months; for the medial cuneiform, two years, and for the intermediate cuneiform, three years. The navicular ossifies between the second and fifth years.

The primary centers of ossification of the second and third metatarsals appear at the ninth week of fetal life, whereas those of the fourth and fifth metatarsals appear at the tenth week. The secondary centers of ossification arise at the epiphyses, which are distally located; they are visible between three and four years of age, appearing in a variable order. The epiphyses of the lateral four metatarsals fuse with the diaphyses between the ages of 16 and 18 years. The primary ossific center of the first metatarsal is visible at the twelfth week of fetal life, and the secondary center for the epiphysis (located proximally) appears between three and four years; it fuses with the diaphysis at between 16 and 18 years.

The cartilaginous sesamoids can be distinguished early in the fetal period—between 30 and 45 mm. The ossification of the medial and lateral sesamoids of the big toe usually takes place between 12 and 14 years of age, but sometimes as early as 8 years. The sesamoids of the second and fifth toes are not constant; if present they ossify late, after 15 years of age.

The tibia and fibula can be seen as mesenchymal condensations at the fifth week (about 11 to 13.5 mm.). Soon chondrification commences. At this early stage the fibula is in contact with the calcaneus. At the eighth week the malleoli chondrify. The primary center of ossification of the tibia appears at the ninth week of intrauterine life. Toward the eighth or ninth month of fetal life, the proximal epiphysis of the tibia begins to ossify; the ossific center of the distal tibial epiphysis does not appear until between the sixth and tenth months of postnatal life. The medial malleolus begins to ossify at seven years in girls and at eight years in boys. The proximal tibial tubercle begins to ossify between 7 and 11 years. In the fibula the primary center of ossification appears at the tenth week of fetal life. The distal epiphysis appears between the eleventh and eighteenth postnatal months, and the upper epiphysis begins to ossify between two and five years. Both the upper and lower epiphyses fuse with the diaphysis between 18 and 22 years of age.

Average ages of appearance of centers of ossification and fusion of epiphyses in the lower limbs in males and females are shown in Figures 1–41 and 1–42.

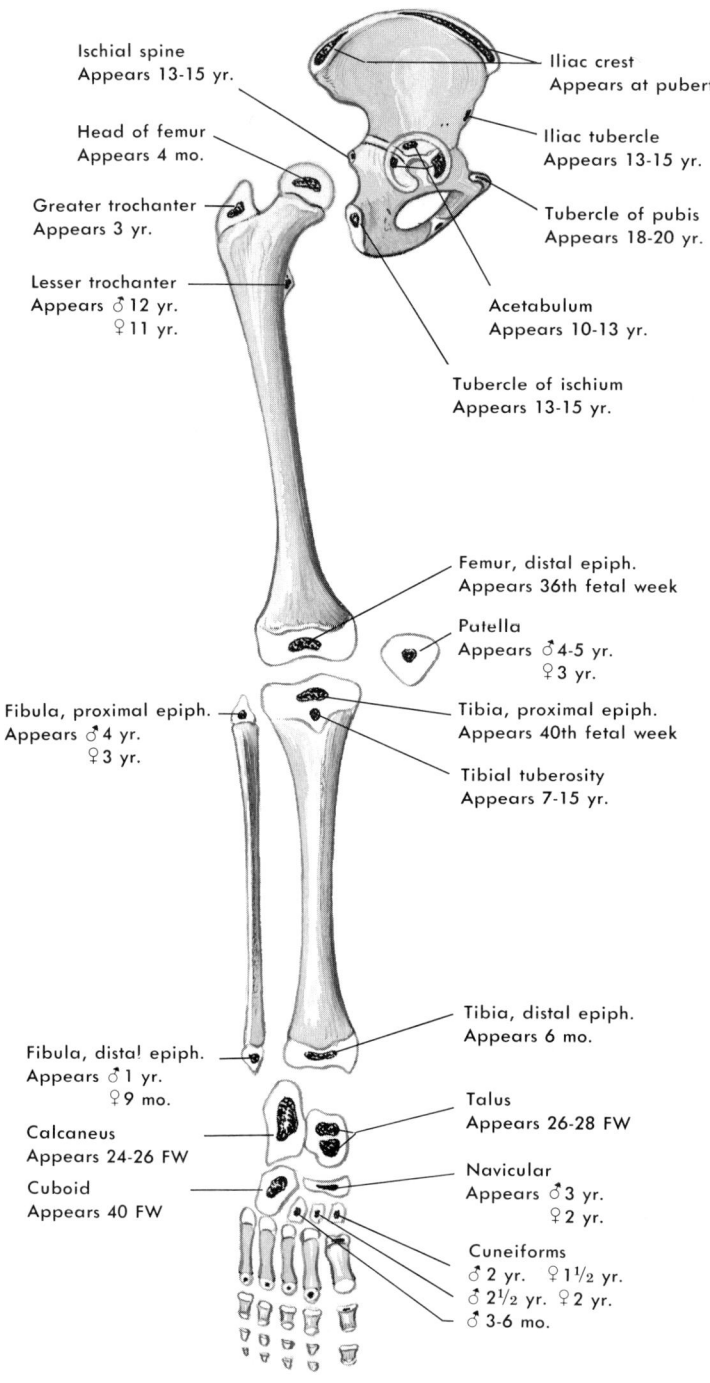

FIGURE 1–41. *Average age of appearance of centers of ossification of epiphyses in the lower limb in males and females.*

(Adapted from von Lanz, T., and Wachsmuth, W.: Praktische Anatomie. Berlin, Julius Springer, 1938, p. 28.)

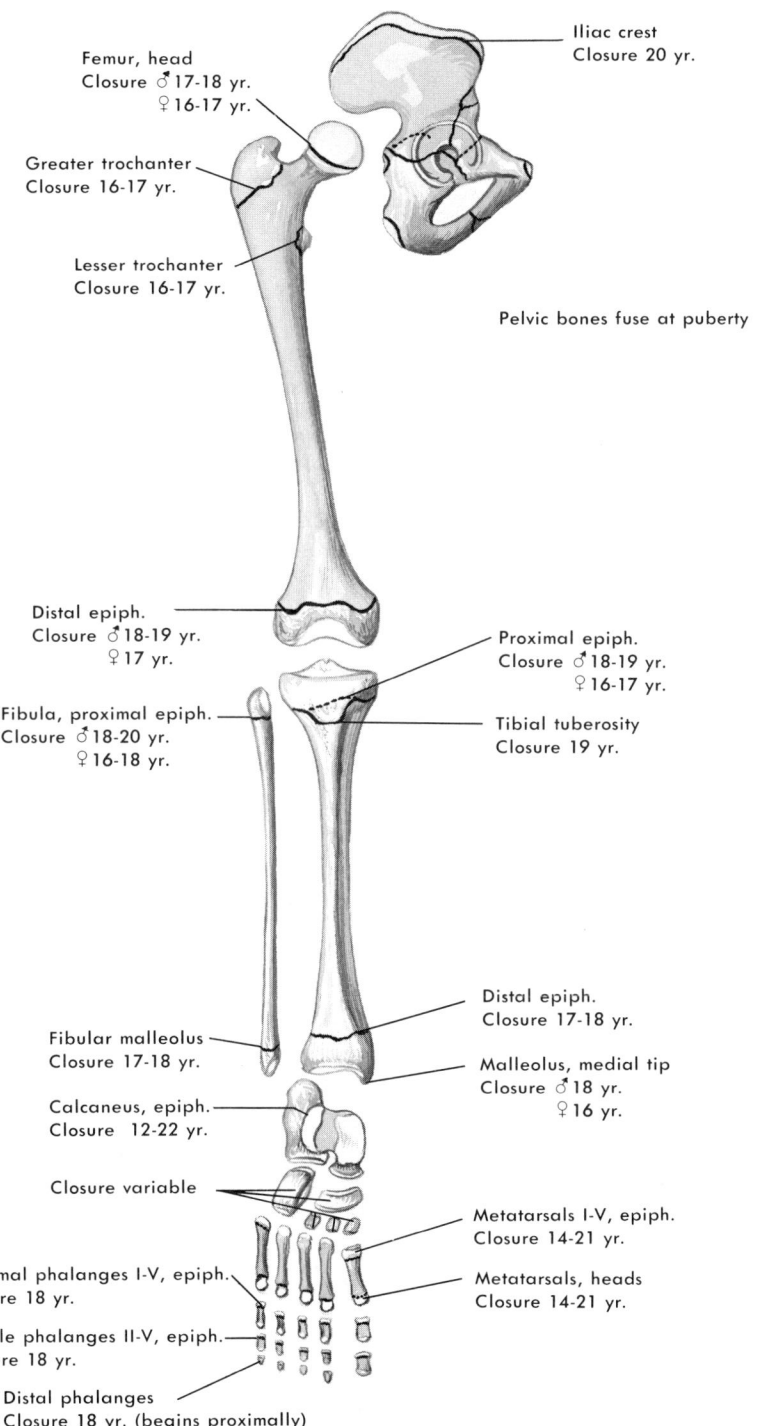

FIGURE 1–42. Average age of closure of the epiphyses in the lower limb in males and females.

(Adapted from von Lanz, T., and Wachsmuth, W.: Praktische Anatomie. Berlin, Julius Springer, 1938, p. 29.)

References

1. Barlow, T. E.: Some observations on the development of the human foot. Thesis. University of Manchester, 1943.
2. Elftman, H., and Manter, J. T.: The evolution of the human foot, with especial reference to the joints. J. Anat., *70*:56, 1935.
3. Gardner, E., Gray, D. J., and O'Rahilly, R: The prenatal development of the skeleton and joints of the human foot. J. Bone Joint Surg., *41-A*:847, 1959.
4. Harris, B. J.: Observations on the development of the human foot. Thesis. University of California, 1953.
5. O'Rahilly, R., Gardner, E., and Gray, D. J.: The skeletal development of the foot. Clin. Orthop., *16*:7, 1960.
6. Straus, W. L., Jr.: Growth of the human foot and its evolutionary significance. Contrib. Embryol., *19*:93, 1927.

DIAGNOSIS

Diagnosis of affections of the foot and ankle and the leg requires not only an evaluation of the entire neuromusculoskeletal system but also a complete general physical examination. A clinical history skillfully obtained and properly analyzed often holds the key to diagnosis. Many misdiagnoses are due to incompleteness of or inaccuracy in the histories. The orthopedic examination should follow a definite order unless the symptoms or status of the patient indicates deviation from it. It is imperative to pay scrupulous attention to minute details. The patient is stripped of all clothing and properly draped to expose the lower limbs and the body in action.

First the shoes are examined. Do they fit? Is there any abnormal wear? If the child has any other appliances such as night splints or orthoses, they also are studied.

Next, the stance and posture of the entire body are inspected. If the child is ambulatory, he is asked to stand, and his natural

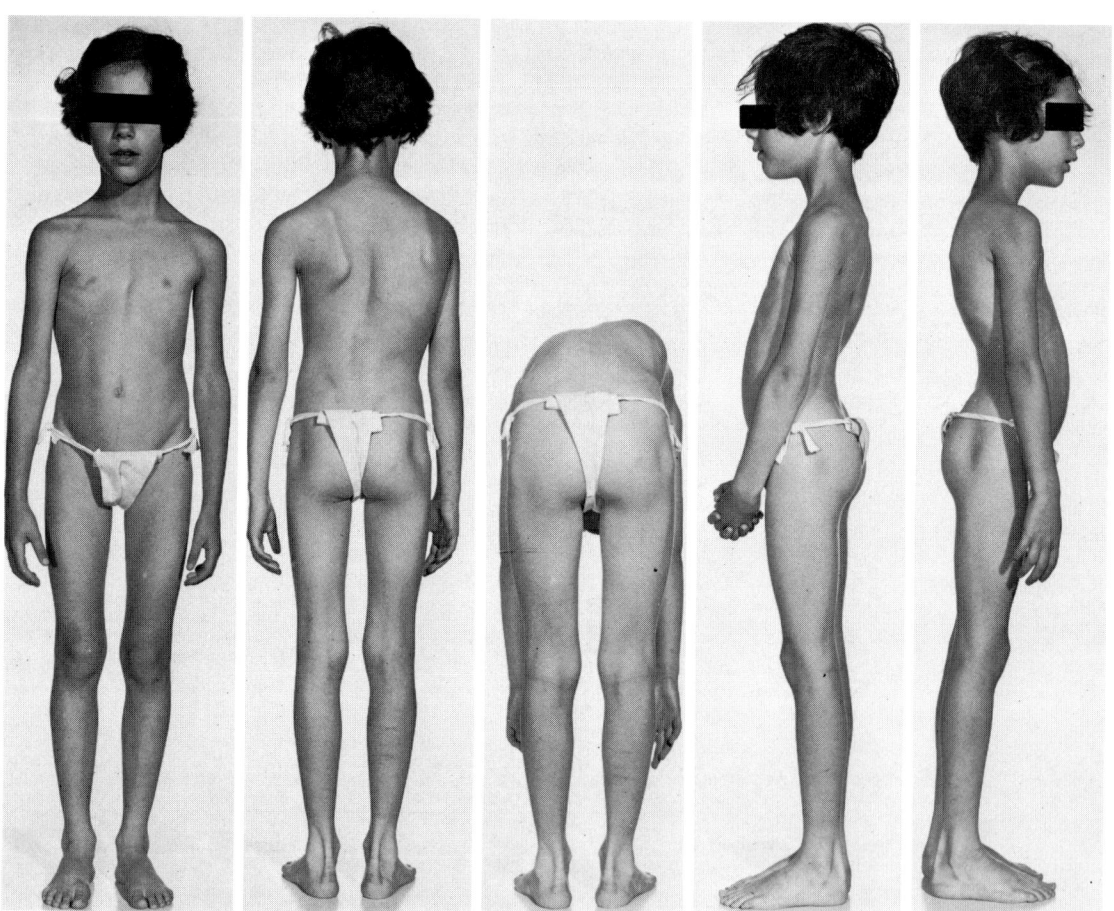

FIGURE 1–43. A girl with structural—right dorsal and left lumbar—idiopathic scoliosis.

When she bends forward the ribs in the right dorsal region are prominent. The rotation of the vertebrae is to the convexity of the lateral angulation.

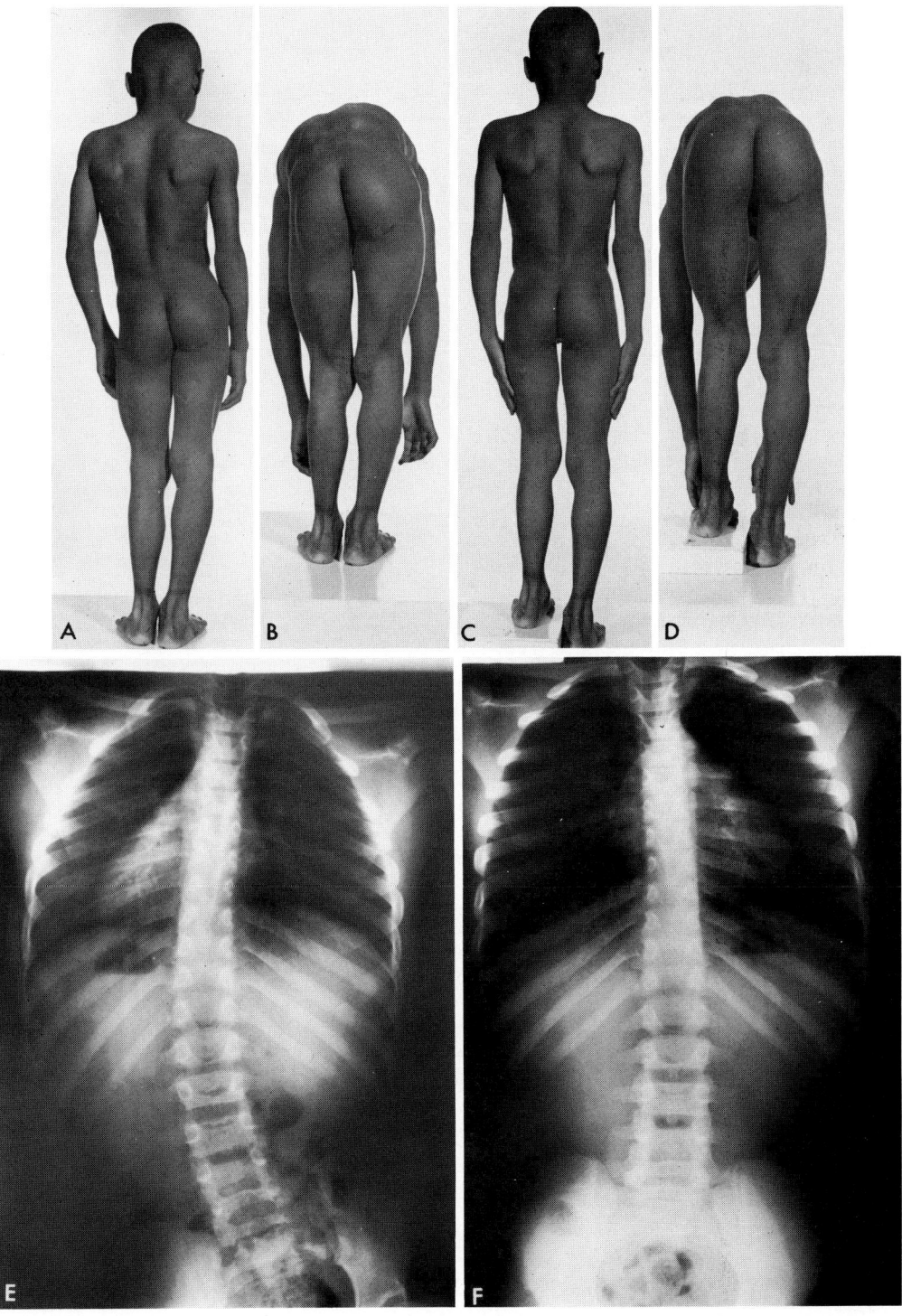

FIGURE 1–44. *Functional left lumbodorsal scoliosis due to a short left lower limb in a ten-year-old boy.*

standing posture and body outlines are observed from the back, front, and side. Are there any obvious defects of the spine or deformities of the limbs? Is there exaggeration or diminution of the normal physiologic anteroposterior curves of the dorsal and lumbar spine? What is the pelvic inclination? Are the shoulders carried behind the pelvis in the lateral view? What is the position of the head, scapulae, shoulders, gluteal and popliteal creases? Are the iliac crests level? Are the shoulders balanced over the pelvis? Is there deviation of the trunk to one side? (A plumb line held over the center of the occiput or over the spinous process of the seventh cervical vertebra should pass through the intergluteal cleft.) Is there any scoliosis? Is one hip more prominent than the other? Are the flank creases symmetrical? If scoliosis is present, the degree and direction of rotation of the involved vertebrae can best be demonstrated by asking the child to bend forward for inspection of his spine from the back (Fig. 1–43). In a structural curve, rotation of the vertebral body is to the convexity of lateral angulation; in a functional curve, it is to the concave side (Fig. 1–44). Is there muscle spasm in the paravertebral muscles? Is there limitation of motion of the vertebral column on forward flexion, extension, lateral bending, or rotation? A Trendelenburg test is performed by asking the patient to stand first on one leg and then on the other. (The hips should be in neutral extension.) Normally, when a person stands on one leg, the contralateral side of the pelvis is elevated with the contraction of the strong ipsilateral hip abductor muscles. When the opposite side of the pelvis drops (a positive Trendelenburg sign) it indicates weakness of the hip abductor muscles (Fig. 1–45).[19]

The general alignment of the lower limbs is also evaluated. Is the child bow-legged or knock-kneed? Is the heel in neutral position, or does it show a valgus or varus inclination (Fig. 1–46)? Are the longitudinal arches normal, high, or flattened? What is the line of weight-bearing in the lower limbs? Normally, the center of gravity of the body lies over the anterior superior iliac spine, and the weight passes to the middle of the patella and the proximal tibial tubercle and falls on the center of the foot, which is the second metatarsal.

If conditions permit, the child is asked to do a deep knee bend, return, and then, standing on one leg, rise to his tiptoes. Next he is asked to walk to demonstrate his gait.

Gait*

The primary objective of human locomotion is translation of the body from one place to another by means of bipedal gait. The act of walking is a dynamic and repetitive performance; it occurs with a definite rhythmic sequence of events that take place during a gait cycle. Normal walking is relatively effortless, performed with minimum expenditure of energy.[21, 28, 37]

Gait is an intricate process affected by a number of bodily mechanisms such as trunk sway, arm swing, and head motion. It is dependent on various reflexes—for example, the postural, labyrinthine, and righting reflexes.

GAIT CYCLE

A complete walk cycle is the period between the time when the foot strikes the ground and the next foot (heel)-strike of the same limb. The phasic events that take place progressively during a single forward step are expressed as a percentage of the walk cycle, the foot-strikes marking 0 and 100 per cent. The gait cycle consists of two phases—stance and swing (Fig. 1–47).

Stance Phase. In the stance phase the foot is in contact with the floor and the lower limb is bearing all or part of the body weight (Fig. 1–47B). This phase begins when the foot strikes the floor and ends when the toes rise off the floor. The stance phase, constituting 62 per cent of the gait cycle, is further subdivided into four periods by five events: foot (heel)-strike, opposite toe-off, reversal of fore-aft shear, opposite foot (heel)-strike, and toe-off. The periods that are delineated by these events are early double support, single limb support (which is divided by reversal of fore-aft shear into midstance and terminal stance), and late double support.

---

*Written with Dr. David H. Sutherland, Professor of Surgery, Division of Orthopedics and Rehabilitation, University of California at San Diego, and Chief of Orthopedic Surgery and Director of Motion Analysis Laboratory, Children's Hospital and Health Center, San Diego, California.

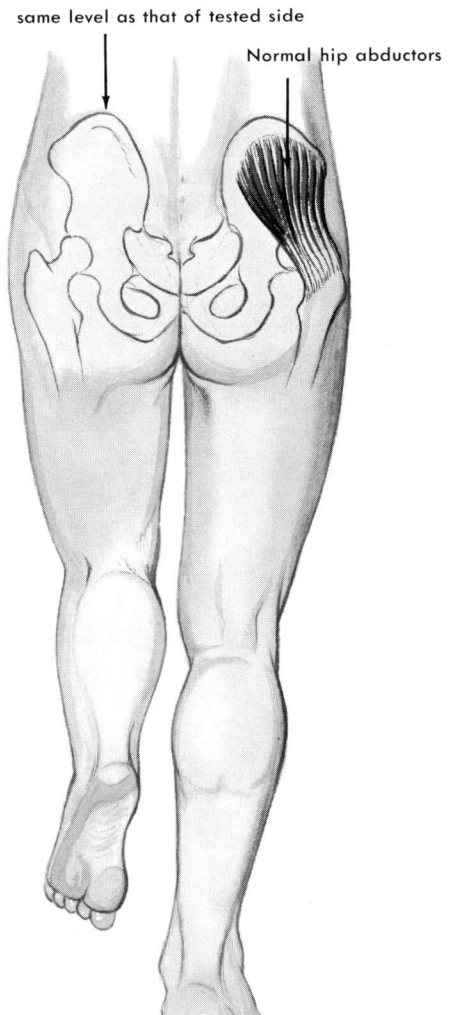 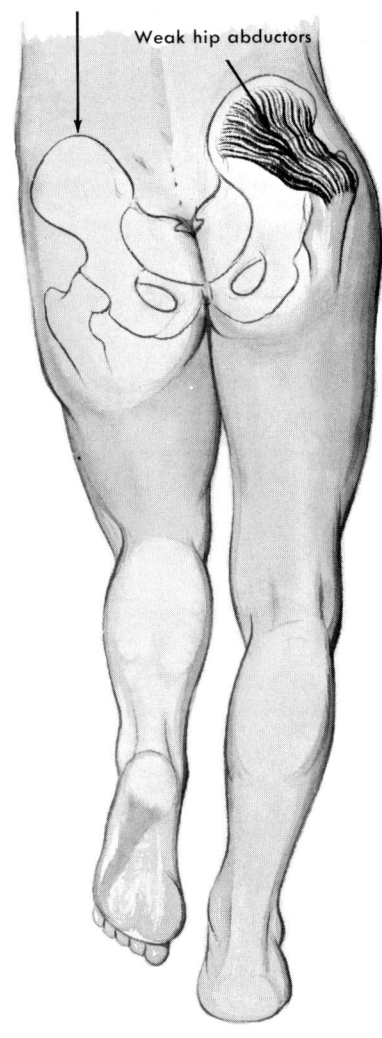

FIGURE 1–45. *Trendelenburg test.*
(Adapted from von Lanz, T., and Wachsmuth, W.: Praktische Anatomie. Berlin, Julius Springer, 1938, p. 167.)

The first period, known as *early double support,* constitutes 12 per cent of the walk cycle. It begins with foot (heel)-strike and terminates with opposite toe-off.

The second period, known as *midstance,* begins with opposite toe-off and ends with absence of forward shear. For visual gait analysis it is necessary to attempt an estimation of the time when the center of mass of the body passes in front of the point of support in the foot. During this period the person is balanced on his weight-bearing leg and the center of mass moves from behind to directly over the center of pressure of the foot.

The third period, *terminal stance,* is initiated by the beginning of aft shear, 35 per cent of the walk cycle, and terminates with opposite foot (heel)-strike, 50 per cent of the cycle. This period constitutes approximately 15 per cent of the walk cycle.

The fourth and final period of stance phase is *final double support.* It begins at opposite foot (heel)-strike, 50 per cent, and

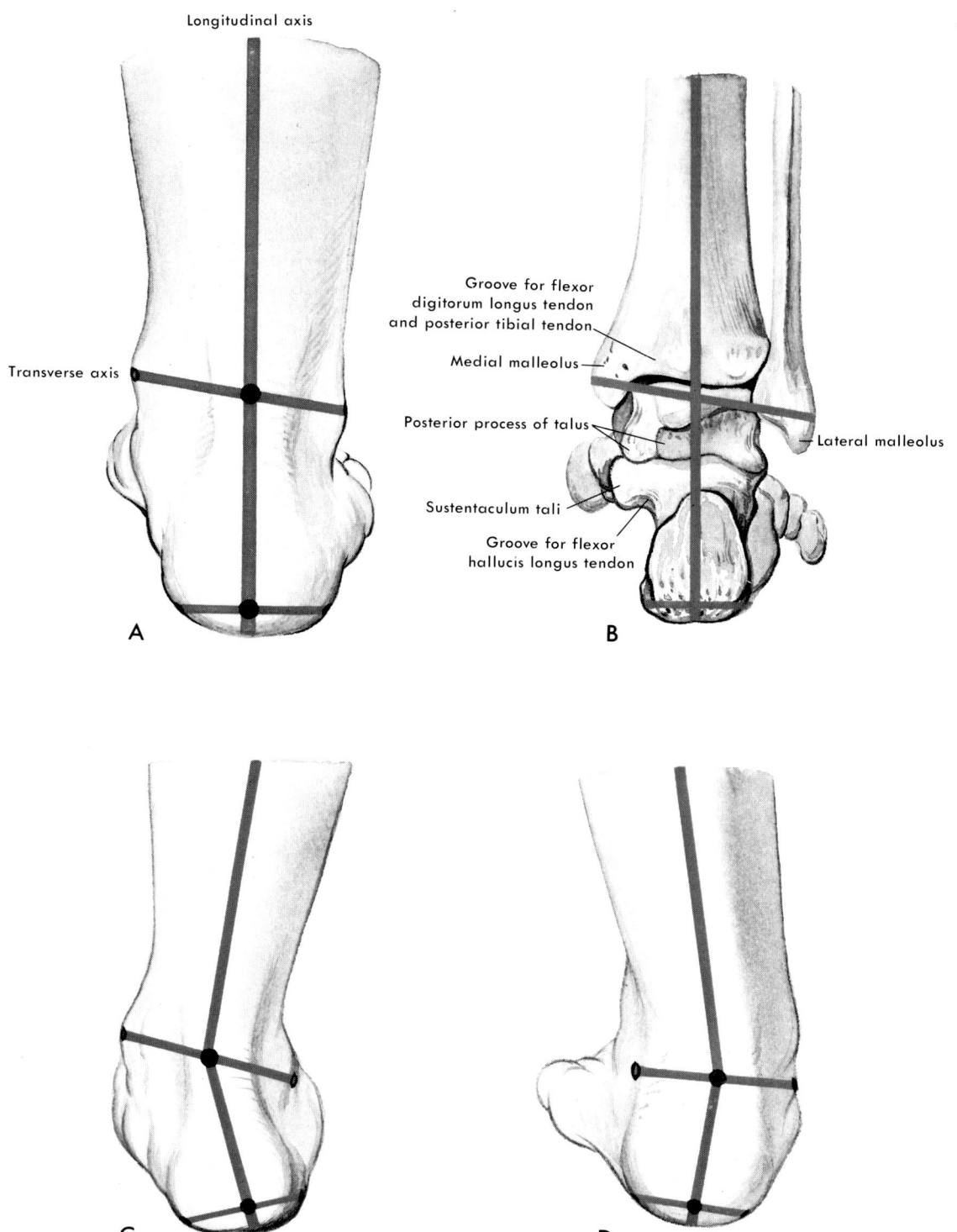

FIGURE 1–46. The heel in stance.

A and **B.** Neutral positions. **C.** Valgus inclination. **D.** Varus inclination.

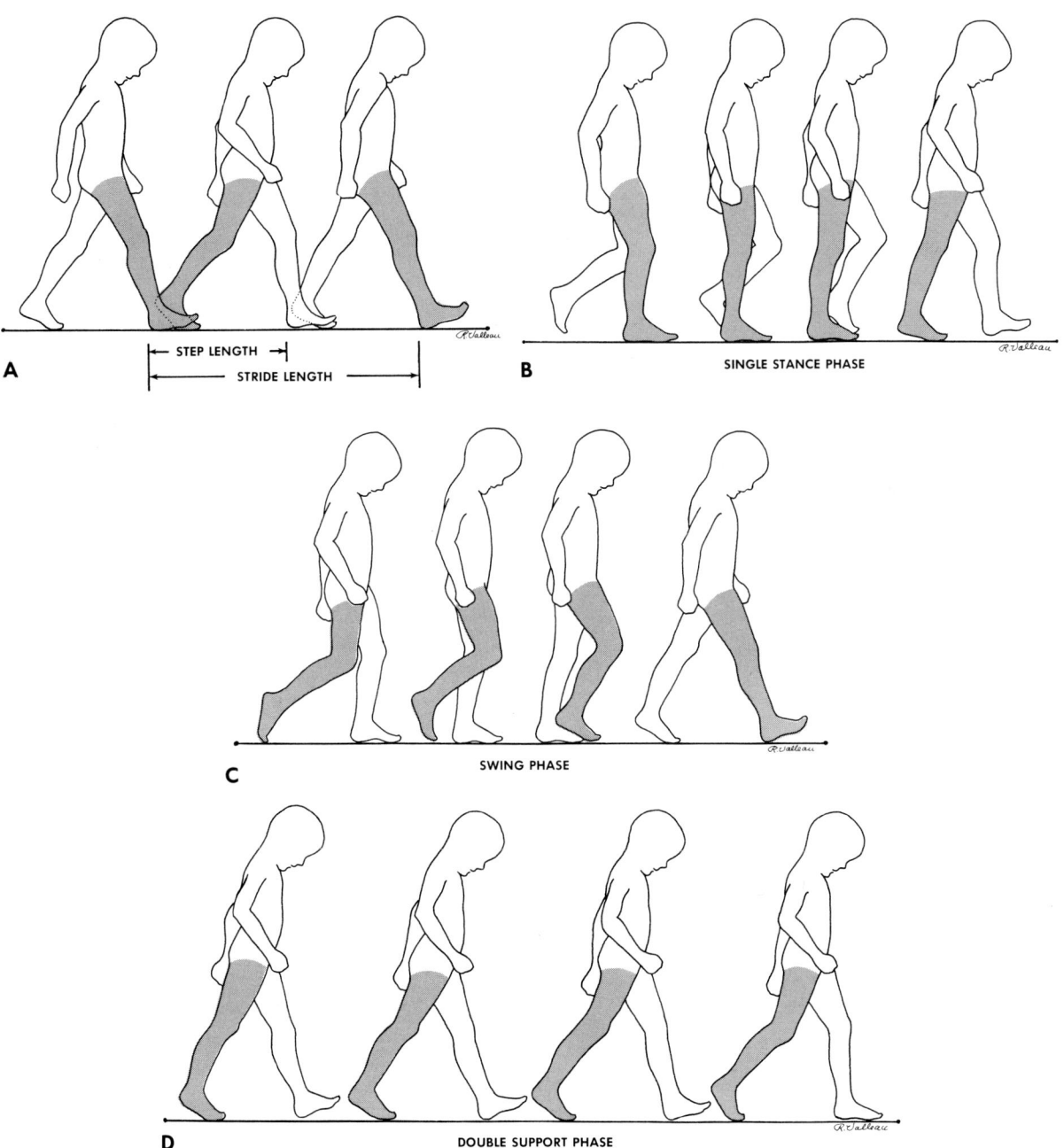

FIGURE 1–47. *The gait cycle.*

A. *Step length* is measured from the heel of one foot to the heel of the opposite foot during double support. *Stride length* is the distance from foot-strike to foot-strike of the same limb. **B.** Single-stance phase is the period (or time) of support by a single limb. **C.** Swing phase is the period in which the foot is off the floor. **D.** Double-support phase is the period in which both feet are on the floor.

ends at toe-off, 62 per cent. During this period weight is transferred to the opposite limb, and knee and hip flexion begin in the original stance limb.

The time in which both limbs are on the floor simultaneously, known as double support time (zero to 12 per cent and 50 to 62 per cent) in normal walking), diminishes with increased walking velocity and disappears during running.

Swing Phase. In the *swing phase* the foot is not touching the floor and the body weight is borne by the opposite limb (Fig. 1–47C). Beginning at toe-off and ending at foot (heel)-strike, this phase occupies approximately 38 per cent of the walk cycle (from 62 per cent to 100 per cent). It is subdivided into three periods—initial swing, midswing, and terminal swing.

Initial swing begins at 62 per cent of the cycle and ends when the trailing limb moves to the plane of the supporting foot, at approximately 78 per cent of the walk cycle.

Midswing begins when the swing limb passes the opposite limb in stance and ends when the tibia is vertical—at 87 per cent of the walk cycle.

Terminal swing is the period in which the limb continues to advance and decelerates and contacts the floor for the beginning of another gait cycle. The deceleration period usually occupies the final 13 per cent of the walk cycle. The force of gravity and the musculature of the limbs break the forward motion of the swing limb smoothly; the foot strikes the ground, and the full sequence of the gait cycle is completed at 100 per cent. This sequence of the cycle is continually repeated with the limbs alternating during normal walking on level ground.

Gait may be described as an interplay between loss and recovery of balance in which the center of gravity of the body shifts constantly. As one pushes forward on his weight-bearing limb, the center of gravity of his body shifts forward, and he tends to fall forward, only to be stopped by the swinging leg, which arrives in its new position just in time.

Other terms are used in analysis of gait. *Stride length* is the distance traveled in the same time span as the gait cycle; *step length* is the distance from the heel of one foot to the heel of the opposite foot during the double-support phase (Fig. 1–47 A). *Cadence* is the number of steps per minute. *Walking velocity* is the speed of movement in a single direction in centimeters per second. *Angular rotation* is rotation of the joint in degrees plotted against percentage of the walk cycle.

A number of forces act upon and modify the human body in forward motion—gravity, counteraction of the floor, muscle forces, and kinetic energy developed with the movement of body mass.

GRAVITY

The location of the center of gravity of the adult body has been estimated to be just anterior to the second sacral vertebra within the true pelvis at a level that is about 55 per cent of the total height of the individual.[31] In normal human gait, the pathway followed by the center of gravity of the body is a smooth, regular curve moving up and down in the vertical plane with an average rise and fall of about 2 inches. The low point is reached at the double-support phase when both feet are on the ground, and the high point at midstance. The center of gravity of the body is also displaced laterally in the horizontal plane during locomotion; the total side-to-side distance traveled is about 2 inches. The motion is toward the weight-bearing limb and reaches its lateral limit in midstance. When the vertical and horizontal motions of the center of gravity of the body are combined, they are found to describe a double sinusoidal curve.

Reactions Between Foot and Floor. Friction between the floor and the foot affects gait. The force of gravity stabilizes the contact of the foot with the ground, modifying acceleration and deceleration.

The *force plate* is a complex device that measures the magnitude and direction of the forces of vertical loading, fore-and-aft shear, medial and lateral shear, and medial and lateral torque.[26, 29, 36, 38] The center of pressure is the instantaneous location of the center of the vertical force on the force plate. The line of application of the floor reaction force (vector $\bar{R}$) is the result of the vertical force (vector $\bar{F}v$) and fore-aft shear (vector $\bar{F}s$) (Fig. 1–48 side view). The termination of the floor reaction force vector $\bar{R}$ is at the center of pressure (Fig. 1–48 top view).

Immediately after heel-strike there is a forward peak in the fore-and-aft shear that

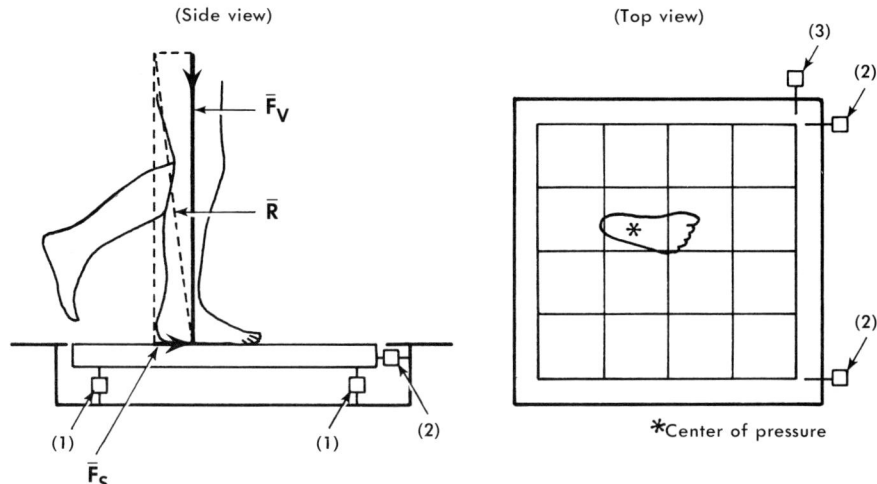

FIGURE 1–48. Force plate.

Side view shows subject in single-limb support phase. Vertical force vector $\bar{F}_v$, fore-aft shear vector $\bar{F}_s$, and line of application of the floor reaction force, $\bar{R}$, are shown. The center of pressure (calculated) is illustrated in the top view.

quickly reverses as the foot pushes backward on the floor.

Lateral and medial shear recordings demonstrate the lateral shift of the center of gravity in gait.

DETERMINANTS OF GAIT

The six basic determinants of gait as defined by Saunders, Inman, and Eberhart in 1953 are as follows:[33]

Pelvic Rotation—the First Determinant. In normal level locomotion, the pelvis rotates in the horizontal plane 4 degrees forward on the swing limb and 4 degrees backward on the stance limb with a total magnitude of rotation of approximately 8 degrees (Fig. 1–49). Since the pelvis is rigid, the rotation acutally occurs at the hip joint, which passes from medial to lateral rotation during the stance phase. The pelvis and two lower limbs during double-stance phase (swing limb at heel-strike and stance limb at heel-off) form an isosceles triangle. The apex of this triangle determines the height of the center of gravity from the ground. The sides of the bipod intersect the plane of the floor at an angle. Rotating the pelvis in the horizontal plane decreases this angle between the limbs and the floor, thereby relatively "lengthening" the limbs and propping up the bipod. This has the effect of flattening the arc of the pathway of the center of gravity by elevating the extremities of the arc. The stride is lengthened without increasing the drop of the center of gravity at the instant of heel-strike. In this way, the expenditure of energy in locomotion is greatly reduced.

Pelvic Tilt—the Second Determinant. The pelvis also tilts during normal locomotion, listing downward in relation to the horizontal plane on the side opposite to that of the weight-bearing limb (positive Trendelenburg sign). The angular displacement occurs at the hip joint and is, on the average, 5 degrees (Fig. 1–50). To permit pelvic tilt, the knee joint of the non-weight-bearing limb must flex to allow toe clearance for the swing-through of that limb. Pelvic tilt causes the center of gravity to lower by approximately half. By cutting the vertical displacement of the center of gravity in half and by shortening the pendulum of the limb by knee flexion in the swing phase, energy is saved.

Knee Flexion After Heel-Strike in Stance Phase—the Third Determinant. The supporting lower limb enters the stance phase at heel-strike with the knee in full extension, after which the knee joint immediately begins to flex until the foot is flat on the ground. The average degree of knee flexion at this time is 15 degrees (Fig. 1–51). Shortly after midstance, the knee joint passes into

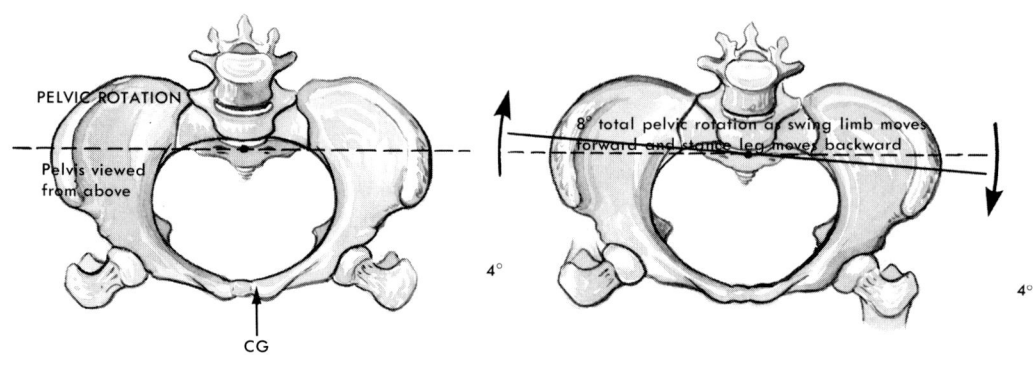

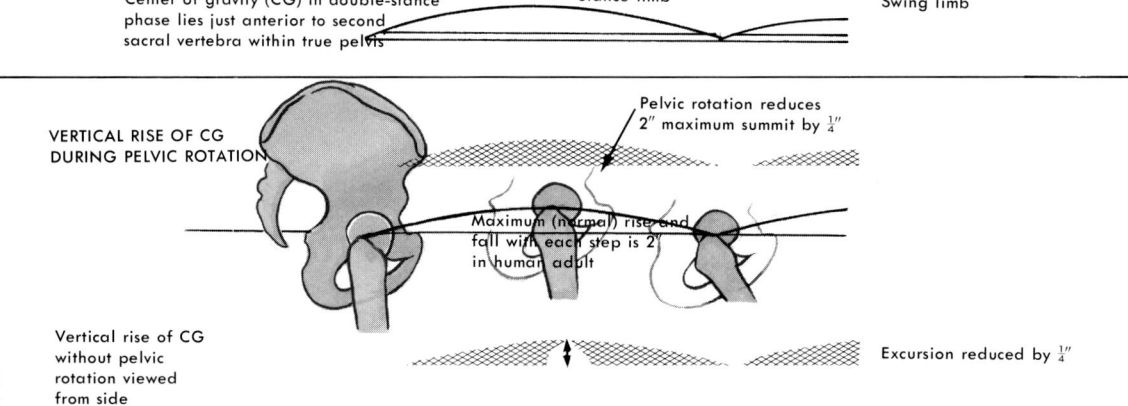

FIGURE 1–49. Pelvic rotation—the first determinant of gait.

The pelvis rotates in the horizontal plane 4 degrees forward on the swing limb and 4 degrees backward on the stance limb with a total magnitude of 8 degrees. This pelvic rotation spreads apart the apex of the isosceles triangle formed by the pelvis and the two lower limbs in double stance. The angle formed by the sides of the bipod is diminished, the length of the limbs is "increased," and the amplitude of the displacement of the center of gravity located at the apex of the isosceles triangle is decreased. A 2-inch amplitude of center of gravity displacement is decreased by ⅛ inch to 1¾ inch. The result is reduction in the expenditure of energy in locomotion.

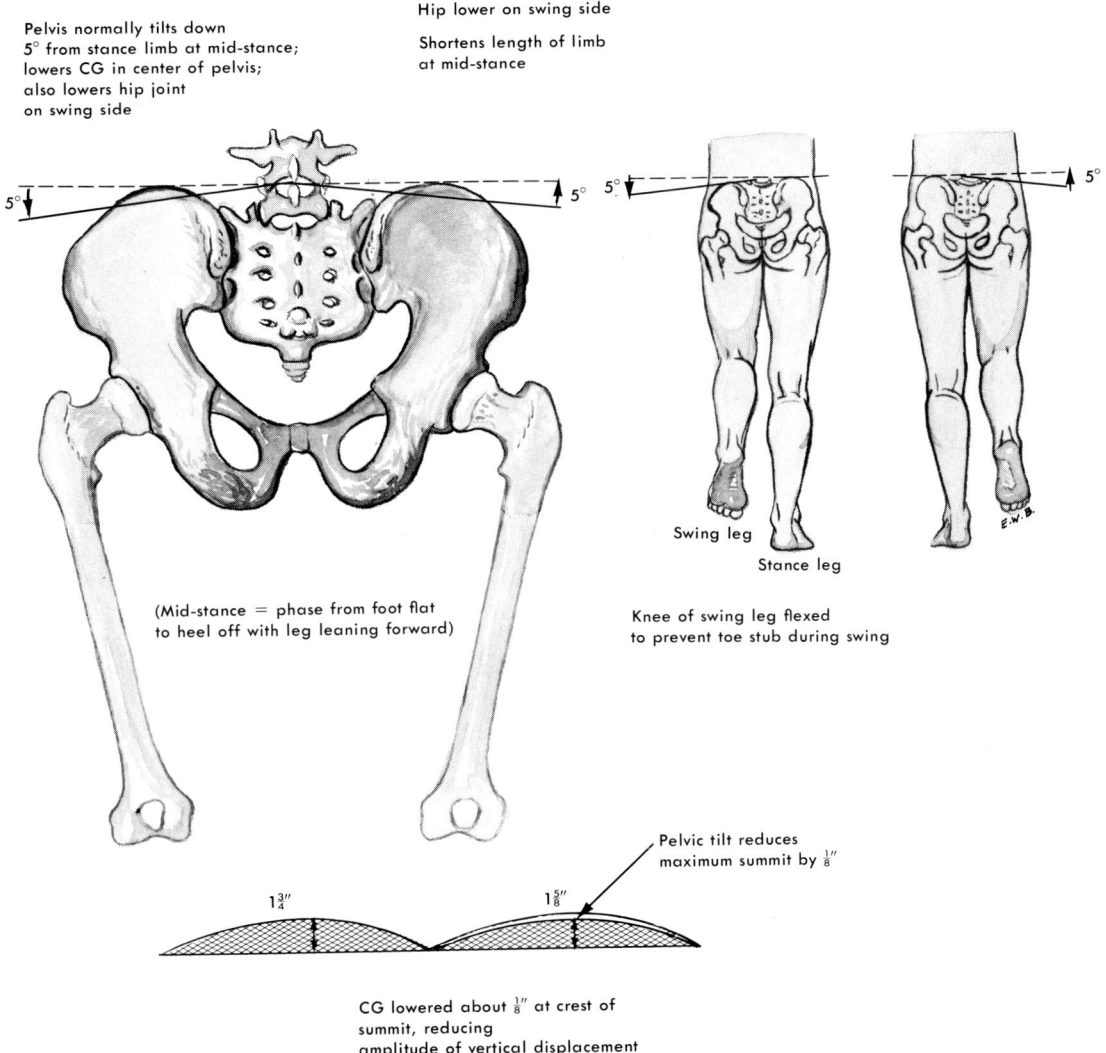

FIGURE 1–50. *Pelvic tilt—the second determinant of gait.*

The pelvis tilts down 5 degrees in relation to the horizontal plane on the side opposite to that of the weight-bearing limb (positive Trendelenburg sign). The knee on the swing limb must flex (as the hip is lowered) to clear the toes. The center of gravity at the crest of the summit is lowered by 3/16 inch, thereby diminishing the amplitude of vertical displacement from 1¾ inches to 1 9/16 inches.

KNEE FLEXION

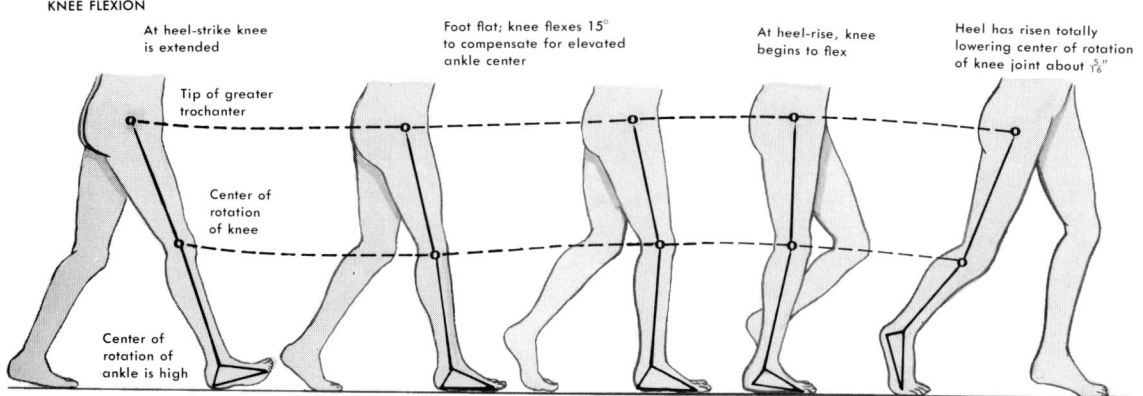

FIGURE 1–51. Knee flexion after heel-strike in the stance phase—the third determinant of gait.

At heel-strike the knee is fully extended, and at foot-flat the knee is flexed 15 degrees, thereby in midstance the path of the center of gravity is depressed. This provides a diminution in the rise of the center of gravity summit by about 5/16 inch.

extension once more, and this is immediately followed by the second flexion of the knee, beginning simultaneously with heel-rise as the limb is carried into the swing phase. This period of the stance phase in which the knee is first locked in extension, unlocked by flexion, and again locked in extension prior to its final flexion is referred to as the period of *double knee-lock*. This pattern of repeated knee flexion results in reduction of vertical displacement of the center of gravity as the body weight is carried forward over the stance leg, again conserving energy.

It is apparent from the foregoing discussion that pelvic rotation, pelvic tilt, and knee flexion in stance (all three determinants) flatten the arc through which the center of gravity of the body is translated. Pelvic tilt and knee flexion act to depress the summit of the arc, whereas pelvic rotation elevates the extremities of the arc.

Foot and Ankle Motion—the Fourth Determinant. The motions of the foot, ankle, and knee are intimately related in smoothing out the pathway of the center of gravity in the plane of progression. The center of rotation of the ankle joint is located approximately at a point connecting the tips of the medial and lateral malleoli; it traverses an

ANKLE ROTATION

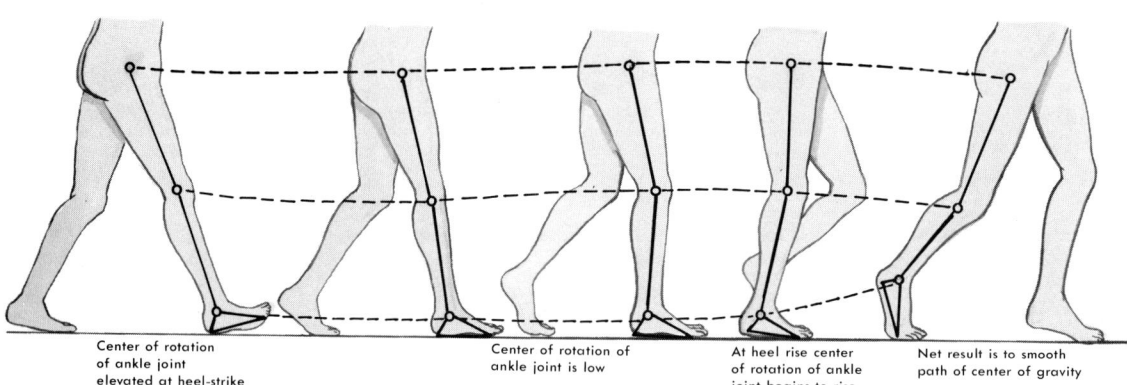

FIGURE 1–52. Foot and ankle motion—the fourth determinant of gait.

At heel-strike the foot is dorsiflexed and the center of rotation of the ankle is elevated; at foot-flat the foot plantar flexes and the center of rotation of the ankle is lowered. At push-off the heel lifts from the floor and the center of rotation of the ankle rises again. The total effect is to make the pathway of the center of gravity smooth. The motions of the foot, ankle, and knee are intimately associated; they should be considered in relation to each other.

KNEE EXTENSION

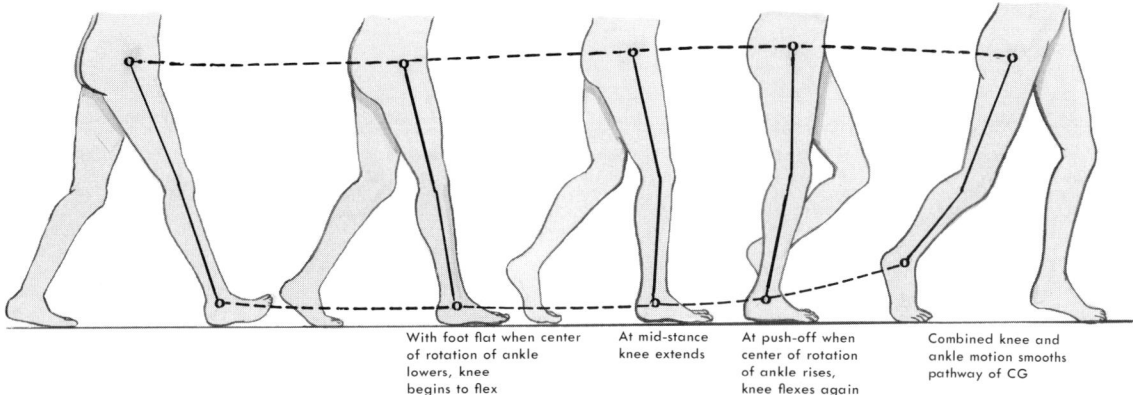

With foot flat when center of rotation of ankle lowers, knee begins to flex

At mid-stance knee extends

At push-off when center of rotation of ankle rises, knee flexes again

Combined knee and ankle motion smooths pathway of CG

FIGURE 1–53. Knee motion—the fifth determinant of gait.

At heel-strike, when the center of rotation of the ankle is high, the knee joint begins to flex. During midstance when the ankle center of rotation is low the knee joint flexes a second time. The net effect of this close relation between the motions of the foot, ankle, and knee is to smooth the pathway of the center of gravity.

arc formed by the level arm of the calcaneus. At heel-strike, the foot is dorsiflexed and the center of rotation of the ankle is elevated; the knee is in full extension (Fig. 1–52). Next, rapid plantar flexion of the foot takes place, and when the foot is flat on the ground through midstance, the center of rotation of the ankle is lowered. The knee is flexed 15 degrees at foot-flat. Then the heel rises from the ground, elevating the center of rotation of the ankle again. These motions of the foot and ankle smooth out the path of the center of gravity when coupled with knee motion, which thus acts as the fifth determinant of gait.

Knee Motion—the Fifth Determinant. The center of rotation of the knee is considered to be a point on the axis connecting the greatest prominences of the medial and lateral femoral condyles. The knee flexes just after heel-strike when the center of rotation of the ankle is elevated, and thereby the center of rotation of the knee is lowered. During midstance the knee is fully extended and its center of rotation raised when that of the ankle is lowered (Fig. 1–53). At pushoff the knee flexes again when the center of rotation of the ankle is rising the second time. The foot-ankle and knee motions are combined in such a manner that the ankle rise is largely cancelled out by the knee flexion.

Lateral Displacement of Pelvis—the Sixth Determinant. In bipedal gait the center of gravity of the body must shift from the second sacral vertebra over the supporting foot while the contralateral limb swings forward. As the weight of the body is being shifted from one limb to the other, the pelvis moves laterally in the horizontal plane (Fig. 1–54). If the two limbs were parallel to one another, the necessary shift would be half the interval between the axes of the hip joints, approximately 4 inches. The femoral and tibial axes do not drop vertically from the hip joints, however; the femora are inclined medially at the hip, and the tibiae are aligned vertically at the knee joint. This tibiofemoral relationship narrows the support base and provides sufficient balance. Therefore, the lateral movement of the center of gravity toward the stance foot is reduced to only 1 inch, or a total of about 2 inches displacement per gait cycle.

The final result of the combination of the six determinants of gait is containment of rise and fall of the center of gravity (vertical displacement), and of side-to-side motion of the pelvis (horizontal displacement) within a 2-inch-square box. Exaggerations in the range of any one of these six basic determinants of locomotion are compensated for by reductions in another. The interaction of the six determinants of gait creates a smooth pathway for the forward displacement of the center of gravity of the body.

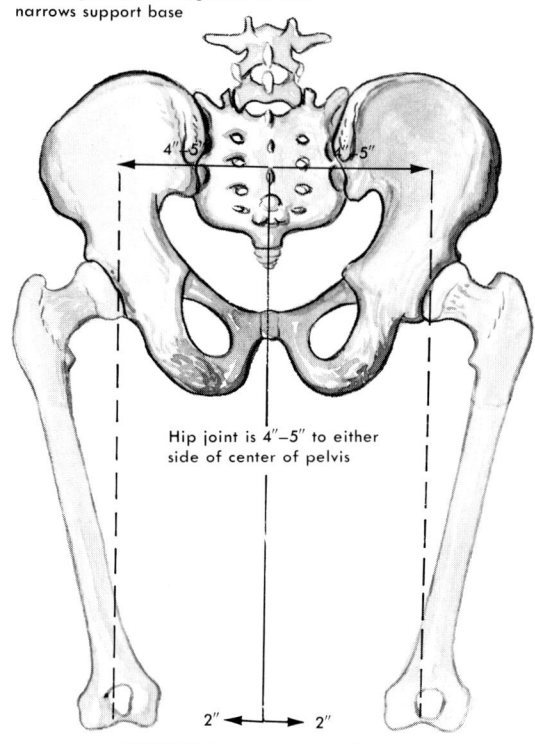
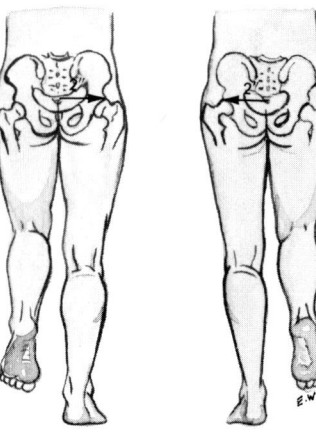

FIGURE 1–54. *Lateral displacement of the pelvis—the sixth determinant of gait.*

The center of body gravity must shift over the stance foot to provide balance; otherwise the person will fall over the unsupported limb. If the lower limbs dropped vertically straight, parallel to each other, from the hip joints, the center of gravity would have to be displaced 3 to 4 inches side to side over the supporting foot. The medial inclination of the femoral shafts and the valgus inclination of the tibiae at the knees narrow the support base and provide a more secure balance. Thereby the center of body gravity shifts only 1 inch toward the stance foot or a total of 2 inches per gait cycle.

AXIAL ROTATIONS

During walking the various segments of the lower limb rotate around their long axes.[24, 25, 30] In general, from the swing phase to foot-flat the rotation is medial, and when the foot prepares to leave the floor the rotation is reversed laterally. In gait analysis, a stick attached to the anterior aspect of the pelvic belt is used to measure pelvic rotation. Viewed from the front, the tip and base of the stick are lined up when pelvic rotation is zero degrees. When the tip of the stick is to the right of center, the right side of the pelvis is rotated medially and the left side laterally. As stated previously, the pelvis rotates anteriorly 4 degrees during swing and posteriorly 4 degrees during stance. During the swing phase, the femur rotates laterally about 5 degrees at the hip joint; in the stance phase it rotates medially 3 to 4 degrees. Its total rotation is 8 to 9 degrees during a full gait cycle. Femoral torsion is measured from the front; it is zero when the hip, patella, and ankle are in a straight line; when the patella is facing the body midline from the hip to ankle line, the femur is rotated medially.

At heel-strike with the foot in neutral position the tibia rotates medially to align the ankle with the foot. At completion of foot-flat it begins to rotate laterally against the fixed foot, and it is at its maximum lateral rotation when the foot leaves the ground. It then begins to rotate medially in preparation for heel-strike. The total rotation of the tibia on the femur is 9 degrees.

In summary, during the act of walking,

the weight of the body is supported by one lower limb (stance phase—the foot is on the ground), while the other limb executes the movement of progression (swing phase—the limb is carried into its new position). Normal locomotion represents a heel-toe sequence of support and progression, i.e., the weight of the body is first supported by the heel of the advancing lower limb, next by the foot, until the heel is lifted, and then by the ball of the forefoot. In addition to associated motions of the pelvis, hip, and knee, there are normal swinging movements of the upper limbs—as one lower limb is advanced, the upper limb of the opposite side advances.

MUSCLE ACTION IN GAIT

A source of energy is required for locomotion. The initial energy to start, accelerate, and decelerate the leg segments is supplied by muscle action (Fig. 1–55). Other factors that enter into the cycle are momentum and gravity.

Muscles are grouped about joints as primary extensors, flexors, abductors, adductors, and medial and lateral rotators. Some muscles cross only one joint, whereas others span two or three articulations. Their function changes according to positions of the limb.

In general, the muscles of the lower limb are used to stabilize, accelerate, or decelerate the leg. These muscles function while contracting, lengthening, or maintaining the same length. Electromyographic studies of muscle action during gait have shown that muscles act over very short periods and that during long intervals of the gait cycle they are relaxed, the limb being propelled forward by the pendulum like action of its own momentum. Concentric contraction of a muscle shortens the distance between its origin and insertion and generates *motor power* to move or lift a part. The force exerted and the work performed can be readily calculated. Another major function of muscles in the lower limb during walking is to act as *shock absorbers* by decelerating a moving limb. Progressive elongation of a muscle by eccentric contraction serves to resist the passive forces that act to move a limb segment in the opposite direction. Muscles also function as stabilizers by isometric contraction and by maintaining a limb in a given position by locking the joints. Therefore, in gait, the muscles of a limb may contract concentrically (shorten the distance between origin and insertion) to provide motor power, contract eccentrically (lengthen the distance between origin and insertion) to perform as shock absorbers, or contract isometrically (no change in the distance between origin and insertion) to act as stabilizers.

Muscle activity is measured by wire electromyography of the lower limb during walking; the electromyograph does not, however, distinguish between the various forms of the muscle's activity of lengthening, shortening, or isometric contraction.

The quadriceps femoris shows muscle action potential during the terminal period in swing and during the early stance phase (90 per cent to 22 per cent of the gait cycle). It contracts eccentrically, lengthening and acting as a shock absorber. It permits flexion of the knee until the foot reaches a foot-flat position. It should be noted that the duration of quadriceps activity is short. When the ankle rises at push-off, the knee is again flexed to counterbalance further heel-rise and make the path of the center of gravity smooth. During this very brief period of acceleration of the stance phase and the beginning of swing phase after toe-off, the rectus femoris and vastus intermedius portions of the quadriceps femoris fire again, contracting eccentrically to act as shock absorbers.

At heel-strike the pelvic balancer and trunk supporter groups of muscles (gluteus medius, gluteus minimus, gluteus maximus, erector spinae, and tensor fasciae latae) are active. They contract eccentrically, allowing the pelvis to drop 5 degrees. They complete their function by heel-off. The next group of muscles to become active are the plantar flexor muscles—the triceps surae, posterior tibial, long toe flexors, and peroneus longus. The soleus and gastrocnemius, the most powerful and vital, provide the greatest force. They begin firing immediately after foot-flat, contracting eccentrically and lengthening to stabilize the tibia and allow extension of the knee. Toward the end of midstance they contract concentrically and plantar flex the ankle from 10 degrees of dorsiflexion to neutral position.

Next, the rectus femoris, tensor fasciae latae, adductor longus, and adductor mag-

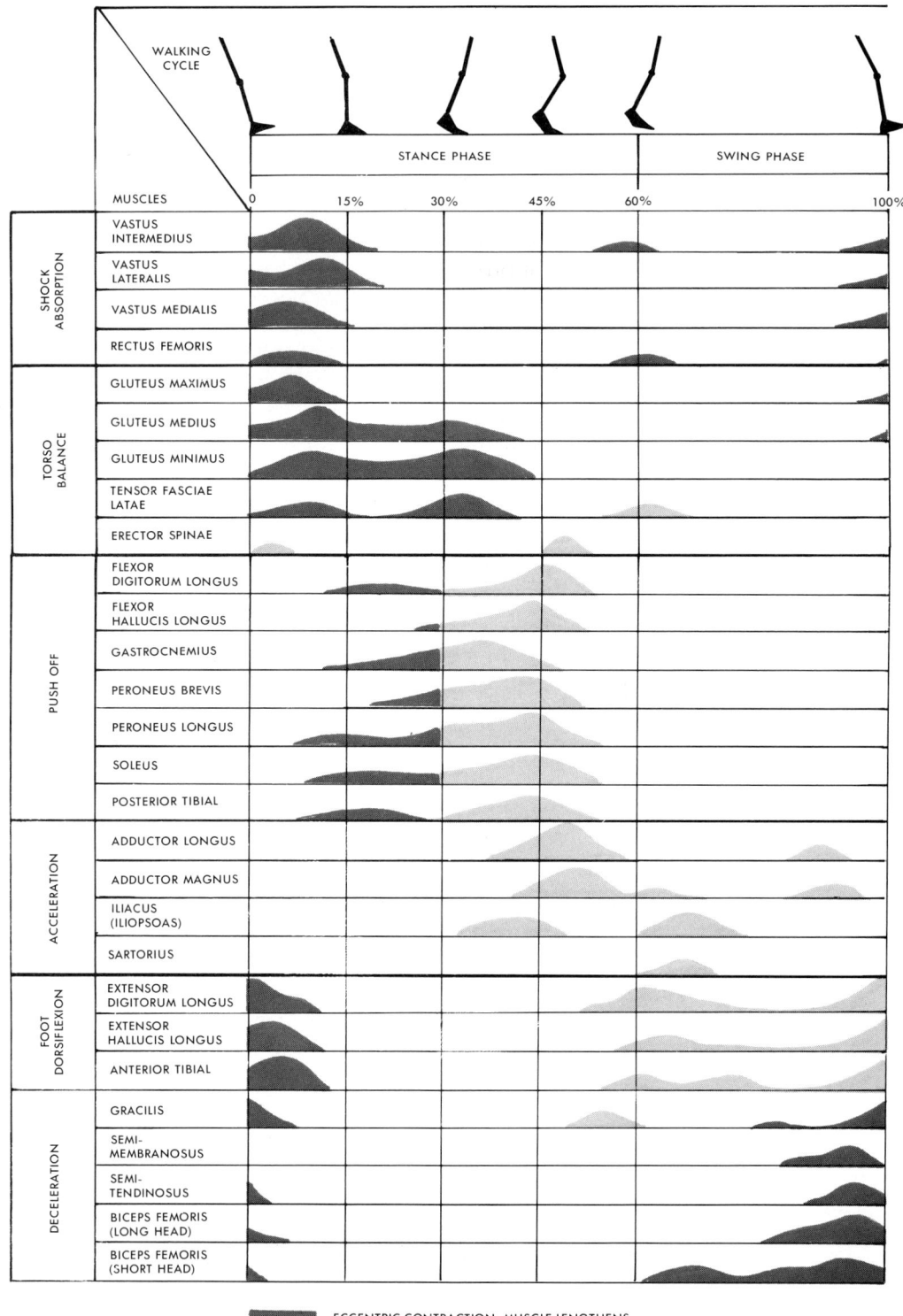

FIGURE 1–55. Electromyograph of lower limb during walking.

(Adapted from Charles O. Bechtol. *In* Bowke, J. H., and Hall, C. B.: Normal human gait *in* Atlas of Orthotics. American Academy of Orthopedic Surgeons. The C. V. Mosby Co., St. Louis, Mo., 1975, p. 141.)

nus contract concentrically during late double support. The iliopsoas acts during early swing.

The foot dorsiflexors (anterior tibial, long toe extensors, and extensor hallucis longus) contract concentrically during swing phase to provide enough force for the foot to clear the floor. They also contract eccentrically after heel-strike to make the descent of the forefoot to the ground smooth.

The decelerator group of the muscles consists of the gracilis, semimembranosus, semitendinosus, and biceps femoris. They contract eccentrically during the last 10 to 20 per cent of the gait cycle just prior to heel-strike to decelerate the swinging limb. The brief period of contraction during the initial stance phase provides limb stability.

DEVELOPMENT OF MATURE GAIT

The average milestones of development of locomotion are as follows: the infant sits at 6 months of age, crawls at 9 months, cruises and walks with assistance at 12 months, walks independently at 15 months, and runs at 18 months.[22, 23, 34, 35] On gross inspection the independent gait of the infant has a wide base, the hips and knees are hyperflexed, the arms are held in extension and abduction, and the movements are brisk. With maturation of the neuromuscular system, gradually the width of the base diminishes, the movements become smoother, reciprocal swing of the upper limbs begins, and step length and walking velocity increase. The adult pattern of gait develops between three and five years of age.[39]

The development of mature gait depends upon maturation of the central nervous system, which progresses cephalocaudally.

Sutherland, Olshen, Cooper, and Woo performed gait studies in 186 normal children between one and seven years of age. Electromyograms were obtained by surface electrodes; 12 joint angle and 9 linear measurements were recorded in each lower limb throughout a gait cycle. The data were gathered and processed by high-speed movies, Graf-pen sonic digitizer, and computer and plotter. These investigators found that, from two years and on, sagittal plane angular rotations in gait are very similar to and more closely related to those of the adult. Children under two years of age exhibited greater knee flexion and ankle dorsiflexion in stance phase, a decrease in knee flexion waves, and pronounced lateral rotation of the hips. By 18 months of age reciprocal arm-swing and heel-strike were present. Major determinants indicating maturity of gait are single-stance percentage (an index of limb stability), walking velocity, cadence, and step length. As the child gets older and acquires an adult gait pattern the cadence decreases and walking velocity and step length increase. According to these criteria gait maturity is established by three years of age.[39]

PATHOLOGIC GAIT

Clinical appraisal of the gait is important. Abnormalities of gait are often specifically diagnostic. The child is usually asked to walk normally, then to walk on his toes and on his heels, then to run. He may be asked to climb stairs. When disorders of the neuromuscular system are suspected, he may be asked to walk "tandem," i.e., to place one heel directly in front of the toes of the other foot; to follow a line on the floor; to walk forward and backward six steps with eyes open and then with eyes closed; to walk sideward and around a chair. He may be asked to walk rapidly and stop suddenly.

In neurologic diseases one may gain some information by listening to the patient walk. The flopping sound of the gait of a person who has a foot drop, the dragging or scraping characteristic of spasticity, and the stamping in ataxia are well known. Inspection of the patient's shoes, noting the worn places, is of great value. When a patient has appliances, such as crutches or braces, he should be observed walking with their aid.

Abnormalities of gait may be caused by muscle weakness (source of motion), structural deformity of bones and joints (the articulated levers), neurologic disorders (which disturb awareness of need for, action of, and control of motion), and cardiopulmonary diseases (which will affect oxygen supply and energy).

Muscle Weakness. A common cause of pathologic gait is muscle weakness. The type of limp depends upon the location of the weakness and its degree.

The *gluteus medius* is the principal hip abductor. Normally, when one stands on one leg, the gluteus medius of the same side elevates the pelvis on the opposite side, balancing the trunk over the weight-bearing hip. If the gluteus medius is paralyzed and the patient stands on the paralyzed lower limb, the opposite side of the pelvis drops (positive Trendelenburg test) (see Fig. 1–45). As he walks and bears weight on the weak limb, because the paralyzed gluteus medius cannot stabilize the pelvis over the weight-bearing leg, the patient, at each stance phase of gait, lurches his trunk over toward the side of the weak gluteus medius (Fig. 1–56). By lurching his trunk toward and over the hip with gluteus medius paralysis, he brings the center of gravity of the body weight over and beyond the femoral head in order to compensate for the abductor weakness. In gaits in which muscle weakness exists, as a rule, the center of gravity of the body is shifted toward the paralyzed muscle in the stance phase.

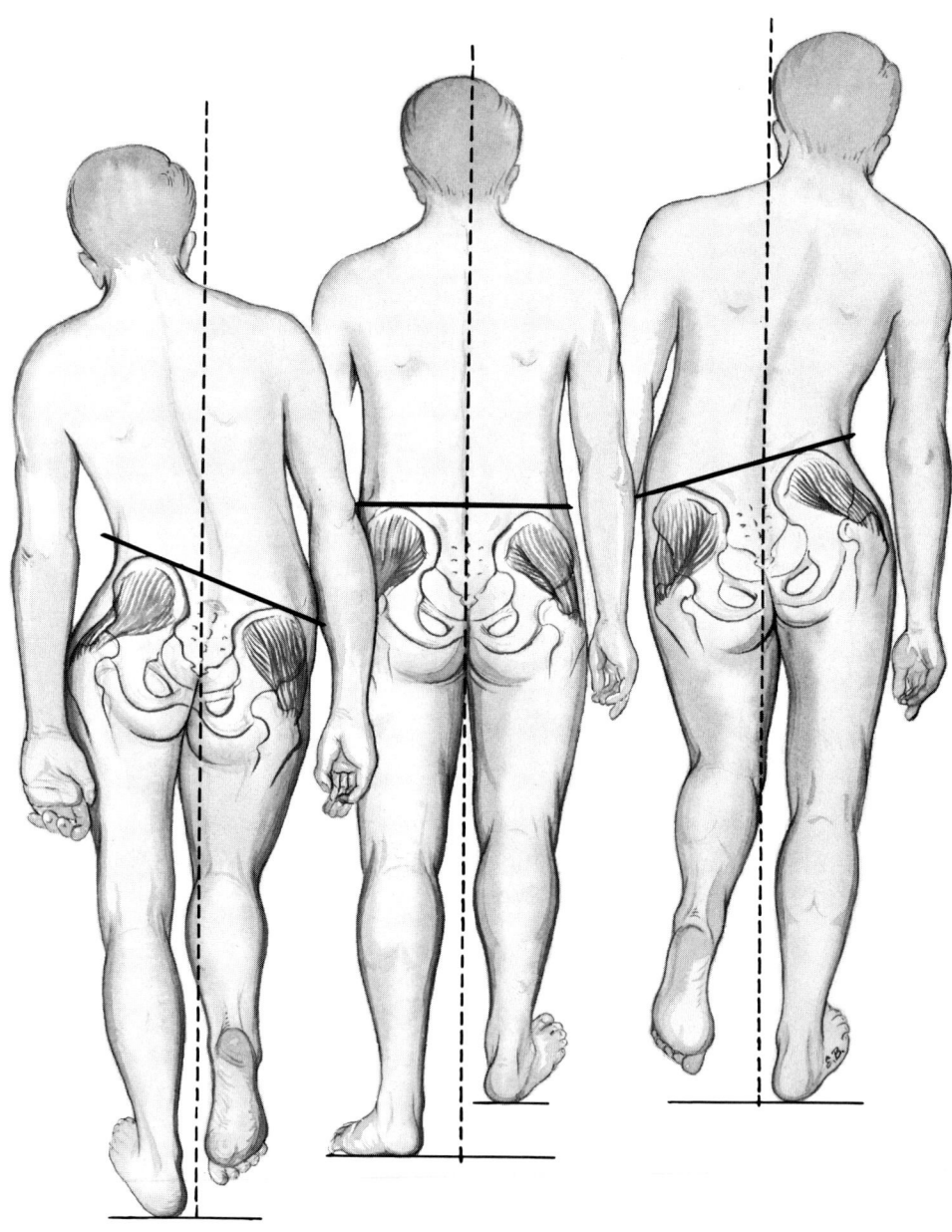

FIGURE 1–56. Gluteus medius lurch.

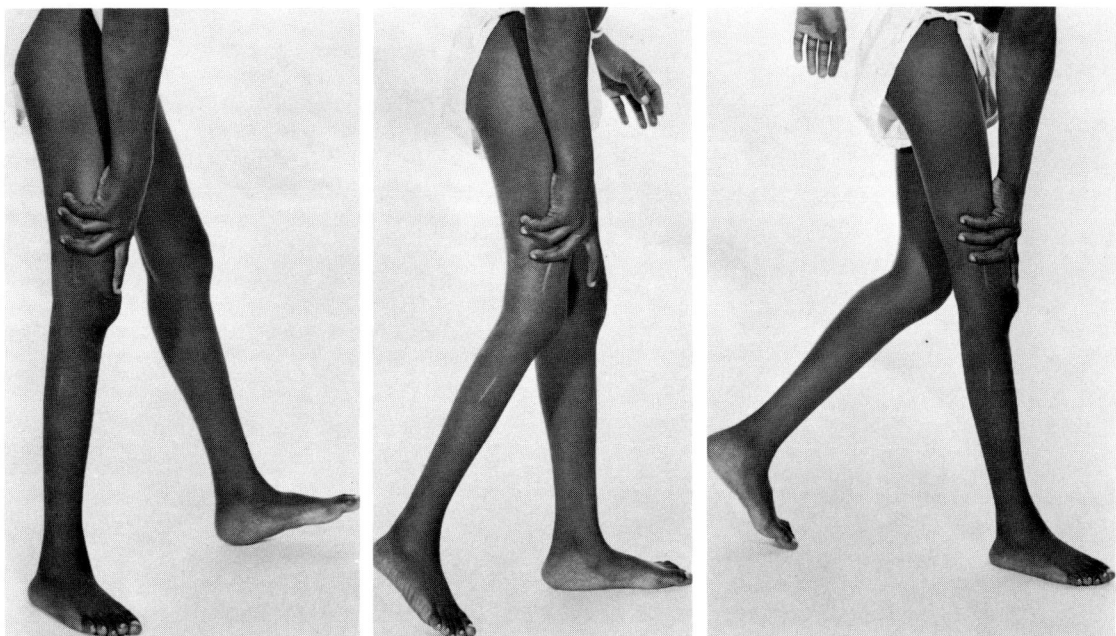

FIGURE 1–57. Quadriceps paralysis.

In quadriceps paralysis associated with flexion deformity of the knee and a poor gluteus maximus, the only way the patient can walk is by supporting the front of his thigh with his hand.

The *gluteus maximus* is the principal hip extensor. The patient with paralysis of the gluteus maximus hyperextends his trunk at the hip joint when bearing weight on the affected limb, bringing the center of gravity posterior to the axis of the hip joint. This compensatory mechanism prevents the hip from giving way on flexion.

The *quadriceps femoris muscle* is the principal knee extensor. Strength of the quadriceps muscle is essential for climbing stairs and establishing stability of the knee; however, a patient with a poor quadriceps can walk almost normally on level ground, provided he does not have flexion deformity of the knee. If there is flexion deformity of the knee, it will give way unless he lurches his trunk forward. In this way, the line of weight-bearing through the knee joint is displaced anteriorly so as to lock the knee in the stance phase of gait. This is another example of shifting the center of gravity and of balance to counteract the effect of weak muscles. With zero strength of the quadriceps in the presence of flexion deformity of the knee and a poor gluteus maximus, often the only way the patient can bear weight is by supporting the front of the affected thigh with his hand (Fig. 1–57). This represents an awkward and poor substitute for the paralyzed muscle.

The *gastrocnemius-soleus* (*triceps surae*) *muscles* are responsible for the final forward propulsion in the push-off portion of the stance phase. When the gastrocnemius-soleus muscles are paralyzed, the patient has a *calcaneus gait*. There is lack of push-off, and the tibia shifts anteriorly over the talus in the final portion of the stance phase when the limb is trying to take off (Fig. 1–58). In order to be functionally effective, the gastrocnemius-soleus muscle must be able to lift the body weight. A normal triceps surae muscle is one that enables the patient to rise up on his toes through the full range of motion of the ankle at least ten times without either flexing his knees or leaning his trunk forward.

In *drop-foot* or *steppage gait* there is paralysis of the muscles that dorsiflex the foot. In the swing phase, as the patient brings his leg forward, he cannot hold his foot against gravity in dorsiflexion. The pull of gravity and the unopposed action of the antagonist muscles of the calf cause the foot to go into plantar flexion—it drops. In order to clear his toes, the patient externally rotates and raises the whole lower limb to a higher level

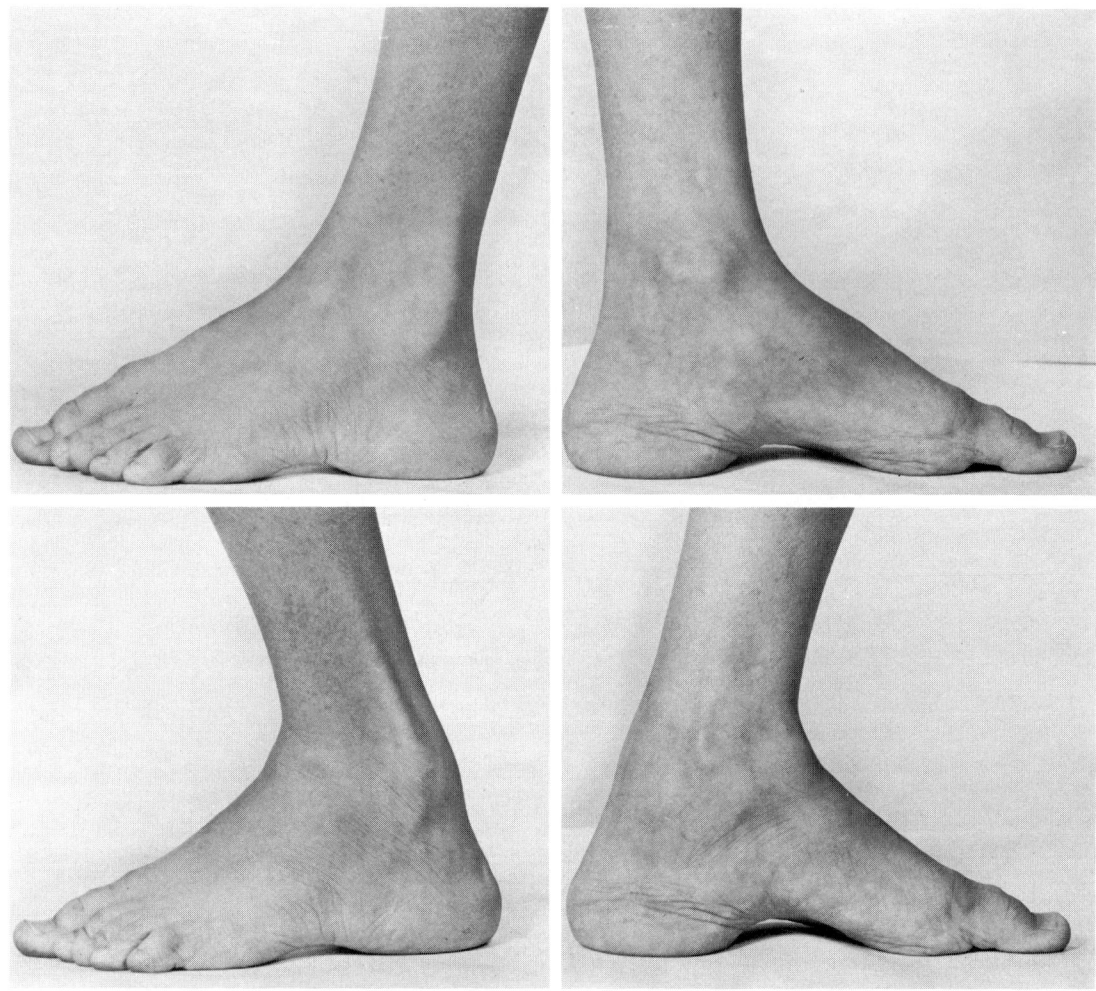

FIGURE 1–58. Calcaneus gait.

Note the posterior shift of the tibia over the talus.

than normal by flexing the knee and hip. A drop-foot gait is an illustration of abnormality in which the disturbed muscular action is in the swing phase.

Structural Deformities of the Bones and Joints. A *short leg*, depending on its degree, may produce a limp. A leg length discrepancy of one half inch or more may be well hidden by the tilt of the pelvis, as demonstrated by the low shoulder, low iliac crest, and low anterior superior iliac spine on the short side. Other means of compensation for leg length discrepancy are to hold the foot and ankle of the short limb in equinus posture, and the knee and hip of the longer leg in flexion. In *short-leg limp*, the patient's head, shoulder, and pelvis *dip down* as the body weight is borne on the short lower limb.

Ankylosis of the joints of the lower limb will cause a pathologic gait. The type of limp depends upon the joint involved and the position of fusion. When the hip is ankylosed, there is greater motion of the pelvis on the lumbar spine during the swing phase; and when the knee is stiff, the pelvis is elevated (hiked) to clear the foot, again during the swing phase. These are easy to diagnose. The gait resulting from an ankylosed ankle, however, may be difficult to distinguish from the normal.

In an *antalgic limp*, because of the painful affection of the bones or joints of the extremity, the duration of single limb stance on the affected side is shortened. On weight-bearing the patient will take quick, soft steps with the painful limb.

In *congenital dislocation of the hip,* the head of the femur does not have a fixed position in the acetabulum and rides high on the side of the pelvis; thus, the action of the gluteus medius is impaired, and its motor strength weakened. The child walks with a gluteus medius limp and Trendelenburg gait.

Neurologic Disorders. Neurologic disorders may cause various abnormalities of gait, some of which may be pathognomonic of certain disease processes. Only the more important and more characteristic of these as seen in pediatric orthopedics are described here.

SPASTIC GAIT. In spasticity there are hypertonicity, hyperreflexia, exaggerated muscle stretch reflex, an imbalance of muscle action of certain predisposed muscle groups, and deformity. The distribution of spastic paralysis may be unilateral or bilateral. The resulting abnormalities of gait are typical. The child may have a toe-toe, toe-heel, or plantigrade gait. The anterior tibial muscle may be cerebral zero in motor strength and does not contract. When there is associated spasticity of the posterior tibial muscle, the foot may be bent inward (pes varus); when the peroneals are spastic, the foot will be bent outward (pes valgus). The extensor hallucis longus may be hyperactive in an attempt to substitute for the weak anterior tibial muscle. The knee and hip may be held in flexion, or the knee may hyperextend after foot-strike because of overactive plantar flexor muscles.

In spastic paraplegia the child walks with a "scissorlike" gait—because of exaggerated adduction and internal rotation of the hips due to spasticity of the hip adductors and medial hamstrings, the knees may cross one in front of the other, rubbing together and rolling around each other. There may be a Trendelenburg gait with a drop of the opposite side of the pelvis in stance phase. When walking, the patient does not swing his arms normally. The posture of the upper limb is typical—the elbow is flexed, the shoulder is adducted and internally rotated, the forearm pronated, the wrist flexed, the thumb adducted, and the fingers flexed in the palm. In acquired spastic paralysis the shoulder may be held in abduction, and the anterior tibial muscle in the leg may be hyperactive. Balance and coordination may be impaired. In mild cases, this is demonstrated by the inability of the patient to walk tandem; in severe involvement, the child may be able to walk only with the assistance of crutches or parallel bars. Presence or absence of a reciprocal pattern of locomotion should be noted. One may have to observe the way in which a child crawls. The worn areas of the shoes may suggest toe walking. A shuffling, scraping sound may be characteristic.

ATAXIC GAIT. Ataxic gait may be of two types. The gait of *spinal ataxia* is caused by interruption of the proprioceptive pathways in the spinal cord or brain stem. In children, this is encountered in peripheral neuritis and in lesions of the brain stem; in adults, it is commonly seen in tabes dorsalis and in posterolateral and multiple sclerosis. The ataxia results from loss of appreciation of the senses of position and motion of the parts of the body and from lack of spatial orientation. The gait may not be too abnormal when the child walks with his eyes open, as he correlates his visual impulses with proprioceptive ones; however, if there is severe involvement, the child walks with a broad base, throwing out his feet, which come down first on the heel and then on the toes with a slapping sound or "double tap." The sound of the double tap produced by the noisy stamping of the hypotonic feet in two phases is so characteristic that one may diagnose the gait of spinal ataxia merely by hearing the patient walk. Upon close inspection, it is evident that the child is keeping his eyes on the floor and watching his feet while walking. When asked to walk with his eyes closed, he staggers, becomes unsteady, his feet shoot out, and he is unable to walk.

In the gait of *cerebellar ataxia,* ataxia is present with the eyes open or closed. It is caused by disease processes that involve the coordinating mechanisms in both the cerebellum and its connecting systems. The gait is wide-based, unsteady, and irregular. The child staggers and is unable to walk tandem or to follow a straight line on the floor. There may be tremors or oscillatory movements of the entire body. This form of ataxia is encountered in cerebellar lesions. If the disease process is localized in one cerebellar hemisphere, there is persistent deviation or swaying toward the affected side.

In *Friedreich's ataxia*, the ataxia is both spinal and cerebellar in type, as there is involvement of the posterior columns, spinocerebellar tracts, lateral columns, and cerebellum. The absence of the patellar reflex, the presence of a Babinski response, marked nystagmus, and other associated musculoskeletal findings will help to establish the diagnosis.

DYSTROPHIC GAIT. The dystrophic gait is encountered in various myopathies. It is most typical of muscular dystrophy. The child is usually brought to the physician with the presenting complaints of difficulty in running and trouble in ascending steps. He stands and walks with marked exaggeration of his lumbar lordosis. There is a pronounced "waddling" element in his gait; he has difficulty in fixing his pelvis. The child throws or rolls his hips from side to side with the stance phase of every forward step to shift the weight of the body. The exaggerated lateral tilting and rotation of the pelvis are largely to compensate for the weakened gluteal muscles. Overuse of the trunk and upper limbs in dystrophic gait has led to its being called a "penguin gait." The child has difficulty in getting up from a supine position on the floor; he has to roll to a prone position and "climb up on himself" by placing his hands first on his knees, then on his thighs, and finally on his hips to brace himself. He has marked difficulty in going up steps except with the help of hand pressure on his knees. This is caused by the weakness of the quadriceps and gluteus maximus in particular. In climbing stairs, he often needs a hand rail to pull himself up with his hands.

GAIT ANALYSIS

Gait analysis is performed in special centers in the United States and throughout the world as a research tool and, also, to assist in planning an effective therapy program. The following studies are carried out in the analysis. Muscular activity is measured by electromyography. Indwelling electrodes identify the activity of specific muscles; their use is indicated when muscle transfers or releases are contemplated. Surface electrodes measure activity of groups of muscles during a movement. Inspection and traditional testing of muscles by slow stretching is not as reliable as electromyography; this is especially true in cerebral palsy.[27] Perry and Hoffer have clearly demonstrated the value of electromyography in planning surgery in cerebral palsy.[32] Their preoperative and postoperative dynamic electromyographic studies showed that when deforming muscles act exclusively in one portion of a gait cycle or movement of an upper limb, appropriate tendon transfer should be performed; whereas if there is continuous muscle activity, tendon lengthening is indicated. This evaluation is discussed in detail in the section on cerebral palsy.

Other data obtained in the gait laboratory include measurements of movements of the

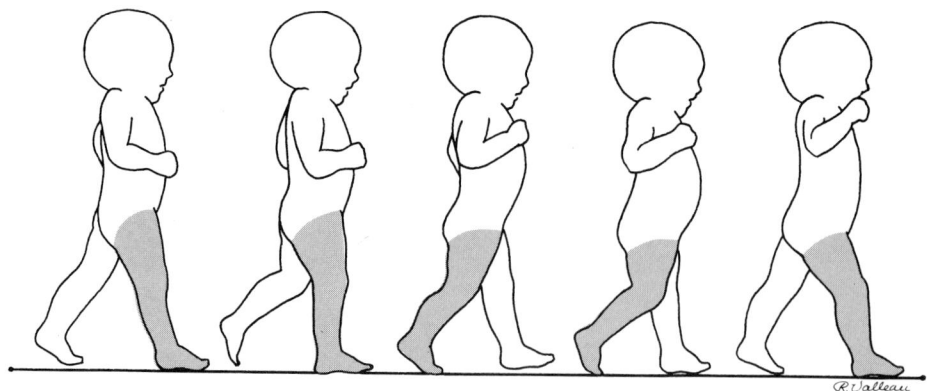

NORMAL 1 YEAR OLD

FIGURE 1–59. Normal gait in one-year-old.

Note the flexed elbows; absence of arm swing, plantar flexion at foot-strike, and increased shoulder sway in this one-year-old girl.

NORMAL 1 YEAR OLD

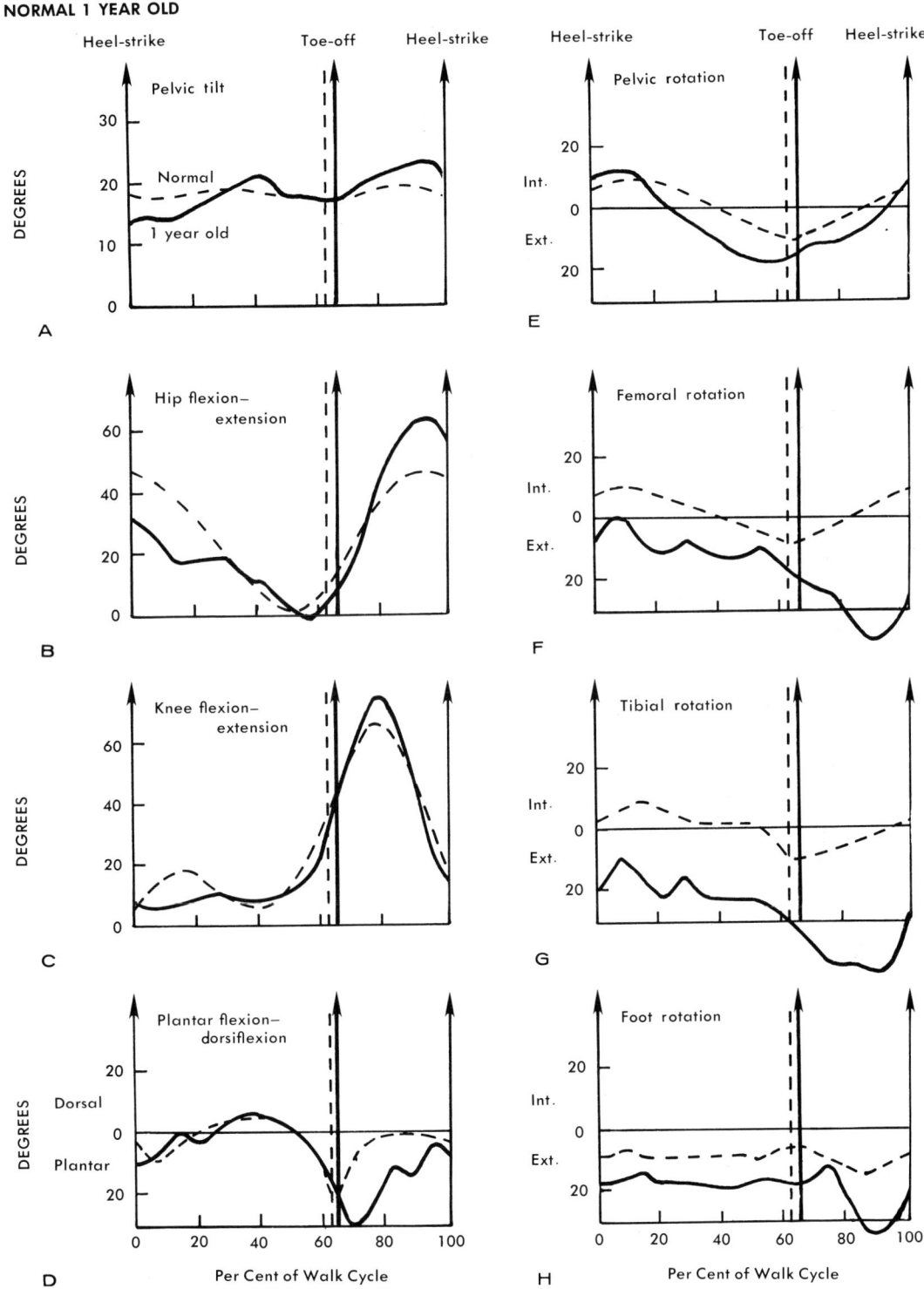

FIGURE 1–60. *Joint angular rotations in normal one-year-old.*

A. Slightly increased sagittal plane pelvic oscillation. **B.** Increased swing phase hip flexion. **C.** Extended knee throughout stance. **D.** Plantar flexion at foot-strike and drop foot in swing. **E** to **H.** Exaggerated lateral rotation of pelvis, femur, tibia, and foot.

lower limbs in three planes, foot-floor reaction (force plate), joint torque, foot switch, and energy consumption. Gait analysis findings in various affections of the neuromuscular skeletal system are presented in the appropriate sections.

The following examples of normal gait pattern in one-year-old, three-year-old, and six-year-old children are presented by courtesy of Dr. David H. Sutherland of San Diego, California.

A normal one-year-old child walks in a staccato manner (Fig. 1–59). The walking cadence is rapid, but the steps are very short. Walking velocity is approximately half that of an average adult. The elbows are kept flexed, and reciprocal arm movements are not yet present. In the frontal plane a wide base of support can be observed. Foot-strike occurs without initial heel-strike.

GENERAL MEASUREMENTS

	Right	Left
Opp. toe-off (per cent cycle)	12	16
Opp. foot-strike (per cent cycle)	50	48
Single stance (per cent cycle)	38	32
Toe-off (per cent cycle)	66	61
Step length (cm.)	21	21
Stride length (cm.)	42	42
Cycle time (sec.)	.7	.7
Cadence (steps/min.)	171	171
Walking velocity (cm./sec.)	60	60
(m./min.)	36	36

In comparison with a composite of normal adult control subjects, the child has greater hip and knee flexion in the swing phase (Fig. 1–60). Plantar flexion is present at foot-strike, but dorsiflexion is impaired in the early swing phase. There is excessive external rotation of pelvis, femur, tibia, and foot in both stance and swing phases.

All these variations from mature gait are normal initial adaptations to the demands of independent walking.

The gait of a normal three-year-old boy resembles mature gait (Fig. 1–61). Reciprocal arm movements are present. The dynamic base of support is normal. Cadence is slower than that of the normal one-year-old girl, and walking velocity is greater. Limitation of step length still prevents achievement of mature walking velocity.

GENERAL MEASUREMENTS

	Right	Left
Opp. toe-off (per cent cycle)	18	17
Opp. foot-strike (per cent cycle)	52	49
Single stance (per cent cycle)	34	32
Toe-off (per cent cycle)	68	67
Step length (cm.)	29	32
Stride length (cm.)	61	61
Cycle time (sec.)	.76	.76
Cadence (steps./min.)	158	158
Walking velocity (cm./sec.)	80	80
(m./min.)	48	48

While angular rotations of hip and knee are very similar to a composite of those of normal adults, ankle dorsiflexion in stance phase is greater (Fig. 1–62). Fully mature gait will be gained when better control of ankle musculature brings about the normal plantar flexor activity necessary to increase step length.

A normal six-year-old girl walks with a mature gait pattern (Fig. 1–63). Walking

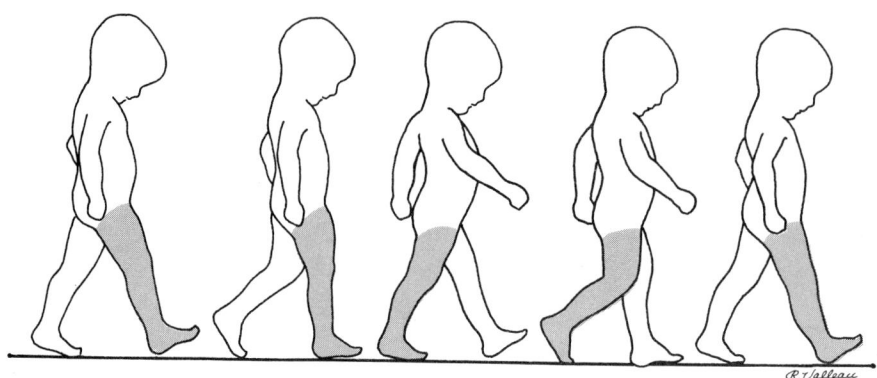

NORMAL 3 YEAR OLD
FIGURE 1–61. Normal gait in a three-year-old boy.

Synchronous arm swing and heel-strike, and apparent trunk stability are indicators of considerable gait maturity.

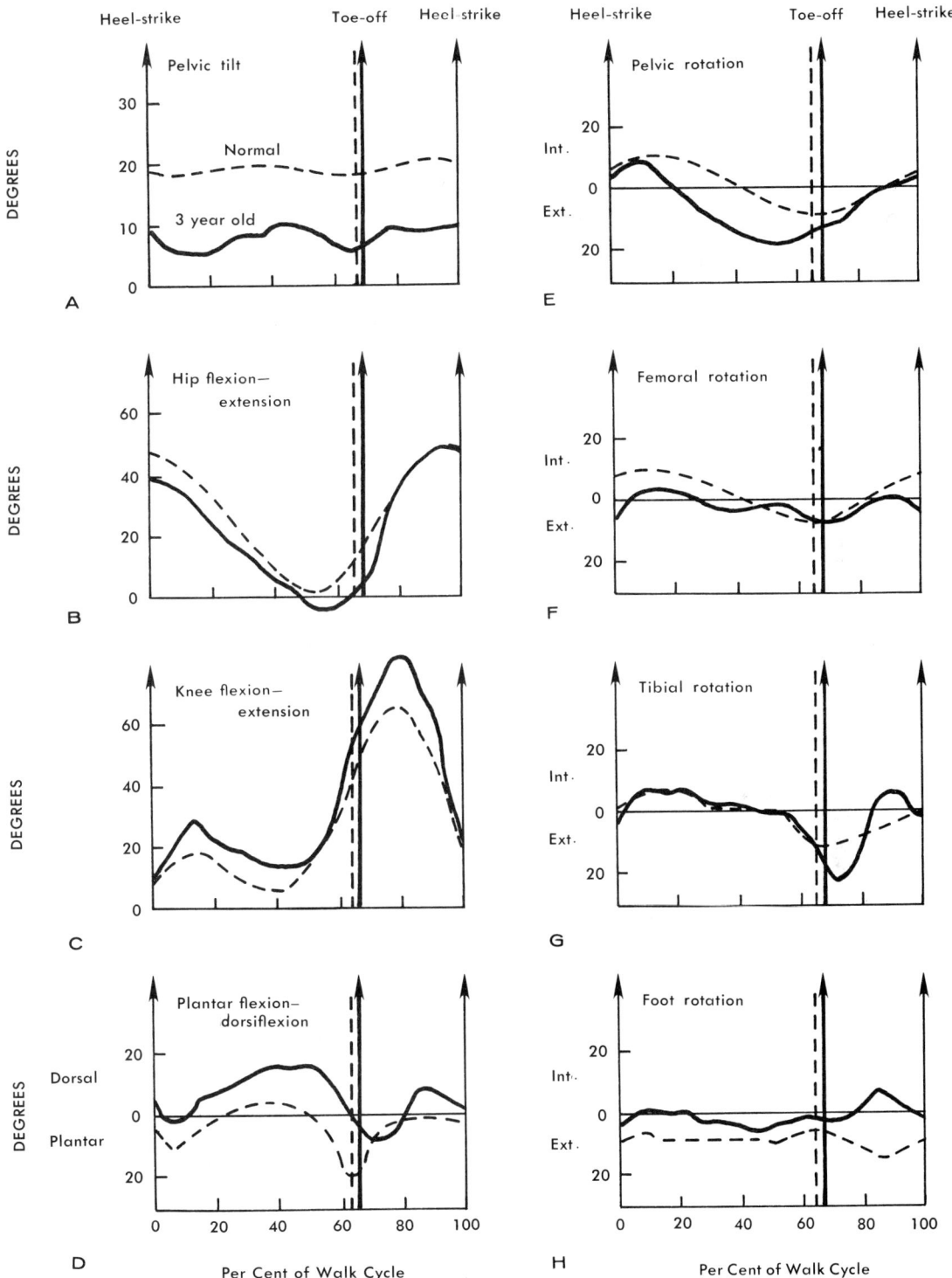

FIGURE 1–62. *Joint angular rotations and force plate curves in normal three-year-old boy.*

A to **D.** The sagittal plane joint angular rotations of this three-year-old boy are comparable to those of normal young adult controls. **E.** Pelvic rotation shows mild exaggeration of stance phase external rotation. **F** to **H.** With the exception of some irregularities of foot and tibial rotations in swing phase, femoral tibial foot rotations are similar to those young adult controls.

Illustration continued on following page

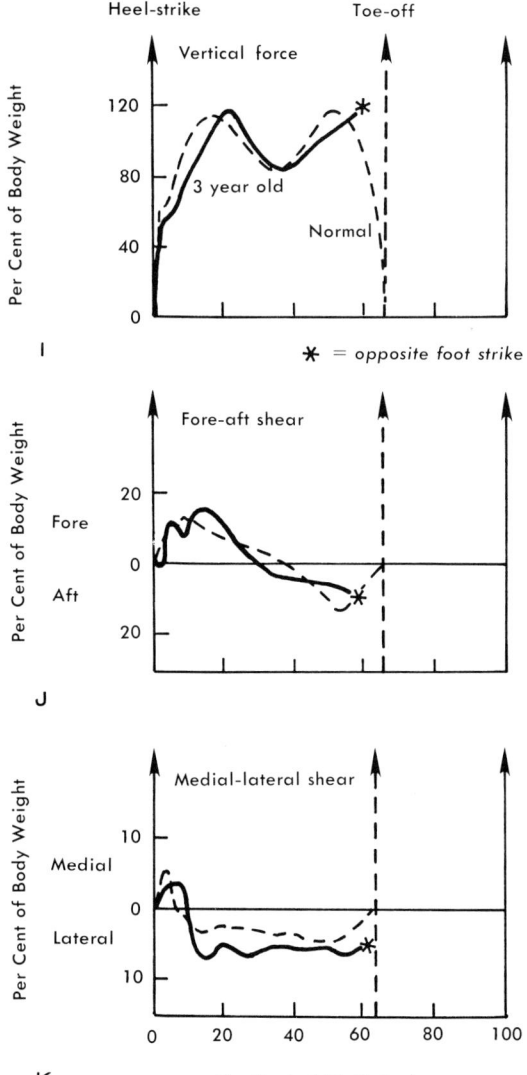

FIGURE 1–62 Continued. *Joint angular rotations and force plate curves in normal three-year-old boy.*

I, J, and **K.** Force plate curves show that vertical force, fore-aft shear, and medial-lateral shear duplicate adult control values. The curves are terminated at the asterisk because of opposite foot-strike on the plate.

velocity, step length, and cadence are appropriately related.

GENERAL MEASUREMENTS

	Right	Left
Opp. toe-off (per cent cycle)	10	11
Opp. foot-strike (per cent cycle)	49	52
Single stance (per cent cycle)	39	40
Toe-off (per cent cycle)	60	63
Step length (cm.)	49	49
Stride length (cm.)	98	98
Cycle time (sec.)	.7	.7
Cadence (steps/min.)	171	171
Walking velocity (cm./sec.)	140	140
(m./min.)	84	84

The increase in pelvic rotation is attributable to rapid free cadence. The first peak vertical force and midstance valley are also increased for the same reason. The rapid cadence is also responsible for increases in fore-aft and lateral shear (Fig. 1–64). Electromyography reveals normal phasic activity of the vastus medialis, vastus lateralis, gluteus maximus, gastrocnemius-soleus, medial and lateral hamstrings, and anterior compartment muscle groups.

The gait of this child differs in no significant qualitative manner from that of a young adult.

Deformities

The type and actual site of a deformity is now determined. Is it in the soft tissues, the bones, or the joints? How severe is it? Is it fixed, or can it be passively or actively corrected? What are the factors producing it? Is there muscle spasm with the deformity? Is there local tenderness or pain on motion?

The angular deformities are measured in degrees and expressed in the same manner as that used for recording joint motions. Other objective measurements are used when indicated. In genu valgum, for example, the amount of knock-knee may be measured by the distance between the medial malleoli with the knees in full extension, and patellae facing exactly forward, and the medial condyles of the femur brought together with moderate firm pressure to compress excessive subcutaneous fat (Fig. 1–65). Another way to measure the degree of knock-knee is to determine the angle between the lateral surfaces of the thigh and leg. Atrophy of the calf, especially of the medial head of the gastrocnemius, and excessive subcutaneous fat on the thigh exaggerate the clinical appearance of knock-knees.

The degree of genu varum is determined in a way similar to that used to measure knock-knees; the distance between the medial femoral condyles is measured with the medial malleoli brought together and firmly compressed. It is imperative for the patellae to face exactly forward, as medial rotation of the lower limbs at the hips will cause apparent bowlegs.

It is often best to make a tracing or photograph of the deformity for subsequent comparison.

Special tests are useful to demonstrate a

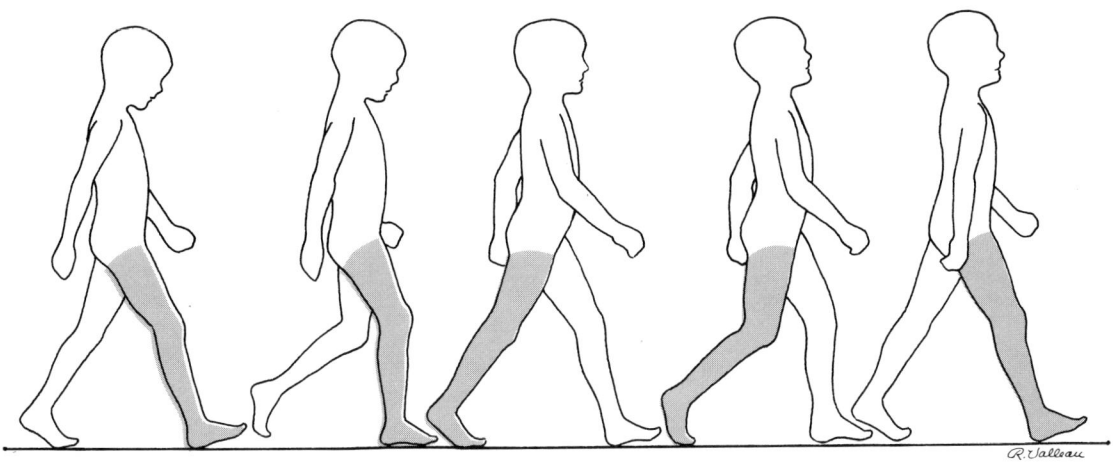

NORMAL 6 YEAR OLD
FIGURE 1–63. The gait pattern of a normal six-year-old girl.
This gait pattern resembles very closely that of a young adult.

deformity, particularly in the detection of fixed deformities of the hip, in which limitation of movement may be obscured by motion of the pelvis. It is imperative to observe the pelvis carefully while examining passive motion of the hip joint. A flexion deformity may be masked by a forward tilt of the pelvis and excessive lumbar lordosis. In the *Thomas test,* the patient is supine, and the limb opposite to the one tested is completely flexed until the knee touches the chest and the lumbar spine is flattened; this rotates the pelvis, and the angle taken by the tested hip is the degree of flexion deformity (Fig. 1–66).[41] If the spine is stiff or the flexion deformity of the hip is considerable in the standing posture, or both, the knee of the same side is held in flexion, and only the toes touch the ground, giving the appearance of shortening.

Ober's test is performed to determine the degree of abduction contracture of the hip (Fig. 1–67).[40] The child lies on the side opposite to the one being tested, and the underneath hip and knee are maximally flexed to flatten the lumbar spine. The hip to be tested (with the knee flexed to a right angle) is first flexed to 90 degrees, then fully abducted, and next brought into full hyperextension and allowed to adduct maximally. The knee of the tested limb should always be kept at 90 degrees of flexion. The angle that the thigh makes with a horizontal line parallel to the table represents the degree of abduction contracture. Normally, the limb drops well below the horizontal.

INEQUALITY OF LENGTH

On inspection, disparity in the length of the lower limbs can be detected by the difference in the level of the popliteal and gluteal creases, the two sides of the pelvis, and the shoulders as the child stands with both feet together, heels on the ground, and knees fully extended. Next, the examiner places the radial border of his index fingers on the uppermost portion of each iliac crest and his thumbs on the anterior superior iliac spines, and compares the height of the pelvis on the two sides. Blocks of wood of various thicknesses are placed under the foot of the short limb to align iliac crests and anterior superior iliac spines horizontally. Possible sources of error are bony abnormalities of the pelvis such as atrophy of the ipsilateral ilium in poliomyelitis.

The difference in the length of the limbs is then measured with a tape with the patient in the supine position. To ensure accurate measurements, it is essential to place the limbs in comparable positions. The *actual leg length* is measured from the under side of the anterior superior iliac spine to the lowest point of the medial malleolus or the plantar surface of the heel—for this, both ankles must be in neutral and identical positions. This is an index of the real length of the lower limbs. The *apparent length,* an index of the functional length of the lower limbs, is measured from the umbilicus to the lowest point of the medial malleolus,

Text continued on page 74

NORMAL 6 YEAR OLD

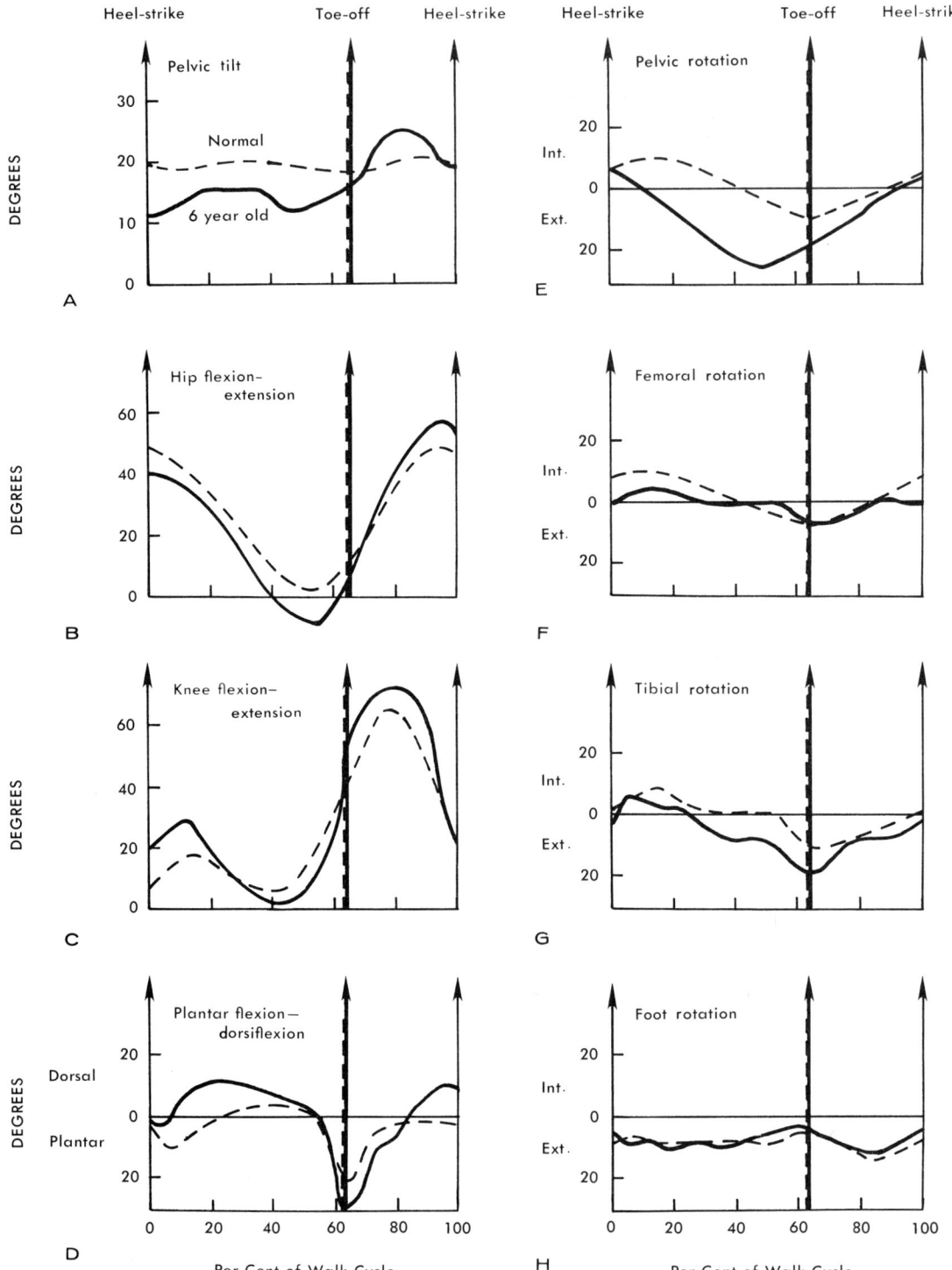

FIGURE 1–64. Joint angular rotations and force plate curves in normal six-year-old girl.

A to **D.** The sagittal plane joint angular rotations of this six-year-old girl differ in no significant manner from a composite of curves for young adult controls. **E.** Pelvic rotation is increased by rapid cadence and increased walking velocity. **F** to **H.** Femoral, tibial, and foot rotations are normal.

Illustration continued on opposite page

Introduction

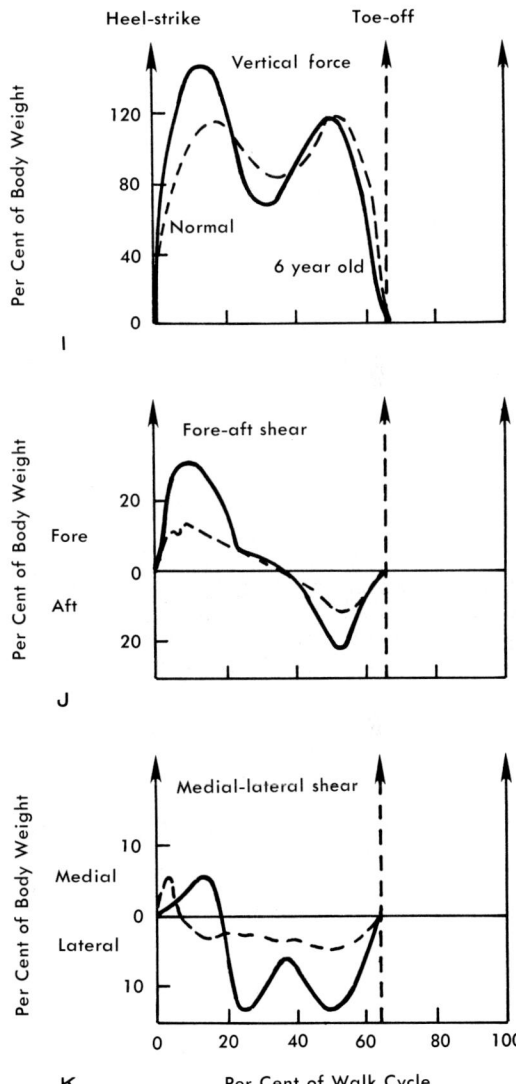

FIGURE 1–64 Continued. *Joint angular rotations and force plate curves in normal six-year-old girl.*

I. Vertical force first peak and midstance valley are increased because of rapid cadence and walking velocity. **J.** Fore-aft shear is increased for the same reason. **K.** Lateral shear is increased because of rapid cadence and walking velocity.

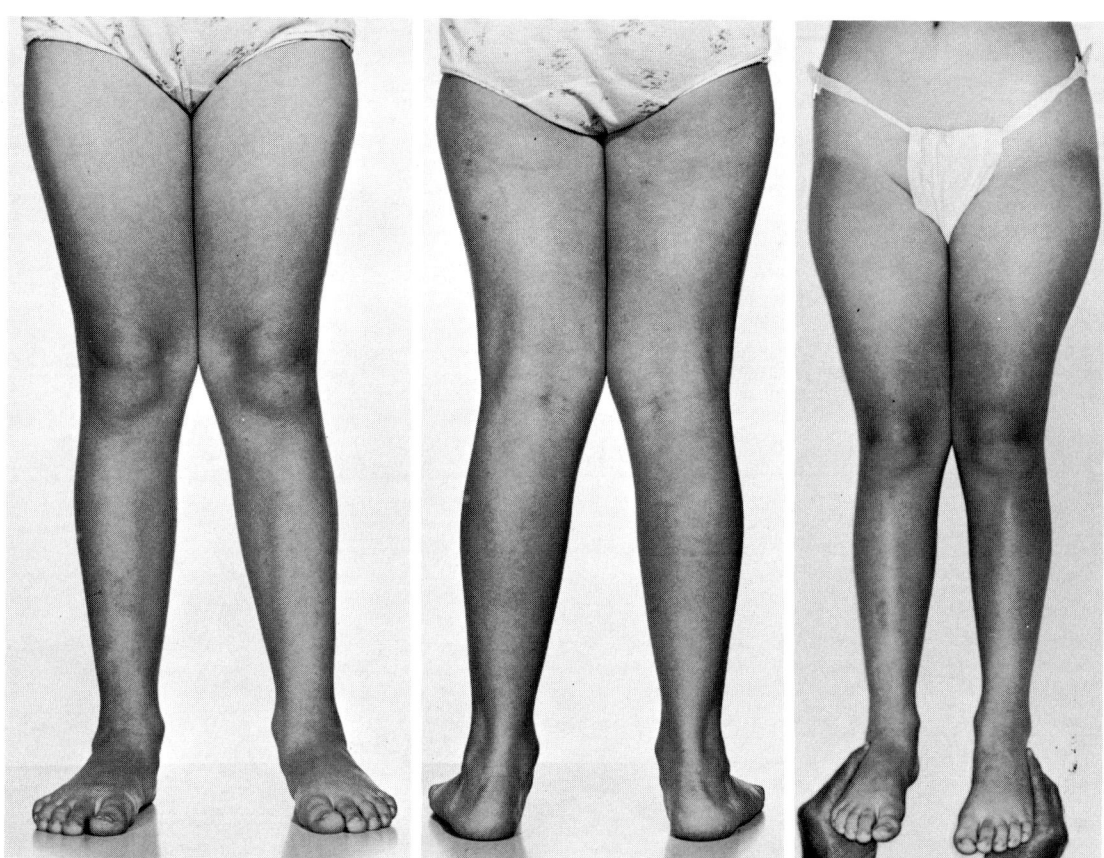

FIGURE 1–65. Measurement of degree of genu valgum.

Introduction

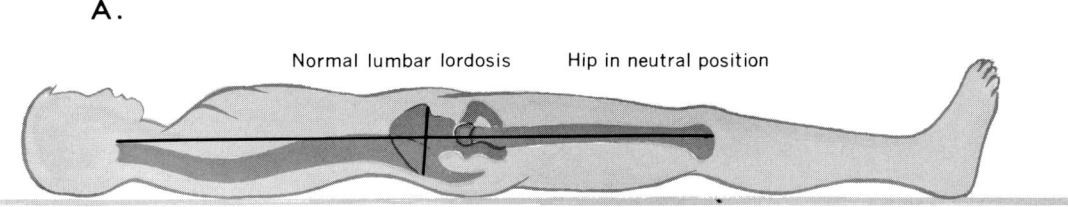

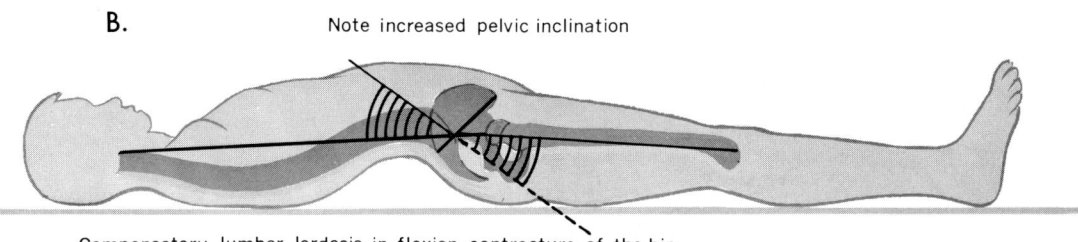

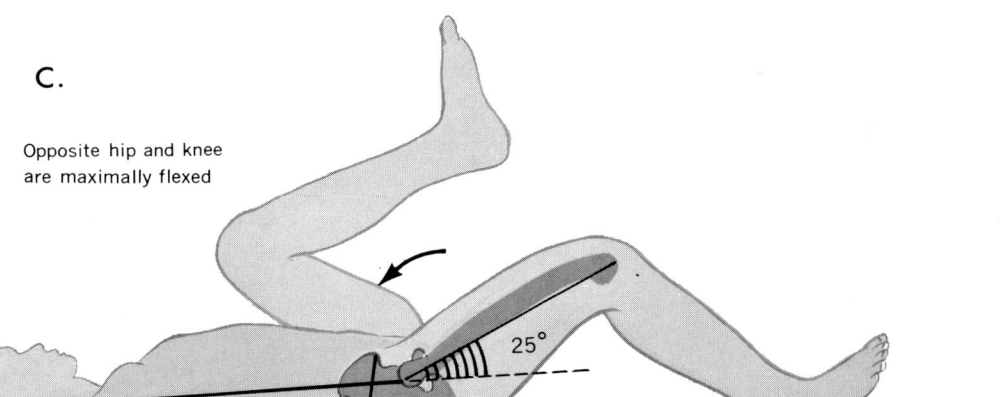

FIGURE 1-66. Thomas test.

(Adapted from von Lanz, T., and Wachsmuth, W.: Praktische Anatomie. Berlin, Julius Springer, 1938, p. 157.)

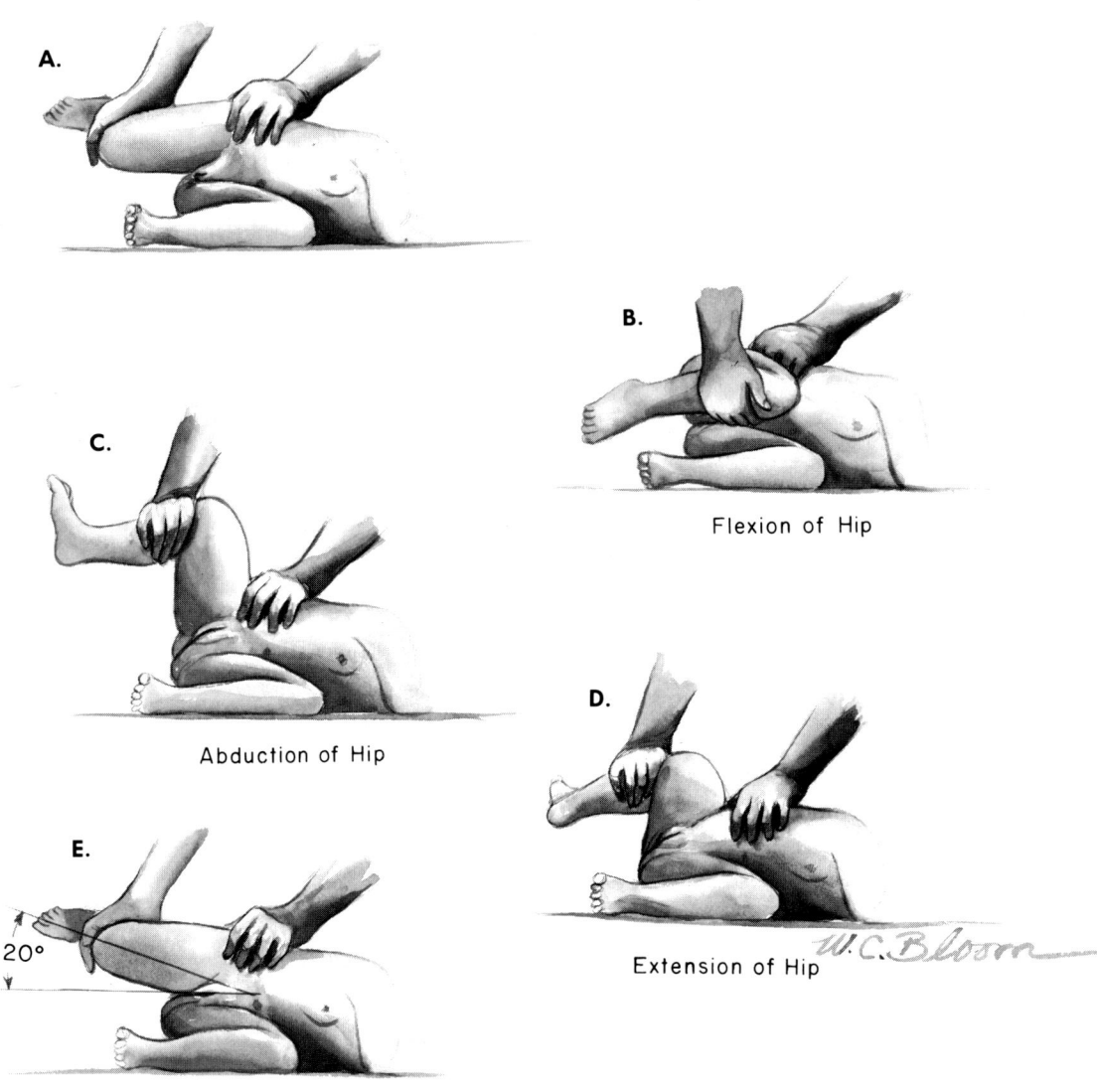

FIGURE 1–67. *Ober's test for determining the degree of abduction contracture of the hip.*

thus taking into consideration the tilt of the pelvis. An adduction deformity of the hip causes an apparent shortening on the side of the contracture, whereas an abduction deformity of the hip produces an apparent lengthening on the same side (Fig. 1–68).

Whenever there is disproportion between the thigh and leg lengths, they should be measured separately. The medial knee joint line is the intermediate landmark; this is easily located by flexing the knee 45 degrees.

The total length of the upper limbs is measured from the posterior tip of the acromion process to the end of the long finger with the elbow, wrist, and fingers in neutral zero degrees extended position. The upper arm is measured from the posterior tip of the acromion to the point of the olecranon; the forearm is measured from the point of the olecranon to the tip of the radial or ulnar styloid process.

The circumference of the calf is measured at its greatest diameter. The thighs are measured at specifically marked identical levels, several inches above the patella or below the anterior superior iliac spine. In the upper limb, the greatest circumfer-

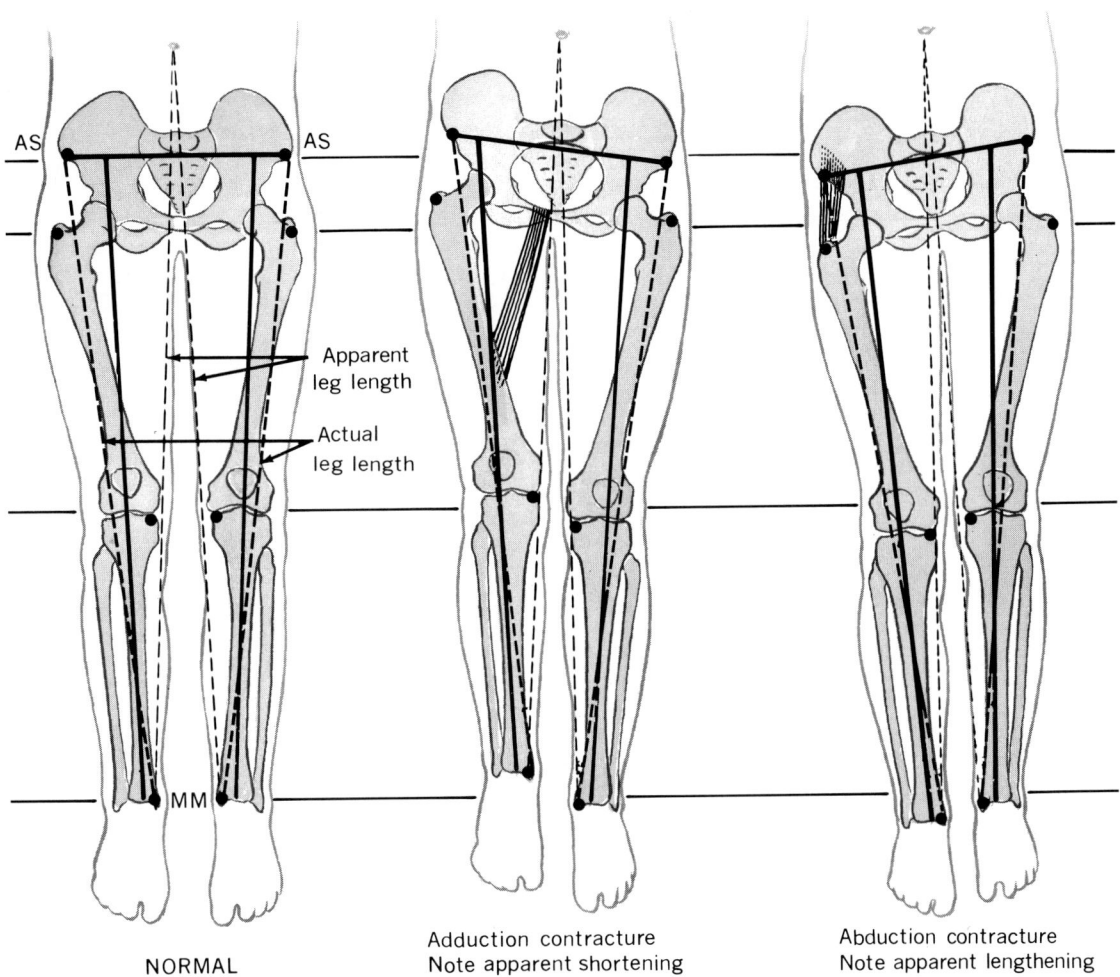

FIGURE 1–68. *Measurement of actual and apparent leg lengths.*

AS, anterior iliac spine; MM, medial malleolus. (Adapted from von Lanz, T., and Wachsmuth, W.: Praktische Anatomie. Berlin, Julius Springer, 1938, pp. 24–25.)

ence of the forearm and midarm are conventional levels of measurement.

ANGULATION OR BOWING

Terms used in describing angular deformities denote the position of the distal segment of the deformity relative to the proximal unit. *Varus* describes an angulation toward the midline of the body distal to the anatomic part named; *valgus* describes angulation away from the midline distal to the part named. For example, in cubitus valgus, the forearm is directed away from the midline of the body. In coxa valga, the angle of the neck and the shaft of the femur is greater than normal, i.e., the distal segment is angulated away from the midline. In coxa vara, it is less than normal.

Range of Motion of Joints

The method of measuring and recording joint motion is standardized by the Committee for the Study of Joint Motion and the American Academy of Orthopedic Surgeons and approved by the appointed committees of the Orthopedic Associations of the English Speaking World.[43] It is based on the principles of the Neutral Zero Method, as described by Cave and Roberts.[44] Motion is measured in degrees of a circle with the joint as its center. The anatomic zero starting position of each joint is defined, and the degrees of motion of a joint are added in the direction in which the joint moves from the zero starting position. In the past, much confusion arose because joint motions were measured from various starting positions. This method eliminates the confusion by accepting the extended "anatomic position" of a limb as zero degrees rather than 180 degrees. For example, when a fully extended elbow joint is bent from the anatomic zero position to a right angle, the range of motion is 90 degrees of flexion.

The range of motion of a joint is determined in both its active and passive ranges. During examination it is important to be gentle, as moving the joint may be painful. The limb should be placed in the position that is most comfortable for the child. It is best for the beginner to use a goniometer until he learns to gauge angles accurately

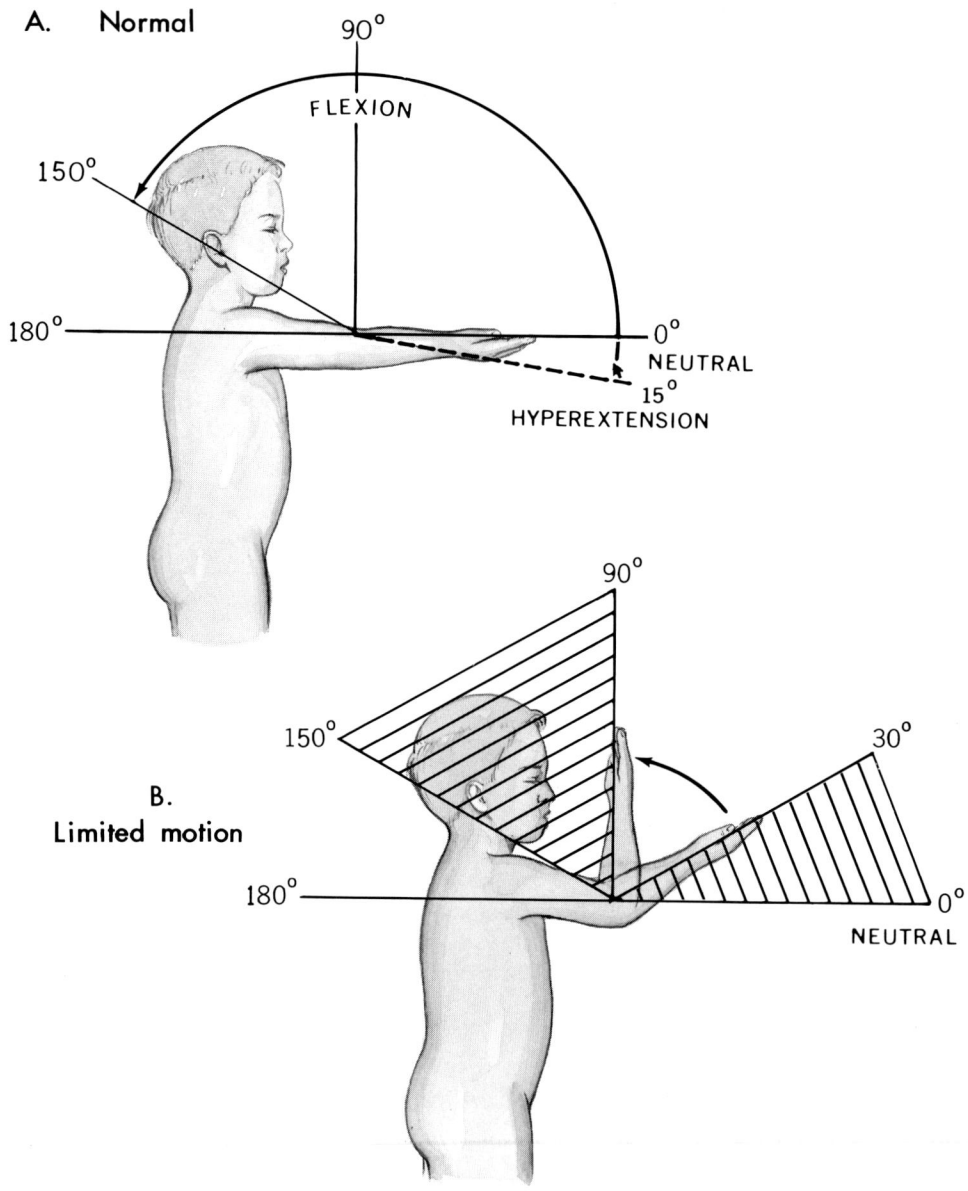

FIGURE 1–69. Measurement of the range of motion of the elbow joint.

by sight. One should remember, however, that the goniometer may give inaccurate information when, owing to excess soft-tissue coverage or other causes, the bony landmarks are not definite.

Flexion is the movement of bending a joint, a motion away from the zero starting position. *Extension* is the act of straightening a joint, the return motion to the zero starting position. A distinction is made between the terms *extension* and *hyperextension*. When the motion opposite to flexion is an unnatural one, as it may be at the knee or elbow, the term used is *hyperextension*. *Adduction* is the drawing of the part toward the axis of the body; *abduction* is motion of the part away from the axis of the body. At the wrist joint, *ulnar deviation* and *radial deviation* are used. *Supination* is the act of turning the palm of the hand or the side of the foot toward the anterior surface of the body or facing upward. *Pronation* is the turning of the palm of the hand or the sole of the foot toward the posterior surface of the body or facing downward. *Inversion* is a term applied to an inward turning motion seen primarily in the subtalar joint of the foot. *Eversion* is the opposite motion. *Medial rotation* and *lateral rotation* are self-explanatory.

A typical hinge joint in which there is one-plane freedom of motion is the elbow. The zero starting position is extended straight elbow (zero degrees). The normal range of motions of the elbow, shown in Figure 1–69A, are: (1) flexion—zero to 150 degrees; (2) extension—150 degrees to zero (from the angle of greatest flexion to zero starting position); and (3) hyperextension—measured in degrees beyond the zero starting position and varying from 5 to 15 degrees. Hyperextension is not present in all persons. Limited motion in the elbow joint is expressed as follows: (1) the elbow flexes 30 degrees to 90 degrees, or (2) the elbow has a flexion deformity of 30 degrees with further flexion to 90 degrees (Fig. 1–69).

Examinations of the motions of the hip are more complicated, as it is a ball-and-socket joint capable of three-dimensional, compound, or rotatory motion. A common pitfall in determining hip motion is the failure to observe that the pelvis does not rotate or tilt during examination. The examiner should always place one hand on the iliac crest to note the point at which the pelvis begins to move. First the patient lies supine on a firm flat surface with the opposite hip held in full flexion to flatten the lumbar spine and bring out flexion contracture of the hip, if present. The normal range of flexion is from zero to 110 to 120 degrees. Limited motion in the hip is expressed in the same manner as is that in the elbow or knee, i.e., (1) the hip flexes from 30 to 90 degrees, or (2) the hip has a flexion deformity of 30 degrees with further flexion to 90 degrees.

Next, rotation of the hip in flexion is determined with the patient still lying supine. The hip and knee of the limb to be examined are each flexed 90 degrees; the thigh is perpendicular to the transverse line across the anterior superior iliac spines of the pelvis. Internal (inward, medial) rotation is measured by rotating the leg away from the midline of the trunk with the thigh as the axis of rotation, thus producing internal rotation of the hip (Fig. 1–70). External (outward, lateral) rotation of the hip is produced by rotating the leg toward the midline of the trunk with the thigh as the axis of rotation.

For testing abduction of the hip, it is imperative that the anterior superior iliac spines be level. The pelvis may be held fixed by abduction of the opposite hip and steadied by the examiner's hand, which will detect pelvic motion (Fig. 1–70C). Abduction is measured in degrees as the outward motion of the extremity from the zero starting position. In measuring adduction, the examiner should elevate the opposite limb so that the tested leg can pass under it. Rotation of the hip in extension can be measured with the patient supine, but it is best for him to turn over into prone position. His knee is flexed to 90 degrees; the leg is perpendicular to the transverse line across the anterior superior iliac spines. The leg is rotated outward to measure internal rotation, and inward for external rotation (Fig. 1–70B). Extension of the hip may be determined with the patient lying face down with a small pillow under the abdomen or with the opposite limb flexed over the end of the table. The lower limb may be extended with the knee flexed or straight. Motion of the lower part of the spine may be reflected to some degree in the test for hip extension.

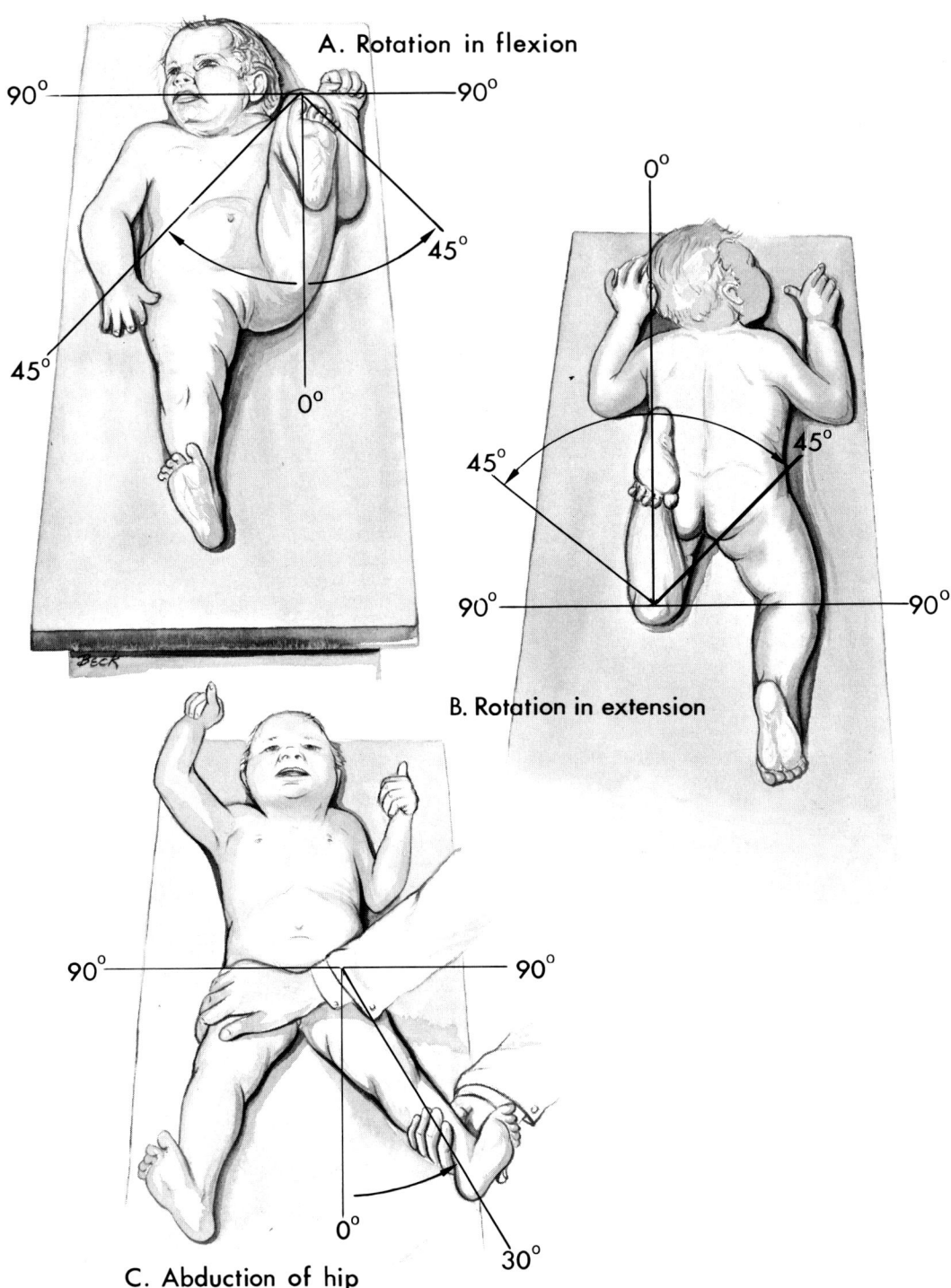

FIGURE 1-70. *Measurement of the range of motion of the hip.*

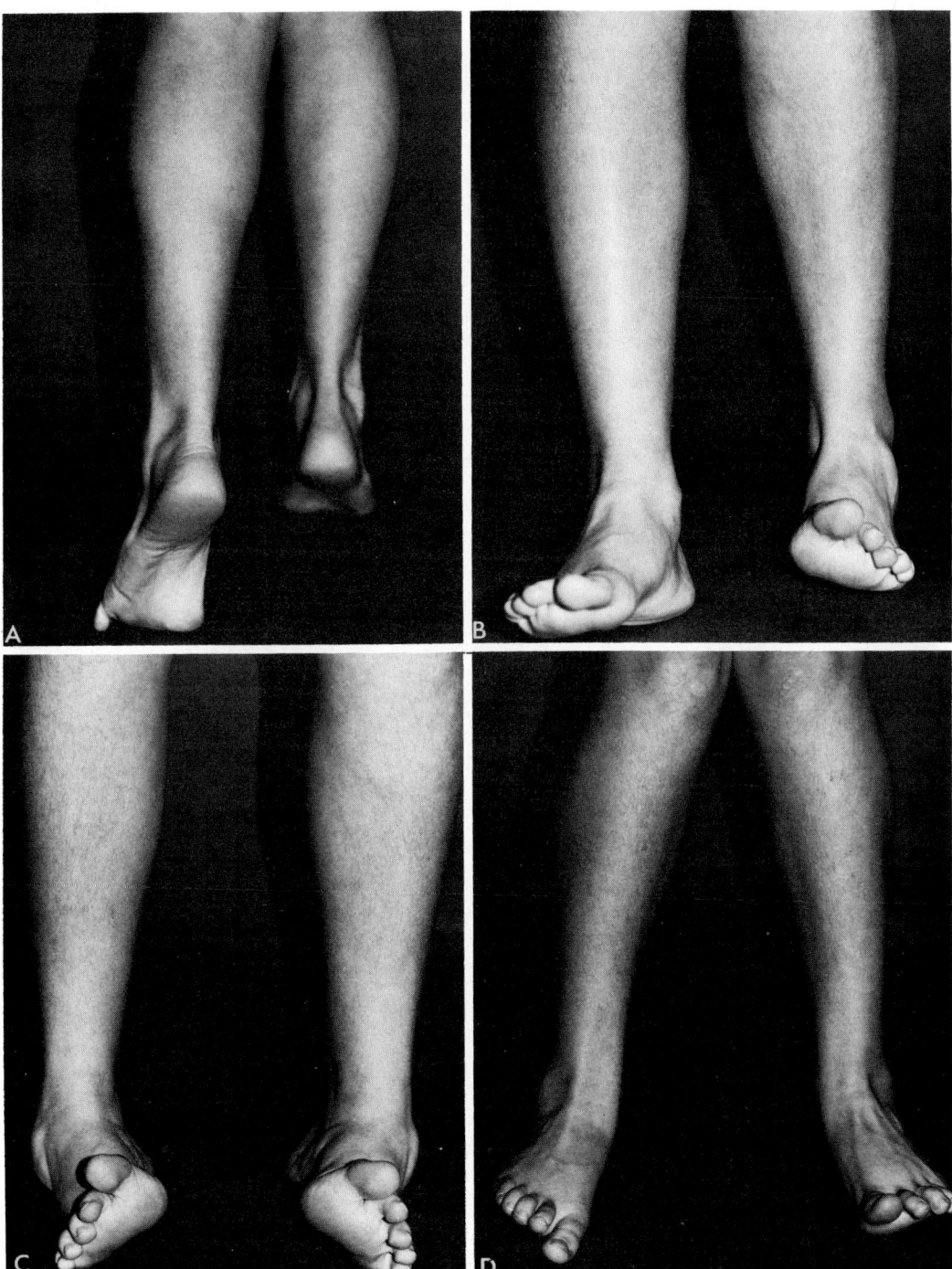

FIGURE 1–71. An expedient way to test range of motion of the foot and ankle, and the motor strength of muscles of the lower leg.

Ask child to walk first on his toes, **A,** and then on his heels, **B,** next have him walk on the lateral and medial borders of his feet, **C** and **D.**

To examine the foot and ankle it is expedient to ask the child to walk on his toes and then on his heels; next have him walk on the lateral and medial borders of his feet (Fig. 1–71). This will quickly demonstrate any gross limitation of foot and ankle range of motion as well as motor weakness and muscles of the lower leg.

Next, the passive range of motion of the ankle and foot is determined. The child is instructed to lie on the examining table or sit on a chair, dangling his legs. He should be relaxed. There should not be any active contraction of muscles. For example, when range of dorsiflexion of the ankle is being tested, active contraction of the anterior tibial and toe extensor muscles will cause reciprocal relaxation of the triceps surae.

Passive dorsiflexion of the ankle joint is tested first with the knee extended and then

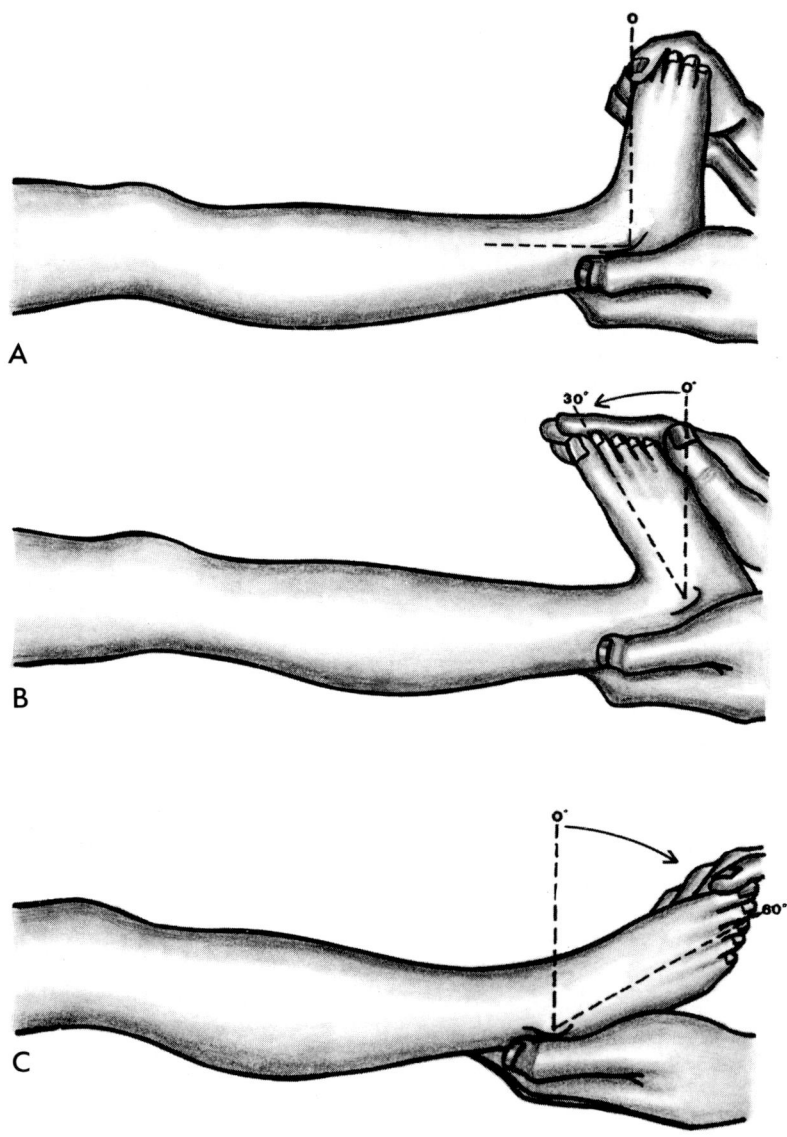

FIGURE 1–72. Testing of passive range of ankle motion.

A. Neutral, or zero, position. The foot is at right angles to the longitudinal axis of the leg. **B** and **C.** The range of ankle dorsiflexion and plantar flexion. Note the foot is inverted to lock the calcaneus under the talus and the forepart of the foot to the hindfoot. The range of motion is judged by inspection from the lateral side.

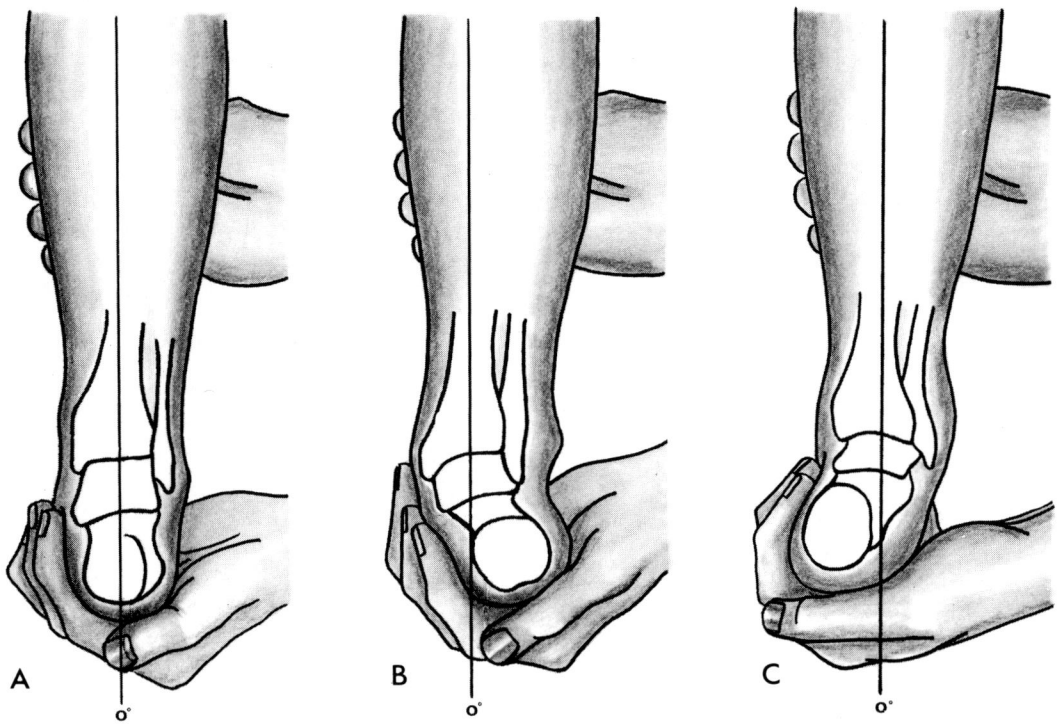

FIGURE 1-73. *Method of testing eversion and inversion of the hindfoot.*
A. Neutral position. **B.** Eversion. **C.** Inversion.

with it flexed. The gastrocnemius portion of the triceps surae originates from the femoral condyles and is, therefore, relaxed when the knee is passively flexed. The subtalar joint is stabilized by holding the calcaneus and inverting the foot; this will lock the calcaneus under the talus and the forepart of the foot to the hindfoot. In the neutral zero position, the foot is at right angles to the longitudinal axis of the leg. The foot is pushed as one unit into dorsiflexion and then into plantar flexion (Fig. 1-72). The range of motion is judged by inspecting from the fibular side. The axis of ankle motion is a line drawn between the midpoints of the medial and lateral malleoli.

The motions of eversion and inversion take place primarily at the talocalcaneonavicular joint. The patient lies prone with the feet dangling free at the edge of the examining table. The tibiotalar joint is stabilized in a neutral or slightly dorsiflexed position. Then the calcaneus is held and moved alternately into eversion and inversion (Fig. 1-73).

The motions of the midtarsal joints are forefoot adduction and abduction; they occur primarily at the talonavicular and calcaneocuboid joints. With one hand the examiner stabilizes the hindfoot, and with the other hand pushes the forefoot medially and laterally (Fig. 1-74). The normal range of forefoot adduction is 20 degrees, and of forefoot abduction, 10 degrees. Precise mensuration of midtarsal motions is difficult. Medial or lateral deviation of the forefoot can be measured in relation to either the second ray or the medial border of the foot.

Inversion usually accompanies adduction (i.e., supination), and eversion is combined with abduction (i.e., pronation) (Fig. 1-75).

The hallux moves at the metatarsophalangeal and interphalangeal joints. To test the passive range of the metatarsophalangeal joint, hold the patient's foot with one hand and with the other hand flex and extend the proximal phalanx of the great toe (Fig. 1-76). The normal range of extension of the metatarsophalangeal joint of the

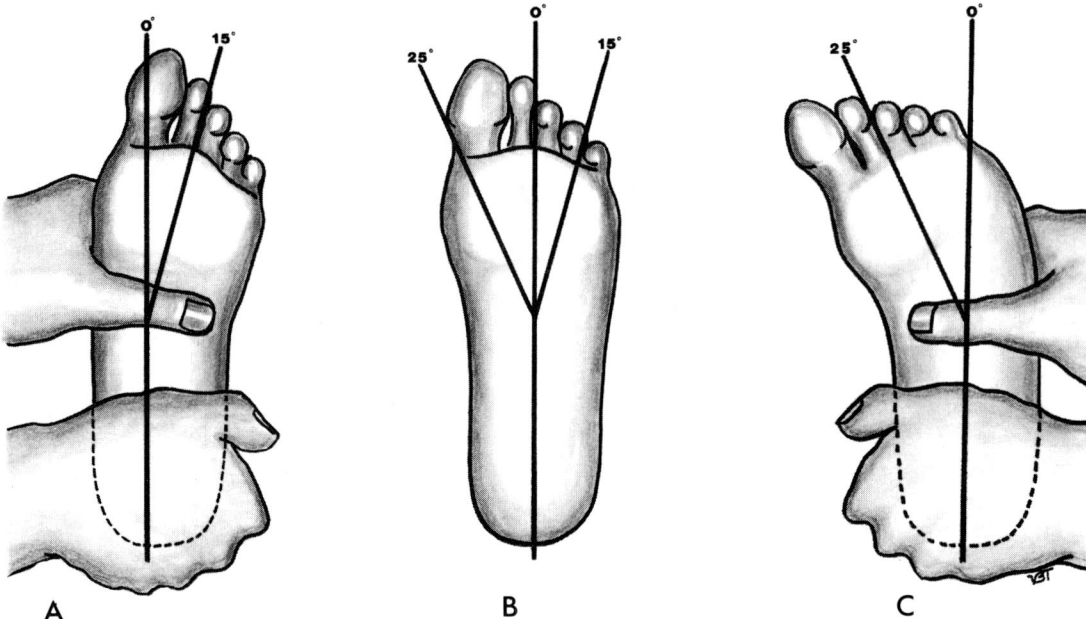

FIGURE 1–74. *Method of testing midtarsal motion.*
A. Forefoot abduction. B. Neutral position. C. Forefoot adduction.

hallux is 70 to 90 degrees, and the range of flexion is 45 to 50 degrees. The interphalangeal joint of the great toe normally flexes 80 to 90 degrees but does not extend (Fig. 1–77).

The second to the fifth toes normally flex at the metatarsophalangeal, proximal interphalangeal, and distal interphalangeal joints. Extension takes place primarily at the metatarsophalangeal joint.

Motor Power

Muscle strength and power may be classified as *kinetic* or *static*, kinetic being the force exerted in changing position, and static being the force exerted in resisting movement. Kinetic power is tested by having the patient carry out movements against resistance provided by the examiner or against the force of gravity. Static power is tested by having him resist active attempts by the examiner to move specific parts. *Paresis* or *weakness* is the term used when there is impairment of strength, while the term *paralysis* denotes total loss of strength.

Muscle weakness is manifested not only by loss of kinetic and static power, but also by fatigability, slowness and irregularity and clumsiness of motion, tremulousness, incoordination, and diminished ability to perform skilled acts.

If muscle weakness is found, one should determine whether it is diffuse or localized. Diffuse (or generalized) muscle weakness is encountered in myopathies such as the dystrophies, electrolyte disturbances, intoxications, deficiency states, and various types of myositis and myasthenia gravis. If localized (or focal) loss of muscle strength is found, one must determine whether it is due to involvement of a specific muscle, of various muscles supplied by one nerve, of a group of muscles supplied by a certain segment of the spinal cord, of a specific movement involving more than one muscle, or of an entire limb. Paralysis of one limb is termed *monoplegia*. More than one limb may be involved, in which case the terms used are: *hemiplegia*—one half of the body; *paraplegia*—the lower limbs; and *quadriplegia* or *tetraplegia*—all four limbs.

If muscle weakness is present one must determine its degree, character, and cause. Is the paralysis flaccid or spastic? Are there associated sensory changes? What are the reflex changes? What is the degree of muscular atrophy? Is there pseudohypertrophy? Is there fibrillation or fasciculation?

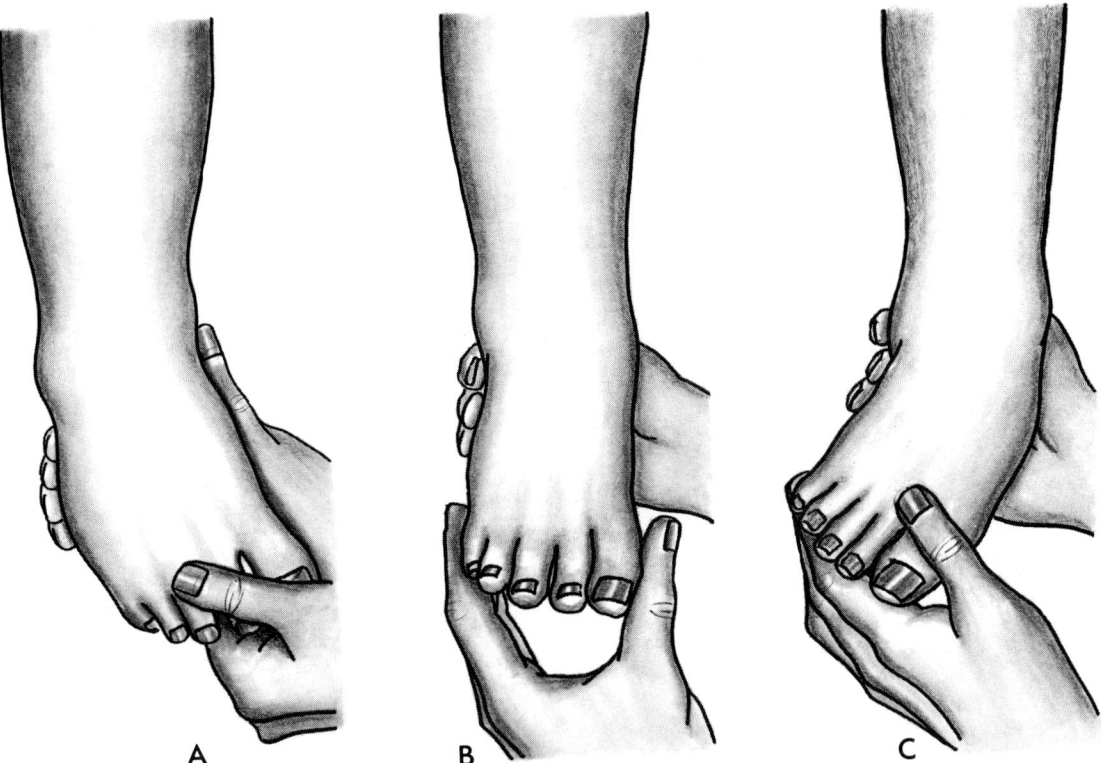

FIGURE 1-75. *Supination and pronation of the foot.*

A. Inversion usually accompanies forefoot adduction-supination. **B.** Neutral. **C.** Eversion is usually combined with abduction-pronation.

When a muscle is maintained in a shortened contracted position for a period of time, a myostatic contracture may develop, and the muscle cannot be stretched to its original normal length. Myostatic contractures may develop because of the overaction of one group of muscles when unopposed by weakened antagonists or following prolonged spasm of muscles, as seen in acute poliomyelitis or in association with spastic paralysis. Contractures may cause deformities of the bones and joints. One should determine whether the deformity itself is increasing the muscle weakness. Is there any pain associated with active or passive motion? Every effort should be made to determine whether limitation or absence of motion is the result of paralysis, involuntary or voluntary muscle spasm, swelling of the joint, or fibrous or bony ankylosis. Finally, one

FIGURE 1-76. *Testing range of extension-flexion of the metatarsophalangeal joint of the great toe.*

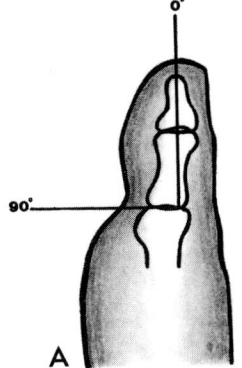
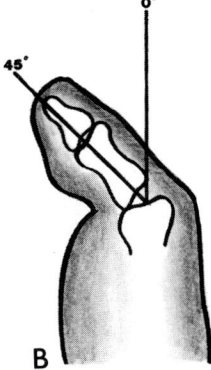

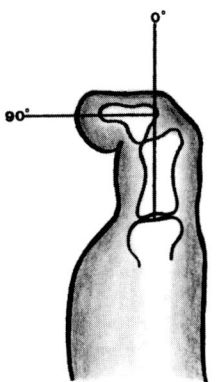

FIGURE 1-77. *Range of flexion-extension of the interphalangeal joint of the great toe.*

should decide whether the muscle weakness is a reversible process or a fixed state, and whether the tendon transfers or transplants can be performed to improve function.

The degree of muscle weakness is objectively graded and recorded on a muscle chart so that the progress of the motor strength can be followed by comparative tests. The original muscle test was developed by Lovett and Martin.[52] The muscle's ability to move the part against gravity or added resistance is used to grade its function. An acceptable classification for grading of muscle strength is given in Table 1-1, and the charts used by the author for recording muscle strength are shown in Table 1-2 for spastic paralysis and in Table 1-3 for flaccid paralysis. The technique of testing the individual muscles controlling the foot and ankle is described and illustrated in Plate 1.

Examination for muscle weakness in infants and small children is difficult. One can, however, readily detect gross defects in movement by observing the spontaneous activity of the infant and watching the small child play. Methods that stimulate reflexes such as the Moro can also be used.[77]

Neurologic Evaluation

A thorough neurologic examination is important in the diagnosis of disorders of the musculoskeletal system. This is especially true whenever there is evidence of muscle weakness, incoordination, or other disturbances in neuromuscular function. The deep and superficial reflexes, sensory function, cranial nerves, and mental and emotional status should be appraised. For details of neurologic examination, the reader is referred to the works of DeJong; Thomas, Chesni, and Saint-Anne; Paine and Oppe; Denny-Brown; and Farmer.[57, 58, 60, 72, 76] An evaluation of the motor development is carried out if the affections of the foot and leg are part of a generalized neuromuscular disorder. The publications of Gesell, Shirley, McGraw, and Zausmer reflect intensive study of this subject.*

Roentgenographic Diagnosis

Roentgenograms are essential for evaluation of the neuromusculoskeletal system, but they should be taken discriminatively. A meticulous history and a thorough phys-

Table 1-1. Grading of Muscle Strength

Grade	Definition
0	No palpable contraction of muscle
Trace	Palpable contraction of muscle, no motion of part that muscle should move
Poor	Muscle moves part through its range, but not against gravity
Fair	Muscle carries part through its range of motion against gravity, but not against added resistance
Good	Muscle lifts part against gravity and added resistance (good minus and good plus used to indicate variations in resistance)
Normal	Normal strength
In practice, certain modified grades may be added:	
Poor minus	Muscle moves part, but not against gravity and not through full range.
Fair minus	Muscle moves part against gravity, but not through full range.

---

*See references 61–63, 66–68, 75, 77–79.

ical examination are needed to determine the area to be x-rayed and the particular views required. On occasion, such as in injuries to joints in children, the contralateral normal side should be roentgenographed for comparison. Often special views are required, and for these, one may have to use the image intensifier for proper orientation.

Details of special roentgenographic examinations of the foot are presented in the appropriate sections of this book.

Bone imaging with radionuclides is of great help in early diagnosis of osteomyelitis, stress fracture, aseptic necrosis, and neoplastic and tumorous lesions.[80]

Computed tomography is of great potential value in the diagnosis and planning of treatment of musculoskeletal lesions.[84] It will, for example, accurately measure femoral antetorsion; however, the reader should be cautioned against the routine use of computed tomography because of excessive exposure to irradiation.[82a, 85]

Electrodiagnostic Methods and Their Use

A meticulous and thorough clinical appraisal of the neuromusculoskeletal system will often lead to correct diagnosis. On occasion, however, various electrical procedures may be utilized to bring out minimal changes of function. This is particularly true in the diagnosis, localization, and prognosis of lower motor lesions. Electrodiagnostic methods may also aid in the discrimination between organic and hysterical paralysis.

It is imperative that one evaluate the results of the various electrical tests as they relate to the total clinical picture. The electrical examination should not be considered a routine procedure in the diagnosis of disorders of the neuromusculoskeletal system.

Electrodiagnostic methods fall into three main groups: tests of neuromuscular excitability by percutaneous stimulation of nerves and muscles; electromyographic studies of motor unit or other muscle action potentials at rest or in action, and nerve conduction velocity studies using both stimulating and recording techniques. In this text, only general principles are outlined. Current references are listed for more detailed information.*

TESTS OF NEUROMUSCULAR EXCITABILITY

Electrical stimulation of nerves and muscles, as described by Erb in 1883, was until just recently the universal method of electrodiagnosis.[90] Though used less frequently now, its importance should not be minimized. Two types of current are used. *Galvanic current* (direct or continuous) stimulates both nerves and muscles, and normally produces momentary unsustained contraction of a muscle upon "making" or "breaking" of the circuit. Muscular contraction is induced through either nerve conduction or direct muscle stimulation. *Faradic current* is induced, interrupted, and rapidly alternating. An induction coil, acting as an interruptor through which a contact is repeatedly made and broken, is used to produce it. Ordinarily, the faradic current is used only in nerve stimulation, and the normal response is a tetantic contraction caused by the rapidly repeated stimuli.

For the electrical examination, the parts of the body to be tested should be relaxed. The limbs should be placed in a proper position for electrical stimulation of the muscle. The stimuli are applied to the *motor nerves* where they are close to the surface of the body and at the *muscle or motor points,* the most excitable parts of the muscles. Motor nerves are usually located over the area where the motor nerve enters the muscle belly or at the site of the greatest concentration of nerve endings. Upon stimulation of a nerve, all the muscles supplied by that nerve contract, and the contraction is appreciated by observing the movement of the part supplied, by palpation of the muscle belly, or by direct inspection.

In lower motor neuron lesions, 10 to 14 days after injury, characteristic electrical changes develop that are known as "reaction of degeneration." In complete reaction of degeneration, no response is obtained from faradic or galvanic stimulation of the motor nerve, whereas galvanic stimulation of the muscle produces a slow, vermicular, long-

Text continued on page 118

---

*See references 86–89, 91–96, 99, 100.

Table 1–2. Chart for Muscle Examination in Spastic Paralysis

**MUSCLE EXAMINATION
CHILDREN'S MEMORIAL HOSPITAL**

Patient Name _____ Chart No. _____

Attending Physician _____ Patient Date of Birth _____

LEFT												RIGHT							
							EXAMINER'S INITIALS												
							DATE												
IP	CC	IP	CC	IP	CC	IP	CC				CC	IP	CC	IP	CC	IP	CC	IP	
							NECK	FLEXORS	STERNOCLEIDOMASTOID										
								EXTENSOR GROUP											
							TRUNK	FLEXORS	RECTUS ABDOMINIS										
								RT. EXT. OBL. / LT. INT. OBL. ROTATORS LT. EXT. OBL. / RT. INT. OBL.											
								TRANSVERSUS ABDOMINUS											
								EXTENSORS	THORACIC GROUP / LUMBAR GROUP										
								PELVIC ELEV.	QUADRATUS LUMB.										
							HIP	FLEXORS	ILIOPSOAS										
								EXTENSORS	GLUTEUS MAXIMUS										
								ABDUCTORS	GLUTEUS MEDIUS										
								ADDUCTOR GROUP											
								EXTERNAL ROTATOR GROUP											
								INTERNAL ROTATOR GROUP											
								SARTORIUS											
								TENSOR FASCIAE LATAE											
							KNEE	FLEXORS	BICEPS FEMORIS / INNER HAMSTRINGS										
								EXTENSORS	QUADRICEPS										
							ANKLE	PLANTAR FLEXORS	GASTROCNEMIUS / SOLEUS										
							FOOT	INVERTORS	TIBIALIS ANTERIOR / TIBIALIS POSTERIOR										
								EVERTORS	PERONEUS BREVIS / PERONEUS LONGUS										
							TOES	M.P. FLEXORS	LUMBRICALES	1										
										2									
										3									
										4									
								I.P. FLEXORS (1ST)	FLEX. DIGIT. BR.	1										
										2									
										3									
										4									
								I.P. FLEXORS (2ND)	FLEX. DIGIT. L.	1										
										2									
										3									
										4									
								M.P. EXTENSORS	EXT. DIGIT. BR.	1										
										2									
										3									
										4									
								I.P. EXTENSORS	EXT. DIGIT. L.	1										
										2									
										3									
										4									
							HALLUX	M.P. FLEXOR	FLEX. HALL. BR.											
								I.P. FLEXOR	FLEX. HALL. L.											
								M.P. EXTENSOR	EXT. HALL. BR.											
								I.P. EXTENSOR	EXT. HALL. L.											
							CHEST	INSPIRATION	(MEASUREMENTS)											
								EXPIRATION											
							ABDOMEN	UMBILICUS TO ANT. SUP. SPINE												
							LOWER	CIRCUMFERENCE – MID CALF												
							EXTREMITY	CIRCUMFERENCE – MID THIGH												
								ANT. SUP. SPINE TO INT. MALLEOLUS												
								UMBILICUS TO INTERNAL MALLEOLUS												

X   Present   Unable to be graded   IP = In Pattern   CC = Cerebral Control   F–   Fair Minus   Incomplete range of motion against gravity
N   Normal   Complete range of motion against gravity with full resistance   P   Poor   Complete range of motion with gravity eliminated
G   Good   Complete range of motion against gravity with moderate resistance   P–   Poor Minus   Incomplete range of motion with gravity eliminated
F+   Fair Plus   Complete range of motion against gravity with slight resistance   T   Trace   Contraction is felt but there is no visible joint movement
F   Fair   Complete range of motion against gravity   0   Zero   No contraction felt in the muscle

Table 1–2. *Chart for Muscle Examination in Spastic Paralysis (Continued)*

		LEFT																RIGHT				
								EXAMINER'S INITIAL														
								DATE														
IP	CC	IP	CC	IP	CC	IP	CC				CC	IP	CC	IP	CC	IP	CC	IP
								SCAPULA	ABDUCTOR	SERRATUS ANTERIOR								
									ELEVATOR	UPPER TRAPEZIUS								
									DEPRESSOR	LOWER TRAPEZIUS								
									ADDUCTORS	⌈ MIDDLE TRAPEZIUS								
										⌊ RHOMBOIDS								
								SHOULDER	FLEXOR	ANTERIOR DELTOID								
									EXTENSORS	⌈ LATISSIMUS DORSI								
										⌊ TERES MAJOR								
									ABDUCTOR	MIDDLE DELTOID								
									HORIZ. ABD.	POSTERIOR DELTOID								
									HORIZ. ADD.	PECTORALIS MAJOR								
									EXTERNAL ROTATOR GROUP									
									INTERNAL ROTATOR GROUP									
								ELBOW	FLEXORS	⌈ BICEPS BRACHI								
										⌊ BRACHIORADIALIS								
									EXTENSOR	TRICEPS								
								FOREARM	SUPINATOR GROUP									
									PRONATOR GROUP									
								WRIST	FLEXORS	FLEX. CARPI RAD.								
										FLEX. CARPI ULN.								
										PALMARIS LONGUS								
									EXTENSORS	⌈ EXT. CARPI RAD. L & BR.								
										⌊ EXT. CARPI ULN.								
								FINGERS	M.P. FLEXORS	LUMBRICALES	1							
											2							
											3							
											4							
									I.P. FLEXORS (1ST)	FLEX. DIGIT. SUB.	1							
											2							
											3							
											4							
									I.P. FLEXORS (2ND)	FLEX. DIGIT. PROF.	1							
											2							
											3							
											4							
									M.P. EXTENSOR.	EXT. DIGIT. COM.	1							
											2							
											3							
											4							
									ADDUCTORS	PALMAR INTEROSSEI	1							
											2							
											3							
											4							
									ABDUCTORS	DORSAL INTEROSSEI	1							
											2							
											3							
											4							
									ABDUCTOR DIGITI QUINTI									
									OPPONENS DIGITI QUINTI									
								THUMB	M.P. FLEXOR	FLEX. POLL. BR.								
									I.P. FLEXOR	FLEX. POLL. L								
									M.P. EXTENSOR	EXT. POLL. BR.								
									I.P. EXTENSOR	EXT. POLL. L.								
									ABDUCTORS	⌈ ABD. POLL. BR.								
										⌊ ABD. POLL. L.								
									ADDUCTOR POLLICIS									
									OPPONENS POLLICIS									
								FACE										

ADDITIONAL DATA:

SIGNATURE_____

Table 1–3. Chart for Muscle Examination in Flaccid Paralysis

Muscle Examination
Children's Memorial Hospital

Patient Name _____ Chart No. _____
Attending Physician _____ Patient Date of Birth _____

Left									(C)₂₃	T₁,₂,₃,₄	T₅,₆	T₇,₈	T₉,₁₀,₁₁	T₁₂	L₁	L₂	L₃	L₄	L₅	S₁	S₂	S₃	Right			
*	*	*	*	* Enter initials of examiner																			*	*	*	*
+	+	+	+	+ Enter date of examination																			+	+	+	+
				Neck	Flexors		Sternocleidomastoid	•																		
					Extensor Group		C₁,₂,₃,₄,₅,₆,₇,₈ T₁																		
				Trunk	Extensors		Thoracic Group		•	•	•	•														
							Lumbar Group		•	•	•	•														
					Flexors		Rectus Abdominis			•	•	•														
					Rotators		Lt. Int. Obl. / Rt. Int. Obl.				•	•	(•)													
							Rt. Ext. Obl. / Lt. Ext. Obl.				•	•	•	1	(2)											
					Pelvic Elev.		Quadratus Abdom.						•	1	2	3										
				Hip	Flexors		Iliopsoas							1	2	3	4									
							Sartorius								2	3	(4)									
					ADDuctor Group										2	3	4									
				Knee	Extensors		Quadriceps								2	3	4									
				Hip	ABDuctors		Gluteus Medius											5	1							
							Tensor Fasciae Latae										4	5	1							
					IR Group												4	5	1							
				Foot	Inv. & Drsfl.		Tibialis Anterior										4	5	1							
					Evertors		Peroneus Brevis										4	5	1							
							Peroneus Longus										4	5	1							
				Hallux	M.P. Ext.		Ext. Hall. Br.										4	5	1							
					I.P. Ext.		Ext. Hall. L.										4	5	1							
					M.P. Flexor		Flex. Hall. Br.										4	5	1							
				Toes	I.P. Flexors		Flex. Digit. Br. 1										4	5	1							
							2										4	5	1							
							3										4	5	1							
							4										4	5	1							
					M.P. Extensors		Ext. Digit. Br. 1										4	5	1							
							2										4	5	1							
							3										4	5	1							
							4										4	5	1							
					I.P. Extensors		Ext. Digit. L. 1										4	5	1							
							2										4	5	1							
							3										4	5	1							
							4										4	5	1							
				Foot	Invertor		Tibialis Posterior										(4)	5	1							
				Toes	M.P. Flexors		Lumbricales 1										4	5	1							
							2										(4)	(5)	1	2						
							3										(4)	(5)	1	2						
							4										(4)	(5)	1	2						
				Knee	M. Flexors		Inner Hamstrings										(4)	(5)	1	2						
				Hip	E.R. Group												4	5	1	2	(3)					
				Toes	I.P. Flexors		Flex. Digit. L. 1											5	1	(2)						
							2											5	1	(2)						
							3											5	1	(2)						
							4											5	1	(2)						
				Hip	Extensor		Gluteus Maximus											5	1	2						
				Ankle	Plantar Flexors		Soleus											5	1	2						
							Gastrocnemius												1	2						
				Hallux	I.P. Flexors		Flex. Hall. L.											5	1	2						
				Knee	L. Flexor		Biceps Femoris											5	1	2	3					

X	Present	Unable to be graded
N	Normal	Complete range of motion against gravity with full resistance
G	Good	Complete range of motion against gravity with moderate resistance
F+	Fair Plus	Complete range of motion against gravity with slight resistance
F	Fair	Complete range of motion against gravity
F–	Fair Minus	Incomplete range of motion against gravity
P	Poor	Complete range of motion with gravity eliminated
P–	Poor Minus	Incomplete range of motion with gravity eliminated
T	Trace	Contraction is felt but there is no visible joint movement
0	Zero	No contraction felt in the muscle

Form No. 77053

Table 1–3. *Chart for Muscle Examination in Flaccid Paralysis (Continued)*

*	*	*	*	* Enter initials of examiner					C_1	C_2	C_3	C_4	C_5	C_6	C_7	C_8	T_1	*	*	*	*
+	+	+	+	+ Enter date of examination														+	+	+	+
					Scapula	Elevator	Upper Trapezius			2	3	4									
						Depressor	Lower Trapezius			2	3	4									
						ABDuctors	Middle Trapezius			2	3	4									
							Rhomboids					4	5								
					Shoulder	ABDuctors	Middle Deltoid					4	5	6							
							Supraspinatus					4	5	6							
						Ext. Rotators	Infraspinatus					(4)	5	6							
							Teres Minor					(4)	5	6							
						Flexor	Anterior Deltoid						5	6							
							Posterior Deltoid						5	6							
					Elbow	Flexors	Biceps Brachii						5	6							
							Brachioradialis						5	6							
					Shoulder	Extensor	Teres Major						5	6	7						
						Horiz. Add.	Pectoralis Major						5	6	7						
						Internal Rotator	Subscapularis						5	5	7						
					Forearm	Supinator	Supinator						5	6	7						
					Scapula	ABDuctor	Serratus Anterior						5	6	(7)	8					
					Wrist	Extensor	Ext. Carpi Rad. L. & Br.						5	6	7	8					
					Forearm	Pronation	Pronator Group							6	7						
					Shoulder	Extensor	Latissimus Dorsi							6	7	8					
					Wrist	Flexors	Flex. Carp. Rad.							6	7	8					
						Extensor	Ext. Carp. Uln.							6	7	8					
					Finger	M.P. Extensor	Ext. Digit. Com.	1						6	7	8					
								2						6	7	8					
								3						6	7	8					
								4						6	7	8					
					Thumb	M.P. Extensor	Ext. Poll. Br.							6	7	8					
						I.P. Extensor	Ext. Poll. L.							6	7	8					
						ABDuctor	ABD. Poll. L.							6	7	8					
					Elbow	Extensor	Triceps							6	7	8	1				
					Wrist	Flexors	Palmaris Longus							(6)	7	8	1				
					Fingers	M.P. Flexors	Lumbricales	1						(6)	7	8	1				
								2													
					Thumb	M.P. Flexor	Flex. Poll. Br.							6	7	8	1				
						I.P. Flexor	Flex. Poll. L.							(6)	7	8	1				
						ABDuctor	ABD. Poll. Br.							6	7	8	1				
						Opponent	Opponens Poll.							6	7	8	1				
					Wrist	Flexor	Flex. Carpi Uln.								7	8	1				
					Fingers	M.P. Flexors	Lumbricales	3							(7)	8	1				
								4							(7)	8	1				
						I.P. Flexors	(1st)	Flex. Digit. Sub.	1							7	8	1				
									2							7	8	1				
									3							7	8	1				
									4							7	8	1				
						I.P. Flexors	(2nd)	Flex. Digit. Prof.	1							7	8	1				
									2							7	8	1				
									3							7	8	1				
									4							7	8	1				
						ADDuctors	Palmar Interossei	1								8	1				
								2								8	1				
								3								8	1				
								4								8	1				
						ABDuctors	Dorsal Interossei	1								8	1				
								2								8	1				
								3								8	1				
								4								8	1				
					Thumb	ADDuctors	ADDuctor Pollicis									8	1				

Muscle Testing

A. TIBIALIS ANTERIOR

Anatomy

Origin. (1) Inferior surface of the lateral condyle of the tibia, (2) upper two thirds to one half of the shaft of the tibia, (3) interosseous membrane, (4) deep surface of the deep fascia, and (5) intermuscular septum between it and the extensor digitorum longus.

Insertion. (1) Medial and inferior surface of the medial cuneiform, and (2) medial and plantar surface of the base of the first metatarsal. *Note*: The insertions of the anterior tibial and peroneus longus muscles are on opposite sides of the medial cuneiform and the base of the first metatarsal (see Fig. 1–36).

Course and Anatomic Relations
- The multipennate muscle fibers converge to a large tendon in the lower third of the leg.
- The tendon passes deep to the superior extensor retinaculum over the anterior aspect of the ankle joint. Over the medial aspect of the dorsum of the foot, however, the upper limb of the inferior extensor retinaculum frequently is thin or absent over the anterior tibial tendon. The anterior tibial tendon becomes prominent on dorsiflexion of the ankle because the upper limb of the inferior extensor retinaculum is absent or thin in front of it. The lower limb of the inferior extensor retinaculum is superficial to the anterior tibial tendon.
- The tendon is invested with a continuous synovial sheath that extends from the upper border of the superior extensor retinaculum to the interval between the divergent limbs of the inferior extensor retinaculum.
- In the upper part of the leg the anterior tibial vessels and deep peroneal nerves are deep to the anterior tibial muscle (see Figs. 1–1 and 1–4).

Nerve Supply. From the deep peroneal nerve, containing fibers from the fourth and fifth lumbar and first sacral nerves, through two or more branches.

Blood Supply. Anterior tibial vessels.

Anatomic Variations
- Tendon may be split into two parts near its insertion, one for the medial cuneiform and the other for the base of the first metatarsal.
- Double tendon—rare.
- Single insertion—to base of first metatarsal only.
- Sends slips to insert to proximal phalanx of hallux or to head of first metatarsal.

Orthopedic Implications

- Especially prone to ischemia because it is encircled in taut fascial compartment and receives all of its blood supply from the anterior tibial vessels (see Fig. 1–7). The other extensor muscles in the leg also derive some circulation from the posterior tibial vessels that penetrate the interosseous membrane.
- Anterior tibial muscle elevates the first metatarsal head, whereas the peroneus longus depresses it. Therefore, paralysis of the peroneus longus muscle with anterior tibial muscle function will result in dorsal bunion, whereas a weak anterior tibial muscle with a strong peroneus longus muscle will cause equinus inclination of the first metatarsal and pes cavus deformity.
- Paralysis—equinus deformity of the ankle.

Method of Testing for Muscle Strength

Position of Patient. Supine or sitting with knee flexed; when muscle strength is poor, side-lying to eliminate gravity.

Stabilization of Limb and Resistance. With one hand hold the back of the leg just above the ankle, and with the other hand on the dorsomedial aspect of the foot, apply pressure toward plantar flexion and eversion.

Movement. Ask the patient to invert the foot and dorsiflex the ankle with the toes, especially the hallux, relaxed.

Plate 1. Muscle Testing

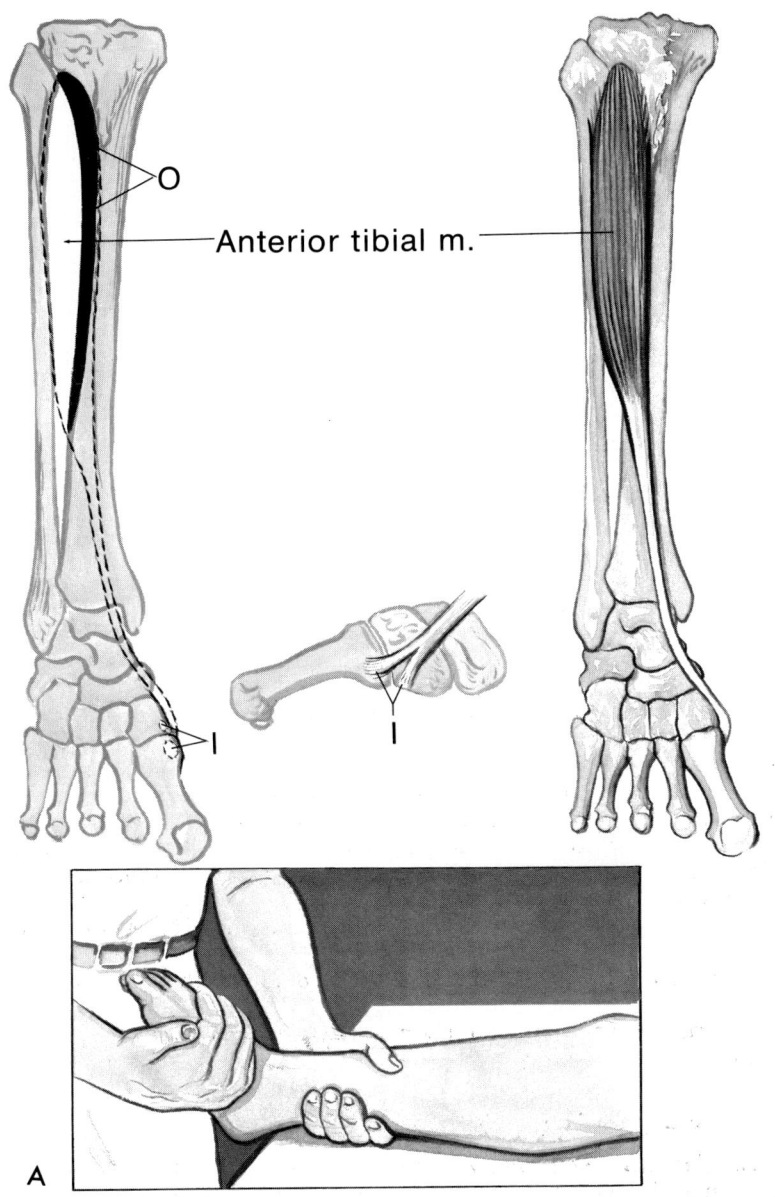

Caution
- The big toe should be relaxed and not go into extension to avoid substitution by the extensor hallucis longus.
- The foot should be in inversion—not neutral position or eversion—to avoid assistance by the extensor digitorum longus and peroneus tertius.
- When the anterior tibial muscle is weak, equinus deformity is common. Be sure there is full range of passive dorsiflexion of the ankle.

Additional Test in an Older Child. Ask him to walk on his heels with the foot inverted and the ankles dorsiflexed.

Muscle Testing (Continued)

B. TIBIALIS POSTERIOR

Anatomy

Origin. Medial part. (1) Lateral part of the posterior surface of the tibia between the soleal (popliteal) line and the junction of the middle and lower thirds of the tibial diaphysis, and (2) posterior surface of the interosseous membrane. *Lateral part:* (3) Medial strip on posterior surface of the upper two thirds of the fibula. *Both parts* also arise from: (4) deep transverse fascia, and (5) intermuscular septa.

Insertion. (1) Tuberosity of the navicular bone. (2) Tendinous bands to the sustentaculum tali of the calcaneus; to the medial, intermediate, and lateral cuneiforms; and to the bases of the second, third, and fourth metatarsals (see Fig. 1–37).

Course and Anatomic Relations

• Deepest muscle of flexor group; located beneath flexor hallucis longus and flexor digitorum longus (see Fig. 1–2).

• A fibrous arch is formed at the upper end of origin—between the tibia and fibula; at this angular interval the anterior tibial vessels cross to enter the extensor compartment.

• Unipennate muscle; tendon lies on its medial side, in contact with the medial edge of the tibia, deep to the flexor digitorum longus (see Fig. 1–5).

• Passes deep to flexor retinaculum, lying against the posterior surface of the medial malleolus. The posterior tibial compartment is the most medial and anterior and is enclosed in its own tendon sheath.

• In the plantar aspect of the foot it is superficial to the plantar calcaneonavicular ligament.

Nerve Supply. Tibial nerve, containing fibers from the fifth lumbar and first sacral nerve.

Action. Primary: Invertor and adductor of the foot. *Secondary:* Weak plantar flexor of the foot.

Method of Testing for Muscle Strength

Position of Patient. Side-lying with the foot resting on its lateral border. When muscle strength is less than fair, change patient's position to supine with the foot hanging free at the end of the table.

Stabilization and Resistance. With one hand gently hold the lower leg and with the other hand apply pressure on the medial border of the forefoot in the direction of eversion and abduction of the foot and dorsiflexion of the ankle.

Caution. To prevent substitution by the flexor hallucis longus be sure the toes are in neutral extension and not actively flexed.

Plate 1. Muscle Testing

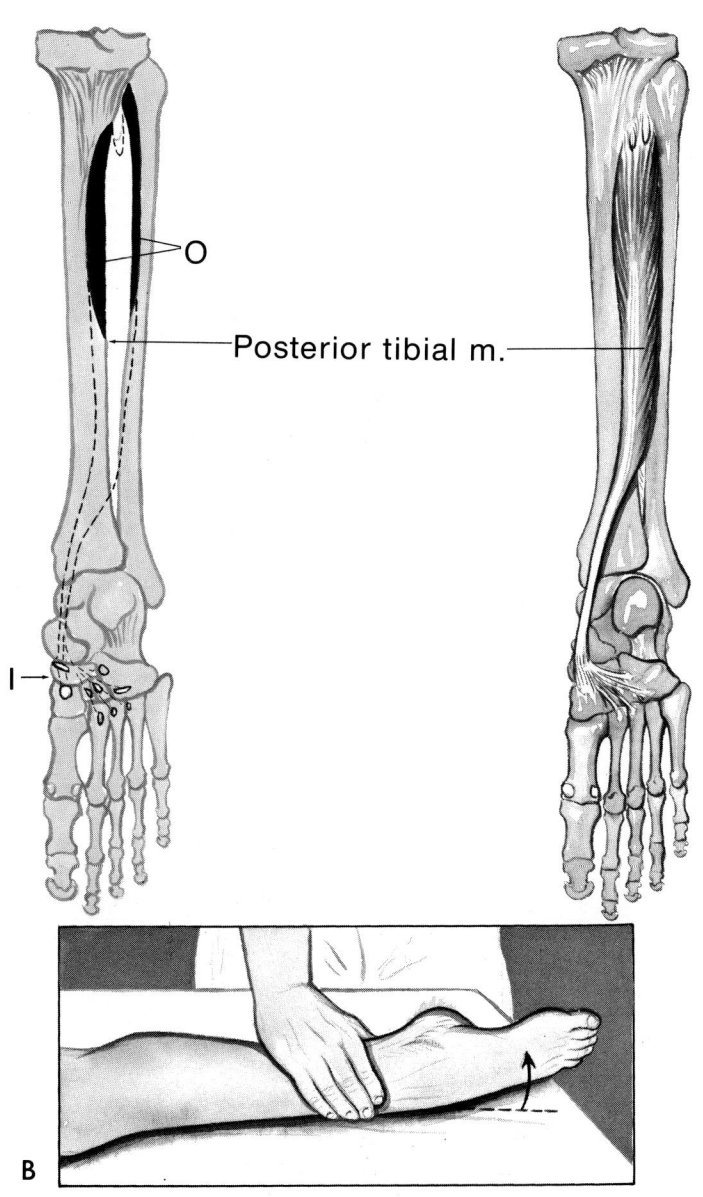

Muscle Testing *(Continued)*

C. EXTENSOR HALLUCIS LONGUS

Anatomy

Origin. (1) From the middle three fifths of the medial surface of the fibula, medial to the site of origin of the extensor digitorum longus; (2) anterior surface of the adjacent interosseous membrane.

Insertion. Dorsum of the base of the distal phalanx of the great toe (see Fig. 1–36).

Course
- In the upper third of the leg it lies deep, between the extensor digitorum longus and anterior tibial muscles (see Fig. 1–1).
- The muscle is penniform. Muscle fibers pass downward to form a tendon, which is situated along its anteromedial border. In the lower part of the leg the tendon becomes superficial between the extensor digitorum longus and anterior tibial muscles.
- The tendon passes deep to the superior extensor retinaculum, occupying the same compartment as the extensor digitorum longus. Beneath the inferior extensor retinaculum it has a separate compartment and requires a separate synovial sheath. The tendon passes distally along the dorsomedial aspect of the foot to its insertion.

Nerve Supply and Anatomic Relations. From several branches of deep peroneal nerve; contains fibers from fourth and fifth sacral nerves. Anterior tibial vessels and deep peroneal nerve are situated between the anterior tibial and extensor hallucis longus muscles, the nerve lying lateral to the artery (see Figs. 1–1 and 1–4). Over the ankle joint the extensor hallucis longus tendon crosses to the medial side of the neurovascular bundle (see Fig. 1–11).

Variation. In about 25 per cent of feet it may also insert to the base of the proximal phalanx through a separate slip.

Action. Primary: Extends the big toe. *Secondary:* Weakly dorsiflexes the ankle. When the anterior tibial muscle is paralyzed the extensor hallucis longus muscle contracts strongly to substitute for it.

Surgical Implications

The motor nerve branches enter the muscle belly of the extensor hallucis longus in the upper third of the leg through its medial and deep surface. During tendon transfer, therefore, elevate the muscle fibers from the medial surface of the fibula and anterior surface of the interosseous membrane from the lateral side.

Method of Testing for Muscle Strength

Position of Patient. Sitting or supine. When strength is less than fair, side-lying to eliminate force of gravity.

Stabilization of Limb and Resistance. With one hand, hold the hindfoot and ankle in neutral position; with the other hand apply digital pressure over the distal phalanx of the great toe in the direction of flexion.

Movement. Ask the patient to dorsiflex the big toe. *Note:* It is difficult to disassociate the action of the extensor hallucis brevis from that of the extensor hallucis longus. When the extensor hallucis longus is paralyzed, however, the extensor hallucis brevis extends the proximal phalanx (not the distal) and pulls it toward the second metatarsal.

Plate 1. Muscle Testing

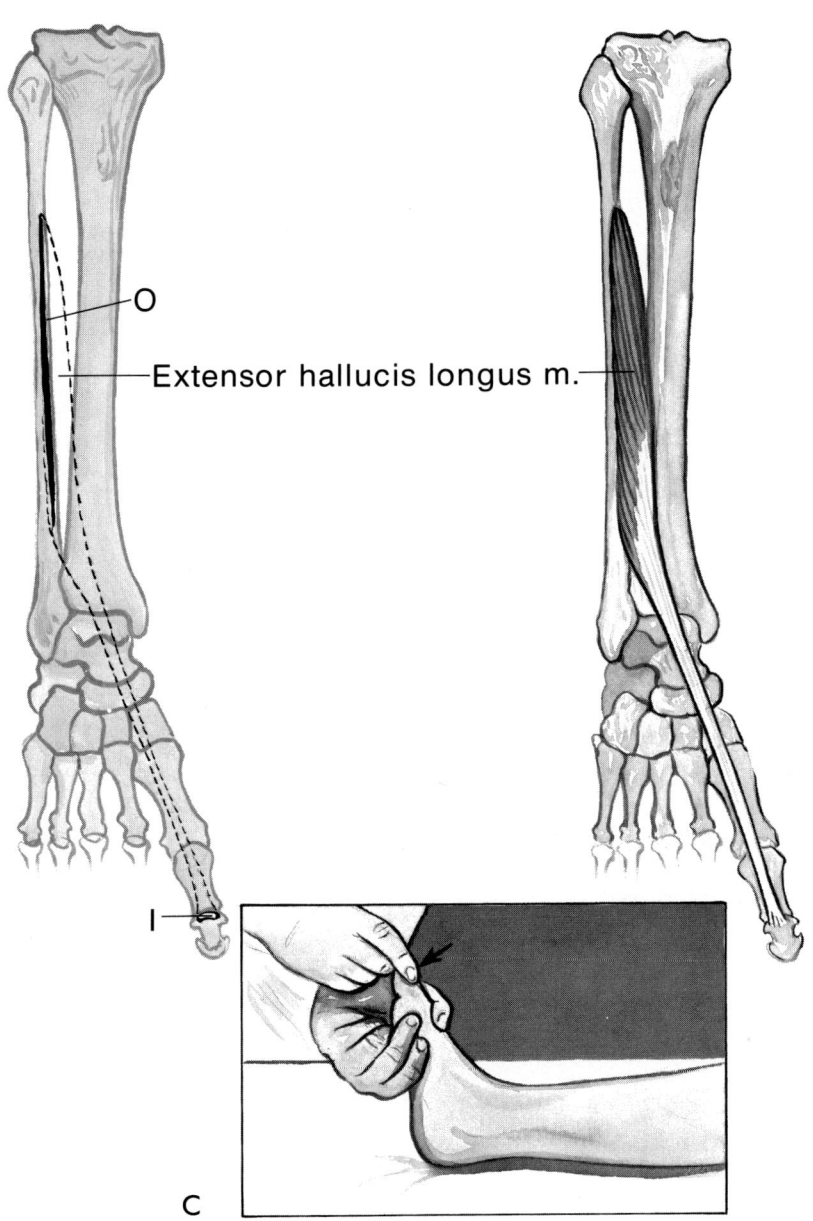

Muscle Testing *(Continued)*

D. EXTENSOR DIGITORUM LONGUS

Anatomy

Origin. (1) Small area on the lateral surface of the lateral condyle of the tibia across the superior tibiofibular joint; (2) Proximal three fourths of the medial surface of the shaft of the fibula; (3) Anterior surface of the interosseous membrane adjacent to its fibular origin; and (4) Adjacent intermuscular septa and the deep surface of the deep fascia.

Insertion. Each tendinous slip inserts to the lateral four toes in the following manner:

- Over the metatarsophalangeal joints the extensor digitorum brevis tendons of the second, third, and fourth toes join the lateral side of the respective tendons of the extensor digitorum longus.
- The combined tendons expand over the metatarsophalangeal joint and the proximal phalanx to form the dorsal part of the capsule and the dorsal digital expansion.
- The lumbricals, and sometimes the interossei, insert to the dorsal digital expansions.
- The tendons then subdivide into three slips: a central one that inserts to the base of the middle phalanx, and two collateral slips that converge to attach to the base of the distal phalanx. It is obvious that the insertions of the extensor digitorum longus are very similar to those of the extensor digitorum communis in the hand (see Fig. 1–36).

Course and Anatomic Relations

- Penniform muscle with tendon forming on its medial border.
- Tendon begins at junction of proximal two thirds and lower one third of the leg.
- Passes deep to superior extensor retinaculum and through loop of inferior extensor retinaculum.
- The tendon widens underneath inferior extensor retinaculum and divides into four slips that diverge and run distally on the dorsum of the foot superficial to the extensor digitorum brevis (see Fig. 1–11).
- The deep peroneal nerve at its origin from the common peroneal nerve runs anteriorly deep to the extensor digitorum longus to the anterior surface of the interosseous membrane, where it comes to lie on the lateral side of the anterior tibial vessels.
- In the upper third of the leg the anterior tibial vessels and deep peroneal nerve are located between the extensor digitorum longus and the anterior tibial muscles.
- In the lower half of the leg the extensor hallucis longus passes between these two muscles. The anterior tibial vessels and deep peroneal nerve, which at first lie between the extensor digitorum longus and the extensor hallucis longus, in the distal 10 cm. of the leg lie anterior to the extensor hallucis longus tendon.
- In its distal part the extensor digitorum longus muscle is continuous with the peroneus tertius on its lateral side—the two muscles are difficult to distinguish.

Variations

- Doubling of tendons to the second and fifth toes.
- Accessory slips may attach to the metatarsals.

Nerve Supply. Three or more branches of deep peroneal nerves, containing fibers from fourth and fifth lumbar and first sacral nerves. Motor points of entry are the medial deep surface of the muscle.

Blood Supply. (1) Anterior tibial vessels, and (2) Perforating branches of posterior tibial vessels through interosseous membrane.

Action. Primary: Extends the interphalangeal joint and metatarsophalangeal joint of the four lateral toes. *Secondary:* Everts foot, dorsiflexes ankle.

The extensor digitorum longus is a weaker dorsiflexor of the ankle than the anterior muscle and abducts the forefoot more strongly than the anterior tibial muscle adducts it.

Plate 1. Muscle Testing

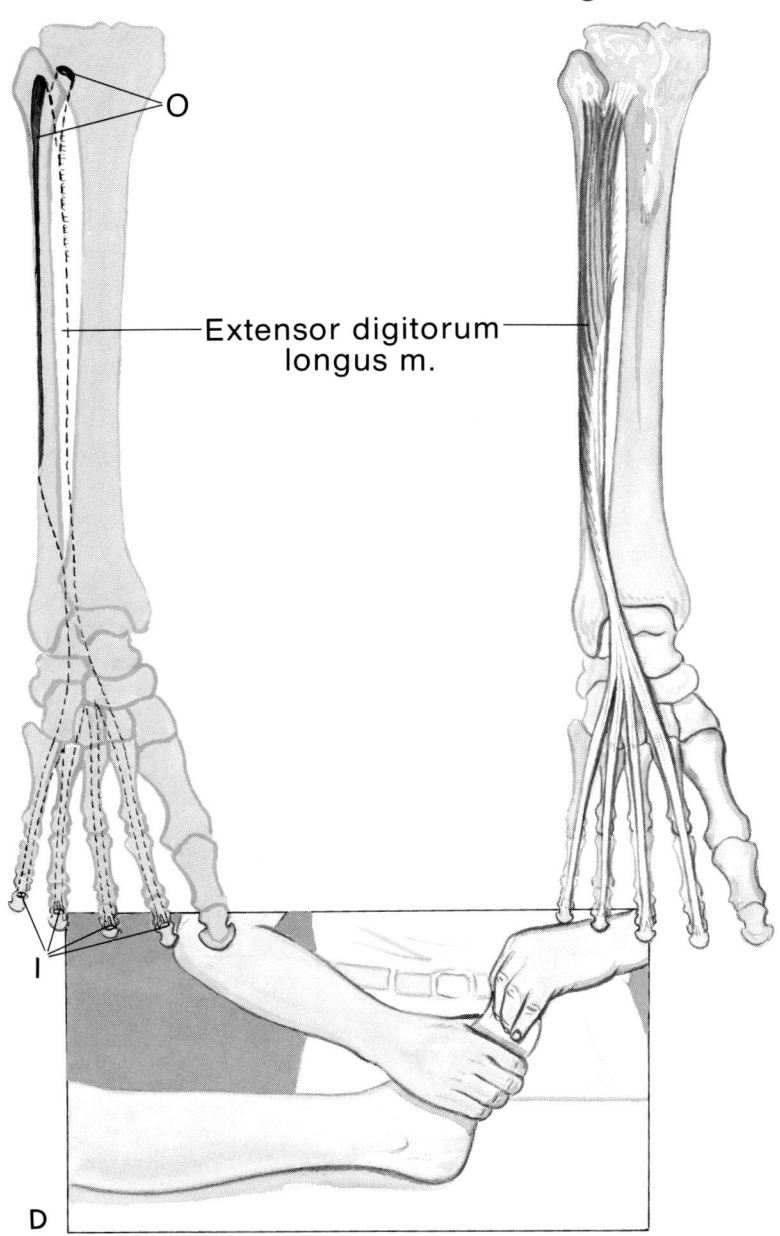

Method of Testing for Muscle Strength

Position of Patient. Supine or sitting.

Stabilization of Limb and Resistance. With one hand hold the ankle and foot in neutral position and with the fingers of the other hand exert pressure on the dorsum of the lateral four toes in the direction of flexion.

Movement. Ask the patient to extend the toes. Each toe can be tested individually if isolated weakness is present.

Muscle Testing *(Continued)*

E. EXTENSOR DIGITORUM BREVIS AND EXTENSOR HALLUCIS BREVIS

Anatomy

Origin. (1) Anterior part of dorsolateral surface of calcaneus in front of the groove for the peroneus brevis, (2) interosseous talocalcaneal ligament, and (3) stem of inferior extensor retinaculum.

Insertion. (1) The medial part to base of proximal phalanx of hallux (sometimes called extensor hallucis brevis muscle); and (2) three lateral divisions attached to the lateral side of the extensor digitorum longus tendons of the second, third, and fourth toes. Sometimes an extra tendon to the fifth toe.

Nerve Supply. Lateral terminal branch of deep peroneal nerve, containing fibers from S_1 and S_2.

Action. Extensor hallucis brevis extends the proximal phalanx of the great toe. Extensor digitorum brevis extends the phalanges of the lesser toes through the tendons of the extensor digitorum longus.

Method of Testing

Position of Patient. Supine or sitting.

Stabilization of Limb and Resistance. With one hand hold the midfoot with the ankle and foot in neutral position and with the fingers of the other hand apply resistance on the proximal phalanges of the toes toward plantar flexion.

Movement. Ask patient to extend toes.

Plate 1. Muscle Testing

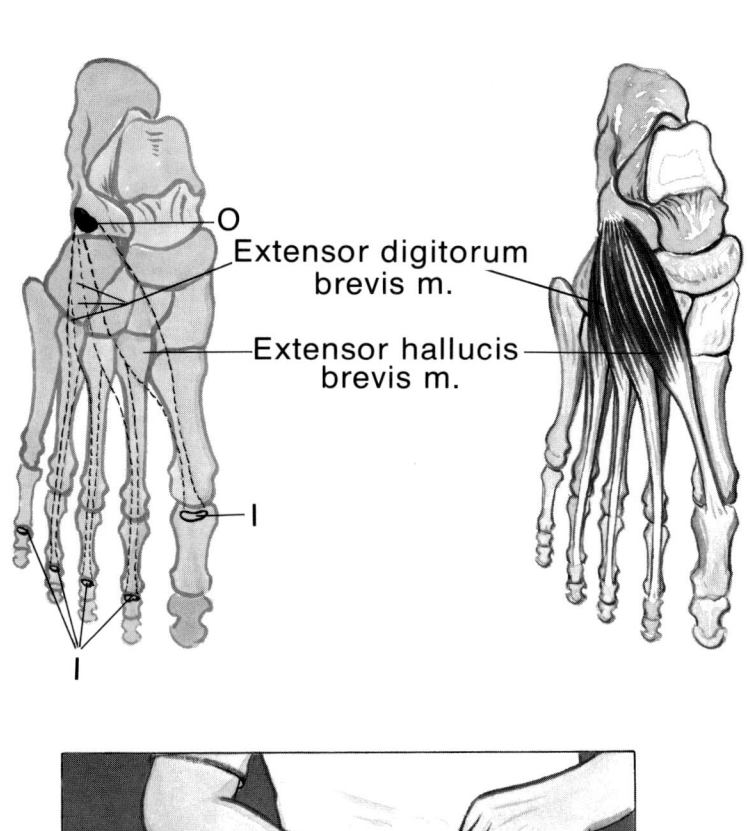

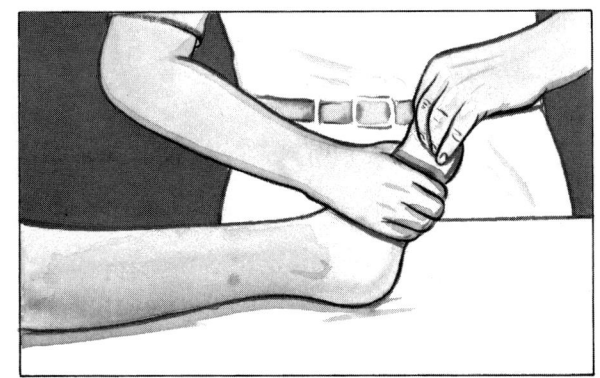

Muscle Testing (Continued)

F. PERONEUS BREVIS

Anatomy

Origin. (1) Lower two thirds of the lateral surface of the fibula (in the middle third of the fibula the origin of the peroneus brevis lies anterior to that of the peroneus longus), and (2) anterior and posterior intermuscular septa adjacent to it.

Insertion. Dorsolateral surface of the base of the fifth metatarsal (see Fig. 1–36).

Course and Anatomic Relations

• Muscle fibers pass distally deep to the peroneus longus and end in a tendon that runs underneath the superior peroneal retinaculum (see Fig. 1–2).

• The peroneus brevis tendon curves forward, lying in a groove on the posterior surface of the lateral malleolus. Here it is anterior to the peroneus longus tendon, and the two tendons are enclosed in a common tendon sheath.

• The peroneus brevis tendon then crosses forward on the lateral surface of the calcaneus above the peroneal trochlea of the calcaneus and deep to the inferior peroneal retinaculum. Here a septum attaches to the peroneal trochlea and subdivides the space into two compartments—a superior canal for the peroneus brevis tendon and an inferior canal for the peroneus longus tendon. Each tendon has its individual tendon sheath.

Nerve Supply. A single branch from the superficial peroneal nerve; contains fibers from the fifth lumbar and first and second sacral nerves.

Action. Everts foot.

Anatomic Variation. A slip from the tendon at its insertion either joins the extensor digitorum longus tendon to the little toe or extends distally to attach to the proximal phalanx of the little toe.

Method of Testing for Muscle Strength

Position of Patient. Semilateral, lying on the side opposite that to be tested, with the ankle joint in neutral position.

Stabilization of Limb and Resistance. With one hand support the lower leg above the ankle joint and with the other hand exert pressure against the lateral border of the foot in the direction of inversion.

Movement. Ask the patient to evert the foot with the ankle in neutral position.

Caution. Be sure that the long toe extensors are relaxed with the toes held relaxed and in some flexion.

PERONEUS TERTIUS

Anatomy

Origin. (1) Distal third of medial surface of fibula, (2) adjacent interosseous membrane, and (3) anterior intermuscular septum.

Insertion. Medial half of dorsal surface of the base of the first metatarsal bone.

Course

• At its origin the peroneus tertius is part of the extensor digitorum longus. The two muscles are indistinguishable.

• The tendon passes deep to the superior extensor retinaculum and courses through the loop of the inferior extensor retinaculum in conjunction with the extensor digitorum longus tendon, which lies on its medial side.

Nerve Supply. Branch of deep peroneal nerve, containing fibers from fourth and fifth lumbar and first sacral nerves.

Action. Dorsiflexes and everts lateral border of the foot.

Variations

• May be absent.

• At its insertion may send a slip to attach to medial border of fifth metatarsal shaft.

Plate 1. Muscle Testing

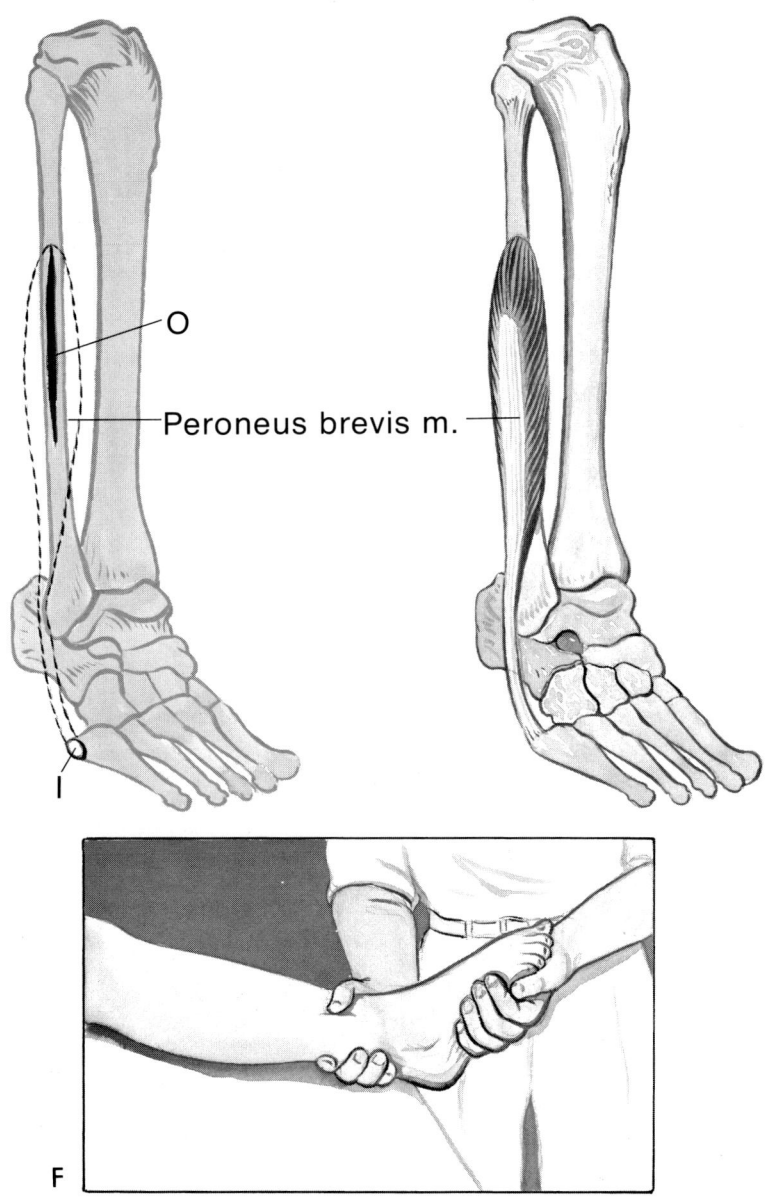

Method of Testing for Muscle Strength

Position of Patient. Supine or sitting.

Stabilization of Limb and Resistance. With one hand hold the lower leg above the ankle joint; with the other hand exert pressure on the dorsolateral aspect of the forefoot in the direction of plantar flexion and inversion.

Movement. Ask the patient to dorsiflex the ankle and evert the foot.

101

Muscle Testing *(Continued)*

G. PERONEUS LONGUS

Anatomy

Origin. (1) Lateral surface of the head of the fibula. (2) Lateral surface of the proximal two thirds of the shaft of the fibula. *Note:* At its origin between the head body of the fibula there is a gap through which the common peroneal nerve winds laterally and anteriorly around the fibular neck (see Figs. 1–1 and 1–4). (3) Deep surface of the deep fascia covering the muscle. (4) Anterior and posterior intermuscular septa. (5) Sometimes a few fibers from a small area on the lateral condyle of the tibia.

Insertion. Lateral side of the plantar aspect of the first metatarsal and medial cuneiform bones (see Fig. 1–36).

Course

• The muscle fibers terminate in a long tendon that is flattened above and rounded near the ankle. In the middle third of the leg the flattened tendon lies superficial to the peroneus brevis muscle.

• The tendon of the peroneus longus changes course at two points; first, behind the fibular malleolus, where it winds around the lateral aspect of the ankle, running in a groove deep to the superior peroneal retinaculum along with the peroneus brevis. The tendon of peroneus longus is thickened here; it lies posterior to that of the peroneus brevis and does not come in direct contact with the lateral malleolus.

• The peroneus longus tendon then passes forward on the lateral surface of the calcaneus inferior to the peroneal trochlea and runs deep to the inferior peroneal retinaculum in a compartment separate from and posteroplantar to the compartment for the peroneus brevis tendon.

• From the lateral surfaces of the cuboid bone the tendon changes its direction for the second time; it plunges into the sole of the foot and crosses obliquely from the lateral to the medial side to its insertion. On the plantar aspect of the cuboid bone the groove (for the peroneus longus tendon) is converted to a canal by the long plantar ligament (see Fig. 1–33). At the plantar and lateral aspects of the cuboid bone the peroneus longus tendon has a sesamoid fibrocartilage that may ossify.

The peroneus longus tendon is enclosed in synovial sheath in the lateral aspect of the ankle; in its upper part the sheath is common to both longus and brevis tendons, but inferiorly each tendon has a separate sheath.

Nerve Supply. Superficial peroneal nerve, containing fibers from the fifth lumbar and first and second sacral nerves. Motor point of entry of nerve is very close to division of common peroneal nerve. Sometimes from two branches, one from the common peroneal nerve and another from the superficial peroneal nerve.

Action. Primary: Everts foot and plantar-flexes first metatarsal head. *Secondary:* Weak plantar-flexor of ankle and abductor of forefoot.

Anatomic Variations

• Peroneus longus and brevis muscles may be fused—*very rare*.

• Insertion may be more diffuse, with tendinous slips to the bases of the second, third, fourth, and fifth metatarsal bones.

Anatomic Relations

• The common peroneal nerve winds around the neck of the fibula in the aperture between the origins of the peroneus longus muscle from the head and body of the fibula.

• The common peroneal nerve bifurcates between the fibula and the peroneus longus muscle (see Fig. 1–4).

• Initially the superficial peroneal nerve is situated deep to the peroneus longus; then it comes to lie between the peronei and the extensor digitorum longus.

• In the lower two thirds of the leg the peroneus longus is superficial and posterior to the peroneus brevis.

• At its insertion the peroneus longus is attached to the lateral part of the plantar aspect of the base of the first metatarsal and the medial cuneiform bones: the extensor tibial tendon is attached to the medial part.

Plate 1. Muscle Testing

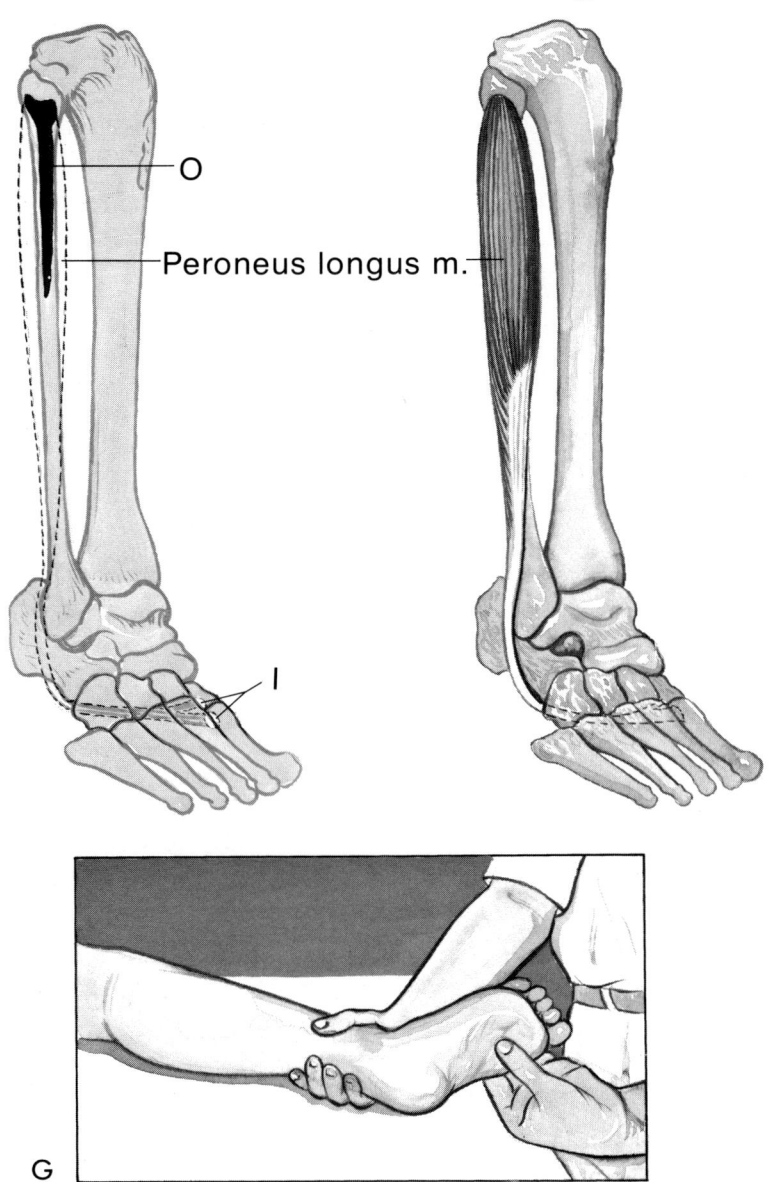

Method of Testing for Muscle Strenth

Position of Patient. Semilateral, lying on the side opposite that to be tested, with the ankle in plantar flexion.

Stabilization of Limb and Resistance. With one hand support the limb by holding the lower leg above the ankle joint; with the other hand exert pressure against the first metatarsal head in the direction of inversion of the foot, dorsiflexion of the ankle joint, and elevation of the first metatarsal head.

Movement. Ask the patient to evert the foot and depress the first metatarsal head from the plantar-flexed position.

Caution. Be sure the common toe extensors are relaxed.

Muscle Testing *(Continued)*
TRICEPS SURAE

The triceps surae consists of two large muscles, the gastrocnemius and the soleus.

H. GASTROCNEMIUS

Anatomy

Origin. By two heads, attached to femoral condyles by flat tendons (see Figs. 1–2 and 1–3).

Medial head: (1) Popliteal surface of femur just above medial condyle, (2) upper part of medial condyle near the adductor tubercle, and (3) posterior aspect of capsule of knee joint (has a sesamoid bone or cartilage in 12 to 15 per cent).

Lateral head: (1) Lateral surface of the lateral condyle of the femur, (2) lateral lip of the linea aspera above the condyle, and (3) posterior capsule of the knee joint (has a sesamoid bone or cartilage—fabella—in about 27 to 29 per cent).

Insertion. Tendo calcaneus into the posterior surface of calcaneus (see Fig. 1–36).

I. SOLEUS

Anatomy

Origin. By two heads that are united by a tendinous arch from which additional fibers arise (see Figs. 1–2 and 1–3).

Lateral head: (1) Posterior surface of the head of the fibula, and (2) proximal third of the shaft of the fibula.

Medial head: (1) Soleal (popliteal) line of the tiba, and (2) middle third of medial border of tibia.

Insertion. Tendo calcaneus into posterior surface of the calcaneus.

Method of Testing for Muscle Strength of Triceps Surae

Position of Patient
- Stands on the limb to be tested (contralateral leg off floor).
- Knee in neutral extension during test.
- Center of gravity of body must be over center of support; child should not lean forward.

Movement. Patient raises heel from floor through complete range of plantar flexion and elevates his body without flexing the knee and without leaning forward.

Grading: Normal—motion completed ten times; *Good*—motion completed five times; *Fair*—motion completed once; *Fair minus*—motion completed once, but not through full range of plantar flexion.

Non–weight-bearing Tests of Triceps Surae. Grades normal and fair should be recorded as hand testing (see position drawing). Always use weight-bearing test if possible.

Position of Patient. Prone, knee in full extension, foot in *neutral position* at ankle and subtalar joints. When muscle strength of triceps surae is poor or less the position of the patient is changed from prone to lateral with the knee in full extension and the ankle and foot in neutral position.

Stabilization and Resistance. With one hand hold the calf and with the other hand hold the posterior surface of the heel; give resistance in the direction of dorsiflexion.

Movement. Ask the patient to plantar-flex the foot.

Caution
- Be sure the foot is in neutral position—when inverted, the tibialis posterior will assist, and when everted, the peroneals will assist.
- Knee should be in full extension. Flexion of the knee will relax the gastrocnemius.

Method of Testing the Soleus

Same as triceps surae, but knee is flexed to relax gastrocnemius.

Plate 1. Muscle Testing

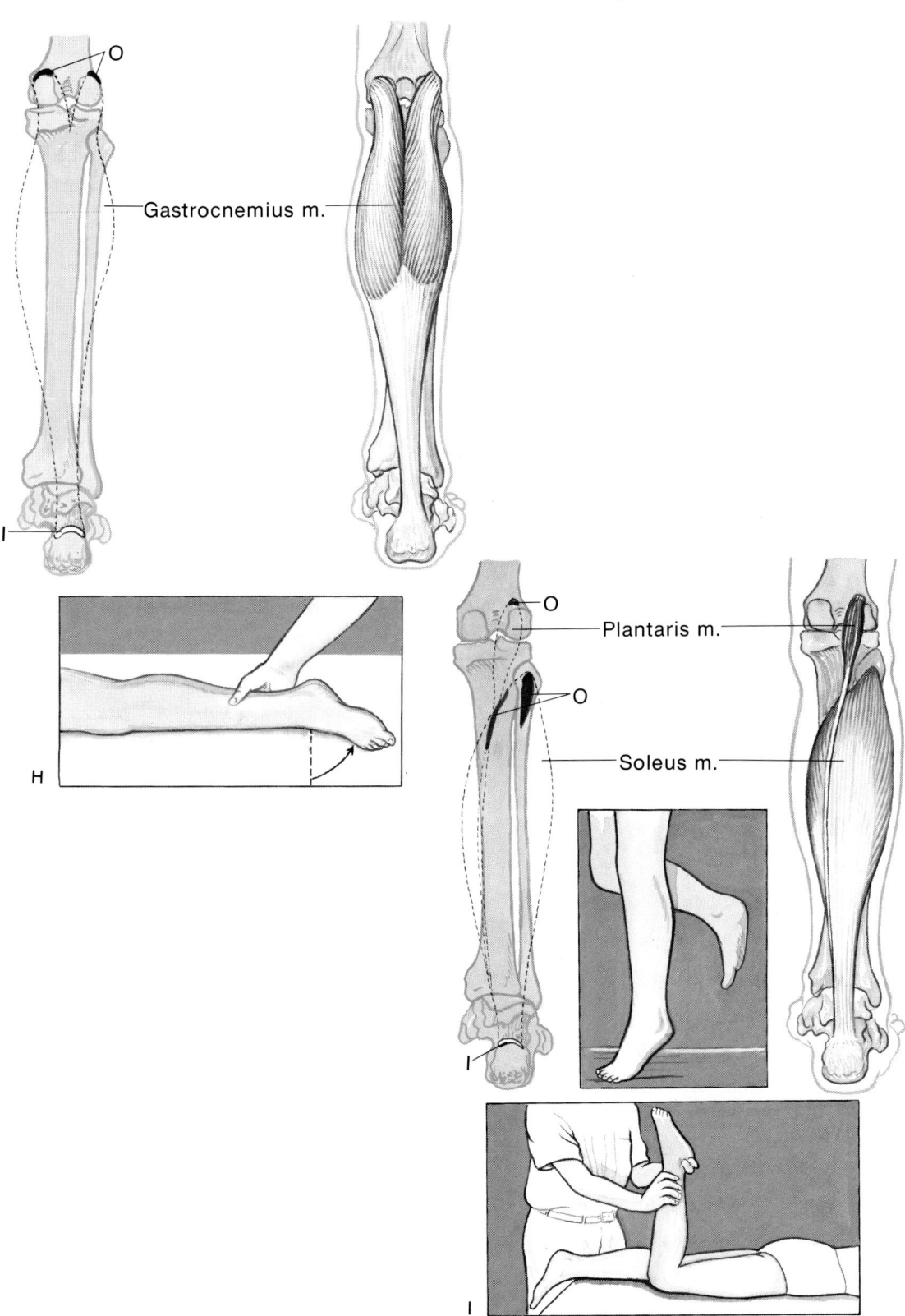

105

Muscle Testing *(Continued)*

J. FLEXOR HALLUCIS LONGUS

Anatomy

Origin. (1) The posterior surface of the distal two thirds of the fibula (except for approximately the lowest 2.5 cm.), (2) the distal part of the interosseous membrane, and (3) the posterior intermuscular septum.

Insertion. Base of the distal phalanx of the great toe (see Fig. 1–37).

Course and Anatomic Relations. The tendon begins high in this bipennate muscle and lies in a broad shallow groove on the posterior surface of the lower end of the tibia. It enters deep to the flexor retinaculum, where it has its own tendon sheath and separate tunnel, which is the most posterolateral of the four compartments. Anteromedial to it is the canal for the posterior tibial vessels and tibial nerves. On the posterior surface of the talus, the tendon passes in the groove between the medial and lateral tubercles. It then runs in a canal on the medial surface of the calcaneus immediately beneath the sustentaculum tali. In the foot, the flexor hallucis longus tendon crosses the upper (or deep) surface of the flexor digitorum longus from the lateral (fibular) to the medial side, taking an obliquely curved course. At the crossing point the flexor digitorum longus and flexor hallucis longus tendons are connected by a fibrous slip—the "master knot of Henry"—which is located one thumb width lateral to the tuberosity of the navicular on the plantar aspect of the foot (see Fig. 1–29). The flexor hallucis longus tendon extends distally on the superficial surface and between two heads of the flexor hallucis brevis muscle, and between the two sesamoids, which protect it from pressure from the first metatarsal head. These large sesamoids bear the entire body weight during take-off.

Nerve Supply. Tibial nerve, containing fibers from fifth lumbar and first and second sacral nerves.

Action. Primary: Flexes distal phalanx of great toe. *Secondary:* Supinates (adducts and inverts) the foot. Adducts with greater force than inverts. Plantar-flexes the foot (weakly). (It will try to substitute for triceps surae when the latter is paralyzed.)

Variations. The tendon may be double with one component inserting into the calcaneus.

Method of Testing for Muscle Strength

Position of Patient. Supine or sitting.

Stabilization of Limb and Resistance. With one hand hold the metatarsophalangeal joint and proximal phalanx of the great toe in neutral position with the ankle at 30 to 40 degrees of plantar flexion; with the other hand apply pressure on the plantar aspect of the distal phalanx of the great toe in the direction of extension.

Movement. Ask the patient to bend the distal phalanx of the great toe.

Caution. Be sure the ankle is not fully dorsiflexed, as the interphalangeal joint of the big toe may flex passively; also complete flexion of the ankle will relax the muscle excessively.

Plate 1. Muscle Testing

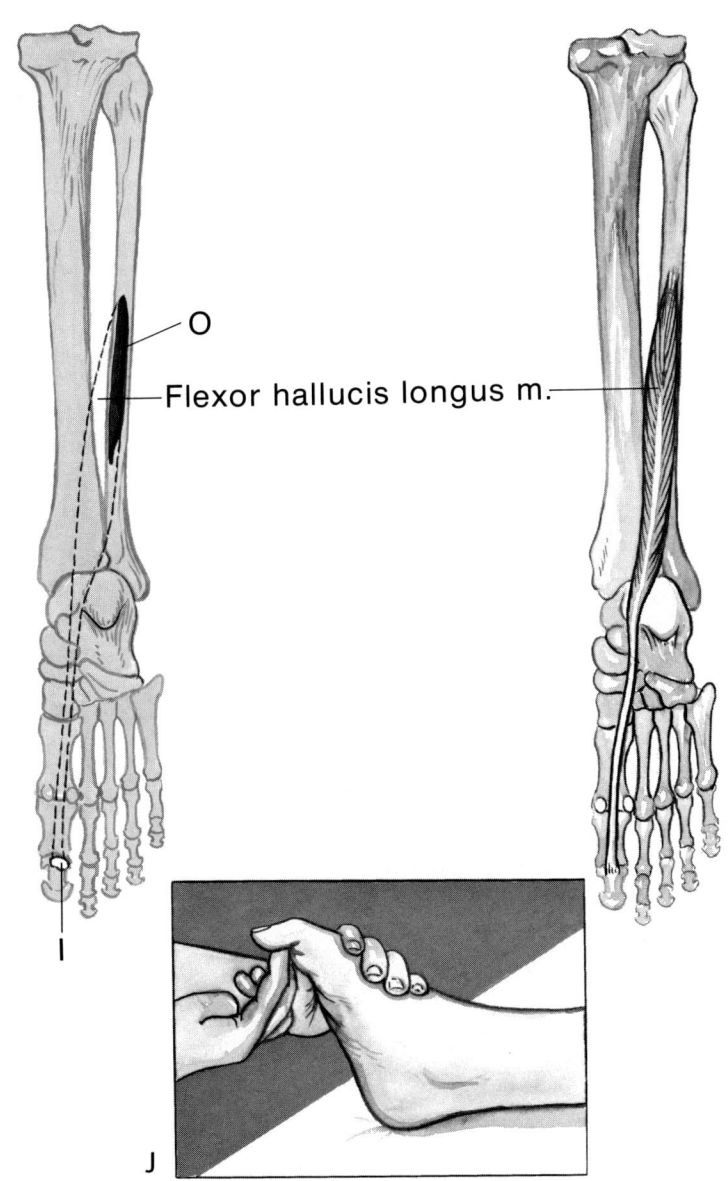

Muscle Testing *(Continued)*
K. FLEXOR HALLUCIS BREVIS

Anatomy

Origin. By a Y-shaped tendon that has rather diffuse attachments: (1) a lateral limb that originates from the plantar aspect of the medial part of the cuboid (behind the groove for the peroneus longus tendon) and the lateral cuneiform, (2) a medial limb attached by a deep part to the slips of the tendon of the tibialis posterior as it spreads out to its insertions in this area, and (3) a superficial part to the medial band of the medial intermuscular septum.

Insertion. (1) The medial tendinous part inserts into the medial sesamoid and the medial side of the base of the proximal phalanx of the great toe in common with the abductor hallucis. (2) The lateral part inserts into the lateral sesamoid and the lateral side of the proximal phalanx of the hallux, blending with the adductor hallucis at its termination (see Fig. 1–37).

Course and Anatomic Relations. The muscular belly, beginning immediately proximal to the tarsometatarsal joint of the great toe, lies on the plantar aspect of the first metatarsal. Distally, near the base of the great toe, the belly of the flexor digitorum brevis divides into two tendons. Proximally the tendon of the flexor hallucis longus lies in a groove in the midline of the muscular belly of the flexor digitorum brevis, and distally it lies between the two tendinous divisions (see Figs. 1–27 and 1–28).

Nerve Supply. A branch of the medial plantar nerve (S_2 and S_3).

Action. Flexes the metatarsophalangeal joint of the great toe.

Method of Testing for Muscle Strength

Position of Patient. Supine or sitting.

Stabilization of Limb and Resistance. With one hand hold the first metatarsal head with the ankle in neutral position; with the other hand apply pressure against the plantar surface of the proximal phalanx of the great toe in the direction of extention.

Movement. Ask patient to flex the proximal phalanx of the great toe.

Plate 1. Muscle Testing

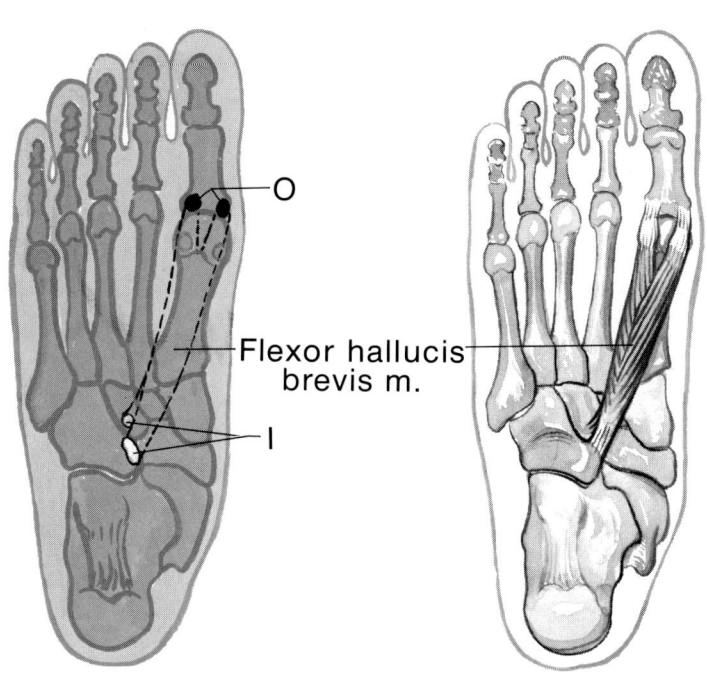

Flexor hallucis brevis m.

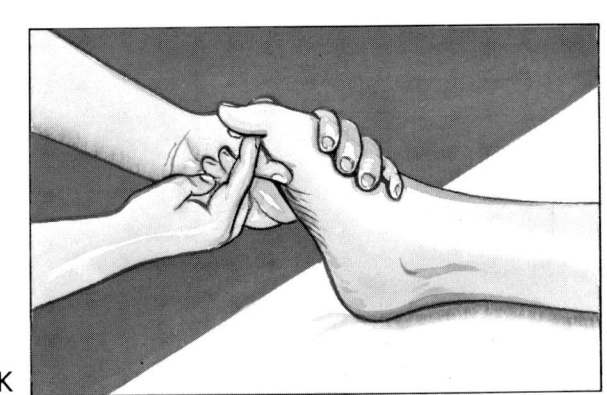

Muscle Testing (Continued)

L. FLEXOR DIGITORUM LONGUS

Anatomy

Origin. The bipennate muscle originates from (1) the middle three fifths of the posterior surface of the tibia (below the soleal line and the origin of the posterior tibial muscle), (2) the fibula by a broad aponeurosis whose oblique fascial fibers are replaced by muscle to form the lateral half of the bipennate muscle, (3) adjacent intermuscular septa and covering fascia.

Insertion. Into the bases of the distal phalanges, after piercing the tendons of the flexor digitorum brevis (see Fig. 1–37).

Course and Anatomic Relations. In the middle of the leg, the flexor digitorum longus is the most medial of the three deep muscles of the calf. In the lower part of the leg, however, its tendon takes an oblique course superficial to the tibialis posterior, which separates it from the tibia. Thus, at the ankle the flexor digitorum longus assumes an intermediate position with the tibialis posterior located anteromedially and the posterior tibial vessels and tibial nerve lying posterolaterally. It then enters the sole, passing deep to the flexor retinaculum, in its own synovial sheath in a separate canal. On the medial aspect of the hindfoot, it lies alongside the free medial margin of the sustentaculum tali of the calcaneus, not beneath it.

In the sole, the tendon of the flexor digitorum longus is covered by the abductor hallucis and the flexor digitorum brevis; it crosses the flexor hallucis longus tendon superficially from the medial to the fibular side to pass to the lateral four toes (see Fig. 1–29). At the crossing the flexor hallucis longus and flexor digitorum longus are bound together by a strong fibrous slip (the "master knot of Henry"), which inserts to the plantar aspect of the navicular. The flexor digitorum longus tendon then divides into four smaller tendons for the lateral four toes (see Figs. 1–28 and 1–29). At the site of its division, the flexor digitorum longus tendon receives on its deep surface the insertion of the quadratus plantae. The oblique course of the flexor digitorum longus is controlled by the straight line of pull of the quadratus plantae. More distally each smaller tendon gives origin to the four lumbrical muscles of the foot. Each tendon passes into a fibrous sheath and courses forward to its insertion.

Nerve Supply. The tibial nerve (fibers from L_5, S_1, S_2).

Action. Primary: Flexes the distal phalanges of the lateral four toes. *Secondary:* Adducts and inverts the foot. Assists in plantar flexion of the foot (weak).

Method of Testing for Muscle Strength

Position of Patient. Supine or sitting.

Stabilization of Limb and Resistance. With one hand hold the middle and proximal phalanges in neutral position and the ankle joint in neutral extension. With the other hand exert pressure on the plantar aspect of the distal phalanges of the lateral four toes in the direction of dorsiflexion.

Movement. Ask the patient to flex the distal phalanges of the lateral four toes. *Note:* The *quadratus plantae* has two heads of origin: (1) a *lateral head* arising from the lateral surface of the long plantar ligament, and (2) a *medial head* arising from the medial surface of the calcaneus and the medial border of the long plantar ligament. It inserts into the lateral border and the dorsal and plantar surfaces of the tendon of the flexor digitorum longus. By modifying the line of pull of the flexor digitorum longus it assists in flexion of the lateral four toes.

Plate 1. Muscle Testing

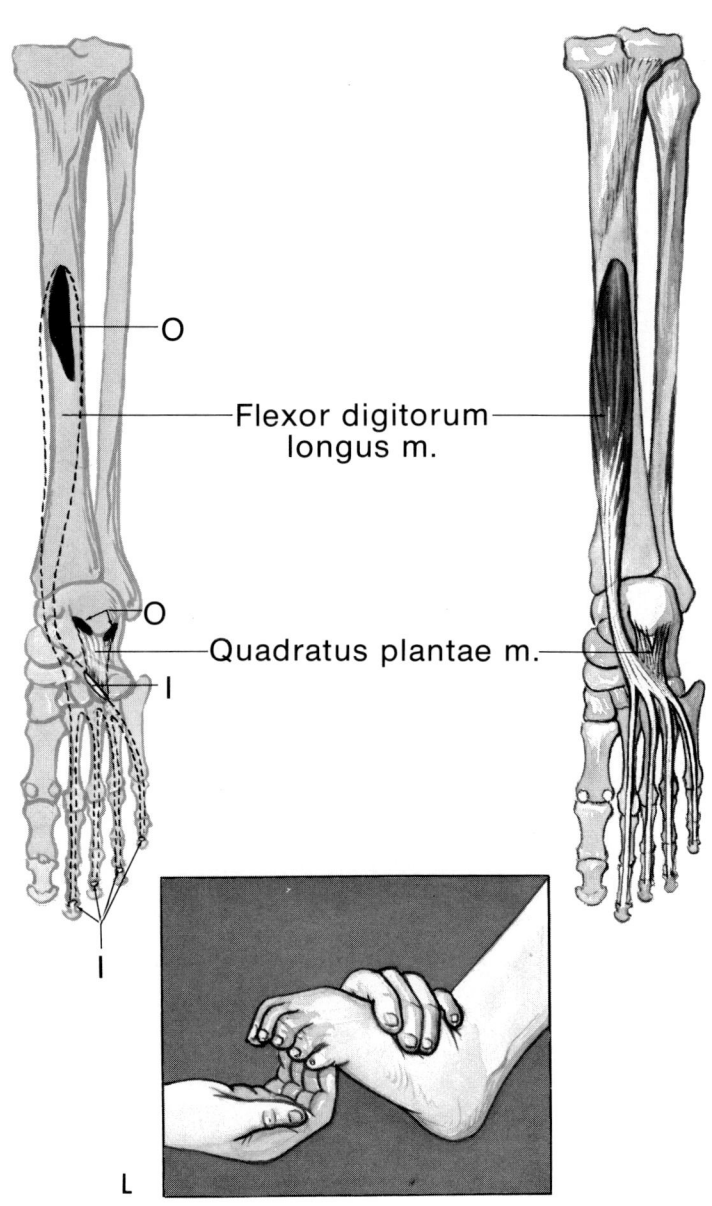

Muscle Testing (Continued)

M. FLEXOR DIGITORUM BREVIS

Anatomy

Origin. (1) By a narrow tendon from the medial process of the tuberosity of the calcaneus, (2) from the middle portion of the plantar aponeurosis, and (3) from intermuscular septa between it and adjacent muscles.

Insertion. At the base of the proximal phalanges each tendon of the flexor digitorum brevis enters the fibrous flexor sheath for the long flexor tendon. It then divides into two slips, one on each side of the corresponding tendon of the flexor digitorum longus, and inserts to each side of the shaft of the middle phalanx (see Fig. 1–37).

Course and Anatomic Relations
• It is covered inferiorly by the middle part of the plantar aponeurosis, to which it is adherent and from which it takes origin.
• On its deep surface is a thin layer of fascia that separates it from the lateral plantar vessels and nerves.
• On either side are two vertical septa that separate it from adjacent muscles.
• As the muscle fibers extend distally, they separate from the overlying plantar aponeurosis and divide into four tendons for the lateral four toes (see Fig. 1–27).

Nerve Supply. Medial plantar nerve (S_2 and S_3).

Action. Flexes proximal phalangeal joints of the lateral four toes.

Method of Testing for Muscle Strength

Position of Patient. Supine.

Stabilization of Limb and Resistance. With one hand hold the proximal phalanges of the lateral four toes in neutral position; with the other hand apply pressure on the plantar aspect of the intermediate phalanges in the direction of extension.

Movement. Ask the patient to flex the lateral four toes.

Plate 1. Muscle Testing

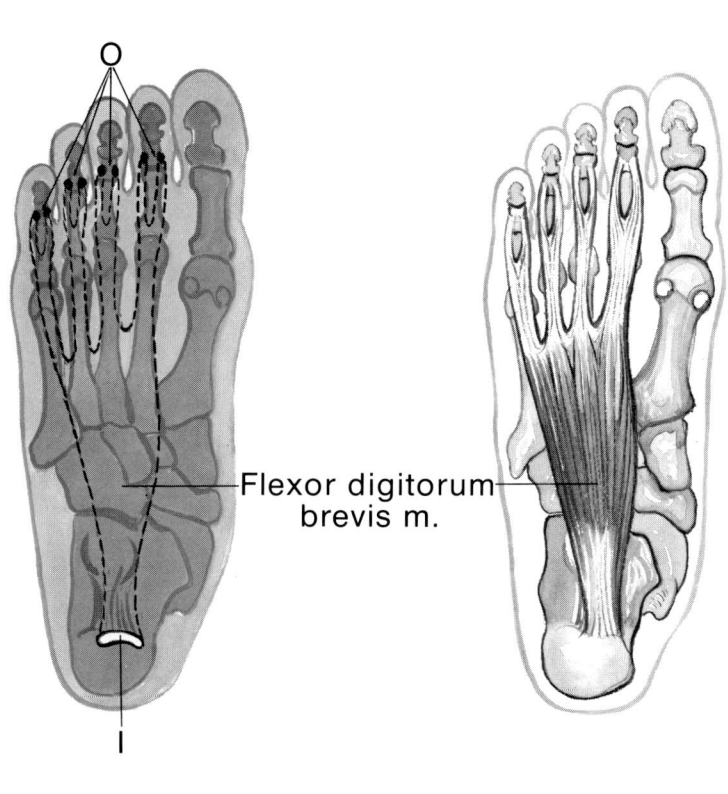

Flexor digitorum brevis m.

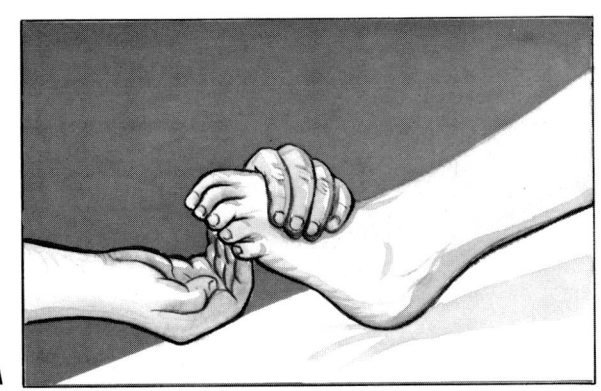

Muscle Testing (Continued)

N. ABDUCTOR HALLUCIS

Anatomy

Origin. (1) Primarily from the flexor retinaculum (lanciniate ligament); (2) the medial process of the tuberosity of the calcaneus; (3) the tuberosity of the navicular; (4) the plantar aponeurosis; and (5) the intermuscular septum that separates it from the flexor digitorum brevis.

Insertion. Along with the tendon of the medial head of the flexor hallucis brevis into the medial aspect of the base of the proximal phalanx of the hallux. Some fibers insert into the medial sesamoid of the great toe (see Fig. 1–37).

Course and Anatomic Relations. The muscle fibers extend forward below the medial longitudinal arch and end in a tendon about two thirds of the way (see Fig. 1–27). Surgically, the foot in stance is like a vaulted cage that opens medially. The cage door is the abductor hallucis muscle.

Nerve Supply. Two branches of the medial plantar nerve (S_2 and S_3). These small branches are located two and three fingerbreadths respectively behind the tuberosity of the navicular. They should not be injured during surgical exposure.

Method of Testing for Muscle Strength

Position of Patient. Supine.

Stabilization of Limb and Resistance. With one hand hold the foot in neutral position, palpating the fibers of the abductor hallucis brevis on the medial side of the forefoot; with the other hand apply pressure on the tibial side of the proximal phalanx of the great toe, pushing it toward the fibular side.

Movement. Ask the patient to abduct the big toe (toward the center of the body, away from the lateral four toes).

ABDUCTOR DIGITI QUINTI (OR MINIMI)

Anatomy

Origin. (1) Lateral process of tuberosity of calcaneus, (2) plantar surface of calcaneus, (3) plantar aponeurosis, and (4) intermuscular septum between it and flexor digitorum brevis.

Insertion. Lateral side of the base of proximal phalanx of the little toe (see Fig. 1–37).

Course and Anatomic Relations
- Lies on lateral margin of foot.
- On its medial aspect are the lateral plantar vessels and nerves.
- Tendon passes distally over a groove on the base of the fifth metatarsal.

Nerve Supply. Lateral plantar nerve (S_2 and S_3).

Action. Abducts the little toe.

Method of Testing for Muscle Strength

Position of Patient. Supine.

Stabilization of Limb and Resistance. Hold the forefoot with one hand and with the other hand give resistance on the lateral side of the little toe in the direction of adduction.

Movement. Ask the patient to abduct the little toe. (The dorsal interossei abduct the third and fourth toes). *Note:* A normal person may be unable to abduct the lesser toes.

Plate 1. Muscle Testing

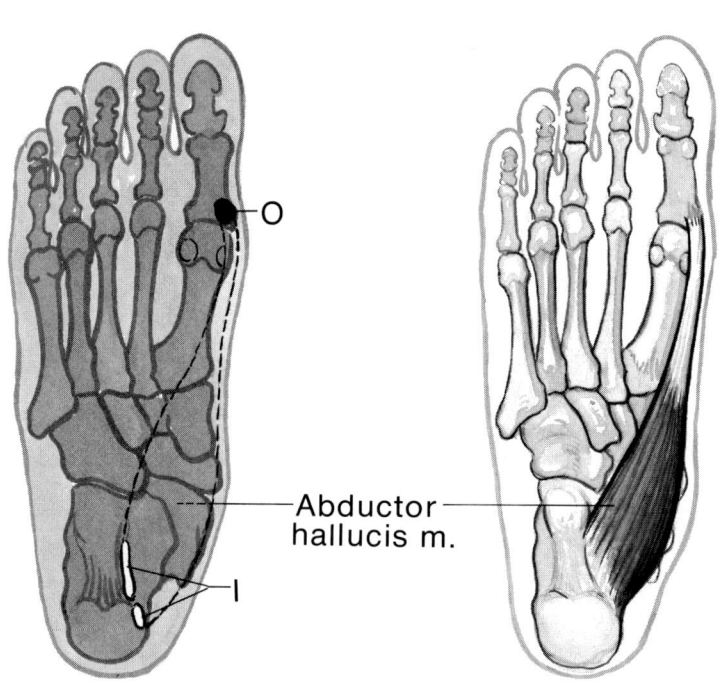

Abductor hallucis m.

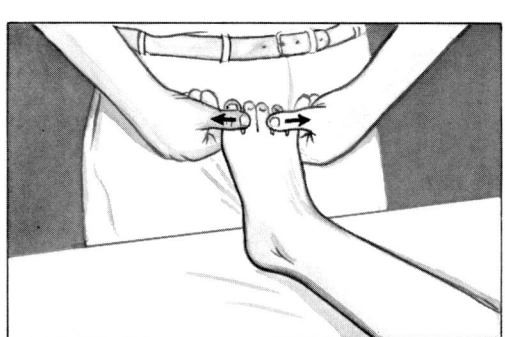

115

Muscle Testing *(Continued)*

O. ADDUCTOR HALLUCIS

Anatomy

Origin. Arises by two heads: *Oblique head,* which comes from the bases of the second, third, and fourth metatarsal bones; and *transverse head,* which takes origin from (1) the plantar ligament of the third and fourth (sometimes the fifth) metatarsophalangeal joints, and (2) the deep transverse metatarsal ligaments.

Insertion. Base of the proximal phalanx of the great toe (see Fig. 1–37).

Nerve Supply. A branch from the deep branch of the lateral plantar nerve (S_2 and S_3).

Action. Adducts big toe.

Method of Testing for Muscle Strength

Position of Patient. Supine or sitting.

Stabilization of Limb and Resistance. Hold toes in abduction and supply pressure on lateral side of big toe.

Movement. Ask patient to adduct the big toe. *Note:* To test the function of plantar on interossei, apply pressure away from second ray on the medial side of the third, fourth, and fifth toes. Ask the patient to hold the toes in adduction.

P. THE LUMBRICALS

Anatomy

Origin. Flexor digitorum longus tendon.

Insertion. Pass distally on the medial sides of the lateral four toes to insert on the dorsum of their proximal phalanges through the expansions of the tendons of the extensor digitorum longus (see Fig. 1–37).

Nerve Supply
• First lumbrical—medial plantar nerve.
• Second, third, and fourth lumbricals—deep branch of the lateral plantar nerve (S_2 and S_3).

Action. Flex the metatarsophalangeal joints and extend the interphalangeal joints of the lesser toes (second through fifth).

Method of Testing of Muscle Strength

Position of Patient. Supine or sitting.

Stabilization of Limb and Resistance. With one hand hold the midfoot with the ankle and foot in neutral position, with the fingers of the other hand apply pressure against the plantar aspect of the proximal phalanx of the four lesser toes toward the direction of dorsiflexion.

Movement. Ask the patient to flex the metatarsophalangeal joints of the lesser toes, avoiding flexion of the interphalangeal joints.

Plate 1. Muscle Testing

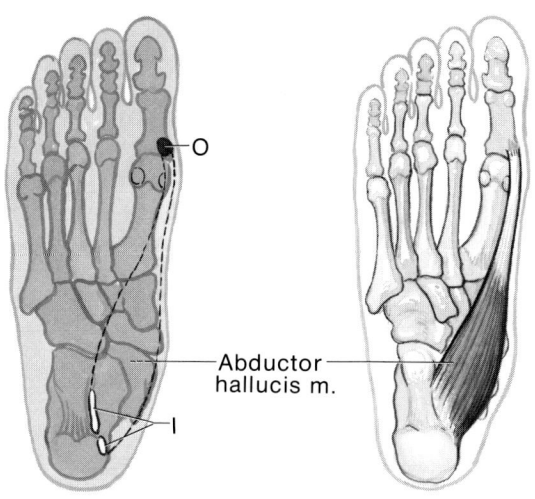

Abductor hallucis m.

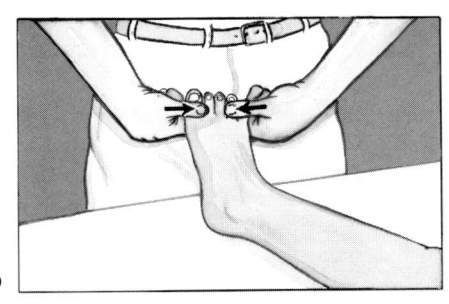

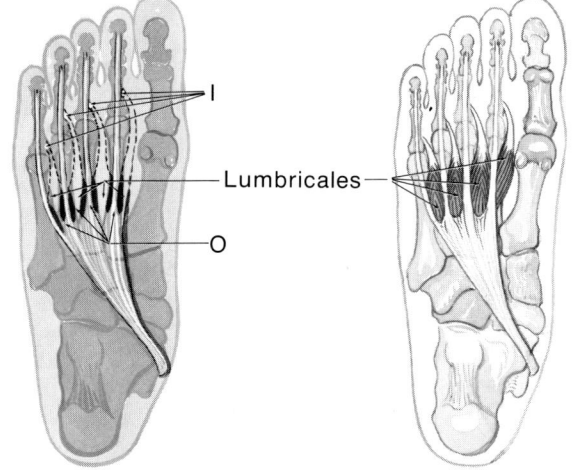

Lumbricales

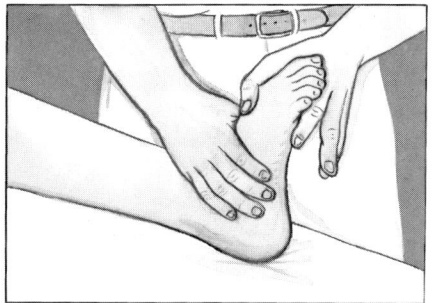

drawn contraction that passes into a continuous tetanus lasting for the entire duration of the current.

Certain disease syndromes are characterized by specific changes in the electrical reactions: in *Thomsen's disease* (myotonia congenita) and *myotonia dystrophica*, the threshold for faradic current is normal, but the contraction obtained is *persistent* and prolonged with delayed reaction. After administration of quinine, this change in the electrical reaction may decrease. In *tetany* there is increased excitability of both nerves and muscles. In *myasthenia gravis*, there is increased fatigability with gradual exhaustion on repeated stimulation. In *familial periodic paralysis* there is cadaveric response with loss of irritability to both faradic and galvanic stimulation during the period of paralysis.

In diseases of the pyramidal, extrapyramidal, or cerebellar systems, and in the paralysis of hysteria or malingering, there are no changes in the electrical reaction. Negative findings in the conditions just mentioned are helpful in differential diagnosis.

Strength-Duration Curve. The curve is obtained by plotting the current in milliamperes necessary to produce a minimal stimulus down to 0.1 msec. In the presence of degeneration, the muscle will be stimulated directly and will require more current to produce a response with pulses of shorter than normal duration. This test will give the earliest possible evidence of impending or actual denervation.

Electromyography. A concentric needle electrode inserted into muscle will pick up the action potentials generated by volitional contraction of neighboring motor units, which can then be amplified and visualized on an oscilloscope, then photographed and recorded. A normal muscle at rest shows no electrical activity, but with volitional contraction, it exhibits a series of action potentials. The muscle fibers supplied by a single anterior horn cell and nerve fiber act together, and their action potentials combine to produce the larger action potentials of the motor unit. In general, normal motor unit discharges are spikelike diphasic or triphasic waves, lasting from 5 to 10 msec. They occur at a rate of 10 to 30 per second, and at an amplitude of up to 4 millivolts. The shape, duration, amplitude, and rate of discharge vary with the choice of muscle and the intensity of volitional activity.

In children, the multiple needle punctures used in electromyography are not often well tolerated, and cooperation may be poor. Experience and rapid analysis are essential for proper interpretation of the findings. In neuromuscular disorders, several types of electrical activity are found. Electromyography is of most use in the diagnosis and prognosis of peripheral nerve lesions.

About one to two weeks after complete denervation of a muscle, spontaneous discharges occur, even at rest, a result of independent, rhythmic contractions of individual muscle fibers. These contractions, or *fibrillations,* are extremely small, have potentials of low voltage (rarely more than 50 mv.), are of short duration (less than 1 or 2 msec.), and occur at a rate of two to ten per second. Fibrillation potentials are present as long as the muscle is not completely degenerated or fibrosed, or until it becomes reinnervated. Polyphasic or complex wave forms appear when a nerve is regenerating. Electromyographic signs of nerve regeneration manifest themselves before it becomes clinically apparent.

Fasciculations, irregular polyphasic discharges, are larger than fibrillations; they are from 0.5 to 1 mv., of 8 to 12 msec. in duration, and occur involuntarily while the muscle is at rest, at a rate of 1 to 30 per minute. With *anterior horn cell degeneration,* such as that in progressive muscular atrophy, the fibrillation potentials are present, but there are also fasciculations. On voluntary muscle contraction, there are isolated motor unit action potentials, which are reduced in number but increased in amplitude. Denervation potentials are seen in poliomyelitis.

In various diseases of muscle there are certain changes in the electromyogram both at rest and on activity. In *myotonia*, immediately upon insertion of the needle electrode into the myotonic muscle, there is a rapid shower of high-frequency action potentials that may continue for a period after relaxation. The sounds emanating from the electromyographic loudspeaker have a crescendo and decrescendo quality. This shower of activity can be reproduced by tapping the electrode or by moving it further into the muscle substance. In muscular dystrophy, the action potentials are polyphasic and are of smaller amplitude and shorter than normal. In *myositis,* there may be fibrillation potentials at rest, and the potentials with voluntary contraction are often polyphasic and are decreased in amplitude and duration.

In the case of upper motor lesions, electromyography is of little assistance in diagnosis.

Nerve Conduction Velocity Determinations. Combined stimulation and recording techniques are used for the determination of motor nerve conduction time. A motor nerve is stimulated at two points, thus defining the latent period between each stimulus and the ensuing muscular contraction. The latency for the propagation of the nerve impulse between the two points stimulated is obtained by subtracting one latency from the other. The result is the nerve conduction velocity. The nerves most often tested are the peroneal, posterior tibial, median, ulnar, and facial. The average conduction time for these nerves has been determined, varying according to the age of the subject. The normal values are 45 to 65 m./sec. in children over the age of five years. At birth the motor nerve conduction velocity may be as low as 25 m./sec.; it gradually increases to 45 m./sec. by the age of three.

In diffuse peripheral neuritis, there is a slowing of conduction velocity—an important finding in differentiation of the lesions of the nerves themselves from diseases of the muscles or anterior horn cells. In locally damaged nerve segments, velocity studies are helpful in localizing the site of the lesion (e.g., as in compression of the ulnar nerve at the elbow). Successive examinations of nerve conduction velocity may give a useful quantitative estimation of the course of the disease.

References

GENERAL

1. Bick, E. M.: Source Book of Orthopedics. 2nd Ed. Baltimore, Williams & Wilkins Co., 1948.
2. Bivings, L.: A new device for footprinting and heel printing without soiling the feet. Amer. J. Dis. Child., *49*:1160, 1935.
3. Dickson, F. D., and Diveley, R. L.: Functional Disorders of the Foot: Their Diagnosis and Treatment. 2nd Ed. Philadelphia, J. B. Lippincott Co., 1944.
4. Fixsen, J. A.: The foot in childhood. *In* Klenerman, L. (ed.): The Foot and Its Disorders. Oxford, Blackwell Scientific Publications, Ltd., 1976, Chapter 4, pp. 51–80.
5. Hauser, E. D. W.: Disease of the Foot. 2nd Ed. Philadelphia, W. B. Saunders Co., 1950.
6. Hensinger, R. N., Cowel, H. R., MacEwen, G. D., Shands, A. R., and Cronis, S.: Orthopaedic screening of school age children. Review of a 10 year experience. Orthop. Rev., *4*:23, 1975.
7. Hoppenfeld, S.: Physical examination of the foot and ankle. *In* Physical Examination of the Spine and Extremities. New York, Appleton-Century-Crofts, 1976, Chapter 8, pp. 197–235.
8. Inman, V. T.: Principles of examination of the foot and ankle. *In* Inman, V. T. (ed.): Du Vries' Surgery of the Foot. St. Louis, C. V. Mosby Co., 1973, Chapter 2, pp. 23–43.
9. Kelikian, H.: Hallux Valgus, Allied Deformities of the Forefoot and Metatarsalgia. Philadelphia, W. B. Saunders Co., 1965.
10. Lake, N. C.: Examination of the foot. *In* The Foot. 3rd Ed. Baltimore, Williams & Wilkins Co., 1943, Chapter 7, pp. 106–117.
11. Lelievre, J.: L'éxamen du pied. *In* Pathologie du Pied. 2nd Ed. rev. Paris, Masson & Cie., 1961, pp. 654–657.
12. Lewin, P.: The Foot and Ankle: Their Injuries, Diseases, Deformities and Disabilities. 4th Ed. Philadelphia, Lea & Febiger, 1959.
13. Liebolt, F. L.: Foot problems in children. Surg. Gynec. Ostet., *90*:461, 1950.
14. Miller, W. R.: Observation on the examination of children's feet. J. Pediat., *51*:427, 1957.
15. Nicholson, J. T., and Qualls, D. M.: Early evaluation of musculoskeletal lesion by the pediatrician. Pediat. Clin. N. Amer., *6*:1163, 1959.
16. Nutt, J. J.: Diseases and Deformities of the Foot. New York, E. B. Treat & Co., 1925.
17. Rapp, I. H.: Foot problems of infancy and early childhood. Med. Times, *86*:272, 1958.
18. Templeton, A. W., McAlister, W. H., and Zim, I. D.: Standardization of terminology and evaluation of osseous relationships in congenitally abnormal feet. Amer. J. Roentgen., *93*:374, 1965.
19. Trendelenburg, F.: Ueber den Gang bei Angeborener Hüftgelenksluxation. Deutsch. Med. Wschr., *21*:21, 1895.
20. Zeide, M. S., and Robbins, H.: Glossary of eponyms: Orthopaedic signs, lines, and tests. Bull. Hosp. Joint Dis., *36*(2):177–206, 1975.

GAIT

21. Gowker, J. B., and Hall, C. B.: Normal human gait. *In* American Academy of Orthopedic Surgeons: Atlas of Orthotics. St. Louis, C. V. Mosby Co., 1975, p. 134.
22. Burnett, C. N., and Johnson, E. W.: Development of gait in childhood. Part I: Method. Develop. Med. Child Neurol., *13*:196, 1971.
23. Burnett, C. N., and Johnson, E. W.: Development of gait in childhood. Part II. Develop. Med. Child Neurol., *13*:207, 1971.
24. Close, J. R., Inman, V. T., Poor, P. M., and Todd, F. N.: The function of the subtalar joint. Clin. Orthop., *50*:159, 1967.
25. Elftman, H.: The transverse tarsal joint and its control. Clin. Orthop., *16*:41, 1960.
26. Hargreaves, P., and Scales, J. T.: Clinical assessment of gait using load measuring footwear. Acta Orthop. Scand., *46*:877, 1975.
27. Holt, K. S.: Facts and fallacies about neuromuscular function in crebral palsy as revealed by electromyography. Develop. Med. Child Neurol., *8*:255, 1966.
28. Inman, V. T.: Conservation of energy in ambulation. Bull. Prosthet. Res., *10*:26, Spring, 1968.
29. Jacobs, N. A., Skorecki, J., and Charnley, J.: Analysis of the vertical component of force in normal and pathological gait. J. Biomech., *5*:11, 1972.

30. Levans, A. S., Inman, V. T., and Blosser, J. A.: Transverse rotation of the segments of the lower extremity in locomotion. J. Bone Joint Surg., *30-A*:859, 1948.
31. Peizer, E., Wright, D. W., and Mason, C.: Human locomotion, Bull. Prosthet. Res., *10*:48, Fall, 1969.
32. Perry, J., and Hoffer, M. M.: Preoperative and postoperative dynamic electromyography as an aid in planning tendon transfers in children with cerebral palsy. J. Bone Joint Surg., *59-A*:531, 1977.
33. Saunders, J. B. M., Inman, V. T., and Eberhart, H. D.: The major determinants in normal and pathological gait. J. Bone Joint Surg., *35-A*:543, 1953.
34. Sheridan, M. D.: The developmental progress of infants and young children. H.M.S.O. (London) Ministry of Health Report No. 102, 1960.
35. Shirley, M.: The First Two Years. Minneapolis, University of Minnesota, Monogram Series No. 4, 1931; No. 7, 1933.
36. Smidt, G. L., and Wadsworth, J. B.: Floor reaction forces during gait: Comparison of patients with hip disease and normal subjects. Phys. Ther., *53*:1056, 1973.
37. Steindler, A.: The pathomechanics of the gait. *In* Kinesiology of the Human Body. Springfield, Ill., Charles C Thomas, 1970, Lecture 28, pp. 665–691.
38. Stott, J. R. R., Hutton, W. C., and Stokes, I. A. F.: Forces under the foot. J. Bone Joint Surg., *55-B*:335, 1973.
39. Sutherland, D. H., Olshen, R., Cooper, L., and Woo, S. L.-Y.: The development of mature gait. J. Bone Joint Surg., *62-A*:336, 1980.

DEFORMITIES

40. Ober, F. R.: The role of the iliotibial band and fascialata as factor in the causation of low-back disabilities and sciatica. J. Bone Joint Surg., *18*:105, 1936.
41. Thomas, H. O.: Diseases of the Hip, Knee, and Ankle Joints with Their Deformities Treated by a New and Efficient Method. Liverpool, J. Dobb & Co., 1875; Boston, reproduced by Little, Brown & Co., 1962.
42. Trendelenburg, F.: Ueber den Gang bei Angeborener Hüftgelenksluxation. Deutsch. Med. Wschr., *21*:21, 1895.

RANGE OF MOTION OF JOINTS

43. American Academy of Orthopedic Surgeons, Committee for the Study of Joint Motion: Method of Measuring and Recording Joint Motion. Chicago, American Academy of Orthopedic Surgeons, Publisher, 1965.
44. Cave, E. F., and Roberts, S. M.: A method for measuring and recording joint function. J. Bone Joint Surg., *18*:455, 1936.
45. Russe, O., Gerhardt, J. J., and King. P. S.: ISOM-International standard orthopedic measurements: S.F.T.R. measuring and recording method. *In* Russe, O. (ed.): An Atlas of Examination. Baltimore, Williams & Wilkins Co., 1972, pp. 45–86.
46. Salter, N.: Methods of measurement of muscle and joint function. J. Bone Joint Surg., *37-B*:474, 1955.

MOTOR POWER

47. Daniels, L., Williams, M., and Worthingham, C.: Muscle Testing: Techniques of Manual Examination. 3rd Ed. Philadelphia, W. B. Saunders Co., 1972.
48. Johnson, E. W.: Examination for muscle weakness in infants and small children. J.A.M.A., *168*:1306, 1958.
49. Johnson, M. K., Zuck, F. N., and Wingate, K.: The motor age test: Measurement of motor handicaps in children with neuromuscular disorders such as cerebral palsy. J. Bone Joint Surg., *33-A*:698, 1951.
50. Kendall, H. W., and Kendall, F. P.: Muscles: Testing and Function. 3rd Ed. Baltimore, Williams & Wilkins Co., 1983.
51. Kop, C. B.: Fine motor abilities of infants. Develop. Med. Child. Neurol, *16*:629, 1974.
52. Lovett, R. W., and Martin, E. G.: Certain aspects of infantile paralysis: with a description of a method of muscle testing. J.A.M.A., *66*:729, 1916.
53. Peterson, H. C.: Diagnosis of hypotonia in children: Types, differential diagnosis and management. Pediat. Ann., *5*(5):229, 1976.

NEUROLOGIC EVALUATION

54. Amiel-Tison, C.: A method for neurologic evaluation within the first year of life. Curr Prob. Pediat., *7*(1):2, 1976.
55. Cahuzac, M., Nichil, J., and Ousset, A.: Principes d'examen d'un infirme moteur cérébral. Rev. Chir. Orthop., *52*:375, 1966.
56. Dargassies, S. S. A.: Neurodevelopmental symptoms during the first year of life. Parts I and II. Develop. Med. Child. Neurol, *14*:235, 1972.
57. DeJong, R. N.: The Neurological Examination. 4th Ed. New York, Hoeber Medical Div., Harper & Row, 1979.
58. Denny-Brown, D.: Handbook of Neurological Examination and Case Recording. Cambridge, Mass., Harvard University Press, 1952.
59. Dohrmann, G. J., and Nowack, W. J.: The upgoing great toe. Optimal method of elicitation. Lancet, *1*(799):339, 1973.
60. Farmer, T. W.: Pediatric Neurology. 3rd Ed. New York, Hoeber Medical Div., Harper & Row, 1983.
61. Gesell, A.: How a Baby Grows. New York, Harper & Brothers, 1945.
62. Gesell, A., and Amatruda, C.: Developmental Diagnosis. New York, Paul B. Hoeber, 1947.
63. Gesell, A., et al.: The First Five Years of Life. New York, Harper & Brothers, 1940.
64. Illingworth, R. S.: The Development of the Infant and Young Child—Normal and Abnormal. 3rd Ed. Baltimore, Williams & Wilkins Co., 1966.
65. Landau, W. M., and Eliasson, S. G.: Disturbances of peripheral nerve function. *In* Eliasson, S. G. (ed.): Neurological Pathophysiology. 2nd Ed. New York, Oxford University Press, 1978.
66. McGraw, M. B.: From reflex to muscular control in the assumption of an erect posture and ambulation. Child Develop., *1–3*:291, 1930–1932.
67. McGraw, M. D. The Moro reflex. Amer. J. Dis. Child, *54*:240, 1937.
68. McGraw, M. B.: The Neuromuscular Maturation of the Human Infant. New York, Columbia University Press, 1943; reprint, New York and London, Hafner Publishing Co., Inc., 1963.
69. Milani-Comparetti, A., and Gidoni, E. A.: Routine developmental examination in normal and retarded children. Develop. Med. Child. Neurol., *9*:631, 1967.
70. Mitchell, R. G.: The Moro reflex. Cerebral Palsy Bull., *2*:135, 1960.
71. Moro, E.: Das erste Tremenon. Muench. Med. Wschr., *65*:1147, 1918.
72. Paine, R. S., and Oppe, T. E.: Neurological Examination of Children. London, Spastics Society/William Heinemann Ltd., 1966.
73. Peterson, H. C.: Neurologic examination of the young child. Pediat. Ann., *4*:8, 1975.
74. Ross, E. D., Vele-Bprras, J., and Rosman, N. P.: The significance of the Babinski sign in the newborn—A reappraisal. Pediatrics, *57*:13, 1976.
75. Shirley, M.: The First Two Years. Minneapolis, University of Minnesota, Monogram Series No. 4, 1931; No. 7, 1933.
76. Thomas, A., Chesni, Y., and Saint-Anne, D.: The Neurological Examination of the Infant. London, National Spastics Society, 1960.
77. Zausmer, E.: Evaluation of strength and motor development in infants. Phys. Ther. Rev., *33*:575, 621, 1953.
78. Zausmer, E.: The evaluation of motor development in children. J. Amer. Phys. Ther. Assoc., *44*:247, 1964.
79. Zausmer, E., and Tower, G.: A quotient for the evaluation of motor development. Phys. Ther., *46*:725, 1966.

ROENTGENOGRAPHIC AND LABORATORY DIAGNOSIS

80. Conway, J. J.: Radionuclide bone imaging in pediatrics. Pediat. Clin. N. Amer., *24*:701, 1977.

81. Curless, R. G., and Nelson, M. B.: Needle biopsies of muscle in infants for diagnosis and research. Develop. Med. Child Neurol., 17:592, 1975.
82. Gamble, F. O., and Yale, I.: Pediatric foot disorders. In Clinical Foot Roentgenology. 2nd Ed. Huntington, N.Y., R. E. Krieger, 1975, Chapter 20, pp. 289–301.
82a. Hernandez, R. J., Tachdjian, M. O., Poznanski, A. K. and Dias, L. S.: CT determination of femoral torsion. Amer. J. Roentgen., 137:97, 1981.
83. Johnson, G. F., Dorst, J. P., Kuhn, J. P., Roche, A. F., and Davial, G. H.: Reliability of skeletal age assessments. Amer. J. Roentgen., 118:320, 1973.
84. Schumacher, T. M., Genant, H. K., Korokbin, M., and Bovill, E. G.: Computed tomography: Its use in space occupying lesions of the musculoskeletal system. J. Bone Joint Surg., 60-A:600, 1978.
85. Weiner, D. S., Cook, A. J., Hoyt, W. A., Jr., and Drovec, C. E.: Computed tomography in measurement of femoral antetorsion. Orthopedics, 1:299, 1978.

ELECTRODIAGNOSTIC METHODS

86. Arieff, A. J., Dobin, N. B.., and Tigar, E. L.: Comprehensive electrodiagnosis. J.A.M.A., 181:1140, 1962.
86a. Aminoff, M.: Electrodiagnosis in Clinical Neurology. New York, Churchill Livingstone, 1980.
87. Buchthal, F., and Clemmesen, S.: On differentiation of muscle atrophy by electromyography. Acta Psychiat. Neurol., 16:143, 1941.
87a. Carr, R. E., and Siegel, I. M.: Visual Electrodiagnostic Testing: A Practical Guide for the Clinician. Baltimore, Williams & Wilkins Co., 1982.
88. Denny-Brown, D.: Interpretation of electromyogram. Arch. Neurol. Psychiat., 61:99, 1949.
89. Eaton, L. M., and Lambert, E. H.: Electromyography and electric stimulation of nerves in disease of motor unit. J.A.M.A., 163:1117, 1957.
90. Erb, W.: Handbook of Electrotherapeutics. 1883. Trans. by L. Putzel. New York, William Wood & Co., 1883.
91. Gilliatt, R. W.: Electrodiagnosis and electromyography in clinical practice. Brit. Med. J., 2:1073, 1962.
91a. Johnson, E. W. (ed.): Practical Electromyography. Baltimore, Williams & Wilkins Co., 1980.
92. Johnson, E. W., and Olsen, K. J.: Clinical value of motor nerve conduction velocity determination. J.A.M.A., 172:2030, 1960.
93. Kugelberg, E.: Electromyography in muscular dystrophies: differentiation between dystrophies and chronic lower motor neurone lesions. J. Neurol. Neurosurg. Psychiat., 12:129, 1949.
94. Licht, S. (ed.): Electrodiagnosis and Electromyography. 2nd Ed. New Haven, Elizabeth Licht, Publisher, 1961.
95. Pollock, L. J., Golseth, J. G., Mayfield, F., Arieff, A. J., and Oester, Y. T.: Electrodiagnosis of lesions of peripheral nerves in man. Arch. Neurol. Psychiat., 60:1, 1948.
96. Rosenthal, A. M.: Electrodiagnostic testing in neuromuscular disease. J.A.M.A., 177:829, 1961.
97. Thomas, P. K., Sears, T. A., and Gilliatt, R. W.: The range of conduction velocity in normal motor nerve fibres to the small muscles of the hand and foot. J. Neurol. Neurosurg. Psychiat., 22:175, 1959.
98. Wagner, A. L., and Buchthal, F.: Motor and sensory conduction in infancy and childhood. Reappraisal. Develop. Med. Child Neurol., 14:189, 1972.
99. Watkins, A. L.: An evaluation of electrodiagnostic testing. New Eng. J. Med., 259:868, 1968.
100. Wynn-Parry, C. B.: Electrodiagnosis. J. Bone Joint Surg., 43-B:222, 1961.

GROWTH OF THE NORMAL FOOT

The pattern of longitudinal growth of the foot is an important consideration in the planning of surgical procedures. Blais, Green, and Anderson have provided normal standards for the length of the growing foot (Fig. 1–78 and Table 1–4).[1] The feet of both boys and girls grow at a sharply

Table 1–4. Length of the Normal Foot*

| Girls Percentile | | | | | | Boys Percentile | | | | |
3	25	50	75	97	Age	3	25	50	75	97
10.5	11.4	12.0	12.3	12.6	1	10.9	11.6	12.0	12.2	13.1
11.6	13.0	13.6	14.0	14.7	2	11.8	12.8	13.6	14.1	15.1
13.2	14.3	14.8	15.4	16.9	3	13.2	14.4	14.9	15.8	16.8
14.0	15.4	16.0	16.4	17.8	4	14.5	15.7	16.2	17.0	17.8
15.0	16.5	17.2	17.6	18.9	5	15.4	16.8	17.2	17.9	19.2
16.1	17.8	18.3	18.9	20.4	6	16.4	17.6	18.2	18.9	20.1
16.8	18.6	19.2	20.0	21.4	7	17.3	18.5	19.2	19.9	21.3
17.3	19.2	20.0	20.7	22.4	8	18.6	19.7	20.2	20.7	22.8
18.3	20.3	20.8	21.5	23.1	9	19.2	20.4	21.1	21.6	23.5
18.9	20.9	21.7	22.4	24.2	10	19.9	21.2	21.9	22.4	24.0
19.9	21.6	22.5	23.4	25.0	11	20.4	21.8	22.6	23.3	24.8
20.6	22.3	23.2	23.9	25.7	12	21.2	22.8	23.5	24.2	25.9
20.9	22.7	23.6	24.3	26.5	13	21.8	23.3	24.2	25.1	27.0
21.4	22.8	23.8	24.5	26.4	14	22.6	24.0	25.1	26.0	27.8
21.5	22.8	23.8	24.7	26.4	15	23.3	24.7	25.7	26.7	28.3
21.4	22.8	23.8	24.7	26.7	16	23.7	25.2	25.9	26.9	28.3
21.1	22.8	23.9	24.7	26.8	17	23.9	25.2	26.1	27.0	28.3
20.8	22.8	24.0	24.7	26.7	18	23.8	25.2	26.2	27.1	28.4

*Caliper measurements in centimeters in weight-bearing position derived from semilongitudinal series of 227 girls and 285 boys.
From Blais, M. M., Green, W. T., and Anderson, M.: Lengths of the growing foot. J. Bone Joint Surg., 38-A:999, 1956. Reprinted by permission.

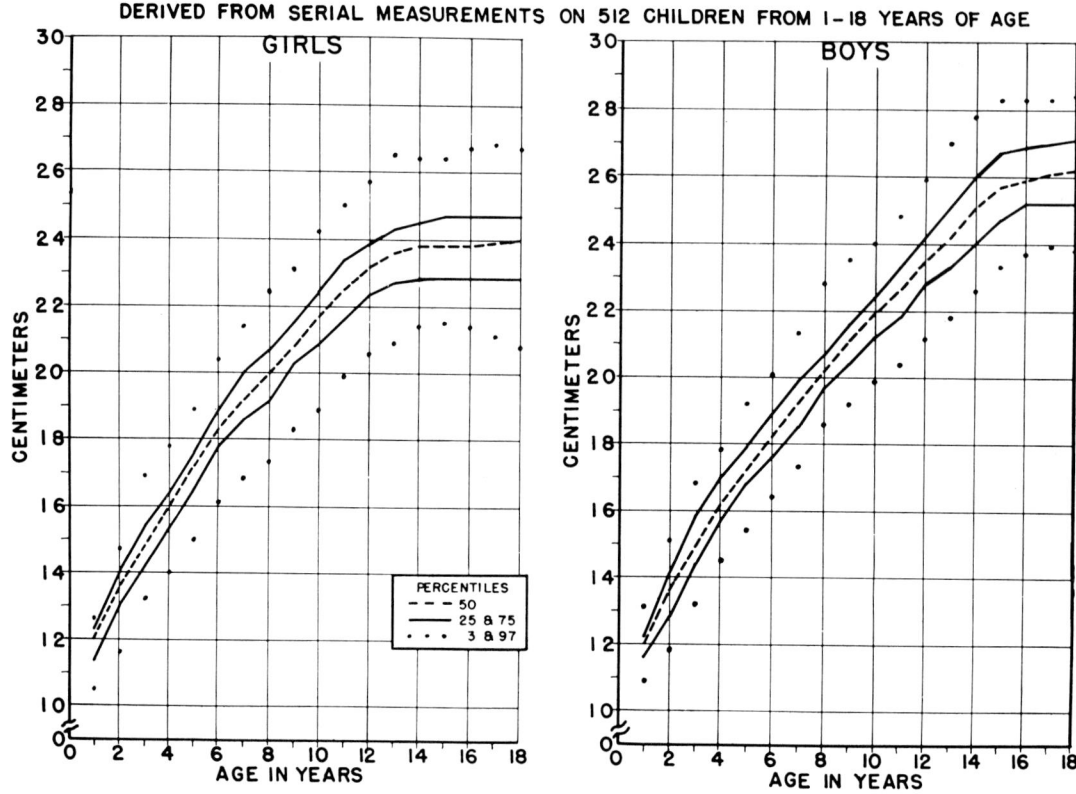

FIGURE 1–78. Length of the growing foot.

Length of normal foot derived from serial measurements of 512 children from 1 to 18 years of age. (From Blais, M. M., Green, W. T., and Anderson, M.: Lengths of the growing foot. J. Bone Joint Surg., *38–A*:998, 1956. Reprinted by permission.)

decreasing rate from infancy through the age of five years. Then from 5 to 12 years of age in girls and from 5 to 14 years of age in boys, the average increase in the length of the foot is 0.9 cm. per year. This rate of growth decreases markedly after 12 years of age in females and after 14 years of age in males, and the foot attains its mature length at the average age of 14 years in girls and 16 years in boys. Blais, Green, and Anderson also observed that at all times during the growth period, the size of the foot is relatively closer to its adult size than is the total height or the length of the femur and tibia of the same individual. For example, at the age of one year in girls and at one and one half years in boys, the foot has achieved half of its mature length. The femur and tibia, on the other hand, reach half their mature length at three years of age in girls and four years in boys. Thus, the factors that would disturb growth would affect the ultimate length of the foot proportionately less than they would the femur or the tibia. If, for example, the linear growth of the foot is completely arrested at the skeletal age of 10 years in girls or at 12 years in boys, the result would be an average reduction in adult length of the foot of only 10 per cent (about 2.5 cm.); or if at the skeletal age of 12 years in girls and 14 years in boys, of only 3 per cent (or about 1 cm.).[1]

Reference

1. Blais, M. M., Green, W. T., and Anderson, M.: Length of the growing foot. J. Bone Joint Surg., *38-A*:998, 1956.

NORMAL VARIATIONS OF THE BONES OF THE FOOT AND ANKLE

The growing tarsal and metatarsal bones are characterized by numerous variations that may simulate pathologic conditions. The orthopedic surgeon should be familiar with these normal anatomic variants in order not to misinterpret them as fractures, osteochondritis, or diseases of bone.

Accessory Bones of the Foot

Numerous accessory bones in the foot have been described. These are shown in the diagrams in Figure 1–79. In the feet of about 22 per cent of children under 16 years of age, one or more accessory bones may be found on roentgenograms.[13] The accessory navicular and os trigonum are described here in detail because of their clinical importance.

ACCESSORY TARSAL NAVICULAR

The accessory tarsal navicular (also referred to in the literature as *os tibiale externum* or *prehallux*) is present as a separate bone in about 10 per cent of human beings. It has been demonstrated to be a separate center of ossification for the tuberosity of the navicular in the fetus. In adolescence it frequently coalesces with the contiguous navicular; in about 2 per cent of the population, however, it persists as a separate ossicle. It is often bilateral, and may be bifid.

The accessory tarsal navicular is located at the medial end of the navicular. The

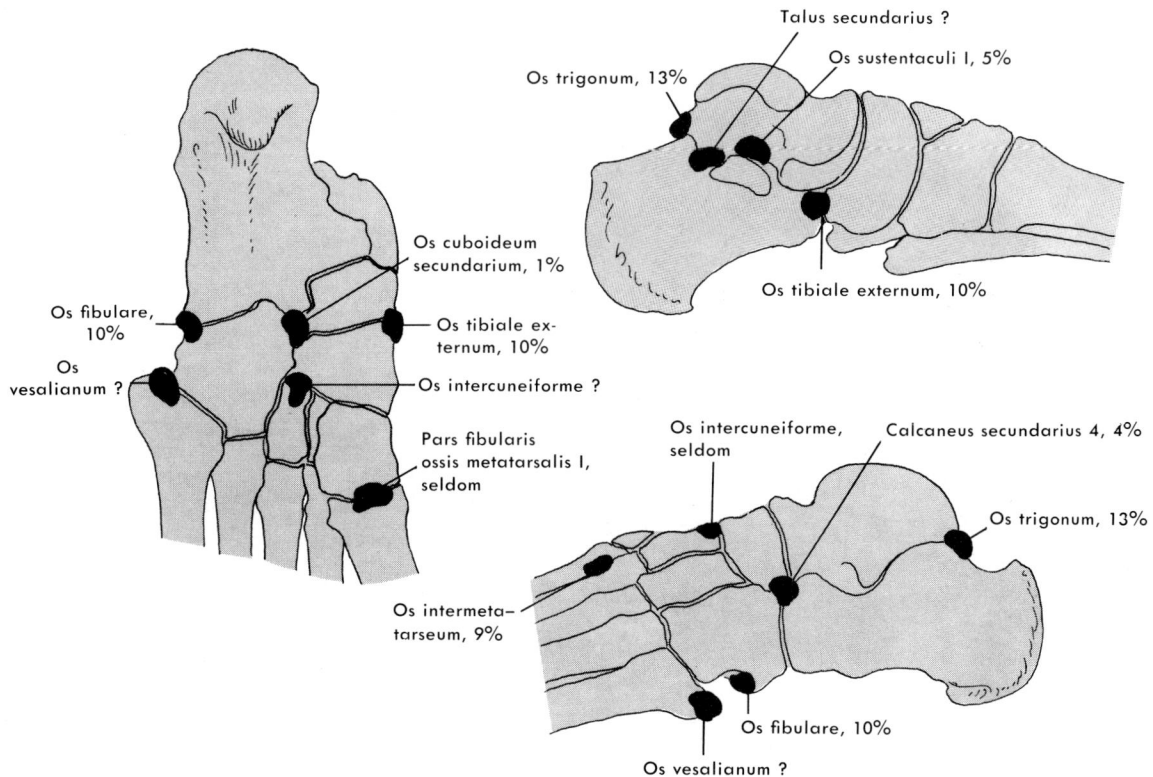

FIGURE 1–79. Accessory bones in the foot.

(Adapted from von Lanz, T., and Wachsmuth, W.: Praktische Anatomie. Berlin, Julius Springer, 1938, p. 359.)

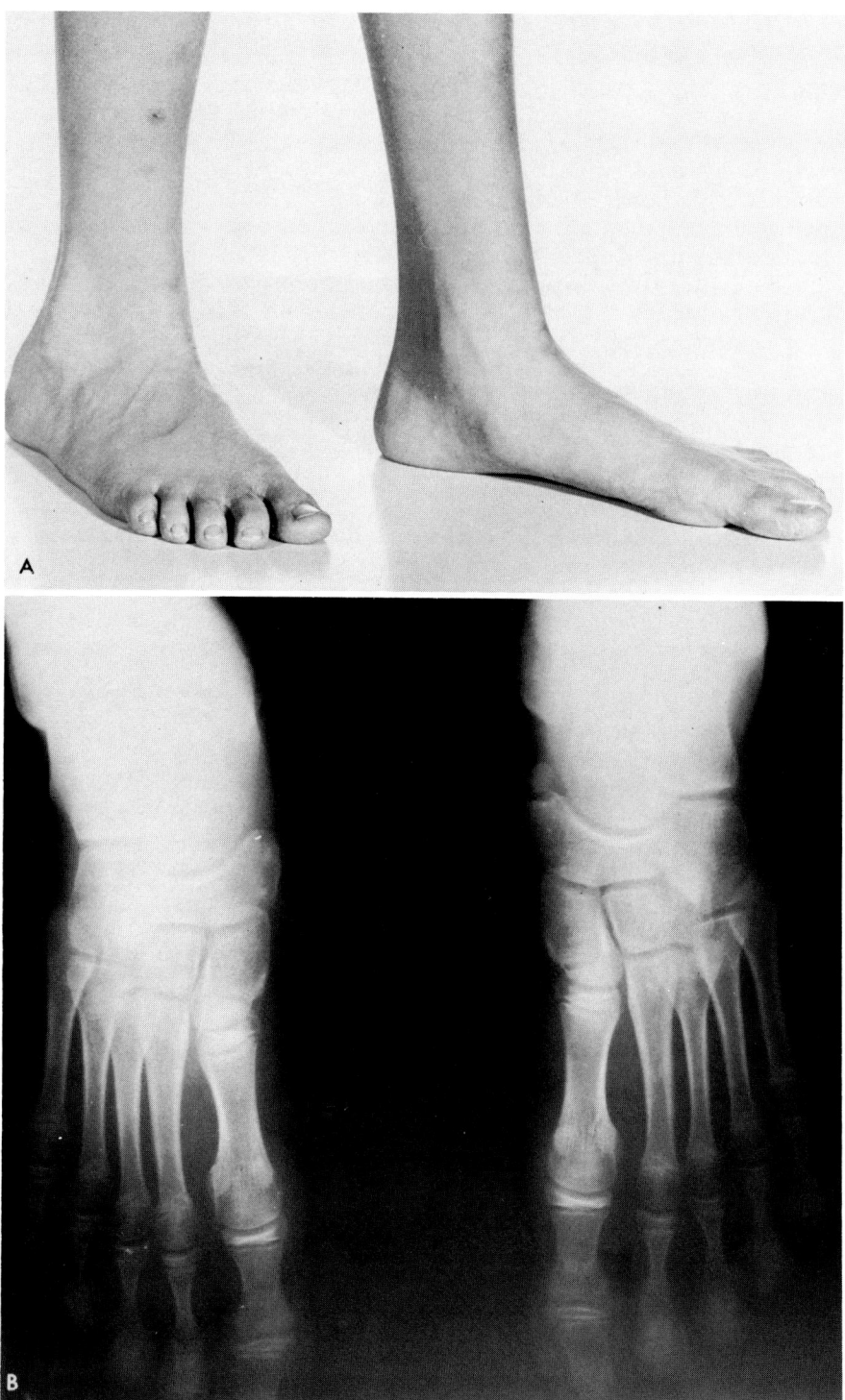

FIGURE 1–80. Accessory navicular of left foot.

A. Clinical appearance—showing the local swelling. **B.** Roentgenographic appearance. Note the smooth and rounded outline of the accessory ossicle.

posterior tibial tendon is attached to it, passing across the medial aspect of the navicular instead of underneath it. Thus, the dynamic support of the longitudinal arch of the foot normally afforded by the posterior tibial muscle is weakened. The result is planovalgus deformity of the foot. Following prolonged walking, the patient will complain of pain in the midfoot. Shoe pressure on the accessory bone may also cause the formation of an inflamed adventitious bursa with local swelling and tenderness (Fig. 1–80A). There may be associated nonspecific tenosynovitis of the posterior tibial tendon.

In the roentgenograms, the accessory bone will be visible medially and proximal to the navicular bone (Fig. 1–80B). Its smooth and rounded outline differentiates it from the irregular margin that characterizes a fracture. In later adolescence, the accessory navicular may fuse with the body of the tarsal bone and present as an abnormally prominent and curved medial end of the navicular (Fig. 1–81). This is referred to as a *cornuted navicular* and produces the same symptoms as the accessory navicular.

Initially, treatment should be conservative. A ⅜-inch felt longitudinal arch support is placed in the shoe. When pain is acute, hydrocortisone may be injected into the adventitious bursa and the inflamed posterior tibial tendon sheath, and the foot immobilized in a below-knee walking plaster cast for a period of three weeks.

If symptoms persist and do not respond to these measures, surgical excision of the accessory navicular with rerouting of the posterior tibial tendon to a point well on the plantar aspect of the navicular (Kidner procedure) is performed.[25, 26]

In the Kidner operation the incision is approximately 5 cm. long and begins 1 cm. inferior and 2 cm. distal to the distal tip of the medial malleolus and extends forward to the base of the first metatarsal bone. The subcutaneous tissue and deep fascia are divided, and the wound margins are retracted to expose the posterior tibial tendon and the medial tip of the navicular bone. The posterior tibial tendon inserts into the tuberosity of the navicular bone, into the plantar surfaces of the three cuneiform bones and of the bases of the second, third, and fourth metatarsal bones, and into the cuboid bone. It is detached only from its insertion to the accessory navicular, its other attachments being left intact.

The accessory navicular bone is excised and the medial surface of the navicular is resected until it is flush with the talus and cuneiform. Bleeding cancellous bone is coagulated with electrocautery. The posterior tibial tendon is transferred laterally and plantarward on the under surface of the navicular, where it is anchored under tension to the periosteum and plantar ligaments with two or three interrupted sutures. Usually it is not necessary to make drill holes through the navicular. The wound is closed, and a below-knee walking cast is applied.

The cast is removed in three to four weeks, following which a longitudinal arch support is used. The result of the Kidner procedure is good. Pain will subside. One should not, however, expect correction of pes planovalgus deformity in the adolescent.

OS TRIGONUM

On the posterior aspect of the talus there is a groove for the flexor hallucis longus tendon. The bony tubercle lateral to this tendon groove is usually larger than the

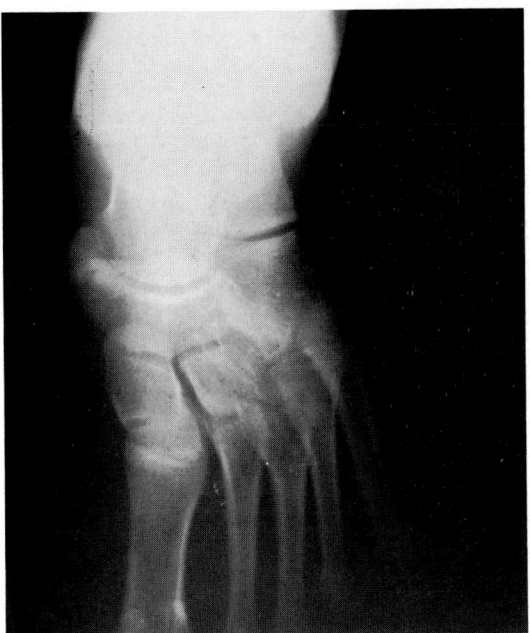

FIGURE 1–81. Accessory navicular fused with the body of the tarsal navicular (cornuted navicular).

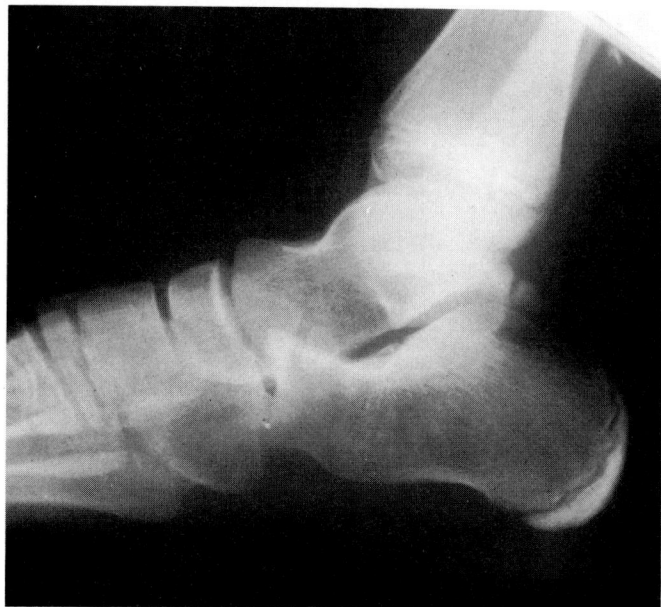

FIGURE 1–82. Os trigonum in a 12-year-old child.

Note also the accessory navicular visible in the lateral projection. The sclerosis of the apophysis of the os calcis is normal.

medial one, and if elongated, it is known as "Stieda's process." Between 8 and 11 years of age, separate centers of ossification appear for the medial and lateral tubercles, and they quickly (usually within a year) fuse with the main body of the talus. The posterior fibers of the lateral ligament of the ankle joint are attached to the lateral tubercle. When the ankle is in full plantar flexion the posterior tubercles of the talus come in full contact with the posterior edge of the distal end of the tibia, serving as a bony block. Repeated minor injury in an active person may cause failure of union of the posterolateral tubercle, which then persists as a separate center of ossification known as *os trigonum* (Fig. 1–82). A fused but large ossicle may be detached by sudden violence, particularly when union of the ossicle to the talus is by synchondrosis (Fig. 1–83). The absence of irregularity between the os trigonum and the main body of the talus distinguishes synchondrosis from a fracture. In doubtful cases, an air arthrogram will settle the diagnosis (Fig. 1–84).[6]

MISCELLANEOUS ACCESSORY BONES

Only a brief listing of the accessory bones and normal anatomic variations of the foot and ankle is given here; for a detailed description the reader should consult the comprehensive reviews of Caffey, O'Rahilly, Trolle, and other cited references.[2, 7, 13, 16]

Medial Malleolus. This may have a separate ossification center (Fig. 1–85). In the literature, the reports of its incidence vary. Selby found it in 47 per cent of girls and 17 per cent of boys, whereas Powell reports 20 per cent.[8, 12] The average age of appearance of a separate center of ossification for the medial malleolus is 7.6 years for girls and 8.7 years for boys; by the twelfth year,

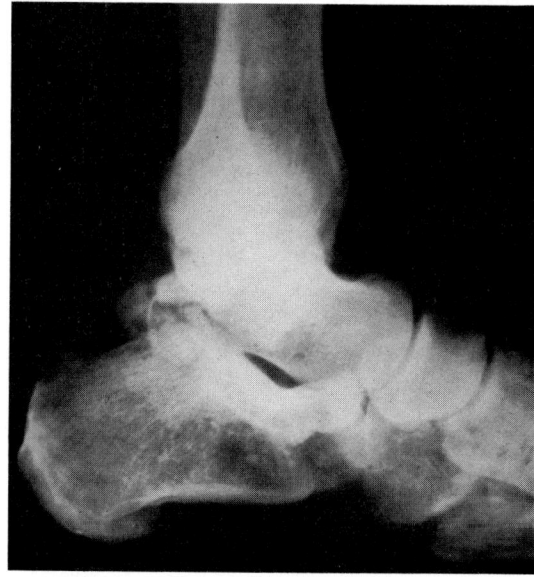

FIGURE 1–83. Fracture of fused os trigonum.

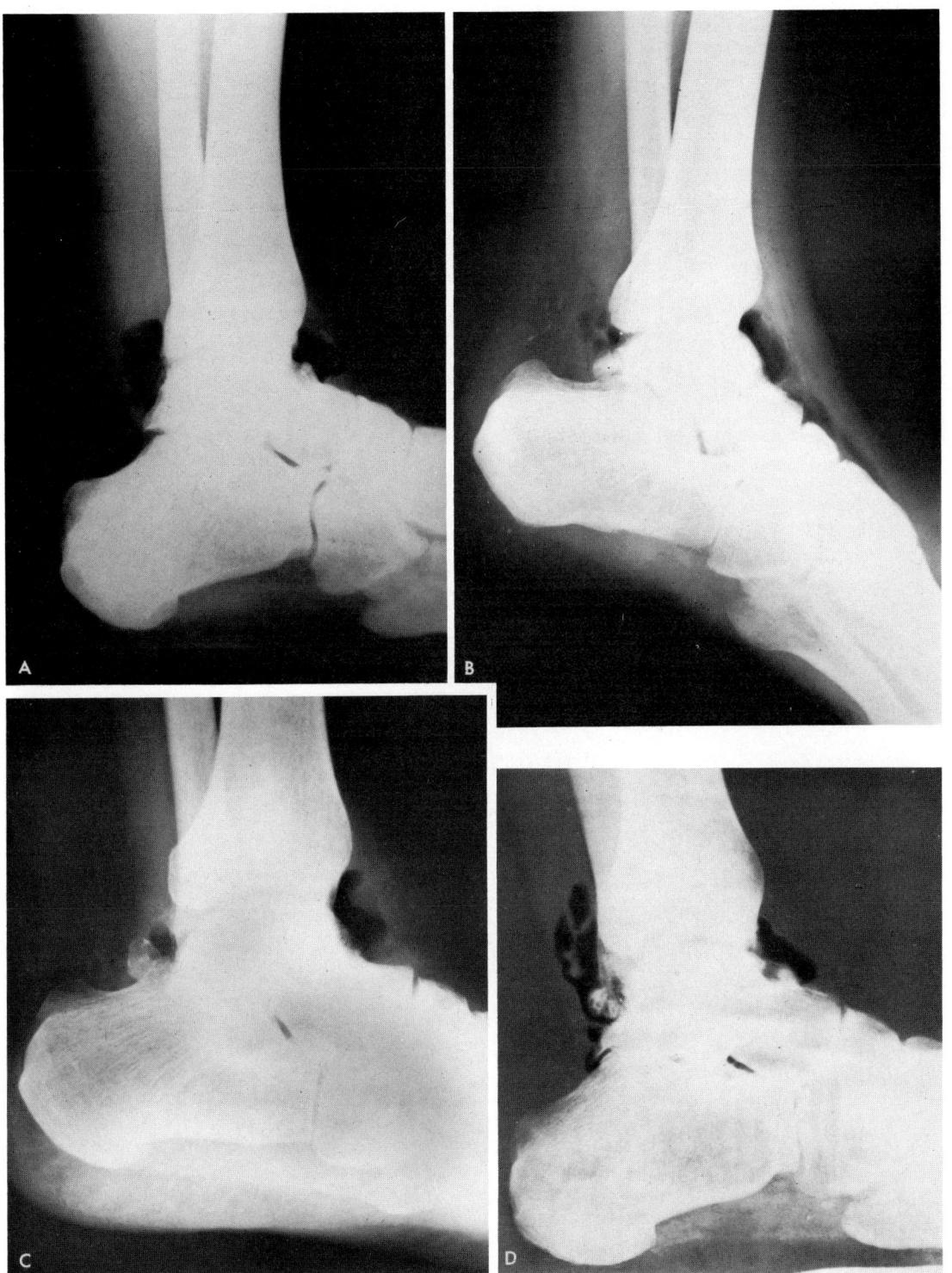

FIGURE 1–84. Arthrogram of the ankle.

A. A normal ankle. **B.** An ankle with os trigonum. Note the radiolucent shadow cast by the air is located superior to the os trigonum. **C.** In a fracture of a fused os trigonum, the air has sandwiched itself between the detached accessory bone and the main body of the talus. **D.** In an osteocartilaginous loose body of the ankle the air shadow surrounds the loose bone. (Courtesy of Dr. H. Kelikian.)

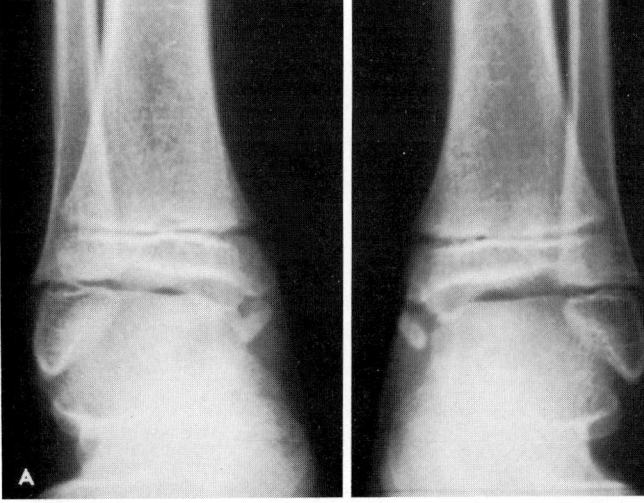

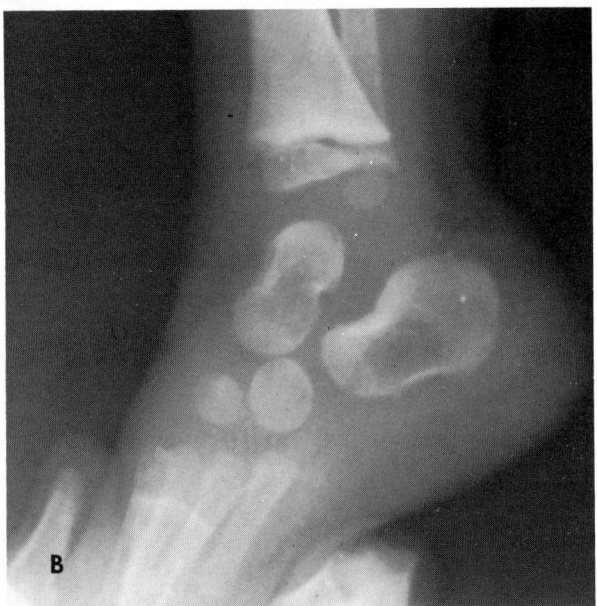

FIGURE 1–85. Normal anatomic variations of the foot and ankle.

A. Accessory ossification center of medial malleolus. **B.** Area of rarefaction in body of os calcis simulating cyst.

the extra center of ossification fuses with the main center.

Distal End of Fibula. The lateral malleolus has a separate center of ossification in 1 per cent of cases. A small accessory ossicle is occasionally present in a notch in the distal fibular metaphysis and should not be mistaken for osteochondritis dissecans; also on oblique views of the lateral malleolus, an area of rarefaction in the medial surface of the distal fibular epiphysis should not be misdiagnosed as a destructive bone lesion.

Talus. In addition to os trigonum, an accessory bone may develop on the dorsal aspect of the head of the talus (os sustentaculare). A separate center of ossification for the head of the talus is a very rare anomaly. *Alfricoid talus* is a developmental anomaly in which the head and neck of the talus are tilted dorsally (Fig. 1–86).

Os Calcis. A triangular or circular area of radiolucency may appear in the inferior half of the body of the calcaneus, suggesting a pseudocyst (Fig. 1–85B). It is a normal variation and not a deficiency of spongy bone, occurring in about 10 per cent of children older than seven years.

The enlarged trochlea of the calcaneus may be mistaken for an exostosis.

The apophysis of the os calcis begins to ossify at four to six years of age in the female and at four to nine years in the male. Often a secondary center of ossification in the calcaneal apophysis develops in

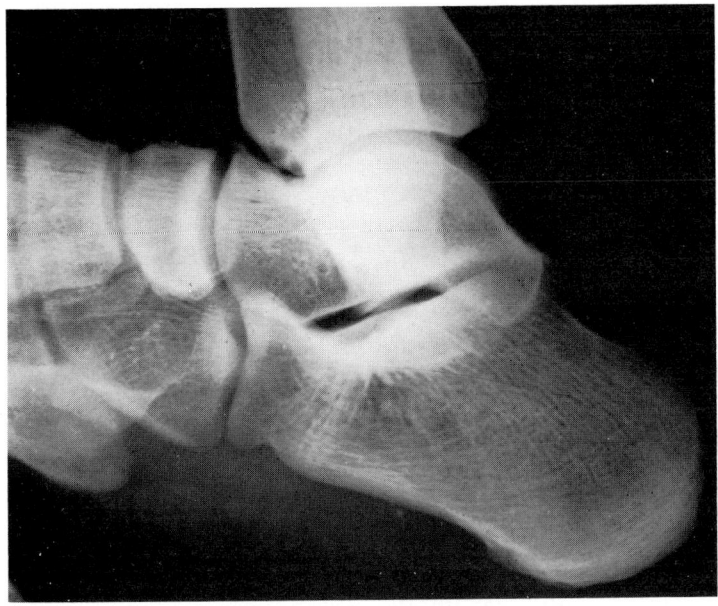

FIGURE 1–86. Africoid talus.

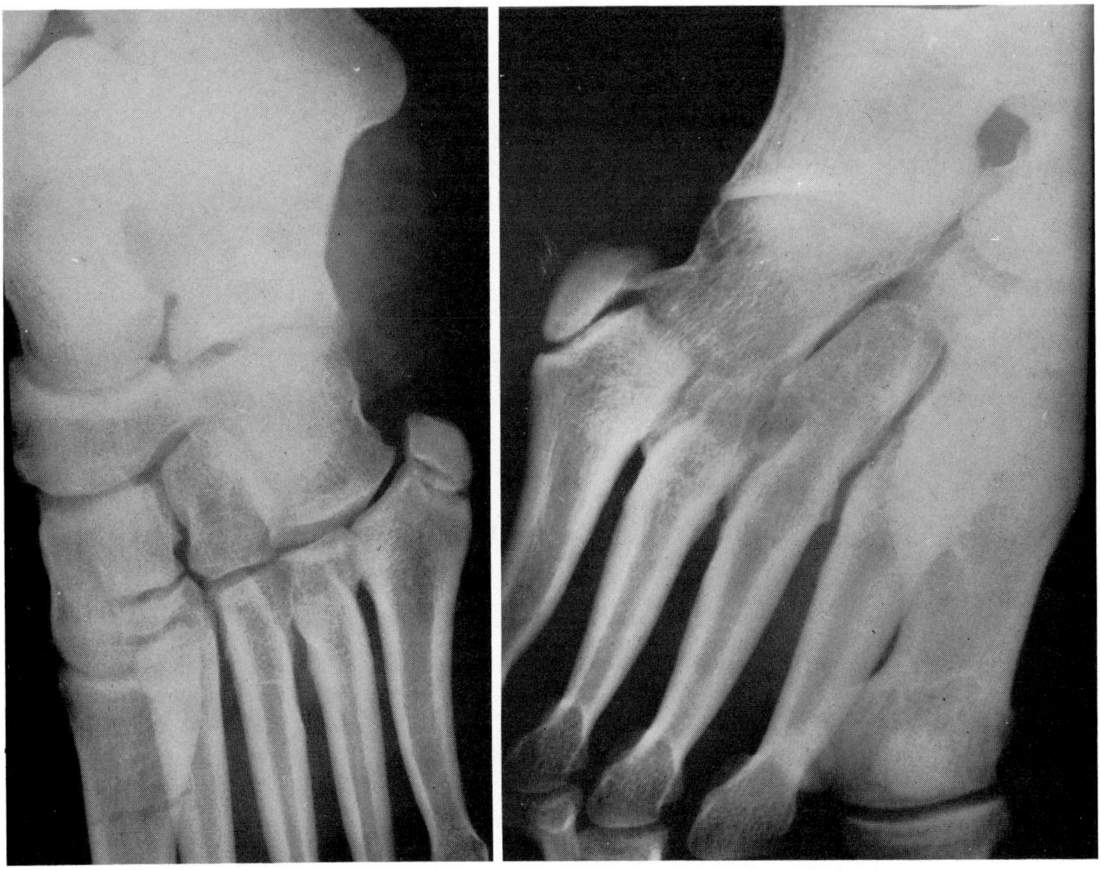

FIGURE 1–87. Accessory ossicle at the base of the fifth metatarsal (os vesalianum).

girls between 10½ and 12 years and in boys between 11½ and 13½ years; it quickly fuses with the body of the calcaneus. A secondary center of ossification may also be present in the tip of the trochlear process on the lateral wall of the calcaneus. Occasionally the body of the calcaneus may ossify from two centers of ossification instead of one, the cartilaginous junction between the two ossific nuclei suggesting a fracture. Sclerosis and fragmentation of the apophysis of the calcaneus are common (see Fig. 1–82).

Cuboid, Navicular, Cuneiforms. Multiple fine ossification centers may be present in the cuboid. In addition to an accessory navicular there may be a small ossicle on the dorsum of the navicular—os supranaviculare. The edges of the cuneiforms may be irregular.

Metatarsals. An accessory ossicle at the base of the fifth metatarsal is quite common (Fig. 1–87); occasionally it may have a fish-scale appearance, simulating a fracture. The distal end of the first metatarsal may have an incomplete synchondrosis.

Phalanges. The skeletal variations of the digits of the foot are numerous. The reader is referred to the statistical study of Venning.[17]

In the hallux the number of phalanges is almost always two, though occasionally a three-phalangeal big toe may be encountered. The lesser toes usually have three phalanges. Not infrequently the fifth toe may have two phalanges, and occasionally the second, third, and fourth toes may have a two-phalangeal form. With the exception of the big toe, toes with two phalanges are nearly always lateral to the toes having three phalanges. The two-phalangeal lesser toes are more preponderant in the female.

The middle phalanx may lack an epiphysis or may be entirely absent. The ossification centers of the epiphyses of the phalanges, particularly the proximal phalanx, may be cone-shaped, invaginating into the diaphysis. Fissuring of the epiphyses of the proximal phalanx of the hallux is another variation. The sesamoid may be bipartite and have to be distinguished from fracture.

References

1. Bjornson, R. G. B.: Developmental anomaly of the lateral malleolus simulating fracture. J. Bone Joint Surg., 38-A:128, 1956.
2. Caffey, J.: Pediatric X-Ray Diagnosis. 5th Ed. Chicago, Year Book Medical Publishers, Inc., 1967, p. 744.
3. Gottlieb, C., and Berenbaum, S. L.: Pirie's bone, accessory ossicle on the dorsum of the astragalus—often bilateral. Radiology, 55:423, 1950.
4. Harding, V. V.: Time schedule for the appearance and fusion of a secondary center of ossification of the calcaneus. Child Develop. 23:181, 1952.
5. Hubay, C. A.: Sesamoid bones of the hands and feet. Amer. J. Roentgen., 61:493, 1949.
6. McDougall, A.: The os trigonum. J. Bone Joint Surg., 37-B:257, 1955.
7. O'Rahilly, R.: A survey of carpal and tarsal anomalies. J. Bone Joint Surg., 35-B:254, 1953.
8. Powell, H. D. W.: Extra centre of ossification for the medial malleolus in children. Incidence and significance. J. Bone Joint Surg., 43-B:107, 1961.
9. Roche, A. F., and Sunderland, S.: Multiple ossification centers in the epiphyses of the long bones of the human hand and foot. J. Bone Joint Surg., 41-B:375, 1959.
10. Ross, S. E., and Caffey, J.: Ossification of the calcaneal apophysis in healthy children: Some normal radiologic features. Stanford Med. Bull., 15:224, 1957.
11. Schlüter, K.: Der "Calcaneus bifidus," eine Ossifikationsanomalie des Fersenbeines im Hackenplattfuss. Fortschr. Roentgenstr., 85:720, 1956.
12. Selby, S.: Separate centers of ossification of the tip of the internal malleolus. Amer. J. Roentgen., 86:496, 1961.
13. Shands, A. R., Jr.: The accessory bones of the foot. Southern Med. Surg., 93:326, 1931.
14. Shands, A. R., Jr., and Wentz, I. J.: Congenital anomalies, accessory bones, and osteochondritis in the feet of 850 children. Surg. Clin. N. Amer., 33:1643, 1953.
15. Sirry, A.: The pseudocystic triangle in the normal os calcis. Acta Radiol., 36:516, 1951.
16. Trolle, D.: Accessory Bones of the Human Foot. Copenhagen, Munksgaard, 1948.
17. Venning, P.: Variation of the digital skeleton of the foot. Clin. Orthop., 16:26, 1960.

ACCESSORY TARSAL NAVICULAR

18. Bautrier: Cited by Meyer, M., Cuny, J., and Trensz, F.: L'os tibial externe et ses divers aspects radiologiques. Strasbourg Med., 85:24, 1927.
19. Dwight, T.: Variations of the Bones of the Hands and Feet. Philadelphia, J. B. Lippincott, Co., 1907.
20. Faber, A.: Os tibiale externum bein erbgleichen Zwillingen. Erbartz, 4:83, 1934.
21. Féré, C. H., and Deniker, M.: Note sur des exostosis symétriques des scaphoides tarsiens. Rev. Chir., 29:544, 1904.
22. Francillon, M. R.: Untersuchungen zur anatomischen und klinischen Bedeutung des Os tibiale externum. Z. Orthop. Chir., 56:61, 1932.
23. Geist, E.S.: The accessory scaphoid bone. J. Bone Joint Surg., 7:570, 1925.
24. Hohmann, G.: Fuss und Bein. 5th Aufl. Munchen, J. F. Bergmann, 1951.
25. Kidner, F. C.: The prehallux (accessory scaphoid) in its relation to flatfoot. J. Bone Joint Surg., 11:831, 1929.
26. Kidner, F. C.: The prehallux in relation to flatfoot. J.A.M.A., 101:1539, 1933.
27. Kienböck, R., and Müller, W.: Os tibiale externum und Verletzung des Fusses. Z. Orthop. Chir., 66:257, 1937.
28. Marti, T.: Kasuistischer Beitrag zum Studium des Os tibiale externum. Praxis, 51:828, 1962.
29. Meyer, M., Cuny, J., and Trensz, F.: L'os tibial externe et ses divers aspects radiologiques. Strasbourg Med., 85:24, 1927.
30. Monahan, J. J.: The human pre-hallux. Amer. J. Med. Sci., 160:708, 1920.
31. Niederecker, K.: Der Plattfuss. Stuttgart, Ferdinand Enke, 1959.
32. Pfitzner, W.: Beiträge zur Kenntnis des menschlichen Extremitätenskeletts. VII. Die Variationen im Aufbau des Fuffskeletts. Schwalbe's Morph. Arb., 6:245, 1896.
33. Trolle, D.: Accessory Bones of the Human Foot. Copenhagen, Munksgaard, 1948.
34. Zadek, I.: The significance of the accessory tarsal scaphoid. J. Bone Joint Surg., 8:618, 1926.
35. Zadek, I., and Gold, A. M.: The accessory tarsal scaphoid. J. Bone Joint Surg., 30-A:957, 1948.

2. Congenital Deformities

POSTURAL DEFORMITIES OF THE FOOT AND LEG
  Talipes Calcaneovalgus
  Talipes Varus
  Postural Talipes Valgus
  Postural Metatarsus Adductus
  Postural Clubfoot

CONGENITAL TALIPES EQUINOVARUS

CONGENITAL CONVEX PES VALGUS

TARSAL COALITION

CONGENITAL METATARSUS VARUS

CONGENITAL METATARSUS PRIMUS VARUS AND HALLUX VALGUS

CONGENITAL BALL-AND-SOCKET ANKLE JOINT

BRACHYMETATARSIA (CONGENITAL SHORT METATARSAL)

CONGENITAL SPLIT OR CLEFT FOOT (LOBSTER CLAW)

POLYDACTYLISM

CONGENITAL HALLUX VARUS

MACRODACTYLISM

MISCELLANEOUS DEFORMITIES OF TOES
  Microdactylism
  Syndactylism
  Divergent or Convergent Toes
  Congenital Digitus Minimus Varus
  Hallux Valgus Interphalangeus
  Congenital Curly (or Varus) Toe

POSTURAL DEFORMITIES OF THE FOOT AND LEG

Confinement of the human fetus in unnatural positions in the uterus may cause a number of postural deformities of the limbs and trunk. In the foot and leg, intrauterine malpostural deformities are talipes calcaneovalgus, talipes varus, talipes valgus, metarsus adductus, and postural clubfoot. Other common sequelae of intrauterine malposture are: in the knee, extension contracture; in the hip, congenital pelvic obliquity with abduction contracture of one

Table 2–1. *Distinguishing Characteristics of Congenital Malformations and Congenital Postural Deformities*

	Malformation	Postural Deformation
Period of development	Embryonic—during organogenesis (teratologic embryopathy)	Postembryonic—after normal formation of the parts (nonteratologic fetopathy)
Incidence at birth	3.6 per cent*	2.0 per cent*
Structural alterations	Common	Very rare
Response to passive manipulation	Not correctable	Correctable
Spontaneous correction	No	Usual

*Data from Dunn, P. M.: Congenital postural deformities: Perinatal associations. Proc. Roy Soc. Med., 65:735, 1972.

hip and adduction contracture of the contralateral hip; in the spine, infantile scoliosis; and in the head and neck, torticollis and plagiocephaly.

Postural deformities are nonteratologic fetopathies, arising in the postembryonic period after organogenesis; they are the result of deformation of a normally formed part. In contrast, malformations are defects that arise during the period of organogenesis—i.e., they are teratologic embryopathies. The distinguishing features of the two groups are shown in Table 2–1.

Historically Hippocrates proposed a causal relation between postural deformations of the limbs and mechanical forces acting in utero.[8] Browne, Chapple and Davidson, and Dunn have studied the problem in detail.[1-5] Malposition may exist only during a particular phase of development of the limbs, i.e., it may be temporal in addition to being spatial.

The incidence of postural deformations has been investigated by Dunn.[3-5] Of 4,754 infants born in the Birmingham Maternity Hospital, 4,486 (94.4 per cent) were normally formed, 170 (3.6 per cent) were malformed (with or without additional deformities), and 98 (2.0 per cent) had postural deformations. Multiple deformities (two or more) were found in 33 per cent of the cases; there was a total of 151 distinct deformations among the 98 infants. These figures indicate that various postural deformities have a common mechanical origin. Dunn also demonstrated a highly significant clinical association between main groups of postural deformities (Table 2–2).

Normal human fetal posture is dependent upon the sequential development of

Table 2–2. *Clinical Association Between Certain Postural Deformations. Statistical Analysis**

	Facial Deformities	Plagiocephaly	Mandibular Asymmetry	Sternomastoid Contracture	Scoliosis (Postural)	Congenital Dislocation of Hip	Talipes
Facial deformities	—	S	S+	S	S+	S+	S+
Plagiocephaly	S	—	S+	S+	S+	S+	N
Mandibular asymmetry	S+	S+	—	S+	N	S+	S+
Sternomastoid contracture	S	S+	S+	—	S+	N	S+
Scoliosis (postural)	S+	S+	N	S+	—	S+	S
Congenital dislocation of hip	S+	S+	S+	N	S+	—	S+
Talipes	S+	N	S+	S+	S	S+	—

N, not significant. S, $P < 0.05$. S+, $P < 0.001$.

*From Dunn, P. M.: Congenital postural deformities. Perinatal associations. Proc. Roy. Soc. Med., 65:736, 1972. Reprinted by permission.

neuromuscular function. The structural development of the central and peripheral nervous systems proceeds in a craniocaudal direction. Consequently, coordinated muscular contractions appear first in the head and neck, then in the upper limbs, the trunk, and the lower limbs. With activation of different muscle groups the limbs assume different postures. In the human the structural development of the lower limb is usually complete by the end of the eighth week of intrauterine life. With the anatomic level of innervation of muscle groups beginning proximally and proceeding distally, the sequential postures of the lower limbs are as follows: first, hip flexion and medial rotation (L_1–L_2 level of innervation of iliopsoas muscle); second, hip adduction (L_2–L_3 level of innervation of hip adductors); and third, knee extension (L_3–L_4 level of innervation of quadriceps femoris muscle). Therefore, the posture of the lower limbs of the human fetus at the twelfth week of gestation is one of hip flexion–medial rotation–adduction and knee extension (Fig. 2–1A). This extended breech posture is normal at this stage of development.

The next stage of development of posture in the human fetus is folding of the extended lower limbs as sustained contraction of the short lateral rotators of the hip (level of innervation L_4, L_5, S_1) is activated and the whole lower limb rotates laterally and the patellae face outward (Fig. 2–1B). Then the knees flex with activation and sustained contraction of the hamstrings (level of innervation L_5, S_1, S_2). Folding of the lower limbs makes room for trunk flexion to take place, which always precedes cephalic version. The activation of the gluteus maximus (L_5, S_1, and S_2) brings the hips into further lateral rotation. Activity of the peroneals, toe extensors, and anterior tibial muscles (L_4, L_5, and S_1) will make the foot assume a dorsiflexed and everted posture; finally, the foot will be drawn into plantar flexion and inversion with activity of the triceps surae and posterior tibial muscles (L_5, S_1, and S_2). Leg folding takes place between 12 and 26 weeks, and vertex posture develops between 26 and 40 weeks of intrauterine life (Fig. 2–1C).

Arrest of development will cause failure of leg folding, which in turn will prevent spinal flexion and cephalic version from taking place. Arrest of lateral rotation of

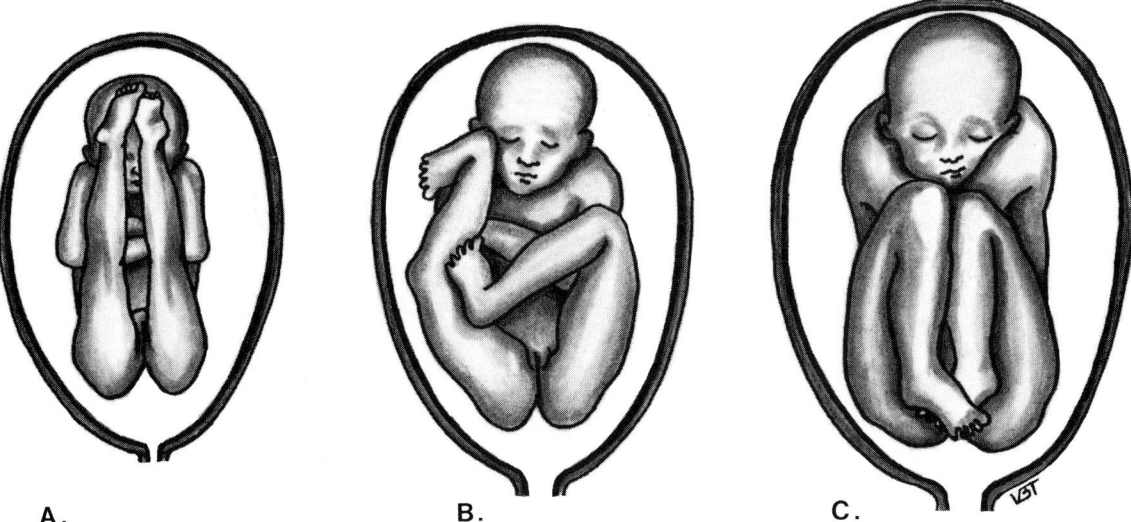

FIGURE 2–1. Development of intrauterine posture.

A. Stage I, extended breech posture. Note the hips are flexed, medially rotated, and adducted, and the knees extended. This is the normal position of the lower limbs in the 8- to 12-week-old human fetus. **B.** Stage II, leg-folding posture. Note the hips are laterally rotated and the knees flexed. Folding of the leg allows trunk flexion to take place, which always precedes cephalic version. The feet are dorsiflexed and everted. This is normal posture for a 12- to 26-week-old fetus. **C.** Stage III, vertex posture. Note the spine is flexed. The ankles and feet are in plantar flexion and inversion. This posture develops between 26 and 40 weeks. (Redrawn from Wilkinson, J. A.: Breech malposition and intrauterine malposition. Proc. Roy. Soc. Med., 59:1107, 1966.)

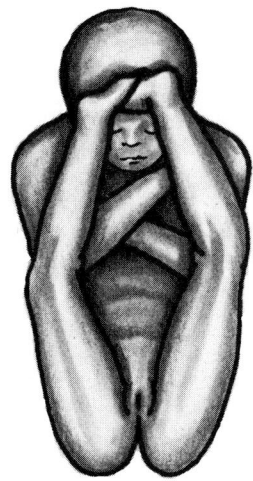

FIGURE 2–2. *Neonatal medial rotation breech malposture.*

Note the hips are flexed and medially rotated, and the knees are extended. (Redrawn from Wilkinson, J. A.: Breech malposition and intrauterine malposition. Proc. Roy. Soc. Med., 59:1107, 1966.)

the hip and flexion of the knee will produce a persistent intrauterine posture in which the hips are flexed and medially rotated and the knees extended (Fig. 2–2). If lateral rotation of the hip takes place but knee flexion is arrested, the hips are locked in flexion and lateral rotation, and the knees

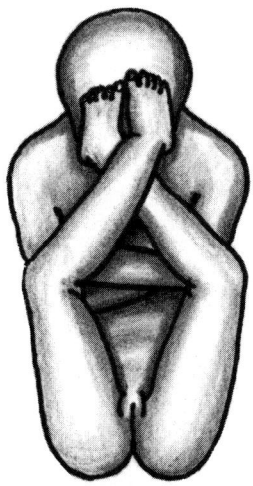

FIGURE 2–3. *Neonatal lateral rotation breech malposture.*

The hips are flexed and laterally rotated, and the knees are in extension. (Redrawn from Wilkinson, J. A.: Breech malposition and intrauterine malposition. Proc. Roy. Soc. Med., 59:1107, 1966.)

in extension (Fig. 2–3). These postures, if present beyond the twenty-eighth week of intrauterine life, constitute breech malposition.

In a survey of 4,000 roentgenograms of the pelves of pregnant women, Vartan found that breech presentation is common and should be considered normal at the appropriate period of development. The breech posture of about 25 per cent of the fetuses persisted at the thirtieth week. Cephalic version did not take place in those with knees completely extended and hips medially rotated, whereas those with semiflexed knees and laterally rotated hips did undergo cephalic version.[13]

Talipes Calcaneovalgus

This postural deformity is characterized by the dorsiflexion and eversion of the entire foot. The soft tissues on the dorsum and lateral aspect of the foot are contracted and limit plantar flexion and inversion (Fig. 2–4). The degree of severity of deformity varies; in severe cases the foot may touch the anterior aspect of the tibia (Fig. 2–5). Roentgenograms of the foot and ankle are normal. There is no subluxation or dislocation of the tarsal joints and no secondary adaptive bone changes or hypoplasia of the ossification centers.

Talipes calcaneovalgus is the most common deformity of the foot seen at birth. Wetzenstein states that the incidence varies between 30 and 50 per cent.[14] Wynne-Davies, in her family studies, found it to be approximately one per thousand live births. It may be higher, however, as some cases may go unnoticed or ignored.[16] Talipes calcaneovalgus is more common in girls than in boys, with a male-to-female ratio of 0.61 to 1. Its incidence is significantly greater among first-born children and children of young mothers. The probable cause is intrauterine malposture—the environmental factor being compression acting late in pregnancy, particularly in the primigravida with a small "tight" uterus and strong abdominal muscles.

It is important to distinguish talipes calcaneovalgus from congenital convex pes planovalgus. In the latter, the talocalcaneonavicular joint is dislocated dorsolaterally;

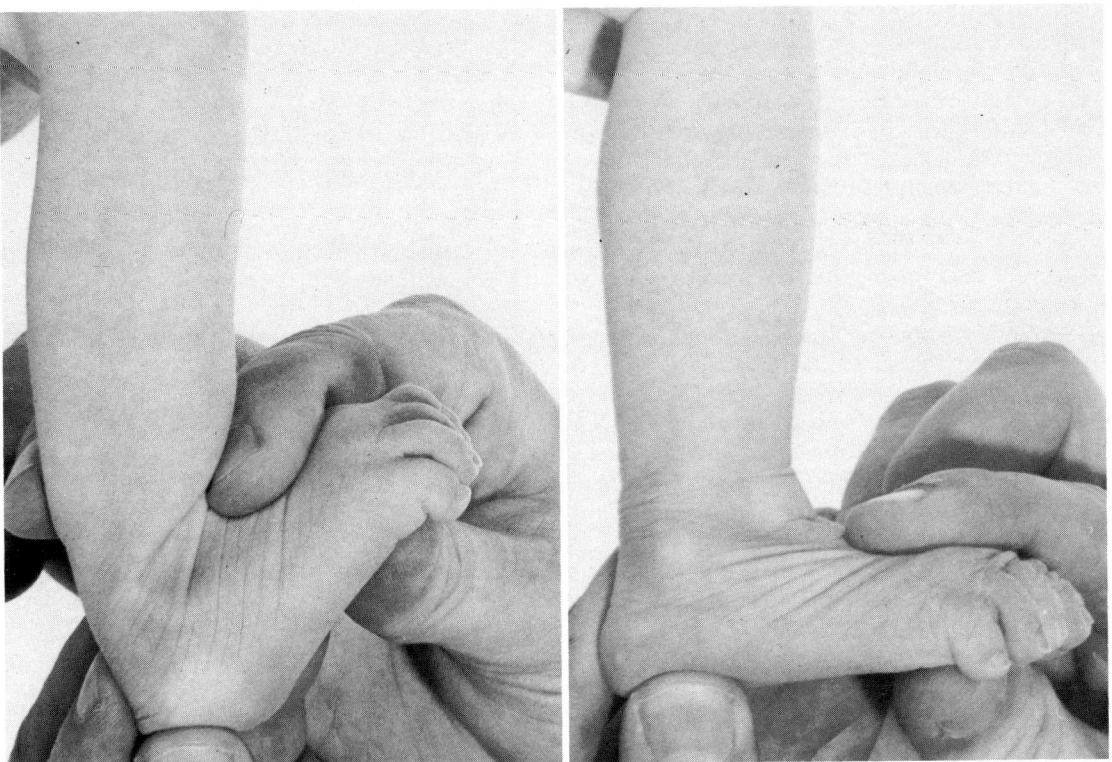

FIGURE 2–4. Talipes calcaneovalgus in an infant.

The foot is dorsiflexed and everted. Note that plantar flexion is limited to neutral position.

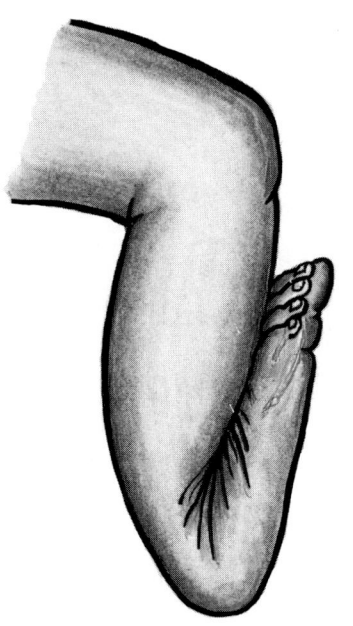

FIGURE 2–5. Severe talipes calcaneovalgus in a newborn.

Note the foot touching the anterior aspect of the tibia. Always examine the hips to rule out congenital dislocations.

the talus is locked in vertical position, the forefoot is in eversion and abduction, and the hindfoot is fixed in equinus position, giving a "rocker-bottom" shape to the sole of the foot. Roentgenograms of the foot should be taken in doubtful cases. Neuromuscular diseases, particularly spina bifida occulta with neurologic deficit, must be excluded. It is important to demonstrate function in the triceps surae, posterior tibial, and long toe flexor muscles. The hips should be examined to rule out congenital dislocation.

The prognosis is excellent. Mild deformities—if the foot can be plantar-flexed and inverted beyond neutral position—require no treatment. Within three to six months the feet resume normal alignment spontaneously. Moderate deformities—i.e., if it is difficult to plantar-flex the foot and invert it to neutral position by passive manipulation—are treated by daily passive stretching exercises performed by the mother. The shortened dorsolateral muscles and soft tissues are elongated by plantar-flexing and inverting the foot, maintaining the stretched position to the count of 10, and then releasing it. The exercises are performed 20 to 30 times in four sessions daily. Severe and resistant deformities are treated by stretching the soft-tissue contractures by manipulation and retaining the foot in the corrected position with plaster casts or Denis Browne splints, both of which hold the foot in equinovarus posture. Within four to six weeks the deformity will be completely corrected.

Larsen, Reimann, and Becker-Andersen investigated the value of treatment in 125 cases of talipes calcaneovalgus of which 49 per cent were treated with manipulation and elastic bandage and 51 per cent were untreated and observed by regular follow-up examinations. The contractural deformity was marked in 39 per cent of the treated group and 28 per cent of the untreated group. On comparison of the results, there was no significant difference between the two groups. The severity of the contractures found at birth appeared to have no influence on the final results. The follow-up period was 3 to 11 years. At the follow-up examination, the majority of the feet were normal. The only residual finding was pronation of the feet when the infants began to stand and walk. In the series of Larsen, Reimann, and Becker-Andersen, the hindfoot valgus deviation was 0 to 10 degrees in 75 per cent and 10 to 20 degrees in 25 per cent. In 45 per cent of the unilateral cases, the residual valgus deviation of the hindfoot was within the normal range but more exaggerated than on the unaffected side.[9] Giannestras has also noted the high degree of correlation between talipes calcaneovalgus in the newborn and flexible flat foot in the older child.[6] Clinical experience of this author concurs with that of Giannestras;

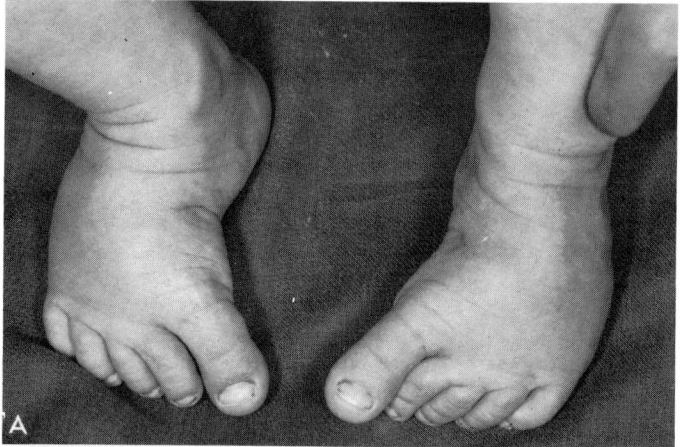
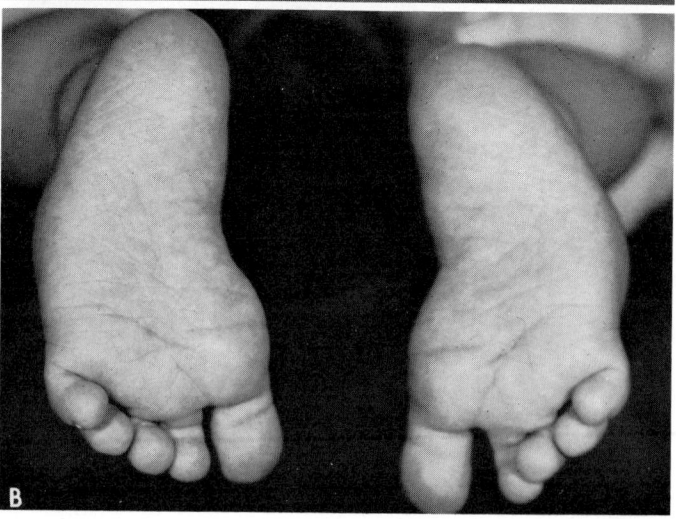

FIGURE 2–6. Bilateral talipes varus.

A. Dorsal view. **B.** Plantar view. The forefoot is inverted and adducted, the hindfoot is inverted, but the range of dorsiflexion of the foot and ankle is normal.

therefore conservative treatment of moderate and severe cases of talipes calcaneovalgus as just outlined is recommended.

Talipes Varus

In postural talipes varus the forefoot is adducted and inverted, and the hindfoot is inverted, but the range of dorsiflexion of the ankle and foot is normal, a feature that differentiates it from postural clubfoot (Fig. 2–6). Palpation reveals the navicular in normal relation to the head of the talus. One or two fingers can be easily inserted between the medial malleolus and the navicular. The talocalcaneonavicular joint is not subluxated medially. There are no adaptive osseous structural changes. The deformity is flexible, and the foot can be easily manipulated into normal position. The contralateral foot may be in valgus posture. The hips should be examined for congenital pelvic obliquity—with adduction contracture of the hip on the side with talipes varus and abduction contracture of the one on the side with talipes valgus. There is frequent association of these combinations of postural deformities. One should also rule out congenital dislocation of the hip, postural scoliosis, and torticollis.

Treatment consists of manipulative stretching of the foot into valgus position and retention in a below-knee cast. The cast is changed at weekly intervals, the foot being manipulated each time before the application of the new cast. The prognosis is excellent. The deformity will usually be completely corrected within two to four weeks. When this has been achieved, in severe cases the use of a polypropylene or other plastic below-knee splint may be indicated to hold the foot in the corrected position. The infant wears the splint only at night. Passive stretching exercises are performed by the mother several times a day. With this regimen of therapy a normal foot can be expected in three to four months.

Postural Talipes Valgus

In this type of postural deformity, both the forepart of the foot and the hindfoot are everted and abducted; the range of dorsiflexion and plantar flexion of the ankle is normal. Treatment consists of passive stretching exercises and retention of the foot in a below-knee cast. Within three to six weeks full correction of the deformity can be expected.

Postural Metatarsus Adductus

In this type of postural deformation of the foot only the forepart of the foot is adducted; the position of the hindfoot is neutral or slightly valgus (Fig. 2–7A). The articular relations of the tarsometatarsal joints are normal. There is no structural deformity. This condition should be distinguished from congenital metatarsus varus, which is a medial subluxation of the tarsometatarsal joint. In postural metatarsus adductus the forefoot can be brought to neutral position easily, whereas in congenital metatarsus varus the forefoot deformity is rigid, resisting passive manipulation (Fig. 2–7 B and C). Usually no treatment is required. Spontaneous correction within three to four months is the rule. The markedly adducted forefeet can be passively manipulated into abduction several times a day by the mother.

Postural Clubfoot

The forepart of the foot is adducted and inverted, and the hindfoot is inverted in this deformation. The whole foot is plantarflexed at the ankle so that the toes are carried lower than the heel. The condition is caused by intrauterine malposture. Anatomically the talocalcaneonavicular joint has normal articular relations and shows neither medial nor plantar subluxation. The head and neck of the talus are *not* tilted medially; i.e., the declination angle of the talus is normal. On examination, the skin creases are normal and there are no furrows on the medial and plantar aspects of the midfoot; the navicular does not abut the medial malleolus. The heel is of normal size. There is no calf atrophy. On manipulation the deformity is not rigid. In the literature, postural clubfoot is referred to as extrinsic type of congenital talipes equinovarus. For the sake of simplicity, however, the author rec-

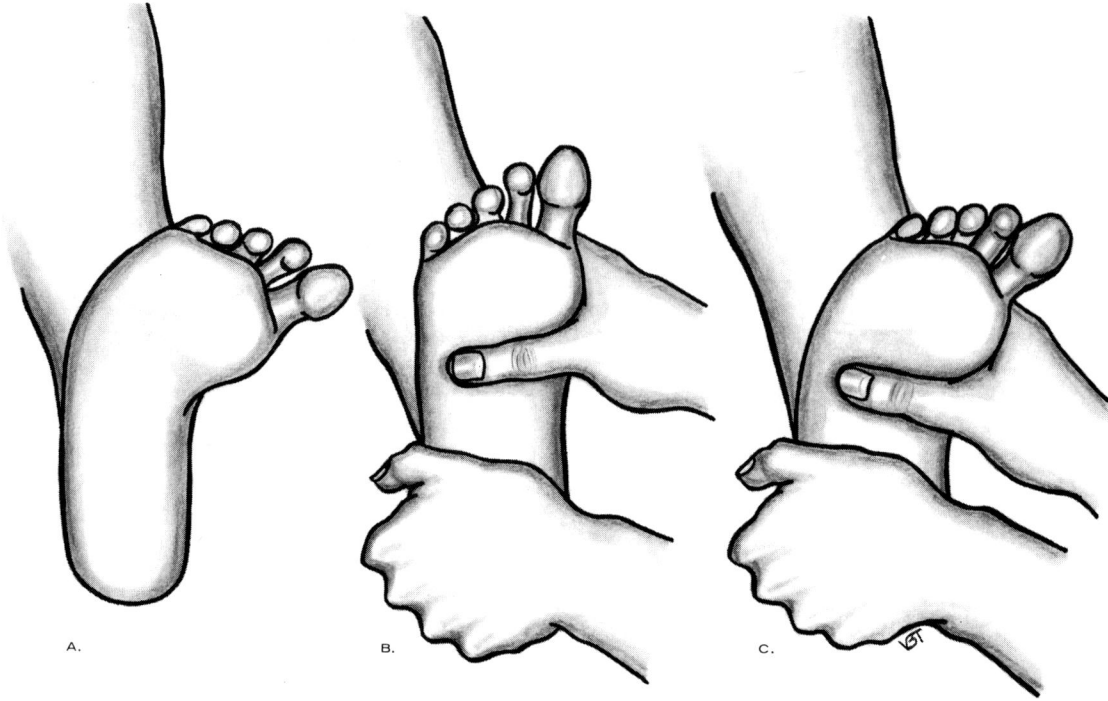

FIGURE 2–7. *Postural metatarsus adductus and congenital metatarsus varus.*

A. In both conditions the forefoot is adducted. In congenital metatarsus varus the varus deviation of the forefoot is greater and the valgus deviation of the heel is greater. **B.** In postural metatarsus adductus the forefoot can be easily manipulated into neutral position. **C.** In congenital metatarsus varus the forefoot deformity is rigid, resisting passive manipulation.

ommends reserving the term *congenital talipes equinovarus* for the true medioplantar displacement of the talocalcaneonavicular joint.

Treatment consists of manipulative stretching of the foot into valgus position and dorsiflexion, and its retention in the corrected position. The choice of retentive apparatus varies with the surgeon's past experience. This author uses a plaster of Paris cast. Others may prefer Robert Jones adhesive strapping or the Denis Browne foot splint. It does not matter which of the aforementioned types of retentive devices is applied.

The prognosis is excellent. With the foregoing regimen of therapy, a normal foot should be obtained within two to three months. The features distinguishing postural clubfoot from congenital talipes equinovarus are given in Table 2–6, page 163.

References

1. Browne, D.: Congenital deformities of mechanical origin, Proc. Roy. Soc. Med., 29:1409, 1936.
2. Chapple, C. C., and Davidson, D. T.: A study of the relationship between fetal position and certain congenital deformities. J. Pediat., 18l:483, 1941.
3. Dunn, P. M.: The influence of the intrauterine environment in the causation of congenital postural deformities, with special reference to congenital dislocation of the hip. M. D. Thesis, Cambridge University, 1969.
4. Dunn, P. M.: Congenital deformation following premature rupture of the membranes. Teratology, 4:487, 1971.
5. Dunn, P. M.: Congenital postural deformities: Further perinatal observations. Proc. Roy. Soc. Med., 67:1174, 1974.
6. Giannestras, N. J.: Recognition and treatment of flatfeet in infancy. Clin. Orthop., 70:10, 1970.
7. Gould, N.: Positional in utero deformities. Amer. J. Orthop., 4:46, 1962.
8. Hippocrates: Vol. 3. Loeb Classical Library. Trans. by E. T. Withington. London, William Heinemann, Ltd.; New York, G. P. Putnam's Sons, 1927.
9. Larsen, B., Reimann, I., and Becker-Andersen, H.: Congenital calcaneovalgus. Acta Orthop. Scand., 45:145, 1974.
10. Støren, H.: Congenital convex pes valgus with vertical talus. Acta Orthop. Scand., Suppl. 94:21, 1967.
11. Templeton, A. W., McAlister, W. H., And Zim, I. D.: Standardization of terminology and evaluation of osseous relationships in congenitally abnormal feet. Amer. J. Roentgen., 93:374, 1965.
12. Timmer, H.: Der Zusammenhang des Pes valgus beim Kinder und des Pes calcaneus beim Neugeborenen. Z. Orthop. Chir., 45:35, 1924.
13. Vartan, C. K.: The behavior of the foetus in utero with special reference to the incidence of breech presentation at term. J. Obstet. Gynaec. Brit. Emp., 52:417, 1945.
14. Wetzenstein, H.: The significance of congenital pes calcaneovalgus in the origin of pes plano-valgus in childhood. Preliminary report. Acta Orthop. Scand., 30:64, 1960.
15. Wilkinson, J. A.: Breech malposition and intra-uterine dislocations. Proc. Roy. Soc. Med., 59:1106, 1966.

16. Wynne-Davies, R.: Family studies of the cause of congenital clubfoot—talipes equinovarus, talipes calcaneovalgus and metatarsus varus. J. Bone Joint Surg., 46-B:445, 1964.

CONGENITAL TALIPES EQUINOVARUS

Traditionally, the definition of congenital talipes equinovarus has been descriptive: The heel is inverted, the forefoot and midfoot are inverted and adducted (*varus*), and the ankle is in *equinus* position—the foot is plantar-flexed with the toes at a lower level than the heel. A definition should, however, be specific, be based upon pathologic findings, and offer greater therapeutic insight. Congenital talipes equinovarus is in utero medial and plantar displacement (subluxation or dislocation) of the *talocalcaneonav*icular (T-C-N) ball-and-socket joint.

Incidence

Congenital talipes equinovarus is one of the more common congenital deformities of the foot. First described by Hippocrates, it has been known since ancient times.[270]

The incidence of talipes equinovarus varies widely with race and sex. In Caucasians, the birth frequency is 1.2 per thousand, with a male-to-female sex ratio of two to one, making the rates 1.6 per thousand in boys and 0.8 per thousand in girls.[712, 715, 717]

Stewart, in 1951, noted the incidence of talipes equinovarus to be 4.9 per thousand in part- or full-blooded Hawaiians.[623] This high incidence in Hawaiians was confirmed by Ching and co-workers, who reported it to be 6.81 per thousand in full-blooded Hawaiians, as compared with 1.12 per thousand in Caucasians, and 0.57 per thousand in Orientals of unmixed blood. They also showed that the incidence of talipes equinovarus increased as the proportion of Hawaiian ancestry increased, indicating the racial effects in the risk of talipes equinovarus to be additive.[111] A high frequency of talipes equinovarus in the Maori—another Polynesian group—has been reported by Elliot, by Alldred, and by Veale and associates.[8, 166, 663] On the basis of these data, Beals concluded the birth frequency to be 6.5 to 7.0 per thousand in the Maori.[32]

The incidence of talipes equinovarus in

Table 2–3. Incidence of Talipes Equinovarus in Various Races*

Race	Cases per Thousand Births
Chinese	.39
Japanese	.53
Malay	.68
Filipino	.76
Caucasian	1.12
Puerto Rican	1.36
Indian	1.51
South African black	3.50
Polynesian	6.81

*From Beals, R. K.: Personal communication; data derived from Ching et al., Chung et al., Pillay et al., and Pompe van Meerdervoort.

South African blacks (3.5 per thousand) is reported by Pompe van Meerdervoort; and that in Malayans, Indians, and Chinese in Singapore, by Pillay, Khong, and Wolfers.[516, 520] The figures for various racial groups are summarized in Table 2–3.

Involvement is bilateral in about 50 per cent of the cases. In unilateral cases the right side is affected slightly more frequently than the left.

Heredity

The pattern of inheritance of talipes equinovarus is polygenic with a threshold effect.[99–101, 716, 717] Single genetic factors or unifactorial disorders show discontinuous variation; that is, an all-or-none phenomenon with the malformation being either present or absent. The pattern of inheritance of unifactoral affections is simple, with ratios illustrating dominant, recessive, or sex-linked traits; however, variations may be encountered in malformations caused by single mutant genes. Multiple gene systems or multifactoral disorders show continuous variation and illustrate polygenic patterns of inheritance. The all-or-none nature of talipes equinovarus is explained by the threshold effect, i.e., an underlying gradation of factors related to the deformity that cause it to be present when the level is beyond a certain threshold and absent when the level is under that point.

The polygenic inheritance of talipes equinovarus is supported by the following evidence. (1) The family studies of Wynne-Davies showed a rapid decrease in incidence

Table 2–4. Proportions of First-, Second-, and Third-Degree Relatives Affected with Talipes Equinovarus*

Index Patient		First-Degree Relative		Second-Degree Relative		Third-Degree Relative	
		Brother	Sister	Uncle	Aunt	Male Cousins	Female Cousins
Male	97	4 of 115	0 of 90	0 of 286	2 of 282	2 of 341	0 of 349
Female	47	2 of 33	2 of 34	1 of 138	2 of 117	0 of 166	0 of 136
Total	144	8 of 272		5 of 823		2 of 992	
Per cent		2.9		0.6		0.2	
Appropriate comparison with general population		× 30		× 5		× 1.5	

*Data derived from family studies of Wynne-Davies, 1964 and 1970.

from first- to second- to third-degree relatives; (about 2.9 per cent of siblings, 0.6 per cent of aunts and uncles, and 0.2 per cent of cousins, as listed in Table 2–4). (2) Female index patients are fewer in number than male index patients (the infrequency of talipes equinovarus in the female may be due to some unknown factor that modifies its manifestation) and they have a greater proportion of affected relatives than do the males, indicating a greater deviance from the norm than in the male. (3) The risk of developing talipes equinovarus in subsequent children is increased when both parents are affected or when there is more than one affected individual in the family. In general, talipes equinovarus is less severe in sporadic cases than in familial ones, and the greater the number of talipes equinovarus cases in a family, the greater the probability of having subsequent children with more rigid deformity.*

In the etiology of talipes equinovarus, besides genetic factors, environmental factors must operate. This is shown by the studies of Idelberger, who compared the incidence of talipes equinovarus in identical (monozygotic) twin pairs with that in fraternal (dizygotic) twin pairs. He found that 13 of 40 (32.5 per cent) of the monozygotic co-twins were affected with talipes equinovarus, in contrast to 4 of 134 (2.9 per cent) of the dizygotic co-twins.[289, 290] These data suggest that both genetic and environmental factors play a role in the genesis of deformity. Little is known about the intrauterine environmental factors.[716]

In genetic counseling, one should consider the sex of the index patient, whether or not the parents are affected by talipes equinovarus, and the race of the family. In a Caucasian family, if both parents are normal and the index patient is a male, the risk of a subsequent child being born with talipes equinovarus is about 2 per cent; if the parents are normal and the index patient is a female, the chances are increased to 5 per cent; however, if a parent has talipes equinovarus and already has one child with talipes equinovarus, the odds are much greater—10 to 25 per cent (accurate figures for this group are not yet available).[716, 717]

In a Maori family, if the index patient is a male and the parents are normal, the risk of a subsequent child having talipes equinovarus is about 9 per cent; if the index patient is a female with normal parents, the chance of a brother being affected is 9 per cent (there were no sisters affected in the series of Beals). If an index patient has a parent affected with talipes equinovarus, the chance increases to 30 per cent. These differences in incidence of talipes equinovarus in the Caucasian and the Maori are explained by the frequency of the gene in the population rather than by its mode of action. By using the Falconer model for the estimate of heritability, it has been shown that the heritability of talipes equinovarus is similar in the Caucasian and the Maori (i.e., 70 ± 8).[32, 176, 663]

Etiology

The exact cause of talipes equinovarus is unknown. It has, in the past, been the subject of much speculation and theorizing based on a striking paucity of facts.

---
*See references 99–101, 112, 113, 491–493, 712, 714–717.

INTRAUTERINE MECHANICAL FACTORS

The mechanical theory, the oldest, was advocated by Hippocrates. He proposed that the fetal foot was forced into the equinovarus posture by external mechanical forces; that consequent to rapid skeletal growth, the ligaments and muscles developed adaptive shortening; and that the tarsal bones, especially the talus, responded by changes in their contour with subsequent articular malalignment.[270] The theory of intrauterine malposture due to mechanical forces was further elaborated by Parker and Shattock in 1884, Nutt in 1925, and Denis Browne in 1933, 1936, and 1955.[77, 79, 81, 477, 499] This theory is not supported by the observation that the incidence of talipes equinovarus is not increased in prenatal environmental conditions that tend to "overcrowd" the uterus—such as twinning, high birth weight, primiparous uterus, hydramnios, and oligohydramnios.[111, 717] At present, the nature of the intrauterine environmental factors has not yet been determined.

NEUROMUSCULAR DEFECT

In the literature, many theories have been put forward about neuromuscular dysfunction as the cause of talipes equinovarus; to mention a few: a peroneal nerve lesion caused by pressure at the intrauterine stage (White, 1929); maldevelopment of the striated muscle (Middleton, 1934); muscle imbalance due to dysplasia of the peroneals (Flinchum, 1953); and relative shortening of the degenerating muscle fibers during growth (Bechtol and Mossman, 1950).*

Irani and Sherman used fetal material to distinguish primary from adaptive changes. They demonstrated by standard anatomic and routine histologic studies that there are no abnormalities in the muscles, nerves, vessels, or tendinous insertions.[298, 299] The same conclusions have been reached by other investigators.[624, 703] Isaacs and coworkers, however, in 1977, presented a histochemical and electron microscopic study of muscles in talipes equinovarus; there was evidence of neurogenic disease in most instances. They proposed abnormal innervation as the prime factor in the development of the deformity. Minor degrees of muscle imbalance evolving during a period of rapid skeletal growth in early intrauterine periods will produce disproportionately severe deformities.[300]

Ritsila was able to produce equinovarus deformity of the foot in 32 young rabbits (mostly six to seven days old) by soft-tissue alterations; namely a combination of Achilles tenodesis, sectioning of the extensor digitorum longus and both peroneal muscles (longus and brevis), and immobilization of the foot and ankle in an extremely rigid equinovarus posture for three to four weeks. Roentgenographic examination and analysis of the anatomic deformities by gross dissection and microscopic studies showed the morphologic changes in the experimental animal to be similar to those in the human. Ritsila concluded that primary soft-tissue changes should be considered a factor in provoking skeletal deformities in talipes equinovarus.[547] The primary cause of soft-tissue contractures remains unknown.

In the literature, there are a number of reports on experimental production of talipes equinovarus in animals. Drachman and Coulombre infused chick embryos with curare for periods of up to 48 hours; at the time of hatching, the chicks consistently had limb deformities. The limbs were deformed in the embryonic position, and there was evidence of the external influences of the calcareous shell. The foot deformity was identical to talipes. Active movement of the embryo is required for normal development of joints. The teratogenic effects of curare are due to its paralyzing action. It seems that even relatively brief periods of immobilization will produce ankylosing of joints.[150] Shoro produced clubfoot deformity in rats (38 of 467 fetuses—8.1 per cent) by temporary, brief periods of paralysis and immobilization with tubocurarine injections.[597]

Jackson immobilized the immature and rapidly growing feet of opossums in a deformed position and produced structural adaptations in muscle, tendon, and bone. When structural changes developed, the de-

---

*See references 35, 190, 448, 691

formity did not resolve spontaneously. The tendency to resolution was inversely related to the duration of immobilization.[303]

Edwards exposed pregnant guinea pigs to hyperthermia by placing them in an incubator set at 43° Celsius for one hour daily between the eighteenth and twenty-fifth days of gestation. Eleven of the forty newborn guinea pigs showed clubfoot deformity; all of them had associated malformations of the spinal cord.[163] In the human, weak peroneal muscles have been incriminated as the cause of clubfoot. Electromyographic studies, however, have shown no lower motor neuron lesion.[487]

ARREST OF FETAL DEVELOPMENT

Over 100 years ago, Hüter regarded talipes equinovarus as the result of an arrest of development of the foot in one of the physiologic phases of its embryonic life.[287] That there are physiologic positions in the embryonic development of the foot that are similar to clubfoot has been demonstrated by Henke and Reyher, by Schomburg, by Bardeen and Lewis, and by Böhm.[24, 65, 259, 577] The four stages in the evolution of the human foot in the first half of prenatal life were delineated by Bohm.[65]

First Stage (Second Month). The form of the foot is characterized by marked equinus inclination (about 90 degrees of plantar flexion) and by severe adduction of the hindpart and forepart of the foot, with the navicular lying in close proximity to the medial malleolus. The plane of the lower leg and the transverse axis of the knee and the plane of the foot (i.e., the one passing transversely through the long axis of the foot plate) are superimposed.

Second Stage (Beginning of Third Month). There is a new development—the foot rotates into a position of marked supination, but remains in 90 degrees of plantar flexion. The first metatarsal is markedly adducted; the lateral four metatarsals are adducted to a lesser extent (Fig. 2–8 A and B).

Third Stage (Middle of Third Month). The equinus inclination decreases to a mild degree, but the marked supination and metatarsus varus persist. In this stage, the long axis of the foot is perpendicular to the plane of the lower leg (Fig. 2–8C).

Fourth Stage (Beginning at Fourth Month). The foot is in midsupination and there is slight metatarsus varus (Fig. 2–8D). In this stage, the foot plate begins to rotate toward pronation on its long axis, the planes of the foot and lower leg gradually assuming the relative positions seen in the adult human.[65]

It is obvious from the preceding observations that the three clinical deformities of talipes equinovarus, namely plantar flexion, adduction, and supination, are normal in the early stages of physiologic embryonic development of the human foot. This relationship is given in Table 2–5. Studies of the pathologic anatomy of severe talipes equinovarus have shown that in its external appearance it resembles an embryonic foot at the beginning of the second month. Böhm had difficulty explaining his theory of medial and plantar subluxation of the talocalcaneonavicular joint in talipes equinovarus, for this medial displacement of the navicular is not observed in any stage of the development of the normal fetus.[65, 98, 673]

Mau objected to the theory that clubfoot is due to arrested fetal development because the embryonic foot does not show distortion of the bones about the tarsal joints, which is found in clubfoot.[440]

Carroll and associates used a dissecting microscope to examine the normal feet of 17 embryos and fetuses. The youngest embryo studied was eight weeks old; up to that

---

FIGURE 2–8. Appearance of lower limbs of human embryo in first half of prenatal life.

A and **B.** Lateral and anteroposterior view of 23 mm. long (vertex to buttocks) human embryo at nine weeks. Note the 90-degree pes equinus, marked supination of the feet, and the adduction of the metatarsals. **C.** Lateral view of 35 mm. embryo (middle of third month). Note the slight pes equinus, marked supination of the entire foot, and moderate metatarsus varus. **D.** An anteroposterior view of 57 mm. long human embryo (end of third month). Note the midsupination of the feet and the slight metatarsus varus. (From Böhm, M.: The embryologic origin of clubfoot. J. Bone Joint Surg., *11*:246, 1929. Reprinted by permission.)

Congenital Deformities

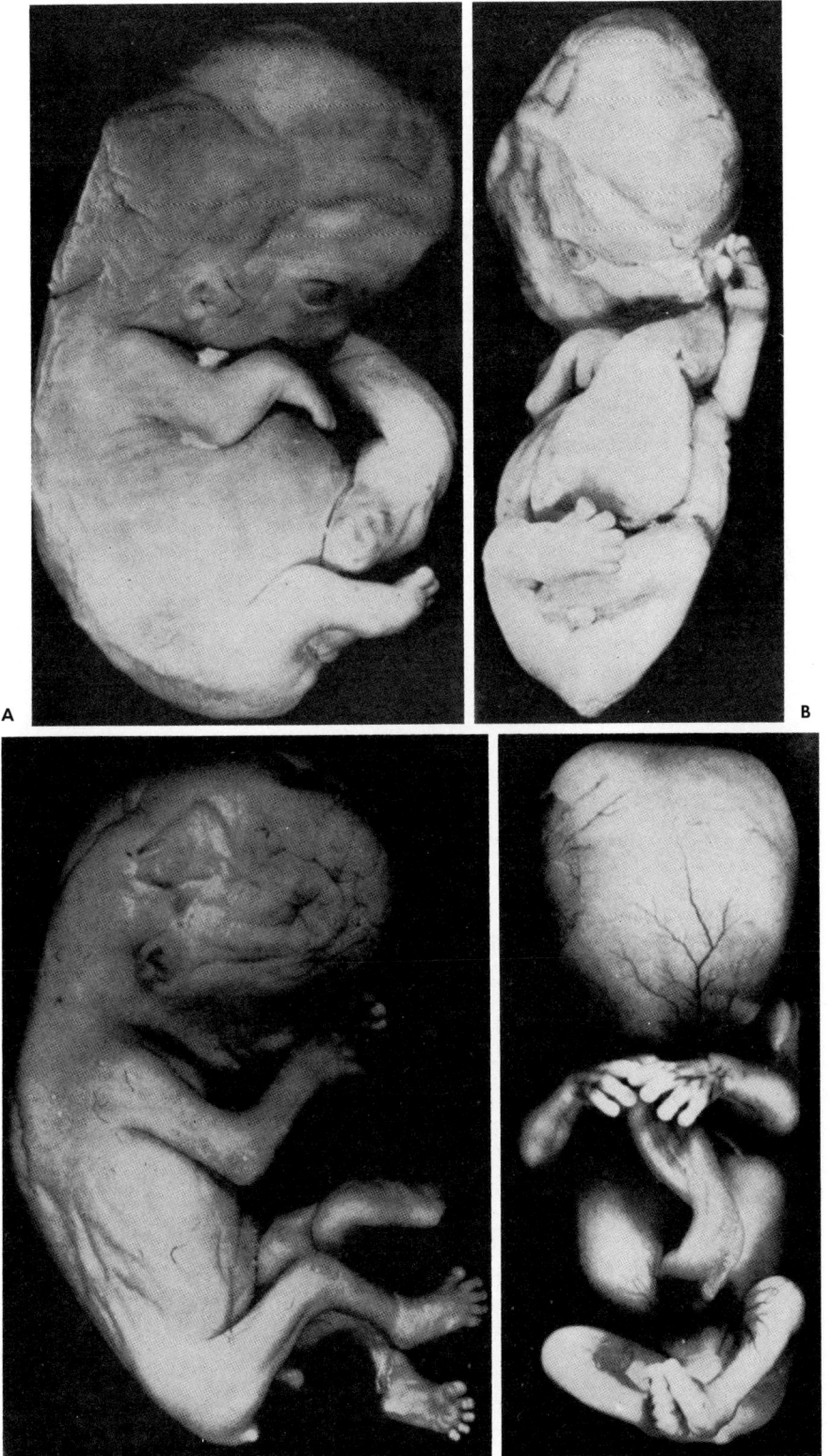

FIGURE 2-8 *See legend on opposite page*

Table 2–5

Stages of Physiologic Embryonic Development	Primary Deformities in Talipes Equinovarus					
	Plantar Flexion		Adduction		Supination	
	Marked	Slight	Tarsus	Metatarsus	Marked	Slight
First stage (second month)	+	−	+	+	−	−
Second stage (beginning of third month)	+	−	−	+	+	−
Third stage (middle of third month)	−	+	−	+	+	−
Fourth stage (beginning of fourth month)	−	−	−	+	−	+

From Böhm, M.: The embryologic origin of clubfoot. J. Bone Joint Surg., *11*:246, 1929. Reproduced by permission of the publisher.

age, the foot was so gelatinous that it could be manipulated into almost any position. In the dissected feet, the mesenchymal condensation or the cartilage model of the navicular had a normal relationship with the head of the talus. The first metatarsal in the younger feet tended to have a varus inclination. These investigators concluded that talipes equinovarus does not reflect persistence of an intrauterine stage of development.[98]

Kaplan studied the comparative anatomy of the talus in relation to talipes equinovarus. He could not find a structure similar to clubfoot in any other species. He concluded that talipes equinovarus does not represent a recapitulation of a pre-existing evolutionary condition.[322]

PRIMARY GERM PLASM DEFECT

The consistent bony deformity in talipes equinovarus is medial and plantar tilting of the head and neck of the talus.[298] Nichols (in 1897) and Elmslie (in 1920) speculated that primary bone dysplasia was the cause of deformation of the talus.[167, 474] The cartilaginous anlagen of the tarsal bones are fully formed by six weeks, and those of the tarsal joints by seven weeks, in the embryo.[213] On the basis of this embryologic fact, Irani and Sherman proposed that talipes equinovarus is the result of a defective cartilaginous anlage produced by a primary germ plasm defect, developing in the first trimester of pregnancy.[298, 299]

In the opinion of this author, there is more than one cause of congenital talipes equinovarus. In some cases it is due to a primary germ plasm defect of the talus and decrease of its angle of declination; under the tethering effect of soft-tissue contracture, the talocalcaneonavicular joint progressively subluxates medially and plantarward. In others, there may be a neuromuscular type of congenital talipes equinovarus in which the paralysis, imbalance, and fibrotic contracture of paralyzed muscles are the primary cause of deformity, the changes in the shape of the talus being secondary. There may be a primary ligamentous disorder with excess of myofibroblasts as the cellular cause of soft-tissue contracture.[549] At present the question of the etiology of congenital talipes equinovarus has not been settled.

Pathology

Upon inspection, the gross pathologic changes of talipes equinovarus are characteristic: the foot is plantar-flexed at the ankle and subtalar joints, the hindfoot is inverted, and the mid- and forefoot are adducted, inverted, and in equinus position (Fig. 2–9). These deformities are the result of medial and plantar displacement and medial rotation of the talocalcaneonavicular joint.[568, 569] The navicular and calcaneus are displaced medially and plantarward around the talus, the cuboid is displaced medially on the calcaneus, and the ankle joint assumes the equinus posture because the mechanics of the foot is disturbed. Fixed contractures of the related soft tissues—i.e., the ligaments, capsules, muscles, and tendons—maintain these articular malalignments.

The pathologic changes observed in talipes equinovarus may be either primary (congenital) or secondary (adaptive), the one being distinguished from the other by study of the morbid anatomy in the fetus. Irani and Sherman carefully dissected 11 fetal limbs with talipes equinovarus deformity, and Settle studied 16 specimens from

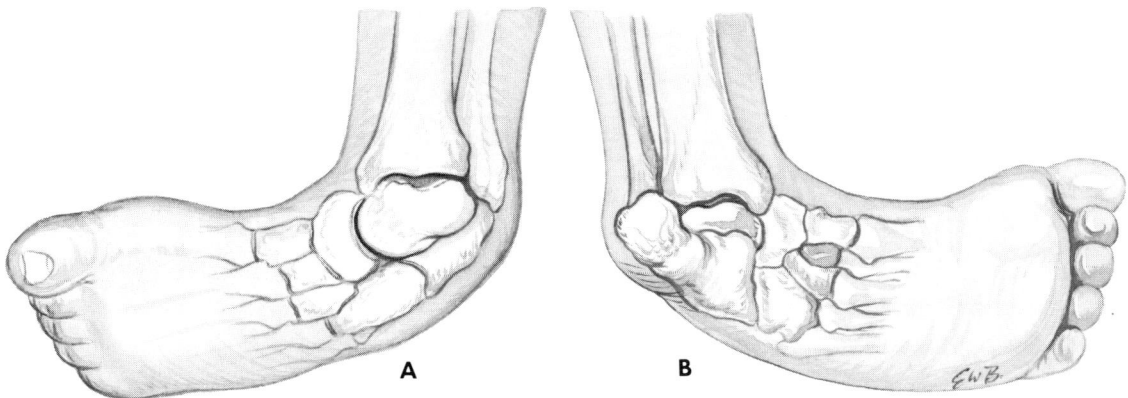

FIGURE 2–9. *The deformity of talipes equinovarus (TEV) on gross inspection.*
A. Anterior view. **B.** Posterior view.

the late fetal period.[298, 299, 587] In 1970, Müller, reviewing the literature of the past 120 years, found reports of 41 dissections of talipes equinovarus in fetuses.[462] Recently, numerous studies of the morbid anatomy of talipes equinovarus in the different stages of fetal development have been reported.[91, 98, 297a, 521, 673] The conclusions reached by these investigators are essentially the same.

BONY DEFORMITIES

The Talus. The primary and basic deformity in talipes equinovarus is medial and plantar deviation of the anterior end of the talus.[298, 299, 588] The angle formed by the long axis of the head and neck of the talus with the long axis of its body is called the "declination angle" of the talus; in the normal adult human foot, it measures between 150 and 160 degrees.[501] In talipes equinovarus, the declination angle of the talus is invariably decreased, measuring 115 to 135 degrees (Fig. 2–10). It is of pathogenetic interest to note that in the young fetus, the head and neck of the talus are tilted toward the medial side of the foot during fetal development; from the sixteenth week onward, the declination angle of the talus increases.[213]

In the literature, medial tilting of the anterior part of the talus is also referred to as obliquity of the neck of the talus.[676] It is measured as follows: the talus is placed with its trochlear articular surface facing superiorly; a horizontal line is drawn across the trochlea between its medial tubercle and lateral process; a longitudinal line is drawn along the center of the trochlear surface,

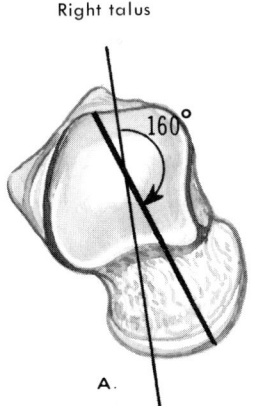
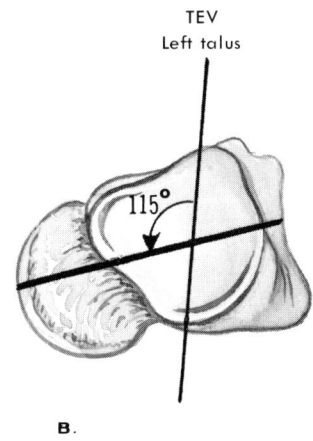

FIGURE 2–10. *Declination angle of the talus.*

A. Normal foot. Note angle of 150 to 160 degrees. **B.** Talipes equinovarus. The angle is decreased to 115 degrees.

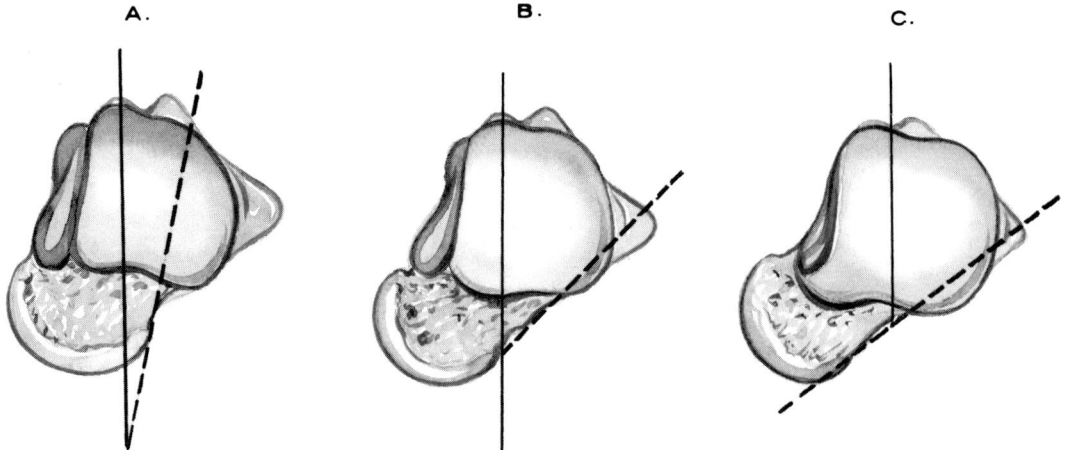

FIGURE 2–11. *Obliquity of the neck of the talus.*

A. In the normal adult. **B.** In the normal fetus. **C.** In talipes equinovarus. (Redrawn from Walsham, W. J., and Hughes, W. K.: Treatment of talipes equinus. *In* The Deformities of the Human Foot. London, Baillière, Tindall & Cox, 1895, Chapter VII, pp. 294–320.)

parallel with its inner border and perpendicular to the horizontal line; then a longitudinal line is drawn parallel to the lateral margin of the neck of the talus. The angle formed between the longitudinal axes of the trochlea and of the neck is the measure of the obliquity of the talar neck. Scudder, combining his figures with those of Parker and Shattock, reported the angle of obliquity to be 12 to 32 degrees in the adult, 35 to 75 degrees in the fetus, and 50 to 65 degrees in talipes equinovarus (Fig. 2–11).[499, 581]

The neck of the talus is shortened, sometimes unidentifiable, so that the head appears to be fused with the body. The normal constriction of the talar neck is absent. The anterior articular surface of the talus in the normal foot faces forward and slightly inward and downward in the frontal plane of its body, whereas in talipes equinovarus it is rotated medially and plantarward, facing almost directly inward and markedly downward. The anterior end of the talus is divided by a ridge into two areas: *an inner part,* which is covered by an articular facet and, in the young fetus, in contact with the navicular; and a *lateral part,* which is devoid of articular surface and is covered with a thin layer of fibrous tissue. The lateral part of the anterior end of the talus is unopposed by bone and is palpable as a rounded prominence on the dorsolateral part of the foot. For practical therapeutic purposes, this lateral part is regarded as the "head" of the talus, and the navicular is reduced to articulate with it.

The posterior articular facet on the inferior surface of the talus is relatively normal. The anterior and middle facets, however, are distorted and fused into a single misshapen, articular surface that is tilted medially and downward; inferolaterally, it articulates with the medial surface of the anterior part of the calcaneus. Thus, as seen from above, the anterior portion of the calcaneus is uncovered and the sinus tarsi is widened.

Normally, the ankle mortise is narrower posteriorly than anteriorly, and the corresponding articular surface of the talus is similarly shaped. In talipes equinovarus, however, the talus is plantar-flexed in fixed equinus posture; consequently, the anterior one quarter to one third of its superior articular surface is uncovered (Fig. 2–12). It may be difficult to reposition the wider anterior part of the dome of the talus into the ankle mortise because there is insufficient space; the talus has forfeited its "right of domicile."[411] In general, the trochlear articular surface is normal; but in long-standing untreated talipes equinovarus there may be a distinct ridge separating its anterior uncovered part from the posterior contained parts, as if it had been indented by the anterior ligament of the inferior tibiofibular joint. The medial surface of the

Congenital Deformities 147

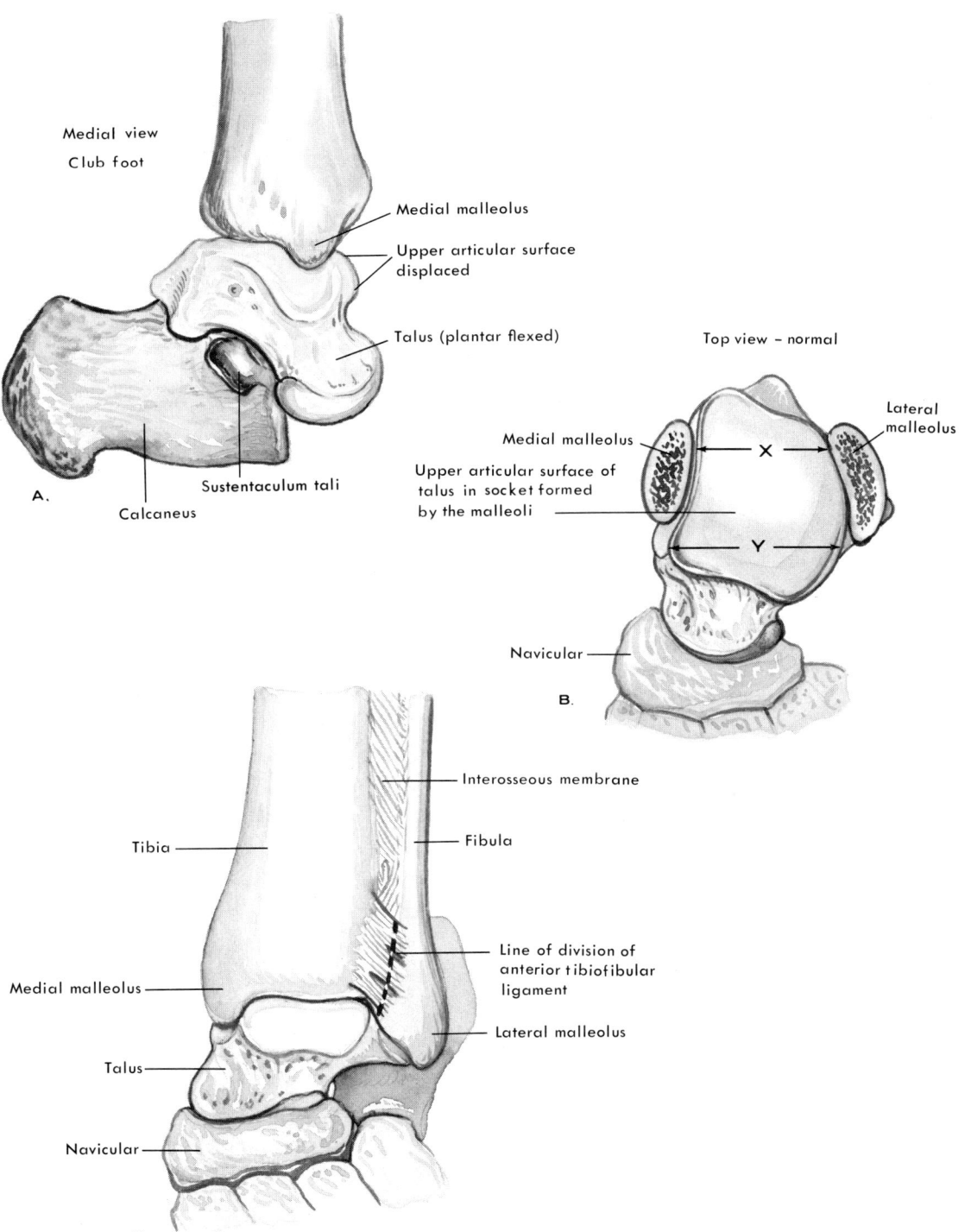

FIGURE 2–12. The anatomic relationships of the talus in the ankle mortise.

A. The talus is plantar-flexed. Note the anterior one fourth to one third of the superior articular surface is uncovered. **B.** The superior articular surface of the talus lying in the mortise formed by the medial and lateral malleoli. Note it is narrower posteriorly than in front. In the older child with talipes equinovarus the plantar-flexed talus may "forfeit its right of domicile," i.e., there may not be room in the ankle mortise to reposition it. **C.** Anterior tibiofibular ligament and lower end of tibiofibular interosseous ligament are sectioned to widen the ankle mortise and make room for the talus.

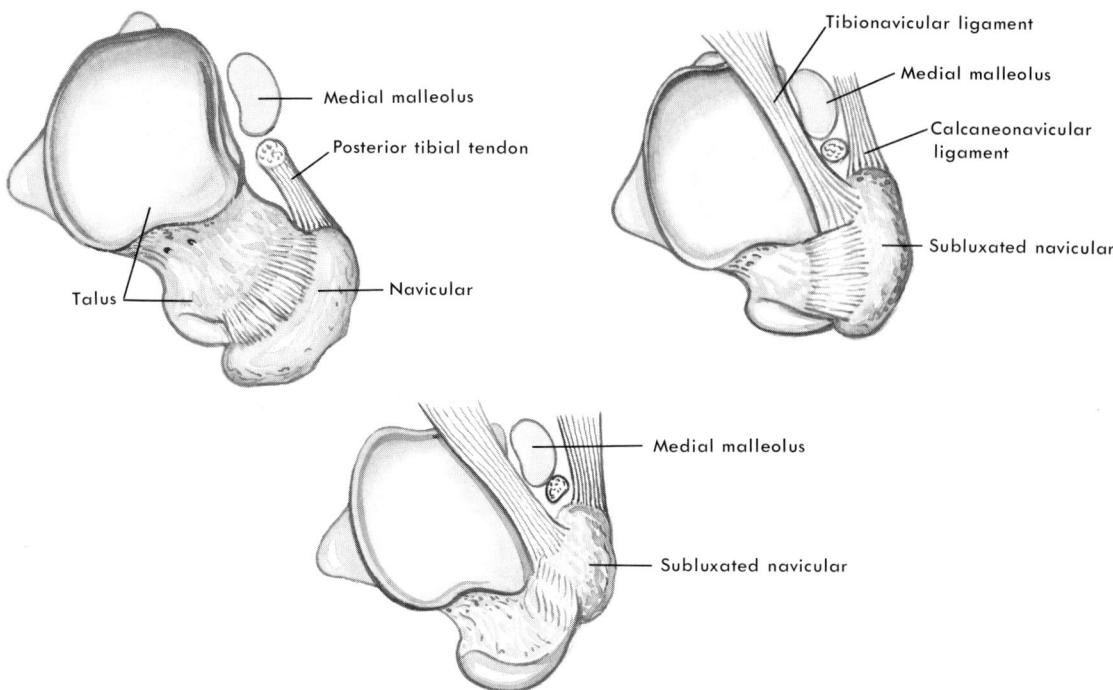

FIGURE 2–13. *Progressive medial and plantar displacement of the navicular in relation to the anterior end of the talus.*

A. In early fetal life the navicular articulates with the medially tilted head of the talus. **B** and **C.** With rapid growth of the foot of the fetus, the pull of the posterior tibial tendon, the plantar calcaneonavicular ligament, and the tibionavicular ligament, the navicular is displaced medially and plantarward and abuts the medial malleolus.

talus is grossly deformed and diminished in size. A large part of it is occupied by the deltoid ligament, which seems to have appropriated the articular facet. In the normal foot of the fetus and the neonate, the medial articular facet is pear-shaped, extends farther distally on the medial wall of the talus, and may be continuous with the anterior articular surface for the navicular. In talipes equinovarus, most of the medial facet is obliterated, and only a narrow, posterior stalk remains.

With the rapid growth of the tarsal bones in the fetus, the pull of the contracted calcaneonavicular and tibionavicular ligaments and the posterior tibial tendon will progressively displace the navicular medially and plantarward toward the medial malleolus (Fig. 2–13). The medial surfaces of the calcaneus and the navicular will abut against the medial malleolus and, in severe cases, even be eroded by it. Accessory articulation may develop between the three bones. The lateral surface of the talus appears to be normal, with a relatively well-developed lateral articular facet.

The deformed talus in talipes equinovarus is small in size, and its ossification center may be delayed in appearing and eccentrically situated in a more anterior and lateral location. The vascular channels are scarcer and arranged in a disorganized fashion.[590, 673] The pathologic changes in the talus are more pronounced than those in any of the other tarsal bones.

The Calcaneus. The os calcis is much less deformed than the talus. In general, its contour is relatively normal, with its articular facets normally oriented on its body. Since these facets articulate with those of the talus, the calcaneus, of necessity, is rotated on its long axis inward and downward beneath the talus. The varus position of the heel disappears upon release of its capsular and ligamentous attachments, indicating that the deformity is secondary and postural. There is minimal medial bowing of the calcaneus, its lateral surface being slightly convex and its medial surface concave. The sustentaculum tali is usually underdeveloped and in close proximity to the medial malleolus. The distal calcaneal articular facet for the cuboid bone slants anteriorly, medially, and plantarward; in the normal foot it faces almost forward. This alteration accounts for the medial inclination of the calcaneocuboid joint.

The Forefoot and Tibia. Smaller than normal, the navicular is normal in shape. Its medial tuberosity may be hypertrophied. In severe cases, it may have an articular facet for the medial malleolus. The cuboid is essentially normal in shape. The cuneiforms, the metatarsal bones, and the phalanges are normal.

Kite states that exaggerated medial tibial torsion is a commonly associated finding in talipes equinovarus.[332, 344] This is not correct. Tibial torsion is normal. The old concept of exaggerated medial tibial torsion as the fourth element of the complex deformity of talipes equinovarus should be discarded.

ARTICULAR MALALIGNMENTS

Relationship of Talus to Distal Tibia and Fibula. The talus has no muscle attachments; it is stabilized by the ankle mortise. The equinovarus posture of the calcaneus and the medial and plantar displacement of the navicular force the talus to tilt out of the ankle mortise, exposing one fourth to one third of its superior articular surface (see Fig. 2–12A). In the literature, there is disagreement about whether the talus also rotates in the ankle mortise. There has been a question whether the medial rotation of the foot in talipes equinovarus is due to the medial rotation of the talus in the ankle mortise or to the medial rotation of the foot at the subtalar joint complex. There has also been much controversy as to the etiology of the posterior position of the fibular malleolus. Is it due to the medial or to the lateral rotation of the talus in the ankle mortise? Adams states that he has never observed medial rotation but that, in contrast, there is lateral rotation in the ankle mortise.[3, 4, 126, 226] Walsham and Hughes point out that, because of the greater convexity of the lateral border of the superior articular surface of the talus and the direction of the trochlea, when the ankle joint is plantar-flexed, the talus inclines medially as well as forward and downward. In talipes equinovarus, the talus is in equinus position, and its head therefore inclines medially as well as downward. Hence, on inspection, one finds the lateral malleolar facet of the talus to be displaced anteriorly in front of the lateral malleolus, while the superior and medial surfaces of the talar neck approximate the anterior border of the medial malleolus. In brief, Walsham and Hughes consider the talus to be plantar-flexed and medially rotated at the ankle joint.[676] McKay states that in 120 clubfeet he has been unable to observe any medial rotation of the talus in the ankle joint or any abnormal plane of motion of the talus relative to the bimalleolar plane of the talocrural articulation.[413]

Relationship of Navicular to Talus. The navicular is displaced medially and plantarward, leaving the lateral part of the anterior globular end of the talus unopposed (see Fig. 2–13). There is some disagreement about terminology—whether this is true subluxation or dislocation. This author believes that it is imperative to restore normal alignment of the talonavicular joint. Otherwise, the hyaline cartilage on the lateral aspect of the talar anterior end will atrophy and the longitudinal growth of the bone will be retarded.

Relationship of Talus to Calcaneus. The calcaneus is rotated medially and tilted into equinus position beneath the talus. Abnormal movements take place in three dimensions—horizontal, coronal, and sagittal. In the horizontal plane, the calcaneus rotates medially so that, anterior to the ankle joint, it slips underneath the head and neck of the talus, whereas posterior to the ankle joint, the calcaneal tuberosity moves toward the fibular malleolus (Fig. 2–14). The calcaneofibular ligament becomes shortened and thickened. In addition the calcaneofibular retinaculum (superior peroneal retinaculum), peroneal tendon sheaths, and posterior talocalcaneal ligament tether the calcaneus to the fibular malleolus.[413]

In talipes equinovarus, the varus appearance of the heel may be difficult to comprehend when, in actuality, the calcaneus is close to the lateral malleolus. This is explained by the rotation of the calcaneus in the coronal plane in addition to the hori-

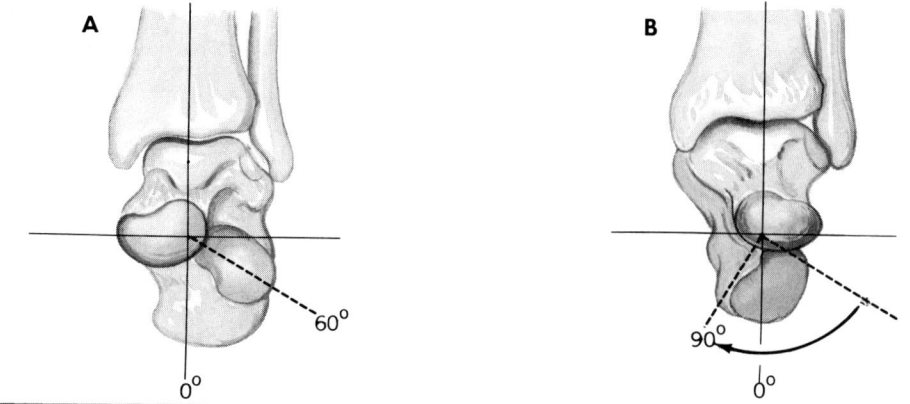

FIGURE 2–14. The articular relationship of the calcaneus to the talus as seen from the front in the left foot.

A. In the normal foot the articular surface of the calcaneus for the cuboid is well to the lateral side of the long axis of the leg. **B.** In talipes equinovarus the medial rotation of the calcaneus in the horizontal plane displaces its posterior tuberosity laterally toward the fibular malleolus and brings the anterior end of the calcaneus beneath the head of the talus instead of lateral to it.

zontal plane. The heel tips into varus inclincation in a fashion very similar to what happens if one takes a banana and rotates it by one end while looking at the other.[413]

Simons and Sarrafian performed a microsurgical dissection on a seven-month-old stillborn fetus with camptomelic dysplasia. The most important pathologic finding was the marked rotation of the calcaneus beneath the talus around a vertical axis. The anterior half of the calcaneus was rotated medially and downward, whereas the posterior half was rotated laterally and upward. A posterior medial and plantar release failed to realign the hindfoot. The bones of the hindfoot could be repositioned only by a complete subtalar release.[603a] The fulcrum upon which the tarsal bones pivot beneath the talus is the interosseous ligament, which is made up of three separate ligaments: the posterior ligament of the talocalcaneal navicular joint, the anterior ligament of the subtalar (posterior talocalcaneal) joint, and the interosseous (cervical) ligament.

Relationship of Calcaneus to Cuboid Bone. The cuboid is dislocated medially in relation to the anterior end of the calcaneus, which is inclined inward. With adduction of the cuboid bone on the os calcis, the bifurcated ligament (calcaneocuboid and calcaneonavicular ligaments), long plantar ligament, plantar calcaneocuboid ligament, naviculocuboid ligament, inferior extensor retinaculum, dorsal calcaneocuboid ligament, and cubonavicular oblique ligament become contracted and thereby supinate and adduct the midfoot and forefoot. The cuboid is translated medially in relation to the anterior facet of the calcaneus, which is inclined inward.

With the medial and plantar subluxation of the talocalcaneonavicular joint, the bones in front of the transverse tarsal joint are adducted, medially rotated, and pitched in an equinus inclination.

Carroll and associates dissected feet of stillborn premature and full-term infants with talipes equinovarus, and demonstrated that the lateral malleolus is directed posteriorly, the head of the talus pointed laterally, and the navicular subluxated medially toward the medial malleolus. The anterior part of the calcaneus is pressed downward by the head of the talus, forced into plantar flexion, and rotated inward (Fig. 2–15). The longitudinal axes of the talus and calcaneus become superimposed and parallel. The equinus deformity and inversion of the calcaneus could not be corrected until the talus was derotated medially. Upon medial rotation of the talus and fixation of the head of the talus to the navicular, the foot assumed a normal appearance. By pushing the head of the talus laterally and fixing the navicular in a medially subluxated position, these investigators were able to produce equinus deformity of the ankle, varus deviation of the heel,

SOFT-TISSUE CHANGES

The soft tissues on the medial and posterior aspects of the foot and ankle are shortened. All the components of the tissues participate in the shortening—ligaments and capsules, muscles, tendons, tendon sheaths, vessels, nerves, and skin.

In talipes equinovarus, there are no gross abnormalities of the muscles, tendons, nerves, or vessels. Routine histologic stains have shown no pathologic changes.

Isaacs and co-workers studied the muscles in talipes equinovarus in 60 children, the majority of whom were under the age of five years. The muscle specimens were taken from the posteromedial and peroneal muscle groups, and occasionally from the abductor hallucis. Histologic and histochemical studies were performed in 111 biopsies, of which 53 specimens were examined by electron microscopy. Evidence of neurogenic disease was present in most instances. These abnormalities were found in both the shortened posteromedial (tibialis posterior, soleus, flexor digitorum longus, and flexor hallucis longus) and the lengthened peroneal muscle groups, indicating affection to a varying degree of all of the musculature between the knee and ankle.[300]

The muscle specimens studied by Isaacs and associates were not taken from fetal material; they were obtained at the operating table. There were, therefore, difficulties in distinguishing between congenital and adaptive changes. The neuropathic changes were more obvious in the older children. Isaacs and his co-workers' patients were treated soon after birth by gentle manipulation and stretching casts, which elongate the posteromedial muscles and relax the peronei. The pathologic changes were similar in both muscle groups and therefore not produced by physical trauma from stretching.[300] Scher, Handelsman, and Isaacs have investigated the effect on muscles of immobilization under tension and relaxation. Four young baboons had one foot immobilized in an extreme calcaneovalgus position. The casts were removed after periods of 8 to 25 weeks. Muscle biopsies were then taken from the posteromedial and peroneal muscle groups of both the immobilized and opposite control legs,

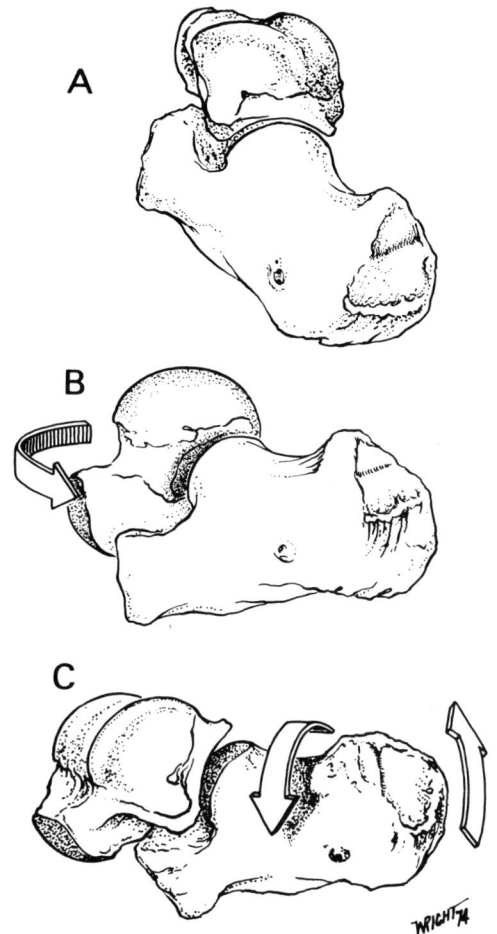

FIGURE 2–15. Pathomechanics of talipes equinovarus.

A. Posterolateral view of the calcaneus and talus of a normal foot. **B.** Lateral rotation of the talus. **C.** The anterior part of the calcaneus is pressed by the head of the talus and forced into plantar flexion, rotation, and varus position. (From Carroll, N., Murphy, R., and Leete, S. F.: The pathoanatomy of congenital clubfoot. Orthop. Clin. N. Amer., 9:227, 1978. Reprinted by permission.)

and adduction of the forefoot in the normal foot of the amputated leg of an eight-year-old boy. They noted the same articular relationships in a one-year-old child with recalcitrant talipes equinovarus. Re-examining patients with residual deformities of talipes equinovarus in the second and third decades of life, they found posterior displacement of the lateral malleolus, lateral direction of the head of the talus, and medial subluxation of the navicular.[98]

and were examined histochemically and under the electron microscope. There were no significant changes in any of the muscle groups. The conclusion was that immobilization and the altered muscle tension produced by serial casts in treatment of talipes equinovarus are not the cause of the reported muscle changes.[572]

Repeated forceful manipulations and bruising of the foot or prolonged immobilization of the foot and leg in extreme positions will lead to fibrosis of soft parts.

In the full-term infant, the leg with talipes equinovarus is atrophic and smaller in circumference than the contralateral normal one; in the young fetus, however, the deformed and the opposite normal limb are of the same size. The atrophic changes are generalized and do not involve any one muscle group. The individual muscles have a normal relationship to each other. The insertion of tendons is normal, but the direction of their course is somewhat altered. The *Achilles tendon* inserts more medially and anteriorly on the calcaneus owing to the medial shift of the posterior part of the heel. The *posterior tibial tendon* is displaced anteriorly; passing from its groove behind the medial malleolus, it courses directly downward to insert into the tuberosity of the navicular and other structures on the plantar aspect of the foot. The *anterior tibial tendon* is displaced medially and is prominent as a tense cord crossing over the medial malleolus to its insertion into the base of the first metatarsal and medial cuneiforms. The peroneal tendons appear to be stretched out on the convex lateral border of the foot. The long toe flexors are contracted. On the plantar aspect of the foot, because of the equinus deformity of the forefoot, the plantar fascia, abductor hallucis, short toe flexors, and abductor digiti quinti are shortened.

The soft-tissue contractures, in order of their importance as obstacles to reduction of the talocalcaneonavicular joint, are as follows: (1) the plantar calcaneonavicular ligament; (2) the tibionavicular ligament; (3) the superior, medial, and plantar parts of the talonavicular capsule; and (4) the posterior tibial tendon with its numerous tendinous slips inserting into the navicular and the plantar aspect of the foot. At their attachment to the navicular, these contracted soft-tissue structures are all fused together into a dense mass of fibrous tissue, tethering the navicular and the sustentaculum tali to the medial malleolus (Fig. 2–16). (5) The master knot of Henry is a fibrous slip that envelops the flexor hallucis longus and flexor digitorum longus tendons as they cross each other; it binds them to the undersurface of the navicular. In talipes equinovarus, this fibrous "knot" is very much thickened and prevents anterolateral mobility of the navicular. It must be sectioned during reduction of the talocalcaneonavicular joint.[70] Additional obstacles are (6) the calcaneofibular ligament, (7) the superior peroneal (calcaneofibular) retinaculum, (8) the posterior talocalcaneal ligament, (9) the posterior capsule of the tibiotalar joint, (10) the tendo Achillis, (11) the interosseous ligament, and (12) the long toe flexors. All these contracted soft tissues are very rigid and prevent concentric reduction of the talocalcaneonavicular joint.

The effect of manipulation on talipes equinovarus in fetal specimens has been reported by Waisbrod. In true talipes equinovarus with deformed tali (decreased angle of declination) the feet could not be manipulated into normal position even by

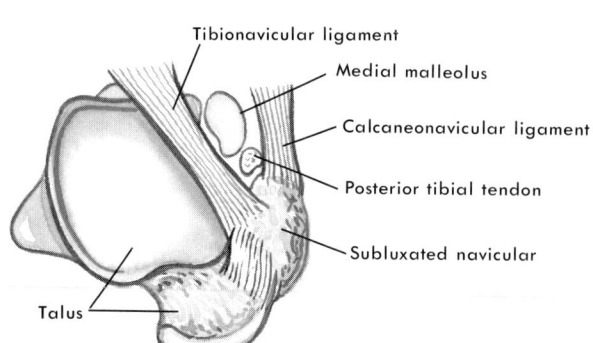

FIGURE 2–16. Primary obstacles to neutral realignment of the navicular on the head of the talus.

(1) The plantar calcaneonavicular ligament; (2) the tibionavicular ligament; (3) the superior, medial, and plantar parts of the capsule of the talonavicular joint; and (4) the posterior tibial tendon with its numerous tendinous slips inserting into the navicular and tethering the navicular to the medial malleolus.

exerting considerable force. When the tali were normal (in postural clubfoot), however, the feet could be manipulated into normal position without difficulty.[673] Irani and Sherman in their study of fetal specimens with talipes equinovarus state that, even after muscles were completely detached from their insertion, the position of the foot could not be corrected by manipulation; it was only after sectioning of all the ligaments between the talonavicular and calcaneonavicular joints together with posterior subtalar joint capsule that the equinovarus deformity could be completely corrected.[298, 299] Repeatedly, the author has observed the same phenomenon; that is, although all the muscles and tendons of the foot and ankle are detached in talipes equinovarus, the deformity of the foot persists; to obtain normal alignment of the talocalcaneonavicular joint, one has to section the ligaments between the talus and navicular, between the talus and calcaneus, and between the navicular and calcaneus, and has to divide the posterior ligaments and capsule of the ankle joint (peritalar release). The talus moves in a plane from anteromedial to posterolateral; therefore, the subtalar joint is always inverted with the talus in plantar flexion. To obtain correction of inversion and to unlock the inverted calcaneus underneath the talus, the equinus deformity must always be corrected.

For better understanding of articular malalignment in talipes equinovarus, the complex mechanism of the talocalcaneonavicular joint is reviewed next. The talocalcaneonavicular joint differs from the ordinary ball-and-socket articulation in that the socket moves around the ball (the head of the talus). The socket is formed anteriorly by the navicular; dorsomedially by the tibionavicular ligament, the capsule of the talonavicular joint, and the posterior tibial tendon; laterally by the calcaneonavicular limb of the bifurcated (Y) ligament; inferiorly by the plantar calcaneonavicular (spring) ligament and the anterior and middle facets on the superior surface of the calcaneus; and posteriorly by the talocalcaneal interosseous ligament. Because of their strong ligamentous connections, the calcaneus and the navicular move as a unit around the talus. The axis of rotation is the interosseous talocalcaneal ligament and the posterior subtalar joint, where minimal motion occurs. Horizontal movements take place at the talonavicular and the anterior and middle subtalar joints. In *eversion*, the navicular and anterior end of the os calcis move *laterally;* whereas in *inversion*, they move medially (Fig. 2–17). Inversion-eversion of the heel cannot take place if the talonavicular joint is internally fixed with a Steinmann pin.[354] Medial rotation of the calcaneus under the talus cannot be corrected unless the navicular is "released" to move distally and laterally on the head of the talus.

Upon plantar flexion and dorsiflexion

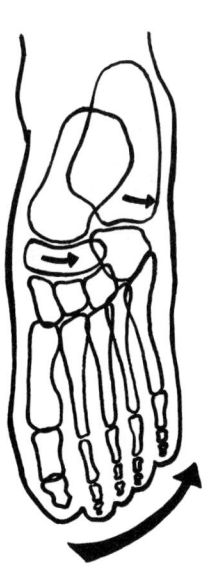 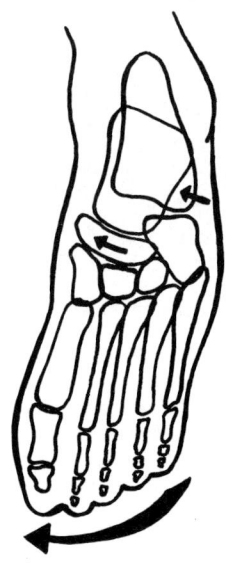

FIGURE 2–17. The calcaneus and navicular move as a unit because of their strong ligamentous connections.

In eversion, the navicular and anterior end of the os calcis move laterally; in inversion, they move medially.

of the ankle, both the tibiotalar and the talocalcaneonavicular joints move. During plantar flexion, the calcaneus supinates under the talus, with the anterior end moving plantarward and medially, while its posterior tuberosity moves dorsally and laterally. Simultaneously, the navicular moves medially on the head of the talus. During dorsiflexion, the calcaneus pronates under the talus with the anterior end of the calcaneus moving dorsally and laterally, while its posteromedial tubercle moves plantarward. Again simultaneously, the navicular moves laterally as the foot dorsiflexes. The talocalcaneonavicular joint expands and contracts because of its partial ligamentous composition. In dorsiflexion the greater portion of the talar head is covered, and the capacity of the talocalcaneonavicular socket is thereby increased; in plantar flexion, however, more of the talar head is exposed laterally, and the talocalcaneonavicular

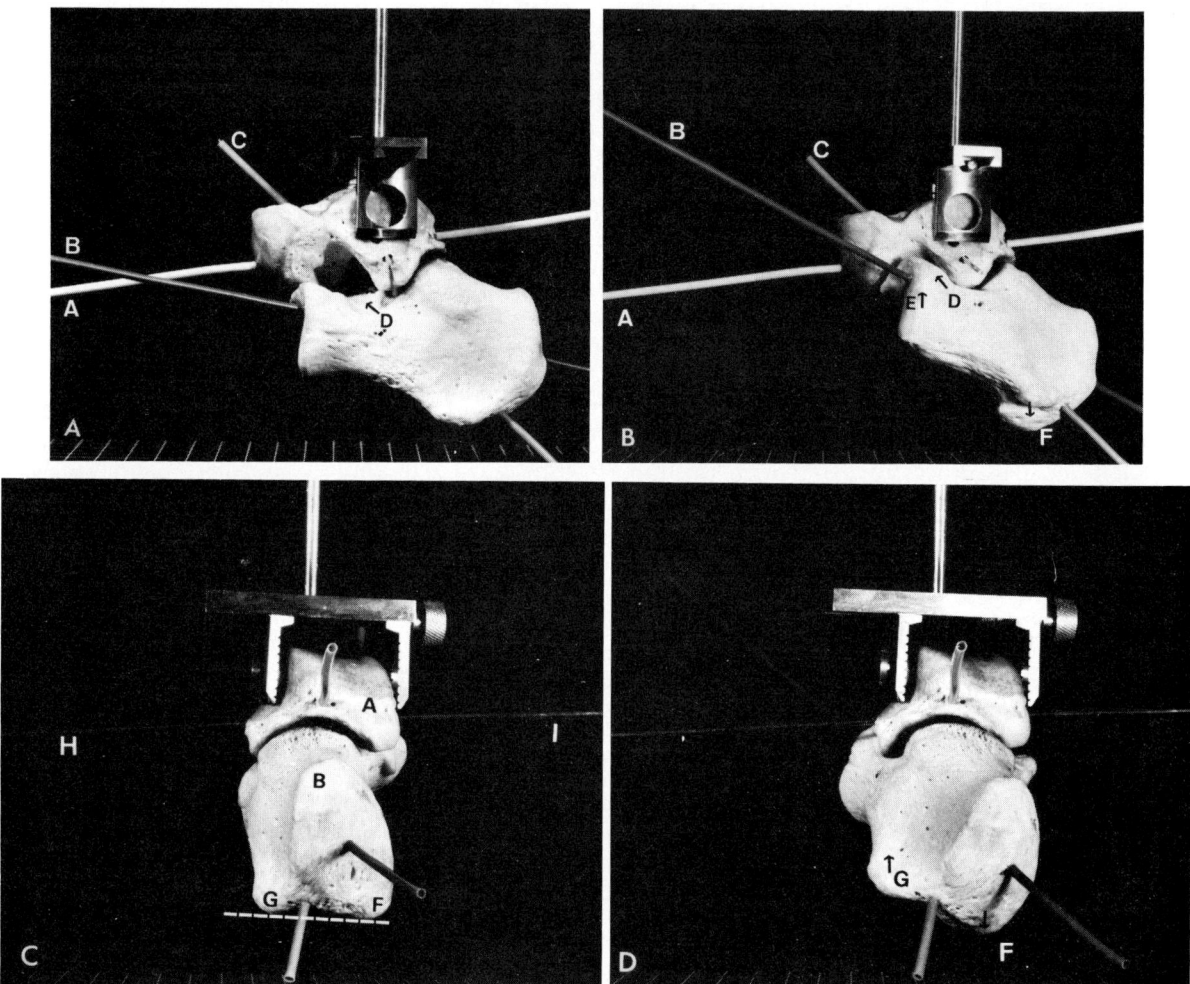

FIGURE 2–18. Movements of the calcaneus under the talus of the left foot.

Kirschner wires mark the longitudinal axes of the talus (A), calcaneus (B), and subtalar joint (C). G is the lateral and F the medial tubercle of the calcaneal tuberosity; E is the anterior end of the calcaneus. D marks the sinus tarsi. **A.** Lateral view in supination. The anterior end of the calcaneus moves in plantar flexion and the sinus tarsi is opened up. **B.** Lateral view in pronation. The sinus tarsi closes, the anterior end of the calcaneus is elevated into dorsiflexion, and the medial tubercle of the posterior tuberosity is displaced into plantar flexion. **C** and **D.** Posterior views of the left foot. In **C,** the cancaneus is in maximal supination—note that the lateral and medial tubercles of the posterior tuberosity of the calcaneus are at the same level. In **D,** the calcaneus is pronated—note the plantar migration of the medial tubercle.

Illustration continued on opposite page

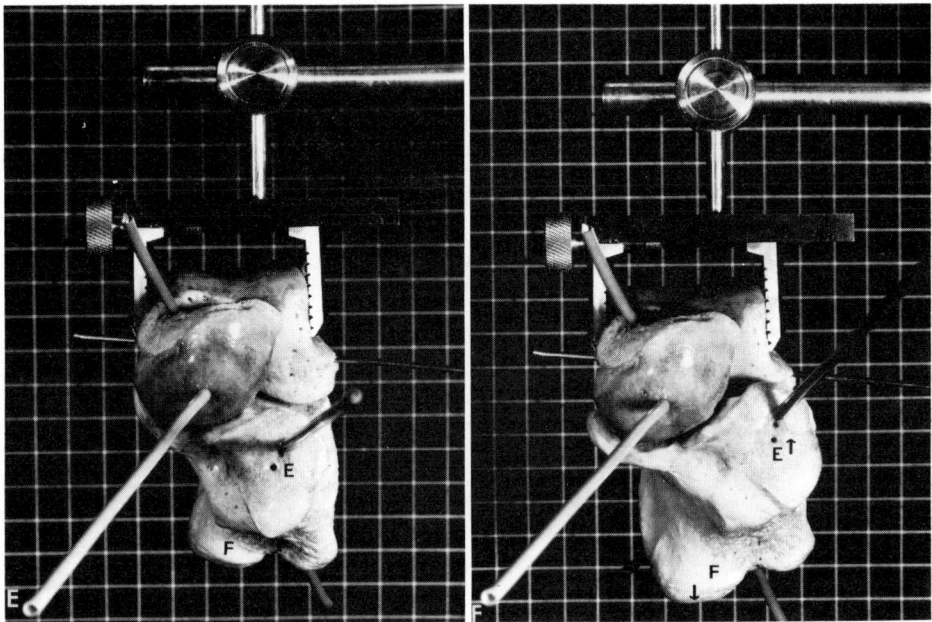

FIGURE 2–18 Continued. Movements of the calcaneus under the talus of the left foot.

E and **F.** Anterior views of the left foot. In **E** the calcaneus is supinated and in **F,** pronated. Note the same movements of the calcaneus under the talus. In transition from supination to pronation, the anterior end of the calcaneus (E) is elevated into dorsiflexion and the medial tubercle of the posterior tuberosity (F) is displaced into plantar flexion. (From Campos da Paz, A., Jr., and De Souza, V.: Talipes equinovarus: Pathomechanical basis of treatment. Orthop. Clin. N. Amer. 9:172–175, 1978. Reprinted by permission.)

socket is decreased in volume.[653–655] The calcaneus navigates under the talus like a boat on ocean waves. Its anterior end (the prow of the boat) pitches as its posterior end (the stern of the boat) plunges; and its body turns on itself.[178]

These complex movements of the calcaneus under the talus have been studied experimentally by Campos da Paz, Jr., and De Souza.[29] Indicating the longitudinal axes of the talus and calcaneus by Kirschner wires and marking the axis of the subtalar joint by a Kirschner wire that penetrates the superomedial aspect of the talar neck, crosses the sinus tarsi, and exits at the posteromedial tubercle of the calcaneus, they suspended the connected talus and calcaneus by a specially designed support and analyzed the movements of the calcaneus. Viewed from the lateral side, supination of the calcaneus opened up the sinus tarsi and lowered the anterior end of the calcaneus into plantar flexion (Fig. 2–18A). Pronation elevated its anterior end into dorsiflexion and depressed the medial tubercle of its posterior tuberosity where the Achilles tendon is inserted (Fig. 2–18B). Seen from behind when the calcaneus is in maximal supination, the lateral and medial tubercles of its posterior tuberosity are on the same level (Fig. 2–18C), whereas in pronation, the medial tubercle is depressed plantarward (Fig. 2–18D). One can best visualize the navigation of the calcaneus under the talus from the front; on transition from supination to pronation, the anterior end is raised superiorly (the pitching of the prow), and the insertion of the Achilles tendon at the medial tubercle of the tuberosity moves inferiorly (plunging of the stern) (Fig. 2–18 E and F). The anteroposterior talocalcaneal angle widens as the calcaneus is shifted from supination to pronation. It is evident, therefore, that to obtain pronation of the calcaneus, the medial tubercle of its posterior tuberosity should move inferiorly into plantar flexion. In talipes equinovarus, this can be accomplished only through lengthening of the triceps surae muscle and sectioning of the posterior contracted soft tissues that restrict dorsiflexion, namely, the posterior capsule of the ankle and subtalar joints, and

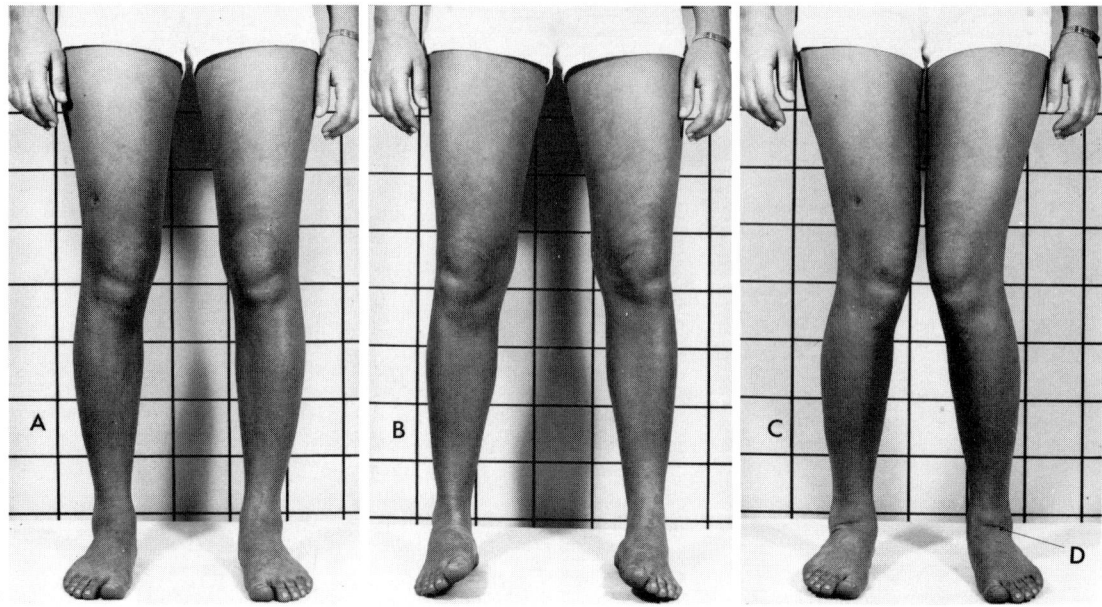

FIGURE 2–19. *The relationship of the calcaneus with the ground and the synchronized movements of the subtalar, ankle, knee, and hip joints.*

A. Normal. **B.** On inversion of the calcaneus, note the corresponding lateral rotation of the hip joints. **C.** On eversion of the calcaneus, the hip joints rotate medially. (From Campos da Paz, A., Jr., and De Souza, V.: Talipes equinovarus: Pathomechanical basis of treatment. Orthop. Clin. N. Amer., 9:177, 1978. Reprinted by permission.)

the posterior talofibular and calcaneofibular ligaments.

With the unified movements of the calcaneus and navicular, the talus and the related joints above the ankle—the knee and hip—move in synchrony. In stance, when the calcaneus of a normal foot is inverted, the anterior part of the calcaneus must first descend plantarward, and then rotate and move medially to lie underneath the head of the talus. Simultaneously, the talar head is elevated into dorsiflexion and moves laterally into lateral rotation; the malleoli rotate, the lateral malleolus moving laterally, and the medial malleolus moving anteriorly. Consequently, the whole leg and the hip rotate laterally, with the patellae facing outward (Fig. 2–19 A and B). On eversion of the calcaneus, a reverse chain of movements takes place—the lateral malleolus moves forward, the patellae face inward, and the hips rotate medially (Fig. 2–19C).

In talipes equinovarus with inversion of the calcaneus, by necessity the malleoli rotate around a vertical axis into lateral rotation. At birth the fibular malleolus is posterior in relation to the medial malleolus. To correct the position of the posteriorly rotated fibular malleolus the anterior end of the talus must be rotated medially (to "unlock" the hindfoot), and the anterior end of the calcaneus must be rotated laterally and elevated dorsally to lie on the lateral side of the head of the talus.

Rotational deformities of the lower limb in talipes equinovarus may be exaggerated during the course of inadequate management. The aggravating and causative factors are improper manipulation and stretching cast, walking on the varus hindfoot, and voluntary compensation at the hip for in-toeing. The levels of lateral rotation are at the ankle, hip, and tibiofibular articulations.

Wynne-Davies and more recently Swann, Lloyd-Roberts, and Catterall have pointed out the effect of improper manipulation and stretching casts on the ankle joint. With fixed contracture of the ligaments (tibionavicular, plantar calcaneonavicular, and talonavicular), correction does not take place at the talocalcaneonavicular joint. The abduction and lateral rotation forces are transmitted to the talus in the ankle mortise. The deformity remains uncorrected in the horizontal plane, and spurious correction

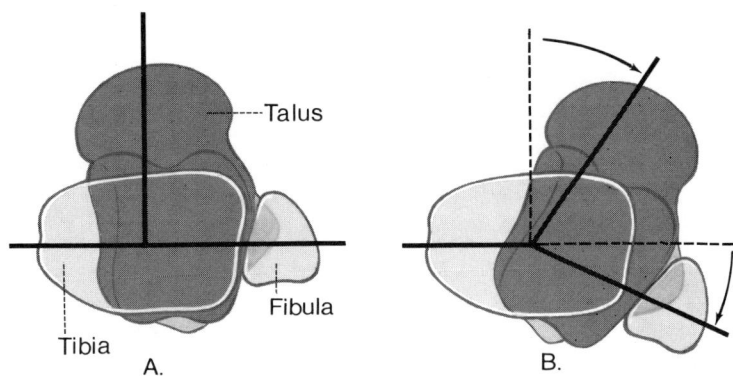

FIGURE 2–20. "Horizontal breach" according to the concept of Swann, Lloyd-Roberts, and Catterall.

A. A cross section through the distal tibia at the level of the ankle shows the normal position of the talus in the ankle mortise. **B.** A cross section through the distal tibia at the level of the ankle shows the position of the talus in the ankle mortise when the "horizontal breach" deformity has occurred. The talus rotates laterally and the fibula moves posteriorly while the tibia remains stationary. (Courtesy of Dr. George Simons.)

takes place at the ankle joint. The talus is rotated laterally in the ankle mortise, carrying the fibular malleolus posteriorly with it (Fig. 2–20). This is called "horizontal breach" by Swann, Lloyd-Roberts, and Catterall.[629, 713]

The already posteriorly positioned lateral malleolus is further displaced posteriorly by premature eversion of the hindfoot. In the lateral roentgenogram of the foot in a standing position this is easily identified by the posterior location of the fibular malleo-

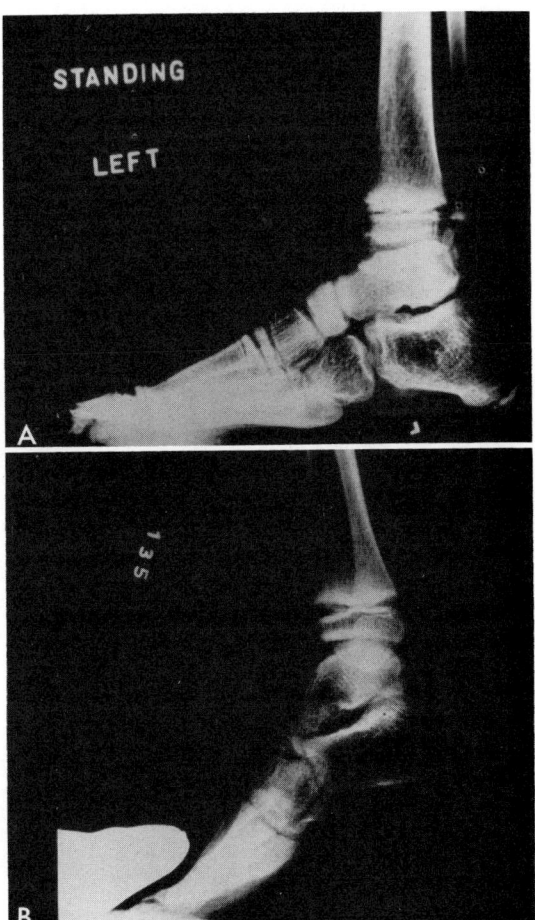

FIGURE 2–21. The roentgenographic appearance of "horizontal breach" in the lateral projection of the foot and ankle.

A. The fibular malleolus appears to have moved to a posterior position in relation to the medial malleolus. The dome of the body of the talus has assumed a "flat-top" appearance. The anteroposterior diameter of the calcaneus is shortened. **B.** In a lateral projection of the same foot and ankle after the foot has been medially rotated 45 degrees, the fibula has returned to its normal position in relation to the tibia, the shadow of the lateral malleolus overlaps that of the medial malleolus, the dome of the talus has been restored to its normal shape, and the anteroposterior diameter of the calcaneus is of normal length.

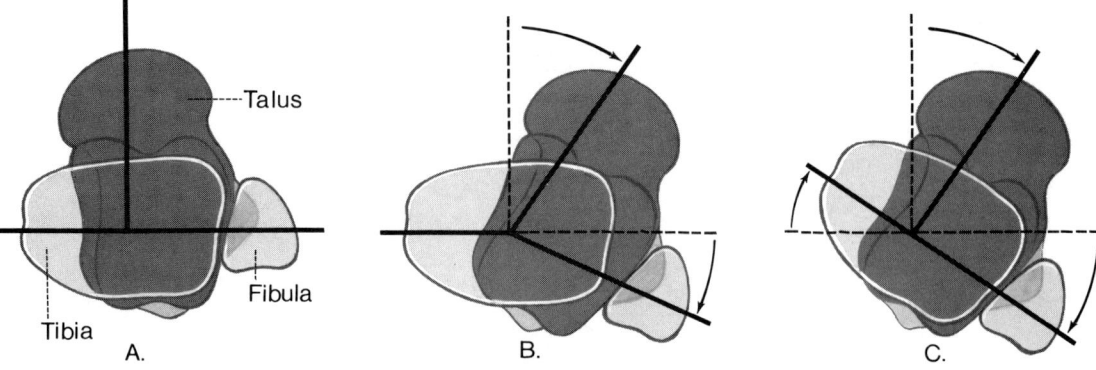

FIGURE 2–22. *Cross section through the ankle.*

A. The normal relationship of the talus in the ankle mortise (*shaded area*). **B.** The relationship of the talus in the ankle mortise when "horizontal breach" takes place. Note that the talus rotates laterally, the fibula moves posteriorly, and the tibia remains stationary. **C.** The relationship of the talus in the ankle mortise when compensatory lateral rotation occurs at the hip. Both the tibia and fibula have rotated laterally through the longitudinal axis of the tibia. The talus has maintained its normal relationship to the ankle mortise. (Courtesy of Dr. George Simons.)

lus in relation to the medial malleolus and the "flat-topped" appearance of the dome of the talus. The x-ray tube is centered on the hindfoot and ankle, with the foot as nearly as possible at a right angle to the leg. The calcaneus will appear shortened and the forefoot will look relatively normal. The flat-topped appearance of the talus is spurious, the result of its lateral rotation and projection in a frontal profile in the lateral roentgenogram. If another roentgenogram is taken with the leg internally rotated, the summit of the talus will be dome-shaped, and the length and contour of the calcaneus will improve. The forefoot varus inclination will be increased, as shown by the overlap of the cuboid and navicular bones on the calcaneus and talus (Fig. 2–21).

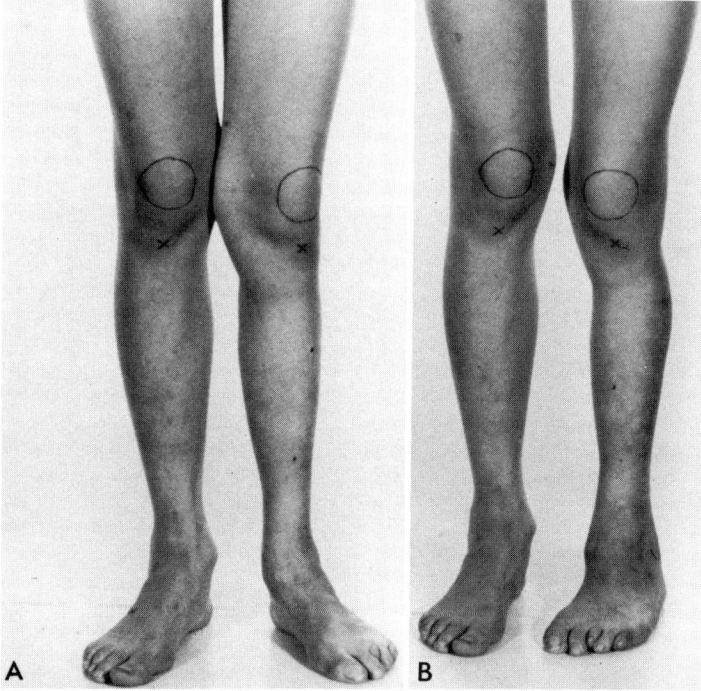

FIGURE 2–23. *Clinical and roentgenographic appearance of the left foot in a seven-year-old child with persistent medial subluxation of the talocalcaneonavicular joint.*

A. The medial border of the left foot is parallel to the sagittal plane and the foot is pointing forward. Note the patella of the affected limb is pointing laterally. The right foot is normal. **B.** Note the varus deformity of the left foot when the limb is medially rotated and the patella is facing straight forward.

Illustration continued on opposite page

Congenital Deformities 159

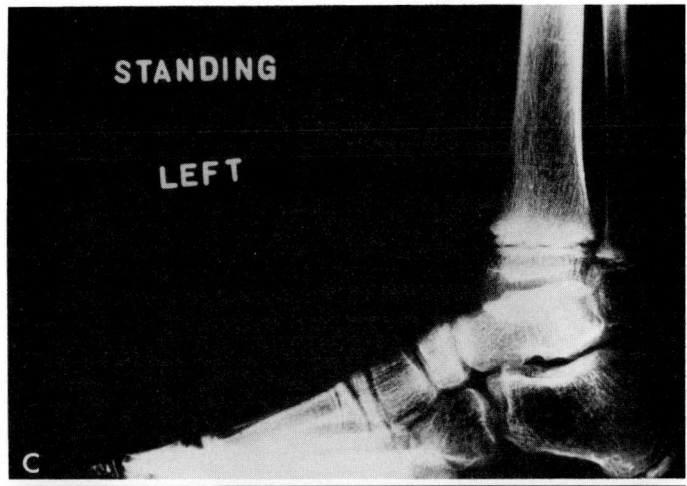

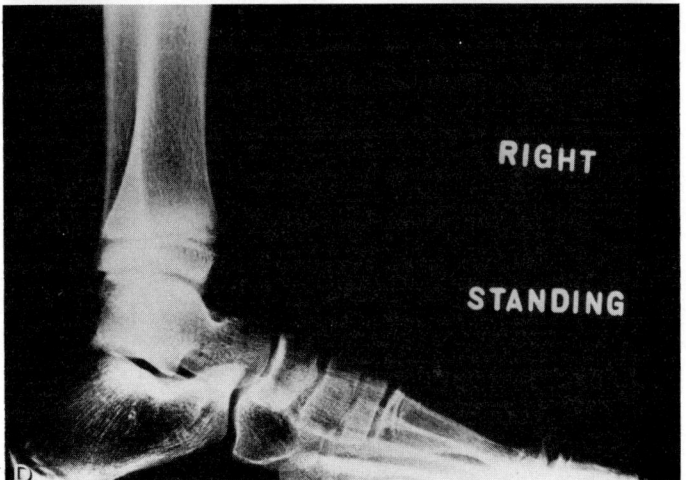

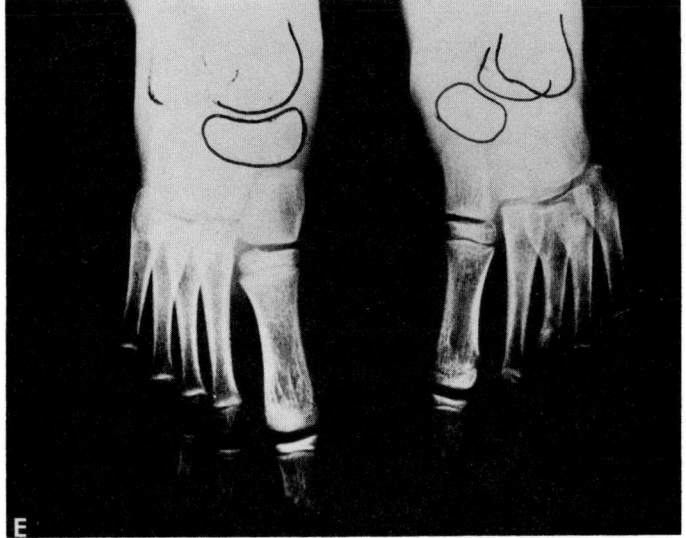

FIGURE 2–23 Continued. Clinical and roentgenographic appearance of the left foot in a seven-year-old child with persistent medial subluxation of the talocalcaneonavicular joint.

C. Lateral roentgenogram of the left ankle and foot with the toes facing straight forward. Note the posterior position of the fibular malleolus in relation to the medial malleolus and the flattening of the talar dome. **D.** Lateral roentgenogram of the normal right foot and ankle. **E.** Anteroposterior roentgenogram of both feet, showing medial subluxation of the navicular.

In addition to lateral rotation at the ankle joint, there may be sufficient rotatory force transmitted vertically along the longitudinal axis of the tibia and fibula to the hip joint to cause the entire lower limb to rotate laterally at the hip (Figs. 2–22 and 2–23). In walking, voluntary lateral rotation takes place at the hip to compensate for in-toeing due to the varus foot. With skeletal growth structural lateral tibiofibular torsion takes place in the older child.[600, 603]

In talipes equinovarus, reduction of medial and plantar subluxation of the talocalcaneonavicular joint is prevented by contracture of soft tissues. It behooves us to remember, when planning surgical division of these soft-tissue contractures, that motions of plantar flexion and inversion at the ankle and talocalcaneonavicular joint take place as synchronized and not as separate isolated movements.

The navicular is fixed to the medial malleolus and the sustentaculum tali of the os calcis by the contracted tibionavicular ligament, plantar calcaneonavicular ligament, dorsal medial capsule of the talonavicular joint, and posterior tibial tendon. For the calcaneus to move from supination to pronation and its anterior end to move from plantar flexion to dorsiflexion, the navicular should be released from these soft-tissue checkreins and positioned concentrically in relation to the head of the talus. This cannot be achieved by manipulative stretching in fetal specimens. It is only after the tissues have been sharply divided with a scalpel that one can position the navicular on the head of the talus.

In order to pronate the calcaneus under the talus and obtain normal divergence of the anteroposterior talocalcaneal angle, the posteromedial tubercle of the calcaneal tuberosity should move plantarward. This is prevented by the calcaneofibular ligament, the calcaneofibular retinaculum, the shortened Achilles tendon, and the contracted posterior capsule and ligaments. In fetal specimens with talipes equinovarus, isolated sectioning of the Achilles tendon will not permit dorsiflexion. One has to divide the posterior capsules of the ankle (tibiotalar) and the subtalar (talocalcaneal) joints, and the calcaneofibular ligament.

The interosseous talocalcaneal ligament is relaxed when the foot is in equinovarus posture. In talipes equinovarus, it may become contracted and may bind the inverted calcaneus under the talus. In such an instance, the interosseous talocalcaneal ligament must be sectioned to achieve reduction of the talocalcaneonavicular joint. The calcaneonavicular limb of the bifurcated, or Y, ligament connects the calcaneus to the lateral border of the navicular. When markedly contracted, it will obstruct lateral mobility of the navicular. It is evident, therefore, that to achieve concentric reduction of the talocalcaneonavicular joint, *all soft-tissue obstacles should be sectioned in one stage by complete peritalar release.*

The pathologic changes vary according to the severity of the bony and articular deformity and the degree of the soft-tissue contracture. The age of the patient and the type of prior treatment are also factors to consider.

Diagnosis

The clinical picture of talipes equinovarus is characteristic; the affected foot and leg have a clublike appearance (Fig. 2–24). The foot points plantarward with the small heel drawn up and rolled in under the talus in an inverted position. There are deep creases at the posterior aspect of the ankle joint. The mid- and forefoot are adducted, inverted, and have an equinus pitch. With the inversion of the entire foot and adduction of the forefoot, the anterior end of the talus is the most prominent subcutaneous bone on the lateral side of the dorsum of the foot. The skin in this convex area of the foot is thinned and stretched, and its creases have disappeared. The lateral malleolus is posterior to and more prominent than the medial malleolus. The skin creases are deeply furrowed on the concave medial and plantar aspects of the foot. The navicular bone abuts the anterior and medial margins of the medial malleolus; on palpation, one cannot insert a finger between the two bones. The forefoot is in equinus position, and the soft tissues on the plantar aspect of the foot are contracted.

On passive dorsiflexion and eversion of the foot, the taut triceps surae and posterior tibial tendon can be palpated. One can also feel the thickened and shortened ligaments and joint capsules on the medial aspect of the foot and the posterior aspect of the

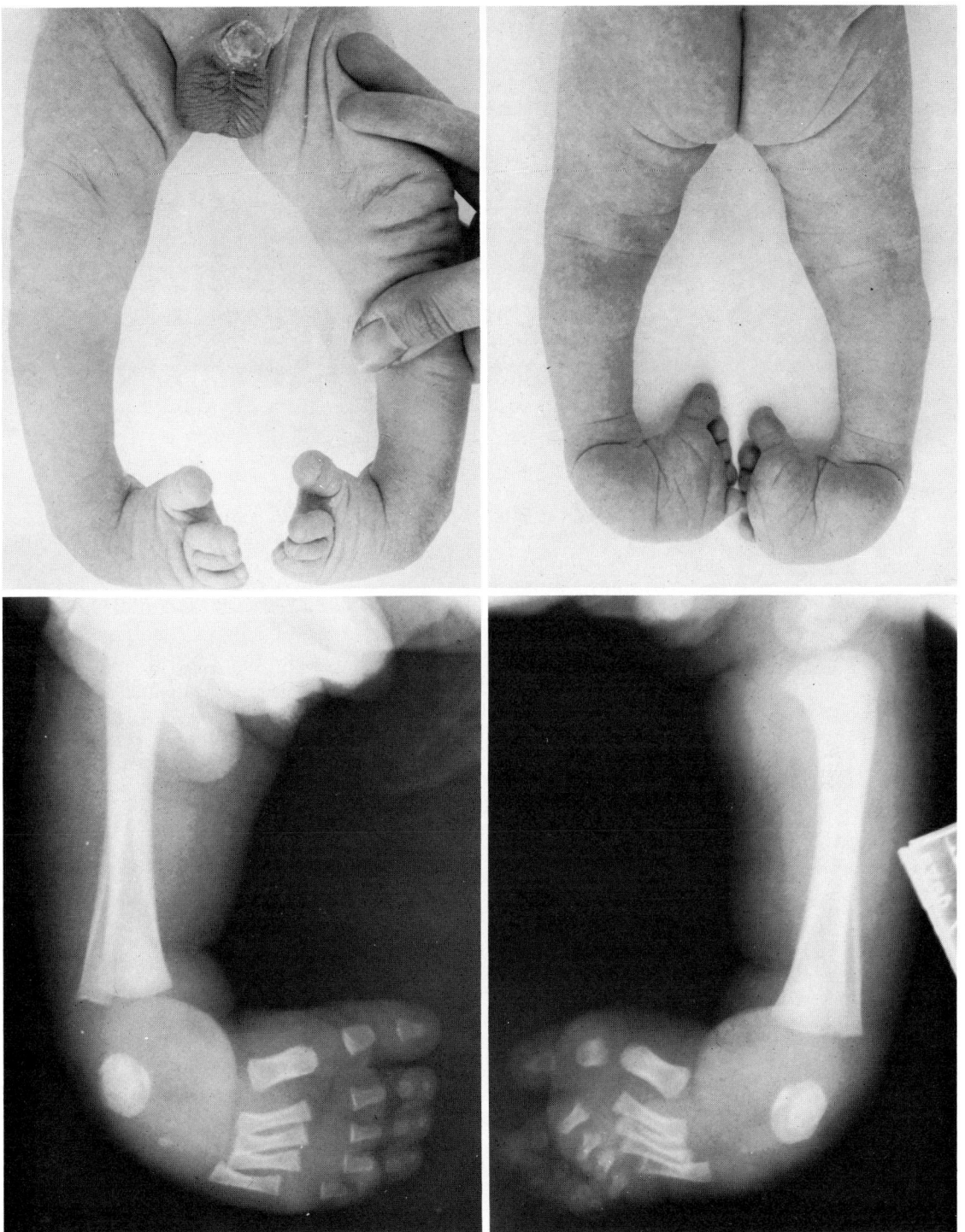

FIGURE 2–24. Bilateral talipes equinovarus in a newborn infant.

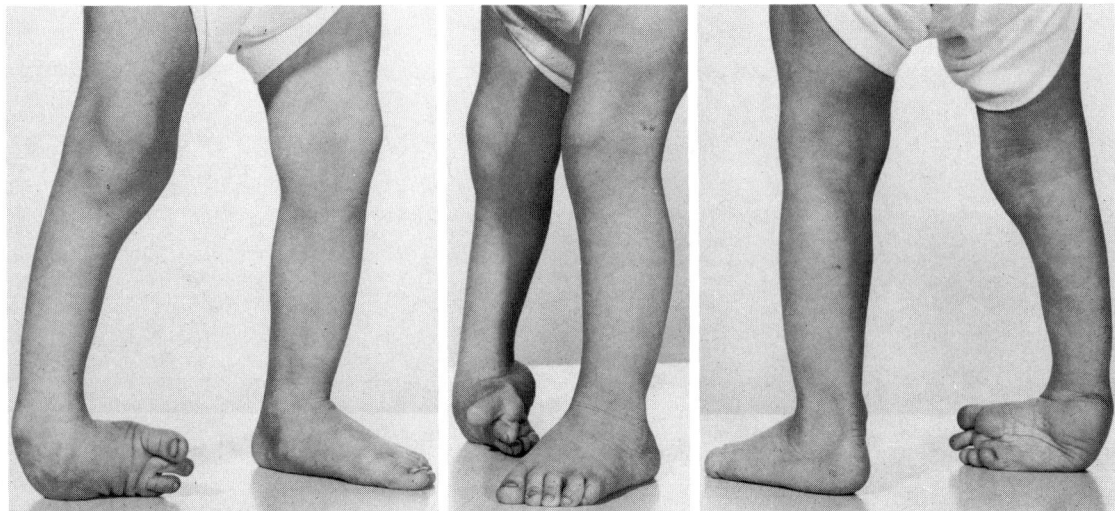

FIGURE 2–25. Untreated severe talipes equinovarus on the right in a three-year-old boy.
The body weight is borne on the lateral border of the foot.

ankle and subtalar joints. There is usually moderate to severe atrophy of the calf and a varying degree of shortening of the affected leg. The equinovarus deformity is fixed and can be corrected only minimally by passive manipulation. If talipes equinovarus remains untreated, the deformity will progressively increase and the contractures will become more rigid. The child will bear weight on the lateral border of the foot and on the fibular malleolus (Fig. 2–25). Ambulation will be difficult and the gait awkward. Soon painful callosities and bursae will develop over the lateral side of the foot.

It is important to differentiate talipes equinovarus from postural clubfoot (Table 2–6). In the latter, the deformity is mild and can be readily corrected to neutral position by passive manipulation. It most probably is caused by intrauterine malposture. Anatomically, the head and neck of the talus are not tilted medially and there is no subluxation or dislocation of the talocalcaneonavicular joint in postural clubfoot. Clinically, the skin creases on the dorsolateral aspect of the ankle and foot are normal, the heel is of normal size, and the leg is of normal circumference or minimally atrophied. On palpation, there is normal space between the navicular and the medial malleolus. The equinovarus deformity is relatively flexible and can be readily corrected to neutral position by passive manipulation. The opposite foot may be in valgus posture, and there may be associated pelvic obliquity with adduction contracture of the contralateral hip and adduction contracture of the ipsilateral hip.

The foot may have a clubfoot appearance in congenital absence or hypoplasia of the tibia and in congenital dislocation of the ankle. Careful palpation of the anatomic relationship of the hindfoot to the medial and lateral malleoli, and roentgenograms will establish the diagnosis.

Talipes equinovarus, a congenital deformity, must also be distinguished from acquired types of clubfoot. In the newborn this is relatively easy, but in the older child it may pose a problem. The spine should be carefully examined for abnormalities, and muscle testing should be performed. Roentgenograms of the entire vertebral column should be made (Fig. 2–26). The neuromuscular system should be carefully assessed to rule out paralytic disease. Paralytic clubfoot is seen in myelomeningocele, intraspinal tumors, diastematomyelia, poliomyelitis, the distal type of progressive muscular atrophy, cerebral palsy, and Guillain-Barré disease.

Not necessarily an isolated deformity, talipes equinovarus may be associated with multiple congenital malformations or be a part of a generalized developmental syndrome. At the Shriner's Hospital for Crip-

Table 2–6. *Differential Diagnosis of Postural Clubfoot and Talipes Equinovarus*

	Postural Clubfoot	**Talipes Equinovarus**
Etiology	Intrauterine malposture	Primary germ plasm defect Defective cartilaginous anlage of the talus
Pathologic Anatomy		
Head and neck of talus	Normal	Medial and plantar tilt
	Declination angle of talus normal 150 to 155 degrees	Declination angle of talus decreased 115 to 135 degrees
Talocalcaneonavicular joint	Normal	Subluxated or dislocated medially and plantarward
Effect of manipulation in fetal specimens	Normal alignment of foot can be restored	Talocalcaneonavicular subluxation cannot be reduced unless ligaments connecting navicular to calcaneus, talus, and tibia are sectioned and posterior capsule and ligaments divided
Clinical Features		
Severity of deformity	Mild and flexible	Marked and rigid
Heel	Normal size	Small, drawn up
Relation between navicular and medial malleolus	Normal space between two bones; can insert finger	Navicular abuts medial malleolus: finger cannot be inserted between two bones
Lateral malleolus	Normal position	Posteriorly displaced with anterior part of talus very prominent in front of it
Skin creases on		
Dorsolateral aspect of foot	Present; normal	Thin or absent
Medial and plantar aspects of foot	No furrowed skin	Furrowed skin
Posterior aspect of ankle	Normal	Deep crease
Calf and leg atrophy	None or very minimal	Moderate to marked
Treatment	Passive manipulation followed by retention by adhesive strapping, splint, or cast	Primary open reduction of talocalcaneonavicular joint often required; surgery is conservative Closed methods of reduction often unsuccessful Prolonged retentive apparatus essential
Prognosis	Excellent; result is normal foot	Poor with closed methods Prolonged cast immobilization results in smaller foot and atrophied leg

pled Children in Mexico City, 14.15 per cent of the 300 patients with talipes equinovarus had other associated congenital anomalies.[665] It therefore behooves us to examine the whole child.

The deformity is commonly encountered in arthrogryposis multiplex congenita. The hips, knees, elbows, and shoulders must be carefully examined for subluxation or dislocation. What is the range of motion of the peripheral joints? Is there any abnormal extension or flexion contracture? A marked decrease of muscle mass and fibrosis are characteristic of arthrogryposis multiplex congenita (Fig. 2–27).

Bartholine, in 1673, was the first to report

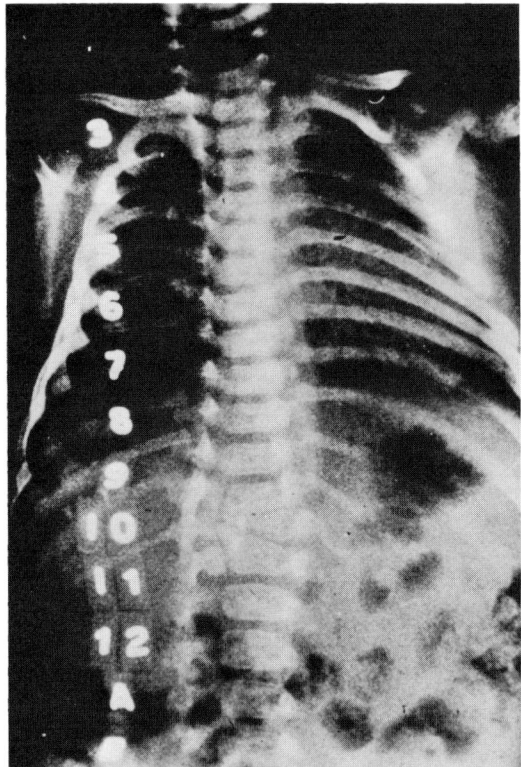

FIGURE 2–26. *Diastematomyelia of the spine at T_{12}–L_1 level in a newborn infant with bilateral severe talipes equinovarus.*

The spine should be carefully examined for abnormalities.

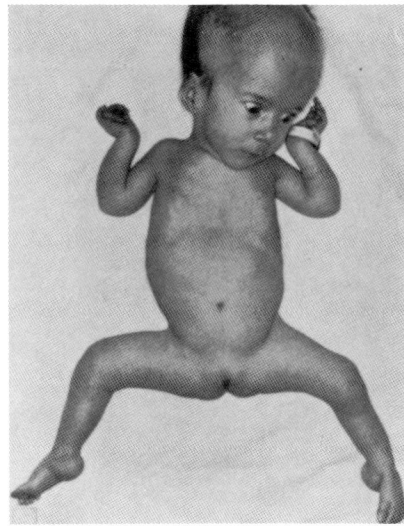

FIGURE 2–27. *An infant with arthrogryposis multiplex congenita.*

Note the bilateral talipes equinovarus. Both hips are dislocated. The knees are fixed in extension. The radial heads are dislocated. The fingers are clenched in the palm and the thumbs adducted.

association of clubfoot with congenital amputation.[28] Clubfoot is also frequently found along with congenital annular constriction bands (Streeter's dysplasia) (Fig. 2–28). Cowell and Hensinger reviewed 25 cases of congenital annular bands of the limbs and found clubfeet in 56 per cent of them.[123] The frequent association of these two congenital malformations can be expained by early rupture of the amnion with formation of amniotic bands and oligohydramnios.[644, 645] In experiments performed on rats, clubbing of the paws was produced by removal of amniotic fluid during gestation.[141]

"Clubfoot" is frequently encountered in other syndromes. *Diastrophic dwarfism* is manifest at birth and is characterized by small stature; soft cystic masses in the auricle, which later develop into hypertrophic cartilage and give cauliflower deformity of the pinnae; cleft palate; marked shortening of the first metacarpals with proximally set hypermobile thumbs; flexion contracture and varying degrees of webbing of the knees, hips, elbows, shoulders, and interphalangeal joints; and progressive kyphoscoliosis (Fig. 2–29). The equinovarus deformity of the feet is severe and bilateral, and there is increased space between the hallux and second toe. In the roentgenograms, the metatarsals and phalanges appear shortened with widened metaphyses; the first metatarsals are particularly short.[355, 361, 675]

In *Freeman-Sheldon syndrome* (craniocarpotarsal dysplasia), the facies is characteristic. The full forehead, deeply set eyes, flattened midface, and small mouth with protuberant lips give a "whistling" appearance (Fig. 2–30). There may be an H-shaped cutaneous crease pattern on the chin. The palate is high and the speech nasal because motion of the palate is limited. The fingers are deviated upward. Associated with the equinovarus deformity is flexion contracture of the toes[86, 107, 196, 235, 413, 684]

Larsen's syndrome is characterized by multiple joint dislocations (especially of the knees, hips, and elbows), a flat facies with depressed nasal bridge, prominent forehead, widely spaced eyes, and shortened

Text continued on page 169

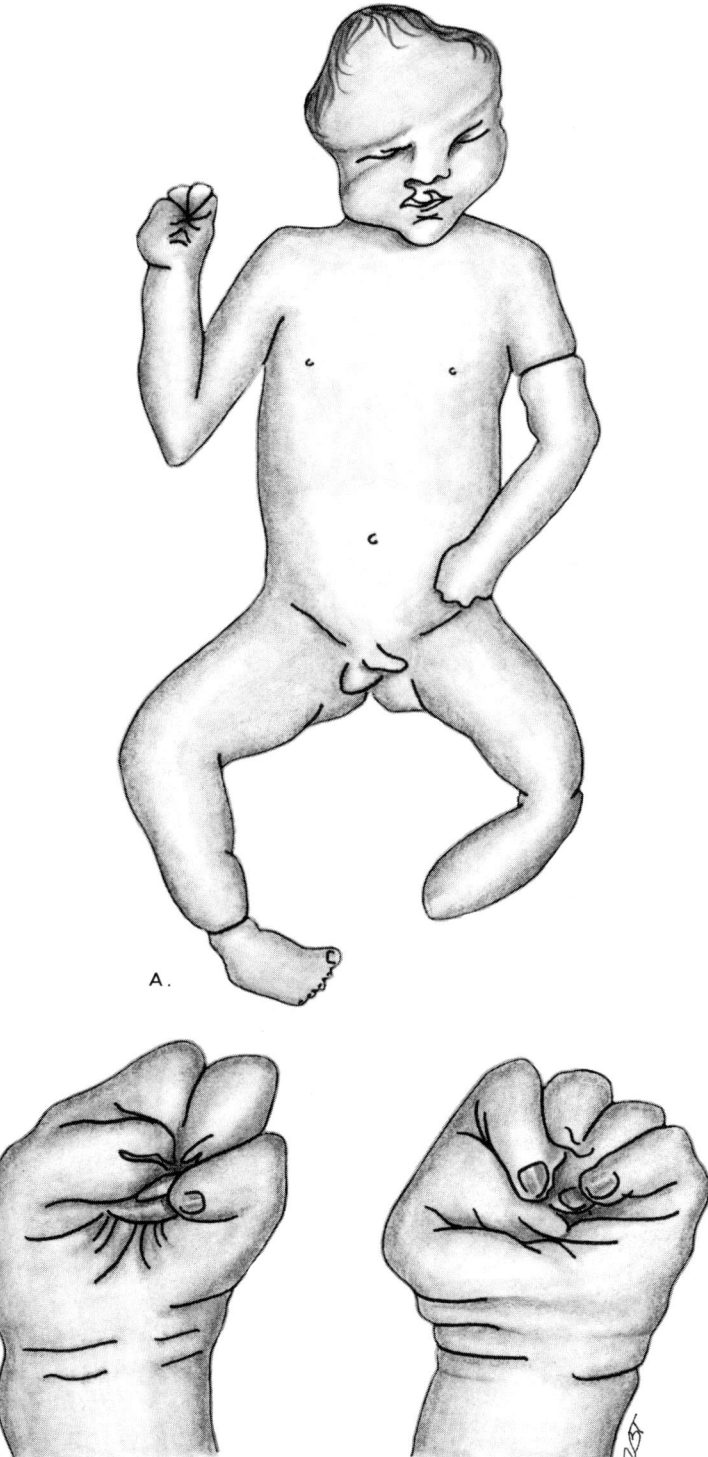

FIGURE 2–28. *Talipes equinovarus in an infant with Streeter's dysplasia.*

A. Note the constriction band on the lower leg on the right. **B** and **C.** Deformities of the hands.

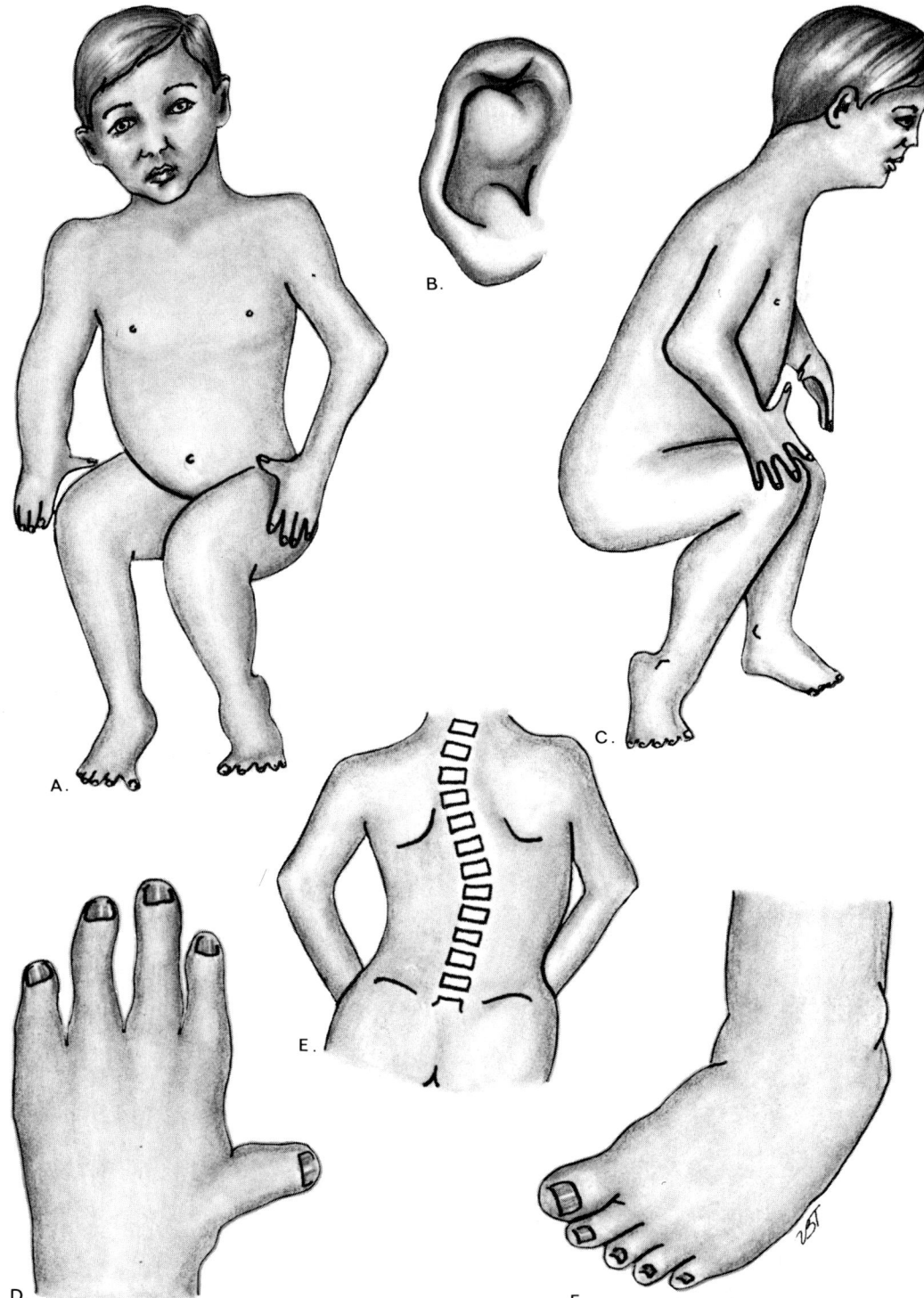

FIGURE 2–29. Diastrophic dwarfism.

Typical physical findings include: **A,** small stature; **B,** auricular masses that give cauliflower deformity of the pinnae; cleft palate; **C,** flexion contracture and varying degrees of webbing of the knees, hips, elbows, shoulders, and interphalangeal joints; **D,** marked shortening of the first metacarpals with proximally set hypermobile thumbs; **E,** progressive kyphoscoliosis; and **F,** severe bilateral equinovarus deformity of the feet.

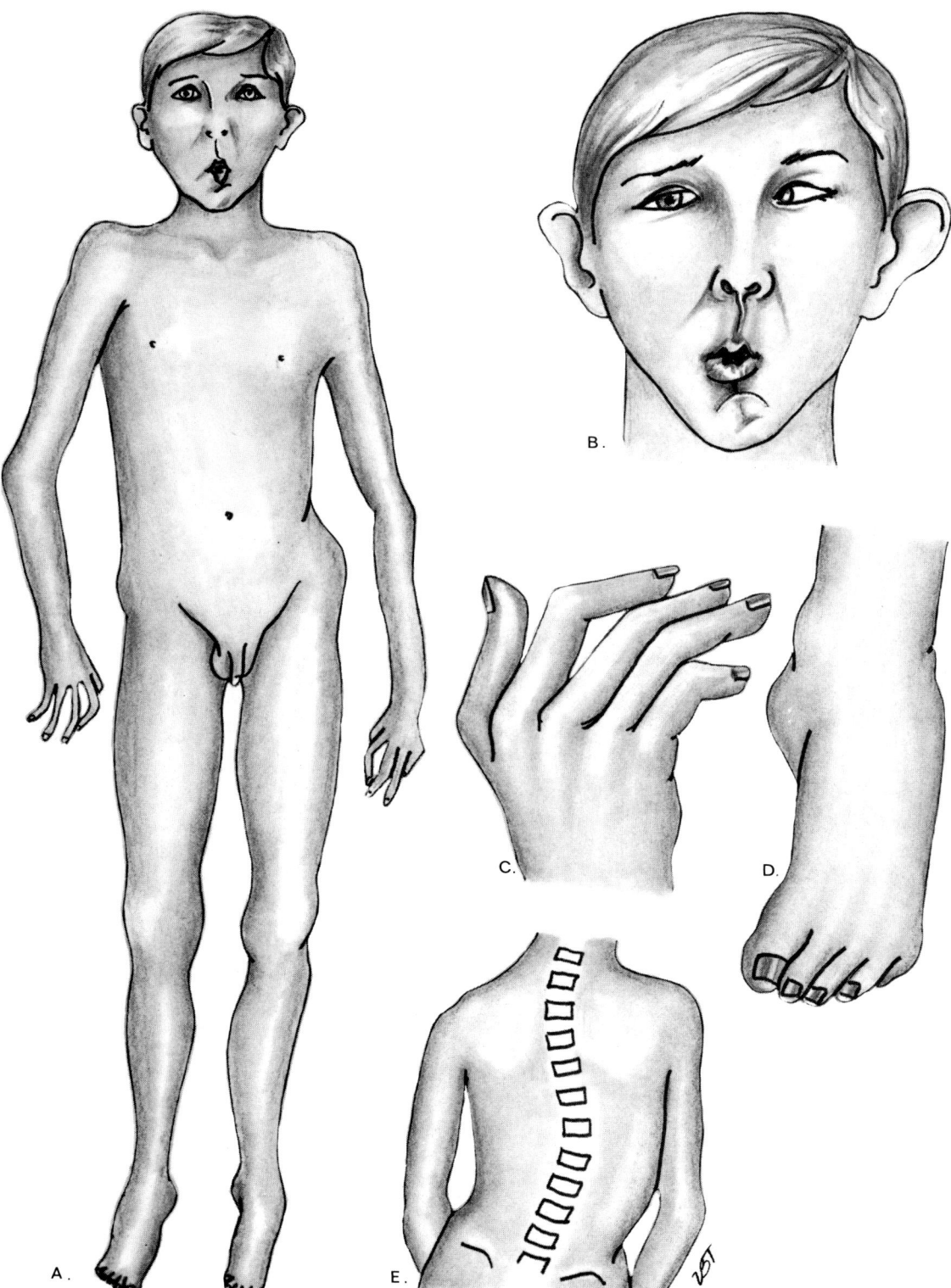

FIGURE 2–30. *Freeman-Sheldon syndrome (craniocarpotarsal dysplasia).*

A and **B.** Characteristic findings include full forehead, deeply set eyes, flattened midface, and small mouth with protuberant lips that give a "whistling" appearance. **C.** The fingers are deviated ulnarward, and there are equinovarus deformity and flexion contracture of the toes, **D,** and scoliosis, **E.**

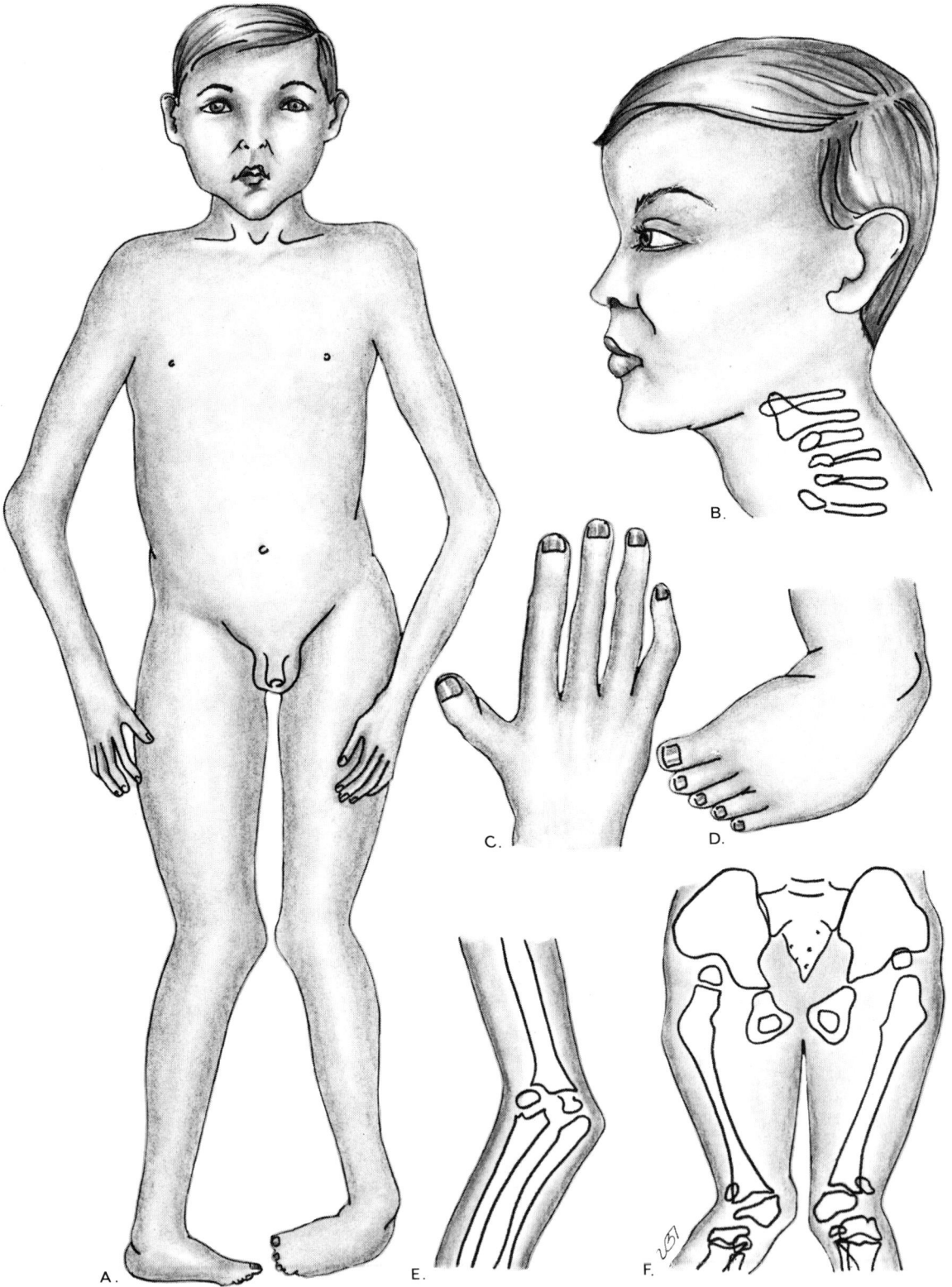

FIGURE 2–31. Larsen's syndrome.

Note the flat facies with depressed nasal bridge and prominent forehead, multiple joint dislocations (knees, hips, and elbows), and vertebral malformations (scoliosis).

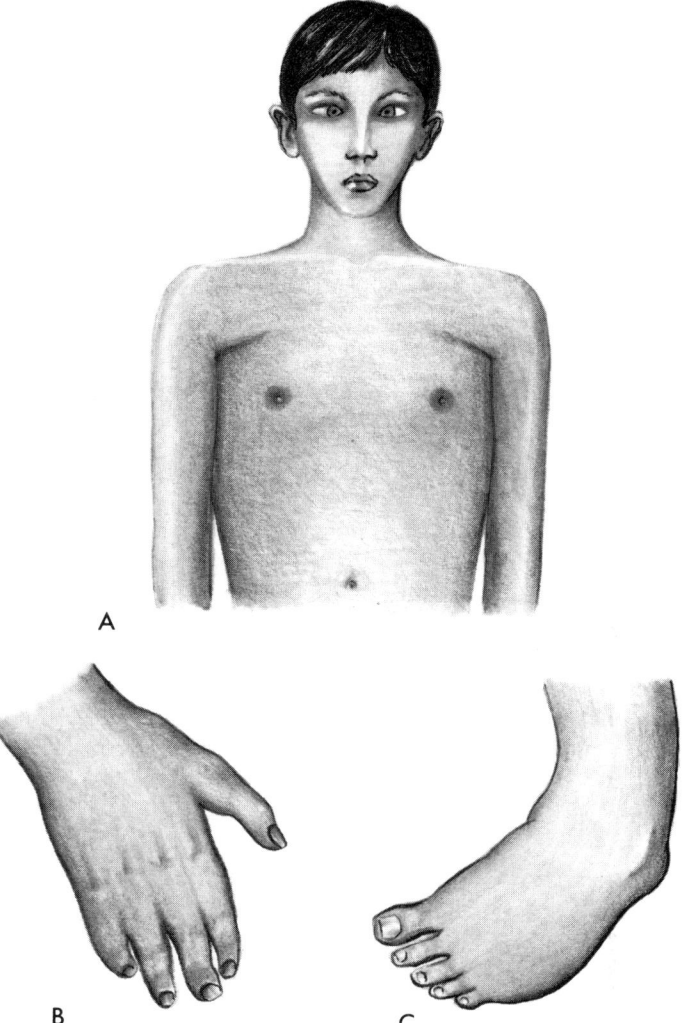

FIGURE 2–32. *Möbius syndrome.*

Note the masklike facies and loss of abduction of the eyes. There is partial or complete facial nerve paralysis. The pectorialis major muscle is absent, and there is syndactyly with bony ankylosis of the proximal interphalangeal joints. One third of the patients have talipes equinovarus.

metacarpals with spatulate thumbs (Fig. 2–31). The ossification centers of the carpus and tarsus may be multiple. Kyphoscoliosis with vertebral malformations is not uncommon.[364, 620]

About one third of the patients with *Möbius syndrome* have talipes equinovarus. The characteristic stigmata of Möbius syndrome are the masklike facies with loss of abduction of the eyes and partial or complete facial nerve paralysis. The affection is usually bilateral and is caused by agenesis or hypoplasia of the sixth and seventh cranial nerve nuclei. Other anomalies of the limbs are syndactyly with bony ankylosis of the proximal interphalangeal joints, absence of the pectoralis major muscle, microdactylia, and failure of development of the three lateral metatarsal rays or absence of all phalanges (Fig. 2–32).[455, 545] *Long arm 18 deletion syndrome* and *aminopterin-induced syndrome* are some other disorders in which multiple malformations, among them talipes equinovarus, are found. (For a complete list, the reader is referred to the textbook of D. W. Smith, *Recognizable Patterns of Human Malformation*).[589] When clubfoot is associated with other anomalies, or the infant does not look otherwise normal, it is advisable to obtain genetic consultation. The initial management of talipes equinovarus in these syndromes follows the same principles outlined for isolated talipes equinovarus. Generally, however, they have a poorer prognosis, and their early detection will guard against future embarrassment.

Roentgenographic Assessment

The purpose of roentgenography is to define precisely the anatomic relationships of talocalcaneonavicular, tibiotalar, midtarsal, and tarsometatarsal joints. Historically, Barwell (in 1896) was the first to propose the value of roentgenography in the assessment of correction of clubfoot; he used both anteroposterior and lateral views, but did not make angular measurements.[30] In 1932, Wisbrun described the use of the talocalcaneal angle in the anteroposterior (dorsoplantar) projection.[707] Kite and Kandel confirmed the method and stressed the importance of the divergence of the longitudinal axes of the talus and the calcaneus.[320, 331-334] Cabanac and associates, and later Heywood, utilized the talocalcaneal angle in the lateral projection, both in plantar flexion and in dorsiflexion.[88, 268]

In the literature, numerous angle measurements for assessing talipes equinovarus have been described. These are summarized in Table 2–7. Special views such as the suroplantar view described by Klieger and Mankin, and the posterior tangential view are utilized, as are the special techniques of tomography, arthrography, arteriography, and recently, computed tomography (CT scan).[38, 51, 275-277, 347, 484, 523, 619]

Roentgenograms are indicated in talipes equinovarus to assess the degree of subluxation of the talocalcaneonavicular joint and the severity of the deformity before commencing treatment; to provide an accurate guide to progress during the course of closed nonoperative treatment; to ascertain whether reduction of the talocalcaneonavicular dislocation and normal articular alignment have been achieved; to analyze the composite deformities preoperatively and to plan operative treatment accordingly; to determine intraoperatively whether concentric reduction of the talocalcaneonavicular joint has been obtained; and to ascertain postoperatively whether normal articular alignment is being maintained.

In infancy, the primary centers of ossification of the talus, calcaneus, and cuboid bone are well-developed and visible in the plain roentgenograms; frequently the third cuneiform may be present. The metatarsals and phalanges are also ossified. The navicular is cartilaginous and, like the nonossified femoral head in the first six months of life in congenital dislocation of the hip, is not visualized in the roentgenograms. The ossification center of the tarsal navicular appears at about three years of age, initially beginning in its lateral quadrant; however, the navicular may not ossify before four years of age or even later.[323] Therefore, lines should be drawn and measurements of angles made to determine the articular relationships in the talocalcaneonavicular joint. It should be remembered that only the small centers of ossification are visualized in the x-ray; the entire bone is not observed, as the surrounding large mass of cartilage has the same density as the soft tissues. An additional difficulty is the delay of skeletal maturation of the tarsus in talipes equinovarus.[375]

TECHNIQUE OF ROENTGENOGRAPHY

In the literature, various methods of roentgenographic assessment of talipes

Table 2–7. Normal Values of Angular Measurements on Anteroposterior and Lateral Projections of Feet

	Normal Range (Degrees)
Anteroposterior View	
Talocalcaneal (T-C)	20 to 50
Talo–first metatarsal (T-MT$_1$)	0 to −20
Talo–fifth metatarsal (T-MT$_5$)	0
Lateral View	
Talocalcaneal (T-C)	25 to 50
Tibiotalar	70 to 100
Tibiocalcaneal (maximal dorsiflexion)	25 to 60
Talocalcaneal Index	
(Sum of T-C angles in anteroposterior and lateral projections)	Greater than 40

equinovarus have been described. It is imperative in these studies that the patient's feet be placed in identical positions and that a standard technique be utilized. This author recommends placing the feet in the maximally corrected position, according to the technique described by Simons.[602] Roentgenograms taken when the feet are not bearing weight or are unstressed do not show the relationship of tarsal bones in the corrected position and are therefore of no value in assessing the correction of deformities.

Positioning. Two persons position the child, preferably a parent and an x-ray technician who is properly instructed by the surgeon. The parent, the child, and the technician should be adequately shielded to minimize the dangers of irradiation. The child is placed in a sitting posture with his knees and hips flexed at right angles; the feet rest on the cassette with their medial borders parallel and touching each other. The forefoot is manually pushed into maximal abduction, and the ankle into maximal dorsiflexion (preferably 15 to 20 degrees), or as close to it as the equinus deformity will allow. If the equinovarus deformity is fixed, or the child is uncooperative, each foot is held manually in a maximally corrected position; often it is necessary to make a separate exposure of each foot. A translucent splint may be used to hold the foot in the maximally corrected position. An anteroposterior roentgenogram is made with the x-ray tube directed craniad 30 degrees from the perpendicular toward the dome of the talus and centered on the hindfoot.

For the lateral projection, the cassette is placed on a slotted board or vertical cassette holder for stability. The patient straddles it with the medial border of his *hindfoot* parallel to the edge of the cassette. A maximal dorsiflexion view is made with the leg flexed forward at the ankle without raising the aligned heel off the cassette (the position of the hindfoot is double-checked to assure that it is not elevated). It is essential to have proper alignment of the ankle mortise. It may be necessary to rotate the limb medially 20 to 50 degrees, depending upon the severity of the varus deformity. The x-ray tube is centered on the hindfoot, perpendicular to the cassette.

Films that are not made by the standardized technique should not be accepted. Clues by which improper technique can be recognized are as follows. In the anteroposterior view, the anterior ends of the talus and the calcaneus are at different levels (difference greater than 2 to 3 mm.). This indicates either that the foot was malpositioned in plantar flexion or that the x-ray tube was not tilted craniad at 30 degrees. When the ankle is dorsiflexed inadequately, the shafts of the tibia and the fibula are visualized. In both instances, there will be a spurious decrease in the talocalcaneal angle. On dorsiflexion of the ankle, the anterior end of the calcaneus moves medially, opening the talocalcaneal angle. Marked overlapping of the metatarsals indicates an inverted foot. This appearance may be due to fixed varus deformity or to inverted posture of the foot during x-ray exposure. An inverted posture of the foot diminished the talocalcaneal angle. The roentgenographic findings and the clinical appearance of the foot should always be compared and double-checked.

In the lateral view, improper technique is suggested by an extreme posterior position of the fibula and the lateral malleolus in relation to the tibia and medial malleolus, which suggests that the ankle mortise and the hindfoot were in lateral rotation. In the presence of varus deformity of both forefoot and midfoot, the whole foot should not be placed parallel to the cassette, as this will force the hindfoot into external rotation. It is the hindfoot that should be placed parallel to the cassette. If the metatarsals do not overlap and are tiered, it means the foot was inverted when the film was made. The tibiotalar angle in the x-ray should be compared with the clinical range of ankle dorsiflexion.

The accuracy of the preceding technique of two-plane roentgenography may be affected by two factors: (1) movement of the foot as a unit with no motion between the individual bones, and (2) movement of the foot with motion taking place between the individual bones. Malpositioning of the foot or change in its position by active motion by the patient prior to film exposure will give a difference between the true angle and the angle that is recorded on the roentgenogram. The experienced technician will see to it that errors in positioning are very minor and will detect and check any significant movement by the patient. Simons has shown mathematically that angle variance (i.e., the difference between the true anatomic angle and the apparent angle on the x-ray) due to minor mistakes of positioning and movement is relatively small and of no practical significance.[602]

During interosseous movement, the true anatomic angle changes; therefore the degree of angle variance due to malposition and the degree due to motion between the individual bones are difficult to determine. Reimann estimated variations in angular measurement from one exposure to another in ten children with talipes equinovarus. Roentgenograms were made twice, either on the same day or on two consecutive days. The difference between measured values was insignificant.[539] Simons believes the accuracy of the technique described is similar to that of Reimann's method.[602]

Measurement of Angles. In the anteroposterior view, the talocalcaneal angle is measured as follows: in the infant, it is best to trace the outline of the ossific nuclei of the calcaneus and talus with a soft lead pencil. The ossified talus is usually pear-shaped, narrower in front than behind. On its medial and lateral margins, two points are made anteriorly and two points posteriorly. The longitudinal axis of the talus is determined by drawing a line between points made midway between each of the two sets of marginal points. The longitudinal axis of the calcaneus is made by drawing a line parallel to its lateral border. Because its medial border is irregular and somewhat indistinct, this is more accurate than drawing a line between the midpoints of the margins of the calcaneus (Fig. 2–33).

In the normal foot, the long axis of the talus points medially toward the first metatarsal and that of the calcaneus laterally toward the fifth metatarsal, forming a V. This talocalcaneal angle normally measures 20 to 40 degrees, as shown in Figure 2–33.

In talipes equinovarus with inversion of the heel, the talocalcaneal angle diminishes and may approach zero. In severe inversion of the hindfoot, the longitudinal axes of the talus and the calcaneus may become superimposed and point laterally to the fourth or fifth metatarsal (Figs. 2–34 and 2–35). As

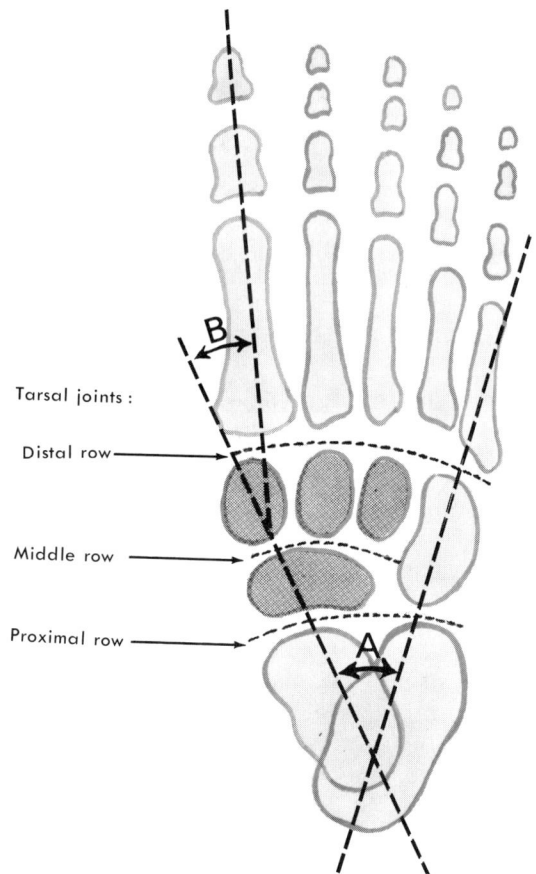

FIGURE 2–33. Measurement of angles in the roentgenogram of the normal foot.

In the anteroposterior view the long axis of the talus points medially toward the first metatarsal and that of the calcaneus laterally toward the fifth metatarsal, forming the talocalcaneal angle, A, which normally measures 20 to 40 degrees. The angle formed between the longitudinal axis of the talus and that of the first metatarsal is called the talo–first metatarsal (or TMT_1) angle, B. It normally measures zero to minus 15 degrees.

the inversion of the heel is corrected, the head of the talus no longer lies on top of the calcaneus, but projects medially, giving a normal talocalcaneal angle.

The longitudinal axis of the first metatarsal is drawn through the center of the bone. The angle formed between the longitudinal axis of the talus and that of the first metatarsal is called the talo–first metatarsal (or $T\text{-}MT_1$) angle. It normally measures zero to minus 15 degrees (cf. Fig. 2–33). A more negative angle than minus 15 degrees indicates varus deviation of the midfoot or forefoot (Fig. 2–34, angles A and B). In the

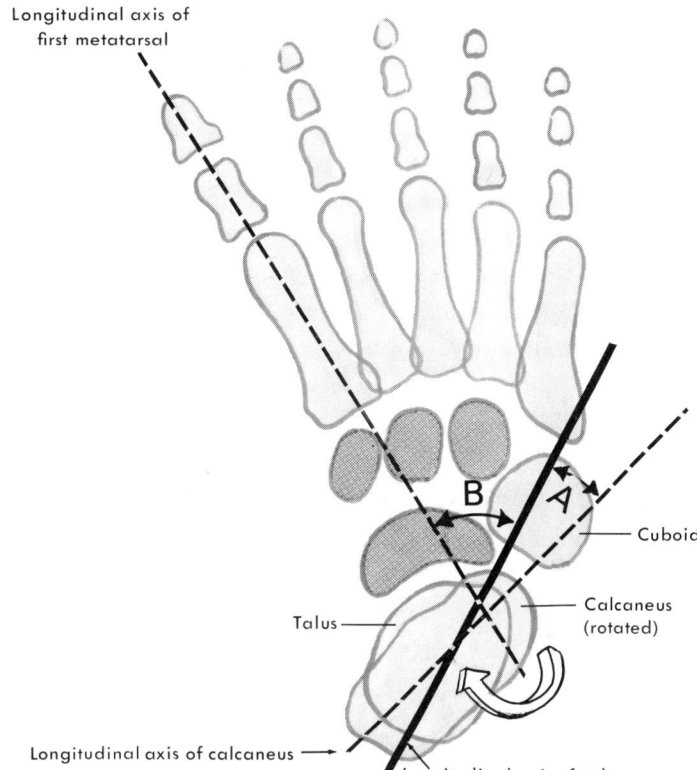

FIGURE 2–34. Measurement of angles in talipes equinovarus.

more skeletally mature foot, one should also note the relationship of the navicular to the cuneiforms and that of the cuneiforms to the metatarsals.[539, 541, 601]

In the normal foot, the lateral margins of the calcaneus and of the cuboid bone form a continuous line. In talipes equinovarus with medial subluxation of the talocalcaneonavicular joint, the cuboid is shifted medially and the calcaneocuboid line is interrupted. On the lateral aspect of the foot, another angle is formed between the longitudinal axis of the calcaneus and that of the fifth metatarsal. Normally the long axis of the calcaneus points toward the fifth metatarsal and the calcaneo–fifth metatarsal angle ($C-MT_5$) measures zero. In talipes equinovarus the angle is decreased and has a minus value.

In the lateral projection, the talocalcaneal angle is measured as follows: the long axis of the talus is aligned by joining the center points of its head and body, which are determined in the same way as in the anteroposterior view. The long axis of the calcaneus is obtained by drawing a line through its plantar surface, joining the calcaneal tubercles and its anterior plantar convexity. In early infancy, the posterior plantar aspect of the calcaneus is not clearly ossified and is irregular in outline. At this young age, it is best to resort to a tracing technique to determine the midline long axis of the calcaneus as described for the talus (see Fig. 2–33).

The talocalcaneal angle in a lateral roentgenogram of the normal foot measures between 35 and 50 degrees as shown in Figure 2–33, whereas in talipes equinovarus it is less than 25 degrees and may reach a negative value of minus 10 degrees as shown in Figure 2–34. On forced dorsiflexion, the lateral talocalcaneal angle is increased in a normal foot because the mobile heel is pulled forward and upward by plantar flexion, but in talipes equinovarus the talocalcaneal angle is decreased further as the calcaneus is tethered in the equinus position by the taut Achilles tendon while the talus moves slightly into dorsiflexion. Therefore,

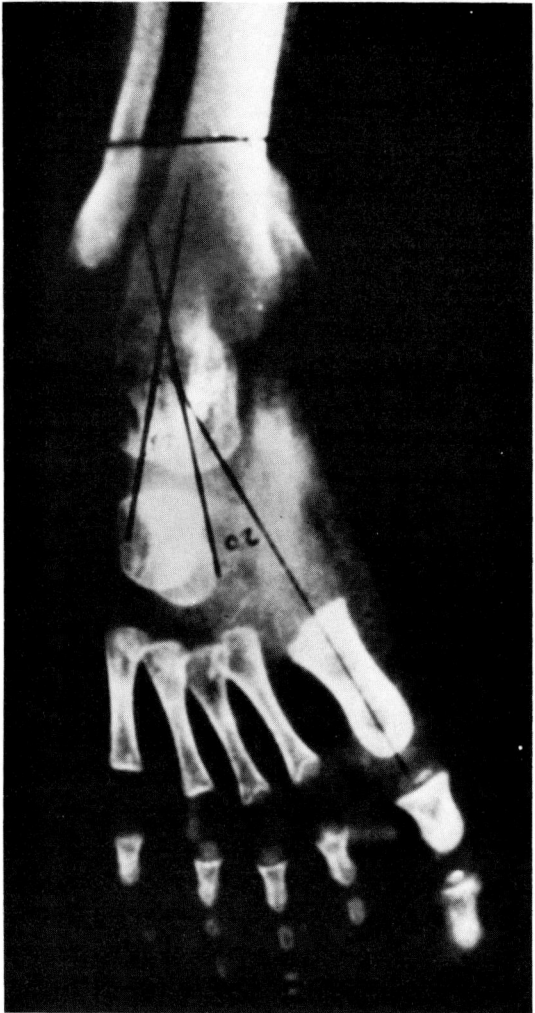

FIGURE 2–35. *Measurement of angle between long axes of the talus and the first metatarsal (note it is 20 degrees).*

minor differences between a normal and an abnormal foot can be accentuated by the maximal dorsiflexion view.

Talocalcaneonavicular subluxation is present when the talo–first metatarsal angle is greater then 20 degrees and the talocalcaneal angle is less than 15 degrees.

Beatson and Pearson have described the talocalcaneal index—i.e., the sum of the talocalcaneal angles in the anteroposterior and lateral projections. According to them, if the talocalcaneal index is less than 40 degrees in a properly positioned foot, talocalcaneonavicular subluxation has not been reduced.[33]

In the lateral view at birth, the ossific nucleus of the talus in talipes equinovarus appears to be displaced anteriorly and plantarward. The degree of equinus inclination of the ankle can also be measured in the lateral projection of the tibiotalar angle formed between the longitudinal axis of the tibia and the long axis of the talus; this normally measures 70 to 100 degrees. Another method of measuring ankle equinus deviation is the tibiocalcaneal angle, which is formed between the longitudinal axes of the tibia and the calcaneus; its value depends upon the degree of dorsiflexion of the ankle in a normal infant in whom the foot may touch the anterior aspect of the leg. The tibiocalcaneal angle may measure as little as 25 degrees. Normally, with marked dorsiflexion of the ankle, it measures 60 to 90 degrees. Both in the lateral and in the anteroposterior view, the contours of the tarsal bones and the articular surfaces should be inspected. The axial view of the calcaneus is helpful in radiographic assessment of a heel varus deformity in the older child who has started walking. Serial roentgenograms will demonstrate correction of the heel inversion.

With improper treatment, certain roentgenographic changes may ensue: "transverse breach," "horizontal or longitudinal breach," and flat-topped talus. A transverse breach in the midtarsal area will give a "rocker-bottom" deformity. This is verified by drawing the longitudinal axis of the sole, which is the line joining the calcaneal tubercle and the head of the third metatarsal. Normally this *sole line* passes below the calcaneocuboid joint; if the line passes through the joint, a "rocker bottom" deformity is present. It is an iatrogenic deformity (Fig. 2–36). A longitudinal breach may occur when medial subluxation of the talocalcaneonavicular joint persists in the horizontal plane, as discussed earlier in the section on pathology.

Ono and Hayashi employed frontal tomography perpendicular to the long axis of the foot in 43 cases of treated talipes equinovarus. Tomograms were made with the patient in the supine position initially, but later the weight-bearing posture was employed. Ono and Hayashi found characteristic changes of the hindfoot, namely, increased inclination of the middle subtalar articular surface of the calcaneus (inversion of the calcaneus), hypoplasia of the sustentaculum tali, and narrowing of the talocal-

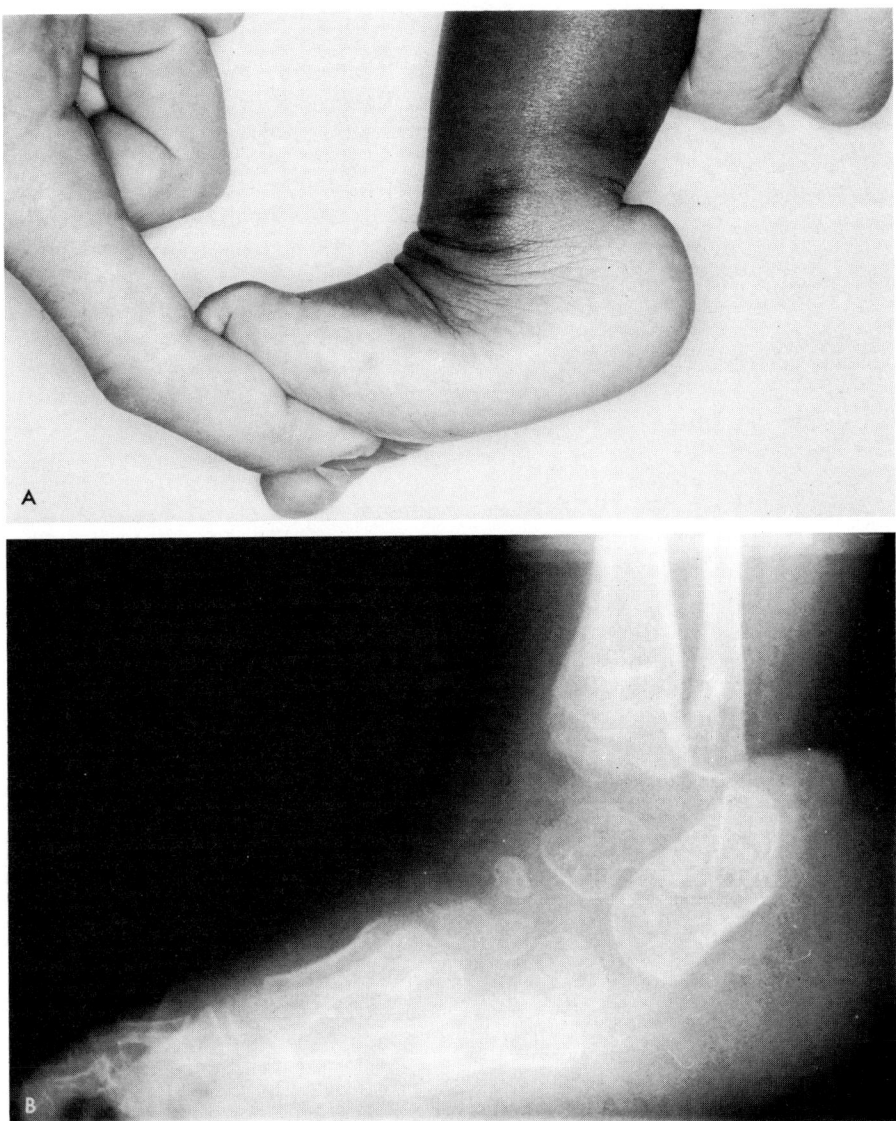

FIGURE 2–36. Rocker-bottom deformity in talipes equinovarus.

Deformity is the result of a transverse breach in the midtarsal area. **A.** Clinical appearance. **B.** Lateral roentgenogram of the foot and ankle.

caneal space. They recommended tomography as a simple and easily available method of determining the anatomic status of the foot in talipes equipnovarus in children over two years of age.[484] This author recommends computed tomography to determine medial spin of the calcaneus and lateral subluxation of the posterior facet of the subtalar joint.[175a]

Arthrography of the ankle joint has been extensively studied by Poulain.[523] Simultaneous arthrography of the ankle and talonavicular joint has been performed by Hjelmstedt and Sahlstedt. They studied 32 autopsy specimens of feet from 19 children of ages up to three years. Measurements of the size and shape of the talus were made on the films, and the results were compared with corresponding measurements made on the anatomic specimens. With respect to the length of the talus and medial declination of the talonavicular joint, there was a fairly good correlation between the radiographic values and the values obtained on the anatomic specimens. These investigators also studied clinically 24 congenital clubfeet in

18 patients and 6 clubfeet in 5 patients with neurologic disorders. In both groups, there were changes in the talus, consisting of medial deviation of the head with flattening of its dome.[275–277] Experience in arthrography is still limited, however, and computed tomography is replacing it.

Treatment

The objectives of the treatment of talipes equinovarus are: (1) to achieve concentric reduction of the dislocation or subluxation of the talocalcaneonavicular joint; (2) to maintain the reduction; (3) to restore normal articular alignment of the tarsus and the ankle; (4) to establish muscle balance between the evertors and invertors, and the dorsiflexors and plantar flexors; and (5) to provide a mobile foot with normal function and weight-bearing. The principles underlying management of congenital dislocation of the hip should be applied to that of in utero dislocation of the talocalcaneonavicular ball-and-socket joint. Treatment of talipes equinovarus is complex and delicate. Nonoperative reduction of talocalcaneonavicular dislocation in true congenital talipes equinovarus is often impossible, and conservative treatment frequently is open surgical reduction.

Treatment should be started as soon as possible, preferably immediately following birth. A frequently quoted adage is that the prognosis in a breech delivery is better than that in a vertex presentation because exercises and treatment can be begun earlier while awaiting delivery of the head. The first three weeks of life are the golden period—because the ligamentous tissues of the newborn are still exceedingly lax under the influence of maternal sex hormones. This is the crucial phase in which contracted soft tissues can be elongated by daily repeated manipulations; if the closed method of reduction will ever succeed, this is the time.

Soon after the baby is born, the orthopedic surgeon should explain to the parents the goals, the nature, and the course of treatment. They should understand that management of the child with talipes equinovarus extends over a period of many years until adolescence, when skeletal maturity of the foot is reached, and that uncompromising care and constant vigilance are required through all stages of skeletal growth.

The parents should realize that a foot with talipes equinovarus can never be completely normal. The deformity is the result of a teratologic malformation—a germ plasm defect. There will always be calf atrophy, and the foot will be smaller than the contralateral normal foot. There may be leg length inequality. A realistic approach initially will prevent much disappointment later.

CLOSED NONOPERATIVE METHOD OF MANAGEMENT

The technique of closed manipulative reduction of the medial and plantar subluxation of the talocalcaneonavicular ball-and-socket joint is as follows: The first phase is *elongation of the contracted soft tissues* by passive manipulation. The sacred rule is to be gentle. The soft tissues—ligaments and capsule—are hard: the hard tissues—physis and articular cartilage—are soft and vulnerable to iatrogenic trauma.[142] Forceful manipulation and stretching cast are more radical than surgery.

First the skin of the infant's foot and lower limb is painted or sprayed with a nonirritative adhesive liquid, such as tincture of benzoin or Ace Adherent. The surgeon should use gloves and a 4- by 4-inch sponge, opened up, for a firm grip. The infant is held in the soft lap of the mother or a gentle nurse.

Elongation of Triceps Surae Muscle, Posterior Capsule, and Ligaments of Ankle and Subtalar Joints. The manipulative technique is as follows: The os calcis, held between the index finger and thumb of one hand, is

---

FIGURE 2–37. *Technique of manipulation to correct talipes equinovarus.*

A and **B.** Elongation of triceps surae muscle and posterior capsule and ligaments of the ankle and subtalar joints. **C.** Elongation of posterior tibial muscle.

See illustration on opposite page

Congenital Deformities

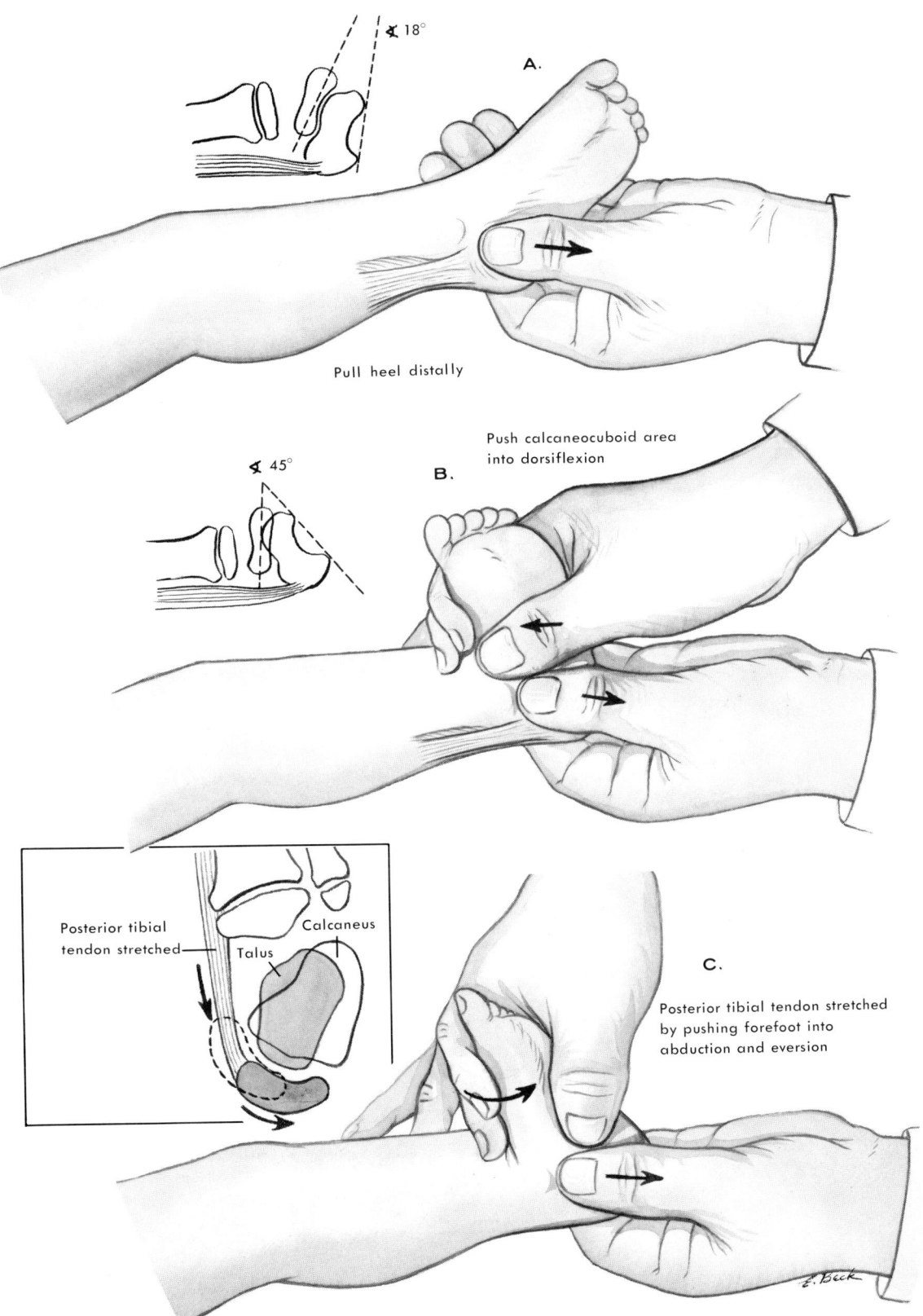

FIGURE 2–37 *See legend on opposite page*

Illustration continued on following page

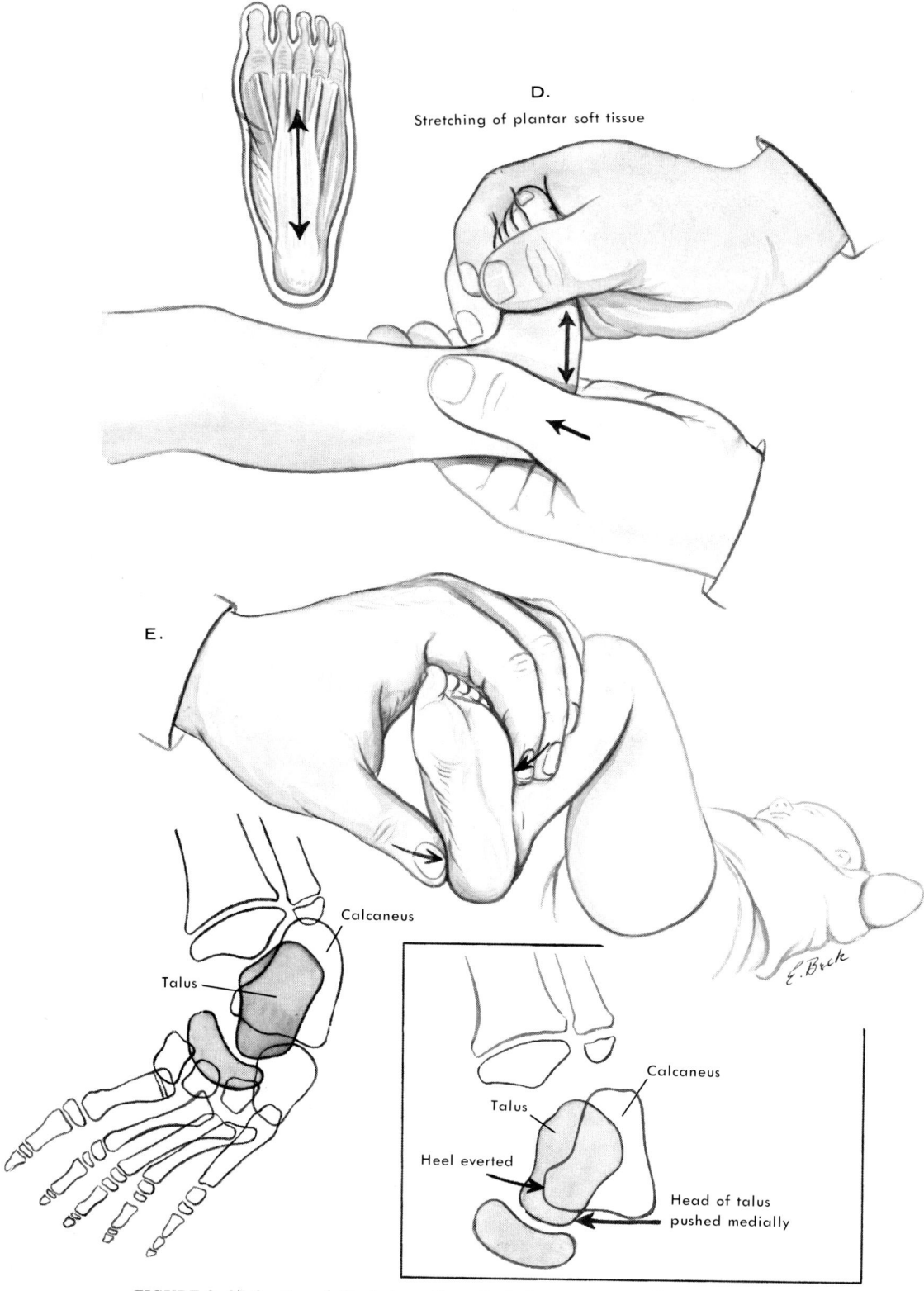

FIGURE 2–37 Continued. Technique of manipulation to correct talipes equinovarus.

D. Elongation of the plantar calcaneonavicular ligament and plantar soft tissue. **E.** Prevention of lateral rotation deformity of the dome of the talus in the ankle mortise. Push the anterior end of the talus medially as the os calcis is everted.

178

Illustration continued on opposite page

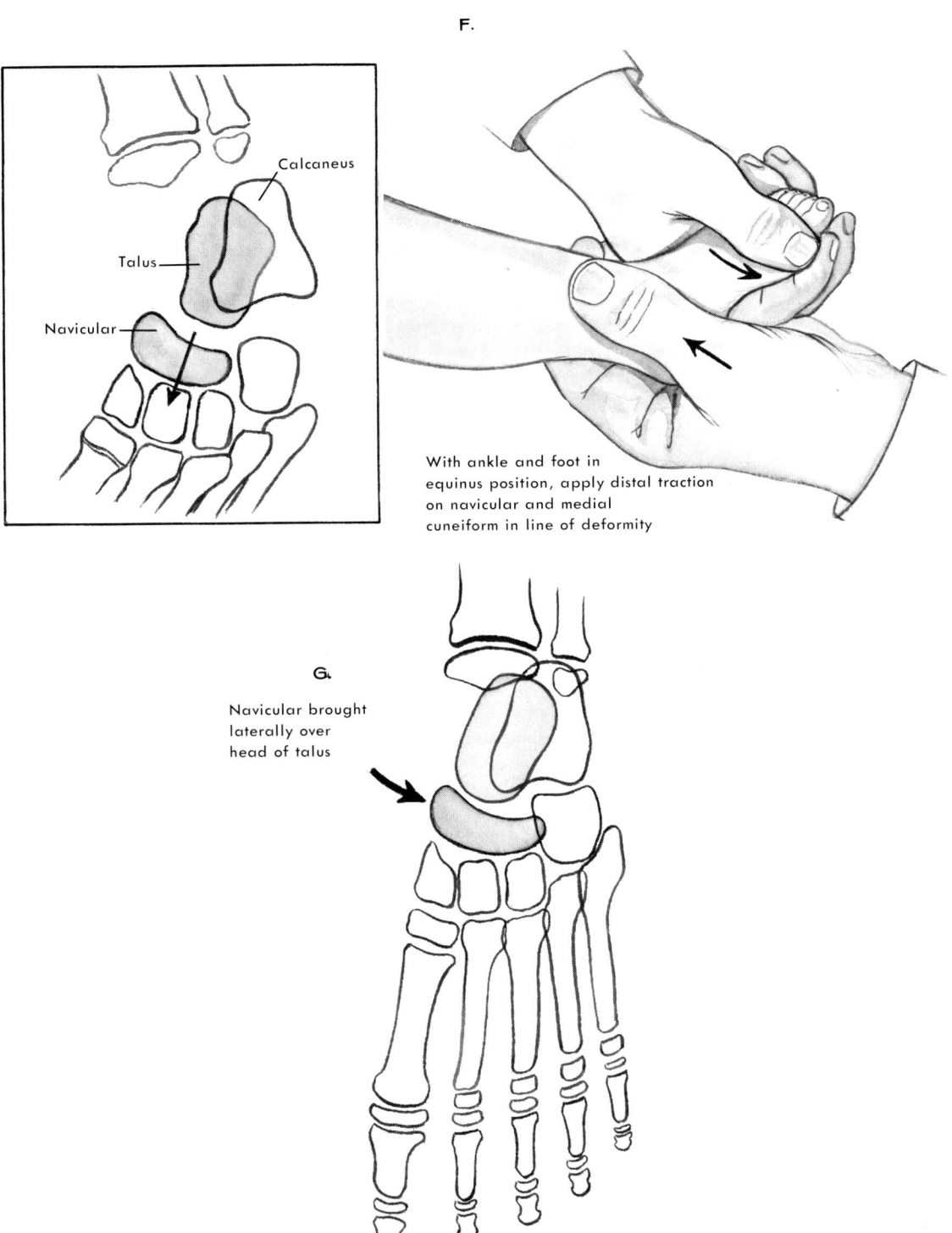

FIGURE 2–37 Continued. Technique of manipulation to correct talipes equinovarus.
F and **G.** Reduction of medial and plantar dislocation of the talocalcaneonavicular joint.

pulled *distally*, bringing the heel down, and pushed medially away from the fibular malleolus; with the other hand, the calcaneocuboid area is pushed into dorsiflexion with the whole foot slightly inverted (Fig. 2–37). One should not stretch the midfoot by forced dorsiflexion of the forefoot, or a "rocker-bottom" deformity of the foot will result owing to a transverse breach (see Fig. 2–36). The stretched position is maintained to the count of 10, and then released. Passive stretching of the taut, posterior soft tissues is repeated 20 to 30 times each session.

Elongation of Posterior Tibial Muscle and Tibionavicular Ligament. The navicular is tethered toward the medial malleolus by the contracted posterior tibial muscle and the plantar calcaneonavicular and tibionavicular ligaments. To stretch them, the os calcis is held between the index finger and the thumb of one hand and pulled down distally; with the other hand, the navicular is gripped between the index finger and thumb, and the navicular and the midfoot are pulled distally toward the big toe and then abducted (Fig. 2–37C). The body of the talus is held steady in the ankle mortise. It is imperative that one does not force the talus into lateral rotation in the ankle mortise and cause horizontal breach (Fig. 2–37 E).

Elongation of Plantar Calcaneonavicular (or Spring) Ligament and Plantar Soft Tissues. Over a hundred years ago, Hugh Owens Thomas stressed the importance of plantar soft tissues as an impediment to correction of talipes equinovarus.[634] It is only recently, however, that we have heeded his advice through the teachings of Wilbur Westin.[595, 690] The plantar calcaneonavicular ligament must be elongated if the navicular bone is to be positioned over the head of the talus. The technique of manipulative stretching is simple. With one hand, the heel is pushed up, and with the other, the midfoot is pushed into dorsiflexion (Fig. 2–37D). The thumb of one hand is over the medial malleolus, and the thumb of the other hand is over the navicular. Again, care should be taken not to cause lateral rotation of the talus in the ankle mortise (Fig. 2–37E). The iatrogenic deformity of "horizontal breach" should be avoided. As in elongation of the triceps surae, each stretched position is maintained to the count of 10, then released and repeated 20 to 30 times.

After manipulation and elongation of the contracted soft tissues, the foot and leg are strapped with adhesive tape, a technique described by Sir Robert Jones in 1900. The strapping provides a dynamic and nonrigid splint that prevents disuse atrophy and encourages the peroneal and ankle dorsiflexor muscles to function in the first few weeks of life.[311] The technique of its application is shown in Figure 2–38. First, the limb is thoroughly washed with soap and water, and cleansed and dried with alcohol. Tincture of benzoin is applied to the foot, the entire leg (between the knee and the malleoli), and the distal thigh for a distance of 3 to 5 cm. above the knee. The tincture of benzoin protects the skin and improves adherence of the strapping. Next, adhesive orthopedic felt, 3 to 5 cm. wide, is smoothly rolled circumferentially, but not completely, around the foot with the edges about 1 cm. apart in the midline on the dorsum of the foot. The circumferential taping as described by Jones is relatively safe in the first two or three weeks of life. It is imperative that the distal edge of the felt (and the adhesive strapping) end at the base of the toes to support the metatarsal head and dynamically stretch the forefoot out of equinus posture. A longer and wider piece of felt is applied over the dorsum of the 90-degree-flexed knee and the lateral and medial sides of the leg, ending 2 cm. proximal to each malleolus. Adhesive strapping is applied over the felt, rolling it against the varus deformity. With the knee always fully flexed, begin at the lateral edge of the dorsum of the foot and cross it from the lateral to the medial side and around the sole, and then upward on the lateral aspect of the leg. As the strapping is rolled against the deformity, the foot is pulled into eversion and dorsiflexion. To increase correction, an additional layer of adhesive tape may be applied on top of the first. The vertical straps on the leg are secured by two transverse pieces of adhesive tape around the calf, applied one on top of the other. Preferably, the tape should not encircle the leg, as it will act as a constrictor and obstruct

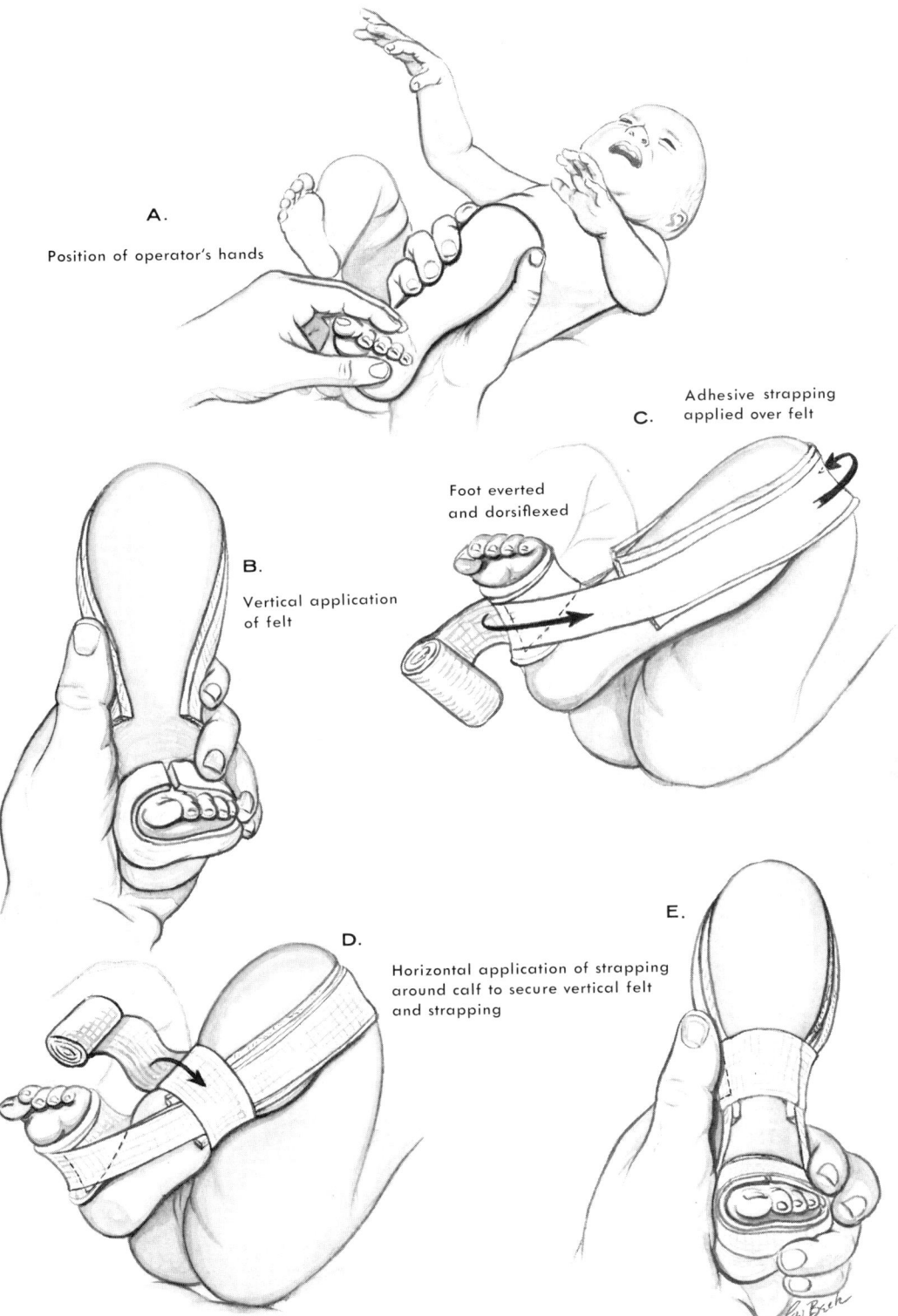

FIGURE 2–38. Technique of application of Robert Jones adhesive strapping for talipes equinovarus. See text for explanation of the steps of the application.

circulation to the distal part; this especially true in the older infant and child. The peripheral circulation is checked, and the mother (or nurse, if the child is an inpatient) is properly instructed in how to check it. If the foot is dusky in color, the straps are adjusted to relieve the vascular impediment. If the circulation is still not completely normal after this, the strapping is gently removed and started over again.

As the infant kicks the fully flexed knee into extension, a dynamic corrective force is transmitted to the foot. Other advantages of the Robert Jones adhesive strapping are that it is inexpensive, can be applied easily, changed readily, and reapplied at frequent intervals; and it is relatively safe, being least likely to cause pressure sores. The strapping is removed daily and, after manipulation of the foot, is reapplied.

During manipulation, all elements of soft-tissue contracture are elongated. This contrasts with the traditional teaching of Kite, which is that the clubfoot should be corrected in sequence from front to back, and that one should not proceed to the next stage until any distal deformity has been fully corrected. Kite first corrects the varus forefoot, then the inverted hindfoot, and then the equinus ankle and subtalar joints. He has constantly alerted us to the dangers of premature dorsiflexion as a cause of transverse breach at the midtarsal joint, which results in a "rocker-bottom" foot.[331-344] Leaving the hindfoot in the equinus position until the varus deformity is fully corrected, however, allows the contracture of the posterior capsule and ligaments of the ankle and subtalar joints, and the tautness of the triceps surae, to become more rigid. This rigidity is an important factor in the pathogenesis of the "rocker-bottom" foot. Another anatomic factor to consider is that full plantar flexion of the ankle is accompanied by varus posture of the foot, and full dorsiflexion by valgus posture. While the hindfoot is left in the equinus position, the subtalar and midtarsal joints are inverted unless the foot is forcibly breached at the midtarsal joint. It is often stated that it is difficult, if not impossible, to manipulate the small, drawn-up heel of an infant with talipes equinovarus. A common error is to apply the dorsiflexion force on the long anterior lever of the forefoot. The correct approach is to paint the small heel and foot with an adhesive liquid and hold it in an opened-up, 4- by 4-inch surgical gauze and *pull the heel down* (see Fig. 2–37 A and B).

Closed Reduction of Medial and Plantar Dislocation of Talocalcaneonavicular Joint. Once the soft-tissue contractures are sufficiently elongated, the next step is closed reduction of the medial and plantar dislocation of the talocalcaneonavicular joint. A basic principle of reduction of overriding both-bone fractures of the forearm is to apply traction *distally in the line of deformity*. The same principle should be applied to the reduction of the talocalcaneonavicular joint in talipes equinovarus. Grasp the hindfoot with one hand, the index finger over the body of the talus above the sinus tarsi, just anterior and distal to the lateral malleolus, and the thumb of the same hand anterior to the medial malleolus, pushing the navicular distally. With the opposite hand, grasp the fore- and midfoot between the thumb and index finger, and apply *longitudinal* traction distally in the line of deformity—that is, with the foot in equinus posture and inversion. This distracts the tarsus and elongates the foot (Fig. 2–37F). Next, reduction of the talocalcaneonavicular dislocation is achieved by abducting the midfoot, displacing the navicular laterally, and pushing the anterior end of the talus medially with the opposite thumb (Fig. 2–37G). The calcaneus is laterally rotated with the cuboid bone as the foot is dorsiflexed at the ankle and subtalar joints. Clinically, reduction is revealed by the normal external contour of the foot in a resting posture. In talipes equinovarus, there is apparent shortening of the hallux; reduction of the dislocation brings the navicular over the distal end of the talus, and the big toe acquires normal length. Digital palpation should disclose a one- or two-fingerbreadth space between the medial malleolus and the navicular.

The success of reduction is confirmed by anteroposterior and lateral roentgenograms of the foot, made in the standardized positions outlined earlier. In the anteroposterior roentgenogram, the talocalcaneal angle should be greater than 20 degrees, and the talo–first metatarsal angle less than 15 degrees; in the lateral view, the talocalcaneal angle should be 30 to 45 degrees. Proper positioning of the foot and correct technique of roentgenography are vital.

Retention of Reduction. Once concentric reduction has been achieved and confirmed by x-ray, an above-knee cast is applied to maintain the reduction. Plaster of Paris cast immobilization is a *static retentive* apparatus. The correct application of a plaster cast to an infant's foot requires considerable skill; it should be applied accurately and with great attention to detail. Three persons working in a harmonious team are necessary: a parent to hold the baby still (the baby may be rebellious, struggling and making every effort to get loose); a trained assistant who will roll the sheet wadding and plaster of Paris cast; and the surgeon, whose responsibility is to hold and mold the cast.

The cast should extend from the toes to the groin with the knee flexed at 60 to 80 degrees to control the heel and prevent the cast from slipping. The infant's lower limb is conical in shape, bulky in the thigh, and

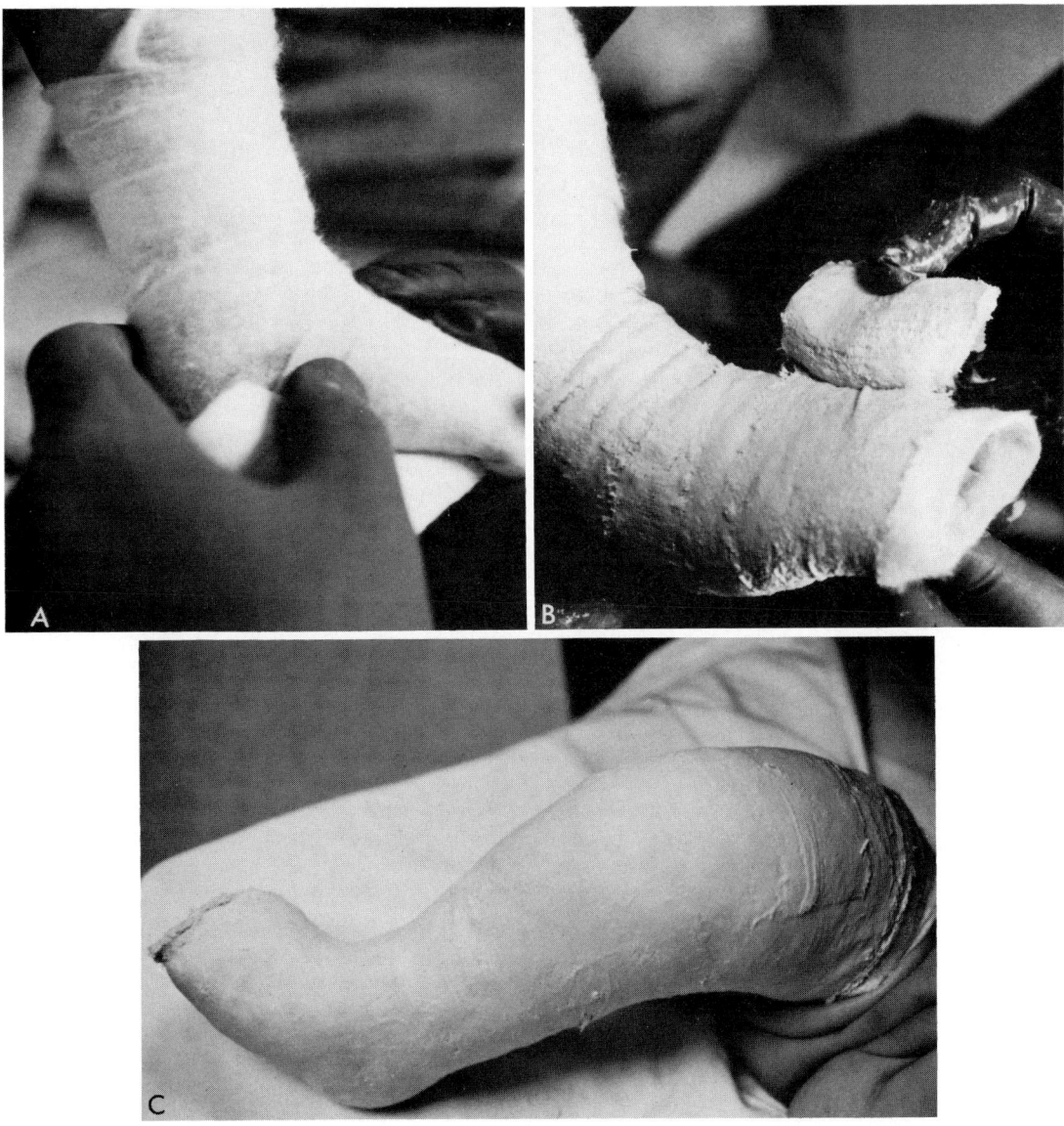

FIGURE 2–39. Technique of plaster of Paris cast application in talipes equinovarus.

A. Rolling of sheet wadding. **B.** Rolling of plaster of Paris cast. **C.** Molding of the cast.

tapered distally in the leg and foot. It is best to paint the skin with a nonirritating adhesive liquid, such as tincture of benzoin or Ace Adherent, to protect the skin and prevent slipping of the cast. Narrow sheet wadding should be used; 1 or ½ inch wide on the foot and lower leg, and 2 inches wide on the upper leg, knee, and thigh. It is rolled snugly against the varus deformity, but not taut and not loose. It should be smooth with no wrinkles. Beginning at the forefoot, the first two turns are applied toward the tips of the toes; then the direction is reversed and the wadding is carried proximally over the rest of the foot, leg, and knee, and up to the upper thigh (Fig. 2–39A). Each succeeding turn overlaps the preceding turn by one half of its width. Two extra turns are applied at the upper thigh to serve as padding. Because the circumference of the calf and thigh is greater above than below, the sheet wadding is torn slightly at its upper edge as the wrapping proceeds proximally so that the lower part lies flat on the limb, not loose and away from the skin. Small tears are made at varying points in the turns to insure exact and smooth conformation to the limb. Three layers of sheet wadding are placed over the heel and extending forward to cover both malleoli.

The surgeon then holds the foot and ankle in the desired corrected position, and the assistant rolls the plaster of Paris cast. A 2-inch-wide roll is sufficient for the foot and lower leg; and a 3-inch roll for the upper part of the leg, the knee, and the thigh. In the bigger infant, or if reinforcement is required because the cast cracks on a restless baby, another 3-inch roll may be used. The plaster should be extra-fast setting. Like the sheet wadding, it is rolled against the varus deformity—that is, it begins on the lateral edge of the foot, onto the dorsum, then on the sole, and onto the lateral side again. Each turn covers two thirds of the width of the preceding turn. As the plaster cast is applied, each turn is rubbed to smooth it. The cast should be of uniform thickness. In the uncooperative infant, the plaster is first carried up to the ankle and the lower third of the leg, and then extended up to the upper thigh (Fig. 2–39B).

Proper and careful molding of the cast is very important. The thenar eminence of one hand is placed over the calcaneocuboid area, pushing the body of the talus medially and also acting as counter pressure. With the other fingers, the back of the heel is molded so that it looks like a normal foot with a prominent, posteriorly displaced heel. The importance of the molding above the heel to give a normal contour to the hindfoot cannot be overemphasized. With the other hand, pressure is applied over the medial and plantar aspects of the mid- and forefoot, not the great toe, pushing it into abduction. The lateral border of the foot should be concave. The midtarsal joint area should be well-molded to prevent a "rocker-bottom" deformity. It should be remembered that the plaster of Paris cast is a retentive, not a corrective, apparatus. Its purpose is to maintain the concentric reduction of the talocalcaneonavicular joint achieved by manipulation. Recently this author has been utilizing a plaster of Paris cast material for the first two layers and then reinforcing it with a synthetic casting tape, which allows a better grip on the infant's foot and firm rapid setting.

Roentgenograms are made through the first cast to ensure concentricity of reduction. The cast is changed at two- to three-week intervals in the young infant, whose foot grows rapidly. When solid casts are left on for long periods of time, the soft tissues and the skin become compressed. Soft-tissue fibrosis, pressure sores, and circulatory embarrassment are inherent dangers.

The solid-cast immobilization is continued for an average period of three months. Before discontinuing retention in the solid cast, roentgenograms are made out of the cast to ensure that concentric reduction is maintained. Then a polypropylene above-knee splint is made to hold the hindfoot in 15 to 20 degrees of eversion, the midfoot and forefoot in 20 degrees of abduction, and the ankle at zero to 5 degrees of dorsiflexion; the knee is flexed 60 degrees. The splint is worn only at night and at nap times. A Reimann dynamic clubfoot splint may be used, if preferred. A prewalker clubfoot shoe is worn during the day (Fig. 2–40). The mother is taught passive stretching exercises to manipulate the mid- and forefoot into abduction and eversion, the heel into eversion, and the foot into dorsiflexion

Congenital Deformities 185

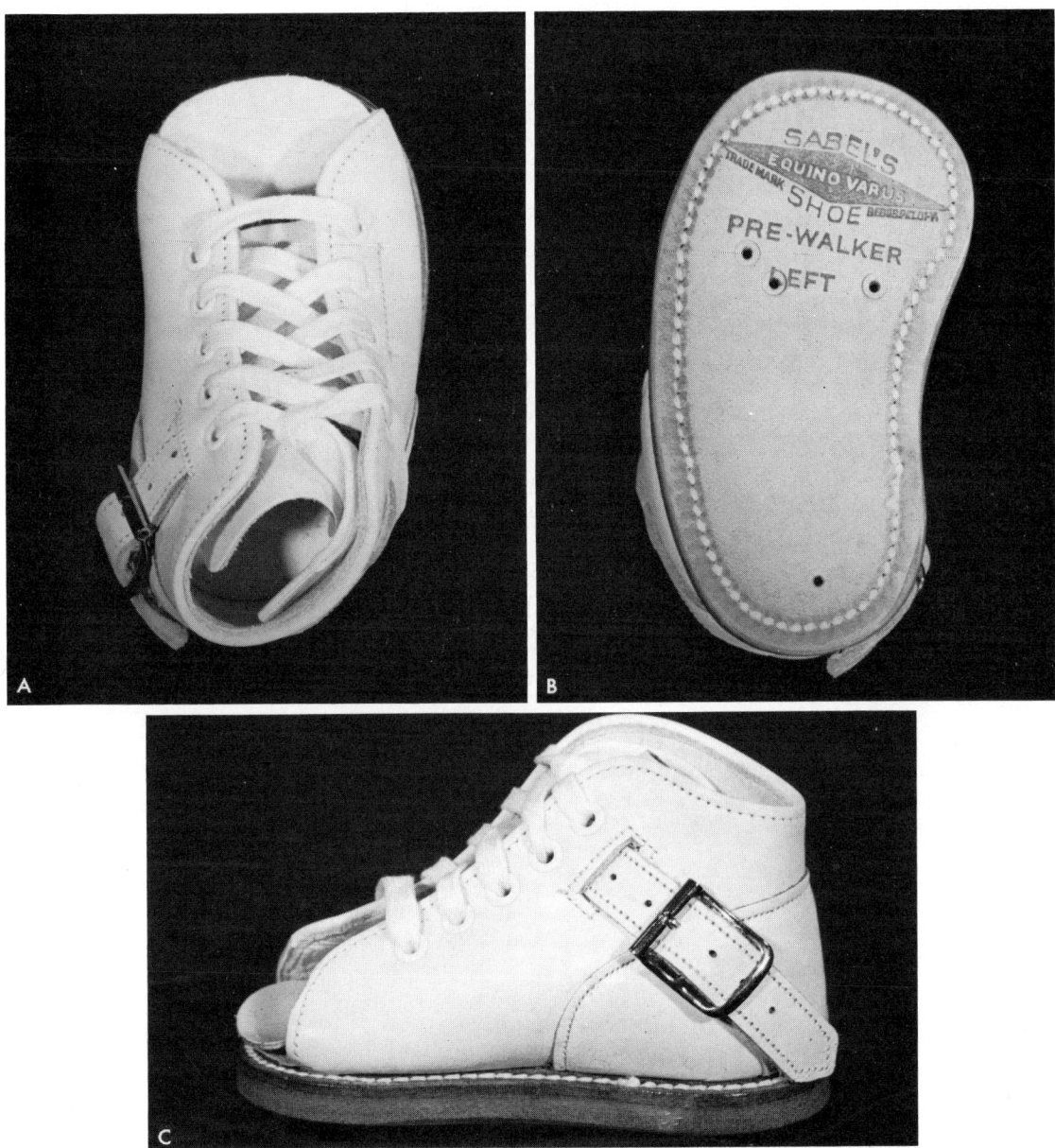

FIGURE 2–40. Prewalker clubfoot shoe with valgus strap.
A. Dorsal view. **B.** Plantar view. **C.** Lateral view.

at the ankle joint by pulling the heel down. Again, the parents should be cautioned over and over again not to stretch the midfoot by forced dorsiflexion of the forefoot. Stimulation techniques are used to elicit active exercises promoting inversion and dorsiflexion of the foot. The exercises are performed 15 times slowly in each direction, four to five times a day.

The follow-up care of talipes equinovarus should be continued until skeletal maturity to ensure that there is no recurrence of the deformity. When the child begins to walk, he should wear outflare (tarsal pronator) high-top shoes with ⅛- to 3/16-inch outer lateral side heel and sole wedges to encourage walking in eversion and abduction (Fig. 2–41). Roentgenograms are made periodi-

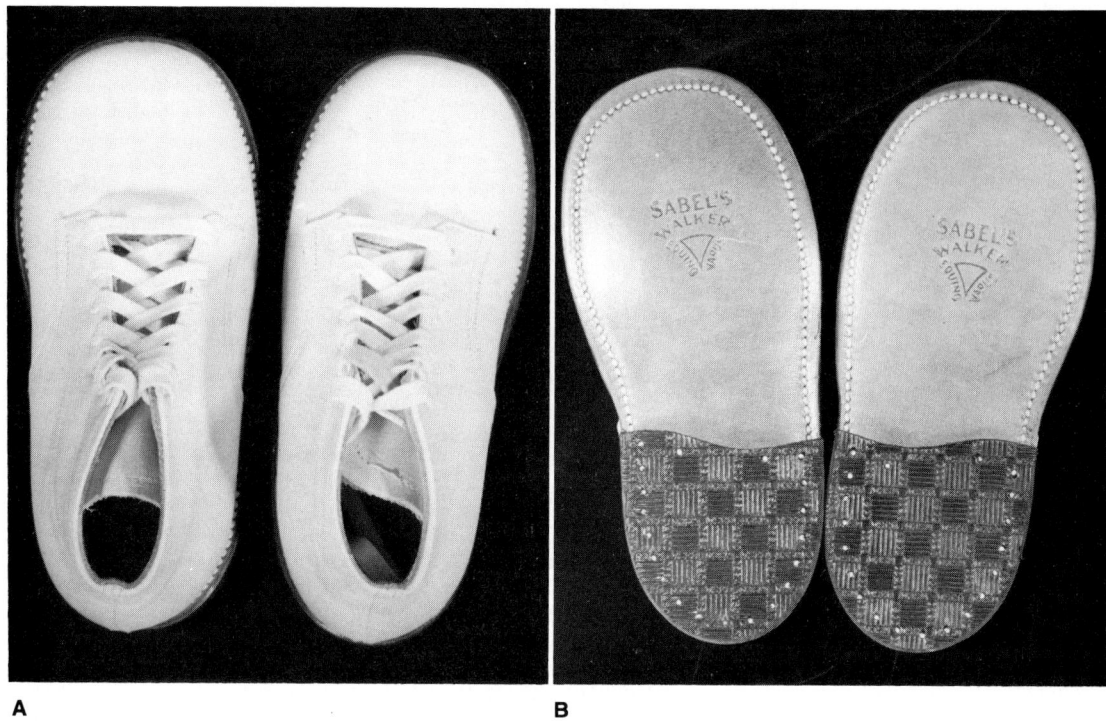

FIGURE 2–41. *Outflare (tarsal pronator) shoes.*

cally. If there is no recurrence of deformity after two years, normal shoes are worn.

REDUCTION OF TALOCALCANEONAVICULAR JOINT BY OPEN SURGICAL METHODS

What are the chances of success of a closed reduction of the in utero dislocation of the talocalcaneonavicular joint in talipes equinovarus? A review of the literature shows a wide range in the rate of success. Kite reported 90 per cent success in correcting deformity with his method of manipulation and cast.[344] Fripp and Shaw reported 19 per cent success with Denis Browne splints and 71 per cent success with manipulation and stretching casts.[200] Dangelmajor reviewed 200 unselected cases and reported 40 per cent success with nonoperative treatment.[130] Persistence or recurrence of the deformity in 46 per cent was reported by Brockman in 1930, and in 56 per cent by Ponsetti and Smoley in 1963.[73, 74, 522] The cause of the confusion and disagreement in the past has been the tendency to group all types of clubfoot into one category. It is imperative that, when discussing the treatment, prognosis, and results of talipes equinovarus, one does not include postural clubfoot. In talipes equinovarus, there is an in utero, rigid dislocation of the talocalcaneonavicular joint that primarily requires open surgical reduction. The likelihood of successful closed manipulative reduction is minimal, probably 5 to 10 per cent. Closed methods of treatment are performed primarily to elongate the contracted soft tissues. Repeatedly it has been demonstrated in fetal specimens that the talocalcaneonavicular dislocation cannot be reduced by forced manipulation. Again, it is impossible to reduce the dislocation by sectioning of the tendo Achillis and posterior tibial tendons alone. It is only upon the additional division of the plantar calcaneonavicular and tibionavicular ligaments and the capsule of the talonavicular joint, and elongation of contracted posterior and lateral soft tissues of the ankle and subtalar articulations that one is able to reduce the medial plantar dislocation of the talocalcaneonavicular joint.

Persistent forceful manipulation and prolonged cast immobilization do more harm

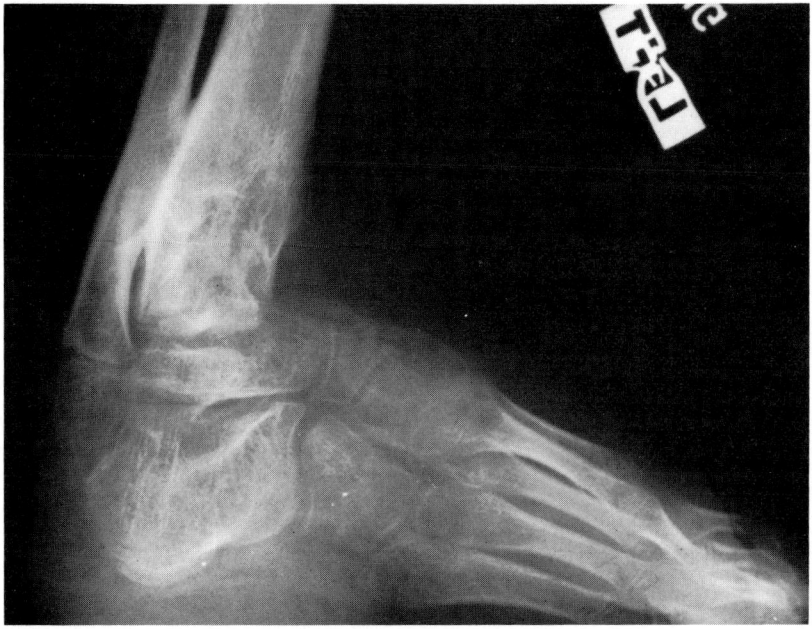

FIGURE 2–42. *Damage to the distal tibial epiphysis and growth arrest caused by forceful manipulation to correct talipes equinovarus.*

Multiple osteochondral compression fractures have resulted in flat-topped talus. Note the overgrown fibular malleolus.

than good. The articular cartilage, physis, and bone will be damaged before ligaments and capsule will yield to stretching. Rigidity of the joints, fibrosis of soft parts, and disuse atrophy of muscles will develop. The osseous complications of nonsurgical management—namely, flat-top talus, distal tibial bowing, metaphyseal compression, distal tibial metaphyseal spur, torus fracture of the distal tibial metaphysis, fracture of the distal fibula, and growth injuries to the distal tibial physis as shown in Figure 2–42—vividly support the thesis that the conservative method of treating talipes equinovarus is by open surgery.

Timing of Surgery. The literature on operative management of talipes equinovarus is extensive, and there is considerable difference of opinion as to the indications for surgery, the age at which to operate, and the procedure to be used. This author strongly recommends that if, by six to ten weeks, depending upon the size of the foot, clinical findings and roentgenograms show that complete correction has not been achieved, open surgical reduction of the talocalcaneonavicular joint be employed. Recently there is increasing evidence to support this position.* The extremely rapid growth taking place in infancy will quickly restore normal articular alignment and architecture of the foot. It should be pointed out, however, that surgery of the small foot of the infant is very delicate, and the smaller the foot, the greater the risk of iatrogenic trauma. The novice should beware! This operation should be performed only by the knowledgeable and experienced surgeon.

Choice of Operative Procedure. The decision depends on (1) the age of the patient, (2) the degree of rigidity, (3) the deformities present, and (4) the extent of correction obtained by previous treatment.

In general, bony procedures are rarely, if ever, indicated in the infant and young child, as they would disturb the normal growth and development of the foot; if surgery is performed on patients in this age category, it should consist only of soft-tissue procedures.

Under four years of age, open reduction can usually be achieved by complete release of the talocalcaneonavicular joint by sectioning or elongation of the contracted soft

---

*See references 246, 272, 417, 526, 541, 614, 724.

Text continued on page 192

Table 2-8. Operative Correction of Talipes Equinovarus by

	Ober	Brockmann	McCauley	Bost, Schottstaedt, and Larsen
Posterior Release				
Achilles tendon	Subcutaneously Do it at end to assist in driving talus back into mortise	Lengthen by Z-plasty 2 weeks after medial release	Lengthen by Z-plasty 8 weeks after medial release	Lengthen (tri-cut method of Hoke)
Posterior capsule of ankle joint	—	Section 2 weeks after medial release	Section 8 weeks after medial release	Section
Posterior talofibular ligament	—	—	—	—
Posterior capsule of subtalar joint	—	Section 2 weeks after medial release	Section 8 weeks after medial release	Section
Calcaneofibular ligament	—	—	—	—
Posterior insertion of deltoid ligament on calcaneus	Section (whole attachment removed from medial surface of calcaneus subperiosteally)	Section	Section	Section
Flexor digitorum longus	—	—	Excise sheath Lengthen by Z-plasty (if necessary)	—
Flexor hallucis longus	—	—	Excise sheath Lengthen by Z-plasty (if necessary)	—
Kirschner wire in os calcis (to be incorporated in cast)	—	—	—	—
Medial Release				
Posterior tibial tendon	Lengthen	Z-plasty lengthening	Z-plasty lengthening	Detach from insertions (tuberosity of navicular, cuneiform, metatarsals)
Tibionavicular ligament (anterior part of deltoid ligament)	Section	Section	Section	Section
Talonavicular capsule	Section	Section	Section	Section
Calcaneonavicular (spring) ligament	Elevate subperiosteally from calcaneus	—	Section	Section
Deltoid ligament (superficial layer)	Elevate subperiosteally from calcaneus	Section	Section	Section
Deltoid ligament (deep layer)	Elevate subperiosteally from talus	Section	Preserve	Section (sometimes)
Capsule of naviculocuneiform joint	—	—	Section (if necessary)	Section
Subtalar Release				
Capsule of medial side of subtalar joint	Lengthen by subperiosteal elevation from calcaneus	Section	Section	Section
Talocalcaneal interosseous ligament	—	—	Section	Section
Bifurcated (Y) ligament (extends from calcaneus to lateral border of navicular and medial border of cuboid)	—	—	—	Section

Soft-Tissue Release and Bony Procedures

Gelman	Turco	Evans	Dwyer
Lengthen 2 months after medial release	Z-technique Detach medial half of insertion on os calcis	Lengthen by Z-plasty	Lengthen by Z-plasty
Section 2 months after medial release	Section	Section	—
Section 2 months after medial release	Section	Section	—
Section 2 months after medial release	Section	Section	—
Section 2 months after medial release	Section	Section	—
Section	Section (retract neurovascular bundle posteriorly for exposure)	Section	—
—	—	—	—
—	—	—	—
—	—	—	—
Z-lengthening	Divide above medial malleolus (use distal stump for traction and identification of navicular, then reinsert)	Lengthen by Z-plasty	—
Section	Section	Section	—
Section	Section	Section	—
Preserve—will prevent rocker-bottom deformity	Detach from sustentaculum tali	Section	Subperiosteally elevated from calcaneus
Section	Section	Section	Subperiosteally elevated from calcaneus
Preserve	Preserve	—	—
—	Section (if necessary)	—	—
Section	Section	Section	Elevate subperiosteally and release
Section through medial approach above sustentaculum tali	Section through medial approach above sustentaculum tali	—	—
—	Section	—	—

Table continued on following pages

Table 2-8. *Operative Correction of Talipes Equinovarus by*

	Ober	Brockmann	McCauley	Bost, Schottstaedt, and Larsen
Plantar Release				
Incision	Subcutaneously	Separate linear incision along anterolateral border of os calcis	—	Medial
Plantar fascia	Section	Excise origin	—	Section
Abductor hallucis Intrinsic toe flexors Abductor digiti quinti	—	Detach all muscles	Superior origin of abductor hallucis detached and displaced downward	Section at origin
Long and short plantar ligaments	—	—	—	Section at the calcaneocuboid joint
Capsule of calcaneocuboid joint	—	—	—	Section
Procedures on Tarsal Bones	No	No	No	No
Internal Fixation	No	No	No	No
Postoperative Care	Change cast at 2 weeks and manipulate foot into overcorrection	Posterior release and heel cord lengthening 2 weeks after medial release	Change cast in 2 weeks and manipulate foot into further correction	Foot held in relaxed position until wound healed
	Change cast monthly, each time manipulating foot into corrected position	Change casts to obtain full correction	Posterior release and heel cord lengthening at 8 weeks (if necessary)	Repeated changes of casts at 2 week intervals to obtain gradual correction
	Total of 4-5 mo. immobilization	Total of 3-5 mo. immobilization	Total of 2-4 mo. immobilization	Total of 5 mo. immobilization
	Some form of clubfoot brace worn night and day 8 months longer	Below-knee orthosis with medial bar and outside T-strap at night	Cross bar splint attached to shoes at night; 1/8" outer sole and heel wedges on shoes during day	Brace at night to hold foot in corrected position
		Outside sole and heel wedges on shoe		Shoe wedges
		Active exercise to strengthen	Active exercises to strengthen peroneals and dorsiflexors	Periodic cast treatment if necessary
Remarks	Subperiosteal elevation of contracted capsule and ligaments (particularly deltoid) provides stability of ankle joint as they heal and reattach in lengthened position Overcorrect every element of deformity Cure not complete until patient actively can put his foot in a position of overcorrection		Release abductor hallucis to decrease its deforming force More extensive sectioning of capsules and ligaments (particularly of interosseous talocalcaneal ligament, which binds talus and calcaneus in varus position) Following sectioning, marked release of deformity occurs	Thorough plantar dissection and release Section of talocalcaneal interosseous and of bifurcated ligaments stressed

Soft-Tissue Release and Bony Procedures (Continued)

Gelman	Turco	Evans	Dwyer
Medial	Separate (3 cm. long on plantar surface of hindfoot)	Medial	Medial
Section	Excise origin	Section	Section
Section at origin	Strip subperiosteally from os calcis	Section	Section
—	—	—	—
—	—	—	—
No	Excise elongated tuberosity of navicular after reduction (to prevent pressure necrosis of skin)	Shorten lateral column of foot by resection and fusion of calcaneocuboid joint	Osteotomy of calcaneus lever inferior segment inferiorly and laterally (held open by wedge of bone graft)
No	Kirschner wire to transfix talonavicular joint	Two staples across calcaneocuboid joint	—
In long leg cast for 2–3 mo.	Cast change under general anesthesia 3 mo. after operation	Immobilize in above-knee cast for 5 mo. Walking in plaster cast permitted in 6 weeks	Immobilize in cast 8 weeks
Posterior release 2 mo. following medial release if necessary to correct equinus deformity	Remove sutures and Kirschner wire at 6 weeks Total of 4 mo. immobilization (last 2½ months can be walking cast in older child) Pronator walking shoes during day Denis Browne splint (25 cm. everting crossbar) at night for 2 yr.		
Preserve calcaneonavicular ligament to prevent rocker-bottom deformity Preserve deep layer of deltoid ligament (tibiotalar portion)	Preserve deep layer of deltoid ligament (it inserts on the body of the talus) Tilting of the talus and pes valgus will develop if tibiotalar ligament is sectioned Calcaneus must be released at both ends to obtain complete correction Internal fixation of talonavicular joint Note: Ingram divides interosseous talocalcaneal ligament and capsule of calcaneocuboid joint through lateral incision He transfixed calcaneocuboid joint with Kirschner wire in addition to talonavicular joint	Shorten lateral column of foot	Corrects fixed bony varus deformity of hindfoot

tissues on the posterior, medial, plantar, and lateral aspects of the articulation. The calcaneofibular ligament and the posterior capsule of the ankle joint are also divided. If the foot is rigid, to prevent dense scar tissue from retethering contracted soft tissues and causing recurrence of deformity, it is wise to excise ligaments, capsule, and tendon sheaths. In arthrogryposis and myelomeningocele, the tendons of nonfunctioning fibrosed muscles are excised.

In the older child, the tarsal and metatarsal bones become deformed and resist correction; in these patients, various bony procedures are performed. In the five- to eight-year age group, posterior, medial, plantar, and lateral soft-tissue release is performed to reduce the talocalcaneonavicular subluxation. The lateral convex column of the foot is overgrown, however, as compared with the medial column. In addition, the anterior articular surface of the calcaneus faces forward and medially; this medial slant of the calcaneocuboid articulation constitutes a lateral obstacle to eversion and prevents lateral translation of the cuboid, and hence of the navicular. Therefore, between five and eight years of age, the lateral column of the foot is shortened by resection of the distal end of the calcaneus (Lichtblau procedure).[379] In the child nine years old or older, the lateral column of the foot is shortened and stabilized by calcaneocuboid resection and fusion (Evans procedure).[170–172] In the older patient with a skeletally mature foot, incongruity of the talocalcaneonavicular joint may be marked and cause instability of reduction, expecially if there is dynamic imbalance of muscles. In such feet and in the paralytic clubfoot in the younger age group, the Evans procedure may be indicated. In the six-year-old or older child, tendon transfers are occasionally performed to provide dynamic balance between the evertors and invertors.

In the ten-year-old or older child, the foot is skeletally mature, and the deformities fixed; therefore, osteotomy of the os calcis, tarsal reconstruction, and triple arthrodesis are required to provide a plantigrade foot; these are salvage procedures. Metatarsal osteotomy at their bases will correct the varus forefoot. Medial rotation osteotomy of the tibia may be indicated to correct severe lateral rotational malalignment of the tibia and fibula. Occasionally, a talectomy is performed. Table 2–8 gives a brief historic résumé of the various operative procedures employed in the treatment of congenital talipes equinovarus.

Procedures on Soft Tissues. The details of open reduction of the talocalcaneonavicular joint are described and illustrated in Plate 2. The surgery should be systematic and performed in sequential steps. The progressive approach will ensure correction of all obstacles to reduction. Clubfeet treated by previous inadequate surgery present a wide spectrum of special problems. Each case should be individualized, the preoperative roentgenograms thoroughly assessed, and the operation planned accordingly. Too little surgery and insufficient correction, or too much surgery and overcorrection, should be avoided.

McKay has described the technique for treatment of talipes equinovarus in which he achieved correction by pushing the calcaneocuboid joint laterally anterior to the ankle joint and the posterior part of the calcaneus medially toward the medial malleolus posterior to the ankle joint. He recommends surgical reduction through the Cincinnati incision with the patient in prone position. McKay preserves the sheaths of the posterior tibial, flexor digitorum longus, and flexor hallucis longus tendons, thereby maintaining flexor tendon function and protecting the ankle joint from fibrosis. Postoperatively, he uses a hinged cast to permit early motion of the ankle joint. In clubfeet in which surgery has previously failed, he transfers the flexor hallucis longus to improve function of the peroneus longus. For details of the operative technique, the reader is referred to the original article.[414]

COMPLICATIONS. Open reduction of the talocalcaneonavicular joint in talipes equinovarus is very delicate surgery, requiring extensive dissection of the small foot of an infant. If meticulous attention to detail is not given, the operative procedure is fraught with hazards and complications, some of which may be disastrous.

Wound Dehiscence. Wound slough is prevented by meticulous surgical technique and gentle retraction of skin margins by silk sutures, not by rakes. By applying the initial cast (more like a compression dressing), with the ankle joint in equinus posture, the

Text continued on page 208

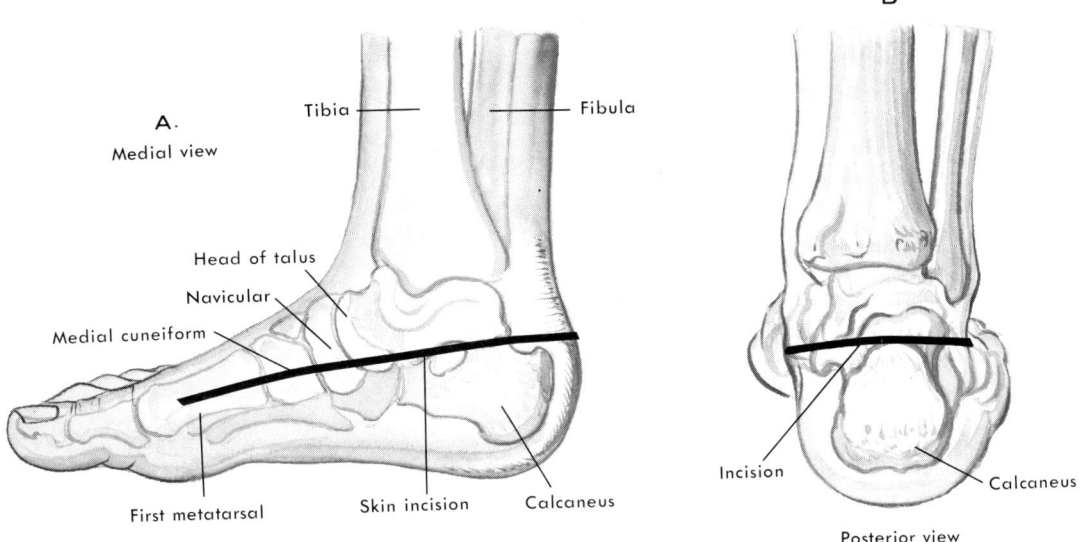
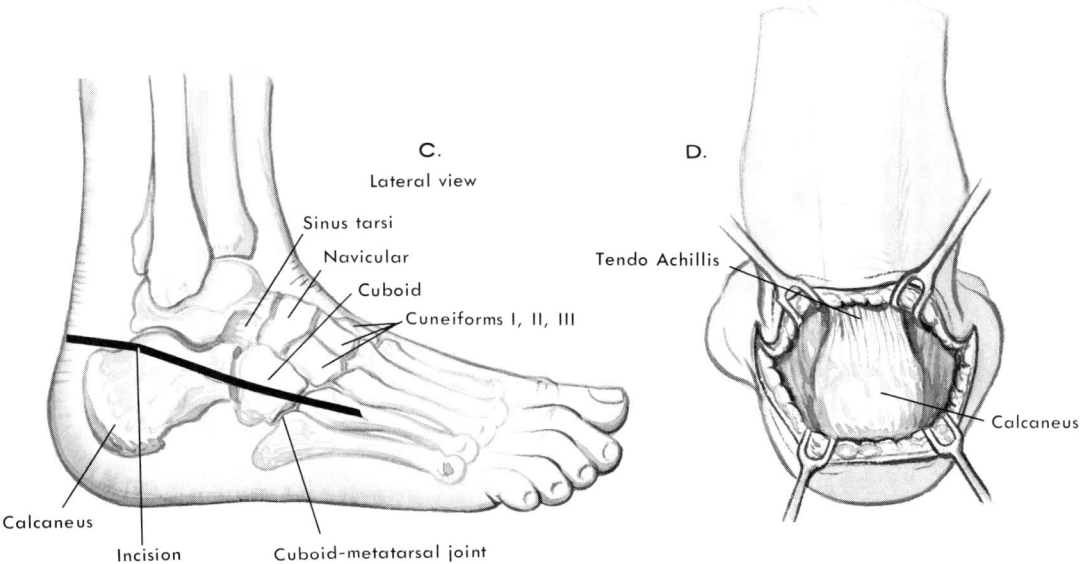

FIGURE 2–43. Cincinnati incision for complete soft-tissue release and open reduction of the talocalcaneonavicular joint in talipes equinovarus.

A to **C.** Transverse incision that starts at the base of the first metatarsal and extends posteriorly 3 mm. superior to the heel crease under the medial malleolus and then posterolaterally to the tip of the lateral malleolus, and distally to the cuboid–fifth metatarsal joint. **D.** Exposure of the Achilles tendon by elevation of subcutaneous tissue proximally and distally. This incision provides an excellent view of the pathologic changes in talipes equinovarus. Its drawbacks are difficulty in dissecting out and exposing the Achilles tendon proximally to permit adequate lengthening of the heel cord, difficulty in supramalleolar lengthening of the posterior tibial tendon, and tautness of the skin posteriorly that does not allow immobilization of the ankle in neutral dorsiflexion.

Open Reduction of Talocalcaneonavicular Joint in Talipes Equinovarus

THE PROCEDURE

The operation is performed in a bloodless field obtained by exsanguinating the limb with an Esmarch bandage and inflating the pneumatic tourniquet to 250 to 300 mm. Hg.

A. A curvilinear posteromedial incision is made, beginning 7 to 10 cm. proximal to the medial malleolus, passing 1 cm. behind the posterior margin of the tibia, and extending inferiorly to a point 1 cm. distal to the tip of the medial malleolus, where it is gently curved distally and anteriorly along the sustentaculum tali to terminate at the base of the first metatarsal bone. The subcutaneous tissue is divided. The wound flaps are undermined and retracted with 00 silk traction sutures. The soft tissues should be handled gently and should not be damaged by vigorous traction with rakes. Injury to veins and cutaneous nerves (the branches of the saphenous nerve and calcaneal branches of the lateral plantar nerve) should be avoided, and if possible, the venous drainage of the foot and leg should be left intact.

An alternative surgical approach is through two separate skin incisions. The medial and plantar aspect of the foot is exposed through a *medial incision,* convex dorsally, starting at the middle of the first metatarsal shaft and continuing proximally along the medial cuneiform and the sustentaculum tali; then swinging plantarward to terminate at the medial aspect of the calcaneal tuberosity. The second incision is for posterior release; it is made lateral to the tendo calcaneus, beginning at the heel and extending proximally for a distance of 7 to 10 cm. Another approach is the transverse Cincinnati incision described by Giannestras and Crawford and illustrated in Figure 2–43. The incision begins at the base of the first metatarsal and extends posteriorly 3 mm superior to the heel crease under the medial malleolus and then posteriorly to the tip of the lateral malleolus and distal to the cuboid–fifth metatarsal joint.

B. The paratenon of the triceps surae is divided longitudinally at the medial margin of the tendo Achillis. Inadvertent injury to the neurovascular bundle should be avoided.

C. Z-plastic lengthening of the tendo Achillis is performed in the anteroposterior plane. With a knife, the Achilles tendon is divided longitudinally into lateral and medial halves for a distance of 5 to 7 cm. The distal end of the medial half is detached from the calcaneus to prevent recurrence of varus deformity of the heel; the lateral half is divided proximally. The medial segment of the divided tendon is reflected proximally, and the lateral segment distally to its insertion to the calcaneal apophysis.

Plate 2. Open Reduction of Talocalcaneonavicular Joint in Talipes Equinovarus

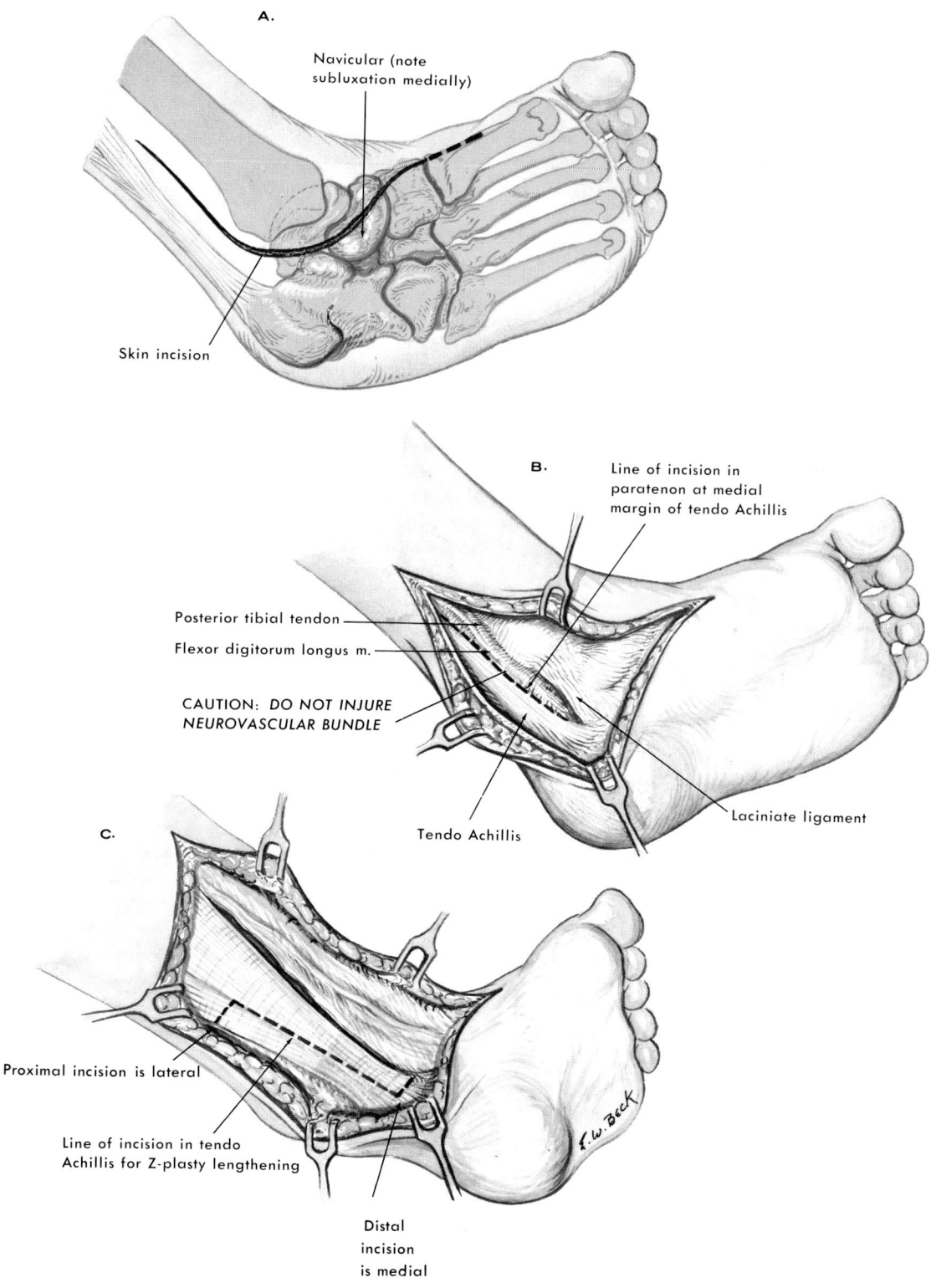

Open Reduction of Talocalcaneonavicular Joint in Talipes Equinovarus *(Continued)*

D and **E**. Next, the following structures are isolated and dissected free. In the distal part of the leg, immediately posterior to the tibia, the posterior tibial tendon is identified; it is deep to the flexor digitorum longus tendon. Pulling on the posterior tibial tendon will invert the midfoot, whereas pulling on the flexor digitorum longus tendon will flex the toes. A length of white Silastic tubing is placed around the posterior tibial tendon and another around the flexor digitorum longus tendon for gentle traction. With a nerve dissector, the neurovascular bundle is freed and traced distally to its canal beneath the laciniate ligament (flexor retinaculum), and a piece of yellow Silastic tubing is passed around it. Next, the flexor hallucis longus tendon is identified and retracted posterolaterally with white Silastic tubing.

The *laciniate ligament* is a strong, fibrous band extending from the medial malleolus above to the calcaneus below. It is the door to the plantar aspect of the foot, converting a series of bony grooves into four canals for the passage of tendons and the neurovascular bundle. Enumerated anteroposteriorly, these canals transmit: (1) the tendon of the tibialis posterior; (2) the tendon of the flexor digitorum longus; (3) the posterior tibial vessels and nerve; and (4) the tendon of the flexor hallucis longus (the latter canal is partly formed by the talus). The abductor hallucis longus muscle fibers take origin from the lower border of the laciniate ligament. With sharp and dull dissection, the abductor hallucis muscle is freed from its extensive origin—the navicular bone, sustentaculum tali, medial process of the calcaneal tuberosity, first metatarsal, and other structures on the medial aspect of the foot—elevated, and reflected distally and plantarward. The nerve supply to the abductor hallucis muscle (medial plantar nerve) should be preserved. In the severely deformed foot, or in the paralytic or arthrogrypotic clubfoot, the entire abductor hallucis muscle may be excised. Next, over a blunt probe, the flexor retinaculum is sectioned near its attachment to the medial malleolus. Do not injure the neurovascular bundle as it enters the plantar aspect of the foot.

Plate 2. Open Reduction of Talocaneonavicular Joint in Talipes Equinovarus

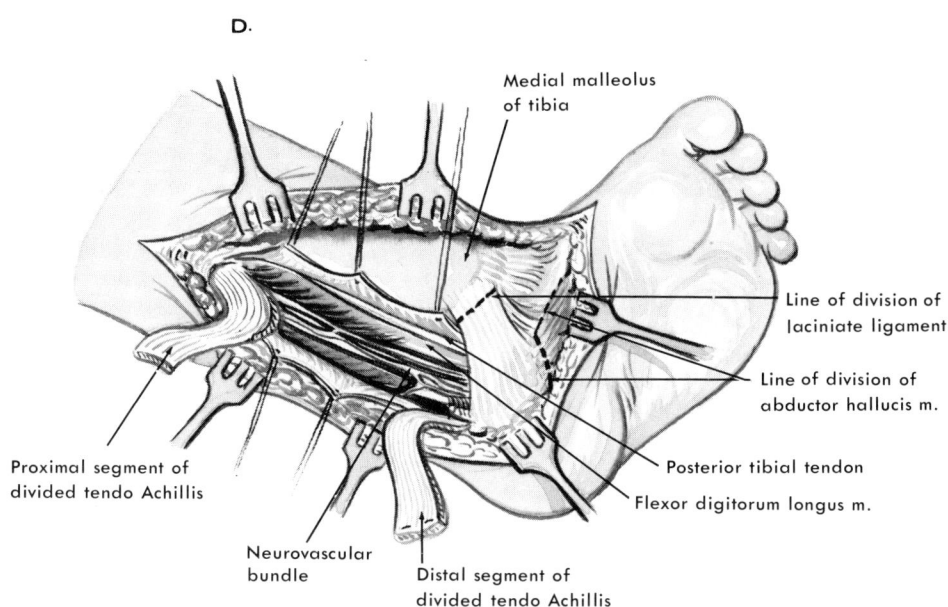

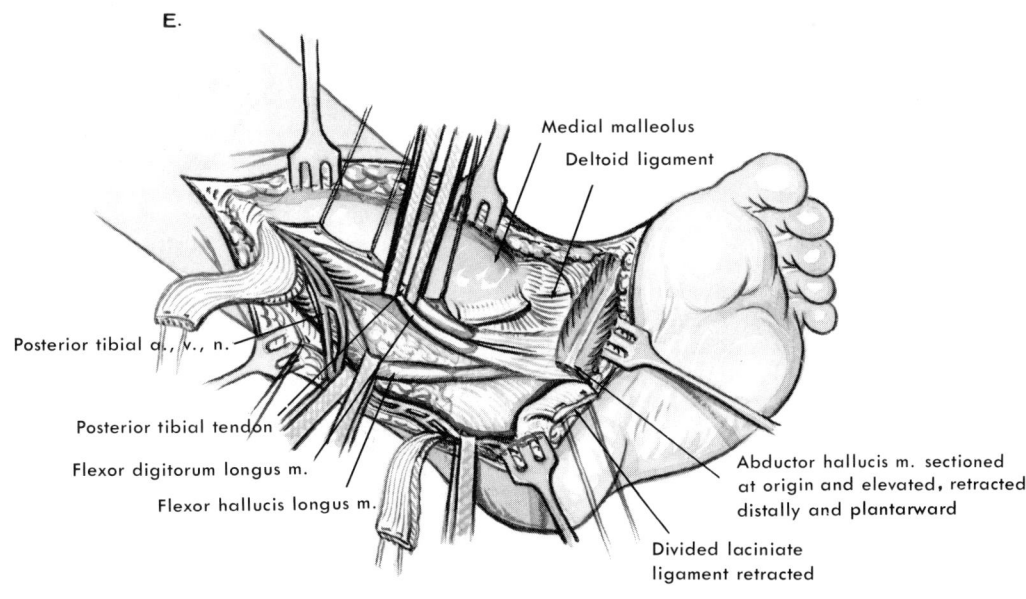

197

Open Reduction of Talocalcaneonavicular Joint in Talipes Equinovarus *(Continued)*

F. The posterior tibial tendon is lengthened by Z-plasty above the medial malleolus. The tendon sheath of the posterior tibial muscle behind the medial malleolus is left intact; its tendon is an important dynamic force in supporting the medial longitudinal arch of the foot, and its function should be preserved. This author does not section and discard it, because overcorrection and pes valgus are definite complications.

G. The proximal segment of the posterior tibial tendon is tagged with 000 Mersilene suture. The distal part of the tendon is pulled out of its sheath distally into the medial aspect of the foot. Traction on the distal posterior tibial stump will locate the navicular bone and talonavicular joint. The navicular will be found displaced medially and plantarward, and tethered to the medial malleolus and the sustentaculum tali by a dense mass of thick fibrous tissue. The joint lines are obscured, and it is easy to damage articular cartilage and bone. In order to avoid injury, dissection should proceed distally and not laterally. Sectioning of the neck or head of the talus and the sustentaculum tali should be avoided. Next, the *tibionavicular ligament* (or anterior part of the deltoid) is sectioned; it is a thickened band that extends from the medial malleolus to the tuberosity of the navicular. By gentle traction on the posterior tibial tendon, the talonavicular joint is identified, and the dorsal-medial parts of the talonavicular capsule are divided. The plantar calcaneonavicular ligament (spring ligament) is a thick band connecting the anterior margin of the sustentaculum tali of the calcaneus to the plantar surface of the navicular. It is shortened and is a fixed obstacle to reduction of the talocalcaneonavicular joint; it should be divided after adequate exposure. Normally, the plantar surface of the spring ligament is supported by the posterior tibial tendon medially and the flexor hallucis longus and flexor digitorum longus tendons laterally. (The posterior tibial tendon has already been divided and dissected free to its insertion.) Next, the flexor hallucis longus and flexor digitorum longus tendons are identified. The flexor hallucis longus tendon lies on the inferior surface of the sustentaculum tali.

H. Distal to the distal end of the sustentaculum tali, the flexor digitorum longus tendon crosses the flexor hallucis longus tendon from the lateral to the medial side in an oblique course dorsal (i.e., deep) to it. At the crossing point, the flexor hallucis longus and the flexor digitorum longus tendons are bound together by a strong fibrous band—the master knot of Henry—which is attached to the plantar surface of the navicular. With sharp scissors, the master knot of Henry is divided and the long flexor tendons are dissected free, mobilized, and retracted plantarward with the neurovascular bundle.

Plate 2. Open Reduction of Talocalcaneonavicular Joint in Talipes Equinovarus

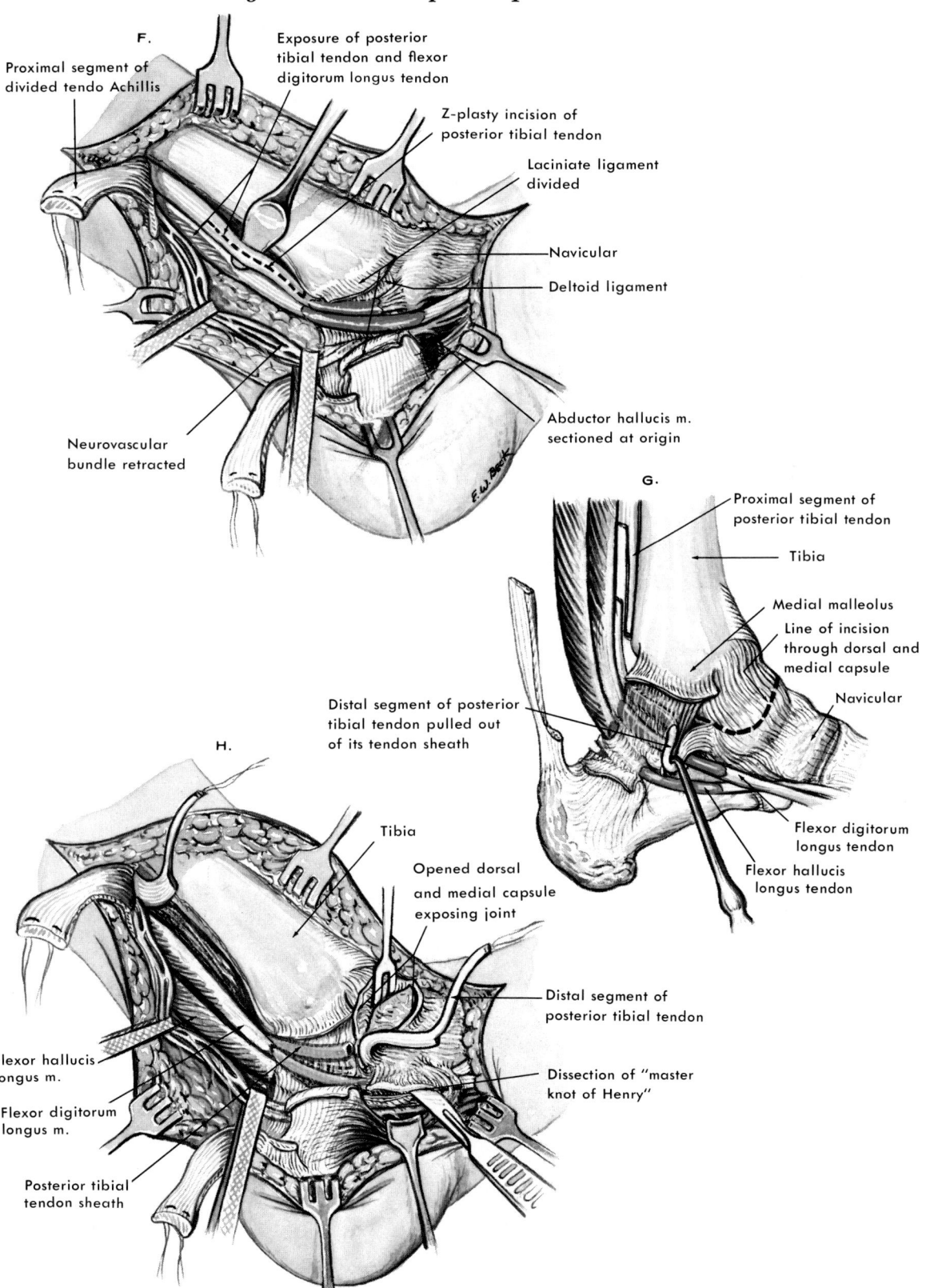

Open Reduction of Talocalcaneonavicular Joint in Talipes Equinovarus *(Continued)*

I. The plantar aspect of the foot is visualized; next, the neurovascular bundle and long toe flexors are retracted inferiorly, and the plantar calcaneonavicular ligament and the plantar part of the capsule of the talonavicular joint are sectioned. Then the calcaneonavicular limb of the bifurcate ligament is sectioned; it attaches the calcaneus to the lateral side of the navicular, and if shortened, will check lateral mobility of the navicular. If on manipulation, the cuboid does not translate horizontally, the calcaneocuboid limb of the bifurcate ligament is also sectioned (it is easier to do this through a lateral incision). The capsule of the naviculocuneiform is left intact.

J. The tibiocalcaneal, or middle, fibers of the superficial deltoid ligament are sectioned near the calcaneus; they descend almost perpendicularly to the whole length of the sustentaculum tali of the calcaneus. Medially, the subtalar joint runs a sinusoidal course; one should take care not to damage articular cartilage. The posterior fibers of the superficial deltoid ligament (posterior tibiotalar), which passes backward and laterally to the medial side of the talus and its medial tubercle, are divided.

K. The deep portion of the deltoid that inserts to the nonarticular portion of the body of the talus must be left intact because if it is divided, the body of the talus will tilt laterally and cause valgus deviation of the ankle. Next, if necessary, the hindfoot is everted and the interosseous talocalcaneal ligament is located above the sustentaculum tali and sectioned under direct vision.

L. The long toe flexors and the neurovascular bundle are retracted dorsally, and the plantar release is completed by partial excision of the plantar fascia and sectioning of the flexor digitorum brevis and quadratus plantae from their origins from the tuberosity of the calcaneus. By staying close to the bone and using a periosteal elevator for extraperiosteal stripping, injury to the neurovascular structures is avoided.

Plate 2. Open Reduction of Talocalcaneonavicular Joint in Talipes Equinovarus

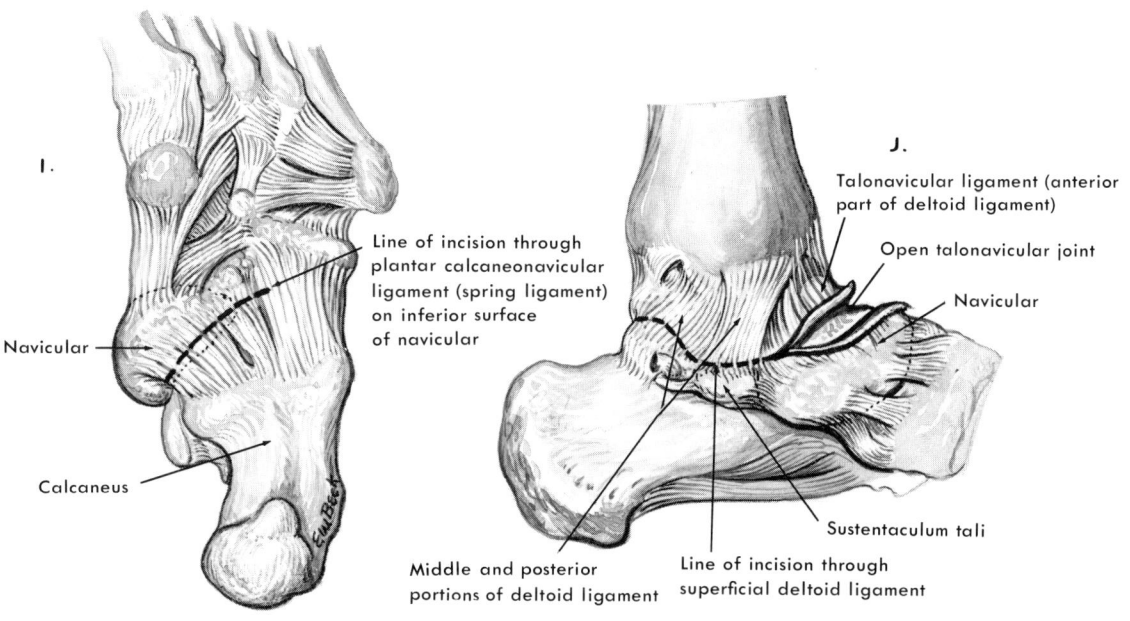

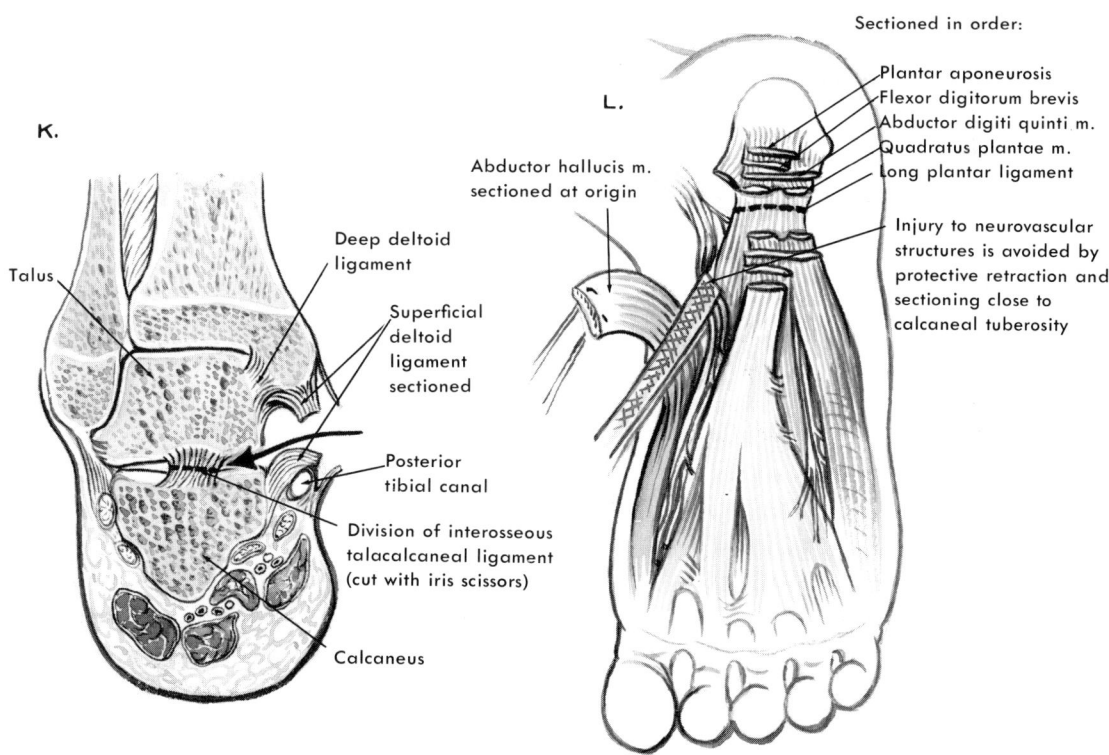

Open Reduction of Talocalcaneonavicular Joint in Talipes Equinovarus *(Continued)*

M. The posterior part of the capsule of the tibiotalar and talocalcaneal joint is exposed by retracting the flexor hallucis longus tendon medially and the peroneal tendons laterally. A Chandler elevator or Davis retractor is used to retract the peroneal tendons and protect them from inadvertent injury. The neurovascular structures behind the medial malleolus are retracted forward. Next, using Mayo or Metzenbaum scissors, completely divide the posterior capsule of the ankle joint by a horizontal incision, and the subtalar joint capsule by a sinusoidal cut. A knife should not be used, as it may damage the articular cartilage. Caution must be exercised so as not to injure the distal tibial physis. If in doubt, roentgenographic control should be utilized.

N. The posterior talofibular ligament holds the talus in a plantar-flexed position; it is divided vertically. In the lateral part of the wound, the calcaneofibular ligament is identified and sectioned, with care taken not to injure the peroneal tendons. This author strongly recommends that a separate lateral incision be used for sectioning of the calcaneofibular ligament and a complete lateral release be performed.

O. A lateral release is performed as follows: A longitudinal incision is made, centered over the sinus tarsi, beginning 2 cm. above and behind the lateral malleolus and ending over the base of the fourth metatarsal. The subcutaneous tissue is divided in line with the other incision; preserve the veins if possible and do not injure the sural nerve. The wound edges are gently retracted. The superior peroneal retinaculum is divided. Identify the peroneal tendons and excise the thickened peroneal tendon sheaths. The peroneal tendons are retracted anteriorly, and the thickened and shortened calcaneofibular ligament is identified and divided by an oblique cut. Next the lateral talocalcaneal ligament and capsule are completely sectioned. Do not disturb circulation of the talus by dissection of the sinus tarsi and inferior aspect of the neck of the talus. The inferior extensor retinaculum is divided and the extensor digitorum brevis is elevated from its origin and reflected distally. Next, divide the dorsal and lateral fibers of the calcaneocuboid capsule and the cubonavicular oblique ligament. This will allow the anterior portion of the calcaneus to rotate laterally.

Plate 2. Open Reduction of Talocalcaneonavicular Joint in Talipes Equinovarus

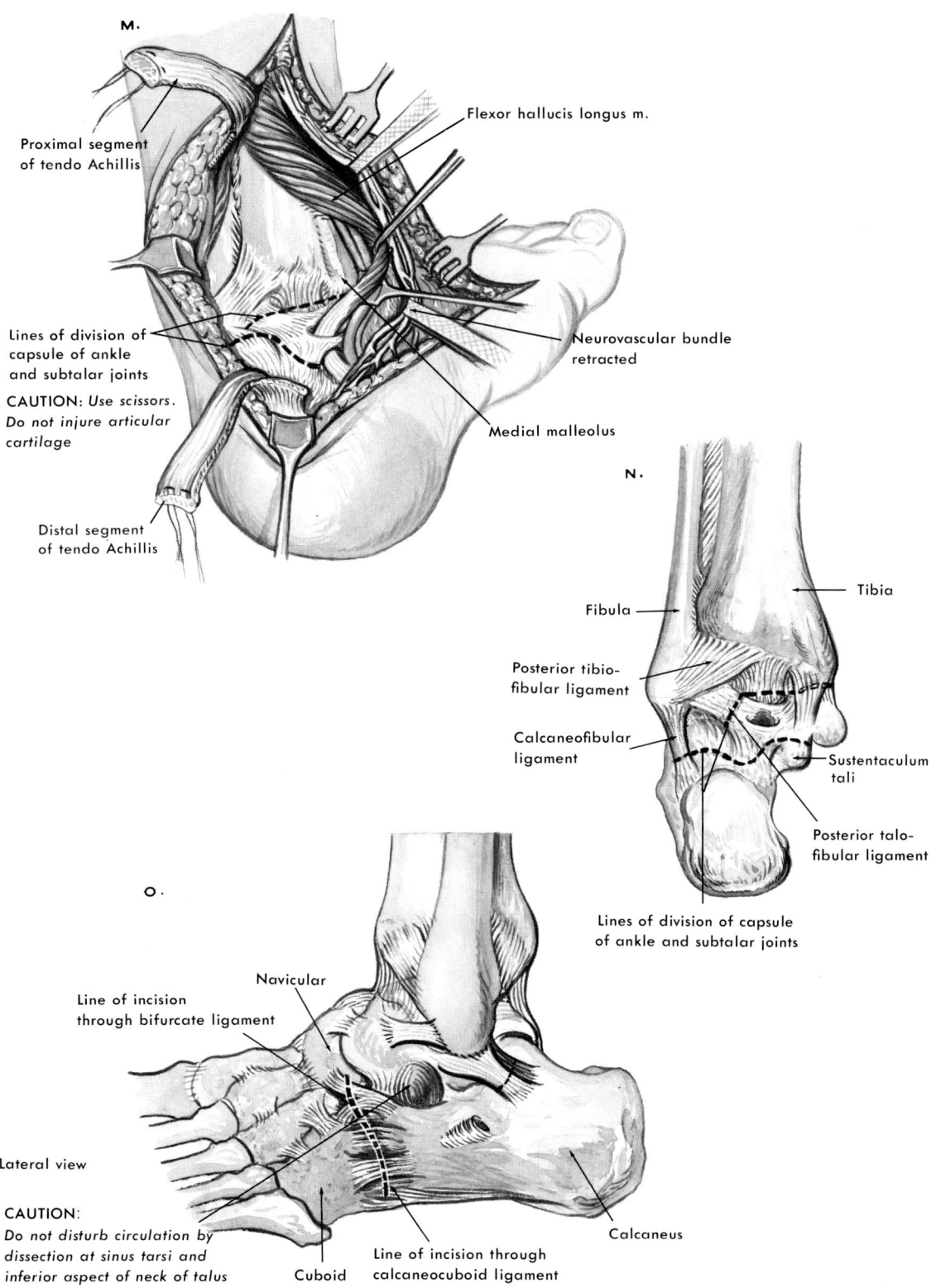

Open Reduction of Talocalcaneonavicular Joint in Talipes Equinovarus *(Continued)*

P. In the older child, or in very rigid talipes equinovarus, the lateral column of the foot is elongated, acting as an obstacle to reduction of the talocalcaneonavicular joint, and therefore it should be shortened. In the child eight years of age or younger, the anterior end of the calcaneus is resected (see Lichtblau procedure). In the child nine years old or older and in paralytic clubfoot or in clubfoot associated with extensive medial scarring and recurrent deformity, the calcaneocuboid joint is resected and fused (see Evans operation).

Q & R. Next, the foot and ankle are gently manipulated into increasing dorsiflexion. The dome of the talus should be repositioned in the ankle mortise, and on dorsiflexion of the ankle, the posterior surface of the body of the talus should be seen. In severe fixed equinus deformity, one may have to section the distal tibiofibular syndesmosis. Fractional lengthening of the flexor hallucis longus and flexor digitorum longus muscles at their musculotendinous junction may be required if the toes are acutely flexed upon neutral dorsiflexion of the ankle. In severe flexion deformity of the hallux, Z-lengthening of the flexor hallucis longus is performed on the plantar aspect of the foot. Next, the anterior end of the talus is rotated medially, and distal traction is applied on the forefoot and midfoot in the equinovarus posture, and then slowly the navicular is repositioned over the anterior end of the talus.

Reduction is facilitated by introducing a threaded Steinmann pin in the longitudinal axis of the talus from the posterior aspect of its body. It should be directed toward the center of the anterior end of the talus. The leverage of the pin is used to rotate the anterior end of the talus medially, and that of the calcaneus laterally, obtaining normal talocalcaneal divergence in the anteroposterior plane. Then distal traction is applied on the forefoot, the navicular is pushed laterally, and the anterior end of the calcaneus rotated laterally, achieving concentric reduction of the talocalcaneonavicular joint. Sometimes the taut interosseous talocalcaneal ligament may have to be sectioned to correct medial spin of the calcaneus. Overcorrection, a common error after extensive soft-tissue release, should be avoided. The Steinmann pin is then drilled distally across the talonavicular joint and out through the forefoot. The drill is changed to the anterior end of the pin, and the pin is withdrawn so that its posterior end is flush with the back of the talus. Anteroposterior and lateral roentgenograms of the foot and ankle are made in the corrected position to verify concentricity of reduction of the talocalcaneonavicular joint. The importance of intraoperative x-rays cannot be overemphasized. If reduction is concentric, the protruding anterior end of the pin is cut off subcutaneously or protruding through the skin 1 cm. If the interosseous ligament is sectioned, it is best to fix the calcaneus to the talus with one or two threaded Steinmann pins to maintain corrected horizontal rotation. The pins are inserted from the plantar surface of the calcaneus, up through the talus but not protruding through the ankle joint. The wounds are irrigated, a compression bandage is applied, and the tourniquet is released. After a few minutes, the compression bandage is removed, and complete hemostasis is obtained.

Plate 2. Open Reduction of Talocalcaneonavicular Joint in Talipes Equinovarus

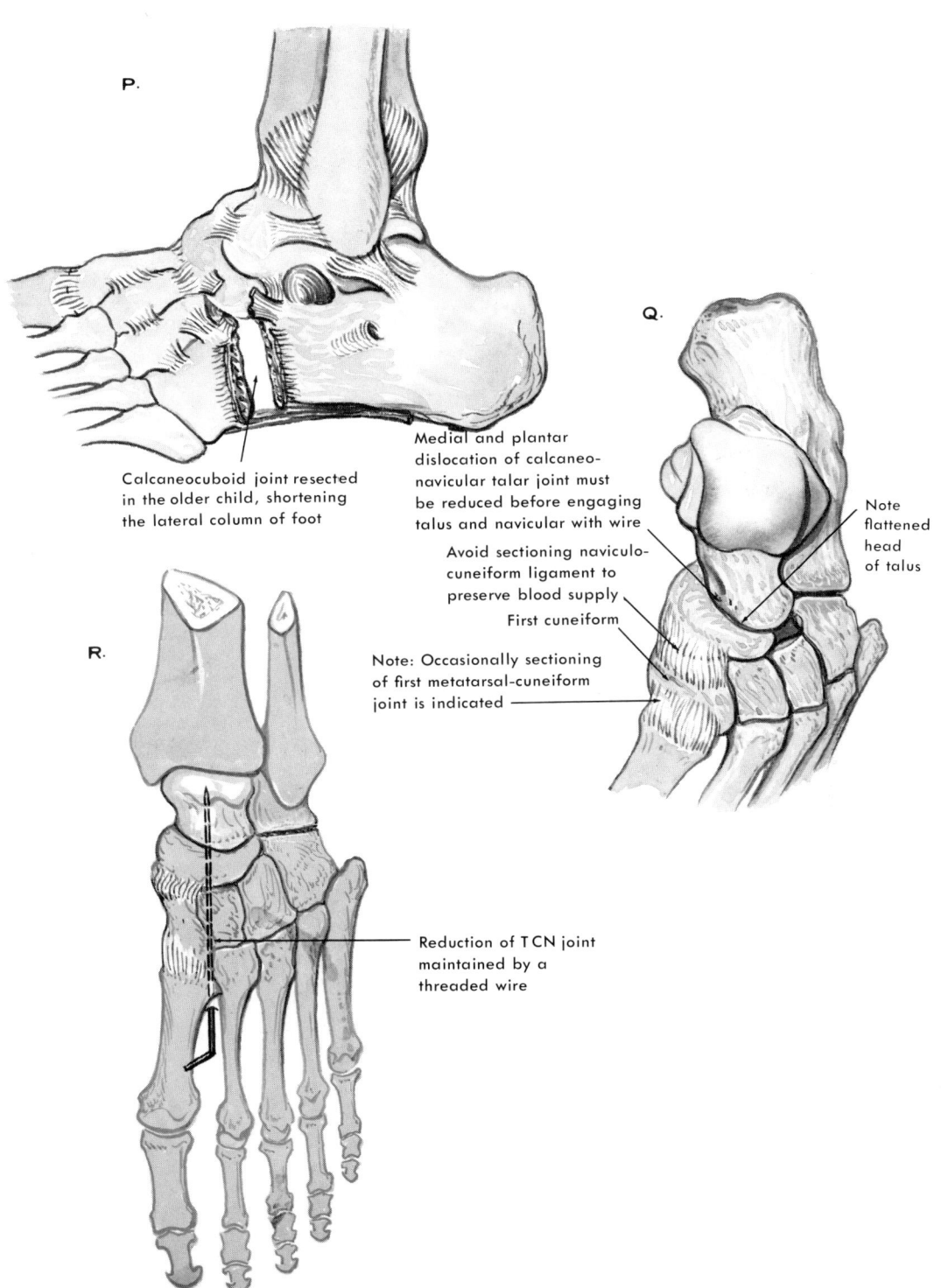

Open Reduction of Talocalcaneonavicular Joint in Talipes Equinovarus (Continued)

S. The distal segment of the posterior tibial tendon is introduced through its canal behind the medial malleolus, delivered into the back of the ankle, and resutured to its proximal segment.

T. The tendo Achillis is resutured with proper tension with the ankle at only 5 degrees of dorsiflexion. Avoid overlengthening of the triceps surae muscle. Do not insert a transverse pin across the os calcis at this time. The skin margins are observed for adequacy of circulation; they may be blanched from tension when the ankle is maximally dorsiflexed. The subcutaneous tissues are closed by interrupted plain catgut sutures, and the skin with intracutaneous Dexon sutures. A few additional interrupted sutures (0000 nylon) are placed behind the medial malleolus and the instep of the foot. A bulky sterile dressing and sheet wadding are applied and reinforced with an above-knee well-padded plaster of Paris cast. The ankle joint is immobilized in plantar flexion to relax the tension on the skin edges. If there is any question about circulation to the skin, the cast is omitted and only a Jones compression dressing with a posterior splint is applied.

POSTOPERATIVE CARE

Ten to fourteen days after surgery, the patient is taken back to the operating room, and under general anesthesia, the dressing is removed and wound healing is assessed. *The sutures are not removed.* The foot is gently manipulated to 10 to 15 degrees of dorsiflexion, and a threaded pin is inserted transversely across the calcaneus. The position of the pins and the articular relations are double-checked by anteroposterior and lateral roentgenograms. The pin ends are cut off with 2 cm. protruding from the skin edge. Sterile Vaseline strips are rolled around the protruding ends of the pin in the os calcis. Insertion of a pin transversely across the os calcis is not always necessary. It is indicated in rigid equinus deformity. An above-knee cast is applied, incorporating the calcaneal pins in the cast; the knee is in 60 degrees of flexion, and the ankle in 10 to 15 degrees of dorsiflexion; the heel and forefoot are at 10 degrees valgus. Avoid excessive valgus inclination and overcorrection; the reduction of the talocalcaneonavicular joint should be concentric.

Two weeks later, the cast may have to be changed if tight. This is done in the office; general anesthesia is not required. At this time, the sutures are removed, but not the pins. The foot is brought into further dorsiflexion (not more than 20 degrees), and a new, well-molded above-knee cast is applied, incorporating the os calcis pin. Again, excessive valgus angulation should be avoided.

The third cast is changed six to seven weeks postoperatively. The skin is cleansed. The sutures and the pins across the talonavicular joint and the os calcis are removed. A new above-knee cast is applied with the ankle at 20 to 25 degrees of dorsiflexion. Thereafter the casts are changed as necessary. The total period of cast immobilization is two to three months. In the older child, the last cast may be a below-knee walking cast. Caution! Place the walking heel under the middle of the foot and not anteriorly. An anterior walking heel will stretch the triceps surae and cause calcaneus deformity.

After removal of the cast, the foot and ankle are held at night in a slightly overcorrected position in an above-knee posterior splint made of polypropylene or some other plastic. The purpose of this retentive apparatus is to maintain correction; it is used for one or two years until skeletal growth remodels and straightens the medial and plantar tilting of the head and neck of the talus, and normal articular relationships are restored. The decreased angle of declination of the talus may be compared to excessive femoral antetorsion in congenital dislocation of the hip; the same principles should be applied.

The Denis Browne splint (with a 10- to 25-cm. everting cross bar between the feet) is not recommended, as it is ineffective in controlling the ankle and hindfoot, and may cause genu valgum and exaggerated lateral tibiofibular torsion.

Plate 2. Open Reduction of Talocalcaneonavicular Joint in Talipes Equinovarus

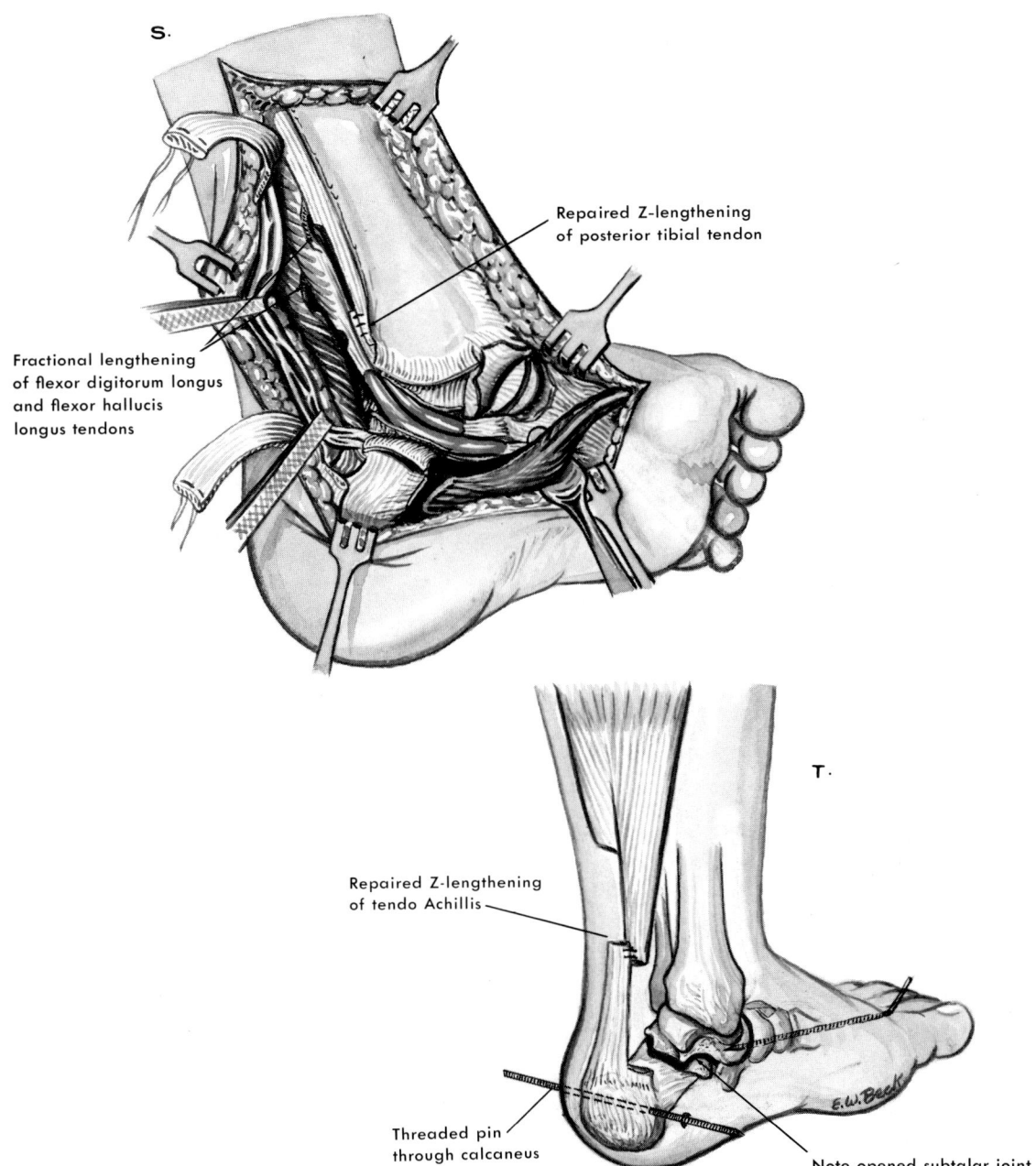

Postoperatively the child wears normal shoes. Special shoes such as outflare lateral heel and sole wedges are unnecessary.

It is vital to provide dynamic muscle forces to act on the foot and ankle. The motor power of the evertors and dorsiflexors is strengthened by *active exercises*. In the infant, stimulation techniques are utilized. *Passive exercises* are carried out to maintain normal range of motion of the ankle and foot. These exercises are performed gently several times a day.

tension on the skin margins is relaxed. The cast is changed 10 to 14 days after the operation, bringing the ankle into dorsiflexion. The sutures are not removed at this time. A transverse pin is inserted in the os calcis if indicated. By paying attention to these details one will obtain primary wound healing.

Wound dehiscence is still a problem in the rigid clubfoot in arthrogryposis multiplex congenita and myelomeningocele. The previously operated on, scarred foot also presents difficulties with wound healing. When wound slough develops, the foot should be maintained in the corrected position in the cast. The wound is allowed to granulate and epithelialize, and Betadine dressings are applied daily through a window in the cast. The cast is changed as necessary. The pin in the talonavicular joint should not be removed; however, one often has to remove the one in the calcaneus. In severe sloughs, consultation with a plastic surgeon may be in order; a split- or full-thickness skin graft may be indicated.

Calcaneus Deformity. This deformity of the ankle and hindfoot is due to overcorrection of the equinus deformity. It can be prevented by not overlengthening the tendo Achillis and by not applying a walking cast with an anterior heel, which will stretch the triceps surae muscle. The walking heel should be put posteriorly under the midfoot near the longitudinal axis of the tibia.

Dorsal Subluxation. Dorsal subluxation of the talonavicular joint or of both the talonavicular and the calcaneocuboid joints may occur (Fig. 2–44). This can be prevented by verifying the concentricity of the talocalcaneonavicular joint by intraoperative roentgenograms.

Overcorrection. Valgus inclination may be produced at either the ankle or the talocalcaneonavicular joint. The tibiotalar portion of the deltoid ligament should not be divided and the foot should not be immobilized in extreme calcaneovalgus position. Valgus distortion of the ankle or foot can be prevented by attention to concentricity of reduction. Function of the posterior tibial muscle should be preserved by lengthening its tendon above the medial malleolus. The posterior tibial tendon should not be resected or transferred at the time of open reduction.

Failure to Achieve (or Loss of) Reduction. To ensure establishment of normal articular relations, it is imperative that intraoperative x-rays of the foot and ankle be made in two planes—true anteroposterior and true lateral. Is there a normal angle of talocalcaneal divergence in the anteroposterior and lateral projections? This author uses a threaded Steinmann pin to transfix the talonavicular joint. At the second cast change, a second threaded pin is inserted across the os calcis and is incorporated in the cast. A smooth pin may slip out. Failure to fix the calcaneus to the cast may allow the heel to slip upward, in which case correction will be lost and a rocker-bottom deformity will result. If the talocalcaneal interosseous lig-

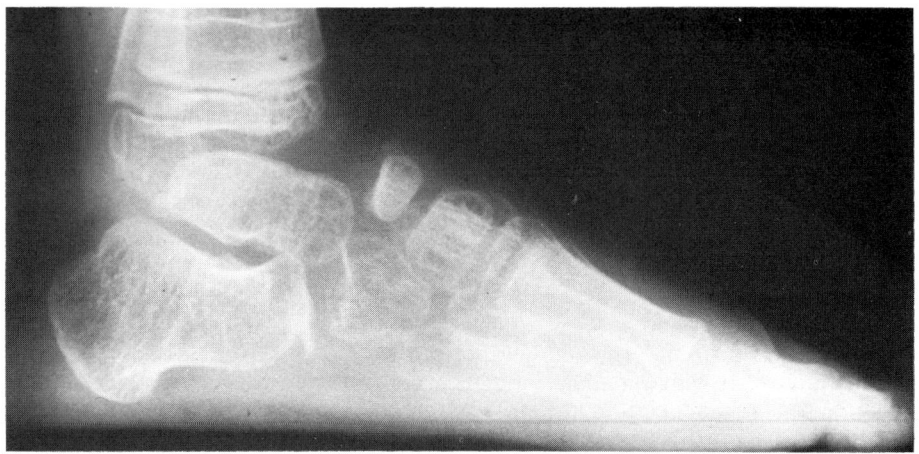

FIGURE 2–44. Dorsal subluxation of the talonavicular and calcaneocuboid joints.

ament is divided, the talocalcaneal joint should be fixed internally with one or two threaded Steinmann pins.

Loss of correction following removal of the cast may be due to failure to maintain reduction in a retentive apparatus for an adequate period. The decreased angle of declination of the talus should straighten to normal, and all articular malalignments should be corrected with skeletal growth and remodeling. It is essential to pay meticulous attention to postoperative care; the foot and ankle should be immobilized in a solid cast for two to three months, followed by splinting at night for another one to two years. Passive exercises are performed to maintain a normal range of joint motion, and active exercises are carried out to establish a dynamic balance of muscles acting on the foot and ankle. Scarring on the medial and plantar aspects of the foot should be avoided.

In some cases talocalcaneal navicular subluxation recurs because of persistent medial and plantar tilting of the head and neck of the talus. Hjelmstedt and Sahlstedt performed a chevron osteotomy to correct the deformity and realign the declination angle to normal.[274, 279, 280] Roberts described an open-up osteotomy of the neck of the talus with bone graft from the ilium.[549a] This author concurs with Roberts and recommends his technique; it should not, however, be a primary procedure and should not be performed on a child under three years of age.

Aseptic Necrosis of Talus. The blood supply of the talus is derived principally from the artery of the tarsal sinus entering from the anterolateral side of the talus, from the artery of the tarsal canal on its posteromedial aspect, and from a rich source from the medial surface distal to the articular facet of the medial malleolus. The major blood supply to the body of the talus enters through the neck of the talus.[242] There is a definite hazard of interruption of the blood supply to the body of the talus when extensive peritalar release is performed. Vascular injury to the three major blood sources proximal to their anastomoses may occur, or one may interrupt circulation at the entrance of the vascular network into the anteroinferior portion of the talar neck. Aplington and Riddle studied 321 congenital clubfeet in 203 patients retrospectively. Thirty-five of these patients had extensive combined medial and lateral release; five of them, or 14.3 per cent, developed aseptic necrosis of the body of the talus. No aseptic necrosis of the talus was found when the medial release was done alone or combined with posterior release, even when the subtalar joint was released from the medial side. In all cases with aseptic necrosis, however, the medial release was combined with extensive lateral dissection, including the sinus tarsi and the subtalar joint, which was released both medially and laterally. The authors strongly urged the surgeon to refrain from lateral dissection of the subtalar joint, particularly of the sinus tarsi, in conjunction with medial release.[13]

This author has avoided aseptic necrosis of the talus by not disturbing the circulation of the inferior aspect of the neck of the talus and by not entering the sinus tarsi.

Aseptic Necrosis of Navicular. This complication is especially likely to occur if the naviculocuneiform capsule is released. It is of no clinical importance, as revascularization of the navicular bone will take place without difficulty.

Wound Infection. If this unfortunate complication develops, the wound is debrided, cleansed, and closed primarily with suction drainage. Do not leave the wound open to granulate; excessive scarring will result. The talocalcaneonavicular joint is kept in the corrected position in a new cast. If possible, the Steinmann pin is left transfixing the talonavicular joint.

Forefoot Varus and Equinus Deformity. Lowe and Hannon reviewed 73 clubfeet in 51 children between the ages of 4 and 14 years to determine the presence or absence of forefoot adduction as a residual deformity. The alignment of the feet was assessed clinically and by weight-bearing anteroposterior roentgenograms. The authors measure the degree of metatarsus varus by relating the position of the first metatarsal to the navicular bone. First, a line is drawn to join the extremities of the proximal articular surface of the navicular; then a central line is drawn through the longitudinal axis of the first metatarsal. The lateral angle formed by the junction of these two lines is the "naviculometatarsal angle" (Fig. 2–45). The authors admit the contribution of the

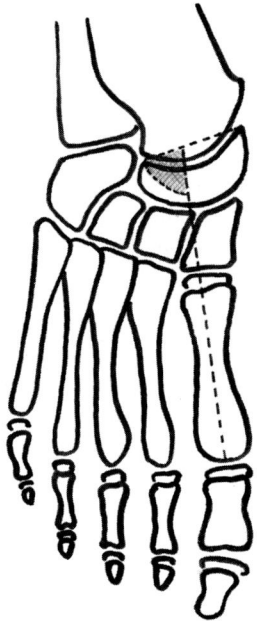

FIGURE 2–45. The naviculometatarsal angle.

The method of measurement is described in the text. (Redrawn after Lowe, L. W., and Hannon, M. A.: Residual adduction of the forefoot in treated congenital clubfoot. J. Bone Joint Surg., 55-B:810, 1973.)

naviculocuneiform and cuneiform-metatarsal joints to this measurement, but state such distinction is of no practical value. The average naviculometatarsal angle of a normal foot is 93.5 degrees, with a range from 86 to 100 degrees. A value in excess of 100 degrees represents some degree of metatarsus varus. On clinical examination, they found forefoot adduction in 38 of 73 treated clubfeet (52 per cent). Roentgenographic study of the group with adduction showed metatarsus varus alone in 45 per cent, and medial subluxation of the talonavicular joint alone in 26 per cent. Meticulous roentgenographic assessment and measurement, therefore, showed that 74 per cent of the group with forefoot adduction had metatarsus varus. In the 35 feet with no residual forefoot adduction, only 45 per cent had normal roentgenographic features; in the remainder, i.e., 55 per cent, there were various forms of spurious correction—metatarsus varus with valgus overcorrection of the talonavicular joint, talonavicular medial subluxation with metatarsus valgus, and talonavicular medial subluxation with outward rotation of the ankle joint. Lowe and Hannon recommended detachment of the origin of the abductor hallucis muscle at the time of extended posterior release, with tenotomy of the tendon of insertion through a separate incision as an additional measure.[392]

The author corrects the overpull of the abductor hallucis and plantar soft tissues at the time of open reduction of the talocalcaneonavicular joint by sectioning the origin of the abductor hallucis and by plantar release. This has obviated the problem of forefoot varus deviation. If metatarsus varus develops, it is corrected by Heymann-Herndon-Strong tarsometatarsal capsulotomies and intermetatarsal ligamentous release if the child is less than seven years of age; in a child eight years of age or over, a valgus osteotomy at the base of the metatarsals is performed.

Rigidity of the Foot. Rigidity is prevented by carrying out very gentle manipulations and avoiding hyaline cartilage compression and cartilage necrosis. During surgery, injury to joint cartilage should be avoided.

Tendon Transfers. The equinovarus position of the foot gives a mechanical advantage to the invertors and plantar-flexors of the foot. The evertors and dorsiflexors are in a relatively weak position as they are stretched over the convexity of the dorsolateral aspect of the foot, whereas the anterior and posterior tibial tendons function in a mechanically advantageous position as they run a straight line to their insertions on the concavity of the medial border of the foot.

Muscle imbalance with motor weakness of the peroneals and toe extensor muscles may be a factor in recurrence of equinovarus deformity in the older child. Occasionally tendon transfers may be indicated to balance the dynamic forces acting on the foot and ankle. The muscles that are available for transfer are the anterior tibial (whole or half), posterior tibial, Achilles tendon, flexor hallucis longus, flexor digitorum longus, and extensor hallucis longus.

ANTERIOR TIBIAL TENDON TRANSFER. Lateral transfer of the anterior tibial tendon was recommended by Garceau.[205-212] Critchley and Taylor, Ponseti and Campos, Raynal and Judet, and Singer and Fripp have also reported their experience with tibialis anterior transfer in congenital clubfoot.[125, 521, 537, 605] In his last report, Garceau stated that the operation is indicated if there have been multiple recurrences of all components of the deformity, if there is weakness or absence of the peroneus longus and brevis muscles, and if "bowstringing" of the anterior tibial tendon and supination of the forepart of the foot are evident in the swing phase of gait. He stressed the importance of correcting fixed deformity prior to tendon transfer. Roentgenograms of the foot should be taken, as clinical evaluation of the foot is not necessarily adequate to assess the amount of correction obtained. Garceau also suggested the possible use of electromyographic studies of the peroneus longus and brevis muscles in order to permit a more accurate assessment of the potential power of these muscles and to minimize the risk of overcorrection.[212] Singer and Fripp found that lateral transfer of the anterior tibial tendon does not increase dorsiflexion power and that relapse occurred in 52 of 76 feet on which the procedure had been performed.[605] Raynal and Judet stated that lateral transfer of all or half of the anterior tibial tendon results in overcorrection, pes cavus, and restriction of plantar flexion. Of the 51 cases they re-examined (with a 9- to 25-year follow-up), only 14 had gained a noticeable benefit.[537]

The author does not recommend lateral transfer of the anterior tibial tendon in talipes equinovarus for the following reasons: (1) with anterior tibial tendon transfer, a varying degree of loss of power of ankle dorsiflexion occurs and causes recurrence of equinus deformity of the ankle; (2) equinus posture of the first metatarsal and clawing of the great toe result because of the unopposed action of the peroneus longus muscle; and (3) when the varus deformity is corrected, peroneal muscle power returns and provides active eversion of the foot. Even when the anterior tibial tendon is transferred only to the third metatarsal, overcorrection and valgus deformity are potential complications. Lateral transfer of the anterior tibial tendon is indicated only very occasionally when (1) there is unquestionable motor weakness of the peroneals; (2) there is definite evidence of motor weakness of the triceps surae muscle as a result of overzealous heel cord lengthening; (3) the foot is completely flexible, with no fixed varus or equinus deformity (i.e., the passive range of ankle dorsiflexion is 10 to 20 degrees, forefoot abduction is 10 degrees, and eversion of the forefoot and hindfoot is 10 to 20 degrees); (4) the anterior tibial tendon is normal in motor strength, and (5) the child is at least four years of age and in a family situation that will provide adequate postoperative training and care. Roentgenograms of the foot should disclose normal alignment of the talocalcaneonavicular articulation preoperatively, because a tendon transfer will not correct a fixed deformity. To prevent overcorrection, the tendon should not be transferred farther laterally than the base of the third metatarsal.

Splitting the anterior tibial tendon into halves and transferring its lateral half to the base of the fifth metatarsal, leaving its medial half intact and attached to its insertion, is useful in treating dynamic calcaneocavovarus deformity of the foot in paralytic conditions. It preserves some function of the anterior tibial as a dorsiflexor of the first metatarsal to balance its antagonist, the peroneus longus, as a plantar-flexor of the first metatarsal. The procedure is not indicated in talipes equinovarus.

POSTERIOR TIBIAL TENDON TRANSFER. The posterior tibial tendon is a strong tethering force in talipes equinovarus.[73, 197] A number of ways of treating it have been recorded in the literature: (1) section and discard; (2) Z-lengthening at the insertion; (3) Z-lengthening above the medial malleolus; (4) anterior transfer through the interosseous route simultaneously with open reduction of the talocalcaneonavicular joint; (5) Z-lengthening at the time of open reduction of the talocalcaneonavicular joint, preserving its motor tendon, and transferring it anteriorly through the interosseous route at a later date if necessary; and (6) sectioning and transferring to the lengthened Achilles tendon.

Fried dissected the insertions of the posterior tibial tendon in 54 clubfeet with recurrent deformity and in two clubfeet that had had no previous treatment. In all the cases, the insertions were abnormal. Beginning at the level of the medial malleolus, the tendon changed to a thick, hard, fibrous mass that encompassed the entire medial side of the tarsus and inserted with thick strands of fibrous tissue to other parts of the foot, namely, the plantar fascia, deep plantar ligaments, anterior tibial tendon, os calcis, navicular, cuneiforms, and cuboid bone. Fried believed the deforming force of the posterior tibial muscle to be the principal cause of recurrence of clubfoot.[197]

The posterior tibial muscle will function as an active dorsiflexor of the ankle when transferred to the dorsum of the foot through the interosseous membrane. This has been demonstrated by numerous authors in various paralytic conditions such as poliomyelitis, leprosy, Charcot-Marie-Tooth disease, Friedreich's ataxia, and spastic paralysis.[96, 237, 304, 454] Fried recommended transferring the posterior tibial muscle to the dorsum of the foot in talipes equinovarus via the interosseous route and suturing it to the third cuneiform bone. Lengthening of the Achilles tendon and capsulotomy of the posterior parts of the ankle and subtalar joints were performed at the same time to achieve correction of equinus deformity. Capsulotomy of the talonavicular, navicular–first cuneiform, and first cuneiform–first metatarsal joints was also carried out. He reported the results to be good in 12 of the 13 patients who were followed for at least four years. In seven patients, the results were excellent, with full correction of the deformity and satisfactory function. In five patients, minor residual deformity persisted, and walking on tiptoes was still not feasible. In one patient, the result was unsatisfactory because of overcorrection resulting from a too lateral transfer of the tendon to the cuboid rather than only as far as the third cuneiform.[197]

Singer, in 1961, reported that anterior transfer of the posterior tibial tendon in 28 congenital clubfeet stabilized the correction obtained by serial wedging casts. The age range of the patients at surgery was two and one half to eight and one half years. The follow-up period was one to three years. There was no relapse in 27 of the 28 feet. In two thirds of the cases, the tendon was too short and was attached to either the peroneus tertius tendon, if present, or to the lateral two tendons of the extensor digitorum longus. In only one third of the cases was the tendon anchored to the bone, either the lateral or the middle cuneiform. Singer did not recommend the operation when soft-tissue release had been previously performed, because in five such feet, when the posterior tibial tendons were exposed, they proved to be thin, atrophic, adherent to surrounding tissues, and unsatisfactory for transfer.[604]

Gartland suggested that muscle imbalance was the primary cause of relapse in clubfoot, and he recommended anterior transfer of the posterior tibial tendon through the interosseous membrane. He published a preliminary report in 1964. The results in 20 feet in 16 patients were given, and the average follow-up was two years.[214] In 1972, Gartland and Surgent reported the results in 26 feet in 22 children with an average follow-up period of seven years. The results were excellent in 14 feet (54 per cent), satisfactory in 8 feet (31 per cent), and unsatisfactory in 4 feet (15 per cent). The result was graded excellent when the foot was plantigrade and normally aligned, with the transferred posterior tibial muscle functioning as a balancing motor unit and the patient wearing normal shoes. A satisfactory result was a foot with minor residual deformities of heel varus deviation or forefoot adduction that was nevertheless balanced and plantigrade, with a functioning posterior tibial transfer and the ability to wear normal shoes. Unsatisfactory feet were those that could not be evaluated as excellent or satisfactory. Analyses of the failures showed the cause to be inadequate surgical technique rather than any basic fault or breakdown of the procedure. In two feet, severe valgus deformity developed; in both, the tendon had been incorrectly transferred to the cuboid instead of the third cuneiform. In two feet, the posterior tibial muscle failed to function because the tendon adhered in a small opening in the interosseous membrane. Gartland and Surgent emphasized the importance of making an aperture in the interosseous membrane large enough to prevent adherence of the tendon at that site. Upon correlating the result with the age at operation, they found that all seven children operated on at three years of age or younger were in the excellent or satisfactory grade (100 per cent). Of the 19 feet of 15 children who were older than three years of age at surgery, however, the result was excellent or satisfactory in 80 per cent, and unsatisfactory in 20 per cent. Gartland and Surgent believed that, when indicated, the procedure should be performed by the age of two or three years in order to forestall adaptive secondary bony changes.[215]

Turner and Cooper reviewed the experience of posterior tibial transfer at the University Hospitals in Iowa City. The operation was performed in seven cases of very difficult recurrent clubfoot; in five the transfer functioned, in four with good result, and in one with poor result; in two the transfer did not function. In the four feet rated good, the correction of equinovarus deformity was maintained and there was active dorsiflexion of the ankle to neutral or slightly beyond. *In none of the cases, however, did the transferred tendon function as a dorsiflexor during gait.* One patient developed calcaneovalgus deformity. They concluded that in difficult recurrent clubfoot, posterior tibial transfer may be beneficial, provided that: (1) its motor strength is good or better before transfer; (2) deformity is fully corrected by soft-tissue release or bony stabilization; and (3) the tendon is transferred to the midline of the foot, to either the second or third cuneiform.[660]

Del Sel and associates divided the posterior tibial tendon at its insertion to the navicular (which facilitates exposure of the talonavicular and subtalar joints) and dissected it free up to its muscle fibers; then they transferred it posteriorly and sutured it to both segments of the lengthened Achilles tendon. The transfer removes the deforming force of the posterior tibial muscle and reinforces the strength of the triceps surae, which may be weakened because of overlengthening in severe neglected cases of talipes equinovarus.[140]

This author strongly objects to the routine primary anterior transfer of the posterior tibial tendon through the interosseous route to the dorsolateral aspect of the foot. In a two- or three-year old child, it is very difficult, if not impossible, to train an out-of-phase tendon transfer (e.g., to teach an invertor and plantar-flexor to function as an evertor and dorsiflexor). As stated previously, in talipes equinovarus, apart from directional changes, there are no primary abnormalities of the muscles and tendons. The posterior tibial muscle is contracted; this strong deforming force can be weakened by Z-lengthening of its tendon above the medial malleolus. Its action should be preserved, however, to prevent pes planovalgus. Therefore, do not section and discard the posterior tibial tendon.

Anterior transfer of the posterior tibial tendon has an extremely limited place in the treatment of talipes equinovarus. Its sole indication is unquestionable muscle imbalance in which the evertors and dorsiflexors of the ankle and foot are weak and the strong invertors and plantar-flexors are pulling the foot into equinovarus position. It is indicated then only when the following prerequisites are met: (1) the deformity of talipes equinovarus and articular malalignment can be corrected with the ankle and foot fully flexible with normal range of passive motion (this basic rule of tendon transfer should not be violated); (2) motor strength of the posterior tibial muscle is good or normal; (3) continuity and length of the tendon are adequate to allow technical feasibility of the transfer; and (4) the age of the child is at least three or four years, i.e., he should be old enough to cooperate in the postoperative re-education program. The tendon should be transferred to the midline of the foot, either to the base of the second metatarsal or to the second or third cuneiform bone, never to the cuboid. The technique of transfer is illustrated in Plate 19. In paralytic equinovarus deformity of the foot, the anterior transfer of the posterior tibial tendon is of definite value in restoring muscle balance.

Other tendon transfers effective in increasing eversion-abduction motor strength of the foot are the extensor hallucis longus to the fifth metatarsal head, and the flexor hallucis longus to the peroneals. This author has had no personal experience with these tendon transfers.

ACHILLES TENDON TRANSFERS

The Switch Operation on the Tendo Achillis. Stewart proposed that inversion of the heel in talipes equinovarus is caused by malinsertion of the tendo Achillis, which is attached on the calcaneus more medially and farther forward than normal. This acts as a positive deforming force, inverting the heel and twisting the os calcis during its growth period. He recommended sectioning the medial and anterior attachments of the tendo Achillis to the calcaneus, leaving a small lateral attachment. Then the tendon is split longitudinally, and its free tendinous part is transferred to the lateral side of the attached remnant and sutured to the os calcis. Stewart states that he has performed this procedure more than 20 times and has been surprised at the degree of eversion and dorsiflexion of the foot obtained. In only two instances was subsequent lengthening of the tendo Achillis necessary.[624]

Settle, in his dissections, found the fibers of the Achilles tendon to be inserted vertically into the calcaneus, which was rotated into a markedly varus position. When the heel was everted into neutral position, the medial fibers of the Achilles tendon were tighter than the lateral ones.[588] Irani and Sherman noted the tendo Achillis to be inserted slightly on the medial side of the calcaneus as a result of the shift of position of the posterior part of the bone. When the os calcis was placed in neutral position following sectioning of its ligamentous attachments, the apparent medial shift of the insertion of the tendo Achillis disappeared completely.[298]

The author finds that he achieves the same results as Stewart by sectioning the medial half or two thirds of the tendo Achillis insertion to the os calcis during sliding lengthening of the heel cord. Correction of equinus deformity is almost always required at the same time as that of the varus heel.

Lateral Transfer of the Achilles Tendon. Axer and Segal transferred the Achilles tendon to the lateral aspect of the calcaneus for correction of paralytic equinovarus deformity. They based the operation on the following pathomechanical consideration: the rotational movements of the subtalar joint take place along an axis that runs obliquely from the neck of the talus downward, laterally, and posteriorly to the posterolateral surface of the os calcis; the Achilles tendon inserts medially to this axis. Therefore, the triceps surae acts as a powerful invertor of the heel and becomes a major deforming force if its antagonists are paralyzed. Through fascial connections with the forefoot, the triceps surae may increase forefoot varus deviation. Axer and Segal devised the operation to maintain the function of the triceps surae as a plantar-flexor of the ankle and to eliminate its action as a supinator of the hindfoot. An L-shaped incision is made on the posterolateral aspect of the Achilles tendon and the heel. The tendon is sectioned at its insertion together with a piece of the calcaneal apophysis. On the posterolateral aspect of the os calcis (at the estimated site of emergence of the axis of the subtalar joint), a bed is prepared, and the Achilles tendon, with the attached bone, is countersunk and fixed with a screw. It is immobilized in a cast for six weeks. Axer and Segal reported the results in 37 feet. The cause of equinovarus deformity was paralytic in 34 feet, congenital in 2 feet, and spastic cerebral palsy in 1 foot. The results were good in 18 feet, fair in 8 feet, and poor in 11 feet. Complications included growth disturbance of the apophysis of the calcaneus, delayed healing, and tenderness over the screw site.[21] The author has no personal experience with the foregoing procedure and does not recommend lateral transfer of the Achilles tendon in the treatment of talipes equinovarus.

Procedures on Bone. Operative procedures on bone used in the treatment of talipes equinovarus are of three types: osteotomy, arthrodesis, and ostectomy. These procedures are often combined with soft-tissue surgery such as section or excision of the ligamentous and capsular structures, tendon lengthening, or tendon transposition. In general, bony procedures are rarely, if ever, indicated in the infant and young child, as they would disturb the normal growth and development of the foot.

SHORTENING OF LATERAL COLUMN OF FOOT. Evans, in 1961, proposed that the essential deformity in talipes equinovarus was medial displacement and rotation of the navicular on the talus, with all other elements of the deformity being secondary and adaptive. He believed relapse of talipes equinovarus is caused by failure to correct this medial dislocation of the navicular on the head of the talus. The medial column of the foot—consisting of the talus, navicular, medial cuneiform, and first ray—is relatively shortened and is held in varus position by the contracted soft tissues. The lateral column of the foot—composed of the calcaneus, cuboid, and fifth ray—gradually adapts by overgrowth in length and distortion in the shape of the calcaneocuboid joint (primarily medial obliquity of its articular surfaces). These adaptive changes provide a resistant barrier to manipulative correction.[171]

The obstruction by the lateral column of the foot has been noted previously. Ogston, in 1902, advocated enucleation of the cuboid bone, of the anterior part of the calcaneus, and of the head of the talus. His operation, however, was not successful because it weakened rather than restored the medial column of the foot.[482] Johanning, in 1958, proposed enucleating the cuboid bone alone.[310] Another procedure designed to shorten the lateral column of the foot included wedge resection of the midtarsal joint between the cuboid and calcaneus.

Evans described a procedure in which, following medial and posterior release of the contracted soft tissues, a wedge resection of the calcaneocuboid joint was performed. He claimed this resection shortened the lateral column of the foot and permitted the released navicular to be placed on the head of the talus so that the axes of the first metatarsal and the talus are aligned. The varus heel was also corrected. Evans emphasized the importance of carrying out the whole procedure in one stage.[170–172]

In the Evans procedure, first an open reduction of the talocalcaneonavicular joint is performed through a posteromedial incision. A lateral incision 4 cm. in length is centered over the calcaneocuboid joint, running parallel to the tendon of the peroneus brevis. The subcutaneous tissue is divided and the skin flaps retracted. The peroneus brevis tendon is retracted plantarward, and the calcaneocuboid joint is fully exposed. A laterally based wedge of the calcaneocuboid joint is resected. If there is associated equinus deformity of the forefoot, the wedge is thicker dorsally; if the foot is rocker-shaped, the wedge is thicker on its plantar surface. With a periosteal elevator, a connection is made between the resected area of the calcaneocuboid joint and the talonavicular joint, ensuring free motion of Chopart's joint as a unit. Next, the foot is manipulated to shift the middle and forepart laterally and align the axes of the first metatarsal and talus. Two staples are inserted to hold the calcaneus and cuboid securely together (one staple is not adequate to prevent rotation). The elongated tendons are then sutured, the incisions are closed, and the limb is immobilized in an above-knee cast, holding the foot in the corrected position. After four to six weeks, a below-knee walking cast is applied. Both Evans and Abrams recommend that immobilization in the cast be continued for about five months.[1, 172]

Initially, Evans routinely transferred the anterior tibial tendon to the lateral side of the foot (26 of 30 feet); this proved unsatisfactory, however, because of the resultant passive dropping of the forefoot. In later cases, he abandoned the tendon transfer as a part of the procedure.[172] Abrams did not transfer the anterior tibial tendon routinely; he found that, with the exception of three cases, there was return of sufficient peroneal power to provide active eversion of the foot.[1]

Evans reported the results of his procedure on 30 feet followed for four to eight years postoperatively. He did not attempt a statistical analysis of the results because the initial factors were too variable and the series was too small. The correction of the deformity obtained at the operation was permanent, and in the experience of Evans, the procedure eliminated all need for aftercare. He also observed that all elements of the deformity, including varus heel, were corrected by the operation.[171]

Abrams reported the results of Evans's operation in 31 feet, with an average follow-up of 44.5 months. The results of his series were roughly comparable to those of Evans; in 74 per cent, good; in 23 per cent, fair; and in 3 per cent, poor. The result was poor when marked scarring and stiffness of the foot were present consequent to extensive or multiple previous surgical procedures. Another important factor determining the outcome of the procedure was the age of the patient. The optimum age, according to both Evans and Abrams, is between four and eight years. They recommended that the operation not be performed before the age of four, as in the immature tarsal bones, wedge resection of the calcaneocuboid joint may remove too much cartilage, and fusion at the site of the joint resection may be difficult to achieve. Abrams also stated that the operation should not be done after the age of nine years. In his experience, the results of this operation were so much better than those following previous soft-tissue procedures performed after the age of two years that he advised using conservative methods to hold the foot between the ages of two and four years, and then performing the Evans procedure. He also warned that the operation does not correct adduction of the forepart of the foot at the tarsometatarsal joints, and that this should be treated separately.[1]

Evans's principal contribution to this procedure is wedge resection of the calcaneocuboid joint, shortening of the lateral column of the foot, and fusion of the calcaneocuboid joint in order to provide fixed stable correction of the articular malalignment. He noted no ill effects on the mechanics of the foot following calcaneocuboid fusion. A review of the Dillwyn Evans procedure has been given by Addison and colleagues.[5]

After a simplified medial release, Lichtblau recommends resection of the anterior end of the calcaneus instead of a wedge resection and fusion of the calcaneocuboid joint.[379] Through a longitudinal incision, about 4 cm. long and centered over the calcaneocuboid joint, the origin of the extensor digitorum brevis is elevated from the os calcis and reflected distally. The capsule of the calcaneocuboid joint is divided. With a single large osteotome, a wedge-shaped segment of the distal end of the calcaneus at the calcaneocuboid joint is resected. The wedge removed includes about 1 cm. of the distal lateral border of the calcaneus and 2 mm. of the distal medial margin. The foot is manipulated to bring the cuboid into contact with the distal, osteotomized end of the calcaneus. If the gap between the cuboid and calcaneus cannot be closed, it usually is because of insufficient excision of the distal medial portion of the calcaneus. In such an instance, or if the correction of varus deviation is inadequate, more of the distal end of the calcaneus is resected. The origin of the extensor brevis is sutured back to the surrounding soft tissues, and the wound is closed in the usual fashion. An above-knee cast is applied for three weeks, and then is exchanged for a below-knee cast.

Follow-up of Lichtblau's cases disclosed a calcaneocuboid joint space in the roentgenograms, and none of his patients had pain on walking. In the experimental animal, it has been shown that when a single side of a joint is resected, the excised hyaline cartilage is replaced by fibrocartilage. This permits maintenance of normal joint function.[89]

The author recommends shortening the lateral column of the foot, if necessary, in fixed talipes equinovarus in a child over four years of age. First, open reduction of the talocalcaneonavicular joint is performed through a peritalar release. In a child between four and eight years of age, a resection of the anterior end of the calcaneus, or Lichtblau procedure, is performed, with care being taken not to disturb the anterior facet of the subtalar joint (Plate 3). If the calcaneocuboid joint is resected and arthrodesis with concentric reduction of the talocalcaneonavicular joint is performed in a child under eight years of age, overcorrection into valgus inclination is a definite hazard (Fig. 2–46).

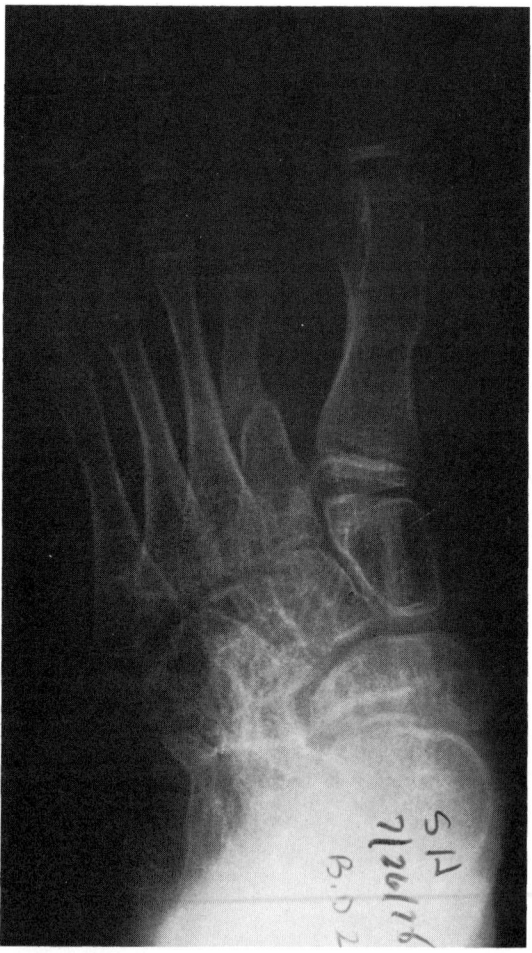

FIGURE 2–46. Valgus deformity of the foot following Evans procedure for correction of talipes equinovarus.

When the child is eight years of age or older, it is relatively safe to fuse the calcaneocuboid joint. Staples are not used for internal fixation at the initial open reduction, however. Initially, the foot and ankle are immobilized in partially corrected position to relax the skin margins and to prevent wound slough. In two weeks, under general anesthesia, the foot is manipulated (without removing the sutures) and brought to full correction. At that time, if necessary, one or two large threaded Kirschner wires are inserted to hold the calcaneus, cuboid, and fifth metatarsal firmly together. Often, the author does not utilize internal fixation.

CALCANEAL OSTEOTOMY. In 1955, Dwyer first described the lateral close-up calcaneal osteotomy for correction of pes cavus.[158, 159] In 1963, he modified his operation for the treatment of resistant talipes equinovarus by performing an open-up medial osteotomy of the calcaneus, grafting a wedge of tibial bone to correct the hindfoot varus deviation. The procedure was combined with Z-lengthening of the Achilles tendon and medial plantar fasciotomy. The results of the operation on 56 feet in 48 patients were good in 27 and fair in 29 feet.[160, 161]

In recalcitrant talipes equinovarus, the heel is in equinus and varus posture. The fibers of the tendo Achillis sweep more medially and anteriorly in relation to the inverted calcaneus and, with the contracted plantar soft-tissue structures, act as a deforming force. In realigning the heel from the varus into a mild valgus deviation and sectioning the medial half of the calcaneus, the "mechanism of correction of the Dwyer calcaneal osteotomy is dependent upon the flexibility of the subtalar and midtarsal joints." Mobility of these joints is a prerequisite. The Dwyer calcaneal osteotomy shifts the weight-bearing surface of the hindfoot laterally; the center of gravity is shifted into a more medial plane, and the body weight is transmitted through the tibia. In gait, the body weight falls medially onto the axis of the subtalar joint. If the subtalar and midtarsal joints have normal mobility, varus deformity of the midfoot and forefoot tends to improve with each step. If the midfoot and hindfoot are rigid, however, Dwyer's calcaneal osteotomy has no effect on the midfoot and forefoot.

By medial division of the tendo Achillis at the Z-lengthening and by plantar release, inversion forces are removed. The height of the heel is increased. Also, the heel is brought down as low as possible by tilting the posterior calcaneal fragment downward and laterally as the bone graft, a wedge of bone that is wider above than below, is placed in the gap.

An essential prerequisite of the Dwyer calcaneal osteotomy is that there is sufficient ossification of the calcaneus for bone grafting. Dwyer felt that the foot of a three-year-old is large enough for insertion of a medial bony wedge. He stressed that the operation should be performed while the child was still young enough for sufficient further skeletal growth and before gross structural deformity had developed.[161]

Dwyer's osteotomy of the calcaneus does not disturb growth of the foot and preserves mobility of the subtalar and midtarsal joints; these are major advantages over triple arthrodesis. Other positive points for a calcaneal osteotomy are a shorter healing period, lesser magnitude of the surgery, and rapid postoperative recovery. It also does not limit the performance of other surgical procedures in the future if necessary. Dwyer's osteotomy of the calcaneus is, however, ineffective in correcting midfoot and forefoot varus and cavus deformities. It satisfactorily corrects varus heel if the osteotomy is accurately placed and properly executed, and if there is no muscle imbalance. This is well-documented in the reports of Fisher and Shaffer and of Dekel and Weissman.[137, 186] This author disagrees with Dwyer's original claims that, with weight-bearing and walking on a plantigrade hindfoot, there are progressive dynamic correction of forefoot equinus and varus deformities and lateral shift of the navicular, the cuboid, and the anterior end of the calcaneus. Dwyer's osteotomy of the calcaneus does not reduce the medial subluxation of the talocalcaneonavicular joint, does not correct articular malalignment in talipes equinovarus, and has no effect on the forefoot or midfoot. Its sole indication is as a salvage procedure in talipes equinovarus that surgery has failed to improve, that requires bony correction of the heel varus deviation, but in which the foot is skeletally immature for triple arthrodesis. In the older child with a rigid varus deformity of the foot, even if

Shortening of the Lateral Column of the Foot

THE PROCEDURE

A. Lateral projection of the foot showing levels of osteotomy. (1) Osteotomy of anterior part of calcaneus. (2) Excision of anterior end of calcaneus (Lichtblau procedure). (3) Excision of calcaneocuboid joint and fusion (Evans operation). (4) Wedge resection and enucleation of cuboid bone.

B. A longitudinal incision about 4 cm. long is made centering over the dorsolateral aspect of the cuboid bone. Subcutaneous tissue and deep fascia are divided in line with the skin incision. The peroneus brevis tendon is identified and retracted plantarward. The extensor digitorum brevis muscle is elevated off the cuboid bone and retracted dorsally and medially. Do not injure the sural nerve.

C. When the calcaneocuboid joint is tilted medially, an osteotomy wedge resection of the anterior part of the calcaneus, based laterally, is performed. The calcaneocuboid joint is left intact.

D. If there is no malalignment of the calcaneocuboid joint, with a sharp osteotome, a ⅜" resection of the anterior end of the calcaneus, including the articular cartilage, is carried out (Lichtblau procedure).

E. Evans operation is indicated when there is paralytic clubfoot and stability of the lateral column of the foot is desired. A wedge resection of the calcaneocuboid joint is performed.

F. When there is varus inclination of the midfoot only, a cuboid decancellation is performed. With an osteotome, a wedge of bone based laterally is excised from the cuboid bone, and with a sharp curet, most of the cancellous bone from the cuboid bone is removed. The foot is then manipulated, bringing the forepart into marked abduction. This author does not recommend the use of staples. The wound is closed and a below-knee cast is applied, holding the forepart of the foot in marked abduction.

POSTOPERATIVE CARE

After two weeks, the cast is changed and a new cast is applied following manipulation of the foot. The foot is immobilized for a total period of six to eight weeks.

Plate 3. Shortening of the Lateral Column of the Foot

SHORTENING OF LATERAL COLUMN OF FOOT
(Six-year-old child)

A. Foot in 20° varus deformity

4 3 2 1
(see below)

B. Skin incision—centered over anterolateral calcaneus and posterolateral cuboid

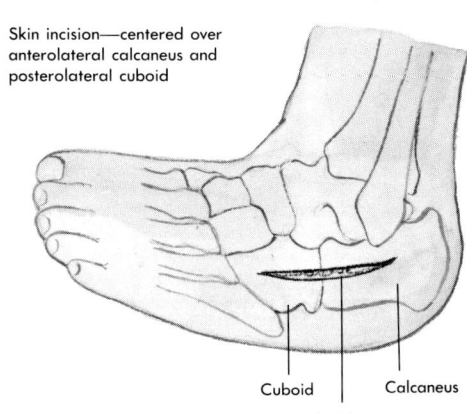

Cuboid — Calcaneus
Incision

C.
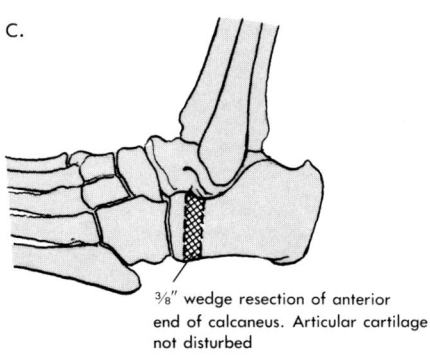
⅜″ wedge resection of anterior end of calcaneus. Articular cartilage not disturbed

D. LICHTBLAU.
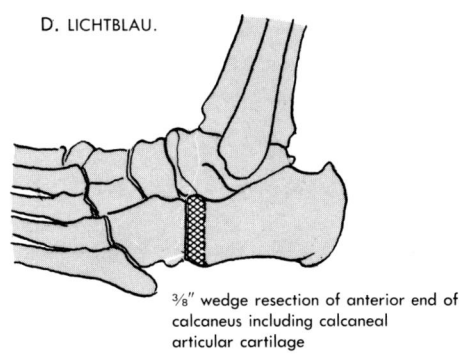
⅜″ wedge resection of anterior end of calcaneus including calcaneal articular cartilage

E. EVANS.
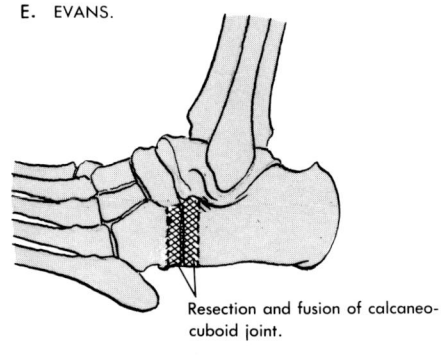
Resection and fusion of calcaneo-cuboid joint.

F. Cuboid decancellation
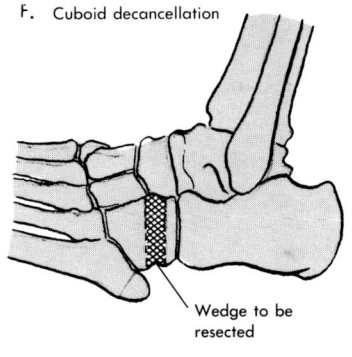
Wedge to be resected

219

the talus and navicular are normally aligned, residual forefoot adduction cannot be corrected. In such an instance, it is best to stage the operation. First, a plantar release is performed to correct the forefoot equinus and varus deformities. In the postoperative period, it is essential that the child walk on a below-knee cast with an anterior heel. At the second stage, a calcaneal osteotomy is performed.

Should one do a close-up lateral or open-up medial osteotomy? Delayed wound healing, dehiscence, and sloughing are the main problems of a medial open-up osteotomy of the calcaneus. Correction of the varus hindfoot invariably increases the distance between the medial malleolus and the posterior tuberosity of the calcaneus; the insertion of a bone wedge on the medial side of the os calcis further widens the gap, making it impossible to close the wound without tension. Originally, Dwyer made a curved incision parallel to the line of osteotomy. This often leaves an oval gap at the apex of the wound whose edges are very difficult to oppose. The wound heals by a hypertrophic scar, which exerts a deforming bowstring effect. Later, Dwyer changed the incision from a single curve to a double curve. The author modified the direction of Dwyer's incision by making it perpendicular to the line of the osteotomy. As the varus heel is corrected, the skin margins are pulled together rather than apart, thus lessening the chances of wound slough (Plate 4).

The problem, however, is complicated by the hypertrophic scar of a previous post-

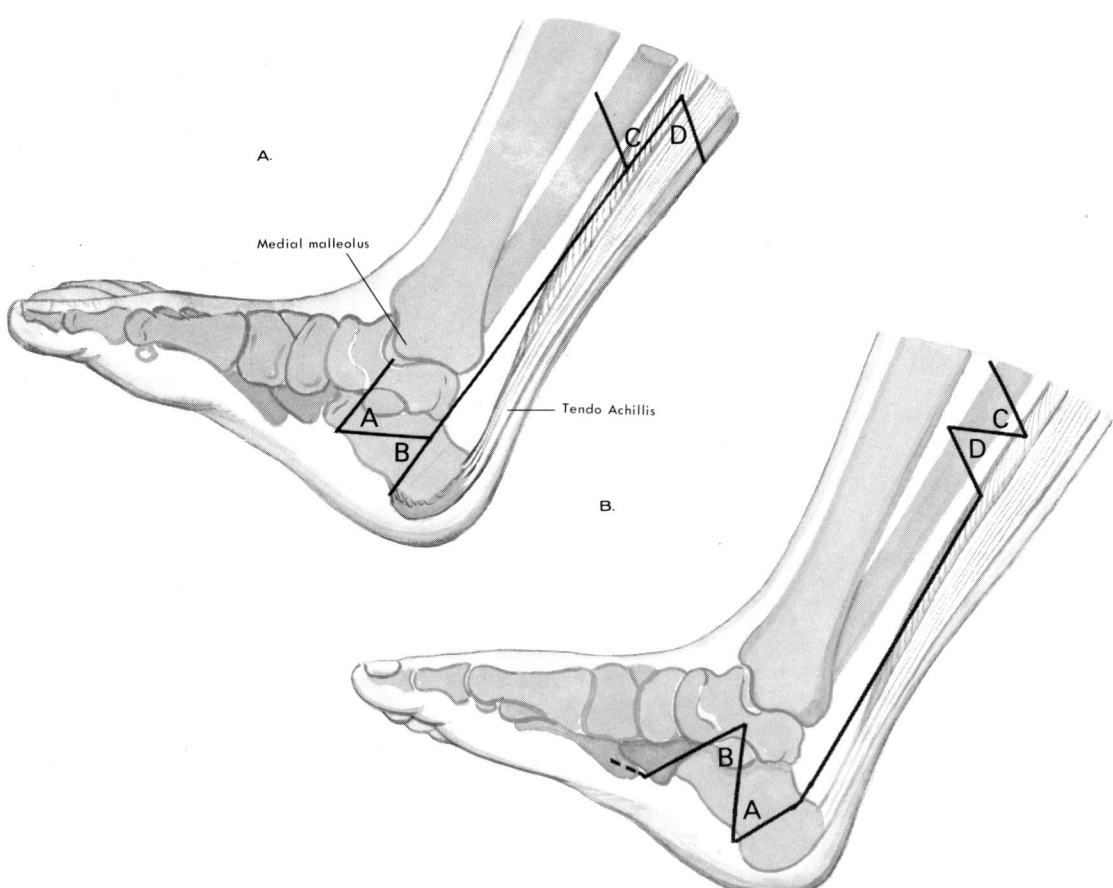

FIGURE 2–47. Z-plasty skin incision for Dwyer os calcis osteotomy in talipes equinovarus.

A. The proximal part of the incision is broken by two oblique limbs at 60 degrees; two 60-degree triangles are constructed in the distal part. **B.** The wound is closed by transposing the flaps.

eromedial release. In such an instance, one should utilize a Z-plasty incision as advocated by Handelsman and associates (Fig. 2–47). A longitudinal incision is made through the old operative scar along the medial aspect of the tendo Achillis. The proximal part is broken by two oblique limbs at 60 degrees. In the distal part, behind the medial malleolus and over the medial aspect of the midfoot, 60-degree triangles are constructed that allow distal extension of the incision as necessary. The wound is closed by transposing the flaps. This technique provides gain in the vertical length and adequate exposure; previous hypertrophic scars can be readily excised and replaced by the Z-plasty. The bowstring effect is checked by the broken lines of the newly healed scar. In some cases, a full-thickness or split-thickness skin graft may be necessary.[249]

In spite of this Z-plasty technique, when a large varus deviation is corrected, the skin usually does not heal by first intention. Therefore, a lateral close-up osteotomy is preferred by most authors.[94, 137, 186]

Fisher and Shaffer reported the correction of heel varus deformity achieved by the Dwyer calcaneal osteotomy in 26 feet with talipes equinovarus in 20 patients as good in 13, fair in 7, and poor in 2; 4 were not rated.[186] Dekel and Weissman, using similar methods of rating, reported results in 12 clubfeet as good in 11 and fair in 1.[137] Masse, Taussig, and Bazin presented an excellent study of the value of lateral close-up calcaneal osteotomy in 32 clubfeet. They regarded the operation as a salvage procedure to correct residual fixed heel varus deviation of 5 degrees or more in a child five years old or older. In their experience, previous medial release did not interfere with the lateral calcaneal osteotomy. They recommended the prone position at surgery for better visualization of correction, which must be technically exact. Poor results were due to insufficient correction of the varus inclination during the operation.[434]

Weseley and Barenfeld recommended the open-up osteotomy of the calcaneus in talipes equinovarus. In their experience, wound healing has not been a problem, and they report excellent results. Posterior release is not performed at the same time as the calcaneal osteotomy. The operation is staged: first, an open-up wedge calcaneal osteotomy is performed, combined with Steindler plantar stripping; second, six to eight weeks later, a posterior release is carried out to correct the equinus deformity. Staging the correction avoids stress on the suture line by the increase in the subjacent bony surface due to downward displacement of the calcaneal tuberosity following correction of the equinus deformity.[685–688]

Weseley and Barenfeld utilize a rectangular graft from the proximal tibia. The graft is notched on either side close to one end, and then is inserted into the open osteotomy so that the notches are grasped by the inferomedial cortex of the calcaneus. The remainder of the graft is wedged between the cancellous surfaces of the calcaneus, providing stable fixation.[688] This author strongly feels that an open-up osteotomy should not be performed. Instead, a lateral displacement osteotomy of the calcaneus is recommended. Occasionally, a close-up lateral osteotomy is indicated.

Should one ever perform an open-up osteotomy?

MEDIAL SUBTALAR STABILIZATION. Shneider and Smith, in a preliminary report, described a method of medial subtalar stabilization with "posterior medial release" in the treatment of unstable varus hindfoot in children six to ten years of age. First, a "posteromedial release" similar to that described by Turco, is performed. They stress the importance of obtaining complete correction by soft-tissue sectioning. Then, with the foot in corrected position, a smooth pin is inserted from the heel across the subtalar joint and usually up into the tibia. With a 7-mm. dowel plug cutter, a trough is fashioned in the sustentaculum tali of the calcaneus and the plantar aspect of the neck of the talus medially. The fusion is intra-articular, in contrast to the Grice extra-articular arthrodesis. Then a double-cortical graft is taken from the iliac crest with an 8-mm. dowel plug cutter and is placed snugly into the previously cut trough. The authors do not use a pin across the talonavicular joint because they have found that fixation by a single pin across the subtalar joint holds the corrected position firmly. The foot and ankle are immobilized in a below-knee cast for 12 weeks. The pin is removed when weight-bearing is begun at six weeks post-

Dwyer Open-Up Medial Osteotomy of Calcaneus with Bone Graft Wedge for Correction of Varus Hindfoot

Through a midline plantar incision, the plantar aponeurosis and short plantar muscles are sectioned near their origin from the tuberosity of the calcaneus, as shown in Plate 23.

THE PROCEDURE

A. The skin incision begins at a point in the midline in the posterior prominence of the heel, along the skin creases, and extends distally to the anterior border of the insertion of the tendo Achillis; then it swings obliquely, dorsally and distally, to a point 2 cm. distal to the lower tip of the medial malleolus. This incision differs from that described by Dwyer; as the varus heel is corrected, the skin margins are pulled together rather than apart, thus preventing delayed wound healing and slough. The subcutaneous tissue is divided in line with the skin incision. The elevated wound flaps are retracted and the plexus of veins is coagulated and divided to prevent bleeding later.

B. Next, the medial one third to one half of the insertion of the Achilles tendon to the calcaneus is sectioned. The laciniate ligament is divided near its insertion to the os calcis, at least 2.5 cm. inferior to the flexor hallucis longus tendon and neurovascular bundle. The medial surface of the calcaneus is subperiosteally exposed. The line of incision in the periosteum is 1.5 cm. inferior and in line with the flexor hallucis longus tendon. Injury to neurovascular structures should be avoided. Chandler elevator retractors are used to partially expose the superior and inferior aspects of the calcaneus.

C. With a wide osteotome, the calcaneus is sectioned just inferior to the flexor hallucis longus tendon. The lateral cortex of the calcaneus is left intact; however, its medial, inferior, and superior aspects should be completely divided.

D. Next, a Steinmann pin is inserted transversely into the os calcis. While the pin acts as a lever, with periosteal elevators and a laminectomy spreader, the site of osteotomy is opened. The width of the bone graft wedge is determined by inserting osteotomes of various sizes between the fragments. An appropriate bone graft wedge is taken from the ilium and, with its base medially, is placed in the gap in the calcaneus. The author finds that bone grafts from the upper end of the tibia are usually inadequate and not sturdy enough. The tension of the tissues will firmly hold the bone graft in position; the Steinmann pin is removed, as special fixation is not required. Roentgenograms are made in the operating room to ensure that the varus deformity of the hindfoot is corrected. The skin is closed with interrupted sutures, and an above-knee cast is applied.

POSTOPERATIVE CARE

The cast and sutures are removed in two to three weeks, and a new above-knee cast is applied. Approximately ten weeks is required for the bone graft to consolidate. Early weight-bearing will result in collapse of the graft and loss of correction. The importance of protecting the foot until the bone graft is fully incorporated cannot be overemphasized.

Plate 4. Dwyer Open-Up Medial Osteotomy of Calcaneus with Bone Graft Wedge for Correction of Varus Hindfoot

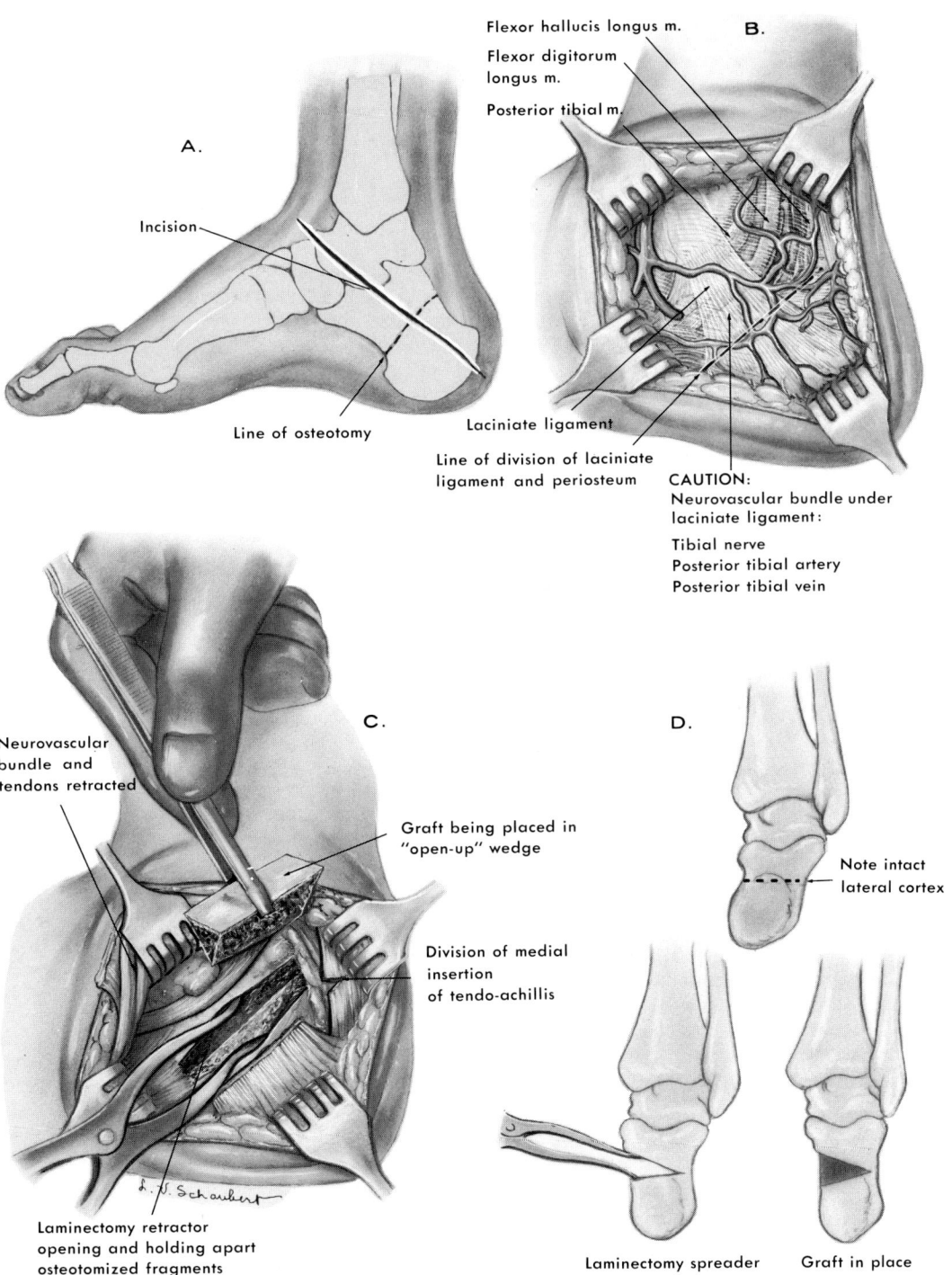

operatively. Short-term results in six patients showed complete correction of the varus deformity in four cases; incomplete correction in two patients was due to the technical failure of inadequate medial release. There were no failures of fusion.[596]

This author has had no experience with medial intra-articular arthrodesis for stabilization of varus hindfoot; it appears, however, to be a sound procedure in a child between six and ten years of age who has marked incongruity and instability of the subtalar joint after open reduction of the talocalcaneonavicular joint.

TRIPLE ARTHRODESIS. Tarsal reconstruction by wedge resection and fusion of the subtalar and midtarsal joints is an operation of last resort, indicated in the skeletally mature adolescent or adult with persistent rigid equinovarus deformity. It is a salvage procedure. The purpose of triple arthrodesis is to provide stability and prevent future arthritis and pain rather than to improve the cosmetic appearance of the foot. Following triple arthrodesis, the foot is smaller and has, of course, no motion at the subtalar and midtarsal joints. With adequate early treatment of talipes equinovarus, triple arthrodesis should rarely be necessary. Some patients with neglected clubfoot may come from underdeveloped countries; others are occasionally encountered in more developed areas with a high rate of immigration. The primary indication for the procedure should be to provide stability in the paralytic equinovarus deformity of the feet in neuromuscular diseases.

Before starting surgical treatment, it is essential to assess the psychological impact of the disability. An older patient may be accustomed to living with his deformities and managing quite well functionally. It is best to correct the deformities only upon the insistence of the patient and his family. Strong motivation and a genuine desire stimulated by social and cosmetic reasons are imperative prerequisites for a successful overall result. The psychological aspects of the problem are well recorded by Weinberg and Halmosh, and by Herold and Torok.[260, 261, 683] Prolonged walking on a deformed foot causes compensatory rotational deformities at more proximal levels: namely, lateral rotation contracture of the hip, exaggerated lateral tibiofibular torsion and lateral rotation of the talus on the tibia in the ankle mortise, and posterior displacement of the fibular malleolus in relation to the medial malleolus. Prior treatment may have caused flattening of the dome of the talus and distortion of the ankle mortise with narrowing of the joint space.

It should be remembered that triple arthrodesis further compromises the biomechanically stressed ankle joint. In the older patient, the osseous and articular deformities at the ankle joint may be so fixed that, after soft-tissue release and before triple arthrodesis, a medial rotation osteotomy of the tibia may be indicated for proper alignment of the ankle mortise in relation to the leg, as is discussed later. This will accentuate the midfoot and forefoot varus deformity.

Details of surgical treatment should be individualized. In general, it consists of four separate steps: first, a short period of gentle manipulation and cast immobilization to elongate the contracted skin and soft tissues; second, surgical soft-tissue release; third, a period of manipulation and cast retention; and fourth, tarsal bone reconstruction.

Soft-Tissue Release. The surgical technique of soft-tissue release is described in Plate 2. The following changes are made in the older patient. (1) The skin incision extends distally to the base of the proximal phalanx of the great toe. (2) The posterior tibial tendon is divided at its insertion to the navicular, transferred, and with one or two sutures, attached to the lateral side of the tendo Achillis. (3) The abductor hallucis muscle is detached from its insertion to the base of the proximal phalanx of the hallux and is totally excised. This facilitates exposure of the neurovascular bundle, permits wound closure with less tension, and diminishes the postoperative incidence of forefoot adduction deformity. (4) The joint capsules are resected rather than incised. During division of the deltoid ligament, the deep part, i.e., the tibiotalar band, should not be disturbed. If divided, it should be repaired. There is compensatory valgus deformity at the ankle in the older patient. Division of the tibiotalar ligament medially will result in a severe valgus deformity at the ankle; it will also cause difficulties in further corrections of the foot deformities by manipulation and plaster cast. It is important to close the skin without tension and to apply the immediate postoperative cast in partial correction. Attention to these technical details is vital.

Manipulation and Cast Retention. Ten to fourteen days after soft-tissue release, the initial cast is removed, and the wound is inspected and re-dressed. It is best not to remove the sutures, as the wound will gape apart at manipulation. Under general anesthesia, the foot and ankle are manipulated to obtain further correction without putting much tension on the skin closure. Manipulation and cast retention are repeated initially at weekly and later at biweekly intervals until maximal correction is achieved. Roentgenograms are made to assess the anatomic result of the soft-tissue release and the need for further bone reconstruction. Muscle testing is performed; it is imperative to provide a dynamic balance of muscle forces acting on the ankle and foot. Overlengthening of the tendo Achillis and consequent triceps surae insufficiency should be avoided.

Tarsal Reconstruction. This stage consists of triple arthrodesis (see Plate 21). If there is any question of the vascular supply to the foot, it is studied by arteriography.[38] It is best to perform the operation through two incisions: an anterolateral one extended distally, and a medial one. Prior soft-tissue release and manipulations achieve enough correction so that a triple arthrodesis can be performed with a minimum of bone resection at the articular surfaces. Bone is added rather than resected. The height of the foot is an important consideration, since low-riding malleoli will be irritated by the shoes and walking will be painful and difficult. The midfoot and forefoot are brought into proper alignment with the hindfoot by closing a laterally based wedge through Chopart's joint (the calcaneocuboid and talonavicular), and by shifting the distal segment laterally on the proximal segment to correct the marked medial displacement of the forefoot.

Internal fixation with heavy threaded Kirschner wires or Steinmann pins may be desired by some surgeons; two threaded pins are used—one drilled through the medial cuneiform, through the navicular and into the talus; and the other drilled through the plantar aspect of the foot and up through the calcaneus to the talus.

Correction of the equinus deformity of the ankle does accentuate that of the forefoot and leads to increased weight-bearing on the metatarsal heads. There may be residual varus deformity of the forefoot. When metatarsalgia and painful pressure keratosis under the prominent metatarsal heads develop, an extension osteotomy of the metatarsals at the base is performed to correct both the equinus and varus deformities of the forefoot.

TALECTOMY. R. Whitman, in 1901, was the first to advocate excision of the talus for paralytic calcaneus deformity; later on, talectomies were performed for a variety of conditions.[696–698]

A. Whitman, in 1922, and T. C. Thompson, in 1939, presented long-term follow-up studies of talectomy and reported varying results. They concluded that the operation is primarily indicated in rigid paralytic deformities of the foot and that best results are obtained in children under four years of age.[635, 693] Young reported a 50-year follow-up in a woman with bilateral talectomy; her feet were most satisfactory.[719]

The operation is a salvage procedure that has a useful place in the management of the severely deformed and rigid foot in some cases of arthrogryposis multiplex congenita, myelomeningocele, and diastrophic dwarfism.[388, 445, 698] Occasionally, it is indicated in a case of surgical failure in talipes equinovarus in which the foot is rigid and deformed, there are multiple scars, and circulation is compromised. Talectomy is unphysiologic and further distorts an already deformed foot; therefore, it is not recommended as a primary operation for rigid talipes equinovarus. When possible, it is best to wait and tide the child over until the age of 10 to 12 years and then to perform a triple arthrodesis to correct the deformity.

The principle of talectomy is that, by excision of the talus, sufficient laxity of soft tissues is provided to correct equinus and varus deformities without tension. It gives a plantigrade foot with a stable and relatively congruous false joint between the calcaneus and the ankle mortise.

The best age for talectomy varies according to the basic disease; in arthrogryposis and myelomeningocele, it is between one and five years; whereas in talipes equinovarus, it is six to nine years. In general, the younger the child, the better the result.

Ablation of the talus does not present any technical problem, but correction of the deformity and internal fixation demand meticulous attention to detail. The incision is curved anterolaterally over the subtalar and talonavicular joints. It begins behind the lateral malleolus and ends over the talonavicular joint. The subcutaneous tissue is divided in line with the skin incision; great care must be taken not to injure the veins. The extensor digitorum brevis muscle is elevated from its origin and reflected distally. The long toe extensors and anterior tibial tendons are retracted medially. The peroneal tendons are divided and tagged with sutures for reattachment. The ligaments and capsule connecting the talus to the distal fibula, tibia, calcaneus, and navicular are divided next. Tenotomy scissors are utilized to avoid damage to hyaline articular cartilage. First, the anterior talofibular ligament is sectioned (it arises from the anterior border of the fibula and runs anteriorly and medially to attach to the neck of the talus). The calcaneofibular ligament is incised proximally at its origin from the lateral malleolus and tagged for resuture later on. Next, the lateral and anterior part of the talocalcaneal ligament is divided. Caution is exercised not to incise the calcaneonavicular and calcaneocuboid limbs of the bifurcate ligament. The dorsal capsule of the talonavicular joint and the interosseous talocalcaneal ligament are sectioned next. At this time, the foot is manipulated into greater equinus and varus inclination, and under direct vision, the medial and posterior ligaments are sectioned. They consist of the medial capsule of the subtalar joint, the tibiotalar (deep part of the deltoid), the posterior tibiotalar and talocalcaneal capsule, and the posterior talofibular ligaments. The talus is grasped with a large towel clip and rotated and displaced in each direction as the dissection proceeds. Usually it can be excised in one piece; if fragments break off, they are removed with bone rongeurs.

The tendo Achillis is sharply divided at its insertion, a small distal segment being left for resuturing later on. Next, the inferior tibiofibular ligament is divided to widen the ankle mortise. Often the lateral malleolus abuts the lateral surface of the calcaneus and prevents a congruous fit of the upper surface of the calcaneus into the ankle mortise. In such an instance, the lower part of the lateral malleolus, distal to its physis, is excised. It is important not to injure the growth plate. With the foot displaced posteriorly, the calcaneus giving a normal contour to the heel, the tip of the medial malleolus should be immediately superoposterior to the navicular, and the lateral malleolus should be just behind the calcaneocuboid joint. It is essential to provide a long lever arm by posterior displacement of the calcaneus to give a mechanical advantage to the triceps surae muscle. If posterior displacement of the hindfoot and correction of the varus inclination is found to be difficult, it is facilitated by partial excision of the cuboid. The foot is laterally rotated 15 to 20 degrees in relation to the leg to stabilize the new articulation. One or two small Steinmann pins are inserted upward through the heel into the tibia for secure fixation. The tendo Achillis is resutured; if it is too lax, a segment is excised. The calcaneofibular ligament is sutured to the lateral malleolus under slight tension. An above-knee plaster of Paris cast is applied with the hindfoot slightly valgus and the ankle in neutral position. The cast and pins are removed after six weeks. Then a below-knee polypropylene orthosis is worn during the day for an additional three to four months. The tendency to rigidity gives stability to the false articulation between the calcaneus and the ankle mortise. It seems that in arthrogryposis, what was an "enemy" working against success turns out to be a "friend."[445]

OSTEOTOMY OF THE TIBIA. Tibial torsion in the newborn with talipes equinovarus is normal, and the old teaching that excessive medial torsion of the tibia is one of the principal deformities in talipes equinovarus should be discarded. The in-toeing one often sees in inadequately treated talipes equinovarus is due to persistence of medial subluxation of the talocalcaneonavicular joint and adduction of the forefoot. Lateral rotation osteotomy of the tibia and fibula should not be performed.

Swann, Lloyd-Roberts, and Catterall have proposed that in improperly treated and uncorrected talipes equinovarus, the talus and the forefoot are laterally rotated in the ankle mortise on the tibia, which has no rotational deformity. The fibular malleolus is displaced posteriorly.[629] Simons has shown that when the child begins to walk with uncorrected talipes equinovarus, compensatory lateral rotation takes place at the hip. In time, structural changes take place with growth, and excessive lateral tibiofibular torsion develops.[600] In the older child, Lloyd-Roberts and associates recommend *medial* rotation osteotomy of the tibia for proper alignment of the ankle mortise in relation to the leg. This will exaggerate the midfoot and forefoot varus deformity, which is corrected at a later stage by open reduction of the talocalcaneonavicular joint, and if necessary, by Evans's procedure.[389]

METATARSAL OSTEOTOMY. Residual forefoot varus deformity in the child over eight years of age may be corrected by valgus osteotomy of the metatarsals at their base. Prior to this age, the Heymann-Herndon soft-tissue procedure described in Plate 7 will give satisfactory results.

References

1. Abrams, R. C.: Relapsed club foot. The early results of an evaluation of Dillwyn Evans' operation. J. Bone Joint Surg., *51-A*:270, 1969.
2. Adam, A.: Tibialis posterior transfer in relapsed clubfoot. J. Bone Joint Surg., *45-B*:804, 1963.
3. Adams, W.: A series of four specimens illustrating the morbid anatomy of congenital club-foot (talipes varus). Trans. Path. Soc. London, *6*:348, 1854–1855.
4. Adams, W.: Club Foot, Its Causes, Pathology and Treatment. London, J & A. Churchill, 1866.
5. Addison, A., Fixsen, J. A., and Lloyd-Roberts, G. C.: A review of the Dillwyn Evans-type collateral operation in severe club feet. J. Bone Joint Surg., *65-B*:12, 1983.
6. Agerholm-Christensen, J.: On Denis Browne's treatment of club-foot. Acta Orthop. Scand., *19*:134, 1949.
7. Albanese, M., Basile, N., and Carbone, C.: Rilievi clinici statistici sul piede torto congenito. Orriz. Ortop. Odierna. Riabilit., *5*:443, 1960.
8. Alldred, A. J.: Early surgery for the correction of congenital clubfoot. New Zeal. Med. J., *65*:665, 1966.
9. Altchek, M.: Molding the talus. A method of treating clubfoot. Clin. Orthop., *84*:44, 1972.
10. Altchek, M., and Bleck, E. E.: Congenital club feet. Clin. Orthop., *130*:303, 1978.
11. Amor, R., Pener, E., and Yannez, P. R.: The treatment of congenital clubfoot. *In* Delchef, J. (ed.): Orthopaedic Surgery and Traumatology. Congenital clubfoot. d. Neglected and inveterate cases. New York, American Elsevier Publishing Co., Inc., 1973.
12. Apley, A. G.: Talipes (clubfoot). *In* A System of Orthopaedics and Fractures. 3rd Ed. New York, Appleton-Century-Crofts, Inc., 1968, pp. 194–220.
13. Aplington, J. P., and Riddle, C. D.: Avascular necrosis of the body of the talus after combined medial and lateral release of congenital clubfoot. Southern Med. J., *69*:1037, 1976.
14. Aranes, A., and Villadot, P.: Clinica y tratamiento de las enfermedades del pie. Pie equino varo congenito. Barcelona, Editorial Científico Médica, 1956, p. 201.
15. Aritamur, A.: Une malformation congénitale rare de pied. Rev. Chir. Orthop., *57*:151, 1971.
16. Ashby, M. E.: Roentgenographic assessment of soft tissue medial release operations in clubfoot deformity. Clin. Orthop., *90*:146, 1973.
17. Assum, H. W.: Untersuchungen über die Erblichkeit des angeborenen Klumpfussleidens. Z. Orthop., *65*:1, 1936.
18. Atlas, S.: The morbid anatomy of clubfoot in the embryo and fetus. *In* Delchef, J. (ed.): Orthopaedic Surgery and Traumatology. Congenital clubfoot. a. Anatomy and pathology of the disease. New York, American Elsevier Publishing Co., Inc., 1973, pp. 753–754.
19. Attenborough, C. G.: Severe congenital talipes equinovarus. J. Bone Joint Surg., *48-B*:31, 1966.
20. Attenborough, C. G.: Early posterior soft-tissue release in severe congenital talipes equinovarus. Clin. Orthop., *84*:71, 1972.
21. Axer, A., and Segal, D.: Transfer of Achilles tendon to the lateral aspect of the calcaneus in the treatment of clubfeet. *In* Delchef, J. (ed.): Orthopaedic Surgery and Traumatology. Congenital clubfoot. c. Surgical treatment in later childhood. New York, American Elsevier Publishing Co., Inc., 1973, pp. 769–771.
22. Bachmann, R.: Klinisches und röntgenologisches Behandlungsergebnis angeborener Klumpfüsse nach 5 Jahren. Zbl. Chir., *78*:1738, 1953.
23. Barcat, J., and Preyssas, J.: Le rôle des tranplantations tendineuses dans le pied bot varus équin congenital. J. Chir., *79*:29, 1960.
24. Bardeen, C. R., and Lewis, W. H.: Development of limbs, body-wall and back in man. Amer. J. Anat., *1*:1, 1901.
25. Barenfeld, P. A., and Weseley, M. S.: Surgical treatment of congenital clubfoot. Clin. Orthop., *84*:79, 1972.
26. Barenfeld, P. A. and Wesely, M. S.: Talipes equinovarus: "Hard" versus "soft" tissues. Clin. Orthop., *123*:109, 1977.
27. Barenfeld, P. A., Weseley, M. S., and Munter, M.: Dwyer calcaneal osteotomy. Clin. Orthop., *53*:147, 1967.
28. Bartholini, T.: De Observationibus Raris Medicorum. Acta Med. et Phil. Hafn., *2*:1, 1673.
29. Bartsolas, C. S.: Hephaestus and clubfoot. J. Hist. Med. Allied Sci., *27*:450, 1972.
30. Barwell, R.: On various forms of talipes as depicted by x-ray. Lancet, *2*:160, 234, 1521, 1896.
31. Batchelor, J. S.: Treatment of the uncorrected clubfoot in childhood. Proc. Roy. Soc. Med., *39*:713, 1946.
32. Beals, R. K.: Club foot in the Maori.: A genetic study of 50 kindreds. New Zeal. Med. J., *88*:144, 1978.
33. Beatson, R. R., and Pearson, J. R.: A method assessing correction in club feet. J. Bone Joint Surg., *48-B*:40, 1966.
34. Beau, A., Prevot, J., and Mathieu, P.: Resultats de l'allongement des parties molles internes et postérieures dans le traitement du pied bot varus équin congenital. Ann. Chir. Infant., *1*:91, 1960.
35. Bechtol, C. O., and Mossman, H. W.: Club-foot; embryological study of associated muscle abnormalities. J. Bone Joint Surg., *32-A*:827, 1950.
36. Bell, J. F., and Grice, D. S.: Treatment of congenital talipes equinovarus with the modified Denis Browne splint. J. Bone Joint Surg., *26*:799, 1944.
37. Belloc, J.: Congenital talipes equinovarus. Bol. Med. Hosp. Infant. Mex., *22*:13, 1965.
38. Ben-Menachem, Y., and Butler, J. E.: Arteriography of the foot in congenital deformities. J. Bone Joint Surg., *56-A*:1625, 1974.
39. Bennet, G. A., and Bauer, W.: Further studies concerning the repair of articular cartilage in dog joints. J. Bone Joint Surg., *17*:141, 1935.
40. Bensahel, H.: Bilan de vingt années de traitement fonctionnel du pied-bot dans le premier âge. *In* Delchef, J. (ed.): Orthopaedic Surgery and Traumatology. Congenital clubfoot. b. Early childhood—conservative and surgical treatment. New York, American Elsevier Publishing Co., Inc., 1973, p. 759.
41. Bensahel, H., Degrippes, Y., and Billot, C.: Comments about 600 club feet. Chir. Pediat., *21*:335, 1980.
42. Bentzon, P. G. K., and Thomasen, E.: On treatment of congenital clubfoot. Acta Orthop. Scand., *11*:129, 1940.
43. Berg, H. W.: Club-foot. Arch. Med., *8*:226, 1882.

44. Bergonzoli, E.: Contributo alla cura del piede torto congenito. Risultati delgi interventi cruenti sulle parti molli del piede torto recidivo. Arch. Ital. Ortop., *56*:378, 1940.
45. Berman, A., and Gartland, J. J.: Metatarsal osteotomy for the correction of adduction of the fore part of the foot in children. J. Bone Joint Surg., *53-A*:498, 1971.
46. Bernardczyk, K., Marciniak, W., and Lempicki, A.: Dwyer's operation in the treatment of equino-varus talipes. Chir. Narzad. Ruchu Ortop. Pol. *43*:179, 1978.
47. Bernbeck, R.: Zur Pathologie des angeborenen Klumpfusses. Das Klumpfussproblem im Lichte der pathologischen Anatomie und Histologie. Z. Orthop., *79*:521, 1950.
48. Bertelsen, A., and Jansen, K.: Treatment of congenital clubfoot. J. Bone Joint Surg., *39-B*:599, 1957.
49. Bertini, S., Guerra, A., and Romano, B.: L'intervento di Codivilla nella cura del piede torto congenito. Chir. Organi Mov., *59*:460, 1970.
50. Bertola, L.: Sindesmocapsulotomia tibio-astragalica posteriore ei allungamento plastico del tendine di Achille nella cura precoce del piede torto congenito. Arch. Ortop., *62*:229, 1949.
51. Bertrand, P.: L'arthrographie dans le pied bot congénital. Rev. Orthop., *33*:548, 1947.
52. Bessel-Hagen, F. C.: Die Pathologie und Therapie des Klumpfusses. Heidelberg, O. Peters, 1889.
53. Bethem, D., and Weiner, D.: Radical one-stage posteromedial release for the resistant clubfoot. Clin. Orthop., *131*:214, 1978.
54. Bick, E. M.: Morphology and genetics. *In* Source Book of Orthopaedics. 2nd Ed. Baltimore, Williams & Wilkins Co., 1948, pp. 140–153.
55. Biezin, A. P.: Modification of the operation of soft tissues in children with congenital clubfoot. Khirurgiia (Moskva), *41*:115, 1965.
56. Bissell, J. B.: The morbid anatomy of congenital talipes equinovarus. Arch. Pediat., *5*:406, 1888.
57. Bjonnes, T.: Congenital clubfoot. A follow-up of 95 persons treated in Sweden from 1940–1945 with special reference to their social adaptation and subjective symptoms from the foot. Acta Orthop. Scand., *46*:848, 1975.
58. Bleck, E. E.: Congenital clubfoot. Pathomechanics, radiographic analysis, and results of surgical treatment. Clin. Orthop., *125*:119, 1977.
59. Blockey, N. J., and Smith, M. G. H.: The treatment of congenital club foot. J. Bone Joint Surg., *48-B*:660, 1966.
60. Blokhin, V. N.: Plastic splints for therapy of congenital clubfoot. Vestn. Khir., *70*:55, 1950.
61. Bluhm, M.: Modification of the Denis Browne splint. J. Bone Joint Surg., *29*:248, 1947.
62. Blumenfeld, I.: The treatment of clubfoot in the newborn by the Denis Browne splint. *In* Delchef, J. (ed): Orthopaedic Surgery and Traumatology. Congenital clubfoot. b. Early childhood—conservative and surgical treatment. New York, American Elsevier Publishing Co., Inc., 1973, pp. 756–758.
63. Blumenfeld, I., Kaplan, N., and Hicks, E. O.: The conservative treatment of congenital talipes equinovarus. J. Bone Joint Surg., *28*:765, 1946.
64. Bogdanov, F. R., and Melikdzhanian, Z. G.: Congenital clubfoot and its surgical treatment. Ortop. Travm. Protez., *35*:33, 1974.
65. Böhm, M.: The embryologic origin of clubfoot. J. Bone Joint Surg., *11*:229, 1929.
66. Böök, J. A.: A contribution to the genetics of clubfoot. Hereditas (Lund), *34*,289, 1948.
67. Boppe and Estève: Le traitement du pied bot varus équin congénital de la deuxiéme ou moyenne. Rev. Chir. Orthop., *34*:403, 1948.
68. Börnbeck, R.: Zur Pathologie des angeborenen Klumpfusses. Z. Orthop., *79*:521, 1950.
69. Bösch, I.: Zur Technik der Klumpfussbehandlung. Z. Orthop., *94*:159, 1961.
70. Bost, F. C., Schottstaedt, E. R., and Larsen, L. J.: Plantar dissection. An operation to release the soft tissues in recurrent or recalcitrant talipes equinovarus. J. Bone Joint Surg., *42-A*:151, 1960.
71. Bostos-Mora, F.: On the surgical treatment of congenital talipes equinovarus. Cir. Ginec. Urol. (Madrid), *19*:265, 1965.
72. Bouvier, H.: Leçons cliniques sur les maladies chroniques de l'appareil locomoteur. Paris, J. B. Ballière, 1858.
73. Brockman, E. P.: Congenital Clubfoot (Talipes Equinovarus). Bristol, John Wright and Sons, Ltd.; New York, William Wood & Co., 1930.
74. Brockman, E. P.: Modern methods of treatment of clubfoot. Brit. Med. J., *2*:572, 1937.
75. Brockway, A.: Surgical correction of talipes cavus deformities. J. Bone Joint Surg., *22*:81, 1940.
76. Brown, L. T.: The treatment of club feet. J. Bone Joint Surg., *18*:173, 1936.
77. Browne, D.: Congenital malformations. Practitioner, *131*:20, 1933.
78. Browne, D.: Talipes equinovarus. Lancet, 2:909, 1934.
79. Browne, D.: Congenital deformities of mechanical origin. Proc. Roy. Soc. Med., *29*:1409, 1936.
80. Browne, D.: Modern methods of treatment of clubfoot. Brit. Med. J., *2*:570, 1937.
81. Browne, D.: Congenital deformities of mechanical origin. Arch. Dis. Child., *30*:37, 1955.
82. Browne, D.: Splinting for controlled movement. Clin. Orthop., *8*:91, 1956.
83. Browne, D.: The pathology and classification of talipes. Aust. New Zeal. J. Surg., *29*:85, 1959.
84. Browne, D.: Talipes equinovarus. (Letter to the Editor.) Lancet, *1*:863, 1962.
85. Burgess, E. M.: Dynamic restoration of muscle imbalance in recurrent club foot. *In* Proceedings. Annual Meeting of the Association of Bone and Joint Surgeons. J. Bone Joint Surg., *38-A*:947, 1956.
86. Burian, F.: The "whistling face" characteristic in a compound cranio-facio-corporal syndrome. Brit. J. Plast. Surg., *46*:140, 1963.
87. Burrell, H. L.: A contribution to the anatomy of congenital equinovarus. Ann. Surg., *17*:293, 1893.
88. Cabanac, J., Petit, P., and Maschas, A.: Le traitement du pied bot varus équin congénital. Reports XXVII Réunion Annuelle de la Société Française D' Orthopédie et de Traumatologie. Rev. Chir. Orthop., *38*:314, 1952.
89. Calandruccio, R. A., and Gilmer, W. S.: Proliferation, regeneration and repair of articular cartilage of immature animals. J. Bone Joint Surg., *44-A*:431, 1962.
90. Camera, U.: Mon expérience dans le traitement de pied bot congénital. Rev. Chir. Orthop., *38*:525, 1952.
91. Campos da Paz, A., Jr., and De Souza, V.: Talipes equinovarus: Pathomechanical basis of treatment. Orthop. Clin. N. Amer., *9*:171, 1978.
92. Capecchi, V., and Casini, E.: Sul trattamento chirurgico del piede torto congenito inveterato. Arch. Putti Chir. Organi Mov., *3*:121, 1953.
93. Capener, N.: Congenital clubfoot. J. Bone Joint Surg., *44-B*:956, 1962.
94. Carlioz, H.: Les ostéotomies calcanéennes et tibiales dans le traitement du pied bot varus. *In* Le pied bot varus équin congénital. Cahiers d'enseignement de la S.O.F.C.O.T. Paris, Expansion Scientifique Française, 1976.
95. Carmack, J. C., and Hallock, H.: Tibiotarsal arthrodesis after astragalectomy. A report of eight cases. J. Bone Joint Surg., *29*:476, 1947.
96. Caroyan, A., Bourges, M., and Touge, M.: Dual transfer of the posterior tibial and flexor digitorum longus tendon for drop foot. J. Bone Joint Surg., *49-A*:144, 1967.
97. Carpenter, E. B., and Huff, S. H.: Selective tendon transfers for recurrent club foot. Southern Med. J., *46*:220, 1953.
98. Carroll, N. C., McMurtry, R., and Leete, S. F.: The pathoanatomy of congenital clubfoot. Orthop. Clin. N. Amer. *9*:225, 1978.
99. Carter, C. O.: Genetics of common disorders. Brit. Med. Bull., *25*:52, 1969.
100. Carter, C. O.: Talipes equinovarus. *In* Sorsby, A. (ed.): Clinical Genetics: The Skeletal System. London, Butterworths, Ind.,1973, pp. 200–201
101. Carter, C. O., and Fairbank, J. J.: Talipes equinovarus. *In* The Genetics of Locomotor Disorder, London, Oxford University Press, 1974, pp. 100–102.
102. Castellana, A.: Lengthening of Achilles tendon and posterior capsulotomy of tibiotarsal joint in therapy of congenital twisted foot. Minersal Ortop., *3*:139, 1952.

103. Cattameo, R.: Development and therapy of tibial torsion in congenital clubfoot. Arch. Ortop. (Milano), 72:1045, 1955.
104. Catterall, R. C. R.: Ex umbris eruditio. J. Bone Joint Surg., 50-B:455, 1968.
105. Caucci, M., and Rocca, I.: La torsione tibiale nel piede torto congenito. Clin. Ortop., 6:345, 1954.
106. Cavanaugh, C. J.: Clubfoot and congenital hand anomalies. J. Hered., 44:53, 1953.
107. Cervenka, J., Figalová, P., and Gorlin, R. J.: Craniocarpo-tarsal dysplasia or the whistling face syndrome. Amer. J. Dis. Child., 117:434, 1969.
108. Cervenka, J., Gorlin, R. J., Figalova, P., and Farkasova, J.: Cranio-carpo-tarsal dysplasia or whistling face syndrome. Arch. Otolaryng. (Chicago), 91:183, 1970.
109. Chapchal, G.: Operative treatment of congenital clubfoot. In Delchef, J. (ed.): Orthopaedic Surgery and Traumatology. Congenital clubfoot. c. Surgical treatment in later childhood. New York, American Elsevier Publishing Co., Inc., 1973, pp. 764–765.
110. Chiappara, P.: La funzione delle articolazioni astragalocalcaneari. Minerva Orthop., 24:6, 1973.
111. Ching, G. H. S., Chung, C. S., and Nemechek, R. W.: Genetic and epidemiological studies of clubfoot in Hawaii: Ascertainment and incidence. Amer. J. Hum. Genet., 21:566, 1969.
112. Chung, C. S., and Myrianthopoulos, N. C.: Racial and prenatal factors in major congenital malformations. Amer. J. Hum. Gent., 20:40, 1968.
113. Chung, C. S., Nemecheck, R. W., Larsen, I. J., and Ching, G. H. S.: Genetic and epidemiological studies of clubfoot in Hawaii: General and medical considerations. Hum. Hered., 19:321, 1969.
114. Clark, J. M. P.: Treatment of clubfoot. Early detection and management of the unreduced clubfoot. Proc. Roy. Soc. Med., 61:779, 1968.
115. Clarke, R. C., and Wenger, R. J. J.: Equinus deformity and haemangioma of calf muscle. Brit. Med. J., 3:283, 1975.
116. Codivilla, S.: Sulla cura del piede equino varo congenito. Nuovo metodo di cura cruenta. Arch. Chir. Ortop., 23:245, 1906.
117. Collburn, R. C.: Flat-top talus in recurrent clubfoot. J. Bone Joint Surg., 44-A:1018, 1962.
118. Commerell, J.: New approach to the untreated or relapsed clubfoot in adults. J. Bone Joint Surg., 45-B:430, 1963.
119. Compere, E. L.: Congenital talipes equinovarus. Surg. Clin. N. Amer., 15:767, 1935.
120. Condon, V. R.: Radiology of practical orthopedic problems. Radiol. Clin. N. Amer., 10:203, 1972.
121. Conrad, A., and Frost, H. M.: Evaluation of subcutaneous heel cord lengthening. Clin. Orthop., 64:121, 1969.
122. Contargyris, A.: Le traitement operatoire précoce du pied bot congénital chez les nouveau-nés. Rev. Orthop. 3e Serie), 18:719, 1931.
123. Cowell, H. R., and Hensinger, R. N.: The relationship of clubfoot to congenital annular bands. In Bateman, J. E. (ed.): Foot Science. Philadelphia, W. B. Saunders Co., 1976, pp. 41–46.
123a. Cowell, H. R., and Wein, L. K.: Genetic aspects of clubfoot. J. Bone Joint Surg., 62-B:1381, 1980.
124. Crabbe, W. A.: Aetiology of congenital talipes. Brit. Med. J., 2:1060, 1960.
124a. Crawford, A. H., Marxsen, J. L., and Osterfeld, D. L.: The Cincinnati incision: A comprehensive approach for surgical procedures for the foot and ankle in childhood. J. Bone Joint Surg., 64-A:1355, 1982.
125. Critchley, J. E., and Taylor, R. G.: Transfer of the tibialis anterior tendon for relapsed clubfoot. J. Bone Joint Surg., 34-B:49, 1952.
126. Curtis, B. H., and Butterfield, W. L.: Surgical treatment of congenital clubfoot. In J. Delchef (ed.): Dixième Congrès International de Chirurgie Orthopédique et de Traumatologie, Paris, 4–9 Septembre, 1966. Bruxelles, Les Publications "Acta Medica Belgica," 1967, p. 1150.
127. Curtis, F. E., and Muro, F.: Decancellation of the os calcis, astragalus, and cuboid in correction of congenital talipes equinovarus. J. Bone Joint Surg., 16:110, 1934.
128. Czernihowski, M.: Tibial torsion in children with congenital talipes equinovarus. Chir. Narzad. Ruchu Ortop. Pol., 44:71, 1979.
129. Dabadie, J.: Intérêt de l'allongement précoce du tendon d'Achille dans le traitement des pieds bots varus équins congénitaux, sévères. Ann. Chir. Infant. (Paris), 12:77, 1971.
130. Dangelmajor, R. C.: A review of 200 clubfeet. Bull. Hosp. Spec. Surg., 4:73, 1961.
131. Davis, L. A., and Hatt, W. S.: Congenital abnormalities of the feet. Radiology, 64:818, 1955.
132. Debeugny, P.: Treatment of congenital clubfoot in the newborn and infants. Lille Med., 10:Suppl.:1103, 1965.
133. Debrunner, H.: Der angeboren Klumpfuss. Stuttgart, Ferdinand Enke Verlag, 1936.
134. Debrunner, H.: De Klumpfuss und andere orthopädische Missbildungen als Erbleiden. Schweiz. Med. Wochschr., 75:981, 1945.
135. Debrunner, H.: Die Therapie des angeborenen Klumpfusses. Stuttgart, Ferdinand Enke Verlag, 1957.
136. Declercq, F.: Talipes equino varus. Etiology patogenèse. Behandelung en resultaten. Acta Orthop. Belg., 33:799, 1967.
137. Dekel, S., and Weissman, S. L.: Osteotomy of the calcaneus and concomitant plantar stripping in children with talipes cavo-varus. J. Bone Joint Surg., 55-A:802, 1973.
138. De Langh, R., Mulier, J. C., Fabry, G., and Martens, M.: Treatment of clubfoot by posterior capsulectomy. Clin. Orthop., 106:248, 1975.
139. Dellapiccola, B., and Capra, L.: Dermatoglyphics in Larsen's syndrome. Lancet, 1:493, 1973.
140. Del Sel, J. M., De Paoli, J. M., Calvo, A., and Espagnol, R. O.: Clubfoot—neglected and resistant cases. In Delchef, J. (ed.): Orthopaedic Surgery and Traumatology. Congenital clubfoot. d. Neglected and inveterate cases. New York, American Elsevier Publishing Co., Inc., 1973, pp. 774–776.
141. DeMeyer, W., and Baird, I.: Mortality and skeletal malformations from amniocentesis and oligohydramnios in rats: Cleft palate, clubfoot, microstomia and adactyly. Teratology, 2:33, 1969.
142. Denham, R. A.: Congenital talipes equinovarus. J. Bone Joint Surg., 49-B:583, 1967.
143. Denham, R. A.: Early operation for severe congenital talipes equinovarus. J. Bone Joint Surg., 59-B:116, 1977.
144. Dessaint, J. J.: Tomographie de pied bots. Presse Méd., 62:183, 1954.
145. DeWet, I. S.: Postero-medial release in clubfoot. 20th Congress of South African Orthopedic Association, 1975. (Abstract) J. Bone Joint Surg., 57-B:257, 1975.
146. Dimeglio, A., and Pous, J. G.: Le pied bot varus équin: Un conflict autour de l'articulation mediotarsien. Du traitement orthopédique au traitement chirurgicale. In Cahiers d'enseignement de la S.O.F.C.O.T. Paris, Expansion Scientifique Française, 1977, p. 73.
147. Dittrich, R. J.: Pathogenesis of congenital club foot. J. Bone Joint Surg., 12:373, 1930.
148. Domeniconi, S., and Perricone, F.: L'operazione di Codivilla nel trattamento precoce del piedo torto congenito. Minerva Ortop., 3:176, 1952.
149. Van Domselaar, F.: Applicacion de las gotieras de Denis Browne para el pie-bot. Bol. Trab. Soc. Argent. Cir. Ortop., 8:95, 1943.
150. Drachman, D. B., and Coulombre, A. J.: Experimental clubfoot and arthrogryposis multiplex congenita. Lancet, 2:523, 1962.
151. DuBois, H. J.: Nievergelt-Pearlman syndrome. Synostosis in feet and hands with dysplasia of elbows. Report of a case. J. Bone Joint Surg., 52-B:325, 1970.
152. Ducci, L., and Grilli, E. P.: Studio clinico-statistico sul piede torto congenito. Arch. Putti Chir. Organi Mov., 5:517, 1954.
153. Dumeau, C. L.: L'astragalectomie temporare subtotale dans le traitement des pieds bots. Thèse Médecine, Bordeaux, 1942.
154. Dunaj, W.: Microscopic examination of muscles in congenital clubfoot. Chir. Narzad. Ruchu Ortop. Pol., 36:197, 1971.
155. Dunn, H. K., and Samuelson, K. M.: Flat-top talus. A long-term report of twenty club feet. J. Bone Joint Surg., 56-A:57, 1974.
156. Dunn, N.: The treatment of congenital talipes equinovarus. Brit. Med. J., 2:216, 1923.
157. Dunn, P. M.: Congenital postural deformities: Perinatal associations. Proc. Roy. Soc. Med., 65:735, 1972.
158. Dwyer, F. C.: A new approach to the treatment of pes

cavus. Société Internationale de Chirurgie Orthopédique. Sixième Congrès International de Chirurgie Orthopédique. Brussels. M. A. Bailleux, 1955, pp. 551–558.
159. Dwyer, F. C.: Osteotomy of the calcaneum for pes cavus. J. Bone Joint Surg., *41-B*:80, 1959.
160. Dwyer, F. C.: The treatment of relapsed clubfoot by the insertion of a wedge into the calcaneum. J. Bone Joint Surg., *45-B*:67, 1963.
161. Dwyer, F. C.: Treatment of the relapsed clubfoot. Proc. Roy. Soc. Med., *61*:783, 1968.
162. Editorial: Club foot. Brit. Med. J., *2*:593, 1962.
163. Edwards, M. J.: The experimental production of clubfoot in guinea-pigs by maternal hyperthermia during gestation. J. Path., *103*:49, 1971.
164. Ehrenfried, A.: The occurrence and etiology of clubfoot. J.A.M.A., *59*:1940, 1912.
165. Eikenbary, C. F.: Congenital equinovarus, report of 114 cases. Surg. Gynec. Obstet., *30*:555, 1920.
166. Elliot, J. K.: Club foot in the Polynesian. J. Bone Joint Surg., *43-B*:190, 1961.
167. Elmslie, R. C.: The principles of treatment of congenital talipes equino-varus. J. Orthop. Surg., *2*:669, 1920.
168. Elsner, H.: Die Osteotomie und zeitweilige Nagelung des Calcaneus bei blutiger Klumpfuss operation. Zbl. Chir., *51*:429, 1924.
169. Erlacher: Totale Tibialisvereisung bei der Behandlung hartnackiger Klumpfusse. Verh. Deutsch. Orthop., *21*:495, 1927.
170. Evans, D.: Treatment of cavo-varus foot and clubfoot. J. Bone Joint Surg., *39-B*:789, 1957.
171. Evans, D.: Relapsed club foot. J. Bone Joint Surg., *43-B*:722, 1961.
172. Evans, D.: Treatment of unreduced or lapsed clubfoot in older children. Proc. Roy. Soc. Med., *61*:782, 1968.
173. Evans, D.: Calcaneo-valgus deformity. J. Bone Joint Surg., *57-B*:270, 1975.
174. Eyre-Brook, A. L.: Talipes equino cavo varus. J. Bone Joint Surg., *45-B*:428, 1963.
175. Eyring, E. J., Earl, W. C., and Brockmeyer, J. F.: Posterior tibial tendon transfers in neuromuscular conditions other than anterior poliomyelitis. Arch. Phys. Med., *55*:124, 1974.
175a. Fahrenbach, G., Kuehn, D., and Tachdjian, M. O.: The use of computerized tomography in assessing residual deformities in talipes equinovarus. To be published.
176. Falconer, D. S.: The inheritance of liability to certain diseases estimated from the incidence among relatives. Ann. Hum. Genet., *29*:51, 1965.
177. Fang, H. S. Y., and Yu, F. Y. K.: Foot binding in Chinese women. Canad. J. Surg., *3*:195, 1960.
178. Farabeuf, cited by Kapandji, I. A.: The physiology of the joints. *In* Annotated Diagrams of the Mechanics of Human Joints. 2nd Ed. Edinburgh, E. & S. Livingstone, Ltd., 1970, Vol. 2, pp. 138–195.
179. Farill, J.: Elongación del tendón de Aquiles. Gac. Med. Mex., *72*:69, 1942.
180. Farill, J.: Splints in talipes equinovarus. Orthopedic correspondence. Club Letter, Dec. 10, 1945.
181. Farill, J.: Tratamiento del pie varus equino-congénito en los niños pequeños. Bol. Med. Hosp. Infant., *2*:252, 1946.
182. Farill, J.: Tratamiento del pie supino fláccido por tenoplastía del tibial anterior. Bol. Med. Hosp. Infant., *10*:123, 1953.
183. Farill, J.: Tibioperoneal tenoplasty for congenital clubfoot with peroneal insufficiency. J. Bone Joint Surg., *38-A*:329, 1956.
184. Favre-Gilly, J.: Correction of talipes equinovarus in the hemophiliac by successive plaster boot. Hemostase, *5*:187, 1965.
185. Feokistov, G. F.: Functional splint for correction of pes equinus and its retention in the position of correction in congenital clubfoot. Ortop. Travm. Protez., *34*:74, 1973.
186. Fisher, R. L., and Shaffer, S. R.: An evaluation of calcaneal osteotomy in congenital clubfoot and other disorders. Clin. Orthop., *70*:141, 1970.
187. Fisk, J. R., House, J. H., and Bradford, D. S.: Congenital ulnar deviation of the fingers with clubfoot deformities. Clin. Orthop., *104*:200, 1974.
188. Fiske, E. W.: The prognosis of congenital clubfoot and its relation to nonoperative treatment. J.A.M.A., *65*:375, 1915.
189. Fjeldborg, O. C., Medfødt Klumpfod. En biomeckanisk analyse af el Klinisk materiale. Arhus, Universitetsforlaget i Aarhus, 1971.
190. Flinchum, D.: Pathologic anatomy in talipes equinovarus. J. Bone Joint Surg., *35-A*:111, 1953.
191. Forrester-Brown, M.: The treatment of congenital equinovarus (clubfoot). J. Bone Joint Surg., *17*:661, 1935.
192. Forrester-Brown, M.: A clamp for stretching congenital club-feet. Lancet, *1*:897, 1936.
193. Fraser, F. C., Pashayan, H., and Kadish, M. E.: Craniocarpo-tarsal dysplasia. Report of a case in father and son. J.A.M.A., *211*:1374, 1979.
194. Frassi, G. A.: Lateral transplant of the tibialis anterior in the treatment of congenital clubfoot and its recurrences. Arch. Ortop., *76*:93, 1963.
195. Fredenhagen, H.: Der Klumpfuss, Vorkommen, Anatomie, Behandlung und Spätresultate. Z. Orthop., *85*:305, 1955.
196. Freeman, E. A., and Sheldon, J. H.: Cranio-carpo-tarsal dystrophy. An undescribed congenital malformation. Arch. Dis. Child., *13*:277, 1938.
197. Fried, A.: Recurrent congenital club-foot. The role of the m. tibialis posterior in etiology and treatment. J. Bone Joint Surg., *41-A*:243, 1959.
198. Fripp, A. T.: The relapsed clubfoot. Proc. Roy. Soc. Med., *44*:873, 1951.
199. Fripp, A. T.: The problem of the relapsed clubfoot (editorial). J. Bone Joint Surg., *43-B*:626, 1961.
200. Fripp, A. T., and Shaw, N. E.: Club-foot. Edinburgh and London, E. & S. Livingstone, Ltd., 1967.
201. Fujii, H.: Early treatment and surgical indication in congenital clubfoot. Shujutsu, *26*:368, 1972.
202. Furmento, A., Silberman, F., and Khoury, S. C.: Pie varo equino congénito evolución y pronostico de acuerdo el estudio radiografico. Presna Med. Argent., *48*:1617, 1961.
203. Fusari, A.: Sul trattamento precoce del piede torto congenito. Arch. Ortop., *62*:208, 1949.
204. Gambier, N.: Les résultats éloignés de l'opération de Codivilla dans le traitement du pied bot congénital. Rev. Chir. Orthop., *38*:531, 1952.
205. Garceau, G. J.: Anterior tibial transposition in recurrent congenital club-foot. J. Bone Joint Surg., *22*:932, 1940.
206. Garceau, G. J.: Talipes equinovarus. A.A.O.S. Instr. Course Lect., *7*:119, 1950.
207. Garceau, G. J.: Recurrent clubfoot. Bull. Hosp. Joint Dis., *15*:143, 1954.
208. Garceau, G. J.: Talipes equinovarus. A.A.O.S. Instr. Course Lect., *12*:90, 1955.
209. Garceau, G. J.: Congenital talipes equinovarus. A.A.O.S. Instr. Course Lect., *18*:178, 1961.
210. Garceau, G. J.: Anterior tibial tendon transfer for recurrent clubfoot. Clin. Orthop., *84*:61, 1972.
211. Garceau, G. J., and Manning, K. R.: Transposition of the anterior tibial tendon in the treatment of recurrent congenital club-foot. J. Bone Joint Surg., *29*:1044, 1947.
212. Garceau, G. J., and Palmer, R. M.: Transfer of the anterior tibial tendon for recurrent clubfoot. A long-term follow-up. J. Bone Joint Surg., *49-A*:207, 1967.
213. Gardner, E.: Prenatal development of the skeleton and joints of the human foot. J. Bone Joint Surg., *44-A*:847, 1959.
214. Gartland, J. J.: Posterior tibial transplant in the surgical treatment of recurrent club foot. A preliminary report. J. Bone Joint Surg., *46-A*:1217, 1964.
215. Gartland, J. J., and Surgent, R. E.: Posterior tibial transplant in the surgical treatment of recurrent club foot. Clin. Orthop., *84*:66, 1972.
216. Gaston, S. R.: Management of club foot deformities. Bull. N.Y. Orthop. Hosp., *2*:12, 1958.
217. Gaul, J. S., Jr.: The evolution of biomechanical analysis in the management of congenital clubfoot. Clin. Orthop., *76*:141, 1971.
218. Geist, E. S.: An operation for the after treatment of some cases of congenital club-foot. J. Bone Joint Surg., *22*:50, 1924.
219. Gelman, W. B.: Soft-tissue releasing procedure for persisting heel varus in the uncorrected clubfoot. Clin. Orthop., *16*:177, 1960.
220. Ghali, N. N., Smith, R. B., Clayden, A. D., and Silk, F. F.: The results of pantalar reduction in the management

of congenital talipes equinovarus. J. Bone Joint Surg., 65-B:1, 1983.
221. Ghinst, Van De H. M., and Claessens, H.: Talipes equinovarus. Verslag by M. Van De Ghinst en H. Claessens. Acta Orthop. Belg., 33:797, 1967.
222. Giaccai, L., and Simonetti, E.: Pathogenetic characteristics of the so-called essential talipes cavus and its treatment with modeling resection-arthrodesis of the mediotarsal joint. Arch. Putti Chir. Organi Mov., 25:303, 1970.
223. Gibson, A.: A universal joint clubfoot splint. J. Bone Joint Surg., 36-A:658, 1954.
224. Gibson, D. A., and Urs, N. D. K.: Arthrogryposis multiplex cogenita. J. Bone Joint Surg., 52-B:483, 1970.
225. Gilles de la Tourette, G.: Pathogénie et traitement des pieds bots. Sem. Méd., 16:517, 1897.
226. Goldner, J. L.: Congenital talipes equinovarus—fifteen years of surgical treatment. Curr. Pract. Orthop. Surg., 4:61, 1969.
227. Goldwny, R. M.: Z-plasty skin closure after lengthening the Achilles tendon. Plast. Reconstr. Surg., 52:431, 1973.
228. Gordon, H., Davies, D., and Bermen, M.: Camptodactyly, cleft palate and club foot. A syndrome showing the autosomal-dominant pattern of inheritance. J. Med. Genet., 6:266, 1969.
229. Gordon, S. L., and Dunn, E. J.: Peroneal nerve palsy as a complication of clubfoot treatment. Clin. Orthop., 101:229, 1974.
230. Gould, N.: Positional in utero deformities. Amer. J. Orthop., 4:46, 1962.
231. Gourdon, R.: Report. Rev. Chir. Orthop., 38:533, 1952.
232. Graham, J.: Treatment of congenital equinovarus (clubfoot). Amer. J. Surg., 36:339, 1937.
233. Grassi, L., and Murari, P.: Il trattamento chirugico del piede torto congenito inverterato mediante intervento sulle parti molli. Arch. Putti Chir. Organi Mov., 22:342, 1967.
234. Greider, T. D., Siff, S. J., Gerson, P., and Donovan, M. M.: Arteriography in club foot. J. Bone Joint Surg., 64-A:837, 1982.
235. Gross-Kieselstein, E., Abrahamov, A., and Ben-Hur, N.: Familial occurrence of the Freeman-Sheldon syndrome: craniocarpotarsal dysplasia. Pediatrics, 47:1064, 1971.
236. Gulledge, W. C.: Skintight casts for the treatment of clubfoot, a follow-up report. Pacif. Med. Surg., 74:28, 1966.
237. Gunn, D. R., and Molesworth, B. D.: The use of tibialis posterior as a dorsiflexor. J. Bone Joint Surg., 39-B:674, 1957.
238. Hadidi, H.: Management of congenital talipes equinovarus. Orthop. Clin. N. Amer., 5:53, 1974.
239. Van Haelst, A.: Traitment du pied bot congénital après deux ans. Rev. Orthop. (3e Série), 18:712, 1931.
240. Hahn, F.: Über der Ätiologie des kongenitalen Klumpfusses. Z. Orthop. Chir., 42:151, 1922.
241. Haicl, A.: Empirical hazards in talipes equinovarus. Acta Chir. Orthop. Traum. Cech., 38:205, 1971.
242. Haliburton, R. A., Sullivan, C. R., Kelly, P. J., et al.: Extra-osseous and intra-osseous blood supply of the talus. J. Bone Joint Surg., 40-A:1115, 1958.
243. Hall, C. B.: Congenital skeletal deficiencies of the extremities. J.A.M.A., 181:590, 1962.
244. Hamada, G.: Orthopaedics and orthopaedic diseases in ancient and modern Egypt. Clin. Orthop., 89:253, 1972.
245. Hamsa, W. R., and Burney, D. W., Jr.: Open correction of recurrent talipes equinovarus. A study of end-result. Clin. Orthop., 26:104, 1963.
246. Handelsman, J. E.: The surgical treatment of clubfoot in later childhood. In Delchef, J. (ed.): Orthopaedic Surgery and Traumatology. Congenital clubfoot. c. Surgical treatment in later childhood. New York, American Elsevier Publishing Co., Inc., 1973, pp. 766–768.
247. Handelsman, J. E., and Isaacs, H.: Aetiology of club foot. Proceedings: 20th Congress of S. Afr. Orthop. Assoc. (abstract). J. Bone Joint Surg., 57-B:262, 1975.
248. Handelsman, J. E., and Solomon, L.: The assessment of correction in club foot. S. Afr. Med. J., 47:1909, 1973.
248a. Handelsman, J. E., and Badalamente, M. A.: Neuromuscular studies in clubfoot. J. Pediat. Orthop., 1:23, 1981.
249. Handelsman, J. E., Youngleson, J., and Malkin, C.: A modified approach to the Dwyer os calcis osteotomy in club foot. S. Afr. Med. J., 39:989, 1965.
250. Harrold, A. J., and Walker, C. J.: Treatment and prognosis in congenital club foot. J. Bone Joint Surg., 65-B:8, 1983.
251. Haudek, M.: Zur Behandlung des angeborenen Klumpfusses beim Neugeborenen und Saugling. Z. Orthop., 25:761, 1910.
252. Hauser, E. D. W.: A manipulative method of treatment for recalcitrant and neglected clubfoot. J.A.M.A., 93:688, 1929.
253. Hauser, E. D. W.: Cohesive bandage for clubfoot in newborn infants. J.A.M.A., 138:19, 1948.
254. Hauser, E. D. W.: Origin and etiology of clubfoot. Quart. Bull. Northwest. Med. Sch., 28:274, 1954.
255. Hauser, E. D. W.: Congenital clubfoot. Springfield, Ill., Charles C Thomas, 1966.
256. Hayashi, H.: Structural deformity and dynamic deformity in congenital club foot. J. Jap. Orthop. Assoc., 46:939, 1972.
257. Hendel, H. L., Wood, G. G., and Arnold, M.: Die Muskulatur beim angeborenen Klumpfuss. Z. Orthop., 108:604, 1971.
258. Hendrix, G., and Marneffe, R. de: Pied bot congénital: Étude radiologique complémentaire. Acta Orthop. Belg., 26:341, 1960.
259. Henke, W., and Reyher, C.: Studies über die Entwicklung der Extremitäten des Menschen insbesondere der Gelenkflächen. Sitzungsberichte d.k. Akademie d. Wissenschaften Wiener Math. Naturwissenschaftliche Klasse, Ed. 3, 50:217, 1874.
260. Herold, H. Z.: Surgical correction of previously untreated clubfeet in older children and adults. In Delchef, J. (ed.): Orthopaedic Surgery and Traumatology. Congenital clubfoot. c. Neglected and inveterate cases. New York. American Elsevier Publishing Co., Inc., 1973, p. 777.
261. Herold, H. Z., and Torok, G.: Surgical correction of neglected club foot in the older child and adults. J. Bone Joint Surg., 55-A:1385, 1973.
262. Hersh, A.: The role of surgery in the treatment of club feet. J. Bone Joint Surg., 49-A:1684, 1967.
263. Hersh, A., and Fuchs, L. A.: Treatment of the uncorrected clubfoot by triple arthrodesis. Orthop. Clin. N. Amer., 4:103, 1973.
264. Herwig, W., and Schiemann, E.: Zur Klumpfussbehandlung nach Scheel und ihren Ergebnissen. Z. Orthop., 90:333, 1958.
265. Heyman, C. H.: The open reduction for congenital clubfoot. Surg. Gynec. Obstet., 49:705, 1929.
266. Heyman, C. H.: The surgical release of fibrous tissue structures resisting correction of congenital clubfoot and metatarsus varus. A.A.O.S. Instr. Course Lect., 16:100, 1959.
267. Heyman, C. H., Herndon, C. H., and Strong, J. M.: Mobilization of the tarsometatarsal and intermetatarsal joints for the correction of resistant adduction of the forepart of the foot in congenital clubfoot or congenital metartarsus varus. J. Bone Joint Surg., 40-A:299, 1958.
268. Heywood, A. W. B.: The mechanics of the hindfoot in clubfoot as demonstrated radiographically. J. Bone Joint Surg., 46-B:102, 1964.
269. Hicks, J. H.: Mechanics of foot; joints. J. Anat., 87:345, 1953.
270. Hippocrates: Vol. 3. Loeb Classical Library. Trans. by E. T. Withington. London, William Heinemann, Ltd.; New York, G. P. Putnam's Sons, 1927.
271. Hirsch, C.: Medfödd Klumpfot och höftledsluxation. Nord. Med., 62:1138, 1959.
272. Hirsch, C.: Observations on early operative treatment of congenital club-foot. Bull. Hosp. Joint Dis., 21:173, 1960.
273. Hjelmstedt, A.: The importance of analysis of skeletal deformities in congenital clubfeet for adequate surgical treatment. Proceedings of the Scandinavian Orthopaedic Society, 37th Assembly, 1974 (abstract). Acta Orthop. Scand., 45:953, 1974.
274. Hjelmstedt, A.: Correction osteotomy of the talus and calcaneus in relapsing or incorrigible clubfeet. Principles and technique. Proc. Scand. Orth. Soc., 37th Assem., 1974 (abstract). Acta Orthop. Scand., 45:978, 1974.
275. Hjelmstedt, A., and Sahlstedt, B.: The anatomy of the talus in clubfeet. Results of an arthrographic study. Proc. Scand. Orth. Soc., 36th Assem., 1972 (Abstract). Acta Orthop. Scand., 44:128, 1973.

276. Hjelmstedt, A., and Sahlstedt, B: Talar deformity in congenital clubfeet. Acta Orthop. Scand., 45:628, 1974.
277. Hjelmstedt, A., and Sahlstedt, B.: Simultaneous arthrography of the talocrural and talonavicular joints in children. II. Comparison between anatomic and arthrographic measurements. Acta Radiol. [Diagn.] (Stockholm), 17:557, 1976.
278. Hjelmstedt, A., and Sahlstedt, B.: Arthrography as a guide in the treatment of congenital clubfoot. Findings and treatment results in a consecutive series. Acta Orthop. Scand., 52:321, 1980.
279. Hjelmstedt, A., and Sahlstedt, B.: Talo-calcaneal osteotomy and soft-tissue procedures in the treatment of clubfeet. I. Indications, principles and technique. Acta Orthop. Scand., 51:335, 1980.
280. Hjelmstedt, A., and Sahlstedt, B.: Talo-calcaneal osteotomy and soft-tissue procedures in the treatment of clubfeet. II. Results in 36 surgically treated feet. Acta Orthop. Scand., 51:349, 1980.
281. Hoeer, N. L., Pyle, S. E., and Krancis, C. C.: Radiographic atlas of skeletal development of the foot and ankle, a standard of reference. Springfield, Ill., Charles C Thomas, 1962.
282. Hoffa, A.: Lehrbuch der Orthopädischen Chirurgie. 5th Ed. Stuttgart. Ferdinand Enke Verlag, 1905, pp. 734–782.
283. Hoke, M.: An operative plan for the correction of relapsed and untreated talipes equinovarus. Amer. J. Orthop. Surg., 9:379, 1911.
284. Holmadhl, H. C.: Astragalectomy as a stabilizing operation for foot paralysis following poliomyelitis: Results of a follow-up investigation of 153 cases. Acta Orthop. Scand., 25:207, 1956.
285. Hopf, A.: Die operative Klumpfussbehandlung im späten Kindesalter und beim Erwachsenen. Verh. Deutsch. Orthop. Ges. 42 Kongress Beil, Z. Orthop., 86:162, 1954.
286. Howorth, M. B.: Textbook of Orthopaedics. Collingdale, Pa., Dorman Printers, 1959, pp. 426–428.
287. Hüter, C.: Zur der Frage über das Wesen des angeborenen Klümpfusses. Deutsch. Klinik, 15:487, 1863.
288. Idelberger, K.: Der angeborenen Klumpfuss. In Schwalbe, E. (ed.): Die Morphologic der Missbildungen des Menschen und der Tierre. Jena, Gustav Fisher, 1958, p. 939.
289. Idelberger, K.: Die Ergebnisse der Zwillingsforschung beim angeborenen Klumpfuss. Verh. Deutsch. Orthop. Ges., 33:272, 1939.
290. Idelberger, K.: Die Zwillingspathologie der angeborenen Klumpfuss. Z. Orthop., Suppl. 69, 1939.
291. Imhäuser, G.: Die Frühbehandlung des angeborenen, muskulären Klumpfusses. Mscher. Kinderheilk., 117:645, 1969.
292. Imhäuser, G.: Die Arthrodese des unteren Sprunggelenkes. Z. Orthop., 111:453, 1973.
293. Inclán, A.: Anomalies of the tendinous insertions in the pathogenesis of club foot. J. Bone Joint Surg., 40-B:159, 1958.
294. Inclán, A.: Las anomalias de las inserciones tendinosas en la patogenia del pié bot varo equino congénito. Rev. Ortop. Trauma., 5:173, 1960.
295. Ingelrans, P.: Report. Rev. Chir. Orthop., 38:535, 1952.
296. Ingelrans, P.: Results of treatment of congenital inturned clubfoot before one year of age by Denis Browne splint. Acta Orthop. Belg., 34:19, 1969.
297. Ingram, A. J., and Sprague, B.: Congenital clubfeet with associated absence of the anterior compartment musculature. In: Delchef, J. (ed.): Orthopaedic Surgery and Traumatology. Congenital clubfoot. a. Anatomy and pathology of the disease. New York, American Elsevier Publishing Co., Inc., 1973, pp. 744–745.
297a. Ippolito, E., and Ponseti, I. V.: Congenital club foot in the human fetus. J. Bone Joint Surg., 62-A:8, 1980.
298. Irani, R. N., and Sherman, M. S.: The pathological anatomy of clubfoot. J. Bone Joint Surg., 45-A:45, 1963.
299. Irani, R. N., and Sherman, M. S.: The pathological anatomy of idiopathic clubfoot. Clin. Orthop., 84:14, 1972.
300. Isaacs, H., Handelsman, J. E., Badenhorst, M., and Pickering, A.: The muscles in club foot—a histological, histochemical and electron microscopic study. J. Bone Joint Surg., 59-B:465, 1977.
301. Ivy, R. H.: Congenital anomalies; as recorded on birth certificates in the Division of Vital Statistics of the Pennsylvania Department of Health, for the period of 1951–1955, inclusive. Plast. Reconstr. Surg., 20:400, 1957.
302. Jackson, C. T., and Weighill, F. J.: A combined peroneal tendon transfer and subtalar fusion using excized fibular bone. Brit. J. Clin. Pract., 27:329, 1973.
303. Jackson, R. K.: Experimental talipes in the Virginia opossum. Clin. Orthop., 81:152, 1971.
304. Jacobs, J. E., and Carr, C. R.: Progressive muscular atrophy of the peroneal type (Charcot-Marie-Tooth disease), orthopedic management and end-result study. J. Bone Joint Surg., 32-A:27, 1950.
305. Jacquemain, B.: Der angeborenen Klumpfuss in therapeutischer Insicht. Z. Kinderchir., 6:80, 1968.
306. Janacek, M., and Liphardt, H. P.: Beitrage zur Therapie des equinovarus congenitus. Beitr. Orthop. Trauma., 12:408, 1965.
307. Jansen, K.: Treatment of congenital club foot. J. Bone Joint Surg., 39-B:599, 1957.
308. Jay, R. M., and Schoenhaus, H. D.: Further insights in the anterior advancement of tendo Achillis. J. Amer. Podiatry Assoc., 71:73, 1981.
309. Jergesen, F. H.: The treatment of unilateral congenital talipes equinovarus with the Denis Browne splint. J. Bone Joint Surg., 25:185, 1943.
310. Johanning, K.: Excochleatio ossis cuboidei in the treatment of pes equinovarus. Acta Orthop. Scand., 27:310, 1958.
311. Jones, R., and Lovett, R. W.: Club-foot. In Orthopaedic Surgery. New York, William Wood & Co., 1926. Chapter 28, pp. 578–598.
312. Jorring, K., and Christiansen, L.: Congenital clubfoot. A follow-up of 58 children treated during 1964–1969. Acta Orthop. Scand., 46:152, 1975.
313. Judet, H., and Judet, J.: La réorientation de l'articulation tibio-tarsienne. Chirurgie, 97:638, 1971.
314. Judet, J.: A propos du traitement des pieds bots. Rev. Chir. Orthop., 28:538, 1952.
315. Judet, J.: Principes et technique de la réposition des os du pied dans le traitement des pieds bots rebelles ou récidivés. Acta Orthop. Belg., 33:876, 1967.
316. Judet, J.: New concepts in the corrective surgery of congenital talipes equinovarus and congenital and neurologic flatfeet. Clin. Orthop., 70:56, 1970.
317. Judet, J.: Le pied bot varus équin de l'adulte. In Cahiers d'enseignement des la S.O.F.C.O.T. Paris, Expansion Scientifique Française, 1977, p. 113.
318. Judet, J., Raynal, L., and Rigault, P.: Traitement des piedes bots varus équin rebelles ou récidivés chez des enfants âgés de 18 mois à 6 ans (préambule). Acta Orthop. Belg., 33:866, 1967.
319. Kalman, E.: Einige Bemerkungen zur operativen Therapie des Klumpfusses. Beitr. Orthop. Trauma., 15:597, 1968.
320. Kandel, B.: The suroplantar projection in the congenital clubfoot of the infant. Acta Orthop. Scand., 22:161, 1952.
321. Kaneda, K.: Posteromedial release operation in congenital clubfoot. Shujutsu, 26:391, 1972.
322. Kaplan, E. B.: Comparative anatomy of the talus in relation to idiopathic clubfoot. Clin. Orthop., 85:32, 1972.
323. Karp, M.: Kohler's disease of the tarsal scaphoid. J. Bone Joint Surg., 19:84, 1937.
324. Keim, H. A., and Ritchie, G. W.: "Nutcracker" treatment of clubfoot. J.A.M.A., 189:613, 1964.
325. Keith, A.: Concerning the origin and nature of certain malformations of the face, head and foot. Brit. J. Surg., 28:173, 1940.
326. Kelly, J. P.: Clubfoot. J. Bone Joint Surg., 44-B:748, 1962.
327. Kendrick, R. E., Sharma, N. K., Hassler, W. L., and Herndon, C. H.: Tarsometatarsal mobilization for resistant adduction of the forepart of the foot. A follow-up study. J. Bone Joint Surg., 52-A:61, 1970.
328. Kerkiacharian, A.: Considérations techniques dans les capsulotomies du coup-de-pied. Presse Méd., 76:1192, 1968.
329. Kilfoyle, R. M., Broome, J. S., Hardy, J. H., and Curtis, B. H.: Talectomy. In Bateman, J. E. (ed.): Foot Science. Philadelphia, W. B. Saunders Co., 1976, p. 162.
330. Kinder, F. C.: Clubfoot. J.A.M.A., 98:1736, 1932.
331. Kite, J. H.: Non-operative treatment of congenital clubfeet. Southern Med. J., 23:337, 1930.
332. Kite, J. H.: The treatment of congenital clubfeet. A study of the results in two hundred cases. J.A.M.A., 99:1156, 1932.

333. Kite, J. H.: The surgical treatment of congenital club-feet. Surg. Gynec. Obstet., 61:100, 1935.
334. Kite, J. H.: Principles involved in the treatment of congenital club-foot: The results of treatment. J. Bone Joint Surg., 21:595, 1939.
335. Kite, J. H.: Treatment of congenital clubfoot. A.A.O.S. Instr. Course Lect., 7:117, 1950.
336. Kite, J. H.: Treatment of congenital clubfoot. A.A.O.S. Instr. Course Lect., 8:181, 1951.
337. Kite, J. H.: Treatment of resistant clubfeet. Discussion of tendon transference. A.A.O.S., Instr. Course Lect., 10:171, 1953.
338. Kite, J. H.: The operative treatment of congenital clubfeet. A.A.O.S. Instr. Course Lect., 12:100, 1955.
339. Kite, J. H.: Congenital clubfeet: Facts designed to aid in providing answers for anxious parents. Amer. J. Orthopsychiatr., 1:58, 1959.
340. Kite, J. H.: Some suggestions on treatment of clubfoot by casts. J. Bone Joint Surg., 45-A:406, 1963.
341. Kite, J. H.: The Clubfoot. New York, Grune & Stratton, Inc., 1964.
342. Kite, J. H.: Errors and complications in treating foot conditions in children. Clin. Orthop., 53:31, 1967.
343. Kite, J. H.: Conservative treatment of the resistant recurrent clubfoot. Clin. Orthop., 70:93, 1970.
344. Kite, J. H.: Nonoperative treatment of congenital clubfoot. Clin. Orthop., 84:29, 1972.
345. Kleiger, B.: Significance of tibiotalar navicular complex in congenital clubfoot. Bull. Hosp. Joint Dis., 23:158, 1962.
346. Kleiger, B.: Anomalies of the posterior tibial tendon observed during medial release operation. Bull. Hosp. Joint Dis., 27:9, 1966.
347. Kleiger, B., and Mankin, H. J.: A roentgenographic study of the development of the calcaneus by means of the posterior tangential view. J. Bone Joint Surg., 43-A:961, 1961.
348. Kocher: Zur Aetiologie und Therapie des pes varus congenitus. Deutsch. Z. Chir., 9:329, 1879.
349. Kovalevich, M. D., and Stavskaia, E. A.: Early surgical treatment of congenital clubfoot. Khirurgia (Mosk.), 47:111, 1971.
350. Kreuz, L., and Stope, H.: Pes equino-varus congenitus. In Hohmann, G. (ed.): Handbuch der Orthopadie. Stuttgart, George Thiem Verlag, 1961, Vol. IV, Part II, pp. 788–821.
351. Kuhlmann, R. F.: Conservative management of congenital clubfoot deformity. Amer. J. Dis. Child., 87:440, 1954.
352. Kuhlmann, R. F.: A survey and clinical evaluation of the operative treatment for congenital talipes equinovarus. Clin. Orthop., 84:88, 1972.
353. Kuhlmann, R. F., and Bell, J. F.: A clinical evaluation of operative procedures for congenital talipes equinovarus. J. Bone Joint Surg., 39-A:265, 1957.
354. Kumar, K.: The role of footprints in the management of clubfeet. Clin. Orthop., 140:32, 1979.
355. Lamy, M., and Maroteaux, P.: Le nanisme diastrophique. Presse Méd., 68:1977, 1960.
356. Lamy, M., and Maroteaux, P.: The genetic study of limb malformations. In Swinyard, C. A. (ed.): Limb Development and Deformity. Springfield, Ill., Charles C Thomas, 1969, pp. 170–175.
357. Landi, F.: L'ereditarieta del piede torto-congenito. Chir. Organi Mov., 34:234, 1950.
358. Lanfranchi, R., and Sabetta, F.: Risultati del trattamento ortopedico e fisiochinesiterapico del P.T.C. nei primi giorni di vita. Chir. Organi Mov., 59:523, 1970.
359. Lange, M.: Orthopädische-Chirurgische. Operationslehre. München, J. Bergman, 1951.
360. Langenskiöld, A., and Ritsalä, V.: Supination deformity of the forefoot. Acta Orthop. Scand., 48:325, 1977.
361. Langer, L. O.: Diastrophic dwarfism in early infancy. Amer. J. Roentgen., 93:399, 1965.
362. Lapidus, P. W.: Congenital bilateral talipes equinus in twins. J. Bone Joint Surg., 21:792, 1939.
363. Larsen, E. H.: Congenital clubfoot. J. Bone Joint Surg., 45-B:620, 1963.
364. Larsen, L. J., Schottstaedt, E. R., and Bost, F. C.: Multiple congenital dislocations associated with characteristic facial abnormality. J. Pediat., 37:574, 1950.
365. Latta, R. J., Graham, B., Aase, J., Scham, S. M., and Smith, D. W.: Larsen's syndrome: A skeletal dysplasia with multiple joint dislocation and unusual facies. J. Pediat., 78:291, 1971.
366. Lauterburg, W.: Zur Behandlung des angeborenen Klumpfusses in Säuglingsalter. Schweiz. Med. Wschr., 75:954, 1945.
367. Lazzareschi, M., Bruschili, S., Verniera, J., and Laredo, J.: Early surgery for resistant congenital talipes equinovarus. In Delchef, J. (ed.) Orthopaedic Surgery and Traumatology. Congenital clubfoot. b. Early childhood—conservative and surgical treatment. New York, American Elsevier Publishing Co., Inc., 1973, pp. 761–762.
368. Leck, J.: Incidence of malformations. In Davis, J. A. (ed.): Scientific Foundations of Paediatrics. Paediatric Aspect of Epidemiology. Philadelphia, W. B. Saunders Co., 1974, pp. 705–726.
369. Leclerc, G. C.: Etude sur les résultats thérapeutiques dans les pieds bots varus équins. Rev. Chir. Orthop., 47:578, 1961.
370. Lelievre, J.: Pied varus équin congénital. In Pathologie du Pied. 2nd Ed. rev. Paris, Masson & Cie, 1961, pp. 154–175.
371. Lemperg, R.: Subastragalar triarticular arthrodesis for congenital clubfoot in children aged 2½–15 years. Acta Orthop. Scand., 36:203, 1965.
372. LeNoir, J. L.: Congenital idiopathic talipes. Springfield, Ill., Charles C Thomas, 1966.
373. LeNoir, J. L.: The long undescribed inverted clubfoot. Southern Med. J., 64:199, 1971.
374. LeNoir, J. L.: A perspective focus on the indicated surgical treatment of resistant clubfoot in the infant. Southern Med. J., 69:837, 1976.
375. Leonard, D. W.: The significance of delayed ossification in the treatment of congenital clubfoot. J. Pediat., 26:379, 1945.
376. Leun, W.: Nachtschiene gegen Klumpfuss. Z. Orthop., 72:250, 1941.
377. Leveuf, J., and Bertrand, P.: La réduction sanglante du pied bot chez le jeune enfant. Rev. Orthop., 34:97, 1948.
378. Lichtblau, S.: Etiology of clubfoot. Clin. Orthop., 84:21, 1972.
379. Lichtblau, S.: A medial and lateral release operation for clubfoot. A preliminary report. J. Bone Joint Surg., 55-A:1377, 1973.
380. Lichtblau, S.: Section of the abductor hallucis tendon for correction of metatarsus varus deformity. Clin. Orthop., 110:227, 1975.
381. Liebermann, B.: Über eine Merkwurdige Exostosenbildung bei Klumpfuss. Arch. Orthop. Chir., 32:16, 1952.
382. Lipmann Kessel, A. W.: The Kite method in the treatment of clubfoot. J. Bone Joint Surg., 33-B:463, 1951.
383. Little, W. J.: A Treatise on the Nature of Club-Foot and Analogous Distortions: Including Their Treatment Both With or Without Surgical Operation. London, W. Jeffs, 1839.
384. Lloyd-Roberts, G. C.: Editorial: "Congenital club foot." J. Bone Joint Surg., 46-B:369, 1964.
385. Lloyd-Roberts, G. C.: Clubfoot. Develop. Med. Child Neurol., 6:507, 1965.
386. Lloyd-Roberts, G. C.: The treatment of clubfoot. Manitoba Med. Rev., 48:198, 1968.
387. Lloyd-Roberts, G. C.: Orthopaedic abnormalities, the foot and ankle. In Norman, A. P. (ed.): Congenital Abnormalities in Infancy. 2nd Ed. Oxford, Blackwell, 1971, pp. 282–287.
388. Lloyd-Roberts, G. C., and Lettin, A. W. R.: Arthrogryposis multiplex congenita. J. Bone Joint Surg., 52-B:494, 1970.
389. Lloyd-Roberts, G. C., Swann, M., and Catterall, A.: Medial rotational osteotomy for severe residual deformity in club foot. A preliminary report on a new method of treatment. J. Bone Joint Surg., 56-B:37, 1974.
390. Lombard, P.: Les bases du traitement dans le pied bot varus équin congénital. Rev. Orthop., 36:46, 1950.
391. Lombard, P.: Note sur la pathogénie et le traitement du pied bot varus équin congénital. Rev. Chir. Orthop., 38:542, 1952.
392. Lowe, L. W., and Hannon, M. A.: Residual adduction of the forefoot in treated congenital clubfoot. J. Bone Joint Surg., 55-B:809, 1973.
393. Lowell, W. W., and Hancock, C. I.: Treatment of congenital talipes equinovarus. Clin. Orthop., 70:79, 1970.
394. Lozano, E., and Padilla, F.: Pié equino varo congénito, Rev. Mex. Pediat. 28:481, 1959.
395. Lubrano di Diego, J. G., Noyer, D., Daudet, M., Kohler,

R., Dodat, H., Vidal, P., Louis, D., and Chappius, J. P.: A new orthopedic apparatus for the treatment of congenital equinovarus clubfoot. The active-passive articulated splint. Critical study apropos of 72 cases treated in our department. Chir. Pediat., 20:371, 1979.
396. Lucas, L. S.: Surgical procedures in treatment of chronic clubfoot. Western J. Surg., 56:542, 1948.
397. Lucas, L. S., and Cottrell, G. W.: Notched rotation osteotomy. A method employed in the corrections of torsion of the tibia and other conditions. Western J. Surg., 57:5, 1949.
398. Lundberg, B. J.: Early Dwyer operation in talipes equinovarus. Clin. Orthop., 154:223, 1981.
399. Lusskin, H.: Nonrigid method of treatment for early clubfoot. J. Int. Coll. Surg., 14:444, 1950.
400. McBride, E. D.: Congenital and hereditary anomalies. In Crippled Children. Their Treatment and Orthopedic Nursing. St. Louis, C. V. Mosby Co., 1937, pp. 278–316.
401. McCauley, J. C., Jr.: Operative treatment of clubfeet. New York J. Med., 47:255, 1947.
402. McCauley, J. C., Jr.: Surgical treatment of clubfoot. Surg. Clin. N. Amer., 31:561, 1951.
403. McCauley, J. C., Jr.: A release operation for problem clubfoot. New York J. Med., 52:2997, 1952.
404. McCauley, J. C., Jr.: Treatment of clubfoot. A.A.O.S. Instr. Course Lect., 16:93, 1959.
405. McCauley, J. C., Jr.: Triple arthrodesis for congenital talipes equinovarus deformities. Clin. Orthop., 34:25, 1964.
406. McCauley, J. C., Jr.: Clubfoot. History of the development and the concepts of pathogenesis and treatment. Clin. Orthop., 44:51, 1966.
407. McCauley, J. C., Jr.: The history of conservative and surgical methods of clubfoot treatment. Clin. Orthop., 84:25, 1972.
408. McCauley, J. C., Jr., and Krida, A.: The early treatment of equinus in congenital clubfoot. Amer. J. Surg., 22:491, 1933.
409. McCollum, R. G.: A functional brace for congenital clubfoot. A preliminary report. Clin. Orthop., 89:197, 1972.
410. MacEwen, G. D., Scott, D. J., Jr., and Shands, A. R., Jr.: Follow-up survey of clubfoot treated at Alfred I. duPont Institute. With special reference to the value of plaster therapy, instituted during earliest signs of recurrence, and the use of night splints to prevent or minimize the manifestations. J.A.M.A., 175:427, 1961.
411. McGregor, A. L.: Congenital clubfoot: An analysis of the deformity and the principles of its treatment. Lancet, 2:20, 1933.
412. McIntosh, R., Merritt, K. K., Richards, M. R., Samuels, M. H., and Bellows, M. T.: The incidence of congenital malformations: A study of 5,964 pregnancies. Pediatrics, 14:505, 1954.
413. McKay, D. W.: New concept of and approach to clubfoot treatment: Section I—Principles and morbid anatomy. J. Pediat. Orthop., 2:347, 1982.
414. McKay, D. W.: New concept of and approach to clubfoot treatment: Section II—Correction of the clubfoot. J. Pediat. Orthop., 3:10, 1983.
415. McKay, D. W.: New concept of and approach to clubfoot treatment: Section III—Evaluation and results. J. Pediat. Orthop., 3:141, 1983.
416. Magnusson, R.: Rotation osteotomy—a method employed in case of congenital club-foot. J. Bone Joint Surg., 28:262, 1946.
417. Main, B. J., Crider, R. J., Polk, M., Lloyd-Roberts, G. C., Swann, M., and Kamdar, B. A.: The results of early operation in talipes equinovarus. J. Bone Joint Surg., 59-B:337, 1977.
418. Malogon Castro, V.: Pié varus equino congénito (factores etiológicos). Rev. Fac. Med. (Bogotá), 22:427, 1955.
419. Marciniak, W.: Guidelines for the evaluation of treatment of congenital clubfoot. Chir. Narzad. Ruchu Ortop. Pol., 36:213, 1971.
420. Marciniak, W.: Results of conservative management of congenital clubfoot in infants in the light of 5-year follow-up. Chir. Narzad. Ruchu Ortop. Pol., 36:333, 1971.
421. Marciniak, W.: Early surgical treatment of residual deformations of congenital clubfoot in infants. Chir. Narzad. Ruchu Ortop. Pol., 36:507, 1971.
422. Marciniak, W.: Single-stage peritalar reposition of congenital club foot in children. Chir. Narzad. Ruchu Ortop. Pol., 37:589, 1972.
423. Marciniak, W.: Reasons for and description of pseudocorrections in conservative treatment of congenital clubfoot. Chir. Narzad. Ruchu Ortop. Pol., 37:679, 1972.
424. Marciniak, W.: Anatomical analysis of deformities in congenital clubfoot and its pseudo-corrections. Selection of surgical method. Chir. Narzad. Ruchu Ortop. Pol., 38:45, 1973.
425. Marciniak, W.: Die anatomische Analyse der Veränderungen beim angeborenen Klumpfuss and bei seinen Pseudokorrektionen als Beitrag zur Auswahl der Methode einer operativen Behandlung. Beitr. Orthop. Trauma., 22:163, 1975.
426. Maresca, A.: Considerazioni sulla lussazione congenital astragalo scafoidea nel quadro del cosidetto piede a dondolo. Orizz. Ortop. Odierna Riab., 4:187, 1959.
427. Marique, P.: La réintegration non sanglante de l'astragale. Méthode nouvelle pour la réduction du pied bot varus équin. Rev. Orthop., 27:37, 1942.
428. Marique, P.: La subluxation du pied bot. Presse Méd., 54:411, 1946.
429. Marique, P., and De Meuter, W.: Le controle radiographique au cours du traitement de pied bot par la méthode de Denis Browne. Rev. Chir. Orthop., 37:250, 1951.
430. Marique, P., and Steebenruggen, C. A.: Le traitement du pied bot varus équin congénital. Acta Orthop. Belg., 13:90, 1947.
431. Marquez Gubern, A.: Some aspects in the treatment of congenital talipes equinovarus (TEV). An. Med. Espec., 51:49, 1965.
432. Martini, G., and Tos, L.: Corrective manual treatment of the congenital talus valgus foot. Gazz. Med. Ital., 124:108, 1965.
433. Massart, R.: Le traitement chirurgical précoce au pied bot congénital. Bull. Mem. Soc. Chir. Paris, June:382, 1931.
434. Masse, P., Taussig, G., and Bazin, G.: External wedge-shaped osteotomy of the calcaneus in the treatment of talipes equinovarus. Rev. Chir. Orthop., 60:Suppl. 2:135, 1974.
435. Masse, P., Taussig, G., and Jacob, P.: Osteotomy of the calcaneus in the treatment of congenital varus equinus clubfoot. Rev. Chir. Orthop., 66:51, 1980.
436. Masse, P., Benichou, J., Dimeglio, A., Morel, J. M., Onimus, M., Padovani, J., and Seringe, R.: Pied bot varus équin congénital. S.O.F.C.O.T. Réunion annuelle, Nov., 1975. Rev. Chir. Orthop., 62:Suppl. 2:37, 1976.
437. Masse, R.: Le traitement du pied bot par la méthode fonctionelle. In Cahiers d'enseignement de la S.O.F.C.O.T. Paris, Expansion Scientifique Française, 1977, p. 51.
438. Match, R. M.: Onycho-osteo-arthrodysplasia with equinovarus. Study of affected family. New York. J. Med., 73:1105, 1973.
439. Matheis, H.: Die Sofortbehandlung des angeborenen Klumpfusses. Wien. Klin. Wschr., 59:55, 1947.
440. Mau, C.: Der Klumpfuss. Ergebn. Chir. Orthop., 20:361, 1927.
441. Mau, C.: Muskelbefunde und ihre Bedeutung beim angeborenen Klumpfussleiden. Arch. Orthop. Unfallchir., 28:292, 1930.
442. Mau, H.: Klumpfuss. Deutsch. Med. Wschr., 98:1782, 1973.
443. Melville, R. S.: Utilization of the body weight in treatment of the residual deformity in clubfeet. J. Bone Joint Surg., 21:456, 1939.
444. Memmi, P.: Lo sviluppo embriologico del piede e i suoi riflessi sulla patogenesi del piede torto congenito. Minerva Ginec., 15:508, 1963.
445. Menelaus, M. B.: Talectomy in equinovarus deformity in arthrogryposis and spina bifida. J. Bone Joint Surg., 53-B:468, 1971.
446. Mezzari, A.: La capsultomia posteriore nella cura del piede torto congenito. Atti Soc. Ital. Ortop. Trauma., 32:354, 1947.
447. Michel, L.: Le pied bot varus équin congénital et son traitement actuel. Rev. Orthop., 35:167, 1949.
448. Middleton, D. S.: Studies on prenatal lesions of striated muscle as a cause of congenital deformity. Edinburgh Med. J., N.S., 41:401, 1934.
449. Migeon, B. R.: Short arm deletions in group E and chromosomal "deletion" syndromes. J. Pediat., 69:432, 1966.

450. Mikyška, V., and Stehlik, V.: Corrective splint with horizontal rotation for follow-up treatment of congenital clubfoot. Beitr. Orthop. Trauma., *14*:403, 1967.
451. Millar, E. A.: Congenital clubfoot. Surg. Clin. N. Amer., *45*:231, 1965.
452. Miller, R.: Zur Erstbehandlung des angeborenen Säuglingsklumpfusses. (Erfahrungen an 48 Säuglingsklumpfussen). Z. Orthop., *79*:552, 1950.
453. Miller, W. E.: Congenital clubfeet. Bull. Univ. Miami Sch. Med. & Jackson Mem. Hosp., *13*:1, 1959.
454. Mimran, R.: Transplantation du jambier postérieur sur le dos du pied. Rev. Chir. Orthop., *52*:681, 1966.
455. Möbius, P. J.: Ueber angeborene doppelseitige Abducens-Facialis-Lähmung. Munch. Med. Wschr., *35*:91, 1888.
456. Moore, J. R.: Clubfoot braces. *In* Orthpaedic Appliances Atlas. Ann Arbor, J. W. Edwards, 1952, Vol. 1, pp. 479–495.
457. Morel, G.: La correction chirurgicale du pied bot chez le grand enfant. *In* Cahiers d'enseignement de la S.O.F.C.O.T. Paris, Expansion Scientifique Française, 1977, p. 91.
458. Morita, S.: A method for the treatment of resistant congenital clubfoot in infants by gradual correction with leverage-wire correction and wire-traction cast. J. Bone Joint Surg., *44-A*:149, 1962.
459. Moroz, P. F.: The method of operative treatment of congenital talipes in children. Ortop. Travm. Protez., *27*:47, 1966.
460. Moroz, P. F.: Recurrence of congenital clubfoot. Ortop. Travm. Protez., *34*:69, 1973.
461. Morris, R. H.: Skeletal traction as a method of treatment for certain foot deformities. Arch. Surg. (Chicago), *46*:737, 1943.
462. Müller, G.: Die morphologischen Ergebnisse der Klumpfussbehandlung aus klinischer und röntgenologischer Sicht. Beitr. Orthop. Trauma., *17*:594, 1970.
463. Müller, G.: Clubfoot therapy. Kinderaerztl. Prax., *41*:7, 1973.
464. Müller, R.: Über das Geschlechtsverhältnis beim angeborenen Klumpfussleiden. Z. Orthop., *72*:237, 1941.
465. Murray, W. R.: Treatment of clubfoot. Postgrad Med., *37*:105, 1965.
466. Musial, W. W.: Results of surgical treatment of pes equinovarus. Folia Med. Cracov., *7*:559, 1965.
467. Myers-Ralfs, M.: Seltene Muskelanomalie bei angeborenem Klumpfuss. Z. Orthop., *111*:801, 1973.
468. Nagura, S.: Zur Ätiologie des angeborenen Klumpfusses. Zbl. Chir., *81*:187, 1956.
469. Nagura, S.: Zur Frage der Vererbung des angeborenen Klumpfusses. Arch. Orthop. Unfallchir., *52*:48, 1960.
470. Neel, J. V., Falls, H. T., and Test, A. R.: Pedigree of club-foot. Amer. J. Dis. Child., *79*:442, 1950.
471. Neff, R. S., Brown, L. P., and Wissinger, H. A.: An unusual complication of a below-the-knee cast. A case report. J. Bone Joint Surg., *52-A*:1651, 1970.
472. Negron, A. J.: Un concepto fundamental en el tratamiento precoz del pié bot congénito, Rev. Hosp. Niño (Lima), *54*:119, 1953.
473. Nemechek, R. W.: Long-term follow-up and family study in congenital talipes equinovarus. J. Bone Joint Surg., *50-A*:1064, 1968.
474. Nichols, E. H.: Anatomy of congenital equinovarus. Boston Med. Surg. J., *36*:150, 1897.
475. Nilsonne, H.: Eine statistische Studie über den kongenitalen Klumpfuss. Z. Orthop. Chir., *48*:219, 1927.
476. Nuñez, E., and Stuardo, M. C.: Cranio-carpo-tarsal dysplasia. Rev. Chil. Pediat., *42*:611, 1971.
477. Nutt, J. J.: Congenital club-foot. *In* Diseases and Deformities of the Foot. New York, E. B. Treat & Co., 1925, pp. 113–173.
478. Nyga, W.: Results of relocating the anterior tibial muscle in treating congenital clubfoot. Beitr. Orthop. Trauma., *26*:44, 1979.
479. Ober, F. R.: An operation for the relief of congenital equinovarus deformity. Preliminary report. J.A.M.A., *65*:621, 1915.
480. Ober, F. R.: An operation for the relief of congenital equinovarus deformities. J. Orthop. Surg., *2*:558, 1920.
481. Ode, A.: Zur histologischen Pathologie des kongenitalen Spitz-Klumpfüsses mit Nachuntersuchungsergebnissen operierter Spitz-Klumpfüsses. Z. Orthop., *82*:102, 1952.
482. Ogston, A.: A new principle of curing club-foot in severe cases in children a few years old. Brit. Med. J., *1*:1524, 1902.
483. Oliver, G.: Formation du sequelette des membres. Paris, Vigot Frères, 1962.
484. Ono, K., and Hayashi, H.: Residual deformity of treated congenital club foot. A clinical study employing frontal tomography of the hind part of the foot. J. Bone Joint Surg., *56-A*:1577, 1974.
485. Ono, K., Hiroshima, K., Tada, K., and Inoue, A.: Anterior transfer of the toe flexors for equinovarus deformity of the foot. Int. Orthop., *4*:225, 1980.
486. O'Rahilly, R.: Morphological patterns in limb deficiencies and duplications. Amer. J. Anat., *89*:135, 1951.
487. Orofino, C. F.: The etiology of congenital club foot. Acta Orthop. Scand., *29*:59, 1960.
488. Otto, F. M. G.: Die "Cranio-carpo-tarsal Dystrophie" (Freeman-Sheldon); ein kasuistischer Beitrag. Z. Kinderheilk., *73*:240, 1953.
489. Paddvani, J. P., Rigault, P., Pouliquen, J. C., Guyonvarch, G., and Durand, Y.: L'astragalectomie chez l'enfant. Rev. Chir. Orthop., *62*:475, 1976.
490. Pages, R.: Treatment of congenital talipes equinovarus. Bull. Soc. Chir. Paris, *59*:252, 1969.
491. Palmer, R. M.: Hereditary club foot. Clin. Orthop., *33*:138, 1964.
492. Palmer, R. M.: The genetics of talipes equinovarus. J. Bone Joint Surg., *46-A*:542, 1964.
493. Palmer, R. M., Conneally, P. M., and Yu, P. L.: Studies of the inheritance of idiopathic talipes equinovarus. Orthop. Clin. N. Amer. *5*:99, 1974.
494. Pandey, S., Jha, S. S., and Pandey, A. K.: "T" osteotomy of the calcaneum. Int. Orthop., *4*:219, 1980.
495. Pansini, A.: Indicazioni e risultati dell'operazione di Codivilla nel trattamento del piede torto congenito. Minerva Ortop., *16*:158, 1965.
496. Papin, E.: Le Phelps-Kirmisson dans le traitement du pied bot congénital après deux ans. Rev. Orthop., *18*:698, 1931.
497. Parker, R. W.: Congenital clubfoot. The part played by the tarsal ligaments in maintaining the deformity and the value of the subcutaneous section in the cure. Brit. Med. J., *2*:10, 1886.
498. Parker, R. W.: Congenital Club-foot: Its Nature and Treatment. London, H. K., Lewis & Co., 1887.
499. Parker, R. W., and Shattock, S. G.: The pathology and etiology of congenital club-foot. Trans. Path. Soc. London, *35*:423, 1884.
500. Pasila, M., and Sulamaa, M.: Early operation on severe club foot. Nord. Med., *66*:1274, 1961.
501. Paturet, G.: Traité d'Anatomie Humaine. Tome II. Paris, Masson & Cie, 1951.
502. Paulos, L., Coleman, S. S., and Samuelson, K. M.: Pes cavovarus. Review of a surgical approach using selective soft-tissue procedures. J. Bone Joint Surg., *62-A*:942, 1980.
503. Pearocca, A.: Contribution of the therapy of congenital clubfoot. Minerva Ortop., *11*:180, 1960.
504. Penners, R.: Muskelanomalien bei angeborenen Klumpfüssen. Z. Orthop., *83*:103, 1954.
505. Pennino, C.: Late therapy of congenital twisted foot. Arch. Chir. Ortop., *19*:47, 1954.
506. Pérez Lorié, J.: Pié varo equino congénito. Cir. Ortop. Trauma., *3*:39, 1935.
507. Perkins, G.: Orthopaedics. London, The Athlone Press, 1961, p. 585.
508. Perugia, L., and Maffucci, M.: Valutazione elettrodiagnostica dello squilibrio muscolare nel piede torto congenito. Orizz. Ortop. Odierna Riab. *4*:219, 1959.
509. Petri, C.: Congenital club-foot. Ther. Umsch., *28*:309, 1971.
510. Petri, C.: The results of the early treatment of congenital clubfoot. Orthopaede, *8*:159, 1979.
511. Pfeiffer, R. A., Ammermann, M., Baisch, C., and Bollhoff, G.: Das Syndrom von Freeman und Sheldon. 3 neue Beobachtung. Z. Kinderheilk., *112*:43, 1973.
512. Phelps, A. M.: The present status of the open incision method for talipes equinovarus. Med. Res., *38*:22, 1890.
513. Picazo, G.: Pié varus equino congenito. IV Cong. Nacl. Soc. Mex. Ortop. Trauma, 1956, p. 59.
514. Picazo, G.: Algunas consideraciones sobre pié equinovaro

congenito o pié bot. Primeras jornadas Nc. de Ortop. y Trauma., 1961, p. 70.
515. Pierre, M.: Subluxation of clubfoot. Presse Méd., 54:411, 1946.
516. Pillay, V. K., Khong, B. T., and Wolfers, D.: The inheritance of club foot in Singapore. Proc. Third Malaysian Cong. Med., 3:102, 1967.
517. Piskorski, Z.: Failures of conservative management of congenital clubfoot. Chir. Narzad. Ruchu Ortop. Pol., 36:221, 1971.
518. Pitanguy, I., and Bisaggio, S.: À chiro-cheilo-podalic syndrome. Brit. J. Plast. Surg., 22:79, 1969.
519. Pizio, Z.: Internal torsion of the tibia and foot as a component of clubfoot. Chir. Narzad. Ruchu Ortop. Pol., 33:215, 1967.
520. Pompe van Meerdervoort, H. P.: Congenital muscularskeletal disorders in the South African Negro. J. Bone Joint Surg., 59-B:257, 1977.
521. Ponseti, I. V., and Campos, J.: Observations on pathogenesis and treatment of congenital clubfoot. Clin. Orthop., 84:50, 1972.
522. Ponseti, I. V., and Smoley, E. N.: Congenital club foot: The results of treatment. J. Bone Joint Surg., 45-A:261, 1963.
523. Poulain, J.: L'arthrographie tibio-tarsienne dans le pied bot varus équin congénital du premier âge. Thèse pour le Doctorat en Médicine. Paris, Libraire Arnette, 1949.
524. Pous, J. G.: La chirurgie de transplantation tendineuse dans le pied bot varus équin. In Cahiers d'enseignement de la S.O.F.C.O.T. Paris, Expansion Scientifique Française, 1977, p. 87.
525. Pous, J. G., and Dimeglio, A.: La chirurgie néonatale du pied bot varus équin: pourquoi pas? In Cahiers d'enseignement de la S.O.F.C.O.T. Paris, Expansion Scientifique Française, 1977, p. 65.
526. Pous, J. G., and Dimeglio, A.: Neonatal surgery in clubfoot. Orthop. Clin. N. Amer. 9:233, 1978.
527. Preston, E. T., and Fett, T. W., Jr.: Congenital idiopathic clubfoot. Clin. Orthop., 122:102, 1977.
528. Pridie, K. H.: Complications of the treatment of club foot. Proc. South-West Orth. Club (Abstract). J. Bone Joint Surg., 35-B:53, 1952.
529. Primrose, D. A.: Talipes equinovarus in mental defectives. J. Bone Joint Surg., 51-B:60, 1969.
530. Prochiantz, A.: La fonction et la forme, double préoccupation du traitement du pied bot varus équin. Ann. Chir. Infant. (Paris), 16:211, 1975.
531. Proppe, P.: Häufigkeit des angeborenen Klumpfusses und der angeborenen Hüftluxation. Z. Orthop., 42:308, 1922.
532. Pyka, R. A., and Coventry, M. B.: Avascular necrosis of the skin after operation on the foot. J. Bone Joint Surg., 43-A:955, 1961.
533. Rabl, C. R. H.: Herunterholen der Klumpfuss-Ferse ohne Tenotomie. Z. Orthop., 82:599, 1952.
534. Rabl, C. R.: Zur Methode der Klumpfussbehandlung. Beitr. Orthop. Trauma., 15:125, 1968.
535. Radke, J., and Janssen, R.: Clinical aspects and therapy of congenital clubfoot. Med. Mschr., 28:293, 1974.
536. Ranieri, L.: Patogenesi e terapia del piede torto congenito. Ar. Organi Mov., 52:64, 1963.
537. Raynal, L., and Judet, J.: Traitement de pied bot varus équin congénital de l'âge de deux à cinq ans. Acta Orthop. Belg., 33:867, 1967.
538. Raynal, L., Judet, J., and Judet, R.: Traitement du pied bot varus équin congénital de l'âge de deux à cinq ans. Acta Orthop. Belg., 25:479, 1959.
539. Reimann, I.: Congenital idiopathic club foot. Thesis. Copenhagen, Munsgaard, 1967.
540. Reimann, I., and Lyquist, E.: Dynamic splint used in the treatment of clubfoot. Acta Orthop. Scand., 40:817, 1970.
541. Reimann, I., and Becker-Andersen, H.: Early surgical treatment of congenital clubfoot. Clin. Orthop., 102:200, 1974.
542. Reimann, I., and Werner, H. H.: Congenital metatarsus varus. Acta Orthop. Scand., 46:857, 1975.
543. Repetto, P.: Early surgery of congenital clubfoot in the first two years of life. Minerva Nipiol. 6:72, 1956.
544. Resnick, D.: Radiology of the talocalcaneal articulations. Radiology, 111:581, 1974.
545. Richards, R. M.: The Möbius syndrome. J. Bone Joint Surg., 41-A:473, 1953.
546. Rigault, P.: Résultats du traitement des pieds bots varus équins congénitaux rebelles ou récidives per allongement ou section des parties molles avec correction de la malposition osseuse. Acta Orthop. Belg., 33:883, 1967.
547. Rintala, A.: Freeman-Sheldon's syndrome. Cranio-carpotarsal dystrophy. Acta Paediat. Scand., 57:553, 1968.
548. Ritsila, V. A.: Talipes equinovarus and vertical talus produced experimentally in newborn rabbits. Acta Orthop. Scand., Suppl. 121, 1969.
549. Roberts, J. M.: Personal communication, 1980.
549a. Roberts, J. M.: Personal communication, 1982.
550. Roetzer, K.: Nachuntersuchungsergebnisse von im kindlichen und jugendlichen alter keilosteotomierten Klumpfüssen. Verh. Deutsch. Orthop. Ges. 36 Kong. (1947) Beil. Z. Orthop., 78:216, 1948.
551. Rogala, E. J., Wynne-Davies, R., Littlejon, A., and Gormley, J.: Congenital limb anomalies: Frequency and aetiological factors. Data from the Edinburgh Register of the Newborn (1964–68). J. Med. Genet. 11:221, 1974.
552. Romanini, L., and Mollica, Q.: I trattamento del piede torto congenito nella storia della medicina. Orizz. Ortop. Odierna Riab., 5:183, 1960.
553. Roper, A.: A simple and effective method of treatment of congenital clubfoot. Cent. Afr. J. Med., 13:226, 1967.
554. Rosa, G.: Deformita del piede da esostosi solitaria dell'astragalo. Orizz. Ortop. Odierna Riab., 8:103, 1963.
555. Rubin, A., and Friedenberg, Z. B.: Clubfoot (talipes). In Rubin A. (ed.): Handbook of Congenital Malformations. Philadelphia, W. B. Saunders Co., 1969, Chapter 5.
556. Rydell, N. W., and Magnusson, A.: A new brace for the treatment of congenital clubfoot. Acta Orthop. Scand., 41:501, 1970.
557. Sahlstedt, B.: Simultaneous arthrography of the talocrural and talonavicular joints in children. I. Technique. (Part II. see Hjelmstedt. A.). Acta Radiol. [Diagn.] (Stockholm), 17:545, 1976.
558. Salle, B., Picot, C., Vauzelle, J. L., Deffrenne, P., Mounet, P., Francois, R., and Robert, J. M.: Le nanisme diastrophique. A propos de trois observations chez le nouveau-né. Pediatrie, 21:311, 1966.
559. Salter, R. B.: Present trends in treatment of club feet. A.A.O.S. Instr. Course Lect. Sound-Slide Program, 1965, No. 7.
560. Salter, R., and Field, P.: The effects of continuous compression on living articular cartilage. J. Bone Joint Surg., 42-A:31, 1960.
561. Salzer, M., and Schwagerl, W.: Die operative Klumpfussbehandlung mit Transfixation des Ruckfusses. Z. Orthop., 106:368, 1969.
562. Savini, R., and Gualdrini, G.: Report on two cases of Freeman-Sheldon syndrome ("whistling face"). Ital. J. Orthop. Trauma., 6:105, 1980.
563. Say, B., Barber, D. H., Thompson, R. C., and Leichtman, L. G.: The Gordon syndrome (letter). J. Med. Genet., 17:405, 1980.
564. Sayre, L. E.: Practical Manual of the Treatment of Clubfoot. New York, Appleton & Co., 1869.
565. Scaglietti, O.: Studio clinico statistico sui casi piede torto congenito oservati all'Instituto Orthopedico Rizzoli dal 1899 al 1933. Chir. Organi Mov., 19:325, 1934.
566. Scaglietti, O.: Considerazioni sulla patogenesi del piede torto congenito. Chir. Organi Mov., 20:25, 1935.
567. Scarlini, G.: Sulla cura del piede torto congenito. Arch. Ital. Chir., 13:726, 1925.
568. Scarpa, A.: Memoria chirugica sui piedi torti congeniti dei fanciulli e sulla maniera di corregger questa deformita. 2nd Ed. Pavia, B. Comino, 1806.
569. Scarpa, A.: A Memoir on the Congenital Club Foot in Children. Translated from Italian by J. W. Wishart. Edinburgh. Constable & Co., 1818.
570. Scheel, P. F.: Beobachtungen bei der Behandlung des kongenitalen Klumpfusses. Z. Orthop., 79:546, 1950.
571. Scheel, P. F.: Fehlerquellen in der operativen Behandlung des Säuglingsklumpfusses. Z. Orthop., 90:343, 1958.
572. Scher. M. A., Handelsman, J. E., and Isaacs, H.: The effect on muscle of immobilization under tension and relaxation. J. Bone Joint Surg., 59-B:257, 1977.
573. Scherb, R.: Zur Ätiologie kongenitaler und Kongenitalbedingter. Fussdeformitäten mit besonderer Berucksichtingung des Pes equino-varus congenitus. Acta Chir. Scand., 67:717, 1930.
574. Scherrer, H., Mumzinger, U., Wiasminitov, M., and

Huber, B.: 10-year-results of club foot therapy (Author's transl.) Orthopaede, 8:151, 1979.
575. Schlicht, D.: The pathologic anatomy of talipes equinovarus. Aust. New Zeal. J. Surg., 33:2, 1963.
576. Scholder, P.: Surgical treatment of congenital clubfoot. Ther. Umsch., 28:315, 1971.
577. Schomburg, H.: Untersuchung der Entwicklung der Muskein und Knochen des Menschlichen Fusses an Serienschnitten und Rekonstruktionen und unter Zuhulfenahme Makrosko-pischer Präparation. Göttingen, Kaestner, 1900.
578. Schulze, H.: Korrekturschiene zur Behandlung eines veralteten angeborenen Klumpfusses und der Innenrotation eines Hüftgelenkes. Beitr. Orthop. Trauma., 18:479, 1971.
579. Schutze, C.: A plastic splint for the treatment of clubfoot in newborn infants. Beitr. Orthop. Trauma, 19:55, 1972.
580. Scolari, F.: Considerazioni sulla cura del piede torto congenito. Arch. Ortop., 62:235, 1949.
581. Scudder, C. L.: Congenital talipes equinovarus. Boston Med. Surg. J., 117:397, 1887.
582. Sell, L. S.: The conservative treatment of congenital clubfeet in infants. Southern Med. J., 32:1199, 1939.
583. Sell, L. S.: Tibial torsion accompanying congenital clubfoot. J. Bone Joint Surg., 23:561, 1941.
584. Semb. H. T.: The treatment of club-foot and its results. Acta Orthop. Scand., 34:271, 1964.
585. Seringe, R.: Anatomie pathologique et physiopathologie du pied bot varus équin congénital. In Cahiers d'enseignement de la S.O.F.C.O.T. Paris, Expansion Scientifique Française, 1977, p. 11.
586. Seringe, R.: Etude clinique et radiologique de pied bot varus équin congénital. In Cahiers d'enseignement de la S.O.F.C.O.T. Paris, Expansion Scientifique Française, 1977, p. 25.
587. Seringe, R.: Traitement du pied bot varus équin congénital chez l'enfant. In Cahiers d'enseignement de la S.O.F.C.O.T. Paris, Expansion Scientifique Française, 1977, p. 57.
588. Settle, G. W.: The anatomy of congenital talipes equinovarus: Sixteen dissected specimens. J. Bone Joint Surg., 45-A:1341, 1963.
589. Shaffer, N. M.: The classic non-deforming club-foot. With remarks on its pathology. Med. Rec., 27:561, 1885; reprinted in Clin. Orthop., 125:2, 1977.
590. Shapiro, F., and Glimcher J. J.: Gross and histological abnormalities of the talus in congenital clubfoot. J. Bone Joint Surg., 61-A:522, 1979.
591. Sharrard, W. J. W., and Grosfield, I.: The management of deformity and paralysis of the foot in myelomeningocele. J. Bone Joint Surg., 50-B:456, 1968.
592. Shaw, N. E.: The primary treatment of congenital talipes equinovarus. Proc. 11th Annual Meeting Brit. Assoc. Paediat. Surg., 1964 (Abstract). Arch. Dis. Child., 40:230, 1965.
593. Shaw, N. E.: Comparison of three methods for treatment of congenital clubfoot. Brit. Med. J., 1:1084, 1966.
594. Shaw, N. E.: The early management of clubfoot. Clin. Orthop., 84:39, 1972.
595. Sherman, F. C., and Westin, G. W.: Plantar release in the correction of deformities of the foot in childhood. J. Bone Joint Surg., 63-A:1382, 1981.
596. Shneider, D. A., and Smith, C. F.: Medial subtalar stabilization with posterior medial release in the treatment of varus feet: A preliminary report. Orthop. Clin. N. Amer. 7:949, 1976.
597. Shoro, A. A.: Club-foot and intra-uterine growth retardation produced by tubocurarine chloride in the rat fetus. J. Anat., 111:506, 1972.
598. Siegel, M. I.: Letters: Reply to "comparative anatomy of the talus in relation to idiopathic club foot." Clin. Orthop., 0:268, 1974.
599. Simons, G. W.: The role of the talo-navicular joint in club foot. Personal communication, 1980.
600. Simons, G. W.: Club feet. Part I. Rotational deformities in club feet. Personal communication, 1977.
601. Simons, G. W.: Analytical radiography of clubfeet. J. Bone Joint Surg., 59-B:485, 1977.
602. Simons, G. W.: A standardized method for the radiographic evaluation of clubfeet. Clin. Orthop., 135:107–118, 1978.
603. Simons, G. W., and Tachdjian, M. O.: Treatment of clubfeet from birth to two years of age. In Cahiers d'enseignement de la S.O.F.C.O.T. Paris, Expansion Scientifique Française, 1977. p. 31.
603a. Simons, G. W., and Sarrafian, S.: The microsurgical dissection of a stillborn fetal clubfoot. Clin. Orthop., 173:275, 1983.
604. Singer, M.: Tibialis posterior transfer in congenital club foot. J. Bone Joint Surg., 43-B:717, 1961.
605. Singer, M., and Fripp, A. T.: Tibialis anterior transfer in congenital club foot. J. Bone Joint Surg., 40-B:252, 1958.
606. Slavik, J.: The clubfoot and its occurrence. Acta Chir. Orthop. Traum. Cech., 34:74, 1967.
607. Slavik, J.: Congenital idiopathic equinovarus as a therapeutic problem. Cesk. Pediat., 21:807, 1968.
608. Smith, D. W.: Recognizable Patterns of Human Malformation. 2nd Ed. Philadelphia, W. B. Saunders Co., 1976.
609. Smith, W. A., Jr., Campbell, P., and Bonnett, C.: Early posterior ankle release in the treatment of congenital clubfoot. Orthop. Clin. N. Amer., 7:889, 1976.
610. Sofield, H. A.: Elastic traction assisting correction of club feet. J. Bone Joint Surg., 13:283, 1931.
611. Soifer, H., and Palew, P.: Proper use of the Denis Browne splint. J. Pediat., 61:648, 1962.
612. Solomon, L., and Handelsman, J. E.: The treatment of club-foot. S. Afr. J. Surg., 5:31, 1967.
613. Solonen, K. A., and Parkkulainen, K. V.: Congenital clubfoot, results of treatment. Ann. Chir. Gynaec. Fenn. (Helsinki), 48:130, 1958.
614. Somppi, E., and Sulamaa, M.: Early operative treatment of congenital club foot. Acta Orthop. Scand., 42:513, 1971.
615. Sonnenschein, A.: Blutige oder unblutige Klumpfuss Behandlung? Acta Orthop. Scand., 18:266, 1949.
616. Sostegni, A., and Paleari, L: Il trattamento precoce chirurgico del piede torto congenito e i suoi risultati a distanza. Arch. Ortop., 62:225, 1949.
617. Sotirow, B.: Congenital club foot, Pathomechanism and treatment. Chir. Narzad. Ruchu Ortop. Pol., 38:337, 1973.
618. Spotorno, A.: Stabilization of congenital equinovarus following surgical and non-surgical therapy by means of transplantation of anterior tibial onto fifth metatarsal. Arch. Ortop., 63:98, 1950.
619. Steel, H. H.: Computerized axial tomography (C-T scan) in assessment of correction of talipes equinovarus. Personal communication; paper read at Sixth Pediatric Orthopedic International Seminar, San Francisco, 1978.
620. Steel, H. H., and Kohl, J.: Multiple congenital dislocations associated with other skeletal anomalies (Larsen's syndrome) in three siblings. J. Bone Joint Surg., 54-A:75, 1972.
621. Steindler, A.: Stripping of the os calcis. J. Orthop. Surg., 2:8, 1920.
622. Steindler, A.: Orthopedic Operations, Indications, Techniques and End Results. Springfield, Ill., Charles C Thomas, 1940.
623. Steindler, A.: Post-Graduate Lectures on Orthopedic Diagnosis and Indications. Springfield, Ill., Charles C Thomas, 1950, Vol. I, pp. 178–196.
624. Stewart, S. F.: Club-foot: Its incidence, cause and treatment. Anatomical-physiological study. J. Bone Joint Surg., 33-A:577, 1951.
625. Steyler, J. C. A., and Van Der Walt, I. D.: Correction of resistant adduction of the forefoot in congenital clubfoot and congenital metatarsus varus by metatarsal osteotomy. Brit. J. Surg., 53:558, 1966.
626. Støren, H.: Operative treatment of club foot in older children and adults. Acta Orthop. Scand., 18:233, 1949.
627. Stover, C. N., Hayes, J. T., and Holt, J. F.: Diastrophic dwarfism. Amer. J. Roentgen., 89:914, 1963.
628. Sutherland, A. D.: Equinus deformity due to haemangioma of calf muscle. J. Bone Joint Surg., 57-B:104, 1975.
629. Swann, M., Lloyd-Roberts, G. C., and Catterall, A.: The anatomy of uncorrected clubfeet. A study of rotation deformity. J. Bone Joint Surg., 51-B:263, 1969.
630. Taylor, H. L.: Treatment of club foot by leverage. Trans. Amer. Orthop. Assoc., 5:178, 1892.
631. Tayton, K., and Thompson, P.: Relapsing club feet. Late results of delayed operation. J. Bone Joint Surg., 61-B:474, 1979.

632. Templeton, A. W., McAlister, W. H., and Zim, I. D.: Standardization of terminology and evaluation of osseous relationships in congenitally abnormal feet. Amer. J. Roentgen., *93*:374, 1965.
633. Terry, R. J.: Sprengel's deformity and clubfoot: An anthropological interpretation. Amer. J. Phys. Anthrop., *17*:251, 1959.
634. Thompson, G. H., Richardson, A. B., and Westin, G. W.: Surgical management of resistant congenital talipes equinovarus deformities. J. Bone Joint Surg., *64-A*:652, 1982.
635. Thompson, T. C.: Astragalectomy and the treatment of calcaneovalgus. J. Bone Joint Surg., *21*:637, 1939.
636. Thomson, S. A.: Treatment of congenital talipes equinovarus with a modification of the Denis Browne method and splint. J. Bone Joint Surg., *24*:291, 1942.
637. Thomson, S. A.: A splint treatment of recurrent club-foot. J. Bone Joint Surg., *28*:778, 1946.
638. Thomson, S. A.: The treatment of congenital club-foot. Nine years' experience with a modification of the Denis Browne method and splint. J. Bone Joint Surg., *31-A*:431, 1949.
639. Thomson, S. A.: Modified Denis Browne splint for unilateral club-foot to protect the normal foot. J. Bone Joint Surg., *37-A*:1286, 1955.
640. Thyes, A.: Le traitement du pied bot varus équin congénital par la méthode de Scheib. Acta Orthop. Belg., *13*:299, 1947.
641. Tokarowski, A.: Osteotomoclasis for tibial detorsion in the treatment of congenital club-foot. Chir. Narzad. Ruchu Ortop. Pol., *38*:173, 1977.
642. Tompkins, S. F.: Millers, R. J., and O'Donoghue, D. H.: An evolution of astragalectomy. Southern Med. J., *49*:1128, 1956.
643. Tönnis, D., and Bikadorov, V.: Untersuchungen über die Ergebnisse verschiedener Behandlungsmethoden bei angeborenen Klumpfuss. Z. Orthop., *104*:218, 1968.
644. Torpin, R.: Fetal Malformations: Caused by Amnion Rupture During Gestation. Springfield, Ill., Charles C Thomas, 1968.
645. Torpin, R., Miller, G. T., Jr., and Culpepper, B. W.: Amniogenic fetal amputations associated with clubfoot. Obstet. Gynec., *24*:59, 1964.
646. del Torto, V.: Arthrodesis for verticalization of astragalus in pes equinus. Rif. Med., *66*:1128, 1952.
647. Treister, M. R.: Letter to the editor. Clin. Orthop., *108*:279, 1975.
648. Treves, A.: Traitement du pied bot varus équin congénital. Rev. Orthop., *18*:393, 1931.
649. Treves, A.: Traitement du pied bot varus équin congénital après deux ans. Rev. Orthop., *18*:695, 1931.
650. Trias, A.: Effect of persistent pressure on articular cartilage. J. Bone Joint Surg., *43-B*:376, 1961.
651. Tripathi, R. P., and Chaturvedi, S. N.: Treatment of clubfoot by one stage medial soft tissue release operation. J. Indian Med. Assoc., *16*:73, 1979.
652. Truscelli, D., Lespargot, A., and Tardieu, G.: Variation in the long-term results of elongation of the tendo Achillis in children with cerebral palsy. J. Bone Joint Surg., *61-B*:466, 1979.
653. Turco, V. J.: Surgical corrections of the resistant congenital club-foot-one-stage release with internal fixation. A.A.O.S. Film Library, Chicago, Ill.
654. Turco, V. J.: Surgical correction of the resistant club foot. One-stage posteromedial release with internal fixation: A preliminary report. J. Bone Joint Surg., *53-A*:477, 1971.
655. Turco, V. J.: Resistant congenital clubfoot. A.A.O.S. Instr. Course Lect., *24*:104–121, 1975.
656. Turco, V. J.: Resistant congenital club foot — one-stage posteromedial release with internal fixation. A follow-up report of a fifteen-year experience. J. Bone Joint Surg., *61-A*:805, 1979.
656a. Turco, V. J.: Clubfoot. *In* Current Problems in Orthopaedics. New York, Churchill-Livingstone, 1981.
657. Turcu, G.: Congenital talipes equinovarus in infants less than 1 year of age. Clinical and laboratory studies. Rev. Med. Chir. Soc. Med. Nat. IASI, *78*:25, 1974.
658. Turcu, G.: Role and value of the footprint in evaluation of development of congenital talipes equinovarus. Rev. Chir., *24*:65, 1975.
659. Turek, S. L.: Orthopedics — Principles and Their Application. 2nd Ed. Philadelphia, J. B. Lippincott Co., 1967.
660. Turner, J. W., and Cooper, R. R.: Anterior transfer of the tibialis posterior through the interosseous membrane. Clin. Orthop., *83*:241, 1972.
661. Valentin, Zucchi Nino: La immovilización enyesada, su tecnica y sus aplicaciones. La immovilizacion del pié equino varo congenito. Buenos Aires, Editorial El Ateneo, 1945, pp. 443–462.
662. Veale, A. M. O.: Polygenic inheritance. New Zeal. Med. J., *67*:344, 1968.
663. Veale, A. M. O., Tapsel, P. W., and Tyler, K. R.: Club foot in Maoris. *In* Proceedings, Third International Congress of Human Genetics, 1966, p. 102.
664. Velasco, A., and Diaz, E.: Pié bot (estudio de 50 casos). An. Orthop. Trauma., *2*:115, 1952.
665. Velasco Polo, G., de, and Ponchener-Lechtman, C.: Surgical treatment of congenital talipes equinovarus adductus. Clin. Orthop., *70*:87, 1970.
666. Vereanu, D., Socolesco, M., and Georgesco, P.: Le traitement chirurgical du pied bot congénital varus-équin par libération des voutes plantaires. *In* Delchef J., (ed.): Orthopaedic Surgery and Traumatology. Congenital clubfoot. a. Anatomy and pathology of the disease. New York, American Elsevier Publishing Co., 1973, pp. 751–752.
667. Vesely, D. G.: A method of application of a clubfoot cast. Clin. Orthop., *84*:47, 1972.
668. Vigliani, F.: Codivilla's operation after seventy years. Ital. J. Orthop. Trauma., *1*:297, 1975.
669. Vilenskii, V. Ia.: Polymeric devices in early conservative treatment of congenital clubfoot (modification of method of therapy). Ortop. Travm. Protez., *34*:24, 1973.
670. Vladimirova, N. A.: Physical therapeutic factors in the complex treatment of congenital clubfoot in radical reconstructive surgery. Ortop. Traum. Protez., *34*:72, 1973.
671. Wagner, L. C., and Butterfield, W. L.: Surgical release of contracted tissues for resistant congenital clubfoot. Amer. J. Surg., *84*:82, 1952.
672. Wahren, H.: Über die Korrektur der Tibiatorsion bei kongenitalen Klumpfuss. Acta Chir. Scand., *67*:928, 1930.
673. Waisbrod, H.: Congenital club foot. An anatomical study. J. Bone Joint Surg., *55-B*:796, 1973.
674. Waisbrod, H.: High medial release operation for resistant clubfoot. Israel J. Med. Sci., *16*:444, 1980.
675. Walker, B. A., Scott, C. I., Hall, J. G., Murdoch, J. L., and McKusick, V. A.: Diastrophic dwarfism. Medicine (Balt.), *51*:41, 1972.
676. Walsham, W. J., and Hughes, W. K.: Treatment of talipes equinus. *In* The Deformities of the Human Foot. London, Bailliere, Tindall & Cox, 1895, Chapter VII, pp. 294–320.
677. Warkany, J.: Clubfoot (talipes equinovarus). *In* Congenital Malformations. Chicago, Year Book Medical Publishers Inc., 1971, pp. 1004–1010.
678. Watkins, M., Jones, J. B., Ryder, C. T., and Brown, T. H.: Transplantation of the posterior tibial tendon. J. Bone Joint Surg., *36-A*:1181, 1964.
679. Watts, A. W.: Anterior transplantation of tibialis posterior tendon. Aust. New Zeal. J. Surg., *34*:284, 1965.
680. Weickert, H.: Ergebnisse konservativer und operativer Klumpfussbehandlung. Beitr. Orthop. Trauma., *15*:753, 1968.
681. Weickert, H., and Stein, V.: Principles of treatment of congenital clubfoot and analysis of results. Beitr. Orthop. Trauma., *26*:409, 1979.
682. Weinberg, H.: Congenital clubfoot. J. Bone Joint Surg., *45-B*:807, 1963.
683. Weinberg, H., and Halmosh, A. F.: Emotional maladjustment in the surgical correction of long-standing deformity. J. Bone Joint Surg., *41-A*:1310, 1959.
684. Weinstein, S., and Gorlin, R. J.: Cranio-carpo-tarsal dysplasia or the whistling face syndrome. Amer. J. Dis. Child., *117*:427, 1969.
685. Weseley, M. S., and Barenfeld, P. A.: Operative treatment of congenital clubfoot. Clin. Orthop., *59*:161, 1968.
686. Weseley, M. S., and Barenfeld, P. A.: Calcaneal osteotomy for the treatment of cavus deformity. Bull. Hosp. Joint Dis., *31*:93, 1970.
687. Weseley, M. S., and Barenfeld, P. A.: Mechanism of the Dwyer calcaneal osteotomy. Clin. Orthop., *70*:137, 1970.
688. Weseley, M. S., and Barenfeld, P. A.: Hard tissue correction of congenital clubfoot. Orthop. Rev., *5*:19, 1976.

689. Weseley, M. S., Barenfeld, P. A., and Barrett, N.: Complications of the treatment of clubfoot. Clin. Orthop., 84:93, 1972.
690. Westin, G. W.: Plantar release in talipes equinovarus. Personal communication, 1975.
691. White, J. W.: The importance of the tibials in the production and recurrence of clubfoot. Southern Med. J. 22:675, 1929.
692. White, J. W., and Gulledge, W. H.: Skin-tight casts for treatment of club-foot. J. Bone Joint Surg., 33-A:475, 1951.
693. Whitman, A.: The Whitman operation as applied to various types of paralytic deformities of the foot. Results in the average cases. Med. Rec., 4:266, 1922.
694. Whitman, A.: Astragalectomy and backward displacement of the foot. An investigation of its practical results. J. Bone Joint Surg., 4:266, 1922.
695. Whitman, A.: Astragalectomy. Ultimate results. Amer. J. Surg., 11:357, 1931.
696. Whitman, R.: The operative treatment of paralytic talipes of the calcaneus type. Amer. J. Med. Sci., 192:593, 1901.
697. Whitman, R.: Further observation on the treatment of paralytic talipes of the calcaneus by astragalectomy and backward displacement of the foot. Ann. Surg., 47:264, 1908.
698. Whitman, R.: Further observation on the treatment of paralytic talipes, calcaneus and allied distortions. Med. Rec., 81:47, 1914.
699. Wiberg, G.: Tiding behandling av den kongenitala Klumfoten. Nord. Med., 8:2660, 1940.
700. Wickstrom, J., and Williams, R. A.: Shoe corrections and orthopaedic foot supports. Clin. Orthop., 70:30, 1970.
701. Widolf, G. A.: Congenital clubfoot — a better splint for conservative treatment. Med. J. Aust., 1:846, 1973.
702. Wiedemann, H. R., and Dibbern, H.: Larsen's syndrome. Med. Welt., 24:1548, 1980.
703. Wiley, A. M.: Club foot. An anatomical and experimental study of muscle growth. J. Bone Joint Surg., 41-B:821, 1959.
704. Wilhelm, R.: Mangelhafte Entwicklung des os naviculare beim angeborenen Klumpfuss. Fortschr. Roentgenstr., 35:735, 1927.
705. Williams, P.: Principles in treatment of talipes equinovarus. Personal communication: Paper presented at Sixth Pediatric Orthopedic Seminar. San Francisco, 1978.
706. Wiltse, L. L., and Bateman, J. G.: Removing plaster from clubfeet. Clin. Orthop., 103:63, 1974.
707. Wisbrun, W.: Neue Gesichtspunkte zum Redressement des angeborenen Klumpfusses und daraus sich ergebende Schlussfolgerungen dezuglich der Atiologie. Arch. Orthop. Unfallchir., 31:451, 1932.
708. Wolff, J.: Ueber die Ursachen, das Wesen und die Behandlung das Klumpfusses. Berlin, August Hirschwald, 1903.
709. Wolff, J. R., and Tönnis, D.: Elektronenmikroskopische Untersuchungen der Muskulatur bei angeborenen Klumpfuss und angeborener Huftluxation. Arch. Orthop. Unfallchir., 68:95, 1970.
710. Wolff, L. V.: The development of the human foot as an organ of locomotion. Amer. J. Dis. Child., 37:1212, 1929.
711. Wood-Jones, F.: Structure and Function as Seen in the Foot. Baltimore, Williams & Wilkins Co., 1944, pp. 133–135.
712. Wynne-Davies, R.: Family studies and cause of congenital clubfoot. J. Bone Joint Surg., 46-B:445, 1964.
713. Wynne-Davies, R.: Talipes equinovarus. A review of eighty-four cases after completion of treatment. J. Bone Joint Surg., 46-B:464, 1964.
714. Wynne-Davies, R.: Family studies and aetiology of clubfoot. J. Med. Genet. 2:227, 1965.
715. Wynne-Davies, R.: The genetics of some common congenital malformations. In Emery, A. (ed.): Modern Trends in Human Genetics. London, Butterworths, 1970, Chapter 11.
716. Wynne-Davies, R.: Genetic and environmental factors in the etiology of talipes equinovarus. Clin. Orthop., 84:9, 1972.
717. Wynne-Davies, R.: Heritable Disorders in Orthopaedic Practice. Oxford, London, Edinburgh, Melbourne, Blackwell Scientific Publications, 1973, p. 206.
718. Wynne-Davies, R.: A review of genetics in orthopaedics. Acta Orthop. Scand., 46:338, 1975.
719. Young, A. B.: Club foot treated by astragalectomy. 50-year follow-up of a case. Lancet, 1:670, 1962.
720. Zadek, I., and Barnett, E. I.: The importance of the ligaments of the ankle in correction of congenital clubfoot. J.A.M.A., 69:1057, 1917.
721. Zatsepin, T. S.: Operation on tendinoligamentous apparatus in congenital clubfoot in children. Khirurgia, No. 11:59, 1944.
722. Zenker, H.: Ossare Klumpfussbehandlung beim Kleinkind. Arch. Orthop. Unfalchir., 68:255, 1970.
723. Zerbi, E.: Sulla cura del piede torto congenito. Minerva Ortop., 9:1, 1958.
724. Zergollern, J.: Biochemical basis for the need of surgical treatment of pes equinovarus congenitus in resistant cases. Acta Med. Iugosl., 25:91, 1971.
725. Zergollern, J.: Importance of early treatment of pes equinovarus congenitus. Liječ. Vjesn. 93:543, 1971.
726. Zimbler, S.: Practical considerations in the early treatment of congenital talipes equinovarus. Orthop. Clin. N. Amer. 3:257, 1972.
727. Zimmer, J.: Das Geschlechtsverhaltnis beim angeborenen Klumpfuss. Z. Orthop. Chir., 69:126, 1939.
728. Zippel, H., and Gummel, J.: Surgical treatment of crus varum congenitum and congenital pseudoarthrosis of the lower leg. Beitr. Orthop. Trauma., 20:193, 1973.

CONGENITAL CONVEX PES VALGUS

Congenital convex pes valgus is a primary dorsal and lateral dislocation of the talocalcaneonavicular joint, developing in utero at some time during the first trimester of pregnancy. The navicular bone articulates with the dorsal aspect of the talus, locking it in a plantar-flexed vertical position. The deformity is commonly referred to as congenital vertical talus or simply vertical talus—a usage to be discouraged, as it focuses attention upon only one facet of this severe deformity.[57]

The condition was first described by Henken in 1914.[37] Its characteristic features were reviewed by Lamy and Weissman, who also presented a comprehensive study of the literature up to 1939.[48]

The entity is known by various synonyms. Originally, it was called congenital flatfoot due to vertical talus (pied plat congénital par subluxation sous-astragalienne congénitale et orientation vertical de l'astragale) by Rocher and Pouyanne.[65] "Congenital rocker-bottom flatfoot"; "rocker-foot due to congenital subluxation of the talus"; and "rocker-foot, or congenital flatfoot, due to talonavicular dislocation" are other names given the condition. The term *congenital convex pes valgus* was initially proposed by Lamy and Weissman, and later adopted in preference to others by Heyman and Herndon.[33]

Teratologic dorsolateral dislocation of the talo-

calcaneonavicular joint is a more accurate name because it directs attention to the pathogenesis and therapeutic implications.

The condition may occur as an isolated primary deformity or it may occur in association with abnormalities of the central nervous and musculoskeletal systems. Sharrard and Grosfield found the incidence of congenital convex pes valgus to be 10 per cent in a large series of patients with myelomeningocele who had foot deformities.[68] Drennan and Sharrard proposed that a neuromuscular imbalance, i.e., a weak posterior tibial muscle and strong evertors of the foot, is responsible for the development of congenital convex pes valgus in myelomeningocele. They also noted the high incidence of abnormalities of the central nervous system in the reported cases of congenital vertical talus, and emphasized the importance of ruling out such associated anomalies prior to accepting the condition as an isolated primary deformity.[20] Arthrogryposis multiplex congenita, talipes equinovarus, pollex varus, dislocation of the hip, and neurofibromatosis are some of the neuromusculoskeletal abnormalities associated with it, and it may also be one of the numerous anomalies associated with autosomal trisomy, occurring with both trisomy 13–15 and trisomy 18.[77,78] It is common with ischiocalcaneal bands.

The cause of the primary isolated form in unknown. Campos da Paz, Jr., and his associates proposed that congenital convex pes valgus probably is the result of an arrest of prenatal development of the foot.[11] At the seventh week of pregnancy the foot is in dorsiflexion, and the calcaneus is in close proximity to the lateral malleolus; in the twelfth week of pregnancy it moves away from the fibula to lie under the talus (Fig. 2–48).[82] The posture of the foot and leg is dependent upon consecutive development of muscle function and muscular dominance.[83] The structural development of the central and peripheral nervous systems proceeds in a craniocaudal direction, and coordinated muscle contractions appear in the different muscle groups in a sequence corresponding to their anatomic level of innervation. Therefore, as the fourth and fifth

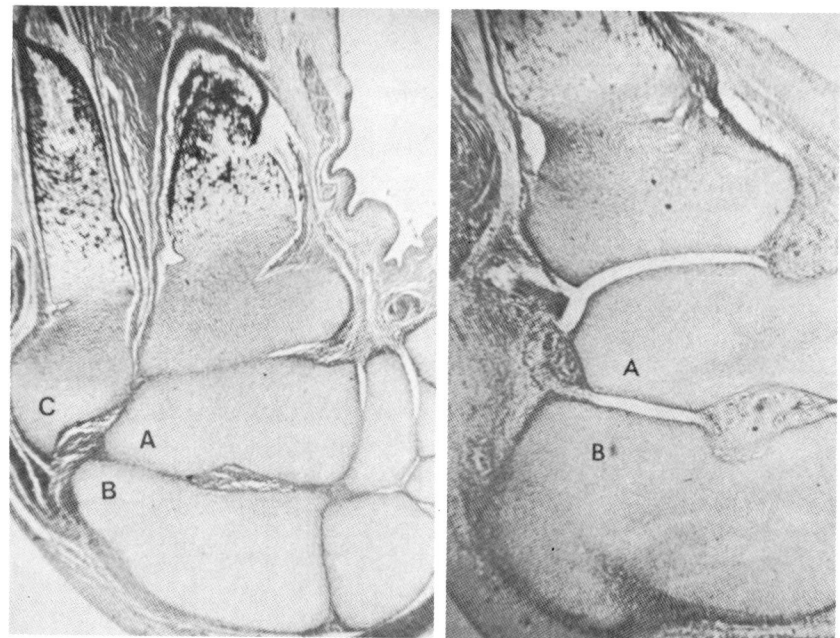

FIGURE 2–48. The relationship of the tarsal bones during development of a normal fetus.

A. At the seventh week of pregnancy, the ossification of the tarsal bones and distal fibula and tibia has commenced. Note the dorsiflexed posture of the foot and the close proximity of the calcaneus (B) to the distal end of the fibula (C). **B.** At the twelfth week of pregnancy, the calcaneus (B) has moved to lie under the talus (A) and away from the fibular malleolus. (From Campos da Paz, A., Jr., de Souza, V., and Conceicao de Souza, D.: Congenital convex pes valgus. Orthop. Clin. N. Amer., 9:207, 1978. Reprinted by permission.)

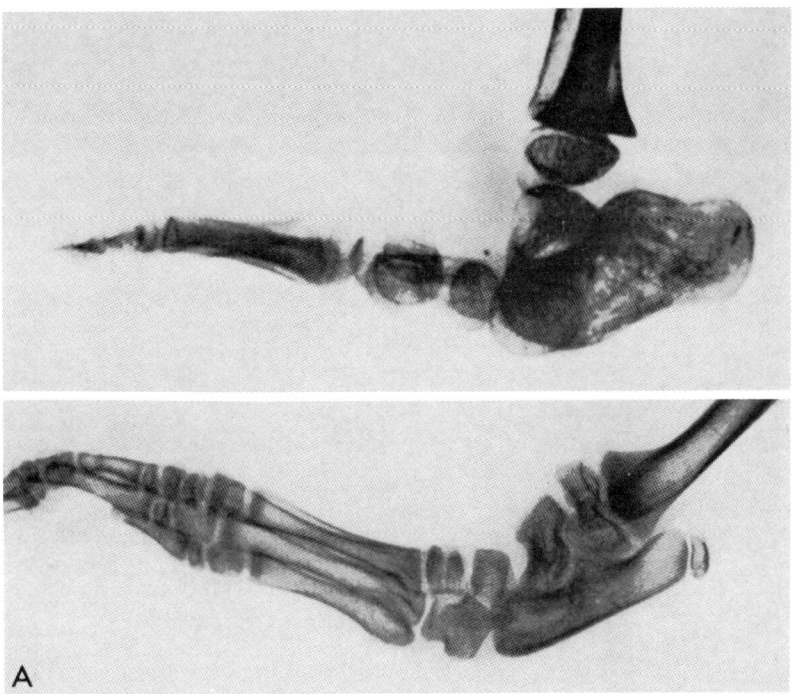

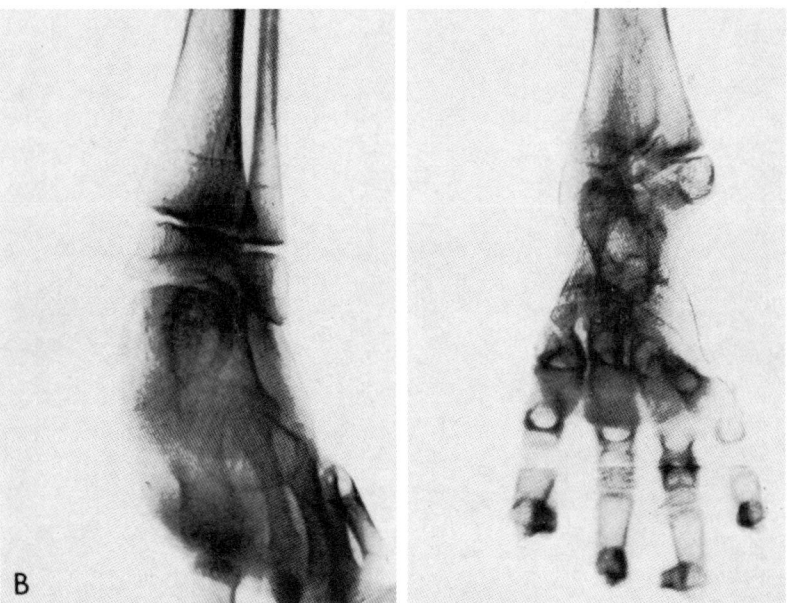

FIGURE 2–49. Congenital convex pes valgus of the "anterior tibial" type.

A. The deformity as seen in lateral roentgenograms in a child *(top)* and in a rabbit *(bottom)*. **B.** Anteroposterior roentgenograms of the deformity in a child *(left)* and in a rabbit *(right)*. (From Ritsila, V. A.: Talipes equinovarus and vertical talus produced experimentally in newborn rabbits. Acta Orthop. Scand., Suppl. 121, 1969, p. 54. Reprinted by permission.)

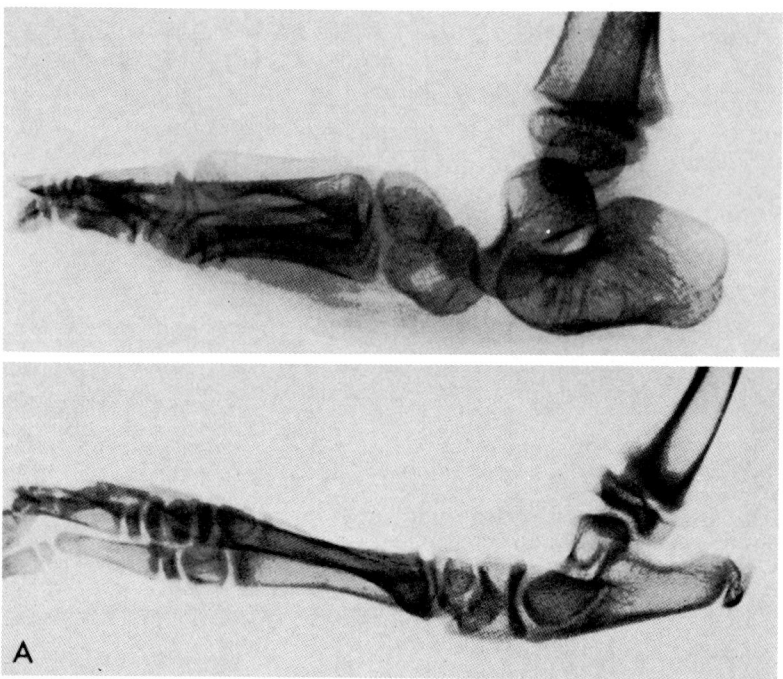

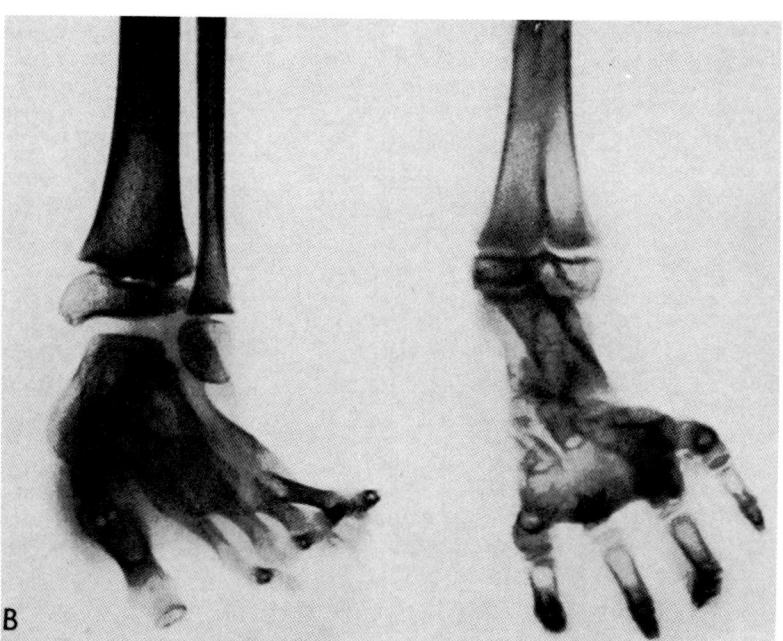

FIGURE 2–50. Congenital convex pes valgus of the "extensor digitorum" type.

A. The deformity as seen in lateral roentgenograms in a child *(top)* and in a rabbit *(bottom)*. **B.** Anteroposterior roentgenograms of the deformity in a child *(left)* and in a rabbit *(right)*. Note abduction and eversion of the forefoot. (From Ritsila, V. A.: Talipes equinovarus and vertical talus produced experimentally in newborn rabbits. Acta Orthop. Scand., Suppl. 121, 1969. p. 54. Reprinted by permission.)

lumbar and first sacral levels are innervated, the foot is in dorsiflexion and eversion; and as the fifth lumbar and first and second sacral levels are innervated, the foot changes its posture to plantar flexion and inversion.

Ritsilä produced vertical talus in rabbits by causing simultaneous shortening of the triceps surae muscle and dorsiflexor muscles of the foot, and sectioning the extensor digitorum longus, the tibialis anterior, and the ligamentum transversum cruris. (The divided tendons of the extensor digitorum longus and tibialis anterior adhered to the dorsum of the foot and acted as the deforming force.) Vertical talus also developed when either the extensor digitorum longus or the anterior tibial muscles were resected in addition to sectioning of the ligamentum transversum cruris and fixation of the Achilles tendon. Two types of vertical talus were produced, an anterior tibial type and an extensor digitorum type. In the *anterior tibial type* the tibialis anterior is taut and is the shortened element on the front of the ankle, whereas in the *extensor digitorum type* the long toe extensor and peroneal tendons are tightened and shortened. In both types as seen in the lateral projection, the sole has the rocker-bottom shape with the forepart of the foot dorsiflexed and the hindfoot in equinus posture, the talus is vertical, pointing to the plantar aspect of the foot, and the navicular articulates with the dorsal surface of the talar neck and not with the head of the talus. The anteroposterior projection shows the forefoot slightly supinated in the anterior tibial type (Fig. 2–49) and definitely pronated in the extensor digitorum type (Fig. 2–50). Ritsilä concluded that primary soft-tissue changes should be considered in the pathogenesis of congenital convex pes valgus.[63]

Heredity may be a factor. Familial incidence in parent and child has been observed by Aschner and Engelmann, by Robbins, and by Lamy and Weissman.[2,48,64] Armknecht found congenital convex pes valgus in identical twins.[1]

The incidence of teratologic dislocation of the talonavicular joint is unknown. The deformity is very rare, as judged by the small number of case reports from major children's hospitals. It is more common in boys than in girls. Involvement may be bilateral or unilateral; in the latter, the opposite foot may have a calcaneovalgus, equinovarus, or metatarsus varus deformity.

Pathologic Anatomy

The gross anatomic and histologic features of congenital convex pes valgus have been described in several investigators: by Güntz in a stillborn with bilateral involvement; by Patterson, Fitz, and Smith in a six-week-old girl who succumbed to congenital heart disease; by Drennan and Sharrard, who reported the findings in an 11-hour-old-girl with myelomeningocele who died of cardiac arrest following spinal osteotomy; and by Campos da Paz, Jr., and his colleagues in an eight-hour-old infant with myelomeningocele who died of atelectasis and hemorrhage.[11,20,29,60] In Patterson and associates' case, the spinal cord was not examined. Observations at operation have also contributed to our knowledge of the deformity's pathologic anatomy. The anatomic abnormalities may be subdivided into those of the bones and joints, those of the ligaments, and those of the muscles and tendons.

BONE AND JOINT CHANGES

The navicular will be found articulating with the dorsal aspect of the neck of the talus, locking it in a vertical position (Fig. 2–51). The proximal articular surface of the navicular is tilted plantarward. The head of the talus develops an abnormal shape and is flattened superiorly, somewhat pointed, and oval rather than spherical. The neck of the talus is hypoplastic and may have an abnormal facet on its dorsal surface that articulates with the navicular. The calcaneus is displaced posterolaterally in relation to the talus, is in close contact with the distal end of the fibula, and is tilted into equinus posture. The anterior part of the calcaneus is deviated laterally, and the talocalcaneal angle (formed by the longitudinal axes of the talus and the calcaneus) is abnormally increased. The sustentaculum tali is hypoplastic and blunted, offering no support to the head of the talus. The calcaneus may be convex on its plantar aspect. There are abnormalities in the facets of the subtalar joint; the anterior articular facet is absent, the middle one is hypoplastic, and

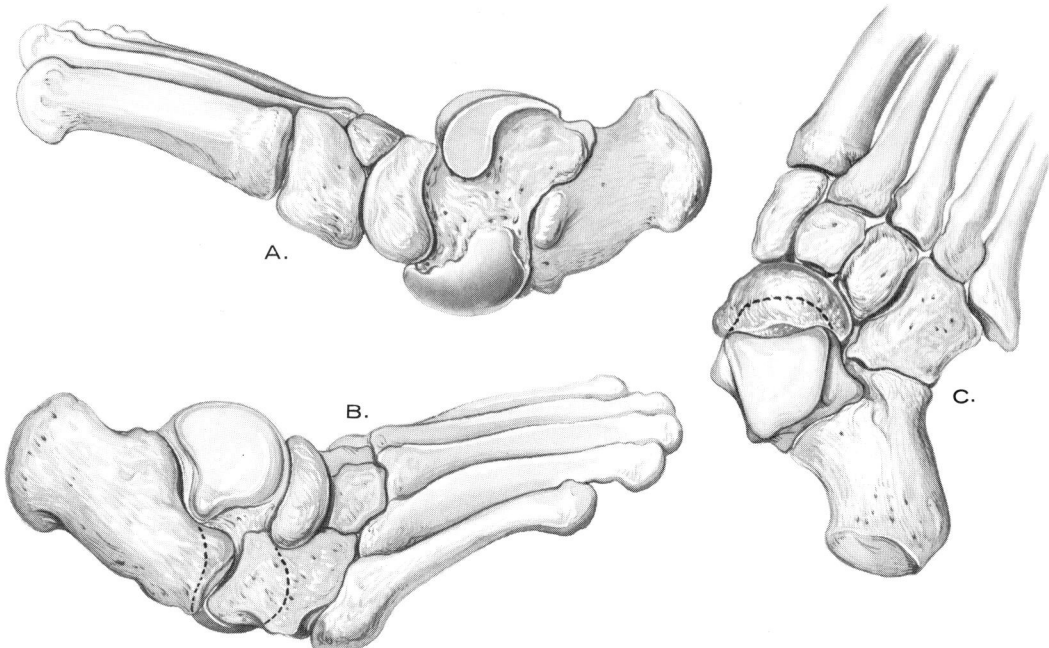

FIGURE 2–51. *Bone and joint changes in congenital convex pes valgus.*

A. Medial aspect of right foot showing dorsiflexion of forefoot at midtarsal joint; vertical talus producing a rocker-bottom convexity; subluxation of the navicular upon the neck of the talus, locking talus vertically; calcaneus 20 to 25 degrees equinus. **B.** Lateral aspect of right foot. Dotted lines indicate displaced head of talus. **C.** Dorsal aspect showing abducted forefoot beginning at midtarsus. Dotted lines indicate head of talus subluxated below navicular bone. (From Tachdjian, M. O.: Congenital convex pes valgus. Orthop. Clin. N. Amer., *3*:133, 1972. Reprinted by permission.)

the posterior one is misshapen and has an increased lateral tilt. These changes are most probably produced by the lack of contact between the normally congruent surfaces of the talus and calcaneus. The lateral column of the foot is concave, and the articular facet of the calcaneus for the cuboid is inclined dorsally and laterally. There is a variable degree of dorsolateral subluxation of the calcaneocuboid joint. The medial column of the foot is elongated, obstructing normal alignment of the navicular over the head of the talus. The anatomic relations of the navicular and cuboid with the cuneiforms and the metatarsals are normal and not disturbed.

LIGAMENTOUS CHANGES

As shown in Figures 2–52, 2–53, and 2–54, the tibionavicular ligament (which is a part of the anterior portion of the deltoid ligament) and the lateral parts of the dorsal medial talonavicular ligament are markedly contracted and present a major obstacle to successful reduction. The bifurcated, or Y, ligament, located between the upper lateral part of the calcaneus and the navicular and cuboid bones, is shortened, causing the forefoot to be held in abduction. Contracture of the interosseous talocalcaneal and calcaneofibular ligaments takes place, preventing reduction of the posterolaterally subluxated os calcis. In untreated cases, the posterior capsule of the ankle and subtalar joints is also shortened.

The plantar calcaneonavicular ligament, or spring ligament, is stretched and moderately attenuated. The capsule of the talonavicular joint is elongated on its medial and plantar aspects.

MUSCLE AND TENDON ABNORMALITIES

The anterior tibial, extensor hallucis longus, extensor digitorum longus, peroneus brevis, and triceps surae muscles are con-

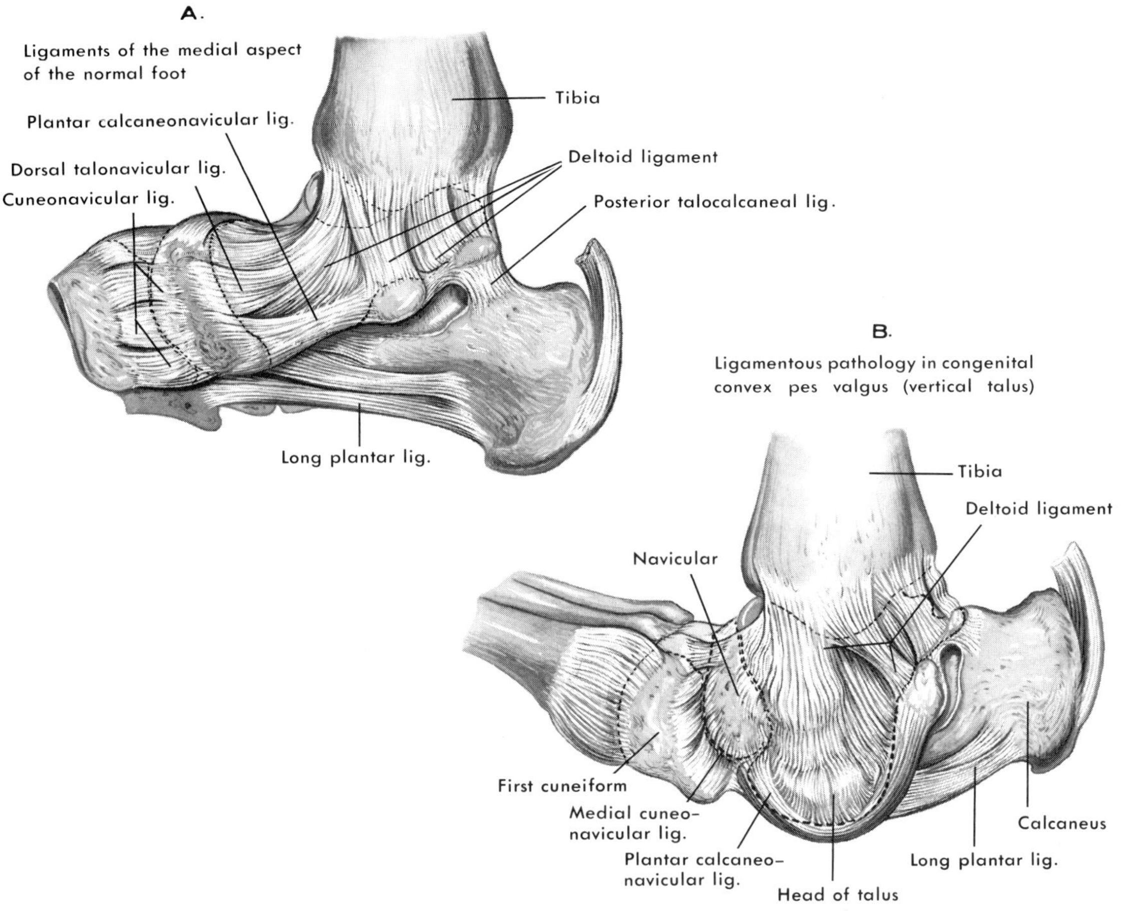

Congenital Deformities   245

FIGURE 2–52. *Ligamentous pathologic changes in congenital convex pes valgus—medial view.*
A. Normal foot. **B.** Malformed foot with congenital convex pes valgus.

FIGURE 2–53. *Ligamentous pathologic changes in congenital convex pes valgus—lateral view.*

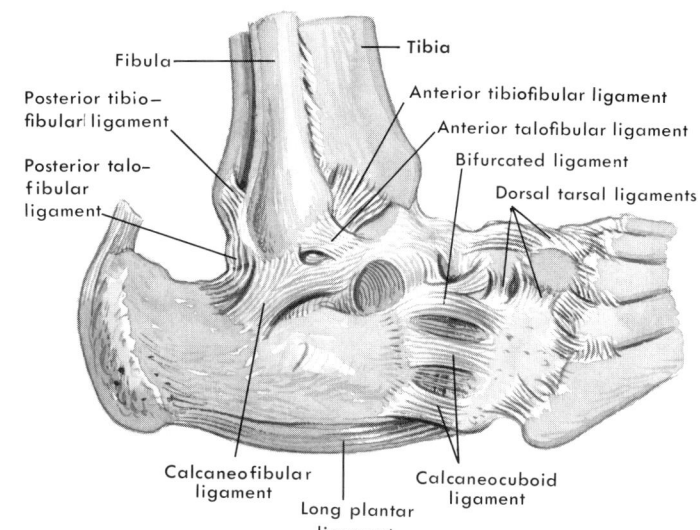

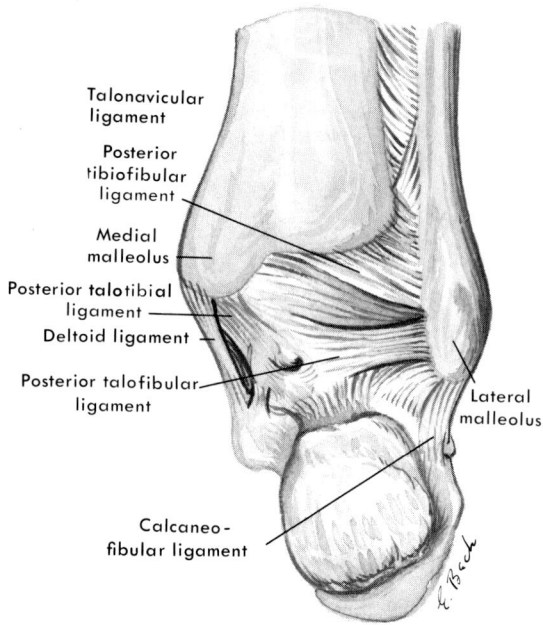

FIGURE 2–54. Ligamentous pathologic changes in congenital convex pes valgus—posterior view.

tracted. The posterior tibial and peroneal tendons are usually anteriorly displaced, lying in grooves on the malleoli and acting as dorsiflexors rather than plantar flexors. In severe cases, they may "bowstring" across the ankle joint (Figs. 2–55 and 2–56). Patterson and co-workers found these muscles to be grossly and histologically normal, and proposed that their contracture is secondary to length deficit.[60] Drennan and Sharrard reported moderate atrophy of the posterior tibial and quadratus plantae muscles and hypertrophy of the extensor digitorum longus muscle; it should be remembered, however, that their anatomic specimen was from a child with myelomeningocele.[20] In an arthrogrypotic child with congenital convex pes valgus, the author has observed fibrosis of the anterior tibial, long toe extensor, and peroneal muscles.

The effect of manipulation in stillborn and fetal specimens with congenital convex pes valgus has been studied by Güntz and

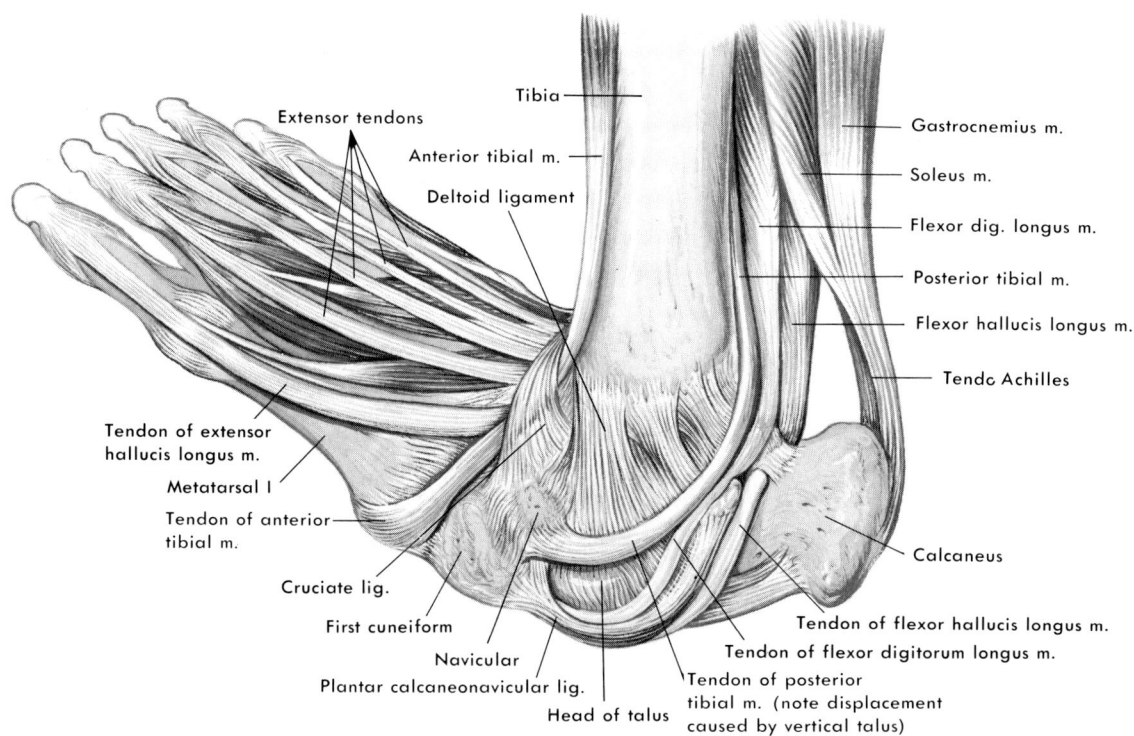

FIGURE 2–55. Abnormalities of muscles and tendons in congenital convex pes valgus.

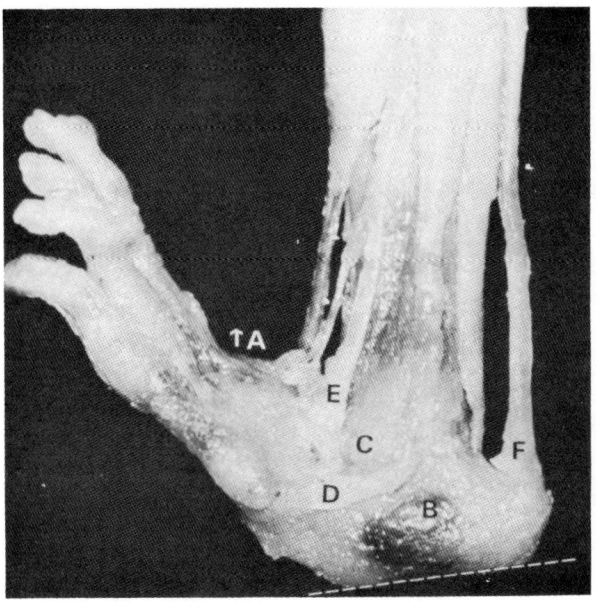 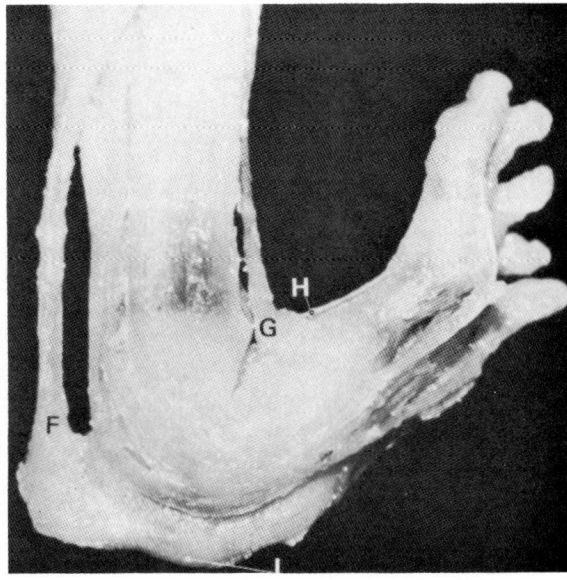

FIGURE 2–56. Pathologic soft-tissue changes in congenital convex pes valgus.

Anatomic findings in an infant who died eight hours after birth. **A.** Lateral view. Note the rocker-bottom foot with dorsiflexion of the forefoot (A) and equinus deformity of the heel. The apex of the angulation of the lateral column is at the calcaneonavicular joint. The calcaneus (B) is displaced laterally under the talus, lying in close proximity to the distal end of the fibula (C). The triceps surae (F) is contracted, holding the calcaneus in plantar flexion. The peroneus longus (D) and peroneus tertius (E) are shortened. **B.** Medial view. The anterior tibial (G) and extensor hallucis longus (H) muscles are shortened. (The extensor digitorum longus is also contracted, but it does not show in this photograph.) The triceps surae muscle (F) is shortened. These musculotendinous contractures are secondary obstacles to anatomic alignment of the talocalcaneonavicular joint. (From Campos da Paz, A., Jr., De Souza, V., and Conceicao de Souza, D.: Congenital convex pes valgus. Orthop. Clin. N. Amer., 9:207, 1978, p. 210. Reprinted by permission.)

by Campos da Paz, Jr., and associates.[11, 29] Talocalcaneonavicular dislocation was not reduced by forceful manipulation; only after division of the aforementioned contracted ligaments and tendons could normal articular alignment be restored.

Clinical Features

The rigid deformity of the foot is present at birth and is so distinct that the condition can be diagnosed at that time. The sole of the foot is convex and has a rocker-bottom appearance (Fig. 2–57). The head of the talus is markedly prominent on the medial and plantar aspects of the foot. The forefoot is abducted and dorsiflexed at the midtarsal joint. The long toe extensor, anterior tibial, and peroneal muscles are markedly shortened. The calcaneovalgus deformity of the forefoot is fixed; the taut muscles and the contracted tibionavicular and talonavicular ligaments resist plantar flexion and inversion of the forefoot. The hindfoot posture is equinovalgus; the triceps surae muscle is contracted, and the calcaneus is everted and tilted downward in plantar flexion. The dislocated navicular may be palpable on the dorsum of the neck of the talus. Deep creases appear on the dorsolateral aspect of the foot near the ankle joint. The deformity is so rigid that on plantar flexion without weight-bearing the fixed convex planovalgus appearance of the foot persists; the longitudinal arch cannot be restored.

Walking is usually not delayed. The older child stands with the involved hindfoot in markedly valgus position with the posterior part of the heel not touching the floor. The forefoot is abducted, and most of the body weight is borne on the head of the talus. The gait is awkward, clumsy, almost peglike, the feet toeing out and rolling into a valgus

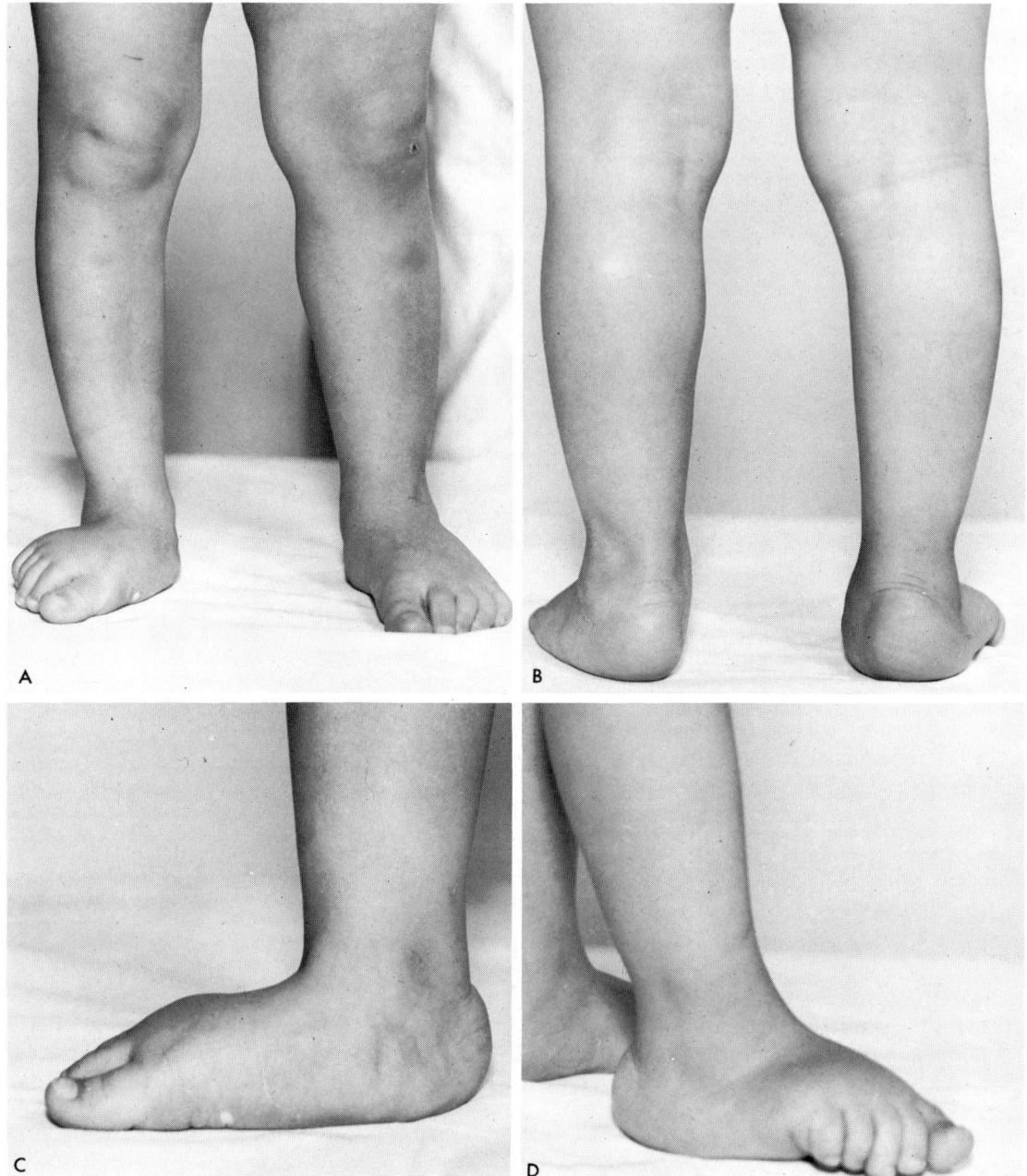

FIGURE 2–57. Congenital convex pes valgus.

A to **D.** Clinical appearance of the deformity in a child.

posture. The balance is poor. Shoes rapidly become distorted, the medial part of the heel and the upper over the longitudinal arch wearing down within a few weeks. Pain is not a symptom in childhood, but it usually becomes a complaint in later adolescence.

Roentgenographic Findings

There is considerable variation in the time for roentgenographic appearance of the ossification centers of the tarsal bones. At birth those of the talus, calcaneus, and metatarsals are clearly visible; however, the ossific nucleus of the cuboid bone may be present or delayed in its appearance until the third to the twentieth day after birth. The cuneiform bones become visible later than the cuboid. The ossification center of the navicular usually appears at three years of age (one and a half to four years); hence it cannot be seen in the roentgenograms at birth. To define their relationships one has to draw lines through the longitudinal axes of the talus, the calcaneus, and the first metatarsal bones as described in the section on roentgenographic investigation of talipes equinovarus.

The roentgenographic findings in congenital convex pes valgus are characteristic, even in the newborn. The talus is vertical, lying parallel with the longitudinal axis of the tibia, and the calcaneus is in equinus position, whereas the forepart of the foot is dorsiflexed and deviated laterally at the midtarsal level. The outline of the soft tissues of the sole is convex. The anteroposterior talocalcaneal angle is abnormally increased. To make the definitive diagnosis, it is imperative to demonstrate that the navicular is dislocated dorsally on the neck of the talus when the foot is maintained in extreme plantar flexion.[23]

The location of the cartilaginous navicu-

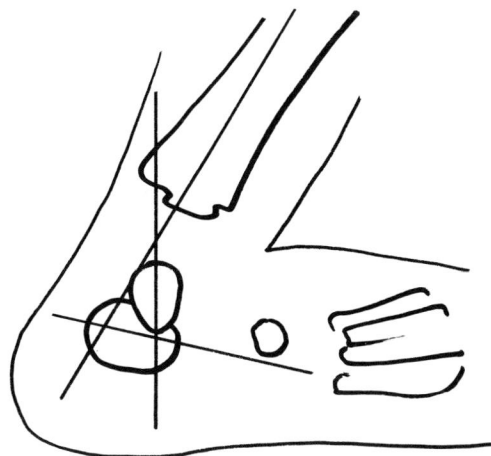

FIGURE 2–59. *Line drawing of the lateral roentgenogram of a foot with congenital convex pes valgus.*

The long axis of the talus passes below and behind the cuboid bone and cuts through the anterior part of the calcaneus, and the long axis of the calcaneus passes plantar to the cuboid.

lar can be determined by drawing the longitudinal axis of the first metatarsal and noting its relation to the head of the talus. In congenital convex pes valgus, on forced plantar flexion, the long axis of the first metatarsal will point dorsally to the head of the talus. In a normal foot it bisects the head of the talus.

The relationship of the long axes of the talus and calcaneus should be noted. In a normal foot the long axis of the talus passes through the lower half of the cuboid, and that of the calcaneus cuts through the upper half of the cuboid (Fig. 2–58). In congenital convex pes valgus the long axis of the talus passes below and posterior to the cuboid and often cuts through the anterior part of the calcaneus or passes very close to its anterior end (Figs. 2–59 and 2–60); and the long axis of the calcaneus passes plantar to the cuboid. By the age of three years, the navicular ossifies and its complete dislocation over the dorsal surface of the neck of the talus is clearly visible (Fig. 2–61).

In paralytic pes valgus in which the feet are severely pronated, the talus may be tilted into vertical position (particularly if there is contracture of the triceps surae), and the navicular will sag on the head of the talus, suggesting subluxation of the talonavicular joint. On close scrutiny, however,

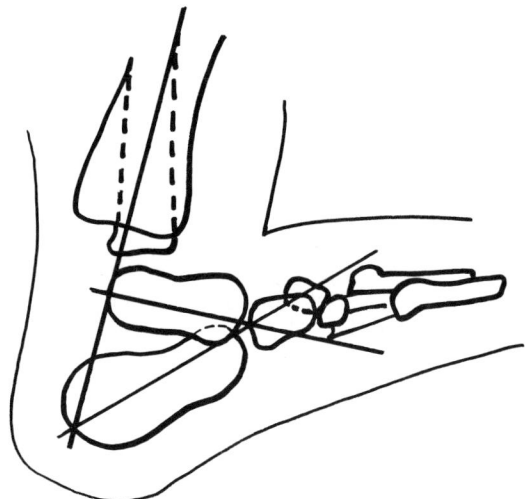

FIGURE 2–58. *Line drawing of the lateral roentgenogram of a normal foot.*

The long axis of the talus cuts the lower half of the cuboid, whereas the long axis of the calcaneus passes through the upper half of the cuboid.

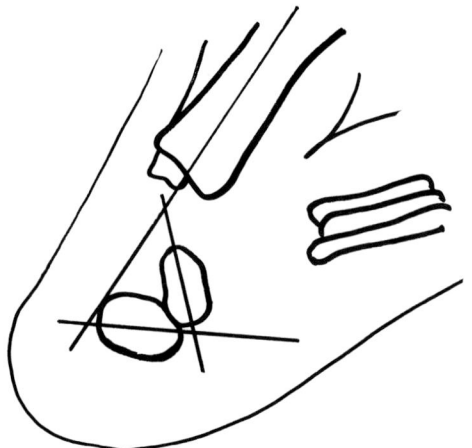

FIGURE 2–60. *Line drawing of the lateral roentgenogram of a foot with congenital convex pes valgus.*

The long axis of the talus passes very close to the anterior end of the calcaneus.

it is evident that there is definite contact between the articular surfaces of the navicular and the head of the talus. On forced plantar flexion of the foot one can restore normal talonavicular relations.

The navicular bone, in congenital convex pes valgus, may be irregularly ossified, suggesting Köhler's disease. With increasing age, it becomes wedge-shaped toward its plantar aspect, and upward tilting of its anterior end gives it a beak-shaped appearance. With dorsal and lateral displacement of the forepart of the foot, dorsolateral subluxation of the calcaneocuboid joint is evident. The first metatarsal is dorsiflexed and the hallux is plantar-flexed at the metatarsophalangeal joint, compensating for the elevated first metatarsal bone.

The talus is underdeveloped, particularly at its waist, resembling an hourglass. In the lateral projection it will be seen that only the posterior portion of the superior surface of the talus is contained in the tibiofibular mortise.

Differential Diagnosis

In early infancy, congenital convex pes valgus is commonly mistaken for talipes calcaneovalgus. In both conditions, the forepart of the foot is dorsiflexed and everted, and there is limitation of plantar flexion and inversion. The heel in congenital convex pes valgus is in equinus position, the sole of the foot convex, and the deformity very rigid, whereas in talipes calcaneovalgus, the os calcis and talus are in dorsiflexion, and the deformity is quite flexible and responds rapidly to stretching exercises and treatment with corrective casts.

The presence of pes valgus with myostatic contracture of the triceps surae muscle may present a problem in differential diagnosis. In stance, the heel position is equinovalgus, and the talus is plantar-flexed with its head prominent on the medial and plantar aspects of the midfoot; the deformity is not rigid, however, and when not bearing weight, the heel can be manipulated into neutral position and the head of the talus

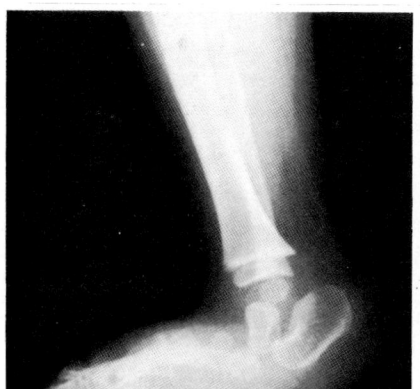
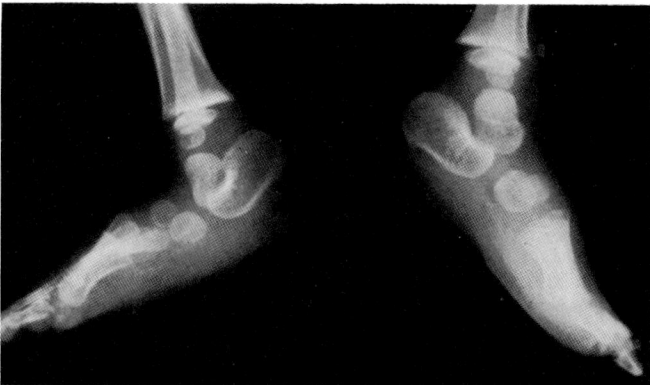

FIGURE 2–61. *Roentgenographic appearance of congenital convex pes valgus in a two-year-old child.*

Lateral projection of the foot and ankle. The navicular is ossified, and its complete dislocation over the head of the talus is clearly visualized.

into dorsiflexion, giving a normal longitudinal arch to the foot. In congenital convex pes valgus, the deformity is fixed and does not improve when not bearing weight. Roentgenograms made with the foot in plantar flexion will establish the diagnosis.

Paralytic pes valgus due to cerebral palsy, myelomeningocele, or poliomyelitis should not be difficult to distinguish from congenital convex pes valgus. Although the clinical appearance of peroneal spastic flatfoot due to tarsal coalition may resemble congenital vertical talus, the roentgenographic findings are distinctive. An accessory navicular produces a prominence on the medial aspect of the foot, which is in a valgus position. Again, roentgenograms should settle the diagnosis.

Table 2–9. Methods of Treatment of Congenital Convex Pes Valgus

---

Procedures on Talus
  Excision of head and neck of talus (Lange, 1912; Nové-Joserrand, 1923)
  Curettage of talus with excision of its cuneiform portion (Camera, 1926)
  Complete astragalectomy (Lamy and Weissman, 1939)
  Open-up wedge osteotomy of neck of talus with insertion of bone graft on its plantar aspect (Hughes, 1957)
Procedures on Navicular
  Excision of navicular (Stone, 1963)
  Excision of dorsal wedge from navicular and placement of the wedge under elevated head of talus combined with open reduction, reefing of spring ligament, and shortening of posterior tibial tendon (Eyre-Brook, 1967)
Procedures on Talonavicular Joint
  Open reduction with or without lengthening of Achilles tendon and release of shortened musculotendinous units, ligaments, and capsules on dorsolateral aspect of foot
  Reduction maintained with plaster cast (Rocher and Pouyanne, 1934)
  Reduction maintained with Kirschner wire across talonavicular joint (Hark, 1950; Heyman, 1959; Herndon and Heyman, 1963)
  Reduction maintained with transfer of peroneus brevis tendon to neck of talus (Osmond-Clarke, 1956)
  Reduction maintained with scarification of talonavicular joint with or without Kirschner wire through navicular into head of talus (Hughes, 1957)
  Reduction maintained with reefing of capsule and rerouting of anterior tibial tendon under neck of talus and fixing to navicular (Grice, 1959)
  Reduction maintained with subtalar arthrodesis (Grice, 1959; Coleman et al., 1966)
  Reduction maintained with plication of calcaneonavicular ligament and reattaching of posterior tibial tendon with shortening (Eyre-Brook, 1967; Harrold, 1967; Støren, 1967)
  Release of capsule of calcaneocuboid joint on its dorsolateral aspect (Coleman et al., 1966)
  Closed reduction in young infant (under 3 mo. of age) following elongation of shortened soft tissues by serial stretching casts (Harrold, 1967; Støren, 1967)
Reconstructive or Stabilization Procedures on Tarsus
  Triple arthrodesis (Hark, 1950; Lloyd-Roberts, 1958; and others)
  Wedge tarsectomy (Lloyd-Roberts, 1958)

Treatment

The objectives of therapy are to place the navicular and calcaneus in a normal anatomic relationship to the talus and to maintain the reduction.

The method of treatment depends upon the age of the patient and the degree and severity of the deformity. A number of methods and techniques of treatment that have been proposed by various authors in the literature are summarized in Table 2–9.

The condition may be diagnosed at birth by the characteristic rocker-bottom convex shape of the foot, the rigidity of the deformity, and its distinctive roentgenographic features. Treatment should begin at birth. The first three weeks of life is the golden period when there may be a chance to achieve and retain reduction of the dorsolateral dislocation of the talocalcaneonavicular joint by the closed method. In general, however, this is extremely difficult, and often one has to employ open surgery to obtain and maintain reduction. Any delay in diagnosis will lead to a crippling deformity of the foot. The older the patient at the time treatment is initiated, the more rigid will be the ligamentous, capsular, and soft-tissue contractures, and the greater the structural osseous changes.

ELONGATION OF CONTRACTED SOFT TISSUES BY MANIPULATIVE STRETCHING

In the neonate and young infant a preliminary period of stretching of the shortened ligaments and muscles by passive manipulation is indicated. As in talipes equinovarus, one should remember that soft tissues are hard and hard tissues are soft. Gentleness is the basic principle. The technique of manipulation is as follows: first, the triceps surae and calcaneofibular ligament are stretched by pulling them distally and medially with one hand and pushing the anterior end of the os calcis (not the cuboid) with the other hand. The stretched position is maintained to the count of 10, then released. The ankle dorsiflexor and evertor muscles are stretched by pulling the forefoot into plantar flexion, inversion, and adduction. Then the tibionavicular and talonavicular ligaments are elongated by applying *distal traction* on the forefoot and navicular bone and gradually bringing them into adduction and inversion. Each time the corrected positions are maintained to the count of 10 and then released. The manipulations are performed for 15 minutes. The skin is then painted with a nonirritating adhesive liquid such as tincture of benzoin to prevent slipping of the cast, and the limb is immobilized in a long leg cast with the foot and ankle in the corrected position— the forepart of the foot in equinus position and inversion, and the heel well molded in the degree of dorsiflexion obtained by passive manipulation. During application of the cast on the foot, thumb pressure is applied on the anterior end of the os calcis. The successive plaster casts are changed twice a week; each time the foot is gently manipulated for 15 minutes to further stretch the soft-tissue contracture.

Following manipulative elongation of the contracted ligaments and muscles over a period of four to six weeks, closed reduction of the talocalcaneonavicular dislocation is attempted. This is performed by applying distal traction on the forefoot and navicular, first in the line of deformity, i.e., into dorsiflexion and eversion. After bringing the navicular over the talar head and the calcaneus under the talus, the forefoot and midfoot are brought into plantar flexion as the head of the talus is pushed into dorsiflexion and the heel is pulled distally and into inversion. Restoration of the normal articular relationship of the navicular with the head of the talus should be verified by roentgenographic examination. As previously stated, because the navicular is not ossified in infancy, the anatomic relationship of the talonavicular articulation is difficult to establish. The exact location of the cartilaginous navicular between the ossified medial cuneiform and the head of the talus is determined. Arthrography of the articulation may be attempted in borderline or doubtful cases.

Occasionally, closed reduction of teratologic dislocation of the talonavicular joint is successful.[34, 73, 74, 80] In such an instance, the author recommends maintenance of reduction by "blind" pinning of the talonavicular joint. Image intensifier roentgenographic control will make the procedure a simple one. A heavy threaded Kirschner wire is inserted in the web interspace between the great and second toes, and is then drilled proximally across the talonavicular joint, holding the forefoot in marked plantar flexion and inversion. Initially, the hindfoot and ankle joint are immobilized in plantar flexion. After two to three weeks, the cast is changed and the foot is brought into increasing dorsiflexion. Immobilization should be continued for at least two months.

OPEN REDUCTION

If closed reduction proves unsuccessful, open reduction should be performed at three months of age (Plate 5).

The reduction of the talonaviculocuneiform joint in congenital convex pes valgus is obstructed by the following structures (in order of priority). *Ligaments:* (1) the dorsal and lateral part of the talonavicular ligament; (2) the tibionavicular ligament; (3) the bifurcated, or Y, ligament (both the calcaneonavicular and the calcaneocuboid limbs); (4) the dorsal and lateral parts of the calcaneocuboid capsule; (5) the calcaneofibular ligament; and (6) the interosseous talocalcaneal ligament. *Musculotendinous tissues:* (1) the triceps surae, (2) the anterior tibial, (3) the long toe extensors, and (4) the peroneals. These permanently shortened muscles serve as secondary obstacles to reduction. In a systematic step-by-step approach these contracted soft tissues should be lengthened by open surgical division under direct vision. In the older child or in the one with very severe rigid deformity, the medial skeletal column of the foot is too long and prevents normal restoration of articular alignment of the talus and navicular; therefore, it is shortened by excision of the dorsally dislocated navicular.

During open reduction it is essential to take measures to maintain the correction. Capsular plication and tightening of the calcaneonavicular (spring) ligament and posterior tibial tendon under the head of the talus by distal transfer should be performed in all cases. Muscle and tendon transfers may be performed to suspend the head of the talus in dorsiflexion; transferring the peroneus brevis as recommended by Osmond-Clarke; splitting the anterior tibial tendon and transferring half of it to the head of the talus as recommended by Grice; or transferring the entire anterior tibial tendon to the head and neck of the talus as recommended by Lloyd-Roberts. In the older child the Grice extra-articular arthrodesis is performed to maintain the reduction and give stability to the subtalar joint.

In the age range of three to six years, and in the rigid dislocation of arthrogryposis or myelomeningocele, the author recommends excision of the navicular. It will effectively reduce the length of the medial skeletal column of the foot and facilitate reduction (Fig. 2–62). The medial cuneiform is aligned with the head of the talus, and with growth and remodeling of the tarsus, the vacant space is gradually filled with the head of the talus.

Eyre-Brook excised a wedge of the navicular and used it to prop up the head of the talus and maintain reduction. He reported the results in four cases; five to ten years after operation, stable reduction was maintained. Eyre-Brook suggested that the entire navicular be excised, at least in the more severe deformities.[23] Earlier, Stone, reporting for Lloyd-Roberts, had described excision of the entire navicular combined with posterior capsulotomy of the ankle, lengthening of the Achilles tendon, and transfer of the anterior tibial tendon through the neck of the talus.[72] Colton followed the technique of Lloyd-Roberts and reported good results in six feet.[17] Clark, D'Ambrosia, and Ferguson performed open reduction and excision of the navicular in 16 feet (12 patients) with true congenital vertical talus.

Text continued on page 260

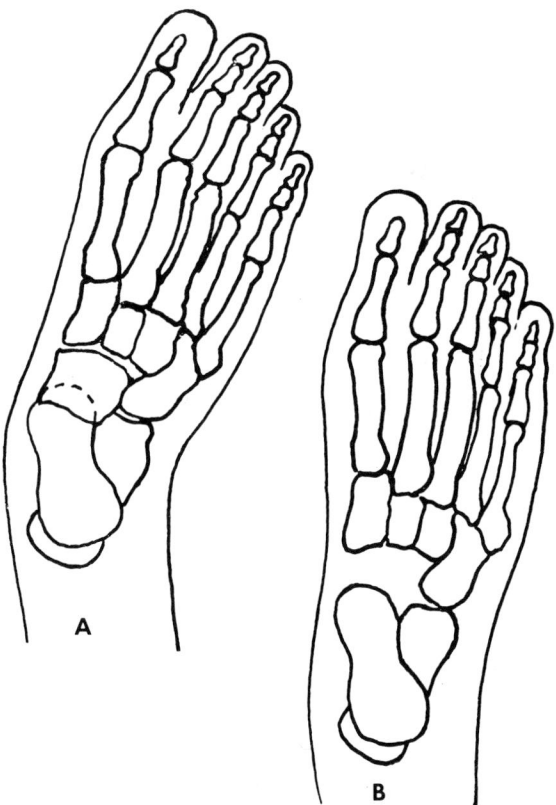

FIGURE 2–62. Principle of excision of navicular in treatment of rigid congenital convex pes valgus.

A. The deformed foot. Note the excessive length of the medial skeletal column. **B.** By excision of the navicular, a vacant space is provided to allow alignment of the forepart of the foot with the hindfoot. The medial cuneiform is brought into line with the talus. With growth and remodeling of the tarsus, the vacant area is filled with the head of the talus. (From Clark, M. W., D'Ambrosia, R. D., and Ferguson, A. B.: Congenital vertical talus. J. Bone Joint Surg., 59-A:816, 1977, p. 822. Reprinted by permission.)

Open Reduction of Dorsolateral Dislocation of Talocalcaneonavicular Joint (Congenital Convex Pes Valgus)

THE PROCEDURE

A. A longitudinal incision is made lateral to the tendo calcaneus, beginning at the heel and extending proximally for a distance of 7 to 10 cm. The subcutaneous tissue and tendon sheath are divided in line with the skin incision, and the wound flaps are retracted, exposing the Achilles tendon.

B. Z-plastic lengthening is performed in the anteroposterior plane. With a knife the Achilles tendon is divided longitudinally into lateral and medial halves for a distance of 5 to 7 cm. The distal end of the lateral half is detached from the calcaneus to prevent recurrence of valgus deformity of the heel; the medial half is divided proximally. When the equinus deformity is not marked, sliding lengthening of the heel cord is performed.

C and **D.** A posterior capsulotomy of the ankle and subtalar joint is performed if necessary. The calcaneofibular ligament is sectioned. The thickened capsule of the calcaneocuboid joint and the bifurcated ligament are divided through a separate lateral incision. The Cincinnati transverse incision shown in Figure 2–43 is an alternative surgical approach; it is preferred by this author.

Plate 5. Open Reduction of Dorsolateral Dislocation of Talocalcaneonavicular Joint (Congenital Convex Pes Valgus)

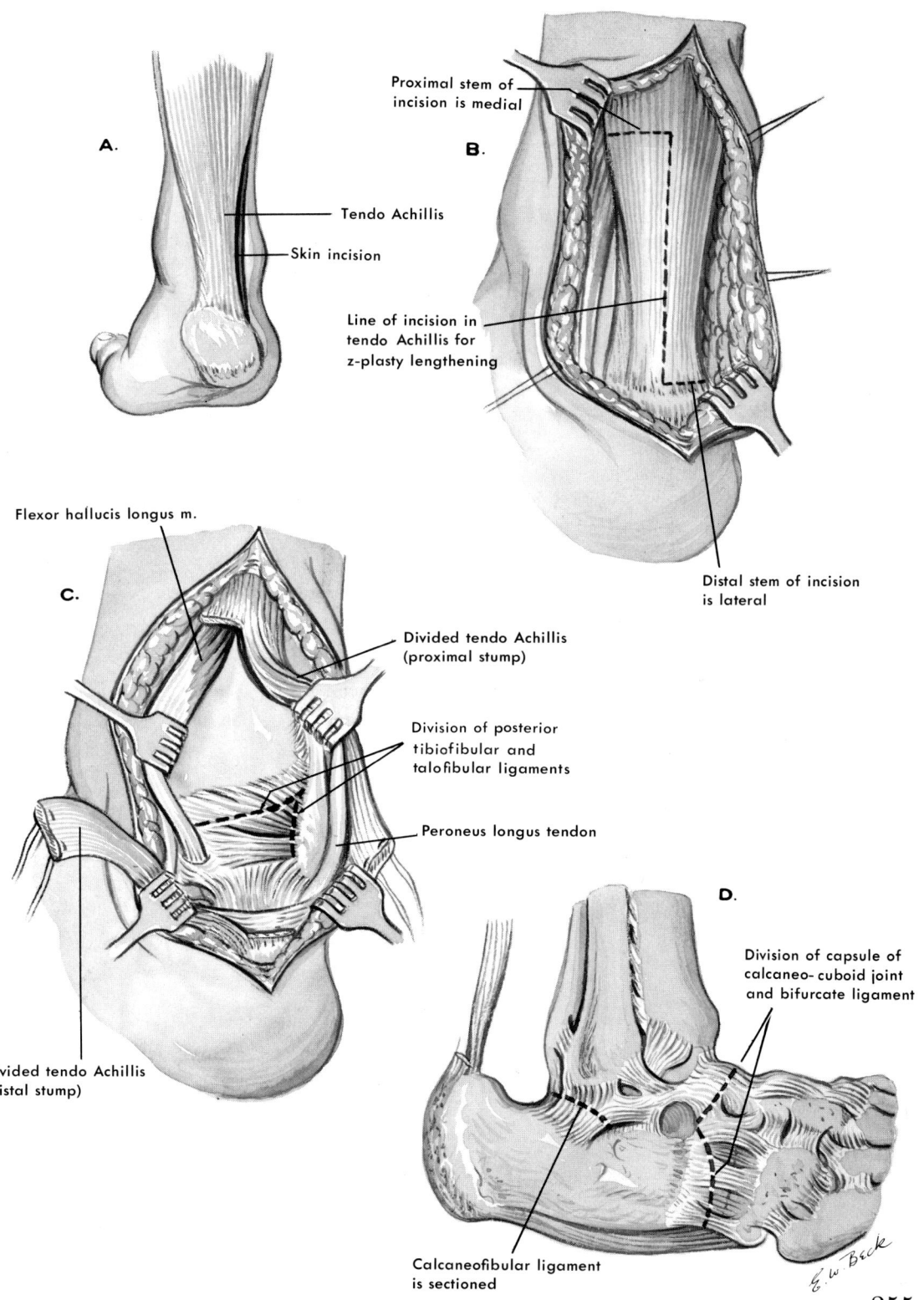

Open Reduction of Dorsolateral Dislocation of Talocalcaneonavicular Joint (Congenital Convex Pes Valgus)
(Continued)

E. The medial skin incision begins at a point 2 cm. posterior and 1 cm. distal to the tip of the medial malleolus and extends distally to the base of the first metatarsal. The subcutaneous tissue is divided. The skin margins are mobilized and retracted to expose the dorsal, medial, and plantar aspects of the tarsus.

F and G. The posterior tibial tendon is identified, dissected, and divided at its insertion to the tuberosity of the navicular. The end of the tendon is marked with 0 Mersilene suture for later reattachment. The articular surface of the head of the talus points steeply downward and medially to the sole of the foot and is covered by the capsule and ligament. The navicular will be found against the dorsal aspect of the neck of the talus, locking it in vertical position. The pathologic anatomy of the ligaments and capsule is noted and the incisions planned so that a secure capsuloplasty can be performed and the talus maintained in its normal anatomic position. Circulation to the talus is another important consideration; it should be disturbed as little as possible by exercising great care and gentleness during dissection. Avascular necrosis of the talus is always a potential serious complication of open reduction. The plantar calcaneonavicular ligament is identified and divided distally from its attachment to the sustentaculum tali, and an 00 Mersiline suture is inserted in its end for later reattachment. The talonavicular articulation is exposed by a T-incision. The transverse limb of the T is made distally over the tibionavicular ligament (the anterior portion of the deltoid ligament) and over the dorsal and medial portions of the talonavicular ligament. A cuff of capsule is left attached to the navicular for plication on completion of surgery. The longitudinal limb of the incision is made over the head and neck of the talus inferiorly.

The articular surface of the head of the talus is identified, and a large threaded Kirschner wire is inserted in its center. With a skid and the leverage of the Kirschner wire, the head and neck of the talus are lifted dorsally and the forefoot is manipulated into plantar flexion and inversion, bringing the articular surfaces of the navicular and head of the talus into normal anatomic position.

Plate 5. Open Reduction of Dorsolateral Dislocation of Talocalcaneonavicular Joint (Congenital Convex Pes Valgus)

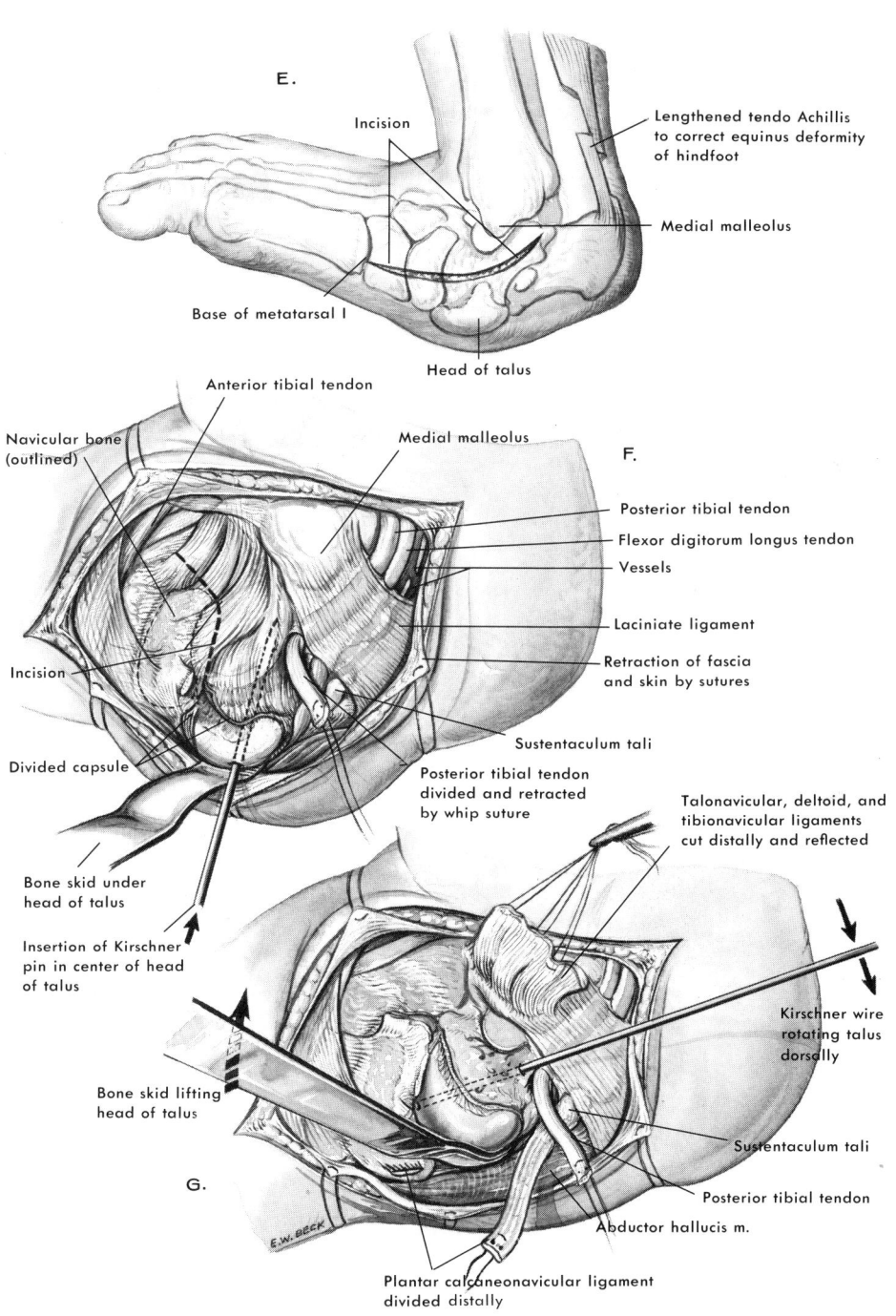

Open Reduction of Dorsolateral Dislocation of Talocalcaneonavicular Joint (Congenital Convex Pes Valgus)
(Continued)

H. The Kirschner wire is drilled retrograde into the navicular, cuneiform, and first metatarsal bones, maintaining the reduction. Roentgenograms of the foot are taken at this time to verify the reduction.

In the older child the calcaneocuboid and talocalcaneal interosseous ligaments may prevent reduction of the laterally subluxated Chopart's and subtalar joints. If necessary, they are divided through a separate anterolateral incision. The anterior tibial, extensor hallucis longus, extensor digitorum longus, and peroneal muscles may also be so shortened that they prevent reduction; if so, they are lengthened. The author prefers fractional lengthening of these muscles through a separate longitudinal incision over the anterior tibial compartment. Others prefer to lengthen them by a Z-plasty over the dorsum of the foot.[329, 330]

I and J. A careful capsuloplasty is very important for maintaining the reduction and the normal anatomic relationship of the talus and navicular. The redundant inferior part of the capsule should be tightened by plication and overlapping of its free edges. First, the plantar-proximal segment of the T of the capsule is pulled dorsally and distally and sutured to the dorsal corner of the inner surface of the distal capsule. Next, the dorsoproximal segment of the T is brought plantarward and distally over the plantar-proximal segment of the capsule and sutured to the plantar corner on the inner surface of the distal capsule. Then, interrupted sutures are used to tighten the capsule on its plantar and medial aspects by bringing the distal segment over the proximal segments.

The plantar calcaneonavicular ligament is sutured under tension to the base of the first metatarsal. To tighten the posterior tibial tendon under the head of the talus, it is advanced distally and sutured to the inferior surface of the first cuneiform.

The anterior tibial may be transferred to provide additional dynamic force for maintaining the navicular in correct relationship to the talus. The tendon is detached from its insertion to the medial cuneiform and first metatarsal bone, and dissected free proximally and medially for a distance of 5 cm. Then it is redirected to pass along the medial aspect of the neck of the talus and beneath the head of the talus, where it is fixed to the inferior aspects of the talus and navicular with 00 Mersilene sutures. Normally the lower end of the anterior tibial tendon may be split near its insertion. Often the author leaves intact the attachment to the first metatarsal, dividing only the insertion to the medial cuneiform. The tendon is split (if not normally bifurcated), and the portion to the medial cuneiform bone is transferred to the head of the talus and the navicular. Sometimes, following adequate capsuloplasty, the reduction of the talonavicular joint is so stable that anterior tibial transfer is not necessary to restore support to the head of the talus.

K. The wounds are then closed in routine fashion. The Kirschner wire across the talonavicular joint is cut subcutaneously. To maintain the normal anatomic relationship of the os calcis to the talus, a Kirschner wire is inserted transversely in the os calcis and incorporated into the cast. An alternate method is to pass the wire from the sole of the foot upward through the calcaneus into the talus. The author prefers the former, as it controls the heel in the cast and prevents recurrence of both equinus deformity and eversion of the hindfoot. An above-knee cast is applied, with the knee in 45 degrees of flexion, the ankle in 10 to 15 degrees of dorsiflexion, the heel in 10 degrees of inversion, and the forefoot in plantar flexion and inversion. The longitudinal arch and the heel in the cast are well molded.

POSTOPERATIVE CARE

The Kirschner wires are removed in six weeks, but the foot and ankle are immobilized in a solid above-knee cast for an additional two to three weeks. After removal of the cast, an above-knee polypropylene splint is worn at night for one to two years. In the splint, the knee is held in 50 to 60 degrees of flexion, the ankle in neutral dorsiflexion, the heel inverted, and the forefoot plantar-flexed and inverted. Passive exercises to develop and maintain range of joint motion and active exercises to develop muscle function are performed several times a day.

Plate 5. Open Reduction of Dorsolateral Dislocation of Talocalcaneonavicular Joint (Congenital Convex Pes Valgus)

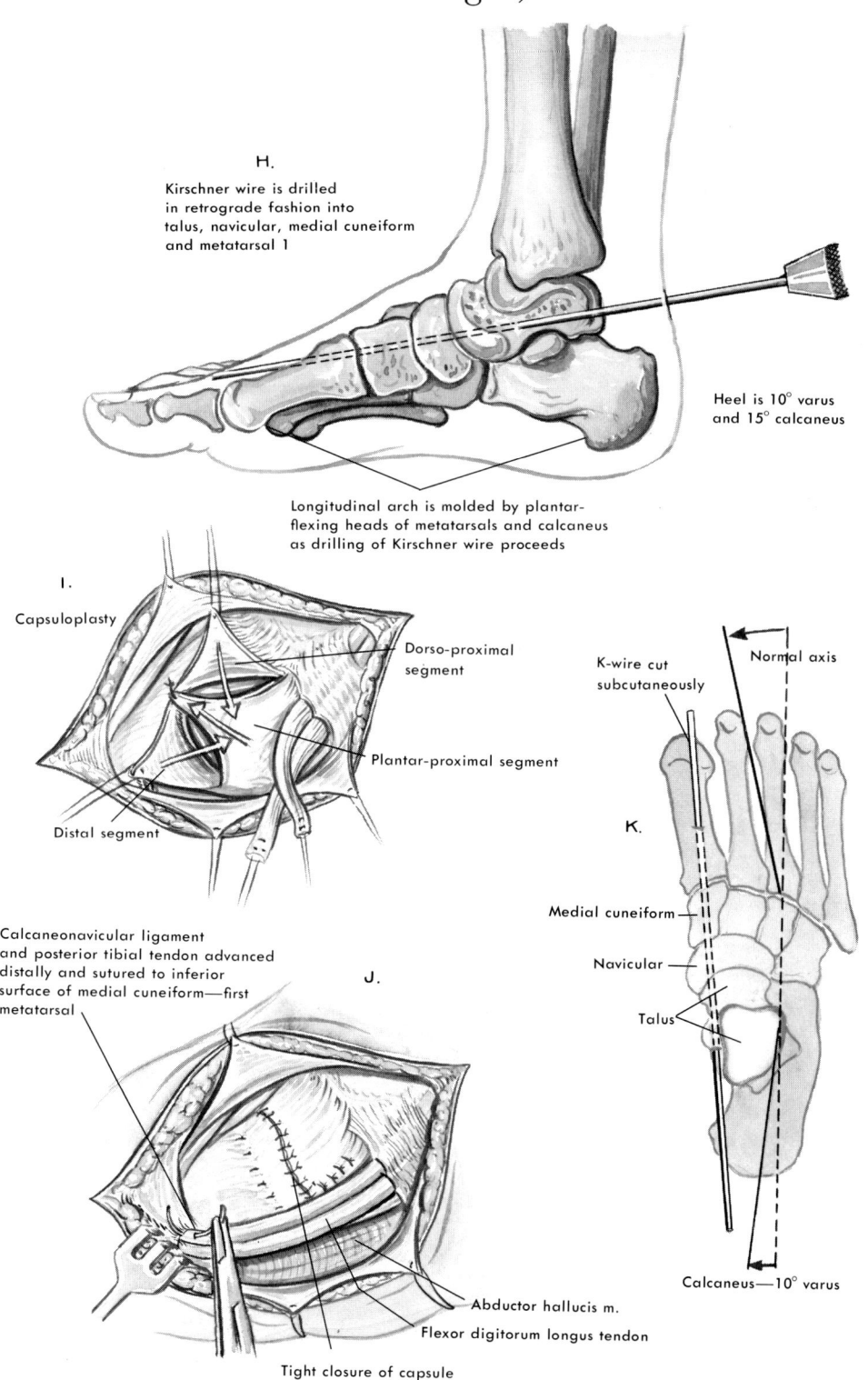

The follow-up was for 2 to 15 years. The anatomic results in 15 of the feet were excellent in 3, good in 7, fair in 4, and poor in 1. Anatomic reduction was best achieved and maintained when the operation was performed in patients less than 18 months of age. Incomplete reductions, however, appeared to be compatible with satisfactory asymptomatic function. In this age group the sustentaculum tali is very hypoplastic and does not support the talar head. Tightening of the calcaneonavicular ligament and dynamic support by the anterior tibial and posterior tibial muscles usually are not sufficient to prevent recurrence of dislocation. The author recommends stabilization of the subtalar joint by the Grice extra-articular subtalar arthrodesis.

In the child over six years of age the deformity is very rigid, and attempts at open reduction are usually unsuccessful. Avascular necrosis of the talus is a definite complication. It is best to wait until the patient is 10 or 12 years old, at which time a reconstructive stabilization procedure on the foot is carried out. Following a preliminary period of corrective casts and soft-tissue lengthening, a triple arthrodesis is performed. The head and neck of the talus and part of the navicular are excised, and appropriate wedges (their bases plantar and medial) are resected at the calcaneocuboid joint to restore the longitudinal arch of the foot. The valgus deformity of the hindfoot is corrected by inserting a bone graft in the sinus tarsi, as in the Grice extra-articular arthrodesis. The excised head of the talus is used as a bone graft. It is not necessary to disturb the posterior subtalar joint.

References

1. Armknecht, P.: Orthopadische Lieden bei Zwillingen. Verh. Deutsch. Orthop. Ges., 26:62, 1931.
2. Aschner, B., and Engelmann, G.: Konstitutionspathologie in der Orthopädie. Erbbiologie des peripheren Bewegungsapparates. Vienna, Julius Springer, 1928.
3. Becker-Andersen, H., and Reimann, I.: Congenital vertical talus. Reevaluation of early manipulative treatment. Acta Orthop. Scand., 45:130, 1974.
4. Bender, G., and Horvath, F.: Uber eine seltene Entwicklungsanomalie des Talus und des Os naviculare pedis. Fortschr. Röntgenstr., 94:281, 1961.
5. Berman, J. L., Rankin, J. K., Harrison, P. A., Donovan, D. J., Hogan, W. J., and Bearn, A. O.: Autosomal trisomy of a group 16-18 chromosome. J. Pediat., 60:503, 1962.
6. Bohm, M.: Der Kongenitale Plattfuss. Zbl. Chir., p. 2987, 1932.
7. Bratberg, J. J., and Scheer, G. E.: Extra-articular arthrodesis of the subtalar joint: A clinical study and review. Clin. Orthop., 126:220, 1977.
8. Browne, D.: Congenital vertical talus in infancy. J. Bone Joint Surg., 48-B:588, 1966.
9. Caffey, J.: Congenital spastic flat feet. In Pediatric X-ray Diagnosis, the Extremities, Diseases of Bones, Congenital Malformations. 4th Ed. Chicago, Year Book Medical Publishers, 1961, Section V, pp. 866–867.
10. Camera, V.: A proposito del piede piatto valgo congenito. Arch. Ortop., 42:432, 1926.
11. Campos da Paz, A., Jr., De Souza, V., and De Souza, D. C.: Congenital convex pes valgus. Orthop. Clin. N. Amer., 9:207, 1978.
12. Canale, G., and Bagliani, G. P.: Considerazioni sull' intervento di Grice per la correzione del piede piatto valgo. Minerva Ortop., 19:442, 1968.
13. Chiappara, P.: Le valgus du talon. Podologie, 4:139, 1965.
14. Clark, M. W., D'Ambrosia, R. D., and Ferguson, A. B., Jr.: Congenital vertical talus. J. Bone Joint Surg., 59-A:816, 1977.
15. Coleman S. S., Martin, A. F., and Jarrett, J.: Congenital vertical talus: Pathogenesis and treatment. J. Bone Joint Surg., 48-A:1442, 1966.
16. Coleman, S., Stelling, F. H., and Jarrett, J.: Pathomechanics and treatment of congenital vertical talus. Clin. Orthop., 70:62, 1970.
17. Colton, C. L.: The surgical management of congenital vertical talus. J. Bone Joint Surg., 55-B:566, 1973.
18. Connolly, J. F., Dornenburg, P., and Holmes, C. D.: Congenital convex pes valgus deformities. In Bateman, J. E. (ed.): Foot Science. A selection of papers from the proceedings of the American Orthopaedic Foot Society, Inc., 1974 and 1975. Philadelphia, W. B. Saunders Co., 1976, Chapter 6, pp. 47–66.
19. Dommisse, F. G.: Flat foot. II. S. Afr. Med. J., 45:726, 1971.
20. Drennan, J. C., and Sharrard, W. J. W.: The pathological anatomy of convex pes valgus. J. Bone Joint Surg., 53-B:455, 1971.
21. Duckworth, T., and Smith, T. W.: The treatment of paralytic convex pes valgus. J. Bone Joint Surg., 56-B:305, 1974.
22. Ellis, J. N., and Scheer, G. E.: Congenital convex pes valgus. Clin. Orthop., 99:168, 1974.
23. Eyre-Brook, A.: Congenital vertical talus. J. Bone Joint Surg., 49-B:618, 1967.
24. Ghisellini, F., and Manaresi, C.: Il piede piatto reflesso congenito. Chir. Organi Mov., 50:37, 1961.
25. Giannestras, N. J.: The congenital rigid flatfoot. Its recognition and treatment in infants. In Proceedings of the American Orthopaedic Foot Society. Orthop. Clin. N. Amer., 4:49, 1973.
26. Gray, E. R.: The role of leg muscles in variations of the arches in normal and flat feet. Phys. Ther., 49:1084, 1969.
27. Gregersen, H. N.: Malformatio congenita articuli talocruralis. Acta Orthop. Scand., 45:462, 1974.
28. Grice, D. S.: The role of subtalar fusion in the treatment of valgus deformities of the feet. A.A.O.S. Instr. Course Lect. 16:127, 1959.
29. Güntz, E.: Die pathologische Anatomie der angeborenen Plattfusses. Z. Orthop., 69:219, 1939.
30. Haliburton, R. A., Sullivan, C. R., Kelly, P., and Peterson, L. F. A.: The extra-osseous and intra-osseous blood supply of the talus. J. Bone Joint Surg., 40-A:1115, 1958.
31. Handelsman, J. E.: Treatment of congenital vertical talus. J. Bone Joint Surg., 50-B:439, 1968.
32. Hansteen, I. L., Schirmer, L., and Hestetun, S.: Trisomy 12p syndrome. Clin. Genet., 13:339, 1978.
33. Hark, F. W.: Rocker-foot due to congenital subluxation of the talus. J. Bone Joint Surg., 32-A:344, 1950.
34. Harrold, A. J.: Congenital vertical talus in infancy. J. Bone Joint Surg., 49-B:634, 1967.
35. Harrold, A. J.: The problem of congenital vertical talus. Clin. Orthop., 97:133, 1973.
36. Haveson, S. B.: Congenital flatfoot due to talonavicular dislocation (vertical talus). Radiology, 72:19, 1959.
37. Henken, R.: Contribution a l'étude des formes osseuses du pied valgus congénital. These de Lyon, 1914.
38. Henssge, J., and Allmeling, W.: Therapeutic experiences in congenital flatfoot with vertical talus. Arch. Orthop. Unfallchir., 59:74, 1966.
39. Herndon, C. H., and Heyman, C. H.: Problems in the

recognition and treatment of congenital convex pes valgus. J. Bone Joint Surg., 45-A:413, 1963.
40. Heyman, C. H.: The diagnosis and treatment of congenital convex pes valgus or vertical talus. A.A.O.S. Instr. Course Lect., 16:117, 1959.
41. Hohmann, G.: Fuss und Bein. Munchen, I. F. Bergann, 1934, pp. 26–33.
42. Hohmann, G.: Pes plano-valgus congenitus. In Hohmann, G. (ed.): Handbuch der Orthopadie. Stuttgart, Georg Thieme Verlag, 1961, Vol. IV, Part II, pp. 832–840.
43. Hughes, J. R.: Congenital vertical talus. J. Bone Joint Surg., 39-B:580, 1957.
44. Hughes, J. R.: Pathologic anatomy and pathogenesis of congenital vertical talus and its practical significance. J. Bone Joint Surg., 52-B:777, 1970.
45. Joachimsthal: Ueber pes valgus congenitus. Deutsch. Med. Wschr., 29:(Vereins-Beilage):123, 1903.
46. Judet, J., Esteve, P., Masse, P., and Rigault, P.: Congenital convex foot. Rev. Chir. Orthop., 60:Suppl. 2:370, 1974.
47. Laburthe-Tolra, Y., and Bensahel, H.: Congenital convex talipes valgus (apropos of 19 cases). Ann. Chir., 26:203, 1972.
48. Lamy, L., and Weissman, L.: Congenital convex pes valgus. J. Bone Joint Surg., 21:79, 1939.
49. Lange, F.: Plattfussbeschwerben und Plattfussbehandlung. Munchen. Med. Wschr., 59:300, 1912.
50. Leveuf, J.: Le traitement du pied convexe valgus congénital. Rev. Orthop., 27:129, 1941.
51. Lloyd-Roberts, G. C., and Spence, A. J.: Congenital vertical talus. J. Bone Joint Surg., 40-B:33, 1958.
52. McFarland, B.: Congenital vertical talus. J. Bone Joint Surg., 39-B:480, 1957.
53. Maresca, A.: Considerazioni sulla lussazione congenita astragalo scafoidea nel quadro del cosidetto piede a dondolo. Oriz. Ortop. Odierna Riab., 4:187, 1959.
54. Mau, C.: Muskelbefunde und ihre Bedeutung beim angeborenen Klumpfussleiden. Arch. Orthop. Unfallchir., 28:292, 1930.
55. Mead, N. C., and Anast, G.: Vertical talus. Clin. Orthop., 21:198, 1961.
56. Nové-Josserand: Formes anatomiques du pied plat. Rev. Orthop., 10:117, 1923.
56a. Ogata, K., Schoenecker, P. S., and Sheridan, J.: Congenital vertical talus and its familial occurrence. Clin. Orthop., 139:128, 1979.
57. Osmond-Clarke, H.: Congenital vertical talus. J. Bone Joint Surg., 38-B:334, 1956.
58. Outland, T., and Sherk, H. H.: Congenital vertical talus. A.A.O.S. Instr. Course Lect., 16:214, 1959.
59. Parrish, T. F.: Congenital convex pes valgus accompanied by previously undescribed anatomic derangements. Southern. Med. J., 60:983, 1967.
60. Patterson, W. R., Fitz, D. A., and Smith, W. S.: The pathologic anatomy of congenital convex pes valgus. J. Bone Joint Surg., 50-A:458, 1968.
61. Pouliquen, J. C.: Pied convexe congénital. Rev. Chir. Orthop., Suppl. 2:370, 1974.
62. Rigault, P., and Pouliquen, J. C.: Le pied convexe congénital. Ann. Chir. Infant., Paris, 11:261, 1970.
63. Ritsilä, V. A.: Talipes equinovarus and vertical talus produced experimentally in newborn rabbits. Acta Orthop. Scand., Suppl. 121, 1969.
64. Robbins, H.: Naviculectomy for congenital vertical talus. Bull. Hosp. Joint Dis., 37:77, 1976.
65. Rocher, H. L., and Pouyanne, L.: Pied plat congénital par subluxation sous-astragalienne congénitale et orientation verticale de l'astragale. Bordeaux Chir., 5:249, 1934.
66. Schulitz, K. P., Schumacher, A., and Parsch, K.: Der angeborene Schaukelfuss. Z. Orthop., 115:55, 1977.
67. Searfoss, R., Bendana, A., King, G., and Miller, G.: Vertical talus of unusual etiology. Case report. J. Bone Joint Surg., 57-A:409, 1975.
68. Sharrard, W. J. W., and Grosfield, I.: The management of deformity and paralysis of the foot in myelomeningocele. J. Bone Joint Surg., 50-B:456, 1968.
69. Silk, F. F., and Wainwright, D.: The recognition and treatment of congenital flat foot in infancy. J. Bone Joint Surg., 49-B:628, 1967.
70. Slavik, M., and Stryhal, F.: Congenital steep talus. (Congenital convex pes valgus, congenital vertical talus.) Acta Chir. Orthop. Trauma. Cech., 37:367, 1970.
71. Specht, E. E.: Congenital paralytic vertical talus. J. Bone Joint Surg., 57-A:842, 1975.
72. Stone, K. H., and Lloyd-Roberts, G. C.: Congenital vertical talus: A new operation. Proc. Roy. Soc. Med., 56:12, 1963.
73. Støren, H.: On the closed and open correction of congenital convex pes valgus with a vertical astragalus. Acta Orthop. Scand., 36:352, 1965.
74. Støren, H.: Congenital convex pes valgus with vertical talus. Acta Orthop. Scand., Suppl. 94:1, 1967.
75. Syntheses Bibliographiques: Pied convexe valgus congénital. Rev. Chir. Orthop., 67:27, 1970.
76. Tachdjian, M. O.: Congenital convex pes valgus. Orthop. Clin. N. Amer., 3:131, 1972.
77. Towns, P. L., Dettart, G. K., Hecht, F., and Manning, J. A.: Trisomy 13-15 in a male infant. J. Pediat., 60:528, 1962.
78. Uchida, I. A., Lewis, A. J., Bowman, J. M., and Wang, H. C.: A case of double trisomy: No. 18 and triple-X. J. Pediat., 60:498, 1962.
79. Wainwright, D.: The recognition and cure of congenital flat foot. Proc. Roy. Soc. Med., 57:357, 1964.
80. Wainwright, D.: Congenital vertical talus in infancy. J. Bone Joint Surg., 48-B:588, 1966.
81. Weiss, P.: Principles of development. New York, Henry Holt & Co., 1939.
82. Wertheimer, L. G.: Personal communication to Campos da Paz, Jr. (see ref. 11).
83. Wilkinson, J. A.: Breech malposition and intra-uterine dislocations. Proc. Roy. Soc. Med., 59:1106, 1966.

TARSAL COALITION

In this congenital abnormality, varying degrees of union occur between two or more tarsal bones, producing a rigid planovalgus foot. Buffon, in 1769, was probably the first to recognize tarsal coalition.[21] Since then, Cruveilhier, in 1829, reported the first recorded example of calcaneonavicular coalition; Zuckerkandl is credited with the first anatomic description, in 1877, of talocalcaneal coalition; and Anderson, in 1880, with that of talonavicular synostosis.[4, 33, 162] Heiple and Lovejoy described bilateral talocalcaneal bridges, one complete and one incomplete, in a pre-Columbian Indian skeleton found in Ohio and dating from approximately A.D. 1000.[68] Their report documents the existence of this anomaly in man in ancient times.

The clinical significance of these intertarsal bridges was not appreciated until 1880, when Holl proposed a possible relationship between flatfoot and intertarsal bar.[71] Sir Robert Jones gave the first clinical description of peroneal spastic flatfoot in 1897; but it remained for Slomann and later Badgley to show that at least some cases of rigid pes planovalgus with peroneal spasm are caused by calcaneonavicular bar.[7, 79, 136, 137] In 1948, Harris and Beath reported the correlation between medial talocalcaneal bridge and peroneal spastic flatfoot.[62]

Table 2–10. Incidence of Tarsal Coalition

Author	Material	Incidence (Per Cent)
Pfitzner[118]	Autopsy	0.38 (2 of 524)
Harris and Beath[61]	Army recruits	0.03 (1 of 3.619)*
Vaughan and Segal[148]	Army personnel	1 (21 of 2,000)
Shands and Wentz[131]	Children's clinic	0.9 (11 of 1,232)

*Of 3,619, 74 (2 per cent) had peroneal spastic flatfoot.

Incidence and Classification

The exact incidence of tarsal coalition in the general population is unknown because the reported studies have been based on selected materials (Table 2–10).[61, 118, 131, 148] Probably it is 1 per cent or less, as in none of the series is it above this figure.

Intertarsal coalition may be of many types. It may occur as an isolated anomaly or sometimes be associated with fusions between other bones (such as those of the carpus or the phalanges). Occasionally tarsal coalitions are part of a generalized syndrome. A classification of the various forms is given in Table 2–11. The coalition may be completely osseous (synostosis), or the bones may be divided by a fissure of varying depth consisting of cartilage (synchondrosis) or fibrous tissue (syndesmosis).

The most common coalitions in the tarsus are between the calcaneus and the navicular, and between the talus and the calcaneus. Harris reported the following distribution of the various types of intertarsal bridges found in 102 patients: medial talocalcaneal bridge in 62, calcaneonavicular bar in 29, posterior talocalcaneal bridge in 4, multiple intertarsal fusions in 4, talonavicular fusion in 1, calcaneocuboid fusion in 1, and cubonavicular fusion in 1.[58–63] In this author's clinical practice, calcaneonavicular coalition is the most common type.

Of the intertarsal coalitions, medial talocalcaneal bridge and calcaneonavicular bar are the more significant clinically, as they are responsible for the majority of cases of peroneal spastic flatfoot and cause the greater disability.

Medial talocalcaneal bridge may take a variety of forms: complete, in which a bony bridge connects the talus and calcaneus, as illustrated in Figures 2–63A, 2–64; incomplete, in which a mass of bone projecting from the talus is united to a mass of bone projecting from the sustentaculum tali by a thin plate of fibrous tissue or cartilage, as shown in Figure 2–63B; or rudimentary, in which only one element of the bridge is present, i.e., the bony mass projects either upward from the posterior margin of the sustentaculum tali or downward from the medial surface of the body of the talus posterior to the sustentaculum tali, in either instance blocking inversion of the os calcis (Fig. 2–63 C and D).[60] The complete and incomplete forms are readily recognizable, but in the rudimentary form the roentgenographic changes are equivocal.

Table 2–11. Classification of Types of Tarsal Condition

Isolated anomaly
  Dual between two tarsal bones
    Talocalcaneal
      Medial
        Complete
        Incomplete
        Rudimentary
      Posterior
      Anterior
    Calcaneonavicular
    Talonavicular
    Calcaneocuboid
    Naviculocuneiform
  Multiple—various combinations of the preceding, e.g., talocalcaneal and calcaneocuboid
  Massive—all major tarsal bones fused into a single block of bone
Part of complex malformation
  In association with other synostoses
    Carpal coalition
    Symphalangism
  As one of manifestations of a syndrome
    Nievergelt-Pearlman
    Apert's
  In association with major limb anomalies
    Absence of toes or rays
    "Ball-and-socket" ankle joint
    Fibular hemimelia
    Phocomelia
    Proximal focal femoral deficiency

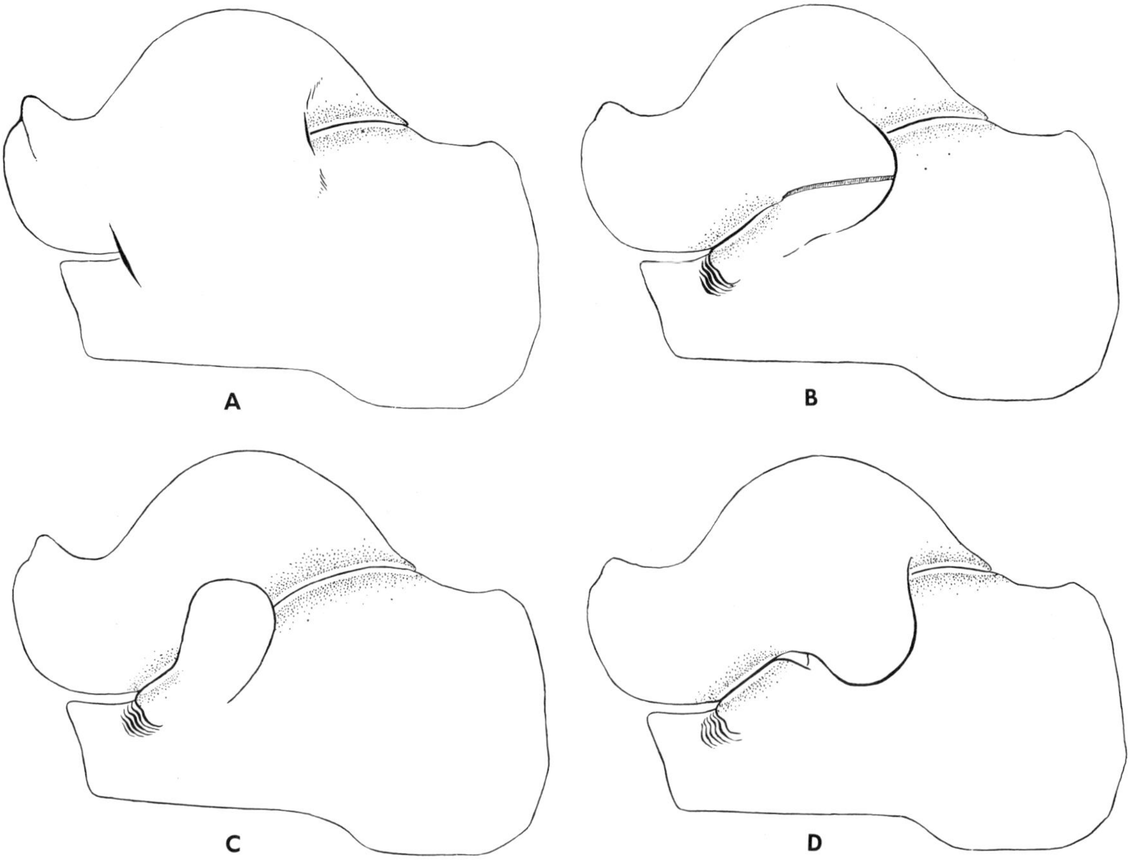

FIGURE 2–63. *Diagrams of variations in medial talocalcaneal coalition (bridge).*

A. Complete medial talocalcaneal coalition. **B.** Incomplete medial talocalcaneal coalition—syndesmosis and synchondrosis. **C.** Rudimentary medial talocalcaneal coalition—sustentacular element. (The bony mass projects upward from the posterior margin of the subtentaculum tali and impinges on the medial side of the body of the talus.) **D.** Rudimentary medial talocalcaneal coalition—talar element. (Bony mass projects downward from the medial surface of the body of the talus posterior to the sustentaculum tali. It impinges on the calcaneus on inversion, though not attached to it.) (From Harris, R. I.: Retrospect—peroneal spastic flat foot (rigid valgus foot). J. Bone Joint Surg., *47-A*:1661, 1965. Reprinted by permission.)

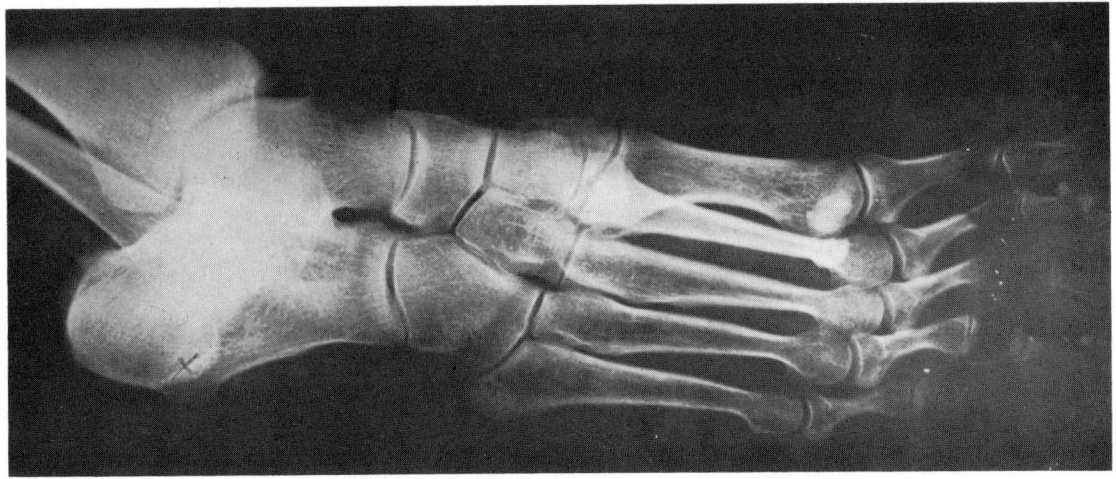

FIGURE 2–64. Complete medial talocalcaneal coalition.

Talonavicular coalition is very rare. The total number of cases reported in the world literature is less than 40; Schreiber has suggested, however, that it may be more common than the literature indicates.[128] Involvement may be unilateral or bilateral, with a definite hereditary factor in the latter.[69, 125]

Calcaneocuboid synostosis was first described by Wagoner in 1928, and isolated case reports have since appeared in the literature.[19, 101, 151] The condition is of ana-

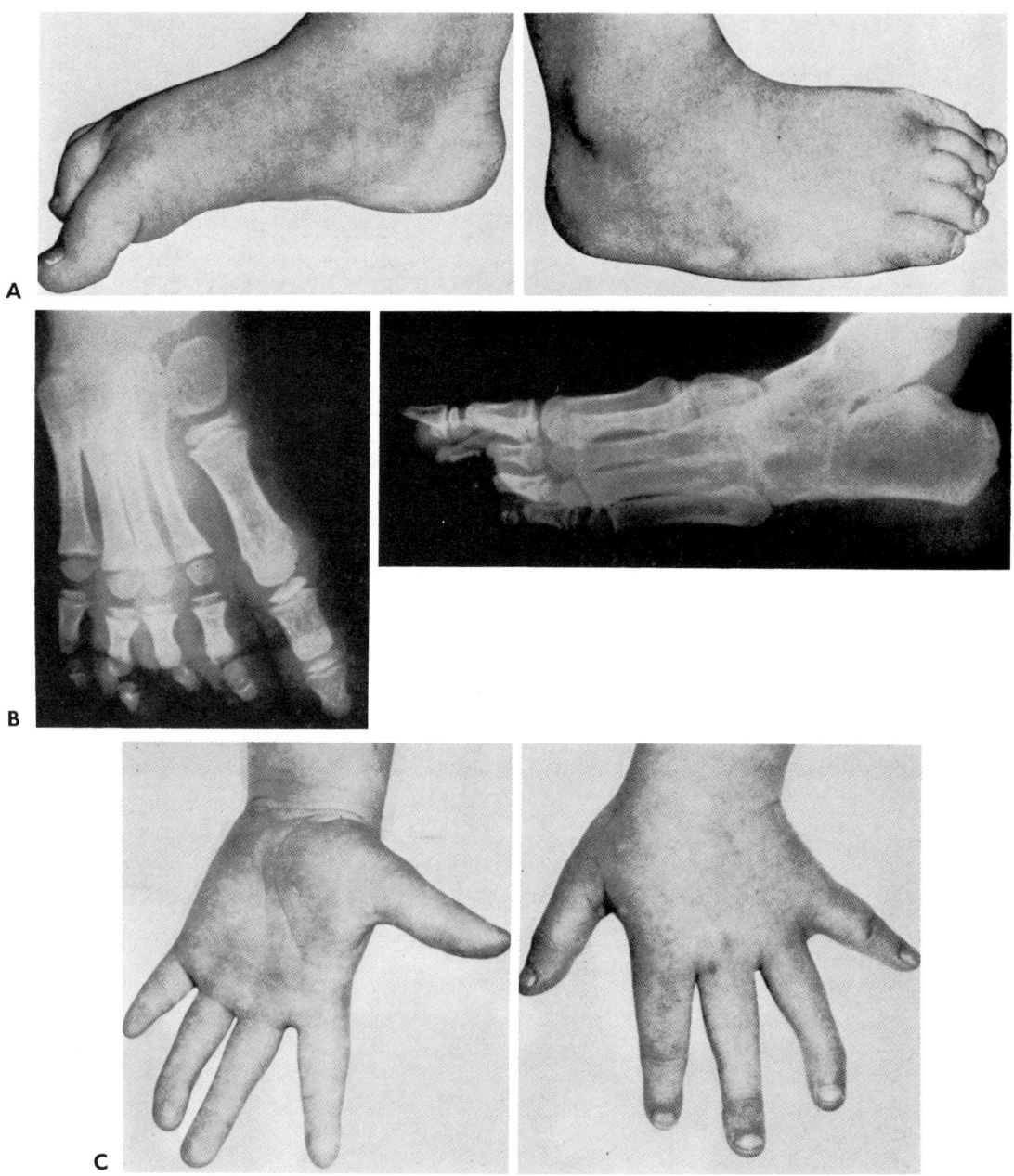

FIGURE 2–65. Nievergelt-Pearlman syndrome—synostoses of feet and hands with dysplasia of the elbows.

A and **B.** Photographs and roentgenograms of feet. There is varus deformity of both feet and massive synostosis of the talus, calcaneus, cuboid, and cuneiform bones. The second, third, and fourth metatarsal bases are fused, with a bony bridge between them and the one tarsal bone. **C.** Photographs of the hands.

Illustration continued on opposite page

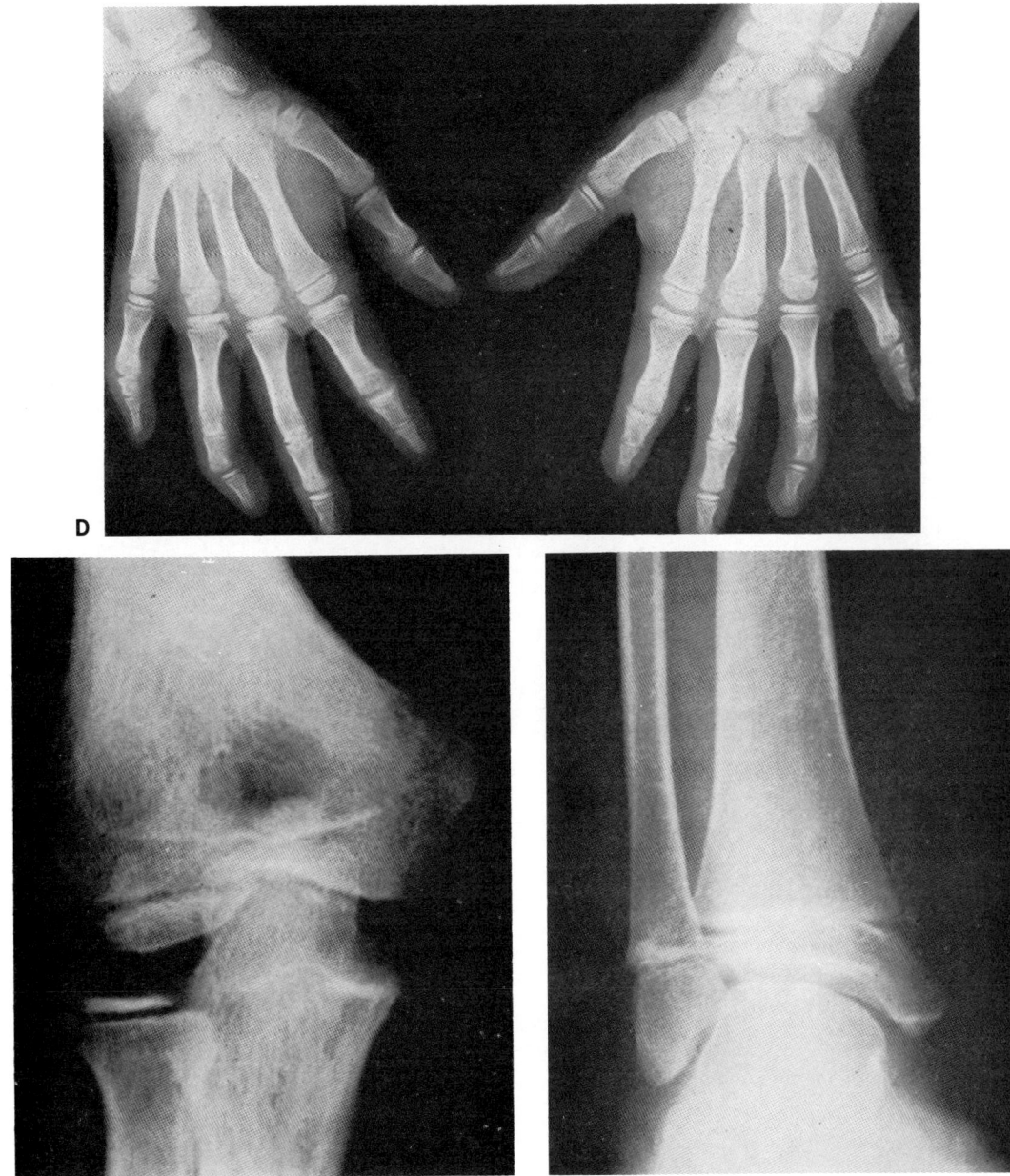

FIGURE 2–65. Continued. Nievergelt-Pearlman syndrome—synostoses of feet and hands with dysplasia of the elbows.

D. Roentgenograms of the hands. The capitate and trapezoid, and the triquetrum and hamate are fused. Note the symphalangism of the proximal interphalangeal joints of the middle and ring fingers and the distal interphalangeal joints of the index and little fingers. **E.** Anteroposterior projections of the elbow and ankle showing dysplasia of the elbow and the typical "ball-and-socket" deformity of the ankle. (From Dubois, H. J.: Nievergelt-Pearlman syndrome. J. Bone Joint Surg., *52-B*:325, 1970. Reprinted by permission.)

tomic interest only, as it is asymptomatic and does not require any orthopedic care.

Cubonavicular synostosis is rare. Waugh reported a case of peroneal spastic flatfoot caused by cubonavicular coalition.[152] Naviculocuneiform synostosis was first described by Lusby; Gregersen reported a bilateral case of symptomatic flatfoot.[54, 100]

Tarsal and carpal coalitions may coexist. Leonard, on clinical and roentgenographic examination, however, did not find any abnormality of the carpus in 69 patients with tarsal coalition. Despite the developmental similarity of the carpus and tarsus, the two conditions seem to be unrelated.[95, 96] Symphalangism (congenital fusion of the proximal or distal interphalangeal joints) may be present in tarsal and carpal coalitions.[6, 22, 41, 56] Tarsal synostoses may occur in phocomelia, fibular hemimelia, or proximal focal femoral deficiency; other anomalies associated with tarsal coalition are "ball-and-socket" ankle joint and absence of toes.[45, 93, 112]

Multiple or massive tarsal coalitions may be part of a more complex syndrome. Nievergelt, in 1944, described a syndrome consisting of tarsal synostosis with clubfeet, bilateral elbow dysplasia with radioulnar synostosis and subluxation of the radial

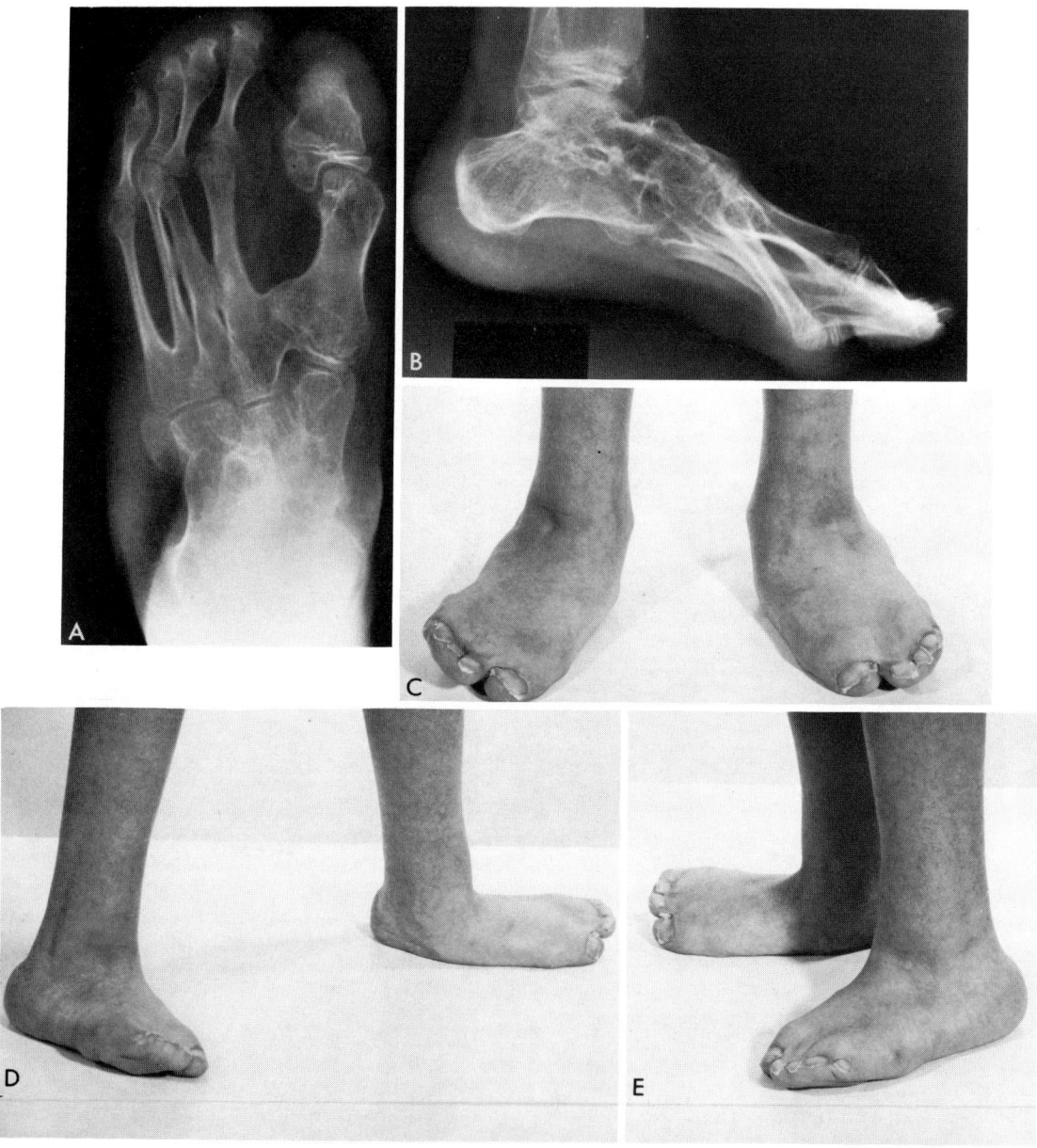

FIGURE 2–66. Massive tarsal coalition in Apert's syndrome.

A and **B.** Roentgenograms of feet. **C, D,** and **E.** Characteristic clinical appearance.

head, and dysplasia of the tibia and fibula with the fibula relatively long because of lesser involvement.[110] Twenty years later, Pearlman, Edkin, and Warren reported a similar combination of deformities in a mother and her daughter; their patients did not have dysplasia of the tibia. The case of Pearlman and associates also presented carpal synostosis, symphalangism, brachydactylia, and clinocamptodactylia. They proposed the name *Nievergelt syndrome*.[117] Dubois reported a case, confirming the descriptions by Nievergelt and Pearlman; the x-rays, in addition, showed a typical ball-and-socket ankle (Fig. 2–65). Dubois suggested that *Nievergelt-Pearlman syndrome* would be more correct.[42] Clinically, when there is dysplasia of the tibia and fibula, the lower legs are short and the deformity is apparent at birth. Roentgenograms will disclose the thick and markedly shortened tibiae, which are triangular in shape. Pronation and supination of the forearms is restricted because of radioulnar synostosis. The syndrome is transmitted as an autosomal dominant trait; it is of interest that Nievergelt's original patient was one of the principal figures in a legal case of disputed paternity—the genetic trait was transmitted to three illegitimate children from three different mothers. Murakami reported three cases of Nievergelt-Pearlman syndrome in a family with impairment of hearing due to bony fusion of the ossicles of the middle ear.[108]

In Apert's syndrome there may be massive synostosis of the tarsal bones (Fig. 2–66). The condition is characterized by craniosynostosis, midfacial hypoplasia, osseous or cutaneous syndactyly of all digits (or commonly, of the second, third, and fourth fingers and toes), and a broad distal phalanx of the thumb and hallux.

Etiology

The exact cause of tarsal coalition is unknown. It seems to arise from failure of differentiation and segmentation of the

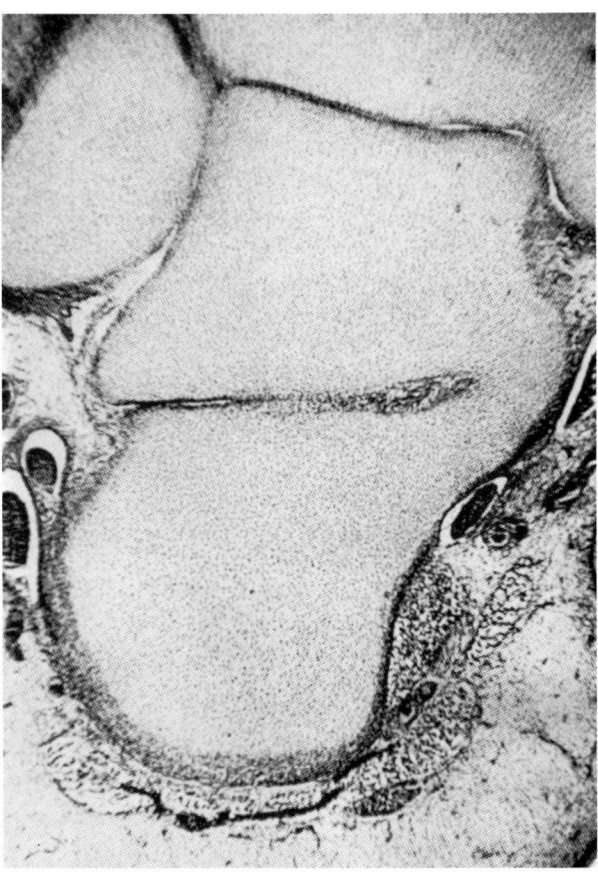

FIGURE 2–67. Complete medial talocalcaneal bridge in the foot of a 72.3 mm. fetus (coronal section).

(Courtesy of Barbara Anne Harris Monie; from Harris, R. I.: Retrospect—peroneal spastic flat foot. J. Bone Joint Surg., 47-A:1658, 1965. Reprinted by permission.)

primitive mesenchyme with resultant lack of joint formation. This theory is supported and confirmed by the finding of intertarsal bridges in fetal feet (Fig. 2–67).[57, 114]

In the past, anatomists such as Pfitzner proposed that tarsal coalition was caused by incorporation of the accessory intertarsal ossicles into the adjacent major tarsal bones.[118] Thus calcaneonavicular coalition was believed to result from the union of the os calcaneus secundarius with the adjacent calcaneus and navicular bones, and incorporation of the os sustentaculare with its neighboring os calcis and talus was believed to cause medical talocaneal coalition. Similarly, one might implicate the os trigonum in posterior talocalcaneal fusion, the os tibiale externum in talonavicular synostosis, the os peroneum in calcaneocuboid fusion, and multiple assessory ossicles in massive tarsal coalition. This hypothesis of incorporation of accessory ossicles is not acceptable, however, as it fails to explain the presence of tarsal coalition in the fetus.

Heredity

In the literature there are several reports of the occurrence of tarsal coalition in several members of the same family. For example, Webster and Roberts described talocalcaneal coalition in two sisters; Boyd reported a family with bilateral talonavicular bars in three generations; Rothberg, Feldman, and Schuster reported familial incidence of bilateral talonavicular synostosis; and Bersani and Samilson reported similar cases involving several tarsal bones.[14, 16, 125, 154] Wray and Herndon, describing the occurrence of calcaneonavicular coalition in three generations of one family, proposed that at least some, perhaps all, cases of calcaneonavicular bar are caused by a specific gene mutation that is autosomally dominant, probably with reduced penetrance.[159] Harris noted calcaneonavicular bars in identical twins and also in a father and son.[60] Glessner and Davis reported monozygotic twins with peroneal spastic flatfoot and tarsal coalition.[52]

Leonard conducted a family survey of 31 patients known to have had treatment for peroneal spastic flatfoot and tarsal coalition (27 calcaneonavicular and 4 talocalcaneal). The pattern of inheritance was studied by clinical and roentgenographic examination of the hands and feet of the 31 index patients and their 98 first-degree relatives—parents, siblings, and children. Some type of tarsal coalition was found in 39 per cent of the first-degree relatives (33 per cent of the parents and 46.5 per cent of the siblings). Of the first-degree relatives of the 27 index patients with calcaneonavicular coalition, 25 per cent had calcaneonavicular fusion, but 14 per cent had talocalcaneal or some other type of tarsal synostosis. In all 11 of the affected first-degree relatives of the four index patients with talocalcaneal coalitions, however, a similar type of fusion was discovered. The findings of Leonard indicate that tarsal coalitions are most probably an inherited autosomal dominant disorder with almost full penetrance. The presence of a different type of tarsal coalition in 14 per cent of the relatives shows that there is no genetic difference in the inheritance of the various coalitions.[97, 98]

Clinical Features

Tarsal coalitions may occur bilaterally or unilaterally. As a rule talonavicular fusions are present in both feet; calcaneonavicular coalition is bilateral in 60 per cent of patients, and talocalcaneal coalition, in 50 per cent.

In infancy and early childhood the condition is usually asymptomatic and is seldom recognized. When the child begins to walk, varying degrees of restriction of motion between the involved tarsal bones may become apparent; during this period, however, the condition is not likely to be suspected, as pain is not a clinical feature, the bar is fibrous or cartilaginous, and the roentgenograms are normal.

Tarsal coalition may be totally asymptomatic and an accidental finding in the roentgenogram. For example, in studying 23 patients with tarsal coalition, Jack found that 5 (22 per cent) were free of symptoms.[75] Leonard was surprised to find that not one of the 38 affected first-degree relatives of the index patients with tarsal coalition had ever had symptoms referable to their feet.[98]

The occurrence of symptoms and the age

of their onset are dependent upon the period at which ossification of the coalition takes place. All coalitions are cartilaginous at birth and may allow motion, whereas a bony union between two or more tarsal bones restricts motion, causing symptoms. According to Cowell, clinical complaints related to talonavicular coalition may develop as early as two years of age; whereas symptoms of calcaneonavicular coalition usually appear between 8 and 12 years of age, and those of talocalcaneal coalition occur during adolescence.[31, 32]

Another factor to consider is the increasing stress and strain exerted on the foot with greater body weight and strenuous physical activity as in sports.

The biomechanics of the foot is disturbed in tarsal coalition. During normal gait the tibia rotates medially 18 degrees during swing phase and the first 15 per cent of stance phase; then lateral rotation of the tibia takes place, reaching its maximum immediately after toe-off, when medial rotation begins again. In the ankle mortise these rotatory motions are transmitted to the talus. The axis of rotation of the subtalar joint is oblique, similar to that of an oblique hinge. Medial rotation of the tibia results in eversion of the calcaneus; conversely lateral rotation of the tibia produces inversion of the calcaneus. With progressive restriction of motion in the subtalar joint, compensatory movement must take place at levels either proximal or distal to it. In the ankle joint the increasing laxity of ligaments predisposes to recurrent ankle sprain; in the transverse tarsal joints the navicular bone

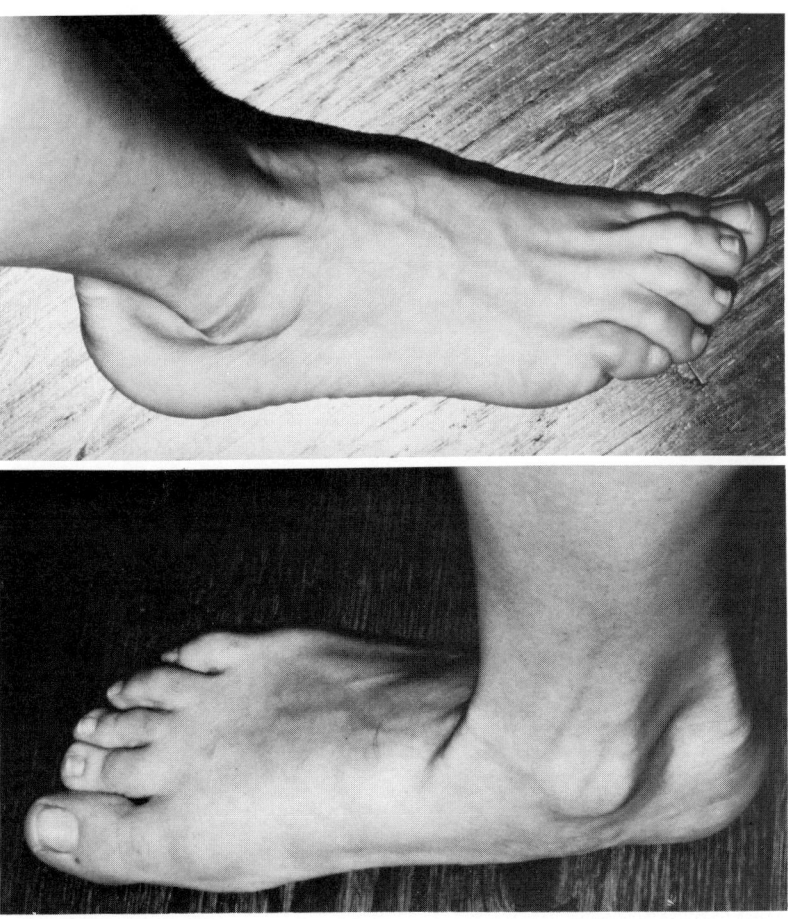

FIGURE 2–68. The clinical findings in peroneal "spastic" flatfoot.

Note the severe pes planovalgus with abduction of the forefoot. The peroneal tendons are taut, and there is marked restriction of subtalar motion.

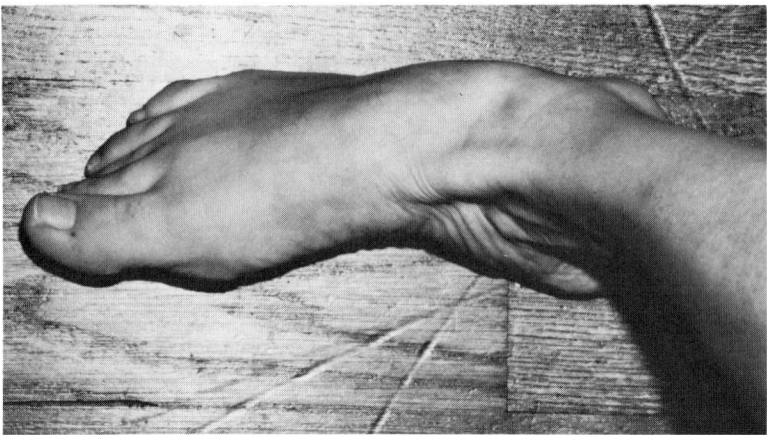

FIGURE 2-69. *Pes varus due to tautness of the anterior tibial muscle in calcaneonavicular coalition.*

gradually becomes displaced dorsolaterally over the head of the talus, causing progressive eversion and valgus deviation of the calcaneus. The peroneal muscles gradually shorten with no true spasticity. When inversion of the hindfoot is attempted, the peroneal muscles are stretched, they contract, and the tautened tendons pull the forefoot into abduction. In medial talocalcaneal coalition, there is progressive restriction of motion on the medial aspect of the joint but not on the lateral aspect, which forces the calcaneus into valgus position, and the longitudinal arch becomes flattened.

The degee of pes valgus varies greatly; it may be very marked or so minimal that it may be overlooked. In general, medial talocalcaneal bridges cause more valgus deformity than do calcaneonavicular coalitions.

Restriction of motion at the subtalar and midtarsal joints is the characteristic physical finding. When the medial talocalcaneal coalition is complete, the hindfoot will be rigidly fixed in some degree of valgus deformity; midtarsal motion may also be restricted. In calcaneonavicular coalitions, motion at the subtalar and midtarsal joints is moderately limited, but usually not completely obliterated.

The most common symptom of tarsal coalition is pain in the subtalar or midtarsal area of the involved foot. It often develops in adolescence, though not in all patients. It is usually noted after some unusual activity or minor trauma, and is aggravated by

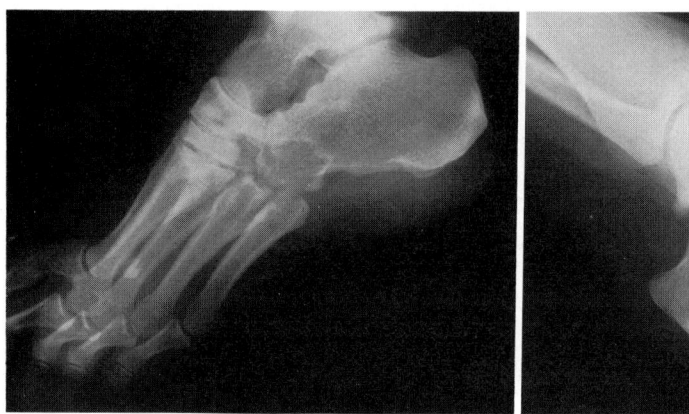 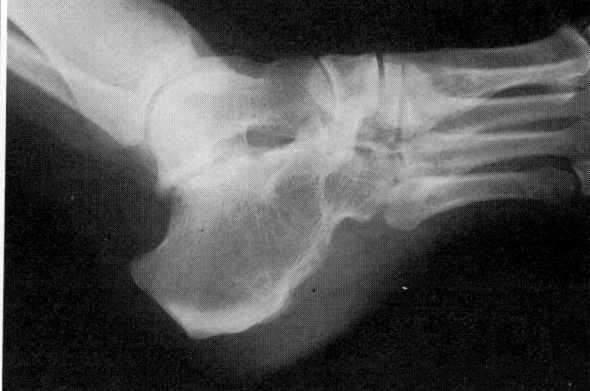

FIGURE 2-70. *Calcaneonavicular synostosis is best visualized in the oblique view.*

Note the bony bridge obliterating the space between the anterior process of the calcaneus and the navicular of both feet.

walking over rough terrain, prolonged standing, jumping, or participating in athletics. Rest relieves the pain. In severe cases the gait may be antalgic.

"Spasm" of the peroneal tendons may develop during the course of the disease. The characteristic findings of peroneal "spastic" flatfoot are restricted subtalar motion, hindfoot valgus deformity, abduction of the forefoot, and tautness of the peroneal tendon. Forced passive inversion of the calcaneus is painful and stretches the peroneal muscles, which contract, increasing the valgus deformity of the foot (Fig. 2–68). In severe cases, the extensor digitorum longus may also be involved. Muscle spasm may occur intermittently or be present continuously in varying severity; overactivity increases it, and rest relieves it.

Occasionally in tarsal coalition, the anterior tibial and posterior tibial muscles are in spasm and cause a varus deformity of the foot (Fig. 2–69).

Peroneal spastic flatfoot may be caused by any condition that restricts the motion and normal biomechanics of the talocalcaneonavicular joint. For example, rheumatoid arthritis may involve the subtalar joint, and it is not uncommon in pauciarticular arthritis for painful peroneal spastic flatfoot to be the presenting complaint. Other conditions include osteochondral fractures involving the anterior or middle facets of the talocalcaneal joint and lesions such as osteoid osteoma or fibrosarcoma.[32]

In talonavicular coalition, the presenting complaint is usually a hard prominence on the medial side of the foot rather than pain. Some cases are discovered accidentally. The longitudinal arch is well maintained. Immobility of the talonavicular joint, however, increases the strain of body weight on the joints adjacent to the fused bones and the cuneiforms. This excess stress may predispose the patient to arthritic changes in adult life. Sanghi and Roby have reported a case

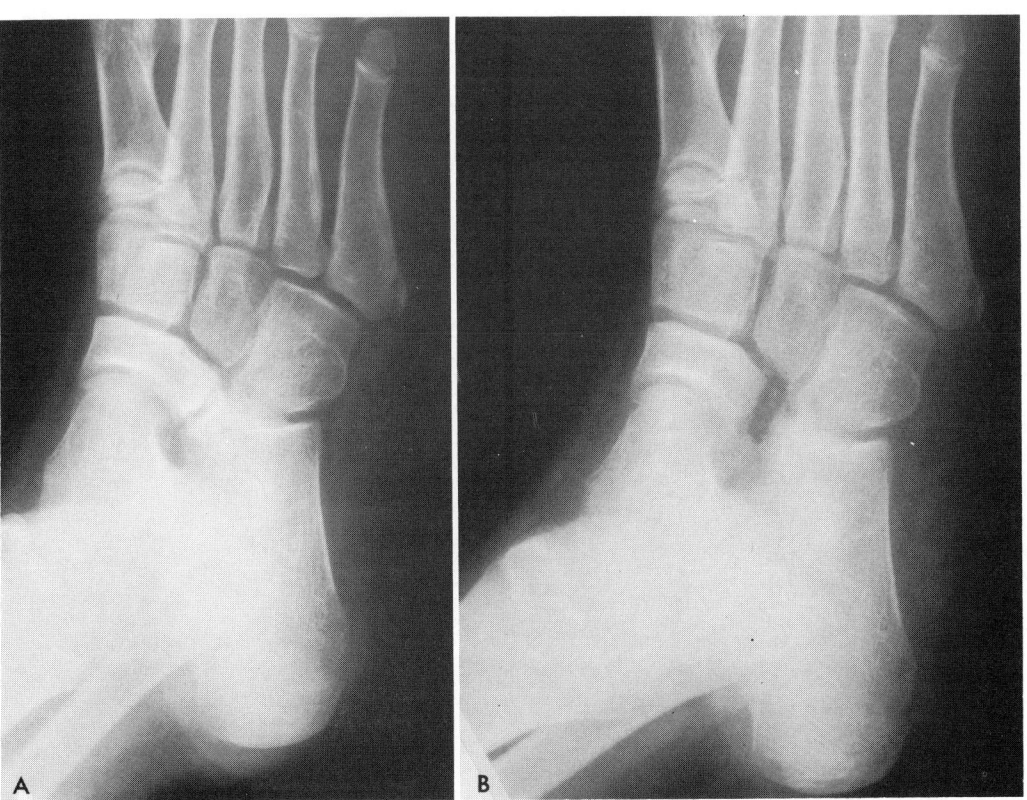

FIGURE 2–71. Calcaneonavicular coalition.

A. Oblique projection of the foot shows a cartilaginous bar; note the flattened ends of the two bones on either side of the cartilaginous bridge. **B.** Postoperative roentgenogram after the bar was excised. Following surgery peroneal spasm disappeared and full range of motion of the subtalar joint was achieved.

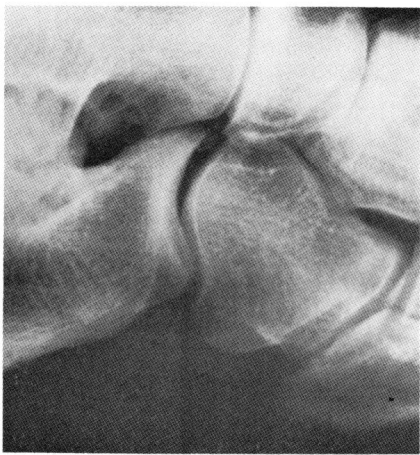

FIGURE 2–72. Oblique roentgenogram of the foot shows os calcaneus secundarius in the calcaneonavicular interspace.

(From Leonard, M. A.: The inheritance of tarsal coalition and its relation to spastic flatfoot. J. Bone Joint Surg., 56-B:522, 1974. Reprinted by permission.)

of bilateral peroneal spastic flatfoot associated with talonavicular coalition.[127]

Roentgenographic Findings

The roentgenographic appearance of tarsal coalition depends upon its site and whether it is bony or fibrocartilaginous. The radiologic examination of the foot should proceed in an orderly manner from the routine and simple to more sophisticated studies. Initial roentgenograms include anteroposterior, lateral, and oblique projections; these will clearly show coalitions between the talus and the navicular and between the calcaneus and the cuboid.

Calcaneonavicular coalitions are best demonstrated in a 45-degree oblique view of the foot made with the patient standing on the film and the x-ray beam projected through the middle of the foot from the lateral to the medial side (Fig. 2–70). Overlap of the tarsal bones may be mistaken for synostosis; in such instances, oblique projections at various angles are necessary for a definitive diagnosis. The importance of these oblique views cannot be overemphasized, as often in the regular anteroposterior and lateral views of the foot, a calcaneonavicular bar may be entirely overlooked.

The connecting bar between the calcaneus and the navicular may be either bony or cartilaginous. When bony, the bridge is at least 1 cm. wide, completely obliterates the space between the calcaneus and the navicular, and is clearly visible in the oblique roentgenogram. When the union is cartilaginous or fibrous, however, diagnosis is not that simple. Such a possibility should be suspected when the anterior medial end of

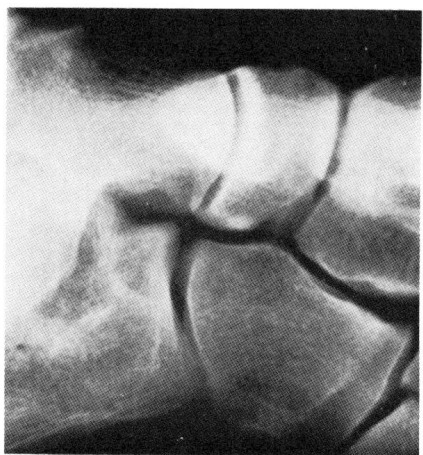 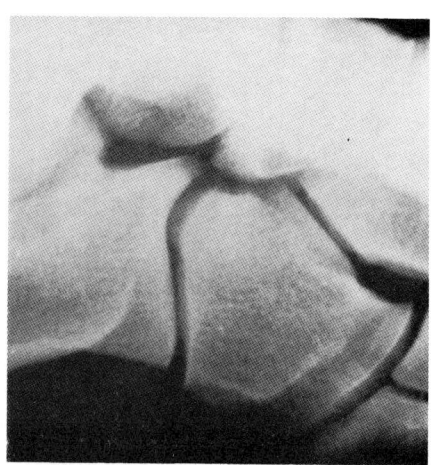

FIGURE 2–73. Slender prolongation of the anterior process of the calcaneus.

A An oblique roentgenogram of a normal foot. **B.** An oblique roentgenogram of the foot showing a slender prolongation of the anterior process of the calcaneus; there may be a cartilaginous bar. (From Leonard, M. A.: The inheritance of tarsal coalition and its relation to spastic flatfoot. J. Bone Joint Surg., 56-B:521, 1974. Reprinted by permission.)

the calcaneus and the navicular are in close proximity and their contiguous cortical surfaces are flattened, having the appearance of a pseudarthrotic joint (Fig. 2–71). Hypoplasia of the head of the talus is another associated finding. Fracture of the anterior process of the calcaneus and the presence of an os calcaneus secundarius should be considered in the differential diagnosis (Fig. 2–72). In chip fracture the bone fragment has a well-delineated trabecular structure, and its surfaces are smooth and clearly demarcated.

Occasionally, the oblique roentgenograms of the foot may show a slender prolongation of the anterior process of the calcaneus; this may contain a cartilaginous bar and be pathologic (Fig. 2–73). To determine whether it is, one may have to resort to arthrography, as described later, or wait until further ossification takes place.

Special projections are necessary to demonstrate talocalcaneal coalitions. Korvin, in 1934, was the first to describe use of the axial view of the calcaneus to reveal talocalcaneal coalition.[90] Harris and Beath, in 1948, emphasized the relation of peroneal spastic flatfoot to talocalcaneal bridge and recommended a 45-degree-angle axial view of the calcaneus for its demonstration.[62]

The subtalar joint is complex, consisting of anterior, middle, and posterior joints that are formed by three separate pairs of facets on the superior surface of the calcaneus and the inferior surface of the talus. The middle and anterior facets are located in the anterior compartment, and the posterior facet is in the posterior compartment (Fig. 2–74). The two compartments are separated by the interosseous talocalcaneal ligament. All three parts of the subtalar joint should be studied to rule out the presence of talocalcaneal coalition. The middle and posterior facet joints usually lie in approximately parallel planes and within the same plane as the sustentaculum (Fig. 2–75). The angle of the sustentaculum (an angle of 30 to 45 degrees to the longitudinal axis of the calcaneus) is determined in the standing lateral roentgenogram, and the axial view of the calcaneus is made at that angle (usually 30, 35, 40, or 45 degrees) (Fig. 2–76). The anterior facet joint is a variable structure; it may be separate and distinct, or it may extend from the middle facet; on occasion it may be absent. When the calcaneus is viewed from above and posteriorly (as in the axial roentgenographic projection) the posterior and middle facets lie in a horizontal plane, but the anterior facet is inclined downward and medially. In the standard lateral roentgenogram of the foot, the middle and posterior facets are clearly visible; the anterior facet, however, is obscured because of its downward and medial inclination. When the foot is rotated so that the projection is not truly lateral, or the x-ray tube is not centered correctly, the middle joint may not be visualized because it is superimposed on the body of the calcaneus. In pes planovalgus, penetrated axial views should be utilized.

A bony coalition across the middle subtalar joint will show continuity of osseous

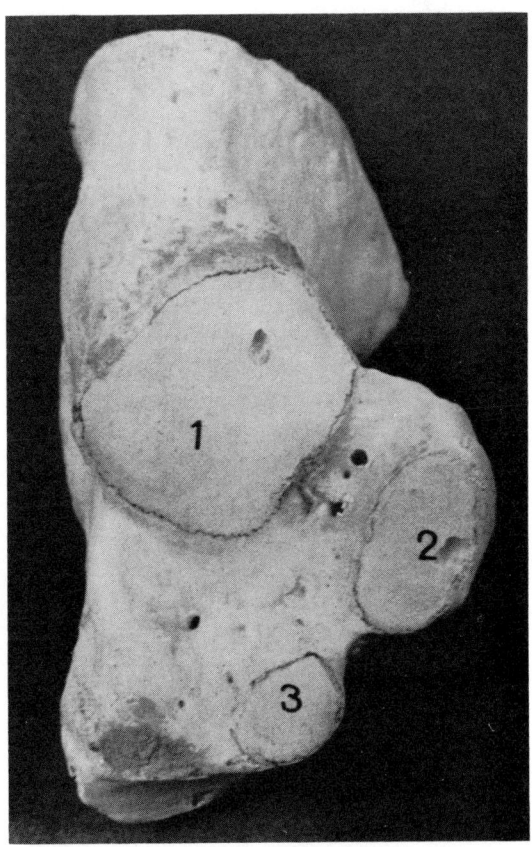

FIGURE 2–74. The dorsal surface of the calcaneus.

Note the three facets of the talocalcaneal joint. The posterior facet (1) is in the posterior compartment. The middle facet (2) and the anterior facet (3) are in the anterior compartment. (Courtesy of Dr. H. Cowell.)

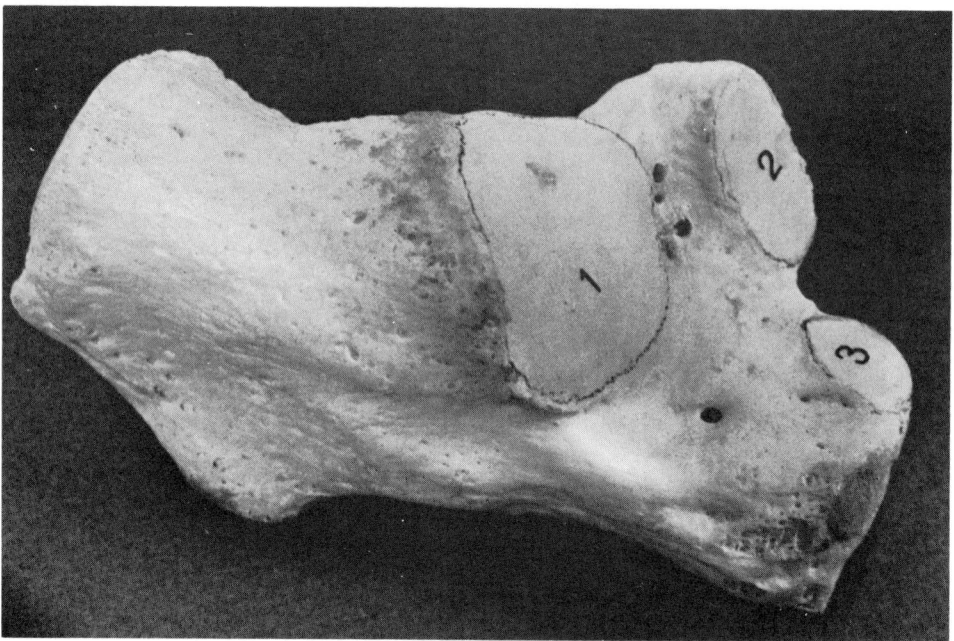

FIGURE 2–75. Facets of the subtalar joint.

In this anatomic specimen the posterior and middle facets (1 and 2) are in the same plane and can be easily visualized in the proper axial projection, whereas the anterior facet (3) is in a different plane and usually is obscured by the head of the talus in the axial view. (Courtesy of Dr. H. Cowell.)

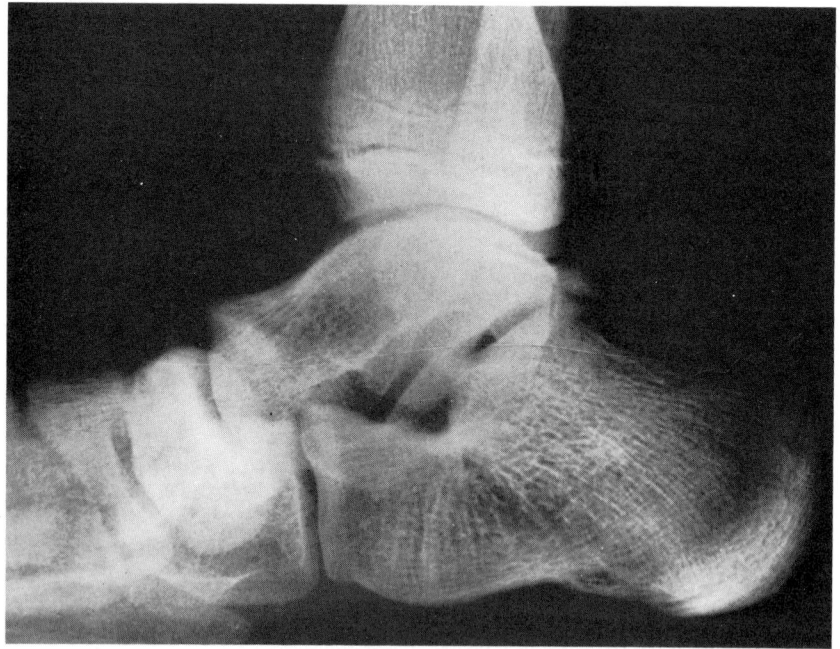

FIGURE 2–76. The proper angle for the axial view of the talocalcaneal joint is determined in the standing lateral roentgenogram.

Note in this extreme example the variation in the plane of the posterior and middle facets; an angle of 40 degrees is necessary to visualize the posterior facet, and an angle of 55 degrees is required for the middle facet. (Ordinarily the middle and posterior facet joints lie within the same plane as the sustentaculum.) (Courtesy of Dr. H. Cowell.)

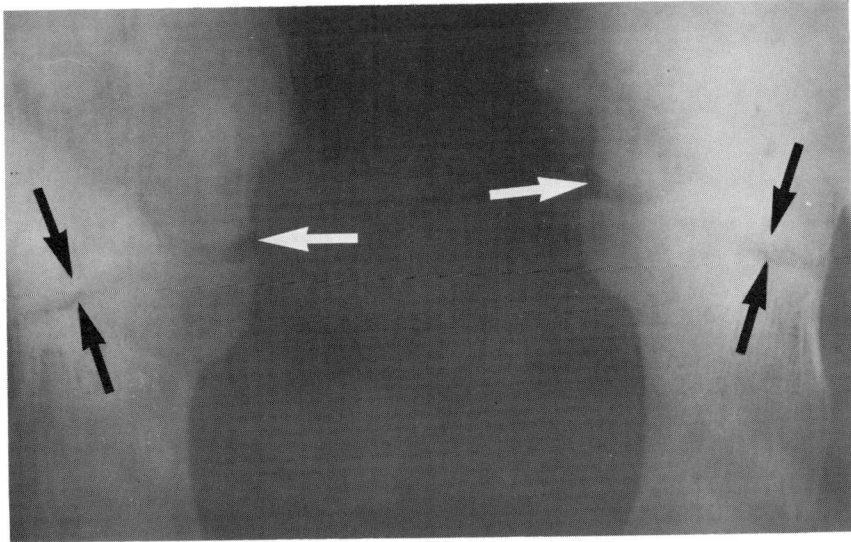

FIGURE 2–77. Penetrated axial view showing a complete bony coalition of the middle facet joint (right) with continuous bony trabeculae between the talus and the sustentaculum.

On the left, there is cartilaginous coalition; note that the radiolucent line lacks normal cortication, is narrowed and inclined downward and medially.

trabeculae between the sustentaculum tali and the talus, obliterating the cartilage space in the axial view (Fig. 2–77). When the coalition is fibrous or cartilaginous a radiolucent line separates the sustentaculum tali from the talus; the margins of this radiolucent line are irregular and lack cortication. In addition, the plane of the radio-

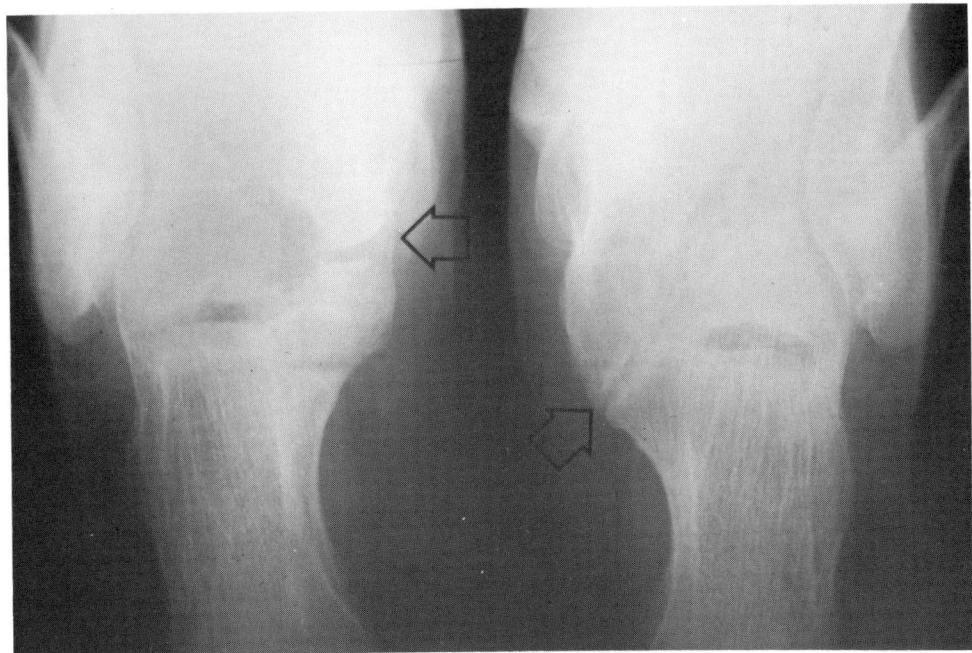

FIGURE 2–78. Penetrated axial view of both feet.

On the left the middle facet joint is normal; note the radiolucent articular cartilage space lies horizontally. On the right there is fibrocartilaginous coalition of the middle facet joint—its radiolucent line is tilted medially and downward with irregular margins that lack cortication.

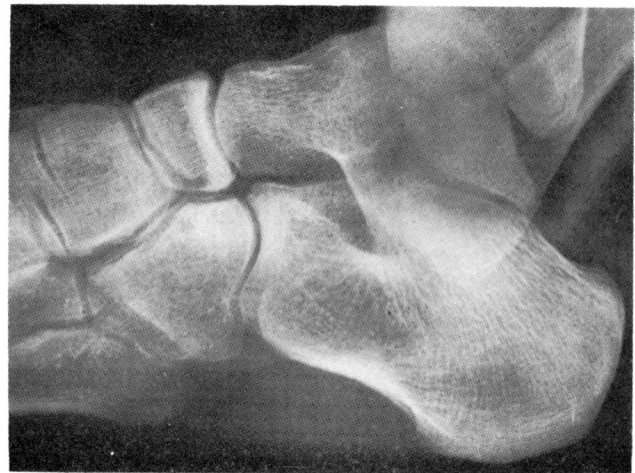

FIGURE 2–79. *The oblique lateral dorsoplantar projection of a normal tarsus.*

Note the clear visualization of the anterior part of the talocalcaneonavicular joint. (From Isherwood, I.: A radiological approach to the subtalar joint. J. Bone Joint Surg., *43-B*:566–574, 1961. Reprinted by permission.)

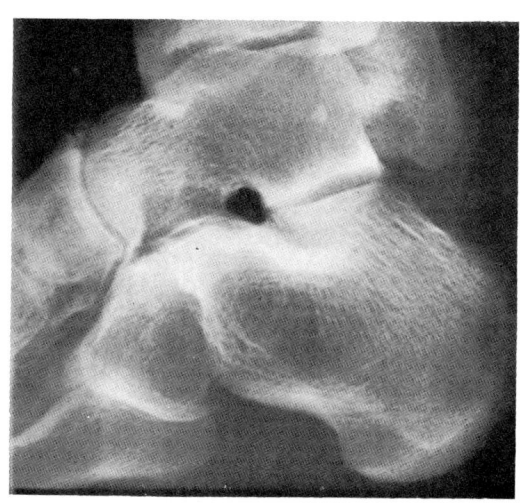

FIGURE 2–80. *Medial oblique axial projection of a normal foot.*

The middle facet joint is well seen. Also depicted is a tangential view of the convexity of the posterior facet joint. (From Isherwood, I.: A radiological approach to the subtalar joint. J. Bone Joint Surg., *43-B*:566–574, 1961. Reprinted by permission.)

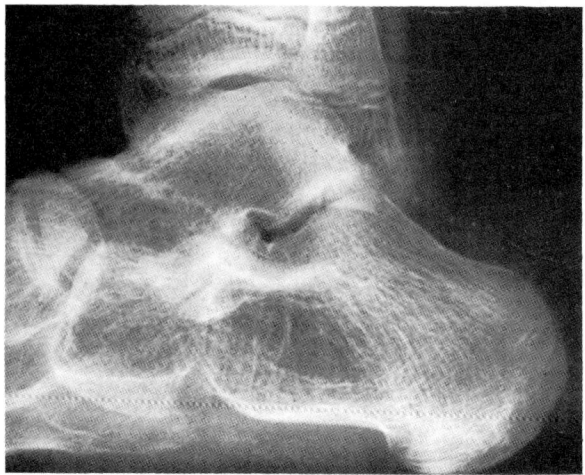

FIGURE 2–81. *Medial oblique axial projection of a foot with talocalcaneal coalition.*

Note the bony union in the posterior aspect of the middle facet joint. (From Isherwood, I.: A radiological approach to the subtalar joint. J. Bone Joint Surg., *43-B*:566–574, 1961. Reprinted by permission.)

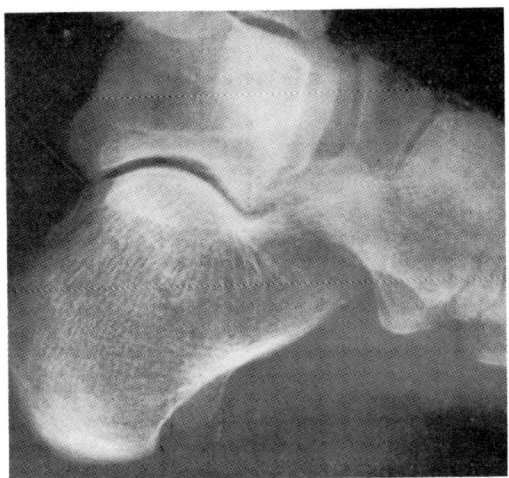

FIGURE 2–82. *Lateral oblique axial projection of a normal foot.*

The posterior facet joint is clearly depicted. (From Isherwood, I.: A radiological approach to the subtalar joint. J. Bone Joint Surg., *43-B*:566–574, 1961. Reprinted by permission.)

lucent line in medial talocalcaneal coalition is inclined medially and downward, in contrast to the more horizontal position of the normal middle facet joint (Fig. 2–78).

Isherwood recommends the following projections for the roentgenographic study of the talocalcaneonavicular joint. The *oblique lateral dorsoplantar view* will often demonstrate the anterior facet joint (Fig. 2–79). The medial border of the foot is placed on the film, with the sole tilted at 45 degrees to the cassette. The tube is centered 2.5 cm. distal and 2.5 cm. anterior to the lateral malleolus.[74]

The *medial oblique axial view* will show the middle joint, and a tangential projection of the convexity of the posterior joint will be depicted (Figs. 2–80 and 2–81). The film is made with the foot dorsiflexed and, when possible, inverted. The position is maintained by strapping with a wide bandage. The limb is rotated 60 degrees medially,

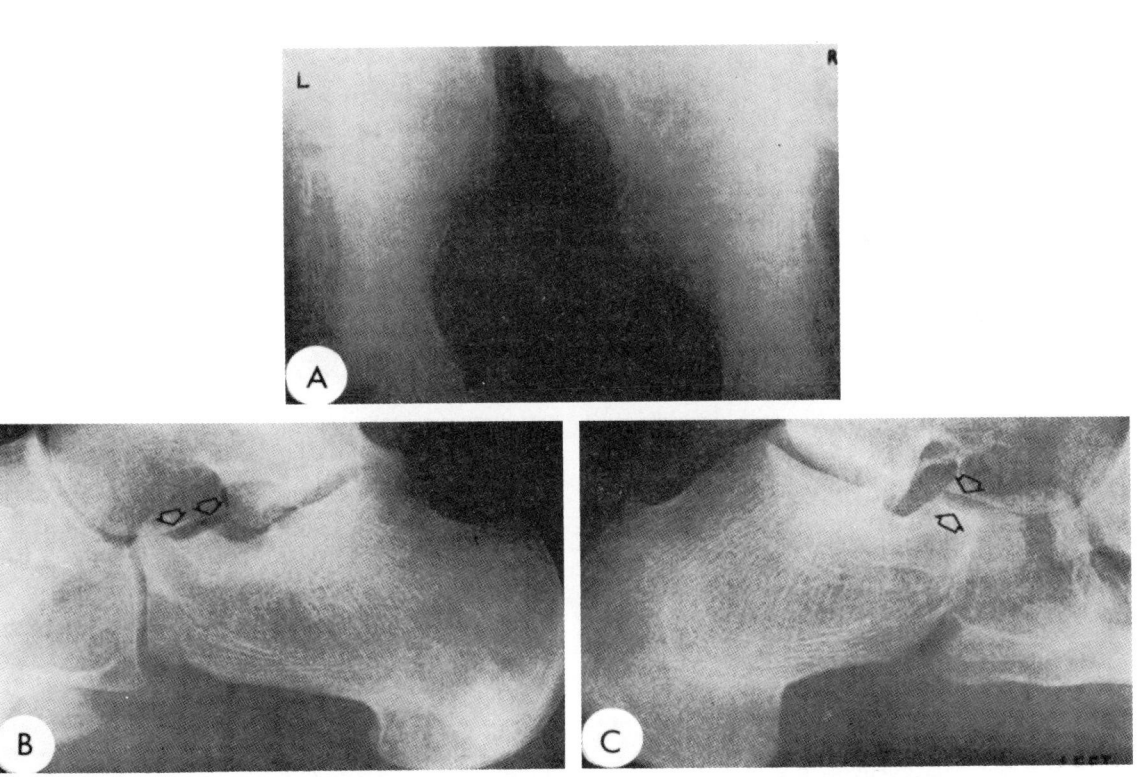

FIGURE 2–83. *Apparent bony coalition between the talus and the sustentaculum.*

A. Penetrated axial projection. Note the absence of the middle joint space. Multiple axial views using different tube angulations failed to show any middle joint cartilage space. **B.** Lateral view of the same foot shows the middle facet joint space. Note the axis of the middle facet joint is more nearly horizontal than usual; it is not in the same oblique plane as the posterior facet joint. **C.** Medial oblique axial view of the same foot clearly demonstrates the middle facet joint space. (From Beckly, D. E., Anderson, P. W., and Pedegana, L. R.: The radiology of the subtalar joint with special reference to talo-calcaneal coalition. Clin. Radiol. *26*:340, 1975. Reprinted by permission.)

and the foot is placed on a 30-degree wedge. The tube is directed axially, tilted 10 degrees cephalad, and centered 2.5 cm. below and 2.5 cm. anterior to the lateral malleolus. The asymmetrical pull of the strapping will maintain inverted posture. The sustentaculum tali is close to the film for bone detail, and an "end-on" view of the tarsal canal is given.[74]

The *lateral oblique axial view* will demonstrate the posterior joint in profile (Fig. 2–82). The foot is dorsiflexed and, when possible, everted, the position being maintained by the asymmetrical pull of the strapping. The limb is rotated laterally 60 degrees, the knee flexed when necessary, and the foot placed on a 30-degree wedge. The tube is directed axially, tilted 10 degrees cephalad, and centered 2.5 cm. below the medial malleolus. Tube direction and tilt may be fixed for both oblique axial views.[74]

When the middle facet joints are more nearly horizontal than usual in the axial view, the articular cartilage space may be obscured and misinterpreted as coalition. Even multiple axial views may fail to demonstrate the middle facet joint, but normal joint spaces will be seen in the oblique, axial, and lateral projections (Fig. 2–83).[10] Occult coalitions of the anterior and middle joints are best demonstrated by tomography (Figs. 2–84 and 2–85). Conway and Cowell have described the tomographic technique for demonstrating the talocalcaneal joint.[28] Computed tomography will clearly visualize the coalition of the talocalcaneal joint (Fig. 2–85).

One should be cautious in interpreting lateral plain tomograms, as obliquity of the anterior joint may give a false appearance of coalition. The anterior facet joint is clearly demonstrated in plain films made in the lateral oblique position; therefore in dubious cases when tomography is indicated, the lateral oblique or the coronal plane should be used.[10]

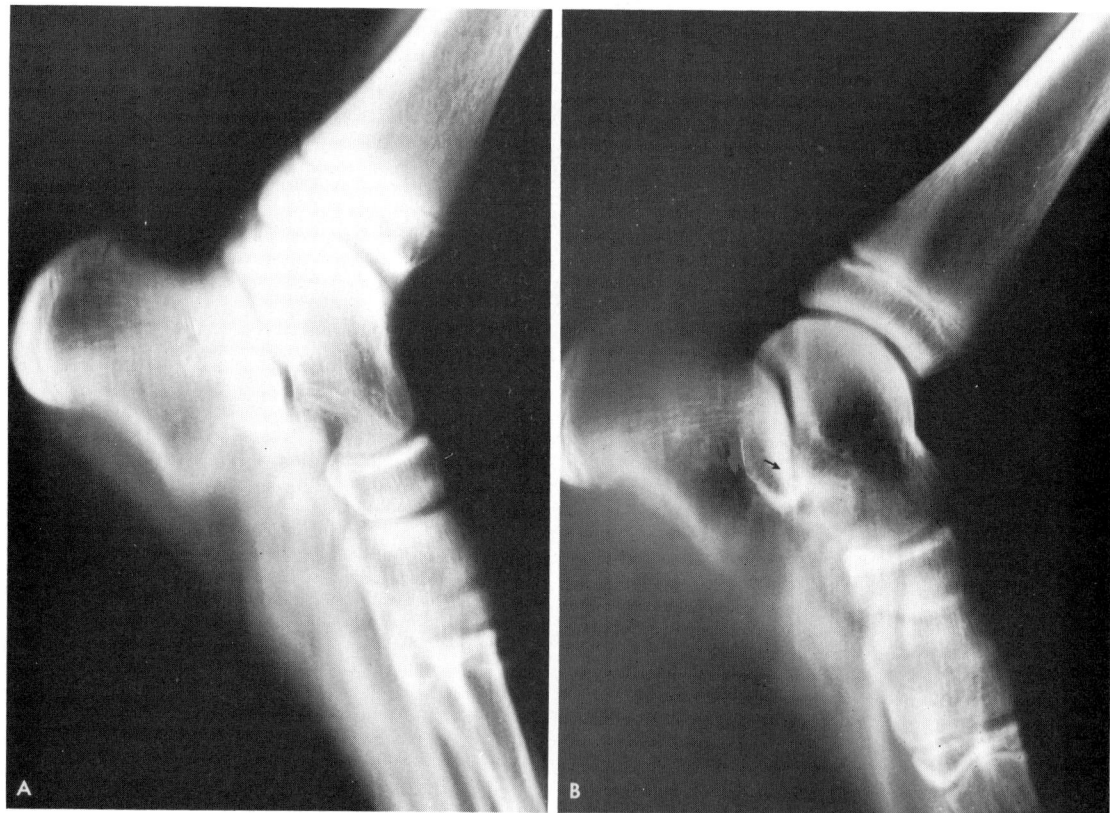

FIGURE 2–84. Coalitions of the middle facet of the talocalcaneal joint.

A and **B**. Simple tomograms. **A**. Normal foot. **B**. Foot with a middle facet coalition.

Illustration continued on opposite page.

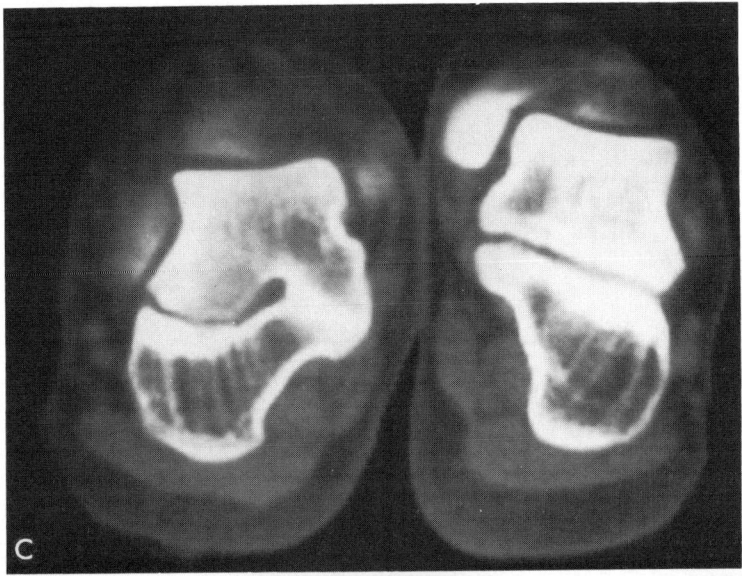

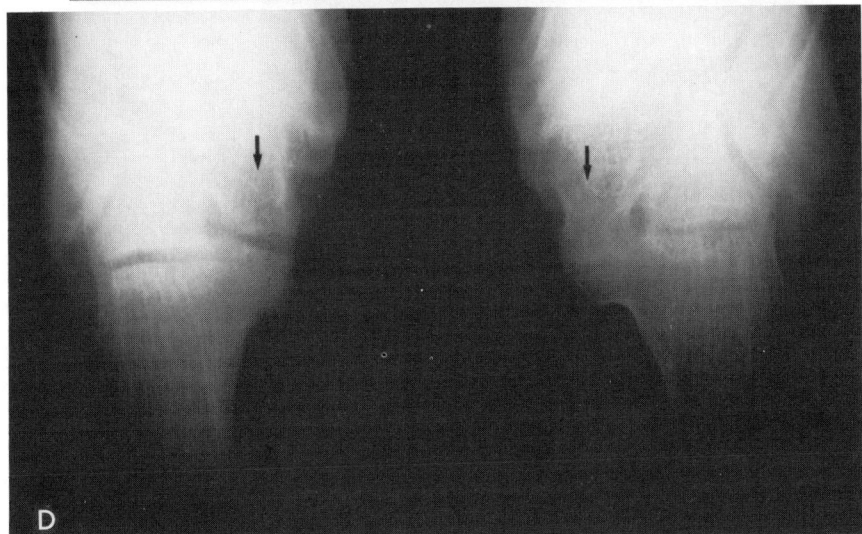

FIGURE 2–84 Continued. Coalitions of the middle facet of the talocalcaneal joint.

C. CT scan of both feet showing medial talocalcaneal coalition of right foot. **D.** Harris axial views of both feet of same patient showing medial talocalcaneal coalition of the right foot. (Courtesy of Dr. H. Cowell.)

Restriction of movement between the talus above and the calcaneus, cuboid, and navicular below results in certain secondary changes visible in the plain roentgenogram. These vary in intensity, depending upon the type of coalition, whether the intertarsal bridge is complete or incomplete, and the age of the patient. They are best seen in standing lateral roentgenograms of the foot (i.e., the patient standing, the film vertical on the medial side of the foot, and the x-ray beam projected from the lateral side with the rays parallel to the ground).

The most striking secondary change is beaking on the dorsal and lateral aspect of the head of the talus adjacent to the talonavicular joint (Fig. 2–86). There is obvious absence of other signs of degenerative arthritis. There are no hypertrophic changes on the navicular, the articular cartilage space is not narrowed, and there is no associated subchondral sclerosis nor any cys-

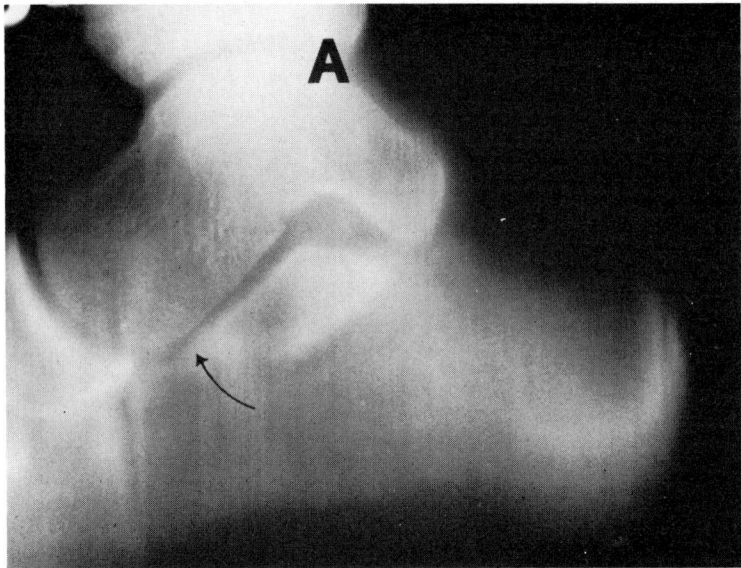
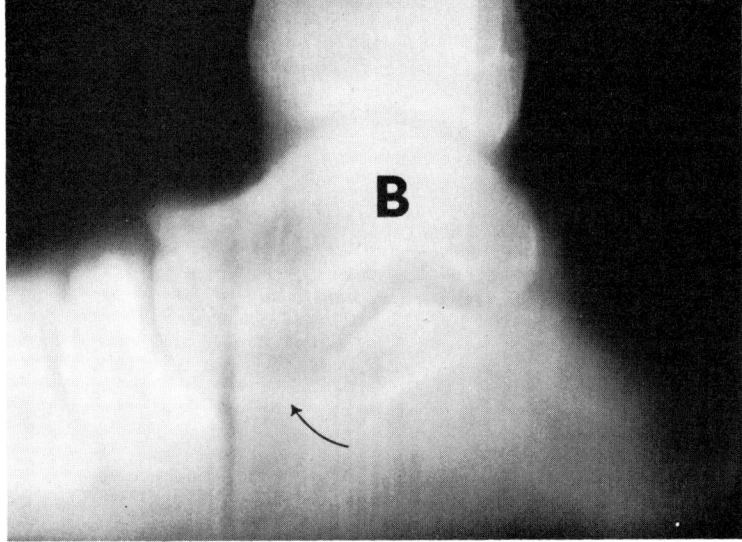

FIGURE 2–85. *Tomograms of anterior facet of talocalcaneal joint.*

A. Normal foot. **B.** Foot with talocalcaneal coalition. Note the talar beak and the irregularity and haziness of anterior facet, indicating coalition. (Courtesy of Dr. H. Cowell.)

tic bony changes. The cause of talar beak is the repeated minute elevation of the talus in response to abnormal mechanics of the subtalar joint; it is not a true degenerative arthritic process, though that may develop later in untreated cases of long standing.

Outland and Murphy proposed that talar beak is produced by impingement of the dorsal part of the navicular on the head of the talus during dorsiflexion. The navicular is rigidly held to the calcaneus by the plantar and lateral calcaneonavicular ligaments. When motion of the subtalar joint is limited, the dorsal aspect of the navicular will impinge on the head of the talus.[115, 116]

Other secondary changes in talocalcaneal coalition are narrowing of the posterior talocalcaneal facet joint space and broadening of the lateral process of the talus, which has a rounded appearance. This may be associated with flattening and even concavity on the undersurface of the neck of the talus on the side with coalition (Fig. 2–86).[26] A ball-and-socket ankle joint may be present.[93]

Talonavicular coalition is readily diagnosed by the evident absence of the talonavicular joint space as seen on the lateral roentgenogram.

Arthrography of the talocalcaneonavicular joint with tangential views of the subtalar

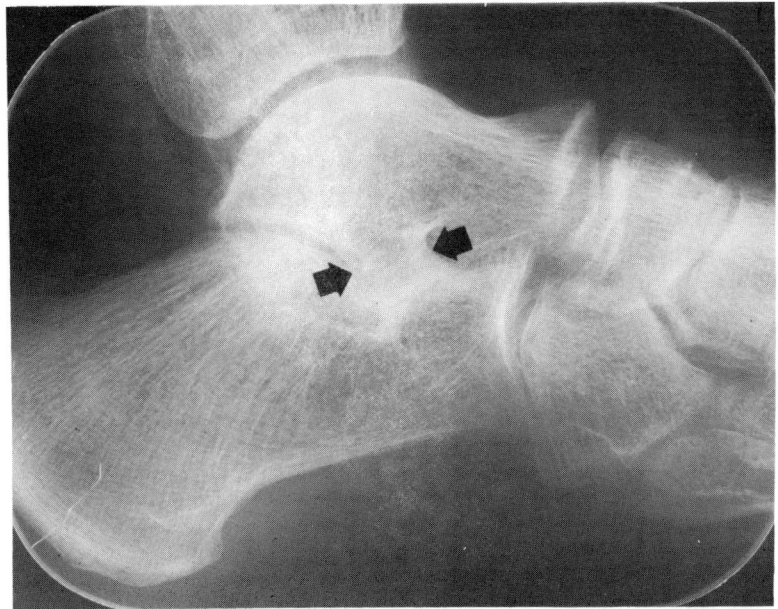

FIGURE 2–86. Secondary signs of calcaneonavicular coalition as seen in the lateral roentgenogram of the foot.

Note the beaking of the head of the talus, the broadening of the lateral process of the talus, and the narrowing of the cartilage space of the posterior subtalar joint.

articulation (Harris views) provides another way to detect talocalcaneal coalition. It is indicated when the routine roentgenograms are normal in painful rigid flatfoot. This author, however, recommends computed tomography of the hindfoot because it is noninvasive and accurate.

The technique of arthrography of the talocalcaneonavicular joint is as follows: the foot and leg are prepared, and sterile drapes are applied. Following local skin anesthesia, 3 to 4 ml. of positive contrast material is instilled through a 22-gauge needle into the talonavicular joint from its dorsal aspect. The site of injection is located 1 cm. lateral to the pulsation of the dorsalis pedis artery. Brief visualization of the lateral projection with image intensification will facilitate correct placement of the needle. Upon entrance into the joint cavity, the contrast material is introduced; it should flow easily, outlining the talocalcaneonavicular joint space. The films taken are the anteroposterior, lateral, and oblique projections of the foot, and tangential Harris views at 35-, 45-, and 55-degree angles from the horizontal.[122]

In the normal foot the talocalcaneonavicular joint space is filled with the contrast material. Therefore, in the lateral view the contrast material can be seen extending above the sustentaculum tali (Fig. 2–87). In the Harris tangential views the thin medial joint space filled by the contrast material can be clearly visualized. These findings exclude a fibrous, cartilaginous, or bony coalition. In the presence of talocalcaneal coalition the arthrogram will fail to show contrast material in the talocalcaneonavicular joint area.

The posterior compartment does not communicate with the anterior compartment, and the posterior joint is clearly visible in standard roentgenograms. Its arthrography is rarely warranted. The injection may, however, be made through a medial approach. The site of insertion of the needle is 1 cm. inferior to the medial malleolus and 1 cm. posterior to the pulsation of the posterior tibial vessels. Under image intensifier control, the needle is advanced distally (toward the toes) and dorsally into the space between the posterior facets of the talus and calcaneus. Care is taken to stay away from the interosseous talocalcaneal ligament and the anterior compartment. Contrast material (1.5 to 2.5 ml.) is instilled, and roentgenograms in the anteroposterior, lateral, and oblique projections are made (Fig. 2–88).[122]

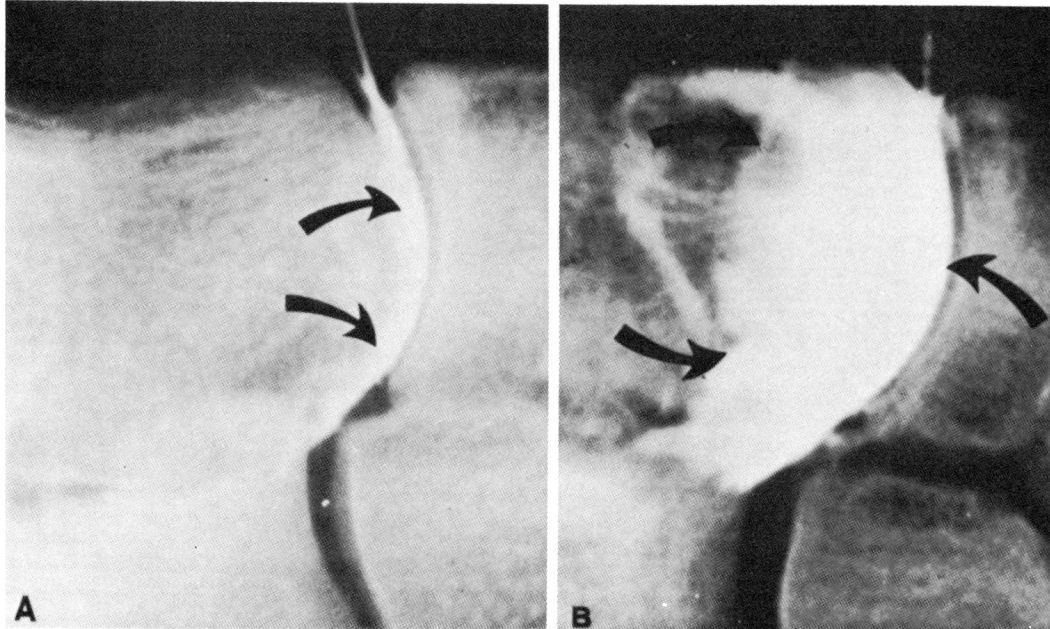

FIGURE 2–87. *Arthrography of the talocalcaneonavicular joint of a normal foot.*

The contrast material is introduced through the dorsal capsule of the talonavicular joint. Oblique projections show, **A**, partial filling and, **B**, complete filling of the synovial cavity *(curved arrows)*. (From Resnick, D.: Radiology of the talocalcaneal articulation. Radiology, *111*:586, 1974. Reprinted by permission.)

Treatment

The treatment varies according to the type of coalition, the age of the patient, the severity of deformity, and the degree of disability caused by pain and muscle spasm.

Many patients with tarsal coalition have little discomfort and will not require treatment. During the growing years, ⅛ to 3/16 inch inner heel wedges on the shoes, Thomas heel, extended medial heel counter, and longitudinal arch support may be used. If the valgus deformity is of significant degree, however, a well-fitted UCBL (University of California Biomechanical Laboratory) foot orthosis will prove more effec-

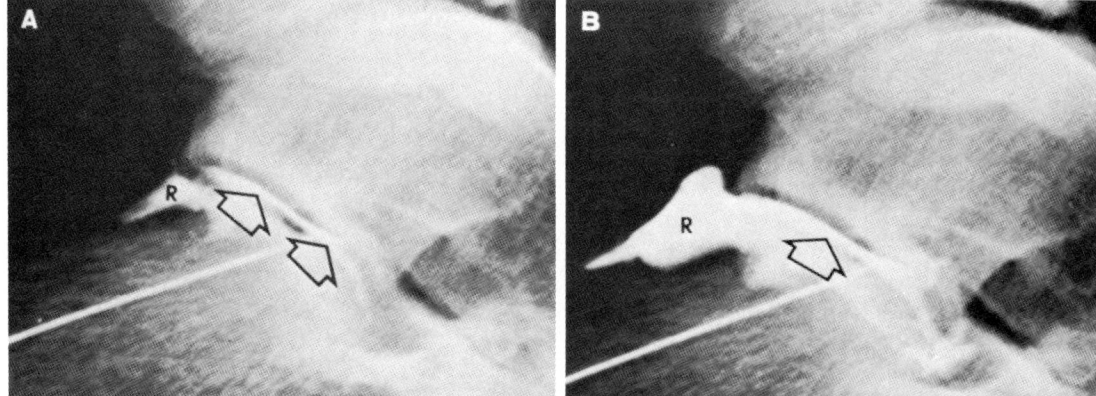

FIGURE 2–88. *Arthrogram of the posterior compartment of the subtalar joint.*

A and **B**. Lateral roentgenograms showing partial and complete filling. (From Resnick, D.: Radiology of the talocalcaneal articulation. Radiology, *111*:586, 1974. Reprinted by permission.)

tive in diminishing stress on the rigid hindfoot.

If peroneal muscle spasm and pain do develop, more aggressive measures are indicated; initially these should be conservative. Acute symptoms following trauma or unusual stress may be relieved by immobilizing the foot and ankle in a below-knee walking cast for a period of three to four weeks.

It is doubtful whether manipulation of the foot under anesthesia is of any value. The hindfoot should not be forced into inversion while the cast is being applied, as it will be uncomfortable and the result will be more spasm. Following removal of the cast the foot is supported in a foot-ankle orthosis made of polypropylene or another plastic for an additional three months. Injection of corticosteroids into the subtalar joint is not recommended.

Braddock studied the natural history of peroneal spastic flatfoot in 28 patients (24 males and 4 females; 15 with bilateral involvement, making a total of 43 feet). The first symptoms appeared during adolescence. In 22 of the feet, tarsal coalition was disclosed in the roentgenograms. These patients were treated with manipulation under anesthesia, a below-knee walking plaster cast, or an orthosis with valgus T-strap. The average period of follow-up was 21 years, the longest being 34 years and the shortest 13 years. About half these patients continued to have minor symptoms for many years, but only 10 per cent were disabled with persistent pain and required operative treatment.[17] An interesting finding in this report was that severe symptoms were more persistent in those patients without apparent tarsal anomalies than in those with obvious bars. Probably more thorough

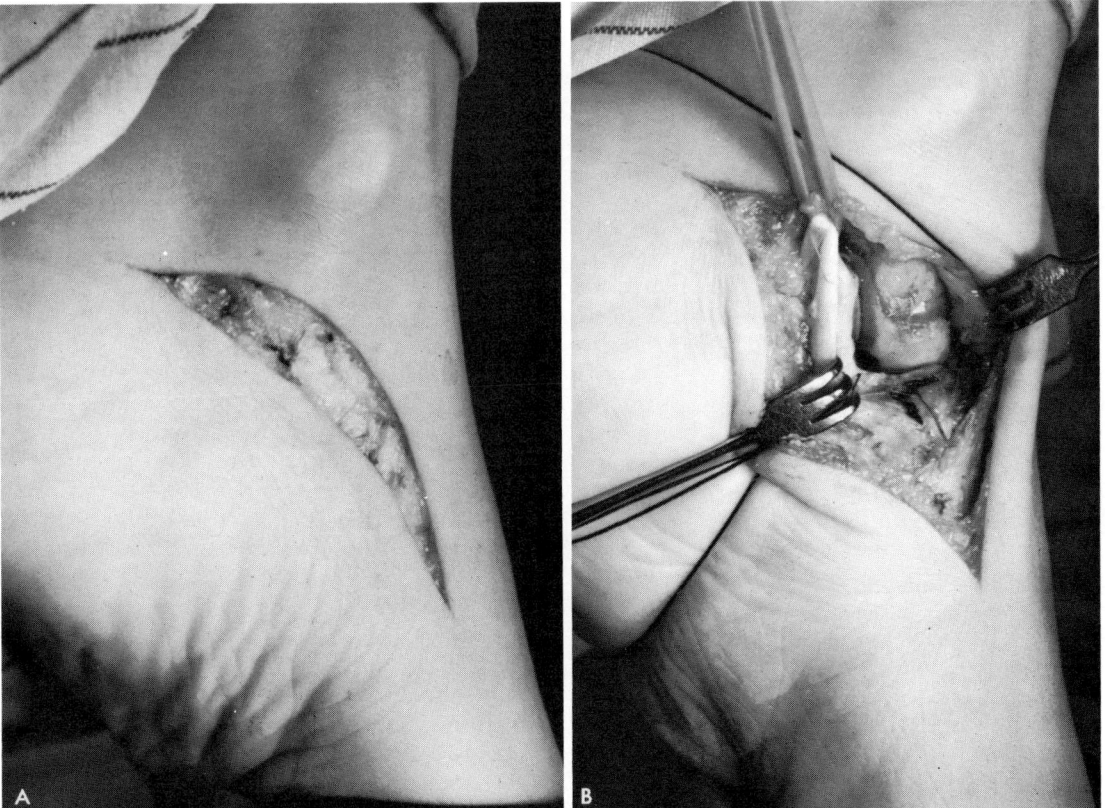

FIGURE 2–89. *Medial approach to subtalar joint.*

A, Skin incision begins at the base of the first cuneiform bone and ends 2 cm. inferior and posterior to the tip of the medial malleolus (the bony prominence in the photograph). **B**. Posterior tibial tendon is elevated and retracted inferiorly and posteriorly, exposing the subtalar joint.

roentgenographic examination including computed tomography (particularly of the anterior and middle facets of the talocalcaneal joint) would have disclosed partial or occult coalitions.

When pain and muscle spasm recur and become chronic or when the deformity is severe, surgical treatment is indicated. The operative procedure employed depends upon the type of coalition and the presence or absence of secondary changes in the talonavicular joint.

MEDIAL TALOCALCANEAL COALITION

For medial talocalcaneal coalition, a medial curvilinear incision is made, beginning at the base of the first cuneiform bone and terminating 2 cm. inferior and posterior to the tip of the medial malleolus. This medial approach, recommended by Harris, provides adequate exposure of the talonavicular joint and the medial aspect of the subtalar joint (Fig. 2–89). It also permits the surgeon to assess the pathologic anatomy of the talocalcaneal coalition, the degree and rigidity of pes valgus, and the changes in the talonavicular joint.[58]

If there is complete union of the medial talocalcaneal articulation, and the fixed valgus deformity of the hindfoot is functionally acceptable (i.e., not exceeding 15 degrees), only the talonavicular joint is fused. It is not necessary to osteotomize and mobilize the synostosis of the subtalar joints, nor is stabilization of the calcaneocuboid joint required. Occasionally the large bony mass of the medial talocalcaneal coalition is partially resected, which diminishes its prominence and prevents irritation from the shoe.

If the talocalcaneal coalition is incomplete, the subtalar joint should be stabilized. Harris recommends fusion of only the talocalcaneal and talonavicular joints; the author, however, prefers to include the calcaneocuboid joint in the fusion (i.e., triple arthrodesis). If the pes valgus exceeds 15 degrees, the intertarsal bony bridge is osteotomized and appropriate wedges are resected, while triple arthrodesis is performed to give the foot a normal configuration. The peroneal muscles usually do not require lengthening, except in an occasional severe long-standing case with marked myostatic contracture. In such an instance, sliding lengthening of the peroneals is performed; i.e., through a separate incision on the lateral aspect of the middle third of the leg, the tendinous fibers are divided at two levels 3 to 4 cm. apart, and the sectioned fibers are slid over the underlying muscles by applying traction distally on the peroneal tendons. Excision of incomplete or rudimentary medial talocalcaneal coalition may be tried. In the experience of this author it was successful in restoring painless subtalar motion in two cases.

The surgical treatment of the rare anterior and posterior talocalcaneal coalitions follows the same principles as those outlined for the medial one.

CALCANEONAVICULAR COALITION

Surgical treatment is indicated when there is persistent pain, muscle spasm, and deformity. Resection of the calcaneonavicular bar was suggested by Badgley and Bentzon more than 50 years ago; their results were disappointing, however, because the operations were carried out in older individuals who had developed degenerative changes in the tarsus.[7, 12]

Mitchell and Gibson recommended excision of the calcaneonavicular bar in children under 14 years of age who showed no roentgenographic evidence of adaptive changes. In their experience, the procedure had an excellent chance of abolishing symptoms and restoring mobility to the foot without any restriction of future activity.[106] In Mitchell's personal series of 13 consecutive selected cases, excision of the bar restored mobility and abolished symptoms in all the cases.[105] In their original communication, Mitchell and Gibson reported their results in unselected series of 41 feet; there were eight failures following excision of the bar—these occurred in feet with long-standing deformity or with adaptive changes in the tarsal joints. They recommended triple arthrodesis in these late cases.[106]

Cowell resected the calcaneonavicular bar, but in addition interposed the extensor digitorum brevis to obliterate the dead space and prevent re-formation of bone. According to Cowell, resection of the bar and extensor brevis arthroplasty are indicated in a patient under 14 years of age who has pain in the foot, limited subtalar motion, and a cartilaginous bar. These procedures should not be performed in the presence of degenerative changes in the talonavicular joint with accompanying talar beak or when there is an additional coalition between the talus and the calcaneus. Cowell reported the results of the procedure on 26 bars in 15 patients. Twenty-three of the twenty-six feet demonstrated no symptoms following surgery, and the patients were able to resume full activity, including participation in sports. According to Cowell, when proper indications are observed, satisfactory results may be expected in 90 per cent of the patients.[30]

This author concurs with Cowell, but he also excises the calcaneonavicular bar when it is ossified in a patient over 14 years of age, provided there are no talonavicular degenerative changes. Instead of interposing the extensor digitorum brevis, he uses adipose tissue from the gluteal region and places it between the resected ends of the calcaneus and navicular as a spacer and to prevent reossification.

The technique of resection of the calcaneonavicular bar with the extensor digitorum brevis arthroplasty or gluteal fat interposition is illustrated in Plate 6.

A triple arthrodesis is performed when there are degenerative changes in the talonavicular joint or when excision of the bar fails to relieve the symptoms.

Talonavicular coalition usually does not require treatment, as the condition is asymptomatic. In adult life, naviculocuneiform fusion may be indicated if hypertrophic changes and pain develop. Subtalar and calcaneocuboid fusion is performed in the occasional case associated with painful and persistent peroneal spastic flatfoot.

Treatment of the other rare tarsal coalitions should be individualized.

References follow on page 292

Resection of Calcaneonavicular Coalition with Interposition of Extensor Digitorum Brevis Muscle or Adipose Tissue

THE PROCEDURE

A. A lateral Ollier approach is made. The incision starts immediately below the lateral malleolus and curves upward to end on the lateral aspect of the talonavicular joint.

B. The peroneal tendons are retracted posteriorly and the long toe extensors are retracted dorsally. The origin of the extensor digitorum brevis muscle is detached and elevated in one piece, and reflected distally.

Plate 6. Resection of Calcaneonavicular Coalition with Interposition of Extensor Digitorum Brevis Muscle or Adipose Tissue

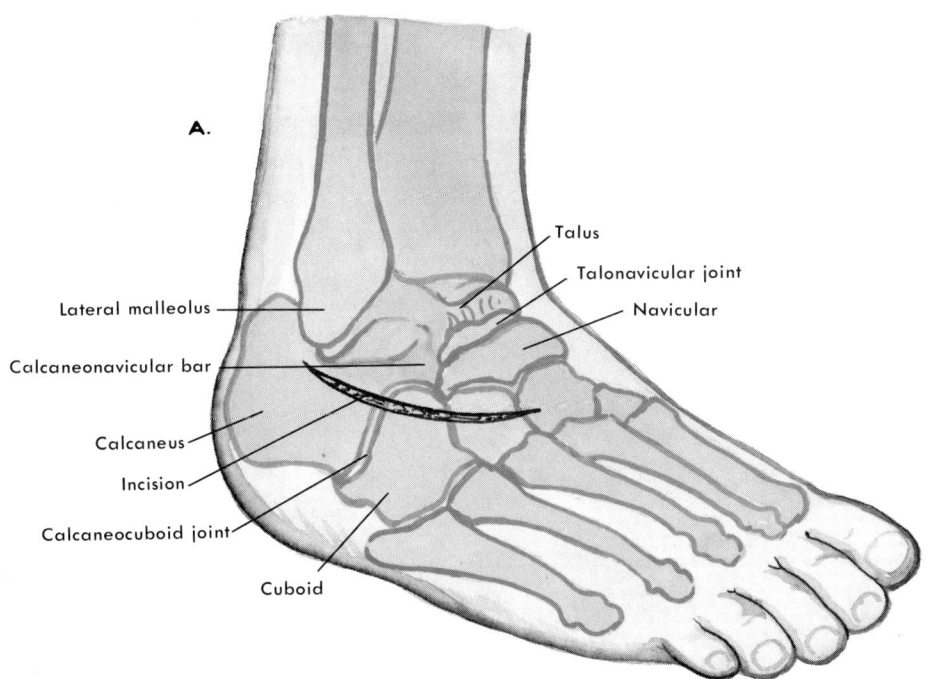

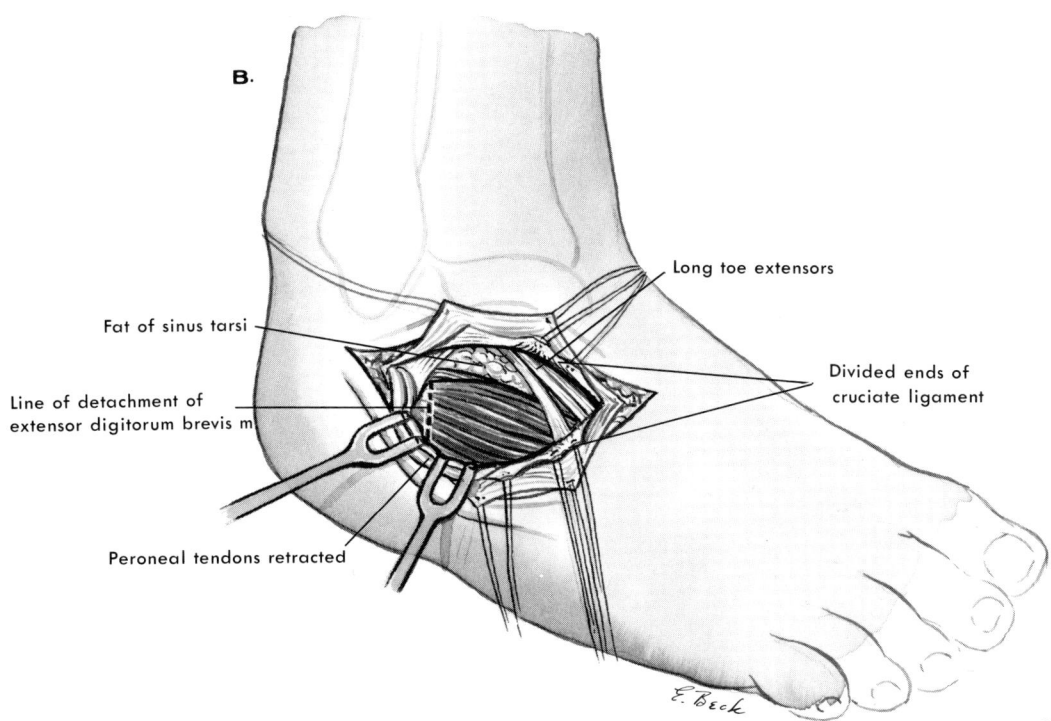

Resection of Calcaneonavicular Coalition with Interposition of Extensor Digitorum Brevis Muscle or Adipose Tissue
(Continued)

C. The calcaneus, cuboid, and navicular bones are identified. The capsule of the calcaneocuboid joint is incised to facilitate exposure of the calcaneonavicular bar. Do not divide the talonavicular capsule, or dorsal subluxation of the navicular on the head of the talus may result. Next, the entire bar is resected as a rectangle, not a wedge, with two straight osteotomes. The osteotome for the calcaneal portion of the bar is directed almost horizontally, whereas the one for the navicular portion is angled plantarward. An oscillating electric saw may be used if preferred.

D. It is imperative to remove the bar adequately, with generous portions of the calcaneal and navicular components. The plantar aspects of the navicular and the talar head should be level. The raw cancellous bleeding bases of the excised bar are coagulated. Caution! Do not disturb the circulation between the talus and the navicular.

Plate 6. Resection of Calcaneonavicular Coalition with Interposition of Extensor Digitorum Brevis Muscle or Adipose Tissue

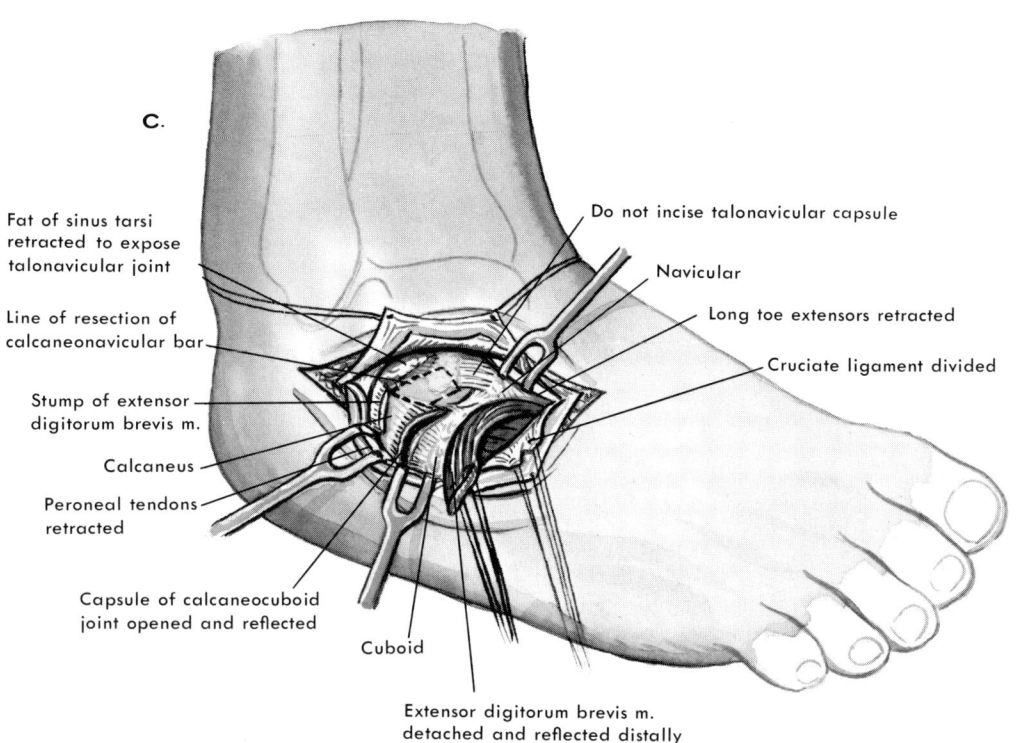

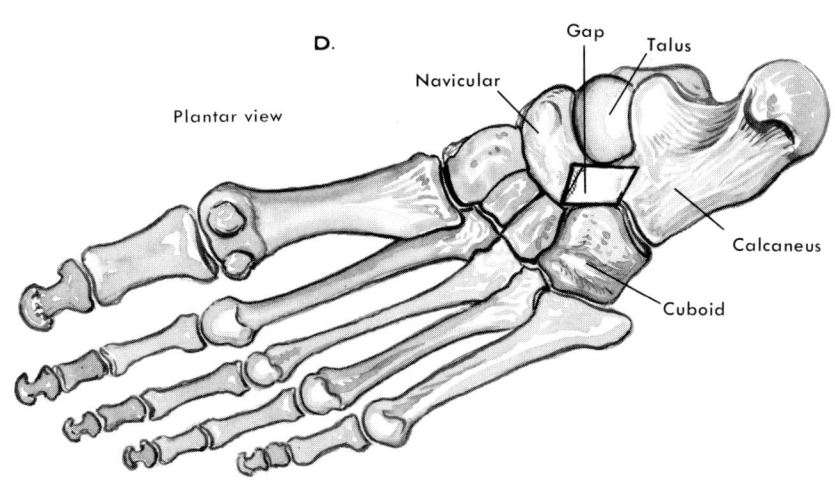

Resection of Calcaneonavicular Coalition with Interposition of Extensor Digitorum Brevis Muscle or Adipose Tissue
(Continued)

E. In Cowell's technique the entire origin of the extensor digitorum brevis muscle is placed in the defect and secured with a chromic suture. Two Keith needles are used, one on each end of the suture; they are pulled out on the medial side of the foot, where the suture is tied over a well-padded button or over a rectangular piece of sterile felt.

F. The author prefers to place adipose tissue from the gluteal area in the gap created by excision of the bar to obliterate dead space and prevent new bone formation. The extensor digitorum brevis is sutured back to its origin. The wound is closed, and the foot and ankle are immobilized in a below-knee cast.

POSTOPERATIVE CARE

In about ten days the cast is bivalved, and passive and active exercises are performed to develop inversion and eversion of the hindfoot. The foot and ankle are supported in neutral position in a posterior splint made of polypropylene or other plastic material. Full weight-bearing is not permitted and the splint support is continued until the patient obtains full active subtalar motion. This will usually require eight to ten weeks.

Plate 6. Resection of Calcaneonavicular Coalition with Interposition of Extensor Digitorum Brevis Muscle or Adipose Tissue

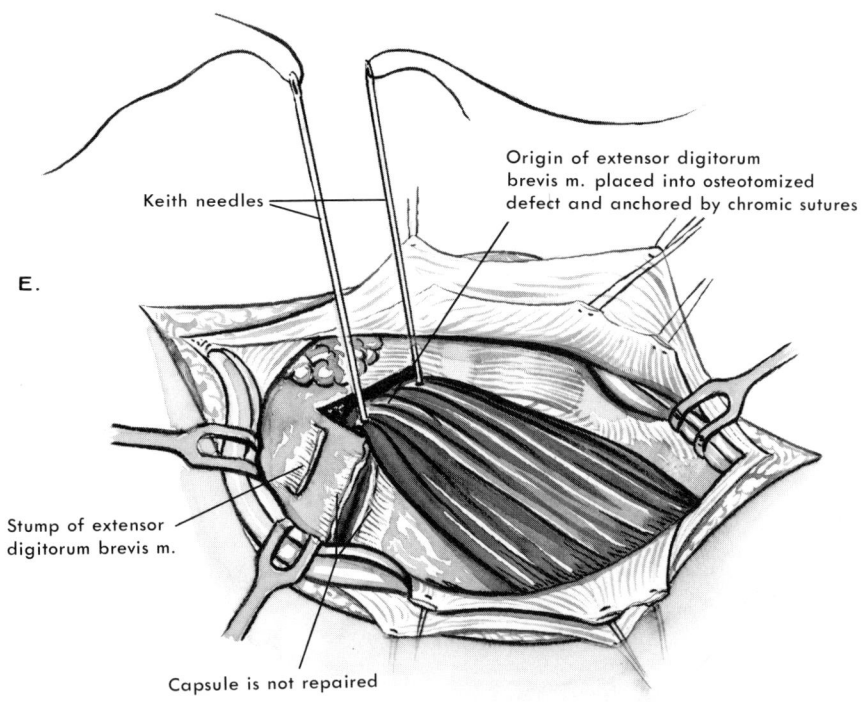

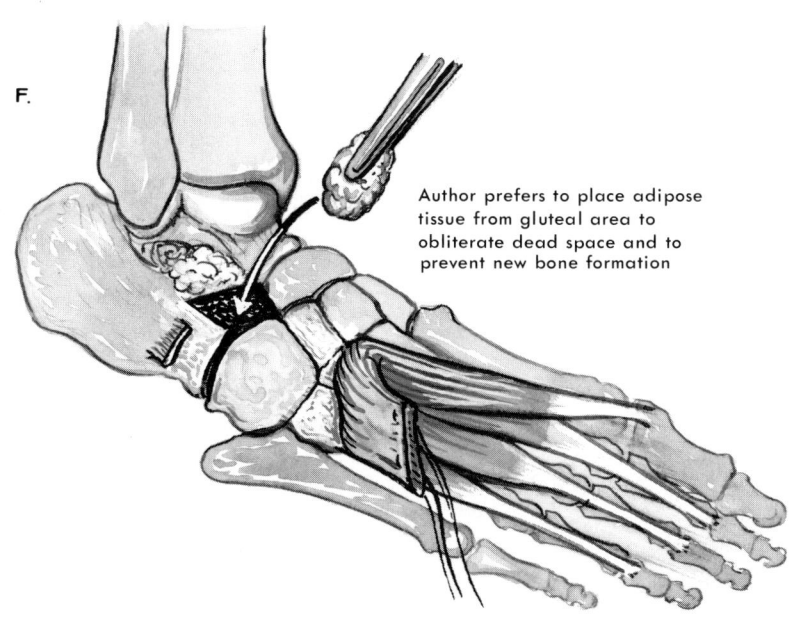

References (Tarsal Coalition)

1. Achterman, C., and Kalamchi, A.: Congenital deficiency of the fibula. J. Bone Joint Surg., *61-B*:133, 1979.
2. Adler, J. B.: Radiologic notes: Case No. 358: Tarsal coalition—calcaneo-naviculo-cuboid. Mt. Sinai J. Med. (N.Y.), *39*:321, 1972.
3. Amr, F., and El-Hadidi, H.: Spasmodic valgus foot: A contribution to its aetiology and treatment. Egyp. Orthop. J., *7*:175, 1972.
4. Anderson, R. J.: The presence of an astragalo-scaphoid bone in man. J. Anat. Physiol., *14*:452, 1880.
5. Anthonsen, W.: An oblique projection for roentgen examination of the talocalcanean joint, particularly regarding intra-articular fracture of the calcaneus. Acta Radiol., *24*:306, 1943.
6. Austin, F. H.: Symphalangism and related fusions of tarsal bones. Radiology, *56*:882, 1951.
7. Badgley, C. E.: Coalition of the calcaneus and the navicular. Arch. Surg. (Chicago), *15*:75, 1927.
8. Bargellini, D.: Fusione calcaneo-cuboidea e piede piatto. Arch. Ital. Chir., *21*:386, 1928.
9. Basu, S. S.: Naviculo-cuneo-metatarso-phalangeal synostoses. Indian J. Surg., *25*:750, 1963.
10. Beckly, D. E., Anderson, P. W., and Pedegana, L. R.: The radiology of the subtalar joint with special reference to talo-calcaneal coalition. Clin. Radiol., *26*:333, 1975.
11. Behr, F.: Ueber eine sym. Synostose der Hand und Fusswurzelnochen. Arch. Orthop. Chir., *32*:12, 1932.
12. Bentzon, P. G. K.: Coalitio calcaneo-navicularis, mit besonderer Bezugnahme auf die operative Behandlung des durch diese Anomalie bedingten Plattfüsses. Verh. Deutsch. Orthop. Ges., *23*:269, 1929.
13. Bentzon, P. G. K.: Bilateral congenital deformity of the astragalo-calcanean joint—bony coalescence between os trigonum and the calcaneus? Acta Orthop. Scand., *1*:359, 1930.
14. Bersani, F. A., and Samilson, R. L.: Massive familial tarsal synostosis. J. Bone Joint Surg., *39-A*:1187, 1957.
15. Blockey, N. J.: Peroneal spastic flat foot. J. Bone Joint Surg., *37-B*:191, 1955.
16. Boyd, H. B.: Congenital talonavicular synostosis. J. Bone Joint Surg., *26*:682, 1944.
17. Braddock, G. T. F.: A prolonged follow-up of peroneal spastic flat foot. J. Bone Joint Surg., *43-B*:734, 1961.
18. Brand, C.: Über die Bedeutung und spec. Diagnostik der Coalitio calcaneonavicularis. Arch. Orthop. Unfallchir., *48*:202, 1956.
19. Brobeck, O.: Congenital bilateral synostosis of the calcaneus and cuboid and the triquetral and hamate bones. Report of a case. Acta Orthop. Scand., *26*:217, 1957.
20. Buffon, G. L. L.: Histoire Naturelle, Géncerale et Particuliere. Tome 3, p. 47. Paris, Panekoucke, 1769.
21. Bullitt, J. B.: Variations of the bones of the foot. Fusion of the talus and navicular, bilateral and congenital. Amer. J. Roentgen., *20*:548, 1928.
22. Calvert, J. P.: A case of symphalangism with associated carpal and tarsal fusions. Hand, *6*:291, 1974.
23. Cavallaro, D. C., and Hadden, H. R.: An unusual case of tarsal coalition: A cuboid navicular synostosis. J. Amer. Podiatry Assoc., *68*:71, 1978.
24. Challis, J.: Hereditary transmission of talonavicular coalition in association with anomaly of the little finger. J. Bone Joint Surg., *56-A*:1273, 1974.
25. Chambers, C. H.: Congenital anomalies of the tarsal navicular with particular reference to calcaneonavicular coalition. Brit. J. Radiol., *23*:580, 1950.
25a. Chambers, R. B., Cook, T. M., and Cowell, H. R.: Surgical reconstruction for calcaneonavicular coalition. Evaluation of function and gait. J. Bone Joint Surg., *64-A*:829, 1982.
26. Christian, J. C., Franken, E. A., Jr., Lindeman, J. P., Lindseth, R. E., Reed, T., and Scott, C. I., Jr.: A dominant syndrome of metacarpal and metatarsal asymmetry with tarsal and carpal fusions, syndactyly, articular dysplasia and platyspondyly. Clin. Genet., *8*:75, 1975.
27. Cobey, J. C.: Posterior roentgenogram of the foot. Clin. Orthop., *118*:202, 1976.
28. Conway, J. J., and Cowell, H. R.: Tarsal coalition: Clinical significance and roentgenographic demonstration. Radiology, *92*:799, 1969.
29. Coventry, M. B.: Flatfoot, with special consideration of tarsal coalition. Minn. Med., *33*:1091, 1950.
30. Cowell, H. R.: Extensor brevis arthroplasty. J. Bone Joint Surg., *52-A*:820, 1970.
31. Cowell, H. R.: Talocalcaneal coalition and new causes of peroneal spastic flatfoot. Clin. Orthop., *85*:16, 1972.
32. Cowell, H. R.: Diagnosis and management of peroneal spastic flatfoot. A.A.O.S. Instr. Course Lect., *24*:94, 1975.
33. Cruveilhier, J.: Anatomie Pathologique du Corps Humain. Tome I, 1829.
34. Del Sel, J. M., and Grand, N. E.: Cubonavicular synostosis: A rare tarsal synostosis. J. Bone Joint Surg., *41-B*:149, 1959.
35. De Marchi, E., Gambier, R., and Vespignani, L.: Les synostoses tarsiennes dans le pied plat valgus douloureux. J. Radiol. Electr., *36*:665, 1955.
36. Devoldere, J.: A case of familial congenital synostosis in the carpal and tarsal bones. Arch. Chir. Neerl., *12*:185, 1960.
37. Diamond, L. S.: A possible new syndrome—clinodactyly, voluntary shoulder dislocation and massive tarsal coalition. Birth Defects, *10*:527, 1974.
38. Domenella, G.: Dimonstrazione ed analisi delle sinostosi calcaneo-scafoidee nel piede piatto-valgo contratto, attraverso una nuova tecnica proiettiva radiografica. Chir. Organi Mov., *52*:501, 1963.
39. Dommisse, G. F.: Flat foot. S. Afr. Med. J., *45*:726, 1971.
40. Drewes, J.: Die angeborenen Synostosen der Fusswurzelknochen. In Kremer, K. (ed.): Die chirurgische Behandlung der angeborenen Fehlbildungen. Stuttgart, Georg Thieme Verlag, 1961, pp. 517–524.
41. Drinkwater, H.: Phalangeal anarthrosis (synostosis, ankylosis) transmitted through fourteen generations. Proc. Roy. Soc. Med. (Section of Pathology), *10*:60, 1917.
42. Dubois, H. J.: Nievergelt-Pearlman syndrome. Synostosis in feet and hands with dysplasia of elbows. Report of a case. J. Bone Joint Surg., *52-B*:325, 1970.
43. Dwight, T.: A Clinical Atlas. Variations of the Bones of the Hands and Feet. Philadelphia, J. B. Lippincott Co., 1907.
44. Ernsting, G.: Zur klinischen Bedeutung der Coalito calcaneo-navicularis. Arch. Orthop. Unfallchir., *48*:433, 1956.
45. Esau, P.: Angeborene Missibildungen der Fuss. (Randdefekt). Deutsch. Z. Chir., *194*:236, 1926.
46. Esau, P.: Angeborene Synostosen im Bereich des Carpus and Tarsus. Roentgenpraxis, *5*:235, 1933.
47. Galinski, A. W., Crovo, R. T., and Ditmars, J. J., Jr.: Os trigonum as a cause of tarsal coalition. J. Amer. Podiatry Assoc., *69*:191, 1979.
48. Garelli, R.: Piede valghi e piatti infantili. Minerva Pediat., *26*:506, 1974.
49. Gaynor, S. S.: Congenital astragalocalcaneal fusion. J. Bone Joint Surg., *18*:479, 1936.
50. Geelhoed, G. W., Neel, J. V., and Davidson, R. T.: Symphalangism and tarsal coalitions: A hereditary syndrome. J. Bone Joint Surg., *51-B*:278, 1969.
51. Geyer, E.: Beitrag zu den Synostosenbildungen der Hand- und Fusswerzel. Z. Orthop., *90*:395, 1958.
52. Glessner, J. R., Jr., and Davis, G. L.: Bilateral calcaneo-navicular coalition occurring in twin boys. A case report. Clin. Orthop., *47*:173, 1966.
53. Grashey, R.: Articulatio talo-calcanea (os sustentaculi). Roentgenpraxis, *14*:139, 1942.
54. Gregersen, H. N.: Naviculocuneiform coalition. J. Bone Joint Surg., *59-A*:128, 1977.
55. Hark, F. W.: Congenital anomalies of the tarsal bones. Clin. Orthop., *16*:21, 1960.
56. Harle, T. S., and Stevenson, J. R.: Hereditary symphalangism associated with carpal and tarsal fusions. Radiology, *89*:91, 1967.
57. Harris, B. J.: Anomalous structures in the developing human foot. (Abstract). Anat. Rec., *121*:399, 1955. (Original thesis in University of California library.)
58. Harris, R. I.: Rigid valgus foot due to talocaneal bridge. J. Bone J. Surg., *37-A*:169, 1955.
59. Harris, R. I.: Peroneal spastic flat foot. A.A.O.S. Instr. Course Lect., *15*:116, 1958.
60. Harris, R. I.: Retrospect: Peroneal spastic flat foot (rigid valgus foot). J. Bone Joint Surg., *47-A*:1657, 1965.
61. Harris, R. I., and Beath, T.: Army Foot Survey. Ottawa, Natl. Res. Council of Canada, 1947, p. 44.

62. Harris, R. I., and Beath, T.: Etiology of peroneal spastic flat foot. J. Bone Joint Surg., *30-B*:624, 1948.
63. Harris, R. I., and Beath, T.: John Hunter's specimen of talocalcaneal bridge. J. Bone Joint Surg., *32-B*:203, 1950.
64. Harold, A. J.: Rigid valgus foot from fibrous contracture of the peronei. J. Bone Joint Surg., *47-B*:743, 1965.
65. Hayd, F. W.: Die Coalitio calcaneo-navicularis und ihre klinische Bedeutung. Z. Orthop., *78*:292, 1949.
66. Hayek, W.: Synostosis talonavicularis. Z. Orthop. Chir., *69*:231, 1934.
67. Heikel, H. V. A.: Coalition calcaneo-navicularis and calcaneus secundarius. A clinical and radiographic study of twenty-three patients. Acta Orthop. Scand., *32*:72, 1962.
68. Heiple, K. G., and Lovejoy, C. O.: The antiquity of tarsal coalition. Bilateral deformity in a pre-Columbian Indian skeleton. J. Bone Joint Surg., *51-A*:979, 1969.
69. Hodgson, F. G.: Talonavicular synostosis. Southern. Med. J., *39*:940, 1946.
70. Hohmann, G.: Angeborene Synostosen zwischen Fusswurzelknochen. Pes planovalgus congenitus. *In* Hohmann, G. (ed.): Handbuch der Orthopädie, Stuttgart, Georg Thieme Verlag, 1961, Part II, Vol. 4, pp. 840–842.
71. Holl, M.: Beitrage zur chirurgischen Osteologie des Fusses. Arch. Klin. Chir., *25*:211, 1880.
72. Holland, C. T.: Two cases of rare deformity of feet and hands. Arch. Radiol. Electrother., *22*:234, 1918.
73. Illievitz, A. B.: Congenital malformation of the feet. Report of the case of congenital fusion of the scaphoid with astragalus and complete absence of one toe. Amer. J. Surg., *4*:550, 1928.
74. Isherwood, I.: A radiological approach to the subtalar joint. J. Bone Joint Surg., *43-B*:566, 1961.
75. Jack, E. A.: Bone anomalies of the tarsus in relation to "peroneal spastic flat foot." J. Bone Joint Surg., *36-B*:530, 1954.
76. James, A. E., Jr.: Tarsal coalitions and peroneal spastic flat foot. Australas. Radiol., *14*:80, 1970.
77. Jaubert De Beaujeu, A., and Benmussa: Synostose astragalo-scaphoïdienne congénitale, bilatérale et isolée. J. Radiol. Electr., *23*:348, 1939.
78. Johansson, S.: A case of congenital ankylosis of the ankle joints and other malformations. Acta Orthop. Scand., *5*:231, 1934.
79. Jones, R.: Peroneal spasm and its treatment. Report of meeting of Liverpool Medical Institution held 22nd April, 1897. Liverpool Med. Chir. J., *17*:442, 1897.
80. Jones, R.: The soldier's foot and the treatment of common deformities of the foot. Brit. Med. J., *1*:709, 1916.
81. Judet, R., Judet, J., and Rigault, P.: Possibilités de correction chirurgical des malformations des os du pied. Presse Méd., *74*:157, 1966.
82. Kadelbach, G.: Ein Beitrag zur den Fusswurzelsynostosen. Arch. Orthop. Unfallchir., *40*:363, 1949.
83. Kaplan, E. G., Kaplan, G. W., and Vaccari, O. A.: Tarsal coalition: Review and preliminary conclusions. J. Foot Surg., *16*:136, 1977.
84. Kaye, J. J., Ghelman, B., and Schneider, R.: Talocalcaneonavicular joint arthrography for sustentacular-talar tarsal coalitions. Radiology, *115*:730, 1975.
85. Kendrick, J. I.: Treatment of calcaneonavicular bar, J.A.M.A., *172*:1242, 1960.
86. Kendrick, J. I.: Tarsal coalition. Clin. Orthop., *85*:62, 1972.
87. Kewesh, E. L.: Über hereditäre Verschmelzung der Hand- und Fusswurzelknochen. Fortschr. Röntgenstr., *50*:550, 1934.
88. Kirmisson, E.: Double pied bot varus par malformation osseuse primitive associée à des ankyloses congénitales des doigts et des orteils chez quatre membres d'une méme famille. Rev. Orthop., *9*:392, 1898.
89. Kolbel, R., and Hermann, H. J.: Ball and socket ankle joint and tarsal synostosis. Z. Orthop., *113*:952, 1975.
90. Korvin, H.: Coalitio talocalcanea. Z. Orthop. Chir., *60*:105, 1934.
91. Kozlowski, K.: Hypoplasie bilatérale congénitale du cubitus et synostose bilatérale calcaneo-cuboïde chez une fillette. Ann. Radiol. (Paris), *8*:389, 1965.
92. LaGrange, M.: Anomalie du pied. Soudure des os du tarse et du metatarse. Progr. Méd. (Paris), *10*:367, 1882.
93. Lamb, D.: The ball-and-socket ankle joint. J. Bone Joint Surg., *40-B*:240, 1958.
94. Lapidus, P. W.: Congenital fusion of the bones of the foot; with a report of a case of congenital tragaloscaphoid fusion. J. Bone Joint Surg., *14*:888, 1932.
95. Lapidus, P. W.: Bilateral congenital talonavicular fusion. Report of a case. J. Bone Joint Surg., *20*:775, 1938.
96. Lapidus, P. W.: Spastic flat foot. J. Bone Joint Surg., *28*:126, 1946.
97. Leonard, M. A.: Inheritance of tarsal coalition and its relationship to spastic flat foot. Proceedings, British Orthopaedic Association, 1973 (Abstract). J. Bone Joint Surg., *55-B*:881, 1973.
98. Leonard, M. A.: The inheritance of tarsal coalition and its relationship to spastic flat foot. J. Bone Joint Surg., *56-B*:520, 1974.
99. Lissoos, I., and Soussi, J.: Tarsal synostosis with partial adactylia. Med. Proc., *11*:224, 1965.
100. Lusby, H. L. J.: Naviculo-cuneiform synostosis. J. Bone Joint Surg., *41-B*:150, 1959.
101. Mahaffey, H. W.: Bilateral congenital calcaneocuboid synostosis. Case report. J. Bone Joint Surg., *27*:164, 1945.
102. Maudsley, R. S.: Spastic pes varus. Proc. Roy. Soc. Med., *49*:181, 1956.
103. Michailow, S.: Über eine angeborene Synostosis zwischen Talus and Kalkaneus. Beitr. Orthop. Traum., *19*:278, 1972.
104. Miller, E. M.: Congenital ankylosis of joints of hands and feet. J. Bone Joint Surg., *4*:560, 1922.
105. Mitchell, G. P., and Gibson, J. M. C.: Excision of calcaneonavicular bar for painful spasmodic flat foot. J. Bone Joint Surg., *49-B*:281, 1967.
106. Mitchell, G.: Spasmodic flatfoot. Clin. Orthop., *70*:73, 1970.
107. Mommsen, F.: Das klinische Bild und die klinische Analyse der Varusdeformitaet des Fusses und hire unblutige Korrektur. Z. Orthop. Chir., *50*:173, 1929.
108. Murakami, Y.: Nievergelt-Pearlman syndrome with impairment of hearing. Report of three cases in a family. J. Bone Joint Surg., *57-B*:367, 1975.
109. Niederecker, K.: Der Plattfuss, Klinik, Pathologie, Konservative und Operative Behandlung. Stuttgart, Ferdinand Enke Verlag, 1959, pp. 53–109.
110. Nievergelt, K.: Positiver Vaterschaftsnachweis auf Grand erblicher Missbildungen der Extremitäten. Arch. Klaus Stift Vererbungforsch., *19*:157, 1944.
111. O'Donoghue, D. H., and Sell, L. S.: Congenital talonavicular synostosis. J. Bone Surg., *25*:925, 1943.
112. O'Rahilly, R.: A survey of carpal and tarsal anomalies. J. Bone Joint Surg., *35-A*:626, 1953.
113. O'Rahilly, R.: Developmental deviations in carpus and tarsus. Clin. Orthop., *10*:9, 1957.
114. O'Rahilly, R., Gardner, E., and Gray, D. J.: The skeletal development of the foot. Clin. Orthop., *16*:7, 1960.
115. Outland, T., and Murphy, I. D.: Relation of tarsal anomalies to spastic and rigid flat feet. Clin. Orthop., *1*:217, 1953.
116. Outland, T., and Murphy, I. D.: The pathomechanics of peroneal spastic flat foot. Clin. Orthop., *16*:64, 1960.
117. Pearlman, H. S., Edkin, R. E., and Warren, R. F.: Familial tarsal and carpal synostosis with radial head subluxation. J. Bone Joint Surg., *46-A*:585, 1964.
118. Pfitzner, W.: Die Variationen im Aufbar des Fussekelts Bertrage zur Kenntniss des menschlichen Extremitatenskelets. VII. Morphol. Arbeit., *6*:245, 1896.
119. Poznanski, A. K.: Foot manifestations of the congenital malformation syndromes. Seminars Roentgen., *5*:354, 1970.
120. Poznanski, A. K., Stern, A. M., and Gall, J. C., Jr.: Radiographic findings in the hand-foot-uterus syndrome (H.F.U.S.). Radiology, *95*:129, 1970.
121. Rankin, E. A., and Baker, G. I.: Rigid flatfoot in the young adult. Clin. Orthop., *104*:244, 1974.
122. Resnick, D.: Radiology of the talocalcaneal articulation. Radiology, *111*:581, 1974.
123. Roger, A., and Meary, R.: Les synostoses congénitales des os du tarse. A propos de 41 cas. Rev. Chir. Orthop., *55*:721, 1969.
124. Rompe, G.: Ankylosen des Unteren Sprunggelenkes nach

Offenem Unterschenkelbruch. Arch. Orthop. Unfallchir., *54*:339, 1962.
125. Rothberg, A. S., Feldman, J. W., and Schuster, O. F.: Congenital fusion of astragalus and scaphoid: Bilateral; inherited. New York J. Med., *35*:29, 1935.
126. Rutt, A.: Zur Genese der Coalitio calcaneo naviculare. Z. Orthop., *96*:96, 1962.
127. Sanghi, J. K., and Roby, H. R.: Bilateral peroneal spastic flat feet associated with congenital fusion of the navicular and talus. A case report. J. Bone Joint Surg., *43-A*:1237, 1961.
128. Schreiber, R. R.: Talonavicular synostosis. J. Bone Joint Surg., *45-A*:170, 1963.
129. Seddon, H. J.: Calcaneo-scaphoid coalition. Proc. Roy. Soc. Med. (Section of Orthopedics), *26*:419, 1932.
130. Shaffer, H. A., Jr., and Harrison, R. B.: Tarsal pseudocoalition—positional artifact. J. Can. Assoc. Radiol., *31*:236, 1980.
131. Shands, A. R., and Wentz, I. J.: Congenital anomalies, accessory bones, and osteochondritis in the feet of 850 children. Surg. Clin. N. Amer., *33*:1643, 1953.
132. Sicard, A., and Moreau, R.: Synostose astragalocalcanéenne bilateral. Rev. Chir. Orthop., *50*:233, 1964.
133. Simmons, E. H.: Spastic tibialis varus with tarsal coalition. J. Bone Joint Surg., *47-B*:533, 1965.
134. Slater, P., and Rubinstein, H.: Aplasia of interphalangeal joints associated with synostosis of carpal and tarsal bones. Quart. Bull. Sea View Hosp., *7*:429, 1942.
135. Sloane, M. W. M.: A case of anomalous development in the foot. Anat. Rec., *96*:23, 1946.
136. Slomann, H. C.: On coalitio calcaneo-navicularis. J. Orthop. Surg., *3*:586, 1921.
137. Slomann, H. C.: On the demonstration and analysis of calcaneo-navicular coalition by roentgen examination. Acta Radiol., *5*:304, 1926.
138. Soeur, R.: Le pied plat contracture. Rev. Chir. Orthop., *45*:817, 1959.
139. Solger, B.: Ueber abnorme Verschmelzung knorpeliger Skelettheile beim Fötus. Zbl. Allg. Path., *1*:124, 1890.
140. Solonen, K. A., and Sulamma, M.: Nievergelt syndrome and its treatment. Ann. Chir. Gynaec. Fenn., *47*:142, 1958.
141. Spoendlin, H.: Congenital stapes ankylosis and fusion of tarsal and carpal bones as a dominant hereditary syndrome. Arch. Otorhinolaryng. (Chicago), *206*:173, 1974.
142. Steinhauser, J.: Further ball-type ankle-joints observed in cases of congenital tarsosynostoses. Z. Orthop., *112*:433, 1974.
143. Sutro, G.: Anomalous talocalcaneal articulation. Cause for limited subtalar movements. Amer J. Surg., *74*:64, 1947.
144. Templeton, A. W., McAlister, W. H., and Zim, I. D.: Standardization of terminology and evaluation of osseous relationships in congenitally abnormal feet. Amer. J. Roentgen., *93*:374, 1965.
145. Tomeno, B.: Flatfoot caused by congenital synostosis of the tarsus. Rev. Chir. Orthop., *63*:783, 1977.
146. Trolle, D.: Accessory Bones of the Human Foot. (Transl. by E. Aagesen.) Copenhagen, Munksgaard, 1949.
147. Umidon, M.: Architettura, topografia e morfogenesi dei retinacoli peroniery e del legamento anulare laterale del tarso, nell'uomo. Chir. Organi Movim., *52*:305, 1963.
148. Vaughan, W. H., and Segal, G.: Tarsal coalition with special reference to roentgenographic interpretation. Radiology, *60*:855, 1953.
149. Veneruso, L. C.: Unilateral congenital calcaneocuboid synostosis with complete absence of a metatarsal and toe. Case report. J. Bone Joint Surg., *27*:718, 1945.
150. Voutey, H.: Traitement chirurgical du pied plat de l'enfant. Rev. Chir. Orthop., *58*:489, 1972.
151. Wagoner, G. W.: A case of bilateral congenital fusion of the calcanei and cuboids. J. Bone Joint Surg., *10*:220, 1928.
152. Waugh, H.: Partial cubo-navicular coalition as a cause of peroneal spastic flat foot. J.A.M.A., *146*:1099, 1951.
153. Weber, V.: Multiple symmetrische Synostosen an Hand und Fuss. Arch. Orthop. Unfallchir., *46*:277, 1954.
154. Webster, F. C., and Roberts, W. M.: Tarsal anomalies and peroneal spastic flat foot. J.A.M.A., *146*:1099, 1951.
155. Weitzner, I.: Congenital talonavicular synostosis associated with hereditary multiple ankylosis arthropathies. Amer. J. Roentgen., *56*:185, 1946.
156. Wheeler, R., Guevera, A., and Bleck, E. E.: Tarsal coalitions: Review of the literature and case report of bilateral dual calcaneonavicular and talocalcaneal coalitions. Clin. Orthop., *156*:175, 1981.
157. Widervank, L. S., Goedhard, G., and Meijer, S.: Proximal symphalangism of fingers associated with fusion of os naviculare and talus and occurrence of two accessory bones in the feet (os paranaviculare and os tibiale externum) in an European-Indonesian-Chinese family. Acta Genet. (Basel), *17*:166, 1967.
158. Wisbrun, W.: Zur morphologie und funktion der articulatio talocalcanea. Arch. Orthop. Unfallchir., *44*:606, 1951.
159. Wray, J. B., and Herndon, C. N.: Hereditary transmission of congenital coalition of the calcaneus to the navicular. J. Bone Joint Surg., *45-A*:365, 1963.
160. Zeidel, M. S., Wiessel, S. W., and Terry, R. L.: Talonavicular coalition. Clin. Orthop., *126*:225, 1977.
161. Zock, E.: Ein Beitrag zu den Synostosen der Fusswurzel. Zbl. Chir., *78*:845, 1953.
162. Zuckerandl, E.: Über eine Fall von Synostose zwischen Talus und Calcaneus. Allg. Wein. Med. Zeit., *22*:293, 1877.

CONGENITAL METATARSUS VARUS

Congenital metatarsus varus is medial subluxation of the tarsometatarsal joints with adduction and inversion deformity of all five metatarsals; the hindfoot is in a slightly valgus or neutral position. The commonly used term *a third of a clubfoot* is a misnomer, as the navicular articulates normally with the head of the talus or is displaced laterally to compensate for the varus deviation of the forefoot; the talonavicular joint is not subluxated medially as seen in talipes equinovarus. The term *congenital metatarsus adductus* is used by the author when the forepart of the foot is adducted as a result of intrauterine malposition. Metatarsus adductus is a postural deformation of the forefoot with an excellent prognosis, correcting itself spontaneously without treatment within a few months; whereas congenital metatarsus varus is an in utero subluxation that will increase in severity without treatment. It is vital to distinguish the two conditions. The term *skewfoot* and *serpentine foot* were suggested by McCormick and Blount to describe the complex deformity of the varus forefoot and valgus hindfoot. The condition may result from delayed and improper treatment of congenital metatarsus varus.[15]

Congenital metatarsus varus was first described by Henke.[4] Its incidence is about one per thousand live births, according to Wynne-Davies, and it occurs more frequently in the female, with a female-to-male ratio of 100:76. Approximately 4.5 per cent of first-degree relatives of a person with metatarsus varus are similarly affected. Thus, if one child is affected, the risk of a second occurrence in a family is about 1 in 20. There is no clear pattern of inheritance, the cause being partly genetic and partly environmental.[22]

Reimann and Werner investigated the pathogenesis of metatarsus varus by means of a series of dissections of 14 normal feet

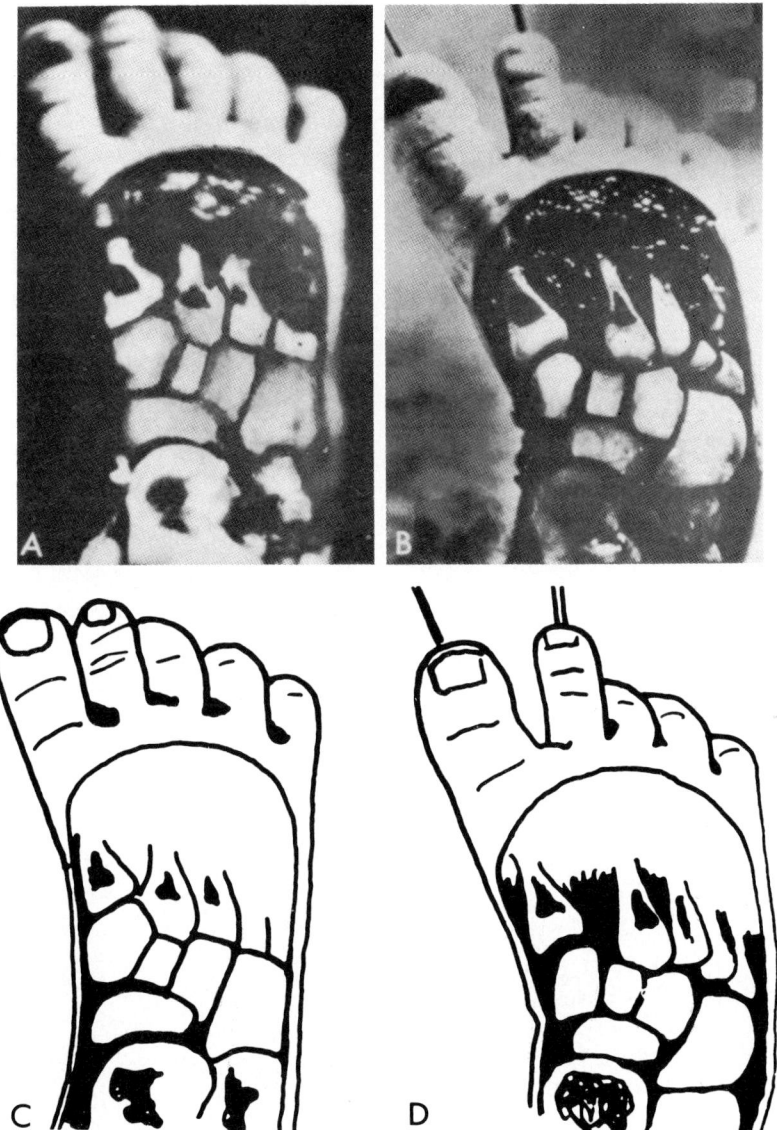

FIGURE 2–90. Experimental production of metatarsus varus in the normal foot of a stillborn infant.

A and **C**. Photograph and diagram of the normal foot. They show the normal articular relations of the bones in neutral position. **B** and **D**. Photograph and diagram of the same foot demonstrating the findings after the hindfoot is fixed in dorsiflexion and the forepart of the foot is adducted and inverted after capsulotomies of all the tarsometatarsal joints and sectioning of all the intermetatarsal interosseous ligaments. Note the medial subluxation of the tarsometatarsal joint; it is most marked between the first metatarsal and medial cuneiform, and there is increased space between the first and second rays. The second to the fifth metatarsals are slightly adducted and inverted. The lateral border of the foot is convex. The navicular is displaced laterally in relation to the head of the talus, and the hindfoot is in valgus position. (From Reimann, I., and Werner, H. H.: Congenital metatarsus varus. A suggestion for a possible mechanism and relation to other foot deformities. Clin. Orthop., *110*:224, 1975. Reprinted by permission.)

of infants who were stillborn or died during the perinatal period. A slight valgus deformity of the hindfoot was produced by maximal dorsiflexion of the ankle. On dissection, the navicular bone was found to be displaced laterally in relation to the head of the talus. The anterior tibial tendon was sectioned. The hindfoot was then fixed in dorsiflexion and experiments were carried out to obtain adduction and inversion of the forefoot—with the following results: (1) traction on the anterior tibial tendon, even with extreme force, could not produce metatarsus varus; (2) capsulotomy of the first metatarsal–medial cuneiform joint and traction on the anterior tibial tendon did not result in the deformity; but (3) only after extensive capsulotomies of all tarsometatarsal joints could the bones be displaced into a position similar to metatarsus varus (Fig. 2–90). Reimann and Werner suggest that congenital metatarsus varus is a primary medial subluxation of the tarsometatarsal joints, taking place in utero when the foot is dorsiflexed. Contracture of the soft tissues and adaptive bony changes are secondary deformities.[20]

Clinical Features

The deformity is present at birth, but may often go unnoticed for as long as several months. Involvement may be unilateral or bilateral.

On inspection of the dorsal and plantar aspects of the foot, all the metatarsals are seen to be adducted and inverted, but the heel is in either valgus or neutral position. The great toe is usually widely separated from the second toe. The base of the fifth metatarsal is prominent. The medial border of the foot is concave, and the lateral border convex. The medial longitudinal arch is high (normally, an infant's foot appears flat because of the presence of a large fat pad under the arch).

There is usually a deep skin crease on the medial aspect of the foot at the tarsometatarsal joint area. Decreased plantar flexion of the ankle and contracture of the anterior tibial muscle are commonly present at birth. On stimulation and contraction of the peroneal muscles, the foot fails to abduct actively, and it cannot be passively abducted to neutral position. The abductor hallucis muscle is taut, pulling the forefoot into varus position. A simple way to demonstrate the tight abductor hallucis tendon is to hold the hindfoot with one hand, with the index finger of the same hand applying counterpressure at the cuboid–fifth metatarsal area, and with the thumb of the opposite hand to push the medial aspect of the first metatarsal head into abduction. The taut tendon of the abductor hallucis is stretched like a bowstring near its insertion and can be seen and palpated with the index finger (Fig. 2–91).[12] Exaggerated medial tibial torsion is often present in metatarsus varus.

When the older child starts to walk, he toes in, his weight being borne on the lateral side of the sole. It is difficult to fit shoes, and shoe wear is noticeably abnormal, with early breakdown of the inner side of the upper of the shoe and the lateral side of the sole.

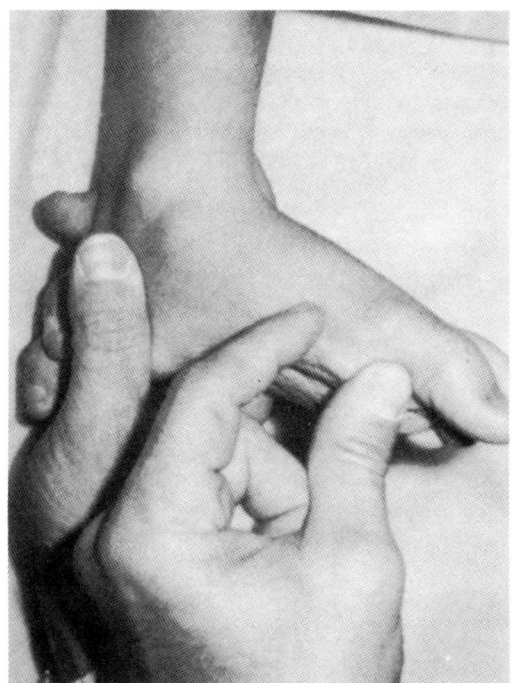

FIGURE 2–91. Lichtblau's test to demonstrate tautness of the abductor hallucis muscle in congenital metatarsus varus.

(From Lichtblau, S.: Section of the abductor hallucis tendon for correction of metatarsus varus deformity. Clin. Orthop., *110*:228, 1975. Reprinted by permission.)

Diagnosis

Functional metatarsus varus may be confused with congenital metatarsus varus. The former is caused by hyperactivity of the abductor hallucis and short toe flexors. All infants have an active plantar grasp reflex and on stimulation will actively hold the forefoot in adduction and the toes in flexion. When the infant is placed at rest in a comfortable prone position, however, the foot has normal contours and range of abduction.

Postural metatarsus adductus is a postural deformation of the forepart of the foot; there is no subluxation of the tarsometatarsal joints. Actively and passively, the forefoot can be brought to neutral position. The varus posture is flexible and not fixed. In addition, in postural metatarsus adductus the foot can be plantar-flexed fully, the anterior tibial is not taut, and the skin creases of the instep are normal.

Congenital metatarsus varus is occasionally misdiagnosed as talipes equinovarus. Clinically, in both conditions the foot is adducted and inverted, but in congenital metatarsus varus the hindfoot is slightly valgus without equinus deformity; in talipes equinovarus the hindfoot is in severe equinovarus position.

Roentgenograms, although they should not be required to establish the diagnosis, will depict the adducted and inverted position of all the metatarsals at the tarsometatarsal joints. The medial angular deformity is greatest at the medial cuneiform–first metatarsal joint area, with a progressive decrease from the first to the fifth tarsometatarsal joints. The talocalcaneal angle in the anteroposterior view is normal or increased (in talipes equinovarus, the talocalcaneal angle is decreased). When the child is over the age of three years and the bone is ossified, the navicular may be either in normal relationship to the head of the talus or lateral to it (in talipes equinovarus, it is displaced medially on the head). In the lateral roentgenogram, the talocalcaneal angle is normal.

Treatment

When a pediatrician makes the diagnosis of congenital metatarsus varus, the infant should be referred to an orthopedic surgeon for immediate treatment. It is very unfortunate that mild deformities are often kept under observation by the pediatrician to see whether they will correct themselves spontaneously. During this period of procrastination the deformity increases and becomes more rigid and progressively more resistant to correction. The importance of treatment of true congenital metatarsus varus within the first week of life cannot be overemphasized.

Certain pitfalls of management should be avoided. (1) Stretching exercises are often poorly and improperly executed by the parents, the entire foot being abducted and pronated. The valgus inclination of the hindfoot is exaggerated, the navicular is displaced dorsolaterally on the head of the talus, which is plantar-flexed, and the metatarsals are fixed in varus position. The resultant "Z" deformity of the foot (fixed varus forefoot and valgus hindfoot) is then much more difficult to treat than the original metatarsus varus. (2) Reversing shoes—putting the left shoe on the right foot—will not correct the deformity. (3) "Swung-out" or tarsal pronator shoes or prewalker clubfoot shoes should not be used, as they accentuate the hindfoot valgus deformity by forcing the heel into eversion. (4) An abduction bar on the shoes (the usual Denis Browne splint or any of its modifications such as the Fillauer bar) should not be used as a corrective device, as the valgus force of the splint is exerted on the hindpart as well as the forepart of the foot.

NONOPERATIVE MANAGEMENT

The only effective way to correct the fixed deformity of congenital metatarsus varus is by manipulative stretching exercises and retention of the foot in the corrected position in an above-knee cast.

The technique of gentle manipulative exercises to stretch the soft-tissue contracture and application of the corrective plaster cast is well described by Kite, by McCormick and Blount, and by Ponseti and Becker.[9–11, 15, 19] It is imperative that the details of technique be followed meticulously (Fig. 2–92).

The tendency is to abduct and evert the whole foot during manipulation and application of the cast. This will increase the

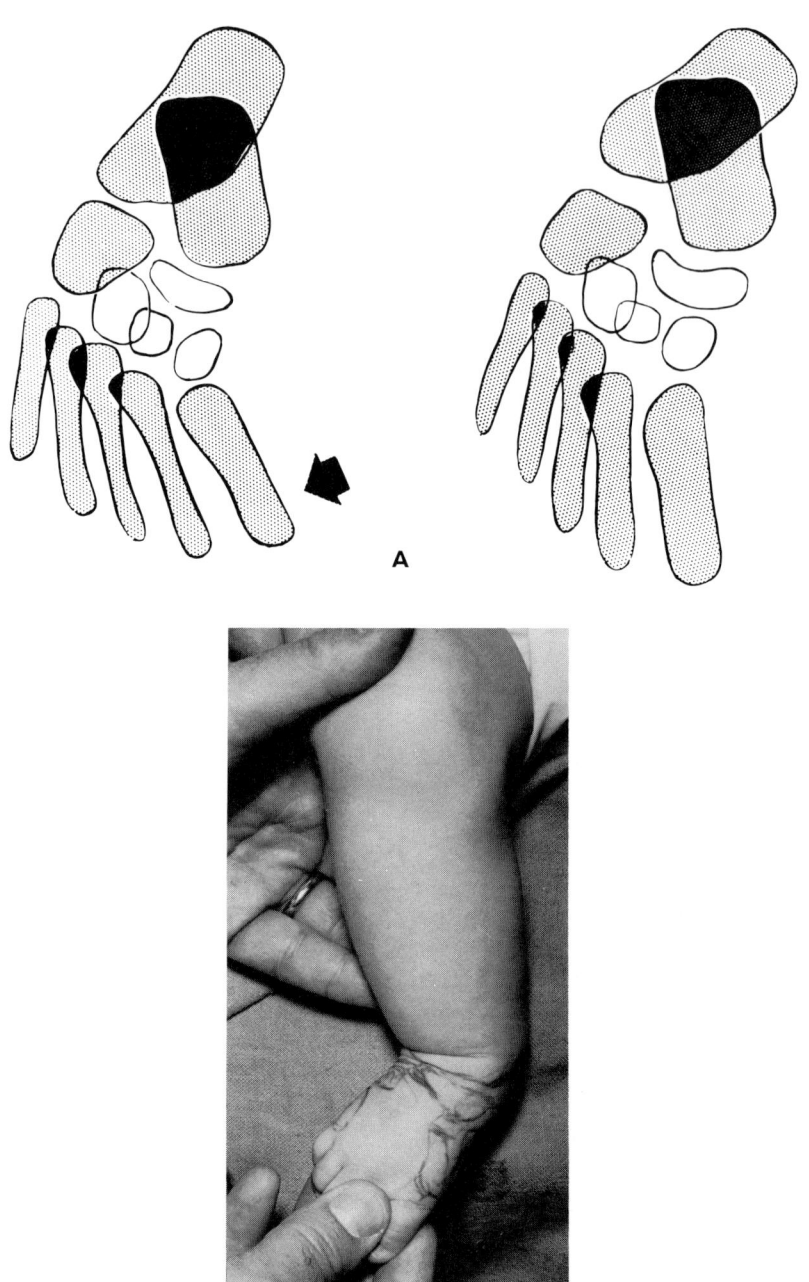

FIGURE 2–92. Correction of congenital metatarsus varus by passive stretching and retention in above-knee cast.

A and **B**. *The incorrect method of manipulation.* The entire foot is abducted and everted by forcefully abducting and everting the forefoot without counterpressure on the hindfoot. The foot is simply being twisted at the ankle, with little corrective force being exerted at the metatarsotarsal joints. The diagram illustrates how the valgus deformity of the heel is increased and shows that the improved appearance of the varus deformity of the forepart of the foot is spurious and not real correction.

Illustration continued on opposite page

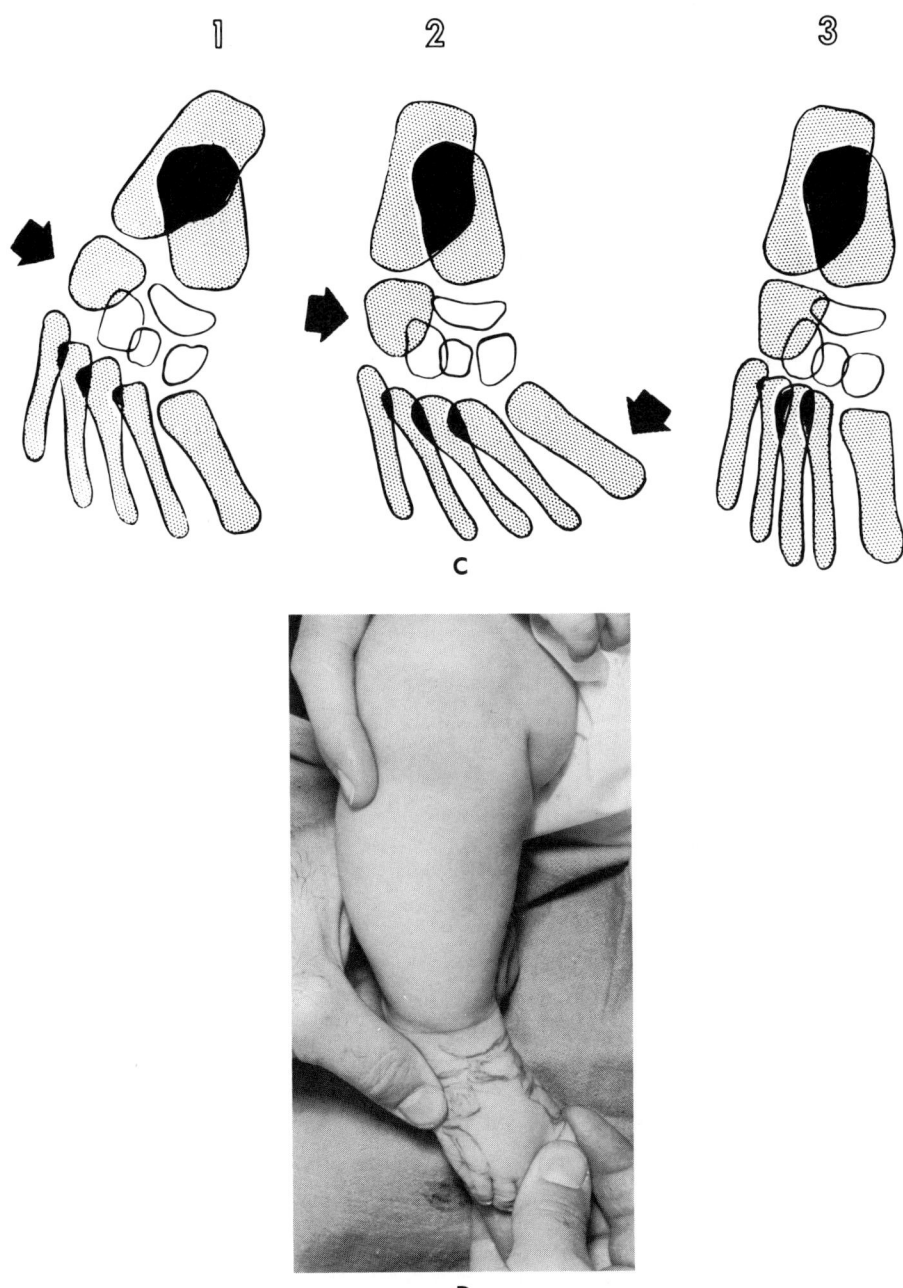

FIGURE 2–92 *Continued. Correction of congenital metatarsus varus by passive stretching and retention in above-knee cast.*

C and **D**. *The correct method of manipulation.* The hindfoot is slightly plantar-flexed, and the anterior process of the talus is displaced medially underneath the head of the talus; the metatarsals are pushed into abduction while counterpressure is applied over the cuboid. The diagram illustrates the proper method.

Illustration continued on following page

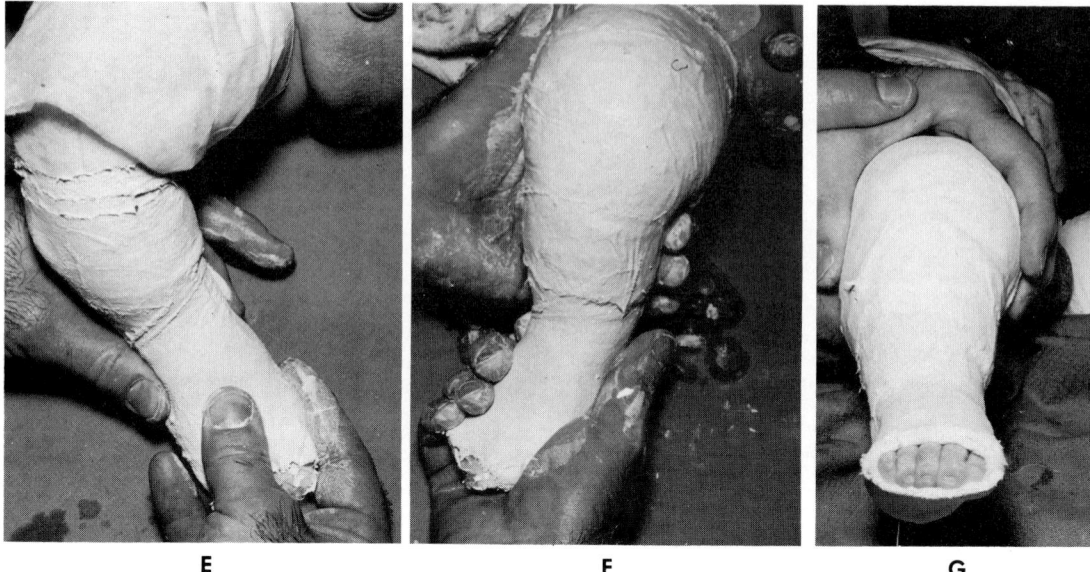

FIGURE 2–92 Continued. *Correction of congenital metatarsus varus by passive stretching and retention in above-knee cast.*

E. The foot points somewhat medialward while the first section of the plaster cast is applied. **F.** The foot and leg are in slight external rotation while the second section of the plaster cast is applied. **G.** Completed plaster cast. The heel and anterior part of the foot are immobilized in a position as near normal as possible. (From Ponseti, I. V., and Becker, J. R.: Congenital metatarsus adductus: The results of treatment. J. Bone Joint Surg., 48-A:706–707, 1966. Reprinted by permission.)

valgus deformity of the heel and provide only minimal corrective force at the tarso-metatarsal joints (Fig. 2–92 A and B). The correct method of manipulation is as follows: (1) The hindfoot is placed in slight plantar flexion and the anterior process of the calcaneus is pushed medially beneath the head of the talus. (2) The metatarsals are forced into abduction while counter-pressure is applied over the cuboid, immediately proximal to the base of the fifth metatarsal. The forepart of the foot is everted (Fig. 2–92 C and D). It is important not to produce an iatrogenic valgus deformity of the hindfoot. The corrected position is maintained to the count of 10 and then released. The exercises are performed for five to ten minutes. The manipulations should be gentle. Then an above-knee corrective cast is applied in two sections (Fig. 2–92 E, F, and G). First the plaster is wrapped over the foot and ankle, and is rolled against the deformity. Again, the hindfoot is maintained in inversion and slight plantar flexion, correcting the valgus deformity of the heel. With pressure over the cuboid bone, the metatarsals are pushed into maximal abduction, but not eversion. Pressure is exerted on the head and neck of the first metatarsal, not on the great toe. After the plaster sets, the cast is extended proximally to include the knee and thigh. Ponseti and Becker laterally rotate the leg when applying the proximal part of the cast to correct the associated medial torsion of the tibia. There is, however, no evidence that immobilizing the leg of an infant in lateral rotation for six to ten weeks will correct exaggerated medial tibial torsion; all it will accomplish is stretching of the soft tissues. If there is associated contracture of the invertors of the foot, the author laterally rotates the leg. In children under the age of one year, below-knee casts are ineffective for controlling the heel in correct position. This author recommends the combined use of the plaster of Paris cast and plastic tape, as it permits better grip and molding. An above-knee cast that holds the knee in 60 to 70 degrees of flexion will provide much better control of the heel and will prevent the cast from slipping. Casts are changed at 10- to 14-day intervals, the total duration of cast treatment varying from four to ten weeks, depending upon the rigidity of the deformity and its resistance to correction.

According to Kite, the following three criteria must be met before cast treatment is discontinued: (1) Complete correction of the convexity of the lateral border of the foot must be achieved (in fact, it is preferable to obtain slight overcorrection so that the convexity is reversed to slight concavity). (2) The prominence at the base of the fifth metatarsal must be no longer palpable. (3) Muscular balance must be restored so that active abduction of the forefoot is just as strong as active adduction.[9-11] In children over one year of age, overcorrection is almost impossible, and in the small infant, it should be avoided, as it will produce a valgus foot. Following cast removal, corrective shoes usually are not required. When the deformity was severe initially or definitive cast treatment was delayed, it is best that the forepart of the foot be held in slight overcorrection in plastic splints during sleep. Again attention should be paid to seeing that the heel is in slight inversion but without valgus distortion. A Denis Browne splint with reversed shoes should *not* be used for this purpose.

SURGICAL TREATMENT

When a patient with metatarsus varus is seen late, i.e., at over one or two years of age, the deformity may have become so fixed that it does not respond to conservative measures. Forceful manipulation in an attempt to correct the deformity of the forepart of the foot may force the heel into valgus position, producing a skewfoot. In such an instance, surgical measures are indicated.

In children under two years of age, the deformity can be satisfactorily corrected by capsulotomy of the first metatarsocuneiform joint and soft-tissue release of the abductor hallucis followed by a stretching plaster of Paris cast for six to eight weeks.

Tarsometatarsal and intermetatarsal soft-tissue release is performed in children between the ages of three and seven years. This procedure is described and illustrated in Plate 7.

Osteotomies at the base of the metatarsals are performed in children over eight years of age. The operative technique is described and illustrated in Plate 8.

Walking on a foot with rigid metatarsus varus forces the hindfoot into valgus position, producing a skewfoot. In such an instance, when only the varus deformity of the forepart of the foot is corrected, a severe pes valgus more disabling than the original skewfoot may be produced. If surgical correction is warranted, a two-stage procedure should be performed: first, a Grice extra-articular arthrodesis to correct the hindfoot valgus deformity; then soft-tissue release or metatarsal osteotomies, depending upon the age of the patient, to correct the forefoot varus deformity.

References follow on page 308

Mobilization of Tarsometatarsal and Intermetatarsal Joints by Capsulotomy and Ligamentous Release for Resistant Varus Deformity of the Forefoot (Heyman, Herndon, and Strong)

THE PROCEDURE

A. A curved transverse skin incision is made, extending from the base of the first metatarsal to the lateral border of the cuboid bone. It runs obliquely across the dorsum of the forepart of the foot just distal to the tarsometatarsal joints.

An alternate method of exposure of the tarsometatarsal joints is to make three longitudinal incisions on the dorsum of the foot—the first overlies the first ray, the second is between the second and third rays, and the third overlies the fourth ray. In the young child, two instead of three linear skin incisions may be made—one between the first and second rays and the other overlying the fourth ray.

B. The subcutaneous tissue and deep fascia are divided. The skin flaps are mobilized and retracted with 00 silk sutures. By meticulous linear dissection the tendons of the extensor digitorum longus, extensor hallucis longus, anterior tibial, and peroneus brevis are exposed and freed. The dorsalis pedis vessels are identified. Meticulous care is taken not to injure the neurovascular structures.

C. The anterior tibial tendon is retracted medially and the extensor hallucis longus tendon with the dorsalis pedis vessels is retracted laterally. The intermetatarsal space between the first and second metatarsals is identified with a small hemostat and the intermetatarsal ligament is divided, beginning distally and progressing proximally. By this method the first metatarsocuneiform joint is located. The epiphyseal plate of the first metatarsal is proximally located; it should not be damaged. The medial and dorsal capsules are divided. The plantar capsule is not sectioned at this time. The anterior tibial tendon should be carefully protected in order to prevent its inadvertent sectioning. The articular cartilage should not be injured.

Plate 7. Mobilization of Tarsometatarsal and Intermetatarsal Joints by Capsulotomy and Ligamentous Release for Resistant Varus Deformity of the Forefoot (Heyman, Herndon, and Strong)

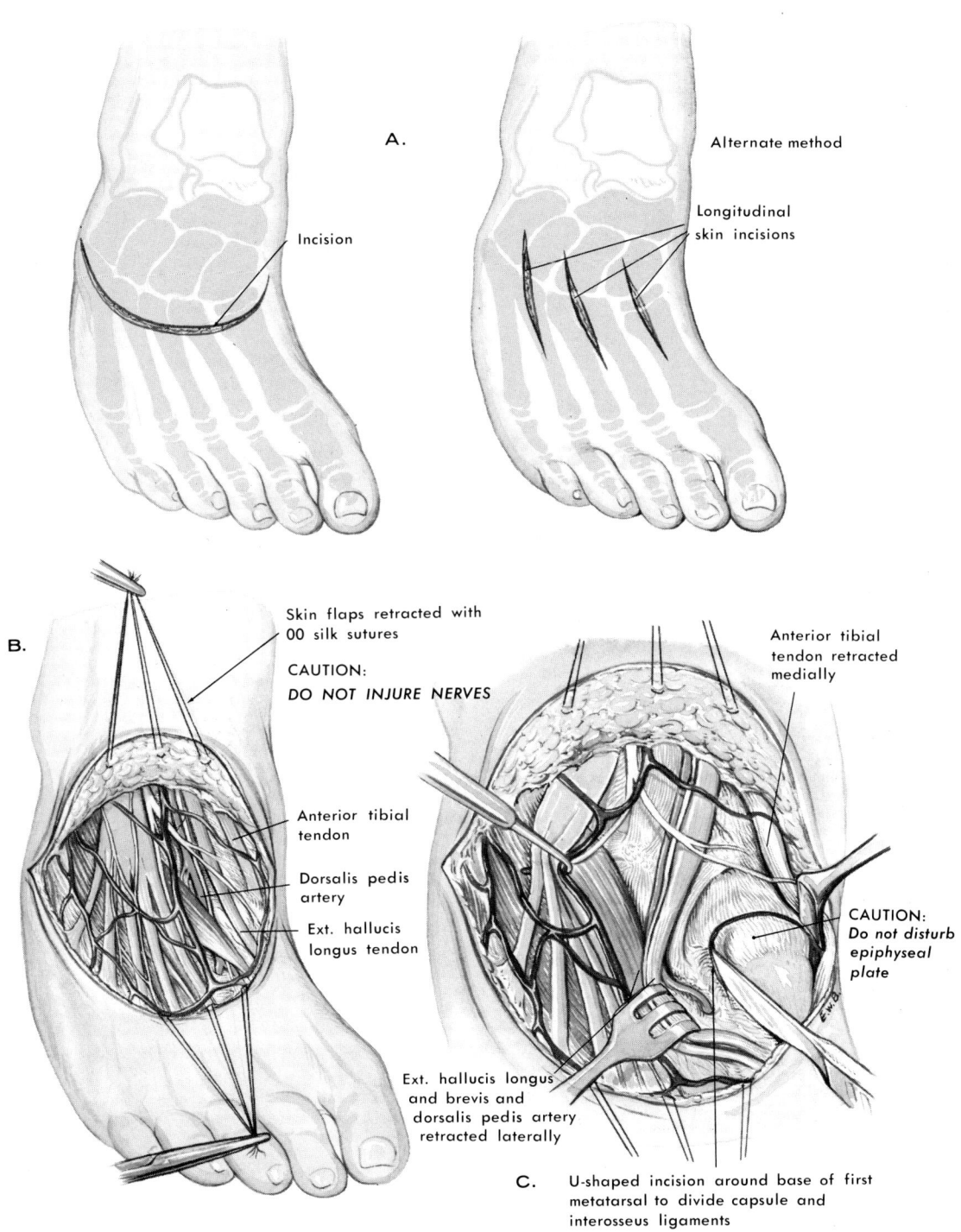

Mobilization of Tarsometatarsal and Intermetatarsal Joints by Capsulotomy and Ligamentous Release for Resistant Varus Deformity of the Forefoot (Heyman, Herndon, and Strong)
(Continued)

D. Next, the second metatarsocuneiform joint is exposed; it is located slightly proximal to the first metatarsocuneiform joint. The intermetatarsal ligaments and dorsal capsule are divided. Then longitudinal dissection is carried out in a plane overlying the third ray, taking care to protect the neurovascular structures and the extensor tendons. Again, with a small hemostat, the intermetatarsal space between the second and third metatarsals is identified, and the intermetatarsal ligaments are sectioned. Dorsal capsulotomy of the second and third metatarsocuneiform joints is completed. The fourth metatarsotarsal joint is essentially at the same level as the second and third; the articulation is readily identified after division of the intermetatarsal ligaments. Dorsal capsulotomy is similarly carried out.

At the fifth metatarsocuboid joint the attachment of the peroneus brevis is protected and the lateral capsule is not disturbed; the latter will serve as a hinge that prevents lateral displacement of the fifth metatarsal as the foot is manipulated.

E. Attention is then directed to the plantar capsule and the plantar ligaments. The metatarsotarsal joints are opened by plantar flexion of the forefoot and distal traction on the individual metatarsals. The medial two thirds of the plantar capsule and ligaments at each joint are divided, leaving the lateral one third intact. This will provide sufficient stability to prevent displacement of the metatarsals while the forefoot is manipulated out of adduction. The intermetatarsal ligaments must be divided completely to permit gliding of the metatarsals as the deformity is corrected.

F and **G.** The forefoot is manipulated into abduction and eversion. After correction is achieved there will be considerable incongruity of the articular surfaces. If there is marked instability of the tarsometatarsal joints Kirschner wires may be inserted to fix the first metatarsal to the first cuneiform and the fifth to the cuboid. The author, however, has not found routine use of Kirscher wires to be necessary.

The tourniquet is released and complete hemostasis is secured. The wound is closed with *interrupted* sutures, and a well-molded above-knee cast is applied, holding the foot in the corrected position.

POSTOPERATIVE CARE

For the first few days after surgery, the leg should be elevated to prevent excessive swelling. In 10 to 14 days, when the reactive swelling has subsided, the cast is changed and a new snug, well-molded one is applied. It is best to carry this out under general anesthesia and to manipulate the foot into the corrected position prior to application of the cast. The skin sutures should not be removed at this time, as the wound edges will separate.

Three weeks later (about four to five weeks after surgery) the cast and sutures are removed, and a carefully molded below-knee walking cast is applied. Immobilization in the cast is continued for a minimum of three to four months; this is important to allow adequate time for remodeling of articular surfaces. The casts are changed every three to four weeks (depending on how robust the child is, as walking is encouraged). Each time the foot is manipulated into the corrected position.

Plate 7. Mobilization of Tarsometatarsal and Intermetatarsal Joints by Capsulotomy and Ligamentous Release for Resistant Varus Deformity of the Forefoot (Heyman, Herndon, and Strong)

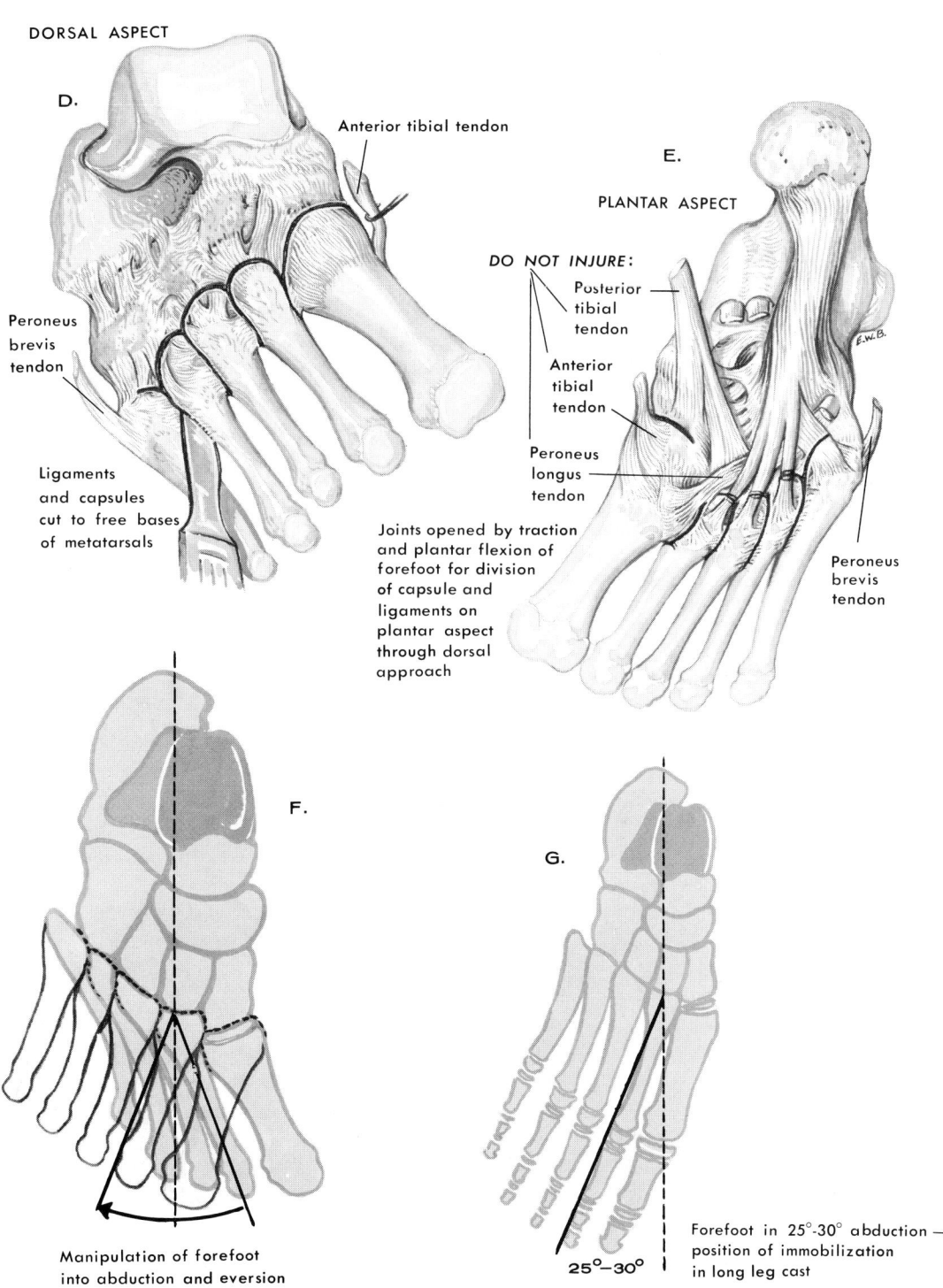

305

Osteotomy of Bases of Metatarsals for Correction of Varus Deformity of Forepart of Foot

THE PROCEDURE

A. The bases of all five metatarsals are exposed by three longitudinal skin incisions, all approximately 5 cm. long—the first on the medial side of the first metatarsal; the second, in the interval between the second and third rays; and the third, between the fourth and fifth rays. The subcutaneous tissue and fascia are divided in line with the skin incisions. The dorsal cutaneous nerves and the dorsalis pedis and metatarsal vessels should be protected from injury. The epiphyseal plate of the first metatarsal, in contrast to the lateral four metatarsals, is proximal in location and should not be damaged. By appropriate retraction of the extensor tendons and the anterior tibial tendon, the bases of all metatarsals are exposed.

B. The lines of osteotomy may be marked with a small starter and drill holes. The osteotomies are dome-shaped, with their apices directed posteriorly. In the first four metatarsals the medial limb is longer than the lateral limb, whereas in the fifth metatarsal the lateral (fibular) limb is longer than the medial one in order to prevent lateral displacement of the distal fragment when the forefoot is manipulated into abduction. In moderate varus deformity, osteotomy of the fifth metatarsal is not necessary. Often a laterally based wedge is excised from the lateral half of the base of the first metatarsal. The osteotomy is completed with a sharp dental osteotome or a small oscillating electric saw.

C. A heavy threaded Kirschner wire is inserted across the distal one fourth of the metatarsal shafts. The wound is closed and the foot is manipulated, swinging the forepart into abduction. An alternate method is internal fixation of the osteotomized fragments with two Kirschner wires—one inserted across the first metatarsal to the medial cuneiform and the other across the fifth metatarsal to the cuboid. A well-molded above- or below-knee cast is applied, holding the forepart of the foot in 5 to 10 degrees of abduction. The heel should be in neutral position. Weight-bearing is not allowed.

Roentgenograms are made in the operating room with the patient under anesthesia to ensure that the desired degree of correction is achieved and that the osteotomized bone fragments are in satisfactory apposition.

POSTOPERATIVE CARE

At three to four weeks, the cast, Kirschner wires, and sutures are removed. A below-knee walking cast is applied while the foot is held in the corrected position. Immobilization in the cast is continued for an additional two to three weeks.

*Plate 8. Osteotomy of Bases of Metatarsals
for Correction of Varus Deformity of Forepart of Foot*

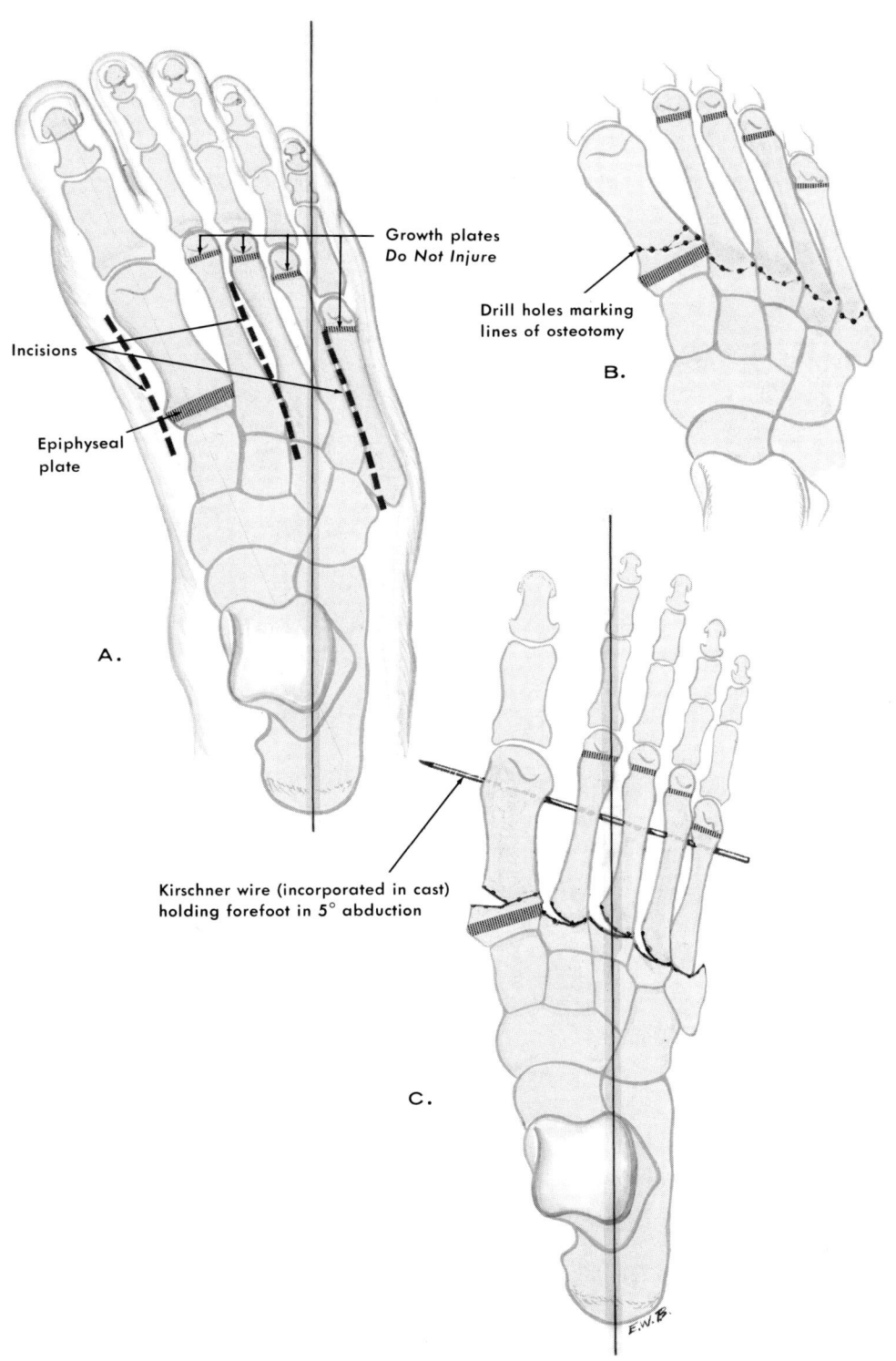

References *(Congenital Metatarsus Varus)*

1. Berman, A., and Gartland, J. J.: Metatarsal osteotomy for the correction of adduction of the forepart of the foot in children. J. Bone Joint Surg., *53-A*:498, 1971.
1a. Bleck, E. E.: Metatarsus adductus: Classification and relationship to outcomes of treatment. J. Pediat. Orthop., *3*:2, 1983.
2. Browne, R. S., and Paton, D. F.: Anomalous insertion of the tibialis posterior tendon in congenital metatarsus varus. J. Bone Joint Surg., *61-B*:74, 1979.
3. Diamond, L. S., Lynne, D., and Sigman, B.: Orthopedic disorders in patients with Down's syndrome. Orthop. Clin. N. Amer., *12*:57, 1981.
4. Henke, W.: Contracteur des metatarsus. Z. Rat. Med., *17*:188, 1863.
5. Herndon, C. H.: Discussion of paper by Berman, A., and Gartland, J. J. J. Bone Joint Surg., *53-A*:505, 1971.
6. Heyman, C. H., Herndon, C. H., and Strong, J. M.: Mobilization of the tarsometatarsal and intermetatarsal joints for the correction of resistant adduction of the forepart of the foot in congenital clubfoot or congenital metatarsus varus. J. Bone Joint Surg., *40-A*:299, 1958.
7. Jacobs, J. E.: Metatarsus varus and hip dysplasia. Clin. Orthop., *16*:19, 203, 1960.
8. Kendrick, R. E., Sharma, N. K., Hassler, W. L., and Herndon, C. H.: Tarsometatarsal mobilizatioh for resistant adduction of the forepart of the foot. J. Bone Joint Surg., *52-A*:61, 1970.
9. Kite, J. H.: Congenital metatarsus varus. Report of 300 cases. J. Bone Joint Surg., *32-A*:500, 1950.
10. Kite, J. H.: Congenital metatarsus varus. A.A.O.S. Instr. Course Lect., *7*:126, 1950.
11. Kite, J. H.: Congenital metatarsus varus. J. Bone Joint Surg., *46-A*:525, 1964.
12. Lichtblau, S.: Section of the abductor hallucis tendon for correction of metatarsus varus deformity. Clin. Orthop., *110*:227, 1975.
13. Lusskin, R., and Lusskin, H.: A metatarsus varus splint for the prewalker. J. Bone Joint Surg., *41-A*:363, 1959.
14. McCauley, J., Jr., Lusskin, R., and Bromley, J.: Recurrence in congenital metatarsus varus. J. Bone Joint Surg., *46-A*:525, 1964.
15. McCormick, D. W., and Blount, W. P.: Metatarsus adductovarus. "Skewfoot." J.A.M.A., *141*:449, 1949.
16. Mitchell, G.: Personal communication, 1978.
17. Mitchell, G. P.: Abductor hallucis release in congenital metatarsus varus. Int. Orthop., *3*:299, 1980.
18. Peabody, C. W., and Muro, F.: Congenital metatarsus varus. J. Bone Joint Surg., *15*:171, 1933.
19. Ponseti, I. V., and Becker, J. R.: Congenital metatarsus adductus: The results of treatment. J. Bone Joint Surg., *48-A*:702, 1966.
20. Reimann, I., and Werner, H. H.: Congenital metatarsus varus. A suggestion for possible mechanism and relation to other foot deformities. Clin. Orthop., *110*:223, 1975.
20a. Reimann, I., and Werner, H. H.: Congenital metatarsus varus. On the advantages of early treatment. Acta Orthop. Scand., *46*:857, 1975.
20b. Rushforth, G. F.: The natural history of hooked forefoot. J. Bone Joint Surg., *60-B*:530, 1978.
21. Thomson, S. A.: Hallux varus and metatarsus varus. Clin. Orthop., *16*:109, 1960.
22. Wynne-Davies, R.: Family studies and the cause of congenital club-foot—talipes equinovarus, talipes calcaneovalgus and metatarsus varus. J. Bone Joint Surg., *46-B*:445, 1964.

CONGENITAL METATARSUS PRIMUS VARUS AND HALLUX VALGUS

Metatarsus Primus Varus

This is a congenital deformity in which the first metatarsal is deviated medially to

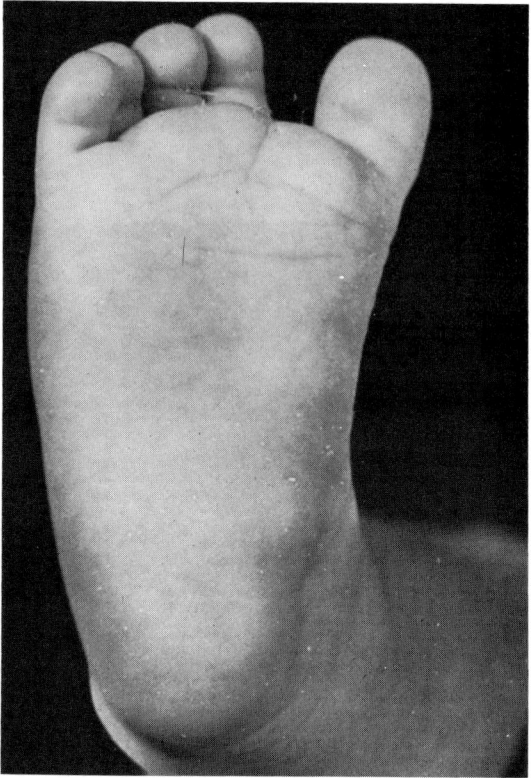

FIGURE 2–93. *Metatarsus primus varus.*

Note that only the first metatarsal is deviated medially to an abnormal degree. The lateral four metatarsals have normal alignment.

an abnormal degree. The lateral four metatarsals have normal alignment (Fig. 2–93). In the standing anteroposterior roentgenogram of the foot, the angle between the first and second metatarsals measures about 7 degrees in the normal foot; an angle greater than 10 degrees is considered pathologic.

The condition is hereditary, with a marked preponderance in girls. Because of the trivial nature of this anomaly, it is often not recognized in infancy and early childhood. This is unfortunate because, in adolescence, the great toe will be gradually pushed into abduction, and the secondary deformities of hallux valgus and bunion will develop (Fig. 2–94). When detected in infancy, metatarsus primus varus is treated by passive stretching and a corrective cast.

Hallux Valgus and Bunion

These two terms, commonly used synonymously, refer to separate elements of the

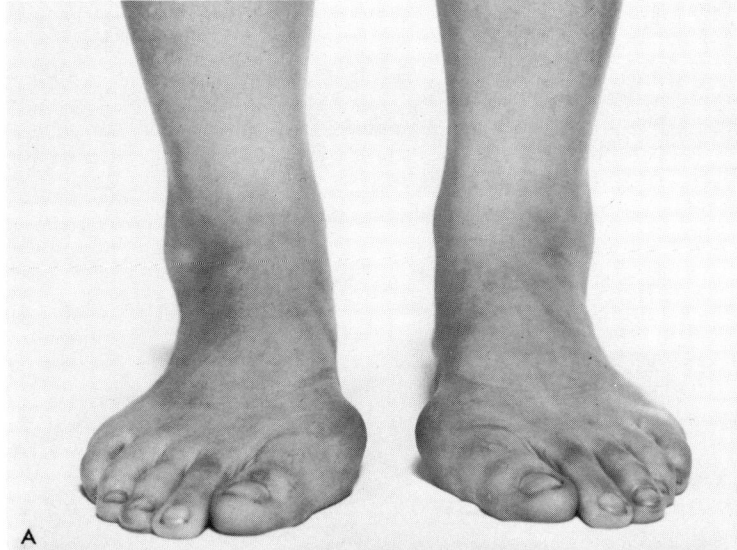
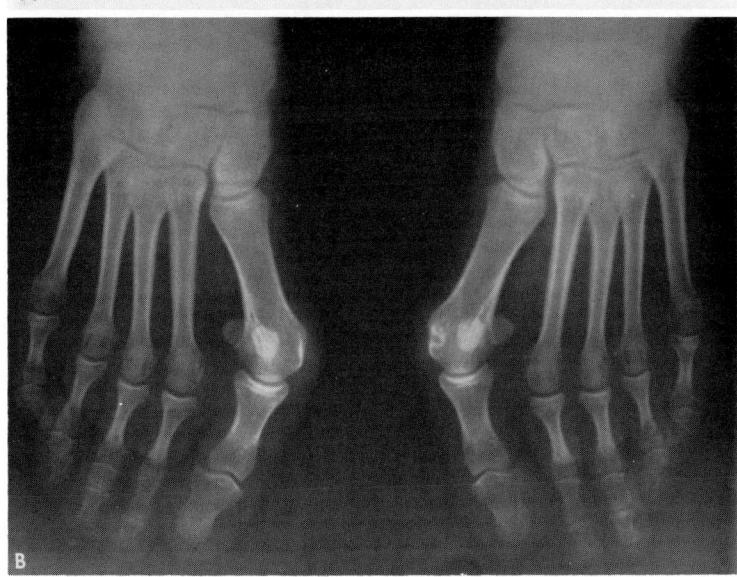

FIGURE 2–94. Severe bilateral metatarsus primus varus, hallux valgus, and bunion in an adolescent girl.

A. Clinical appearance. **B**. Standing anteroposterior roentgenograms.

same syndrome, namely, the lateral deviation of the great toe at the metatarsophalangeal joint and the prominence on the medial aspect of the forefoot produced by the bony deformity together with its acquired bursa. Since the deformity usually causes disability in patients at or past middle age, the pathologic changes are not discussed here, and the presentation of the treatment of hallux valgus is very brief. The literature on the subject is voluminous; one excellent treatise is the monograph by Kelikian.[14]

The symptoms comprise those due to the bunion and those due to the secondary deformities and metatarsalgia. The initial presenting complaint is tenderness over the bunion from pressure and friction against the shoe. The adventitious bursa becomes inflamed and may also be secondarily infected and may suppurate. Metatarsalgia and secondary deformities such as hammertoe and callosities are other causes of discomfort.

Treatment

Conservative measures will provide symptomatic relief, but they will not correct the primary deformity. Shoes of adequate width in the forefoot are provided, the bunion is protected with pads of felt, and a rubber wedge between the great and second toes or special bunion splints to hold the hallux straight are given to be worn at night. Metatarsal arch support in the form of appropriate insole pads is provided to treat metatarsalgia.

Operative treatment is indicated when conservative measures fail to give symptomatic relief and when the deformity is very severe. Surgical methods that have been described are many and include the following general technical features: (1) osteotomy of the first metatarsal at its base or neck to correct the metatarsus primus varus deformity; (2) soft-tissue procedures to correct the hallux valgus deformity at the metatarsophalangeal joint; (3) section and transfer of the adductor hallucis to the first metatarsal head; (4) partial excision of the medial prominence of the first metatarsal head; and (5) resection of the proximal two thirds of the proximal phalanx of the great toe.

In adolescents, degenerative changes in the first metatarsophalangeal joint are usually absent and arthroplasty by the Keller procedure is not indicated. If there is associated hallux rigidus with restriction of dorsiflexion of the great toe, osteotomy of the first metatarsal near its neck, displacing the metatarsal head plantarward as well as laterally, is advisable. One or two Kirschner wires are inserted to maintain alignment of the osteotomy. Otherwise, the author prefers the following technique for correcting metartarsus primus varus and hallux valgus (Fig. 2–95).

A dorsomedial incision is made, extending from the middle of the proximal phalanx of the great toe to the base of the first metatarsal. The subcutaneous tissue is divided in line with the skin incision; the digital nerves are identified, care being taken not to injure them inadvertently. Three sets of silk sutures are placed on the skin edges for retraction; the loops are passed distal to the toes, and the ends of the sutures are tied on the lateral side of the forefoot. A U-shaped incision is made on the medial aspect of the capsule of the first metatarsophalangeal joint; the width of the U should be at least 2 cm. The capsule is divided as close to its metatarsal attachment as possible and is reflected distally, leaving its base attached to the proximal phalanx. With an osteotome, the prominent nonarticular portion of the metatarsal head is resected in one piece and kept sterile in a moist sterile sponge. The big toe is laterally displaced, and with Mayo or tenotomy scissors, the lateral part of the capsule of the metatarsophalangeal joint and the adductor hallucis tendon are sectioned. (The author has not found it necessary to transfer the adductor hallucis to the head of the first metatarsal, the only exception to this being in hallux valgus in a spastic foot—in which instance a separate short dorsolateral incision is made and the adductor hallucis longus tendon is divided under direct vision and transferred to the first metatarsal head.) Then a 00 Mersilene whip suture is inserted on the proximal end of the capsule, which is attached firmly to the distal shaft of the first metatarsal through two drill holes. If the abductor hallucis tendon is displaced plantarward, it is detached at its insertion and transferred to a more dorsal site on the medial aspect of the base of the proximal phalanx. Next, *without stripping the periosteum,* the site of osteotomy is marked with a sharp starter and drill holes at the base of the first metatarsal. The lateral cortex is left intact. The bone is divided transversely with a thin osteotome, and the bone previously removed from the metatarsal head is shaped into a wedge and driven in between the osteotomized bone fragments—with care that the lateral cortex is not broken. Precautions should be taken to avoid elevating or depressing the first metatarsal unless this is indicated. This open-up osteotomy will correct only moderate medial divergence of the first metatarsal. If the metatarsus primus varus is severe, a modified dome-shaped osteotomy with a medial buttress in the proximal segment will more effectively correct the deformity. In such an instance, the alignment of the osteotomized fragments is maintained by fixation with a heavy threaded Steinmann pin that fixes the shaft of the first metatarsal to the lateral metatarsals. The pin protrudes on the lateral aspect of the foot for ease of removal when the osteotomy is healed. The wound is closed in the usual manner, and a below-knee walking cast with a toe cap is applied. Ordinarily the osteotomy will heal in six weeks, at which time the cast and pin are removed and a new below-knee walking cast

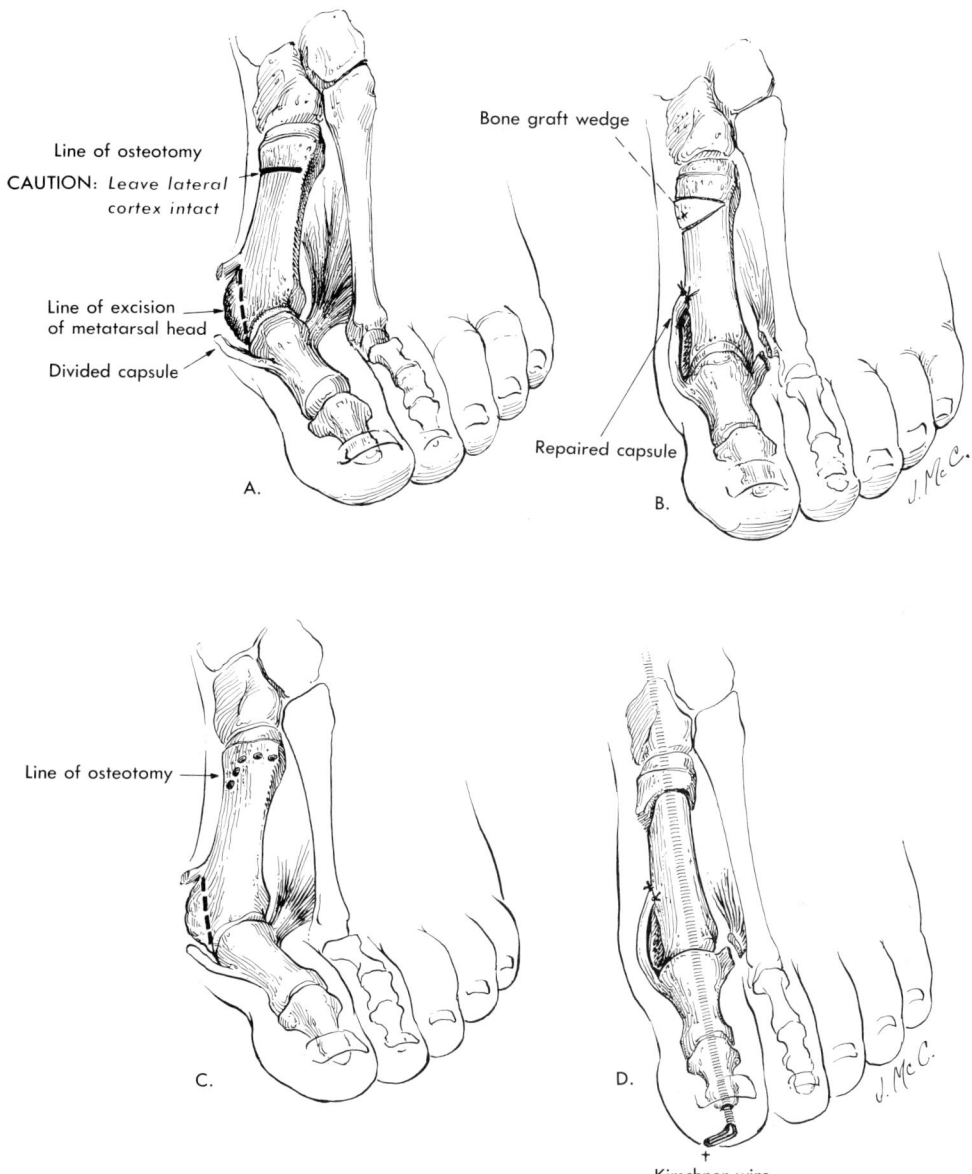

FIGURE 2–95. Correction of hallux valgus and metatarsus primus varus.

Diagrams showing the deformity (**A**) and the postoperative correction (**B**). The hallux valgus is corrected by medial capsular tightening and sectioning of the adductor hallucis longus tendon and lateral capsule. The medial prominence of the first metatarsal head is excised and is used for bone graft. Metatarsus primus varus deformity is corrected by an open-up transverse osteotomy at the base of the metatarsal. The lateral cortex is left intact. **C** and **D**. Correction of metatarsus primus varus and hallux valgus by modified dome osteotomy of the first metatarsal at its base (note the medial buttress) and internal fixation with Kirschner wire. The author, however, recommends that the distal part of the first metatarsal shaft be fixed to the lateral metatarsals with a threaded Steinmann pin.

is applied for 10 to 14 days, and then weight-bearing is permitted without restriction. Passive exercises of the first metatarsophalangeal joint are performed several times a day until full range of motion is obtained.

References

1. Bonney G., and MacNab, I.: Hallux valgus and hallux rigidus. A critical survey of operative results. J. Bone Joint Surg., *34B*:366, 1952.
2. Carr, C. R., and Boyd, B. M.: Correctional osteotomy for metatarsus primus varus and hallux valgus. J. Bone Joint Surg., *50-A*:1353, 1968.

3. Cholmeley, J. A.: Hallux valgus in adolescents. Proc. Roy. Soc. Med. (Section of Orthopedics), 51:903, 1958.
4. Dhanendran, M. Pollard, J. P., and Hutton, W. C.: Mechanics of the hallux valgus foot and the effect of Keller's operation. Acta Orthop. Scand., 51:1007, 1980.
5. Ellis, V. H.: A method of correcting metatarsus primus varus. Preliminary report. J. Bone Joint Surg., 33-B:415, 1951.
6. Glynn, M. K., Dunlop, J. B., and Fitzpatrick, D.: The Mitchell distal metatarsal osteotomy for hallux valgus. J. Bone Joint Surg., 62-B:188, 1980.
7. Haines, R. W., and McDougall, A.: The anatomy of hallux valgus. J. Bone Joint Surg., 36-B:272, 1954.
8. Hardy, R. H., and Clapham, J. C. R.: Observations on hallux valgus. Based on controlled series. J. Bone Joint Surg., 33-B:376, 1951.
9. Hardy, R. H., and Clapham, J. C. R.: Hallux valgus. Predisposing anatomic causes. Lancet, 1:1180, 1952.
10. Houghton, G. R., and Dickson, R. A.: Hallux valgus in the younger patient: The structural abnormality. J. Bone Joint Surg., 61-B:176, 1979.
11. Jones, A. R.: Hallux valgus in the adolescent. Proc. Roy. Soc. Med. (Section of Orthopedics), 41:392, 1948.
12. Keller, W. L.: Surgical treatment of bunion and hallux valgus. New York Med. J., 80:741, 1904.
13. Keller, W. L.: Further observations on the surgical treatment of hallux valgus and bunions. New York Med. J., 95:696, 1912.
14. Kelikian, H.: Hallux Valgus. Allied Deformities of the Forefoot and Metatarsalgia. Philadelphia, W. B. Saunders Co., 1965.
15. Kritsikis, N., Meyer, J. M., and El-Manouar, M.: Long-term follow-up of the surgical treatment of hallux valgus in 100 operated patients. Acta Orthop Belg., 45:186, 1979.
16. Lapidus, P. W.: Operative correction of the metatarsus varus primus in hallux valgus. Surg. Gynec. Obstet., 58:183, 1934.
17. McBride, E. D.: A conservative operation for bunions. J. Bone Joint Surg., 10:735, 1928.
18. McBride, E. D.: Hallux valgus, bunion deformity; its treatment in mild, moderate and severe stages. J. Int. Coll. Surg., 21:99, 1954.
19. McBride, E. D.: The McBride bunion hallux valgus operation. Refinements in the successive surgical steps of the operation. J. Bone Joint Surg., 42-A:965, 1960.
20. Mitchell, C. L., Fleming, J. L., Allen, R., Glenney, C., and Sanford, G. A.: Osteotomy-bunionectomy for hallux valgus. J. Bone Joint Surg., 40-A:41, 1958.
21. Piggott, H.: The natural history of hallux valgus in adolescence and early adult life. J. Bone Joint Surg., 42-B:749, 1960.
22. Silver, D.: The operative treatment of hallux valgus. J. Bone Joint Surg., 5:225, 1923.
23. Simmonds, F. A., and Menelaus, M. B.: Hallux valgus in adolescents. J. Bone Joint Surg., 42-B:761, 1960.
24. Stokes, I. A., Hutton, W. C., Stott, J. R., and Lowe, L. W.: Forces under the hallux valgus foot before and after surgery. Clin. Orthop., 142:64, 1979.
25. Swanson, A. B., Lumsden, R. M., and Swanson, G. D.: Silicone implant arthroplasty of the great toe. A review of single stem and flexible hinge implants. Clin. Orthop., 142:30, 1979.
26. Wiasmitinow, N. P., and Zollinger, H.: 10-year results after Hohmann's operation in hallux valgus. Orthopaede, 8:165, 1979.

CONGENITAL BALL-AND-SOCKET ANKLE JOINT

In this rare malformation, the contour of the ankle joint is abnormal. The proximal articular surface of the normal talus is dome-shaped in the lateral, but not in the anteroposterior, view. In the ball-and-socket ankle joint the upper end of the talus is dome-shaped in both the anteroposterior and lateral projections, and articulates in a reciprocal manner with the concave distal end of the tibia (Fig. 2–96). The fibular malleolus may or may not participate in the ball-and-socket ankle.

Lamb, in 1958, described five cases of this rare entity; four of his patients had associated coalition of the tarsal bones; the fifth patient had congenital shortening of the

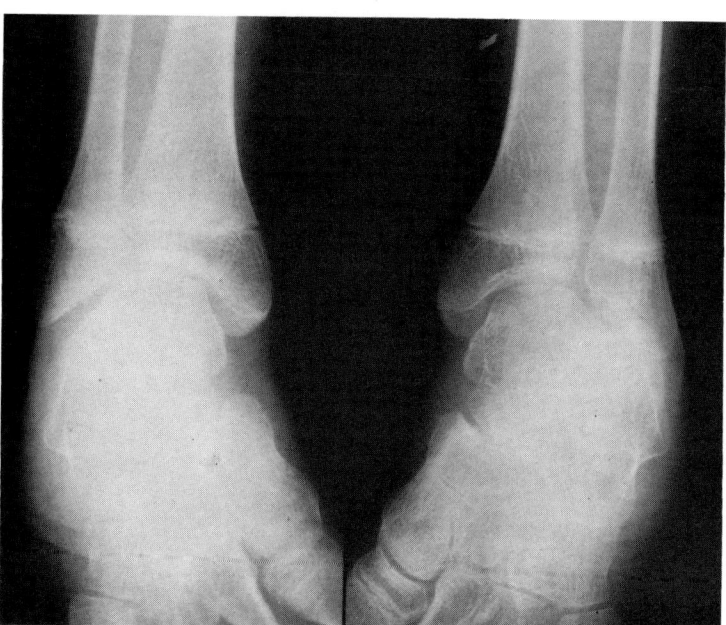

FIGURE 2–96. Roentgenograms of ankle showing ball-and-socket joint.

lower limb without tarsal fusion.[8] Brahme reported another case with bilateral involvement and used the term *upper talar enarthrosis*.[1] Congenital ball-and-socket joint may also be seen in association with congenital hypoplasia or absence of the fibula and failure of segmentation of the vertebrae. Lloyd-Roberts and Clark reported three children with ball-and-socket ankle joints who also had metatarsus adductus varus (S-shaped or serpentine foot).[9] Schreiber reported 27 congenital ball-and-socket ankle joints in 21 patients; the abnormality was found in 10 of 26 cases of congenital shortening of the leg (38 per cent), in 11 of 64 cases of tarsal coalition (17 per cent), and in 4 of 18 cases of congenital hypoplasia or absence of the fibula (22 per cent). No associated deformity of the lower limb could be found with 6 of the 27 congenital ball-and-socket joints (22 per cent).[11]

The condition is twice as common in the male as in the female. Jacobs has reported a familial occurrence in a father and daughter, each of whom had bilateral involvement.[6] The exact cause is unknown.

The basic underlying pathogenetic factor appears to be loss of subtalar joint motion and resultant increased motion and stress at the ankle joint.[7] By means of serial roentgenograms taken from the first month of life to puberty, Imhauser studied three feet with congenital synostosis of the tarsal bones. He demonstrated that the transformation of the ankle joints to spherical shape is a secondary process taking place between the second and fourth years of life. It is a morphologic response to altered function caused by restriction of motion in the tarsus. He also showed that shortening of the fibular malleolus, a roentgenographic finding associated with ball-and-socket ankle joint, is not of pathogenetic significance.[5]

Congenital ball-and-socket ankle joint is usually asymptomatic. The abnormal lateral mobility at the ankle may cause repeated sprains of the joint, and patients often complain of weakness of the ankle. When there is associated loss of subtalar motion, degenerative arthritis of the ankle may develop in adult life because of excessive stress and repeated minor trauma to the joint.

The roentgenographic appearance is characteristic. The trochlear surface of the talus, which is normally convex in the anteroposterior plane and gently concave from side to side, loses its concavity in this deformity and becomes spheroid in shape. The lower end of the tibia is correspondingly molded into a cuplike cavity, forming the socket of a ball-and-socket joint. In infancy and late childhood, it is difficult to determine the exact shape of the ankle joint because of the great amount of cartilage in the unossified tibia, talus, and fibula.

Treatment is not indicated, as the condition is asymptomatic. Ankle fusion is performed if degenerative arthritic changes in late adult life cause the deformity to become very disabling.

An acquired form of ball-and-socket ankle joint is sometimes seen in which the rounding of the talus is not as smooth as in the congenital variety. It is reported to follow subtalar arthrodesis (Grice procedure) performed at an early age and probably represents an attempt to compensate for loss of subtalar motion. It is also found in congenital insensitivity to pain. It seems to be associated with marked abnormal laxity of the ligaments about the ankle joint. Robins studied the ankle joints of 52 patients with poliomyelitis who had had arthrodesis of their feet: triple arthrodesis (42 cases), subtalar arthrodesis (4 cases), Lambrinudi arthrodesis (4 cases), and Campbell's bone block (2 cases). Eight feet (15 per cent) disclosed some compensatory increase in lateral movement of the talus within the tibiofibular mortise, and roentgenograms showed some rounding of the margins of the talus.[10]

References

1. Brahme, F.: Upper talar enarthrosis. Acta Radiol., *55*:221, 1961.
2. Channon, G. M., and Brotherton, B. J.: The ball and socket ankle joint. J. Bone Joint Surg., *61-B*:85, 1979.
3. Fischer, V., and Refior, H. J.: Talo-crurales Kugelgelenk bei Rückfusssynostosen. Arch. Orthop. Unfallchir., *73*:278, 1972.
4. Henssge, J., and Engelke, B.: Die fibulo-ulnare Hypoplasie mit kugelförmigem Knöchelgelenk, Strahlendefekten und Synostosen. Z. Orthop., *107*:502, 1970.
5. Imhauser, G.: Kugelformige Knochelgelenke bei angeborenen Fusswurzelsynostosen. Beitrag zur Form-Funktions-Beziehung. Z. Orthop., *108*:247, 1970.
6. Jacobs, P.: Some uncommon deformities of the ankle and foot. Brit. J. Radiol., *35*:776, 1962.
7. Jensen, J. K.: Ball and socket ankle joint. Clin. Orthop., *85*:28, 1972.
8. Lamb, D.: The ball-and-socket ankle joint. J. Bone Joint Surg., *40-B*:240, 1958.
9. Lloyd-Roberts, G. C., and Clark, R. C.: Ball and socket

joint in metatarsus adductus varus. (S-Shaped or serpentine foot). J. Bone Joint Surg., *55-B*:193, 1973.
10. Robins, R. H. G.: The ankle joint in relation to arthrodesis of the foot in poliomyelitis. J. Bone Joint Surg., *41-B*:337, 1959.
11. Schreiber, R. R.: Congenital and acquired ball-and-socket ankle joint. Radiology, *84*:940, 1963.
12. Steinhäuser, J.: Beitrage zur Umformung des Knöchelgelenkes zum Kugelgelenk bei angeborenen Fusswurzelsynostosen. Z. Orthop., *105*:381, 1968.
13. Steinhauser, J.: Weitere Beobachtungen kugelförmiger Knöchelgelenke bei angeborenen Fusswurzelsynostosen. Z. Orthop., *112*:433, 1974.
14. Vichard, P., Pinon, P., and Peltre, G.: Ball and socket ankle associated with congenital synostosis of the tarsus. Report of a case (Author's transl.). Rev. Chir. Orthop., *66*:387, 1980.
15. Weston, W. J.: Congenital ball and socket ankle joint. Brit. J. Radiol., *35*:871, 1962.

BRACHYMETATARSIA (CONGENITAL SHORT METATARSAL)

Congenital shortening of one or more metatarsals is not uncommon. Frequently the first metatarsal is shortened, a condition known as metatarsus primus atavicus. The

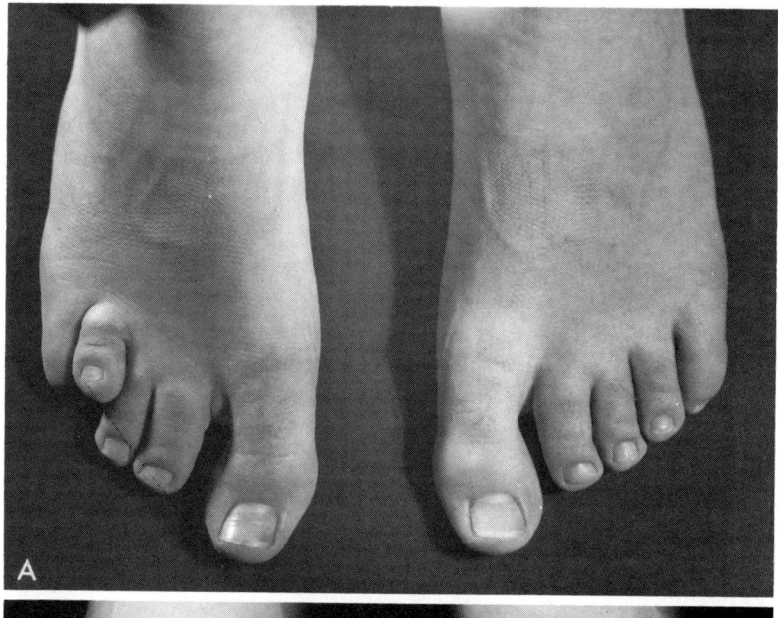

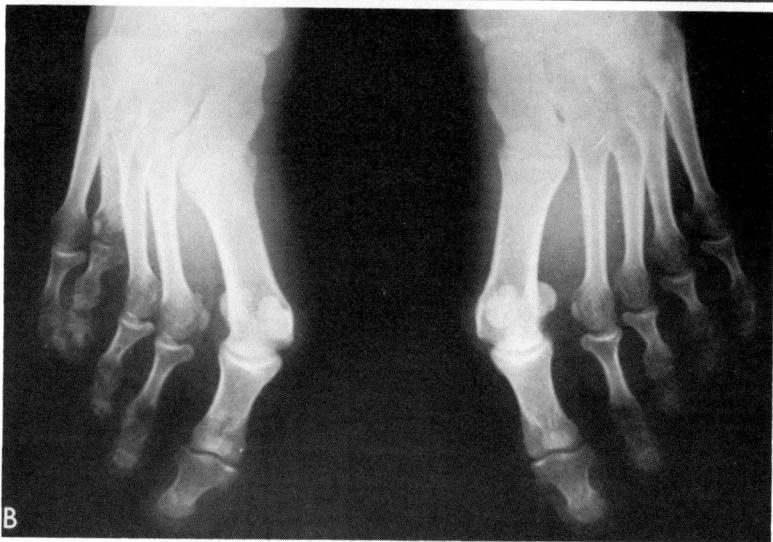

FIGURE 2–97. Congenital shortening of the right fourth metatarsal.

A. Clinical appearance. Note the "apparent" shortening of the right fourth toe. Left foot is normal. **B.** Anteroposterior roentgenogram of both feet, showing the short fourth metatarsal of the right foot.

Congenital Deformities 315

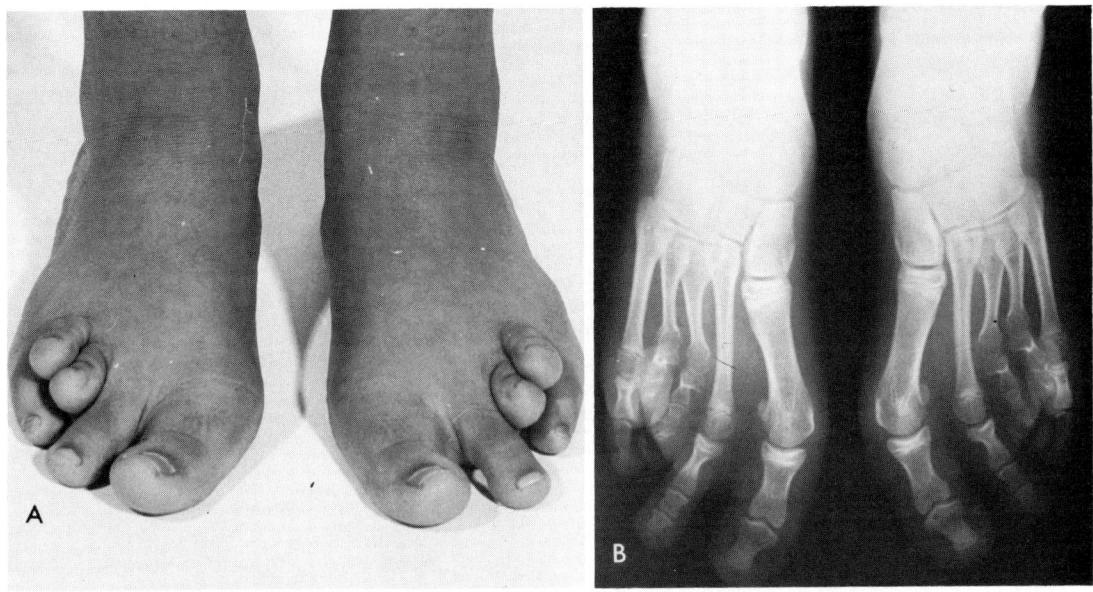

FIGURE 2–98. Congenital shortening of third and fourth metatarsals.
A. Clinical appearance. **B**. Anteroposterior roentgenogram of both feet.

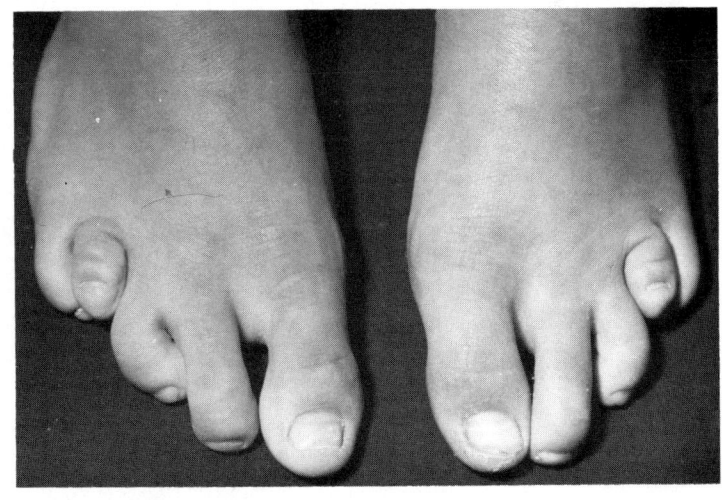

FIGURE 2–99. Bilateral congenital shortening of fourth metatarsals with curly (or varus) third toe on the right.

length of the first metatarsal in relation to that of the second metatarsal may vary considerably in the normal foot. This was determined by Harris and Beath on standardized dorsoplantar roentgenograms that showed all the bones of the foot with equal clarity from the posterior end of the calcaneus to the tips of the distal phalanges. They measured the distance from the posterior end of the calcaneus to the head of the second metatarsal in 7,167 individual feet. In 2,878 feet (40 per cent), the first metatarsal was *shorter* than the second by 1 mm. or more; in 2,693 feet (38 per cent), the first metatarsal was *longer* than the second by 1 mm. or more; and in 1,596 feet (22 per cent), the first and second metatarsals were of equal length (within 1 mm.).[2]

Morton, in 1935, in his monograph *The Human Foot*, proposed that shortness of the first metatarsal can cause disability by disturbing the transmission of weight and thrust forces through the forepart of the foot. According to his thesis, the head of the short first metatarsal does not reach the ground as readily as that of the longer second metatarsal. Hence, the greater part of the body weight that is borne through the forepart of the foot is shifted from the first metatarsal to the second or to the second and third metatarsals. The forefoot pronates in an attempt to put the head of the first metatarsal into a weight-bearing position on the ground. This compensatory mechanism lowers the longitudinal arch, which is then subjected to undue strain. In response to this increased stress, callosities develop beneath the heads of the second and third metatarsals, and the shaft of the second metatarsal may thicken. Morton, however, emphasized that shortness of the first metatarsal is but *occasionally* the cause of foot disability, and then only in adult life.[3] Despite his observations, however, the presence of this anomaly was commonly believed to be the cause of symptomatic flatfoot.

The fallacy of this assumption was proved by Harris and Beath, who found in the Canadian Army Foot Survey that the short

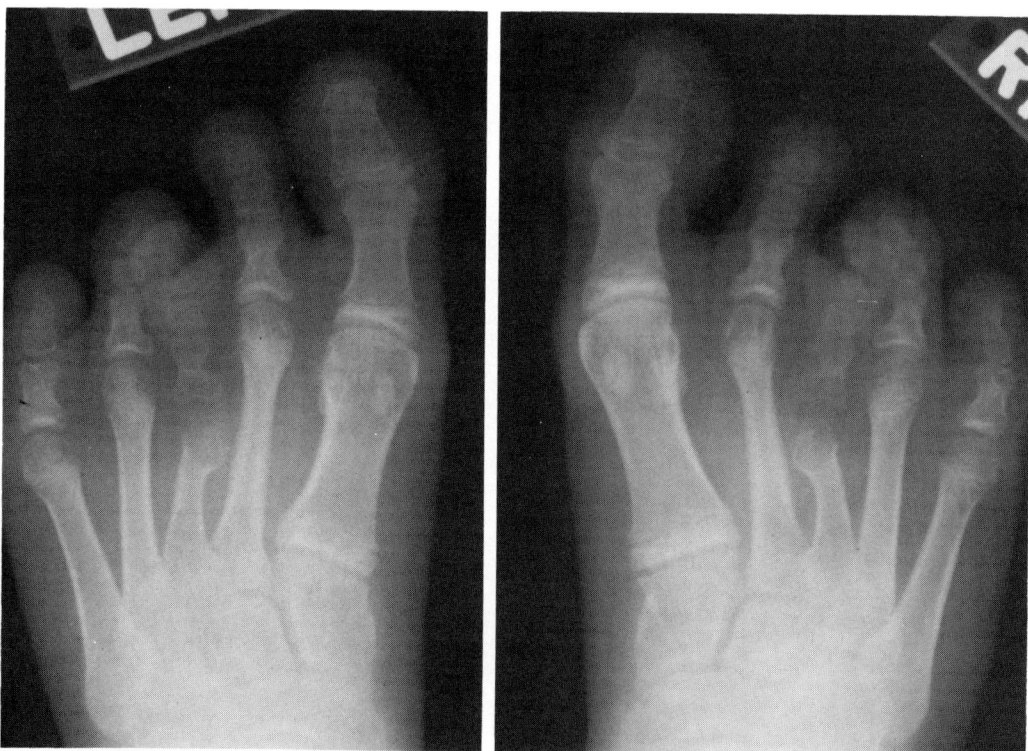

FIGURE 2–100. Congenital shortening of third metatarsal.

Anteroposterior roentgenograms of both feet show congenital shortening of the third metatarsal.

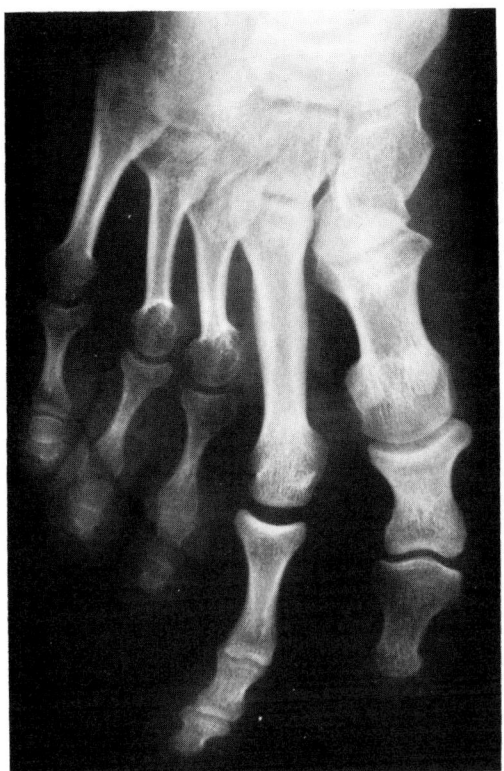

FIGURE 2–101. *Anteroposterior roentgenogram of foot showing congenital shortening of the first, third, fourth, and fifth metatarsals.*

isolated anomaly. It may also occur in association with metatarsus varus and talipes equinovarus. These may lead to abnormal stress and cause painful callosities under the remaining metatarsal heads. Treatment consists of fitting a metatarsal pad that is elongated medially under the first metatarsal to redistribute the body weight.

The next most common shortened metatarsal is the fourth. Other types of shortening of the metatarsals are illustrated in Figures 2–97 through 2–101. Usually no treatment is required unless there is difficulty with pressure from the shoe on the upriding toes. Lengthening of the metatarsals has been performed successfully by using the technique for shortened metacarpals.

References

1. Harris, R. I., and Beath, T.: Report 1574, Army Foot Survey. Ottawa, National Research Council of Canada, 1947.
2. Harris, R. I., and Beath, T.: The short first metatarsal. J. Bone Joint Surg., *31-A*:553, 1949.
3. Morton, D.: The Human Foot, New York, Columbia University Press, 1935.

CONGENITAL SPLIT OR CLEFT FOOT (LOBSTER CLAW)

first metatarsal is seldom if ever the cause of foot disability.[1] They stressed that callus under the heads of the central metatarsals is not specifically related to the short first metatarsal, as it occurred almost as frequently in those feet in which the first metatarsal was longer than the second. That the first metatarsal is short does not necessarily indicate that it cannot reach the ground as readily or that less weight will be transmitted through this bone. The obliquity of the metatarsals in relation to the ground demonstrates that all can share equally in weight-bearing, provided the longer metatarsals are on a higher plane than the shorter. Depression of the central metatarsals and marked pressure under their prominent heads cause the callosity. Limitation of plantar flexion of the toes and fixation of the toes in dorsiflexed position will further exaggerate the depression of the metatarsal heads.

Primary marked shortening of the first metatarsal may be encountered as a rare

Congenital split foot is a form of ectrodactyly characterized by the absence of two or three central digital rays of the foot. The cone-shaped cleft in the forefoot tapers proximally. The first metatarsal may be of normal size, or it may be broad and connected with the intermediate cuneiform at its base, representing fusion of the first and second metatarsals. Valgus deformity of the great toe is common. The lateral digital ray may consist of only the fifth metatarsal or the fifth and fourth metatarsals. The phalanges of the lateral ray usually deviate toward the midline. The hindfoot is normal (Figs. 2–102 to 2–105).

Split foot (lobster claw) is a very rare malformation; it exists in two forms. In the typical form, the deformity is always bilateral and is inherited as an autosomal dominant trait with incomplete penetrance.[2,11] In the less common atypical form, the deformity is unilateral and there is no evidence of familial inheritance.

Text continued on page 322

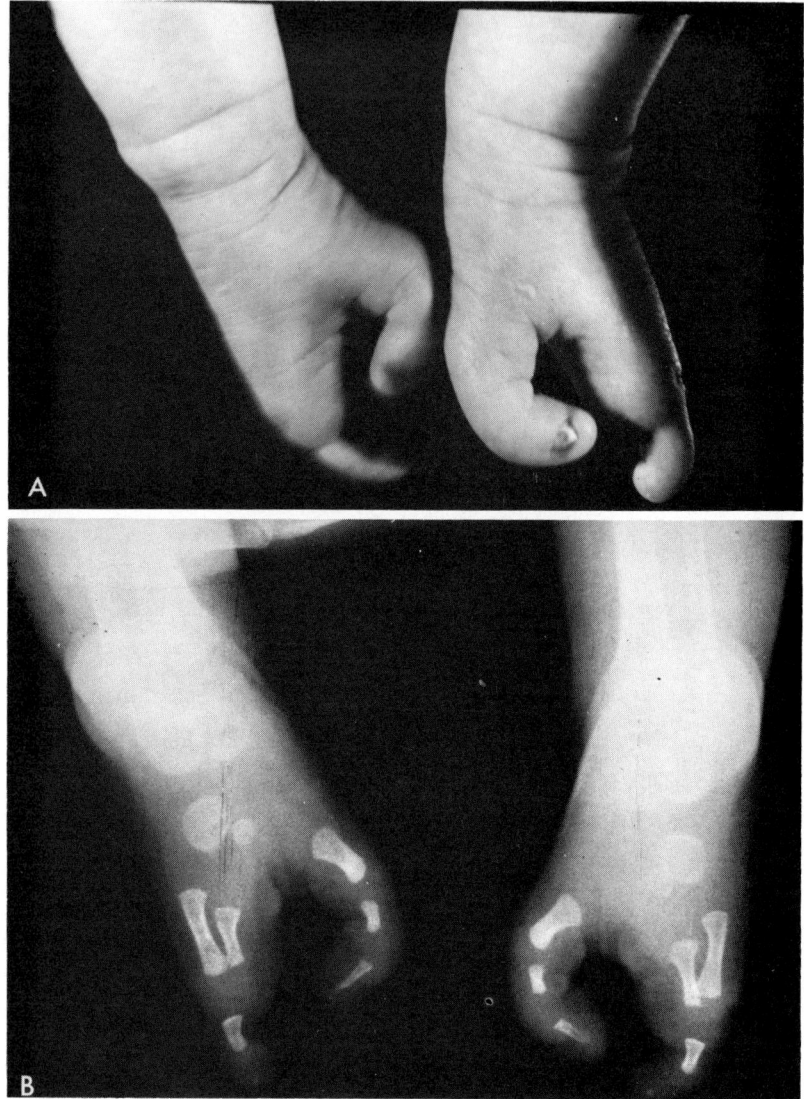

FIGURE 2–102. Congenital split or cleft foot.

A and **B**. Clinical appearance and roentgenogram of both feet in an 18-month-old child.

Illustration continued on opposite page

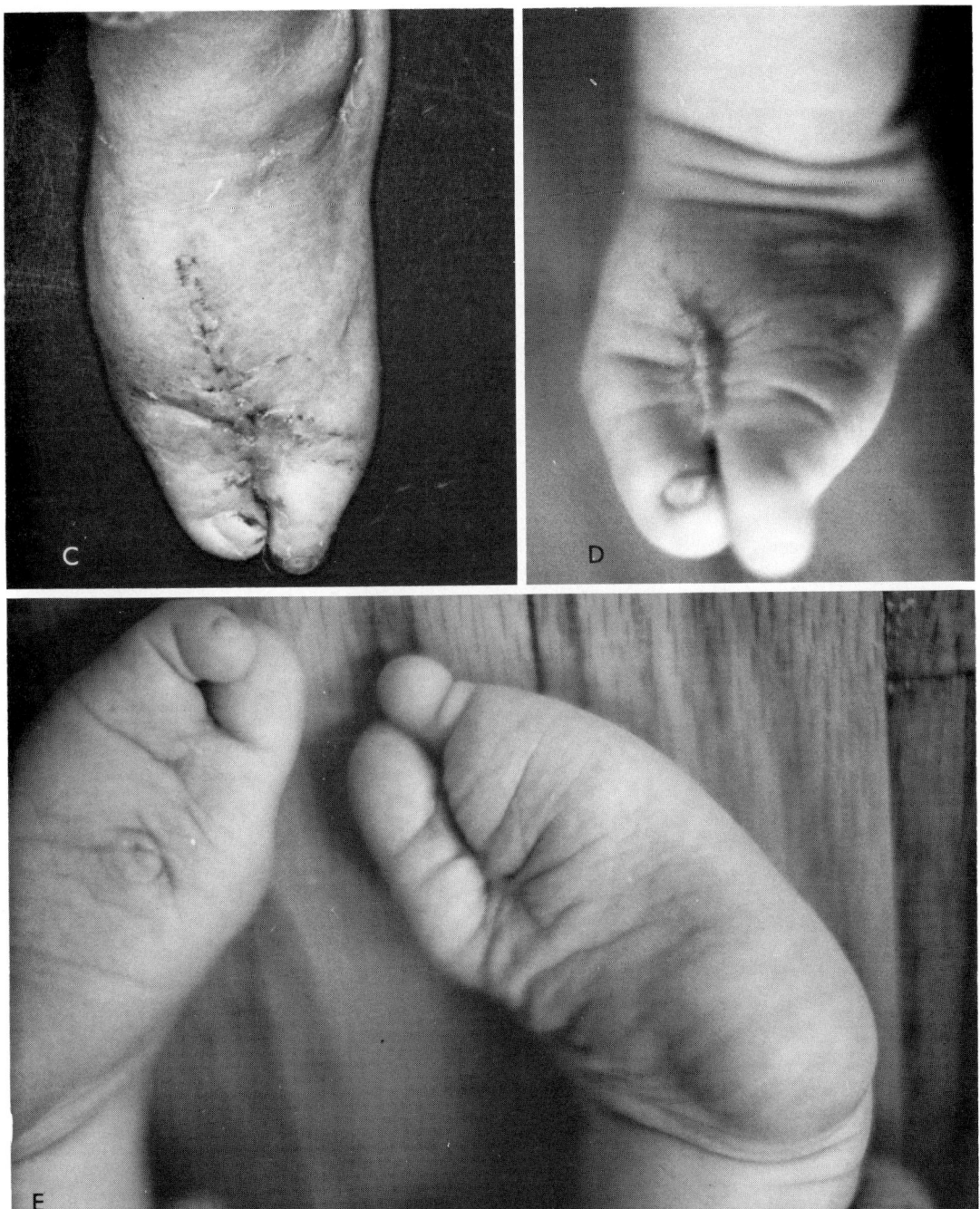

FIGURE 2–102 Continued. Congenital split or cleft foot.

C. Immediate postoperative photograph of left foot. The divergent metatarsals were brought together by osteotomy at their bases, the toes were normally aligned, and the split forefoot was surgically syndactylized to maintain correction. **D.** Dorsal photograph of the left foot six months later. **E.** Plantar photograph of both feet six months postoperatively.

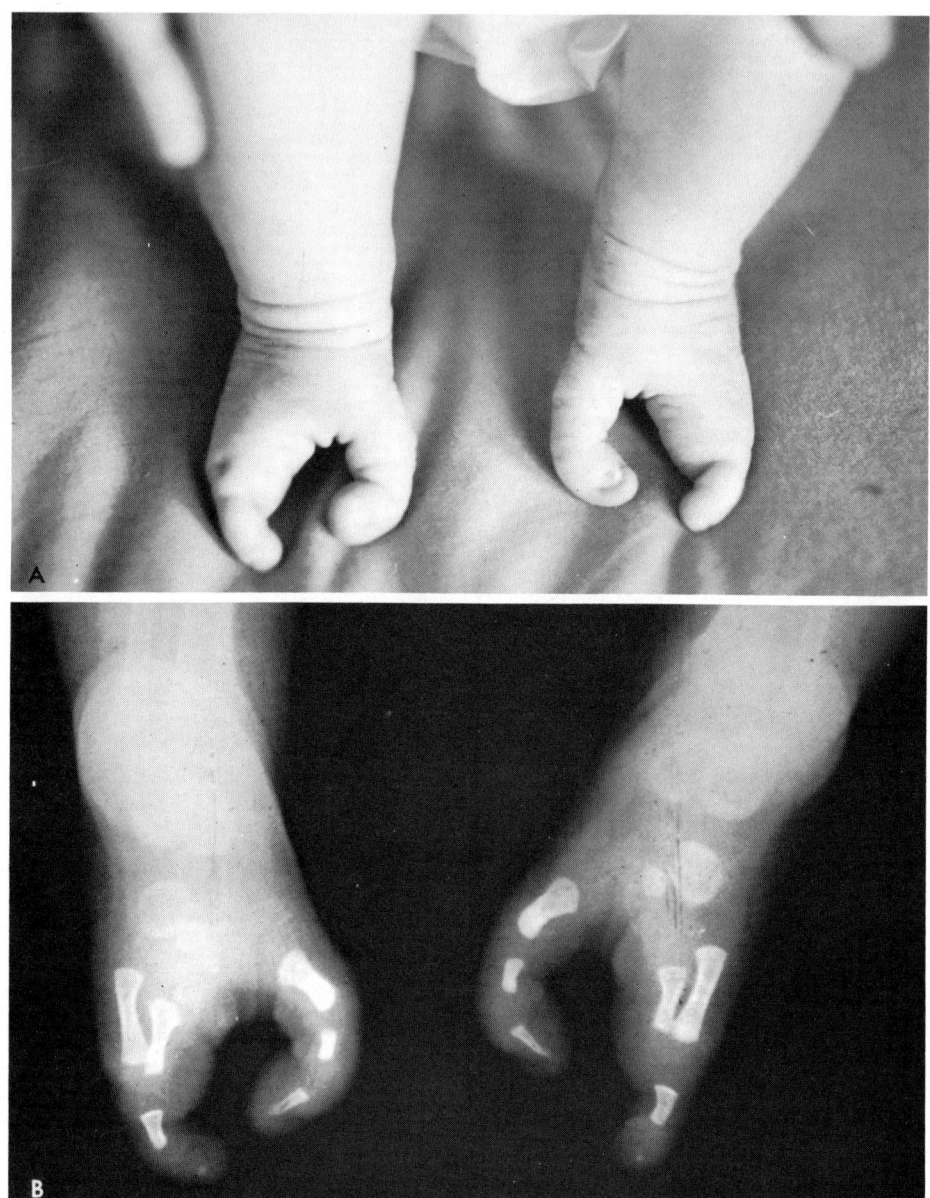

FIGURE 2–103. Congenital split or cleft foot (lobster claw).
A. Clinical appearance in a six-month-old infant. **B.** Roentgenograms of both feet.

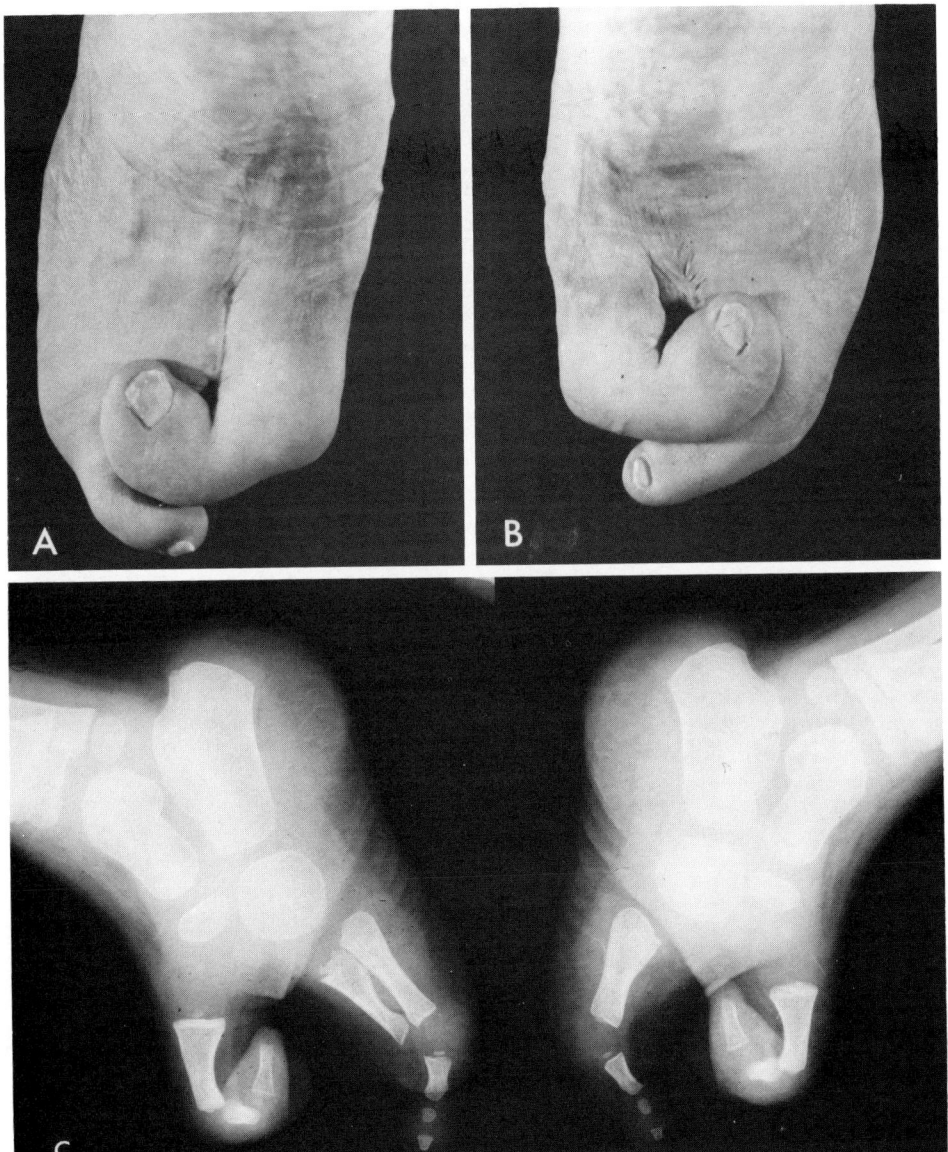

FIGURE 2–104. Lobster or split foot in 12-year-old child.

A and **B**. Clinical appearance of both feet. **C**. Roentgenograms. To facilitate shoe wear, deformity is usually corrected by walking age. Note the adaptation of the toes to the external pressure of the shoes.

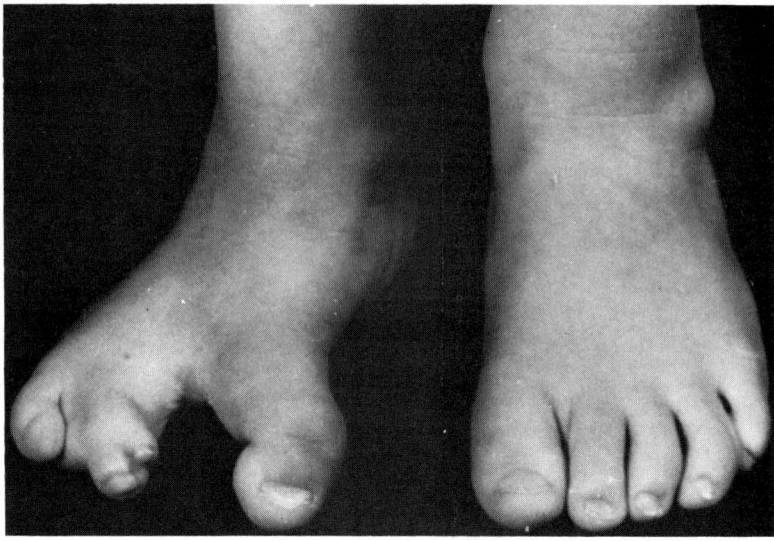

FIGURE 2–105. Atypical form of split foot.

Only the right foot was malformed. The left foot and both hands were normal. (Courtesy of Dr. H. Kelikian.)

Although bilateral split foot may be an isolated deformity, it usually occurs in conjunction with lobster clawing of the hand.[2, 19] Other associated abnormalities are cleft lip and palate, reduction in number and size of phalanges, syndactyly and polydactyly, triphalangeal thumb, and deafness.[10, 14, 15, 23]

Surgical correction of split foot is indicated to facilitate the fitting of shoes and to improve the objectionable appearance. Surgery is performed between one and two years of age. The divergent metatarsals are approximated by osteotomy at their bases, the deformed toes are normally aligned, and the split forefoot and toes are surgically syndactylized to maintain correction.

References

1. Ayer, A. A., and Rao, V. S.: Split hand and split foot. J. Indian Med. Assoc., 24:108, 1954.
2. Barsky, A. J.: Cleft hand: Classification, incidence and treatment. J. Bone Joint Surg., 46-A:1707, 1964.
3. Berndorfer, A.: Gesichtsspalten gemeinsum mit Hand- und Fussspalten. Z. Orthop., 107:344, 1970.
4. Blankenburg, H.: Spalthand- und Spaltfussbildungen in typischen and atypischen Formen. Beitr. Orthop. Traum., 14:209, 1967.
5. Cockayne, E. A.: Cleft palate, hare lip, dacryocystitis, and cleft hand and feet. Biometrika, 28:60, 1936.
6. Cowan, R. J.: Surgical problems associated with congenital malformations of the forefoot. Canad. J. Surg., 8:29, 1965.
7. Eder, H., and Port, J.: Familial cleft foot—a clinical study over 4 generations. (Author's transl.). Z. Orthop., 116:189, 1978.
8. Grand, M. J. H., and Dolan, D. J.: Heredofamilial cleft foot. Amer. J. Dis. Child., 51:338, 1936.
9. Lange, M.: Grundsätzliches über die Beurteilung der Entstehung und Bewertung atypischer Hand- und Fussmissbildung. Z. Orthop., 66:8, 1937.
10. Lewis, T., and Embleton, D.: Split-hand and split-foot deformities, their types, origin and transmission. Biometrika, 6:26, 1908.
11. McMullen, G., and Pearson, K.: On the inheritance of the deformity known as split foot or lobster claw. Biometrika, 9:381, 1913.
12. Meyerding, H. W., and Upshaw, J. E.: Heredofamilial cleft foot deformity (lobster-claw or split foot). Amer. J. Surg., 74:889, 1947.
13. Pfeiffer, R. A., and Verbeck, C.: Spalthand und Spaltfuss. Ektodermale Dysplasie und Lippen-Kiefer-Gaumen-Spalte: ein autosomal-dominant vererbtes Syndrom. Z. Kinderheilk., 115:235, 1973.
14. Phillips, R. S.: Congenital split foot (lobster claw) and triphalangeal thumb. J. Bone Joint Surg., 53-B:247, 1971.
15. Potter, E. L., and Nadelhoffer, L.: A familial lobster claw. J. Hered., 38:331, 1947.
16. Ray, A. K.: Another case of split foot mutation in two sibs. J. Hered., 61:169, 1970.
17. Robinson, G. C., Wildervanck, L. S., Chiang, T. P., and Hyg, S. M.: Ectrodactyly, ectodermal dysplasia, and cleft lip-palate syndrome. J. Pediat., 82:107, 1973.
18. Rudiger, R. A., Haase, W., and Passarge, E: Association of ectrodactyly, ectodermal dysplasia, and cleft lip-palate. Amer. J. Dis. Child., 120:160, 1970.
19. Stiles, K. A., and Pickard, I. S.: Hereditary malformations of the hands and feet. J. Hered., 34:341, 1943.
20. Sumiya, N., and Onizuka, T.: Seven years' survey of our new cleft foot repair. Plast. Reconstr. Surg., 65:447, 1980.
21. Van Den Berghe, H., Dequeker, J., Fryns, J. P., and David, G.: Familial occurrence of severe ulnar aplasia and lobster claw feet: A new syndrome. Hum. Genet., 42:109, 1978.
22. Vogel, F.: Verzögerte Mutation beim Menschen; einige kritische Bemerkungen zu Ch. Auerbachs Arbeit (1956). Ann. Hum. Genet., 22:132, 1958.
23. Walker, J. C., and Clodius, L.: The syndromes of cleft lip, cleft palate and lobster-claw deformities of hands and feet. Plast. Reconstr. Surg., 32:627, 1963.

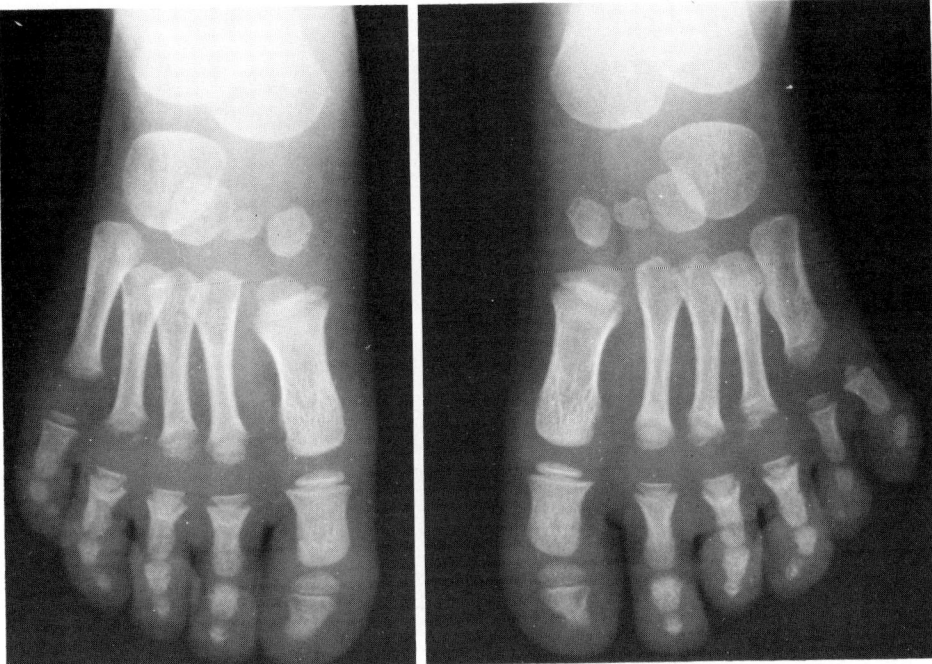

FIGURE 2–106. Unilateral postaxial polydactyly.

The fifth and sixth toes share a common fifth metatarsal.

POLYDACTYLISM

Supernumerary digits are common in the foot; they occur more frequently in the black and in the female. Polydactyly is usually transmitted as an autosomal dominant trait, but sporadic cases are caused by mutant genes. The supernumerary toe may be associated with polydactyly in the hand or other major congenital malformations such as absence or hypoplasia of the tibia. The whole child should be examined to rule out association with syndromes such as Ellis–van Creveld chondroectodermal dysplasia or Jeunes's infantile thoracic dystrophy.

Morphologically the extra digit may be preaxial, on the medial (big toe) side; postaxial, on the lateral (little toe) side; or it may be a duplication of one of the middle toes (central). The various forms of digital duplications of the foot are illustrated in Figures 2–106 to 2–113.

Surgical removal of the supernumerary toes is indicated for cosmetic reasons as well as for the sake of comfort in wearing shoes. The optimum age for surgery is between 9 and 12 months, when the infant begins to stand and walk. In deciding which toe is to

Text continued on page 329

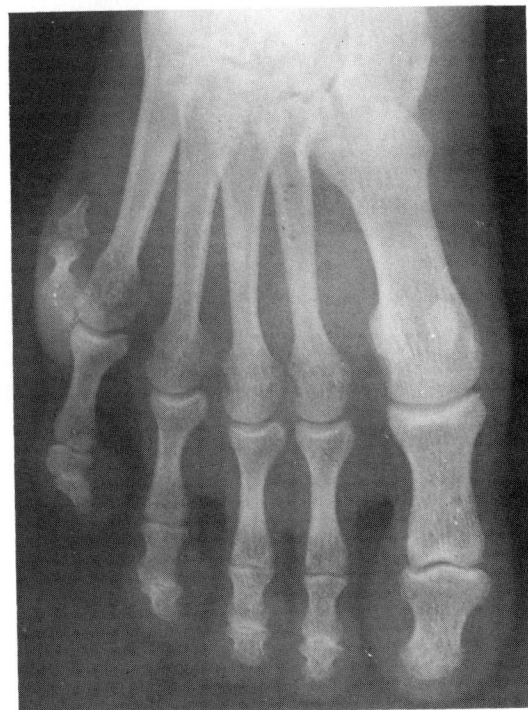

FIGURE 2–107. Roentgenogram of forefoot showing postaxial polydactyly.

Note that the extra little toe is directed posteriorly.

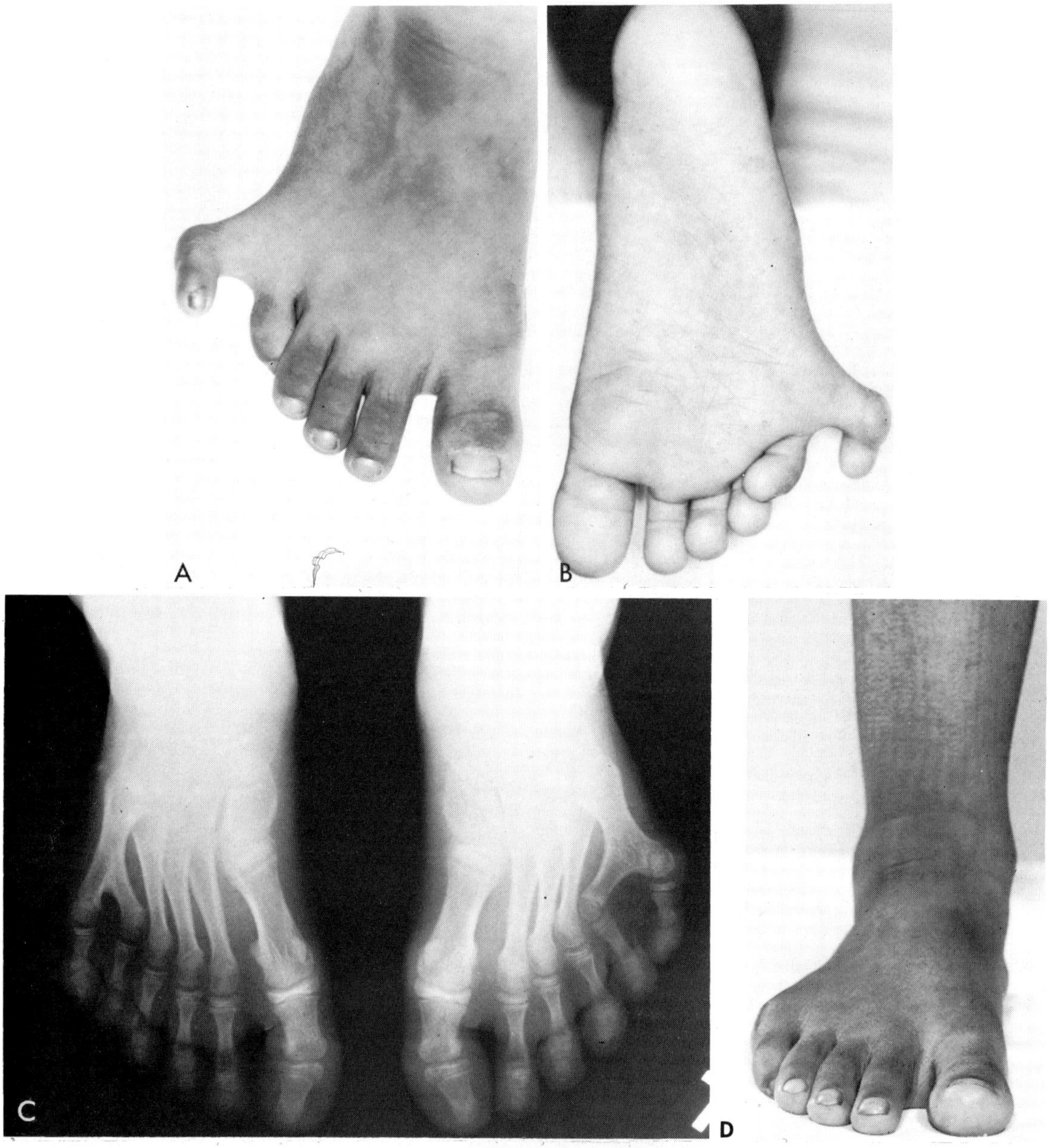

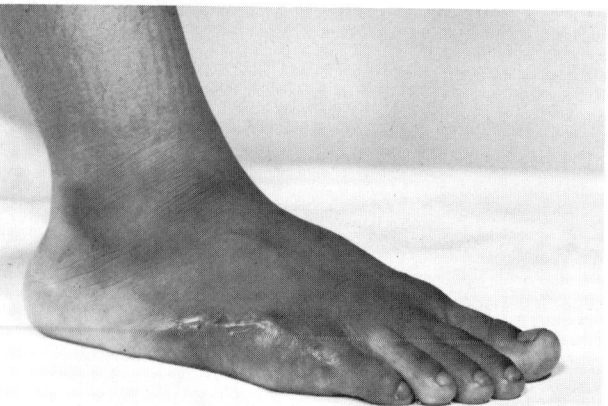

FIGURE 2–108. Postaxial polydactyly.

A and **B**. Clinical appearance of right foot. **C**. Anteroposterior roentgenogram of both feet. Note the bilateral involvement and fusion of the supernumerary metatarsals at their distal third. **D** and **E**. Postoperative photographs of the right foot showing result.

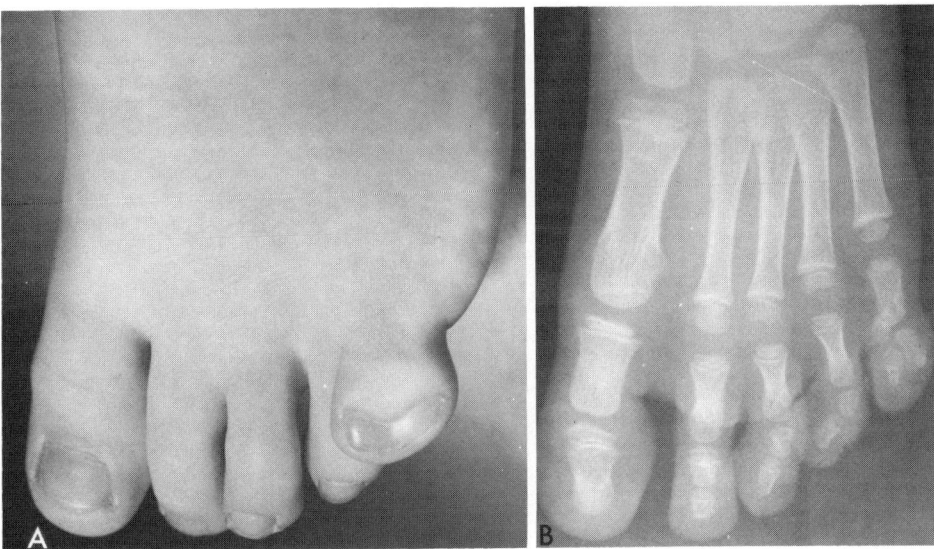

FIGURE 2–109. Postaxial polydactyly with syndactyly of little toe.

A. Clinical appearance. **B.** Roentgenogram showing that only the distal and middle phalanges are duplicated. This is best treated by excision of the distal and middle phalanges of the extra digit on the tibial side and surgical syndactyly of the sixth toe to the fourth toe.

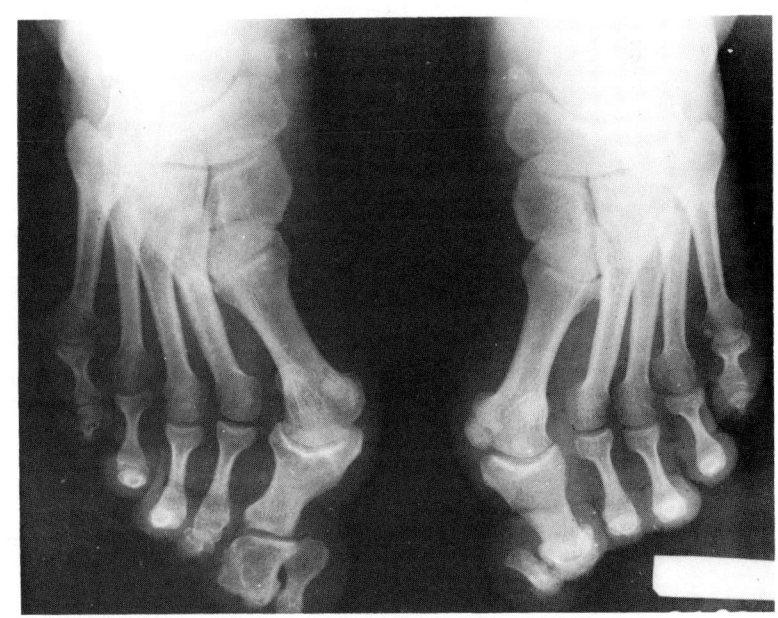

FIGURE 2–110. Bilateral preaxial polydactyly.

The roentgenogram shows that only the distal phalanx of the great toe is duplicated. There is associated hallux valgus and metatarsus primus varus.

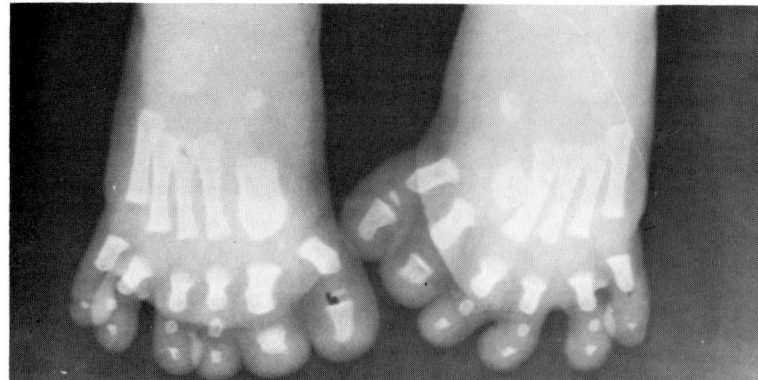

FIGURE 2–111. Bilateral preaxial polydactyly.

Both phalanges of the great toe are duplicated.

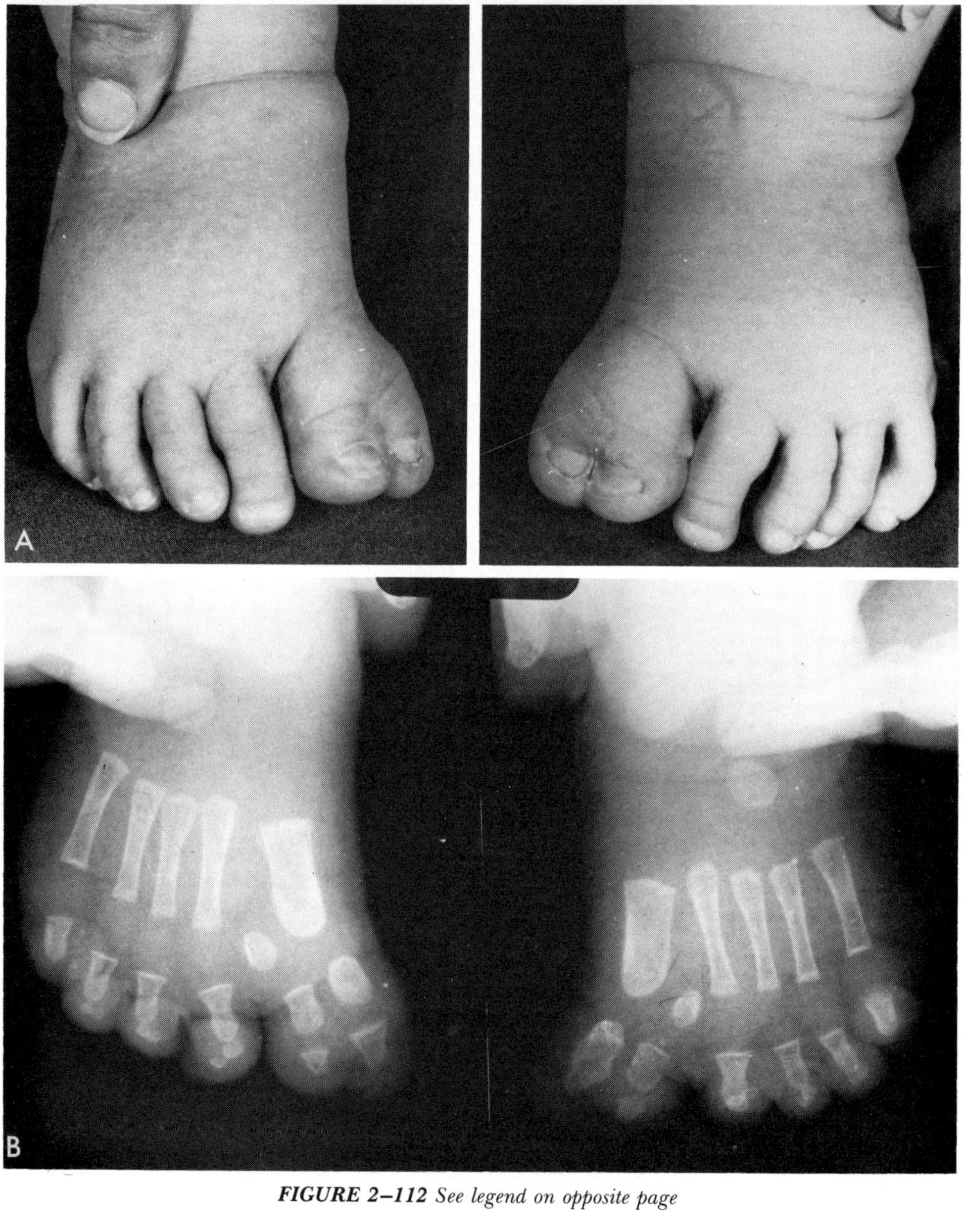

FIGURE 2–112 See legend on opposite page

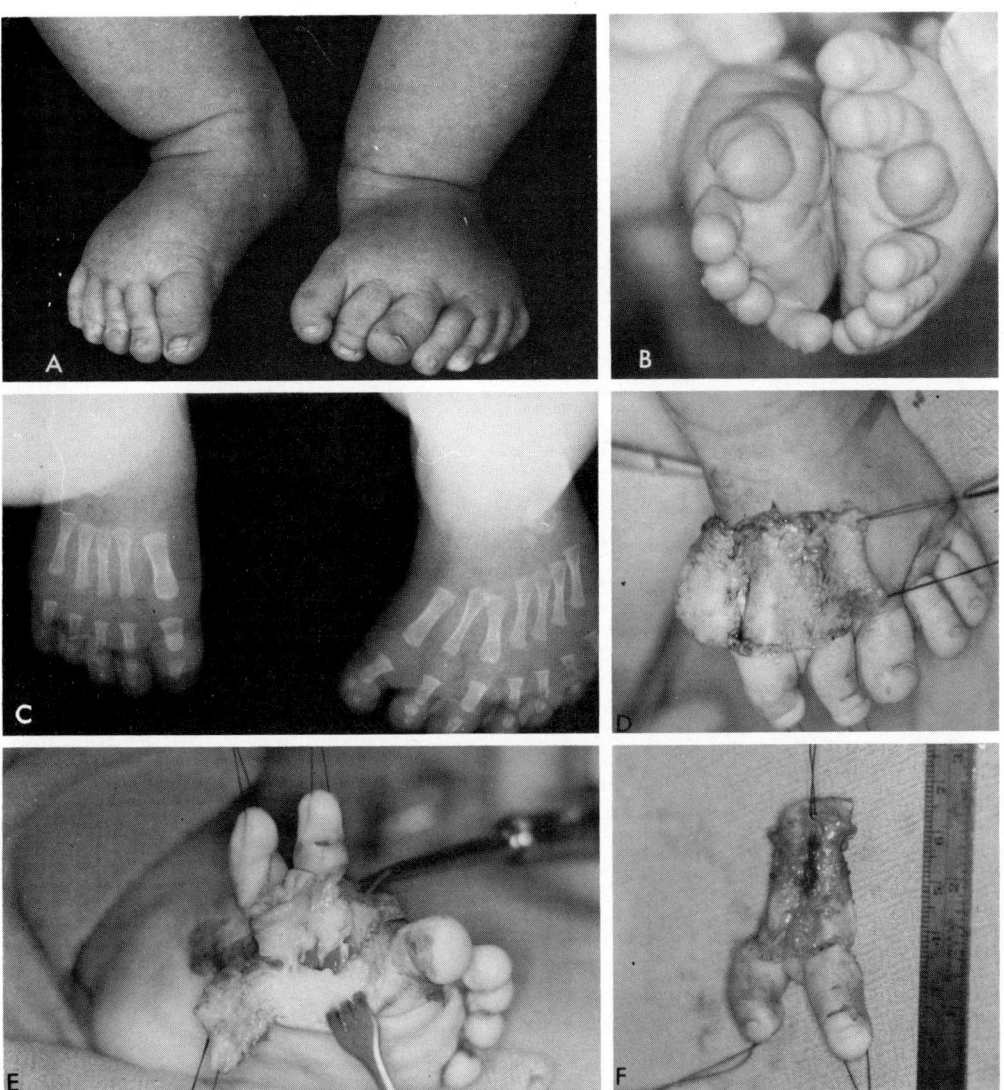

FIGURE 2–113. Polydactyly of left foot.

A and **B**. Clinical appearance. Note the swan toes on the left. **C**. Roentgenogram showing that both the phalanges and metatarsals of the supernumerary digital rays are present. **D**. The skin incision and the raising of the wound flaps. **E** and **F**. The medial two digital rays are dissected and excised.

Illustration continued on following page

FIGURE 2–112. Bilateral preaxial polydactyly.

Both distal and proximal phalanges of the great toes and the distal end of the metatarsals are duplicated. **A**. Clinical appearance. **B**. Anteroposterior roentgenograms of both feet.

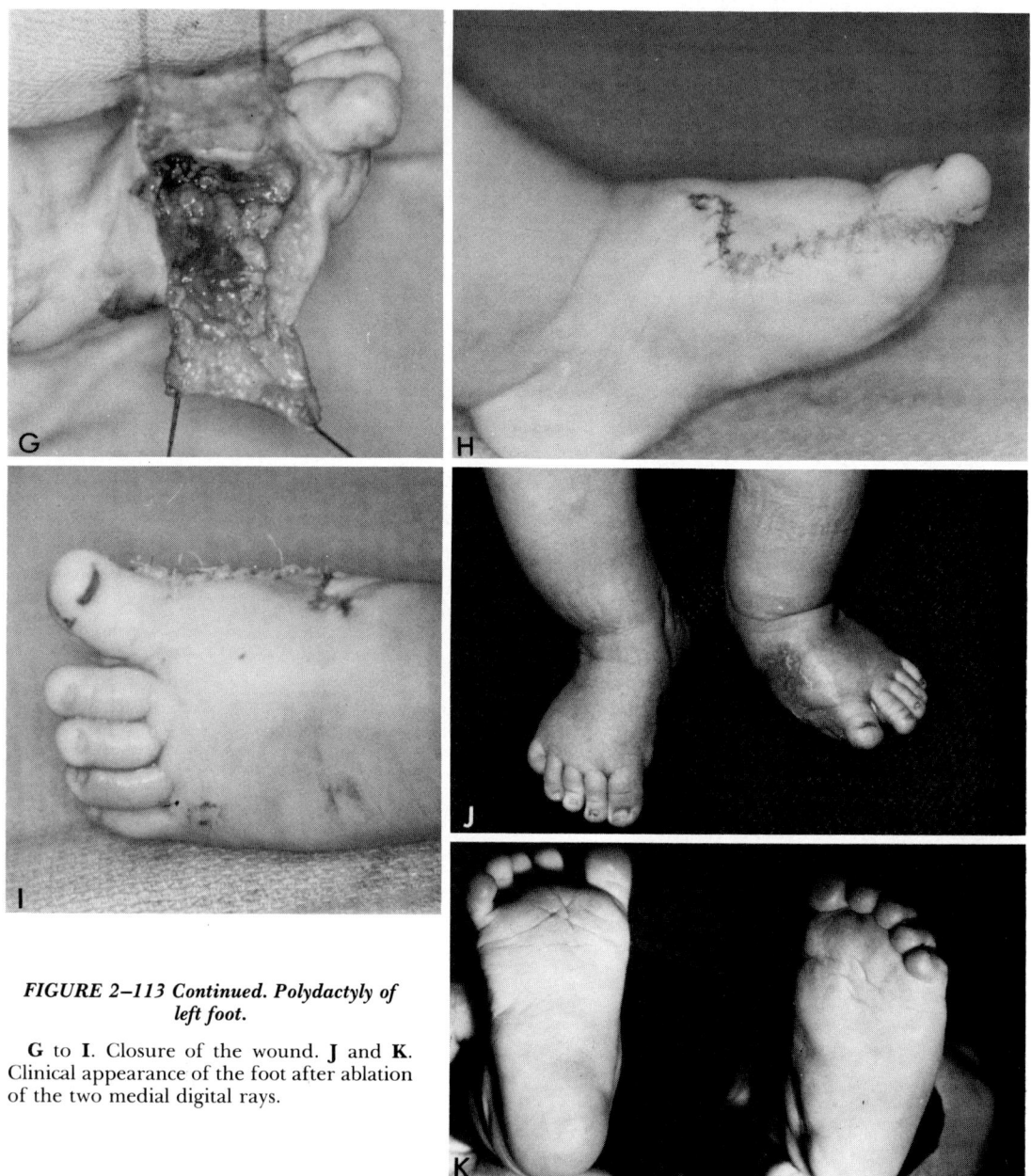

FIGURE 2–113 Continued. *Polydactyly of left foot.*

G to **I.** Closure of the wound. **J** and **K.** Clinical appearance of the foot after ablation of the two medial digital rays.

be excised, the important consideration is the general contour of the foot. Usually the most peripheral toe is amputated, despite the fact that it may be more normal than the one adjacent to it. Roentgenograms of the foot should also be considered in the decision. The extra toe is amputated through a racquet-shaped incision at its base, and the tendons are divided near their insertion and sutured to the adjacent tendon to preserve function. A transverse incision is made in the capsule of the metatarsophalangeal joint, and the toe is disarticulated. Injury to the growth centers of the adjacent digits should be avoided. Any bony protrusion of the common metatarsal is sharply excised; if there is a corresponding supernumerary metatarsal, it is ablated through a proximal extension of the skin incision on the dorsolateral aspect of the foot. The capsule and ligaments are reconstructed to prevent malalignment of the neighboring toes.

References

1. Crawford, M. D., and Saldana-Garcia, P.: Brachydactyly and polydactyly with dermal ridge dissociation and ridge hypoplasia. J. Med. Genet., *16*:402, 1979.
2. Funderburk, S. J., Sparkes, R. S., and Klisak, I.: The 9P syndrome. J. Med. Genet., *16*:75, 1979.
3. Mollica, F., Volti, S. L., and Sorge, G.: Autosomal recessive postaxial polydactyly type A in a Sicilian family. J. Med. Genet., *15*:212, 1978.
4. Pfeiffer, R. A., and Santelmann, R.: Limb anomalies in chromosomal aberrations. Birth Defects, *13*:319, 1977.
5. Schinzel, A.: Postaxial polydactyly, hallux duplication, absence of the corpus callosum, macrencephaly and severe mental retardation: A new syndrome? Helv. Paediat. Acta, *34*:141, 1979.
5a. Venn-Watson, E. A.: Problems in polydactyly of the foot. Orthop. Clin. N. Amer., *7*:909, 1976.
6. Waldrigues, A., Grohmann, L. C., Takahashi, T., and Reis, H. M.: Ellis-Van Creveld syndrome. An inbred kindred with five cases. Rev. Bras. Pesqui. Med. Biol., *10*:193, 1977.

CONGENITAL HALLUX VARUS

In this deformity there is congenital medial angulation of the great toe at the metatarsophalangeal joint. There are several types of congenital hallux varus: (1) a primary type, not associated with any other congenital anomaly, in which a taut fibrous band extends from the medial side of the great toe to the base of the first metatarsal and progressively pulls the great toe toward the midline; (2) a type associated with congenital deformities of the forepart of the foot, namely hallux varus with metatarsus varus, hallux varus with isolated congenital marked shortening of the first metatarsal, and hallux varus with accessory bones or toes, as shown in Figures 2–114 and 2–115; and (3) hallux varus associated with extensive developmental affections of the skeleton, as in diastrophic dwarfism.

The method of treatment depends upon the type of hallux varus. The deformity is satisfactorily corrected by any one of the surgical methods of McElvenny, Farmer, or Kelikian and associates.[2, 3, 5] The contracted fibrous band on the medial aspect of the great toe, the taut abductor hallucis, and the shortened medial capsule of the metatarsophalangeal joint of the big toe are released. Any accessory phalanx or bone is excised, and surgical syndactylism between the great and second toes is carried out to maintain correction. Capsuloplasty on the lateral side of the metatarsophalangeal joint and extensor hallucis tendon rerouting will assist in holding the hallux in proper anatomic alignment. A Kirschner wire is inserted into the great toe, across the metatarsophalangeal joint, and into the first metatarsal for three weeks to maintain correction.

References

1. Bishop, J., Kahn, A. D., and Turba, J. E.: Surgical correction of the splayfoot. The Giannestras procedure. Clin. Orthop. *146*:234, 1980.
2. Farmer, A. W.: Congenital hallux varus. Amer. J. Surg., *95*:274, 1958.
2a. Haas, S. L.: An operation for correction of hallux varus. J. Bone Joint Surg., *20*:705, 1938.
2b. Horwitz, M. T.: An unusual hallux varus deformity and its surgical correction. J. Bone Joint Surg., *19*:828, 1937.
3. Kelikian, H., Clayton, L., and Loseff, H.: Surgical syndactylism of the toes. Clin. Orthop., *19*:208, 1961.
4. Kleiner, B. C., and Holmes, L. B.: Brief clinical report: Hallux varus and preaxial polysyndactyly in brothers. Amer. J. Med. Genet., *6*:113, 1980.
5. McElvenny, R. T.: Hallux varus. Quart. Bull. Northwest. Med. Sch., *15*:277, 1941.
5a. Myginal, H. B.: Surgical correction of congenital hallux varus. Nord. Med., *49*:914, 1953.
6. Thomson, S. A.: Hallux varus and metatarsus varus. Clin. Orthop., *16*:109, 1960.

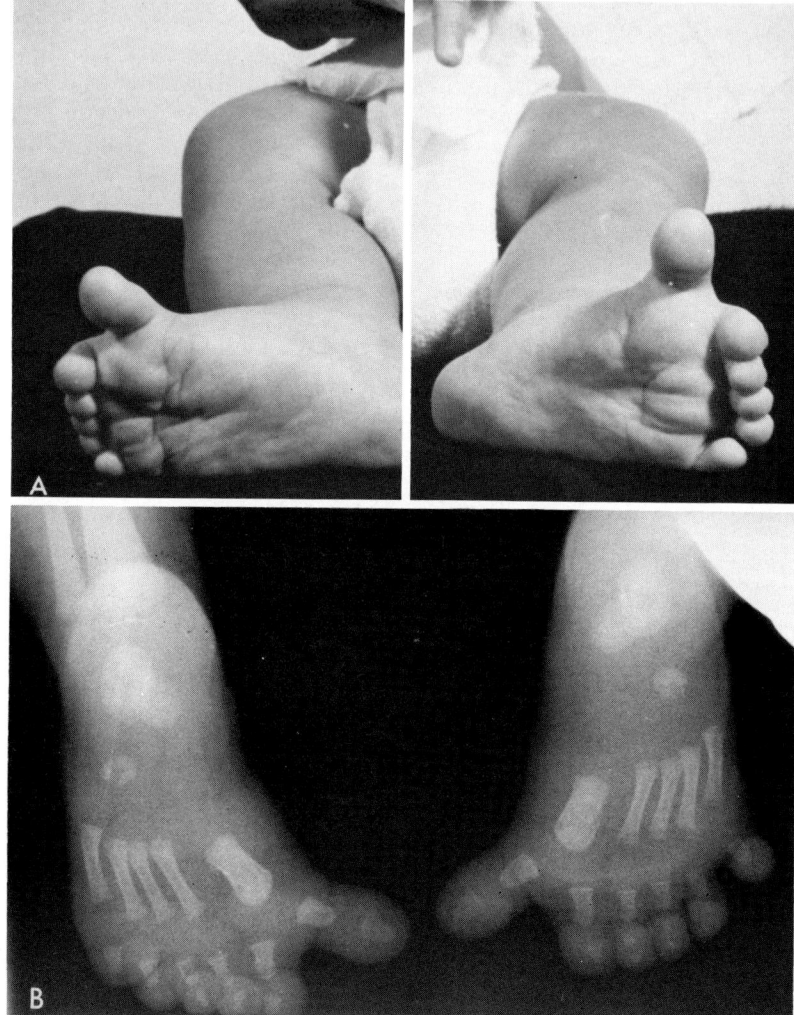

FIGURE 2–114. Congenital hallux varus due to preaxial polydactyly of great toe.

A. Clinical appearance. **B**. Roentgenogram. Only the phalanges of the hallux are duplicated; note also the stout first metatarsal.

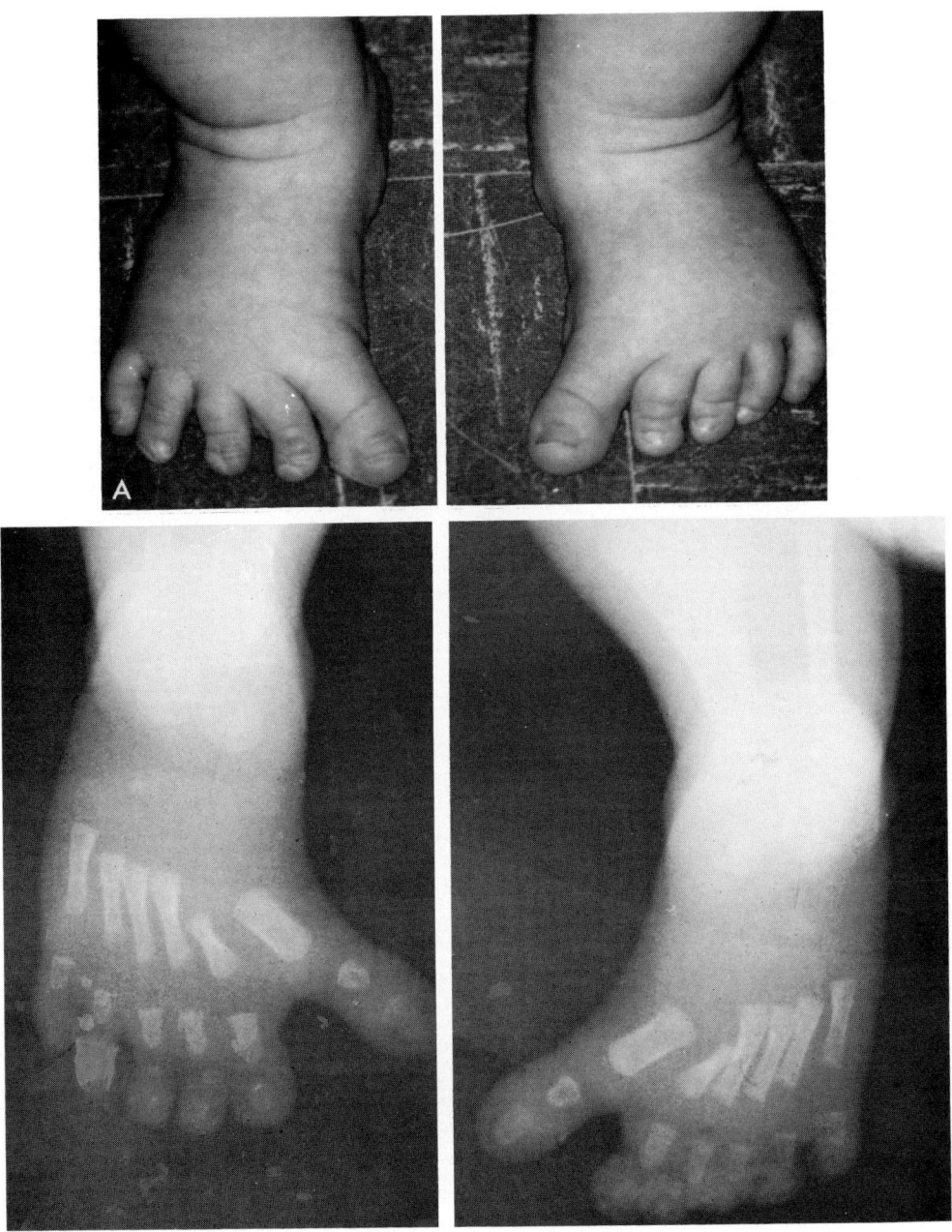

FIGURE 2–115. Bilateral congenital hallux varus due to preaxial polydactyly of great toe.
A. Clinical appearance. B. Roentgenogram of both feet.

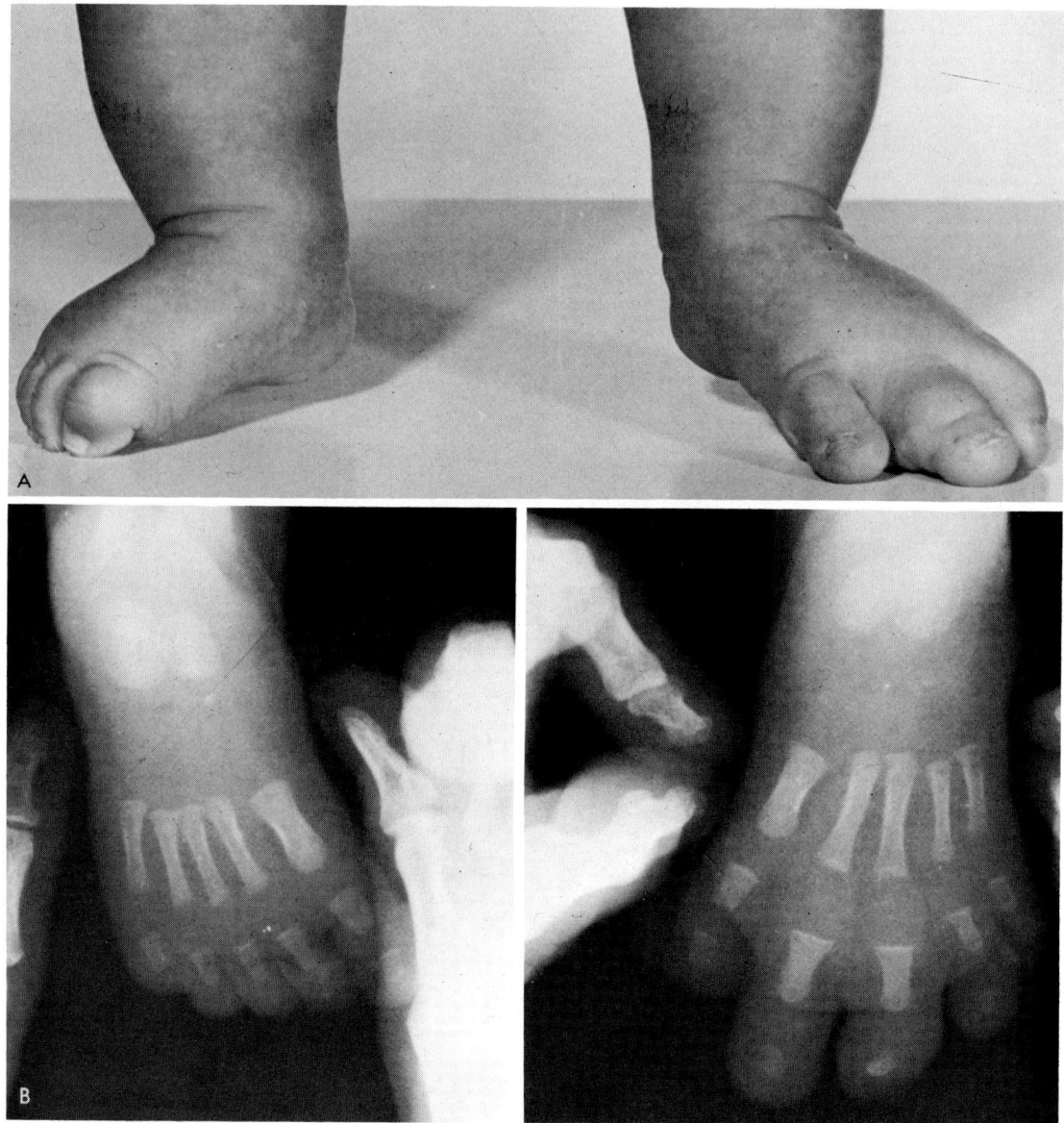

FIGURE 2–116. Macrodactyly of the second and third digits of the left foot.

MACRODACTYLISM

Gigantism of one or more toes is a rare deformity. The hypertrophy is frequently caused either by neurofibromatosis or by congenital hyperplasia of lymphatic and adipose tissue (Figs. 2–116 and 2–117). A grotesque appearance, difficulty in shoe-fitting, and interference with weight-bearing are indications for surgical treatment.

The operation is performed in two or three steps. First, the proximal phalanx is resected, and the toe is partially defatted on one side. The growth plate of the middle phalanx is arrested. Alignment is maintained by syndactyly of the affected toe with its neighboring toe. Several months later, hypertrophied tissue is resected on the opposite side (Fig. 2–118). If the corresponding metatarsal is enlarged, its growth is arrested by epiphyseodesis at the appropriate age. Amputation of a gigantic second toe should not be performed, as its removal will lead to hallux valgus deformity. Severe macrodactyly of the third toe, however, may be treated by amputation of the affected toe, partial resection of the corresponding metatarsal, and surgical syndactyly of the second toe to the fourth toe.

References

1. Bouvet, J. P., Huc de Bat, J. M., Benoit, J., and Ramadier, J. O.: Bilateral symmetrical macrodactyly of the toes (Author's transl.): Rev. Chir. Orthop., 66:331, 1980.
2. Dennyson, W. G., Bear, J. N., and Bhoola, K. D.: Macrodactyly in the foot. J. Bone Joint Surg., 59-B:355, 1977.
3. Devalentine, S., Scurran, B. L., Tuerk, D., and Karlin, J. M.: Macrodactyly of the lower extremity: A review with two case reports. J. Amer. Podiatry Assoc., 71:175, 1981.
4. Ofodile, F. A., and Oluwasanmi, J.: Pedal macrodactyly—report of seven cases. East Afr. Med. J., 56:283, 1979.
5. Perdive, R. L., Mason, W. H., and Bernard, T. M.: Macrodactyly: A rare malformation. Review of the literature and case report. J. Amer. Podiatry Assoc., 69:657, 1979.

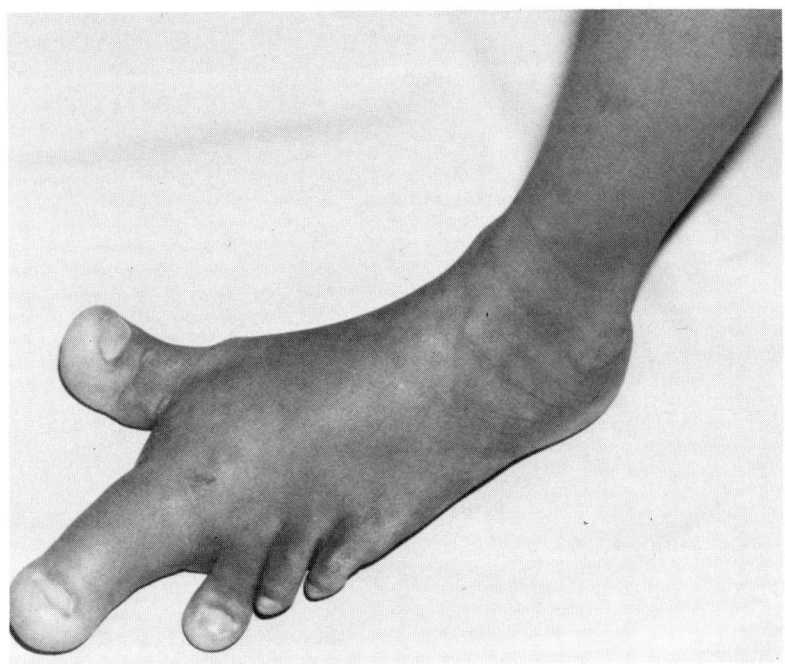

FIGURE 2–117. Macrodactyly of the second toe in an adolescent.

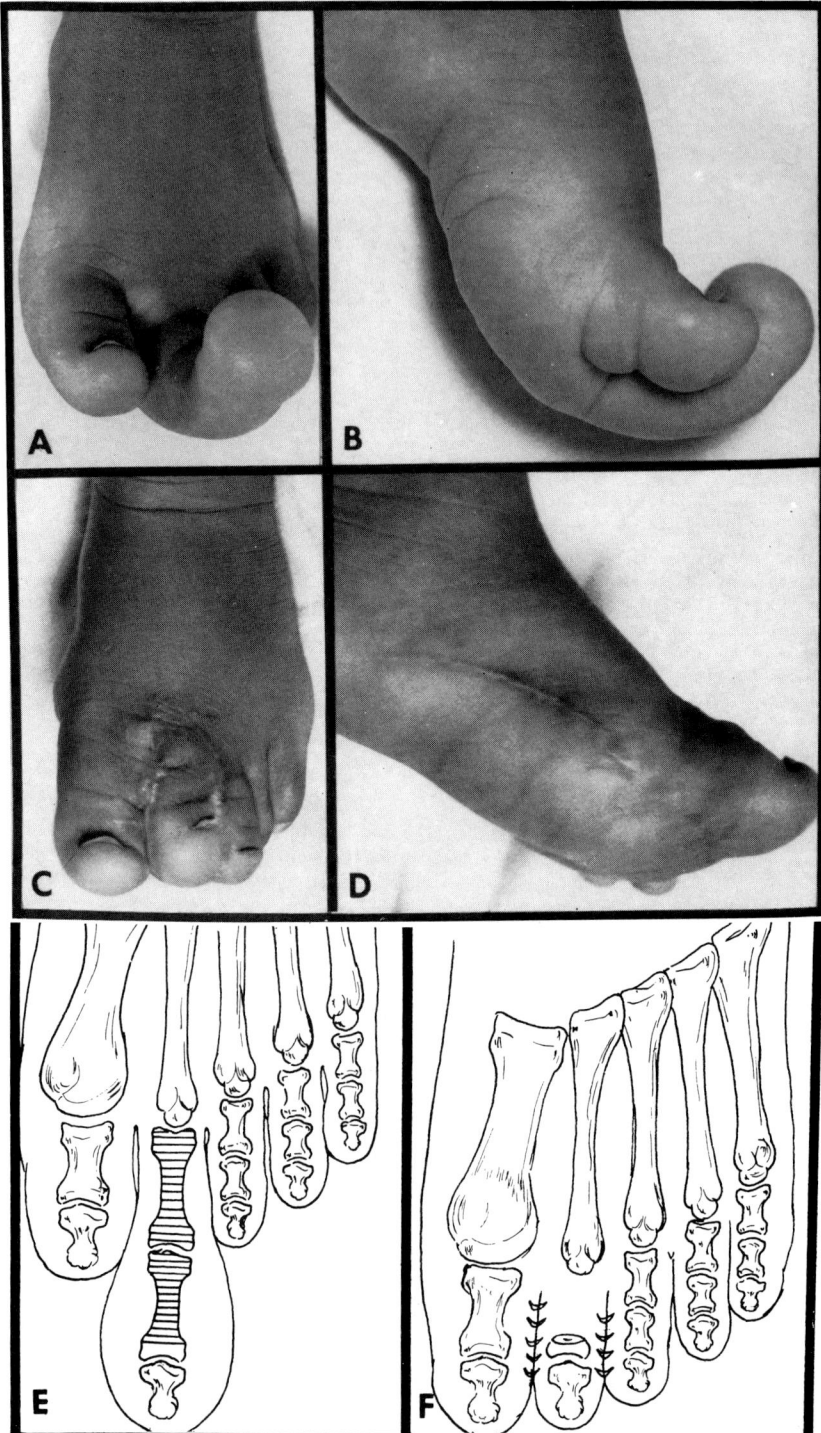

FIGURE 2–118. Severe macrodactyly of the second toe in a young girl.

A and **B**. Preoperative photographs. The deformity was treated in two stages: first the proximal phalanx of the second toe was excised, the toe was defatted from its medial side and syndactylized to the big toe; three months later, the middle phalanx of the second toe was excised, the toe was defatted from its lateral side and syndactylized with the third digit. The medial plantar nerve was normal on exploration. **C** and **D**. Postoperative photographs. **E** and **F**. Interpretive diagrams show the amount of bone resected. Amputation of the second toe should not be performed, as it will lead to hallux valgus. (From Kelikian, H.: Hallux Valgus, Allied Deformities of the Forefoot and Metatarsalgia. Philadelphia, W. B. Saunders Co., 1965, p. 332. Reprinted by permission.)

MISCELLANEOUS DEFORMITIES OF TOES

Microdactylism

Small toes may be an isolated deformity, with or without hypoplasia of the corresponding metatarsals, or may be associated with Streeter's dysplasia. Because they do not usually cause disability, treatment is not required.

Syndactylism

Congenital webbing of the toes neither causes disability nor does it interfere with function. Cosmetically it is usually not objectionable, and no treatment is necessary (Figs. 2–119 to 2–121). If webbing is associated with polydactylism, the most peripheral digit is excised to facilitate shoe wear (Fig. 2–122).

Divergent or Convergent Toes

These may occur as an isolated angular deformity, without flexion contracture of the distal interphalangeal joint (Fig. 2–123). In minimal deformity, treatment is not necessary. In severe cases, when the angulated toe underrides or overrides the adjacent toe, surgical syndactylism of the affected toes is indicated; in adolescents, it is combined with proximal phalangectomy.

Congenital Digitus Minimus Varus

Congenital dorsal overriding of the fifth toe is a common familial deformity in which the fifth metatarsophalangeal joint is subluxated dorsomedially. The fifth toe is hyperextended and adducted, lying across the base of the fourth toe (Fig. 2–124). The capsule of the metatarsophalangeal joint is contracted on its dorsomedial aspect. The

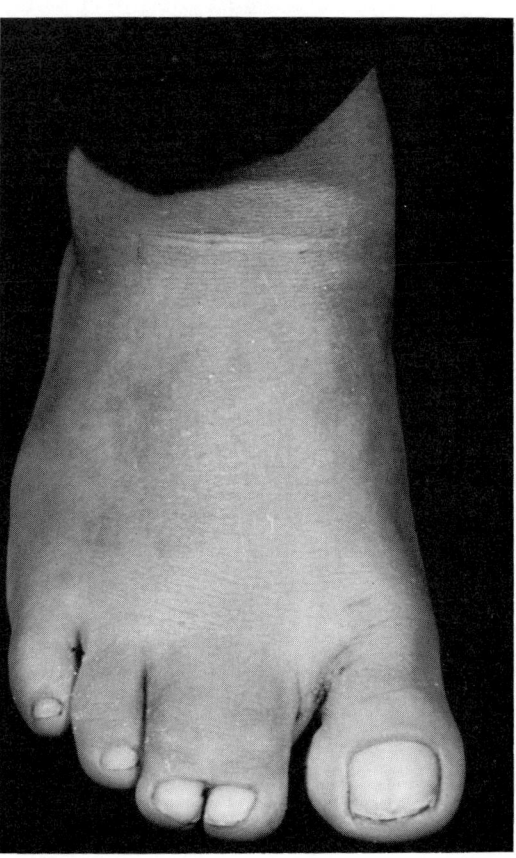

FIGURE 2–119. Syndactyly of the second and third toes.

Congenital Deformities

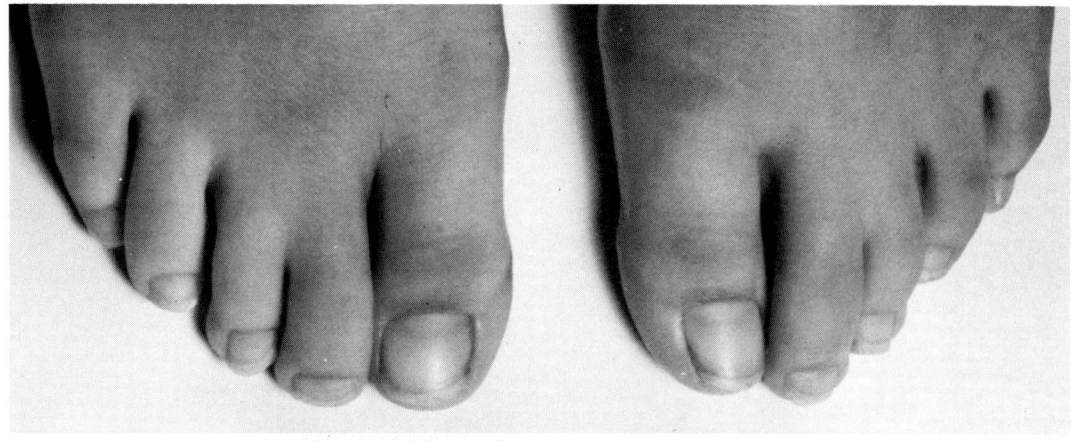

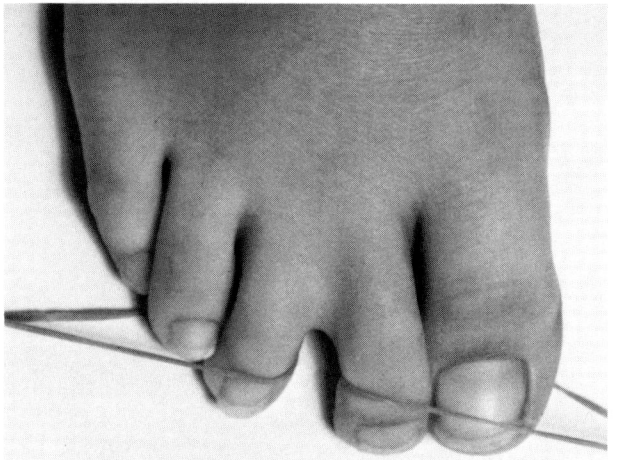

FIGURE 2–120. Congenital webbing of toes.

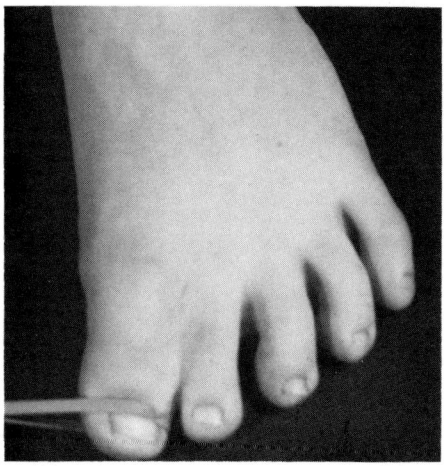

FIGURE 2–121. Congenital syndactyly between the great and second toes.

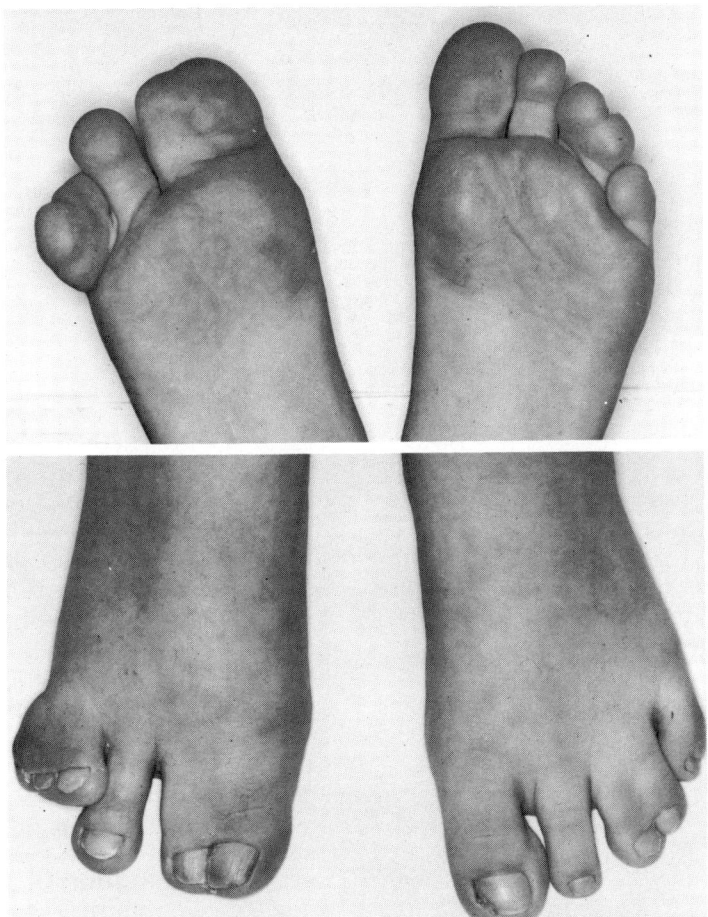

FIGURE 2–122. Congenital syndactylism of the fourth and fifth toes and the first and second toes on the right foot and the third and fourth toes on the left foot.

In the right foot, there is a supernumerary digit. It was surgically excised.

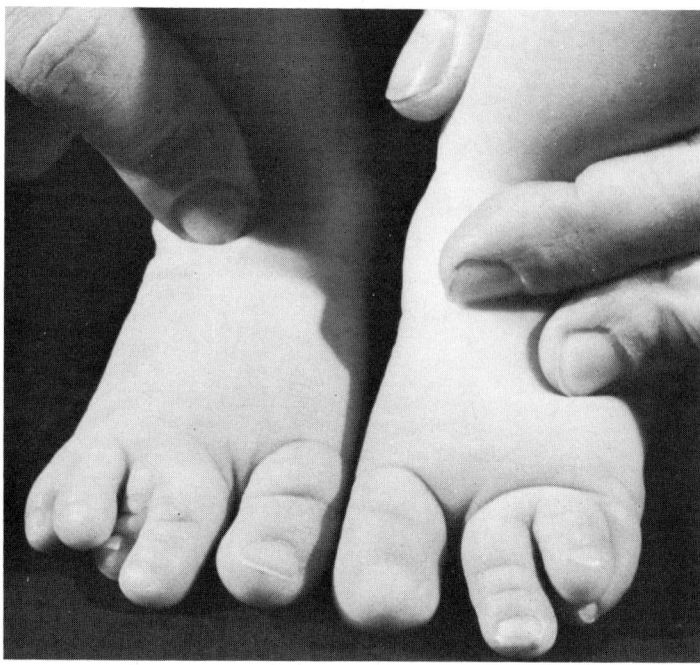

FIGURE 2–123. Angular deformity of toes.

Fourth toe on the right foot overrides the third toe. In the left foot, there are only three lesser toes and metatarsals.

extensor tendon is shortened, and the skin on the dorsum of the fifth and between the fourth and fifth toes is taut. In severe deformity, the fifth toe becomes rotated on its longitudinal axis with its nail pointing laterally. There is no flexion deformity of the interphalangeal joints. A hard callus often develops over the dorsum of the fifth toe because of irritation caused by the shoe. The condition is usually bilateral. It causes disability in about half the affected patients.

TREATMENT

In the infant and the young child, conservative measures are indicated: passive stretching of the little toe in plantar flexion and abduction, and strapping of the little toe in normal alignment with adhesive tape. Usually, however, these methods do not correct the deformity and, in the adolescent, if symptoms warrant it, operative correction is necessary.

Numerous surgical procedures have been proposed in the literature: (1) transfer of the extensor tendon of the fifth toe to the neck of the fifth metatarsal (Lantzounis); (2) division of the extensor tendon of the fifth toe over the dorsum of the midfoot and transfer of its distal segment to the abductor digiti quinti by rerouting the tendon from the medial to the lateral side of the proximal phalanx (Lapidus); (3) Z-plastic lengthening of the extensor tendon, dorsal and medial capsulotomy of the metatarsophalangeal joint, and plastic lengthening of the contracted skin fold (Goodwin and Swisher Y-plasty, Wilson and DuVries V and Y-plasty, Thompson Z-plasty); (4) excision of the proximal phalanx through a lateral incision (Gocht and DeBrunner); (5) excision of the proximal phalanx and surgical syndactyly of the fourth and fifth toes; and (6) amputation of the fifth toe.[10–17, 23]

The author recommends tenotomy of the extensor tendon, dorsal and medial capsulotomy of the fifth metatarsophalangeal joint, excision of the proximal phalanx, and fusion of the skin (surgical syndactylism) of the fourth and fifth toes as shown in Figure 2–125. The operative technique is described and illustrated in Plate 9. In children the proximal phalanx is partially excised, leaving the growth plate at its base intact. The results of the McFarland operation are very satisfactory.[17]

Plastic procedures involving V-Y elongation of the skin and soft tissues are not recommended by the author because they often result in an ugly scar that is cosmetically undesirable. Sometimes a keloid may form, which may be irritated by the shoe.

Cockin recommends the Butler opera-

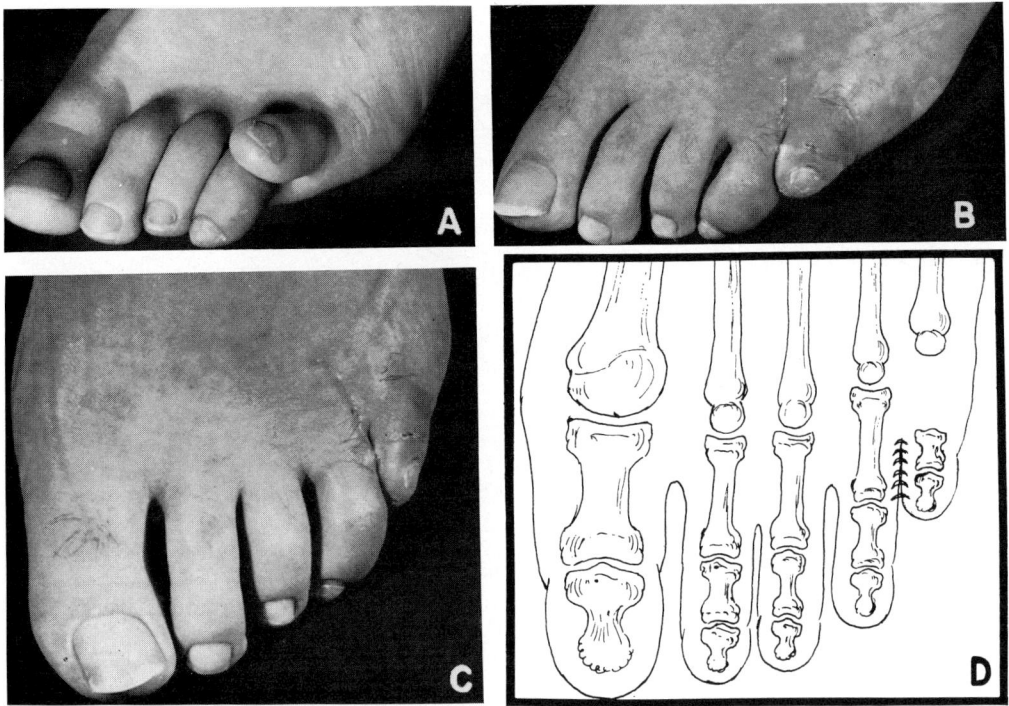

FIGURE 2–124. Digitus minimus varus.

Deformity was treated by excision of the proximal phalanx of the little toe, extensor tenotomy, dorsal capsulotomy of the fifth metatarsophalangeal joint, and surgical syndactyly of the fifth and fourth toes. **A.** Preoperative photograph. **B** and **C.** Postoperative photographs. **D.** Interpretive diagram. (From Kelikian H.: Hallux Valgus, Allied Deformities of the Forefoot and Metatarsalgia. Philadelphia, W. B. Saunders Co., 1965, p. 328. Reprinted by permission.)

tion, as it is safe and simple, and full correction of the deformity is obtained without tension.[8, 9] He reported the results of 70 operations performed on 19 male and 36 female patients; the result was good in 91 per cent, fair in 6 per cent, and poor in 3 per cent. In the failures, the deformity recurred rapidly (within a year) and was then treated by amputation. Circulatory embarrassment to the little toe is prevented by avoiding traction on the neurovascular bundles. In the experience of Cockin, there has been no circulatory damage to the toe, and wound healing has not been a problem. The operative technique of the Butler operation is as follows:

A dorsal racquet incision is made on the skin; then a second handle is added to the racquet on the plantar aspect (the plantar handle inclined laterally and a little longer than the dorsal handle) (Fig. 2–125 A and B). The wound flaps are undermined and elevated, exposing the shortened extensor tendon of the fifth toe (Fig. 2–125C). The neurovascular bundle is identified and carefully protected from injury (Fig. 2–125D). The extensor tendon and the dorsomedial part of the capsule of the metatarsophalangeal joint are sectioned (Fig. 2–125E). The toe can now be manipulated freely downward and laterally into correct alignment. Occasionally, in severe long-standing cases, adhesions on the plantar aspect of the capsule are separated from the metatarsal head by blunt dissection (Fig. 2–125F and G). Now the toe moves into the plantar handle of the incision and dangles in normal alignment without any tension (Fig. 2–125H). The wound is closed so the surrounding skin sutures hold the toe in the corrected position (Fig. 2–125 I and J). Figure 2–125K is a diagrammatic illustration of the mechanics of the operation.

Skin dressing is applied. Splints to im-

Text continued on page 344

Correction of Digitus Minimus Varus (McFarland, Kelikian)

THE PROCEDURE

A. First, a 00 silk whip suture is passed through the pulps of the fourth and fifth toes. The suture ends are clamped with hemostats and the toes are pulled apart, bringing the web space into full view.

B. Three sets of incisions are made: (1) a web-bisecting incision that starts on the dorsum of the forefoot in the groove between the metatarsal heads and extends distally to bisect the web, and then passes plantarward to terminate at about the same point posteriorly on the plantar aspect of the forefoot as it does on the dorsum; (2) two *paradigital incisions,* one for each toe, which begin at the point where the web-bisecting incision begins to dip plantarward and extend lengthwise along the adjacent side of each toe. The paradigital incision for the little toe ends on the side of the distal phalanx at a point plantar and just proximal to the base of the nail, whereas the incision for the fourth toe is the same length as that for the fifth. The paradigital incisions are placed slightly toward the plantar border of the toe to give a semblance of an interdigital groove after surgical syndactylism. (3) Two connecting oblique incisions extend from the terminal point of the paradigital incision on each side to the proximal end of the web-bisecting incision on the plantar aspect.

C. The triangular patches of skin between the paradigital and oblique connecting incisions are excised. In dissection of subcutaneous tissue in this area, care is taken not to injure the plexus of veins. The skin flaps are mobilized and retracted to their respective sides. The digital nerves and vessels should be identified and protected from injury.

D and **E.** The long extensor tendon of the fifth toe is divided at its insertion; a 00 silk whip suture is applied to its distal end. (This end is later transferred to the fifth metatarsal head according to the technique for the Jones procedure described in Plate 24.) Next, the long flexor of the fifth toe is dissected free of the proximal phalanx. Small retractors are placed on the dorsal and plantar aspects of the bone to protect the soft tissues. The capsules of the metatarsophalangeal and proximal interphalangeal joints of the little toe are divided, and the proximal phalanx is excised. The long fifth toe extensor is transferred to the fifth metatarsal head. The wound is packed with moist gauze, the pneumatic tourniquet is deflated, and bleeding vessels are clamped and coagulated.

F. The terminal points of the paradigital incisions are sutured together with 0000 nylon, bringing the toes together. The alignment of the toes is inspected. Care is taken is avoid eversion or inversion of the toes; if necessary, the terminal suture is removed and reapplied. The dorsal wound is closed with 0000 nylon and the plantar skin edges with 0000 plain catgut.

POSTOPERATIVE CARE

A below-knee walking cast is applied. Three to four weeks following surgery, the cast and sutures are removed. The patient is allowed to bear weight and resume normal activities.

Plate 9. Correction of Digitus Minimus Varus (McFarland, Kelikian)

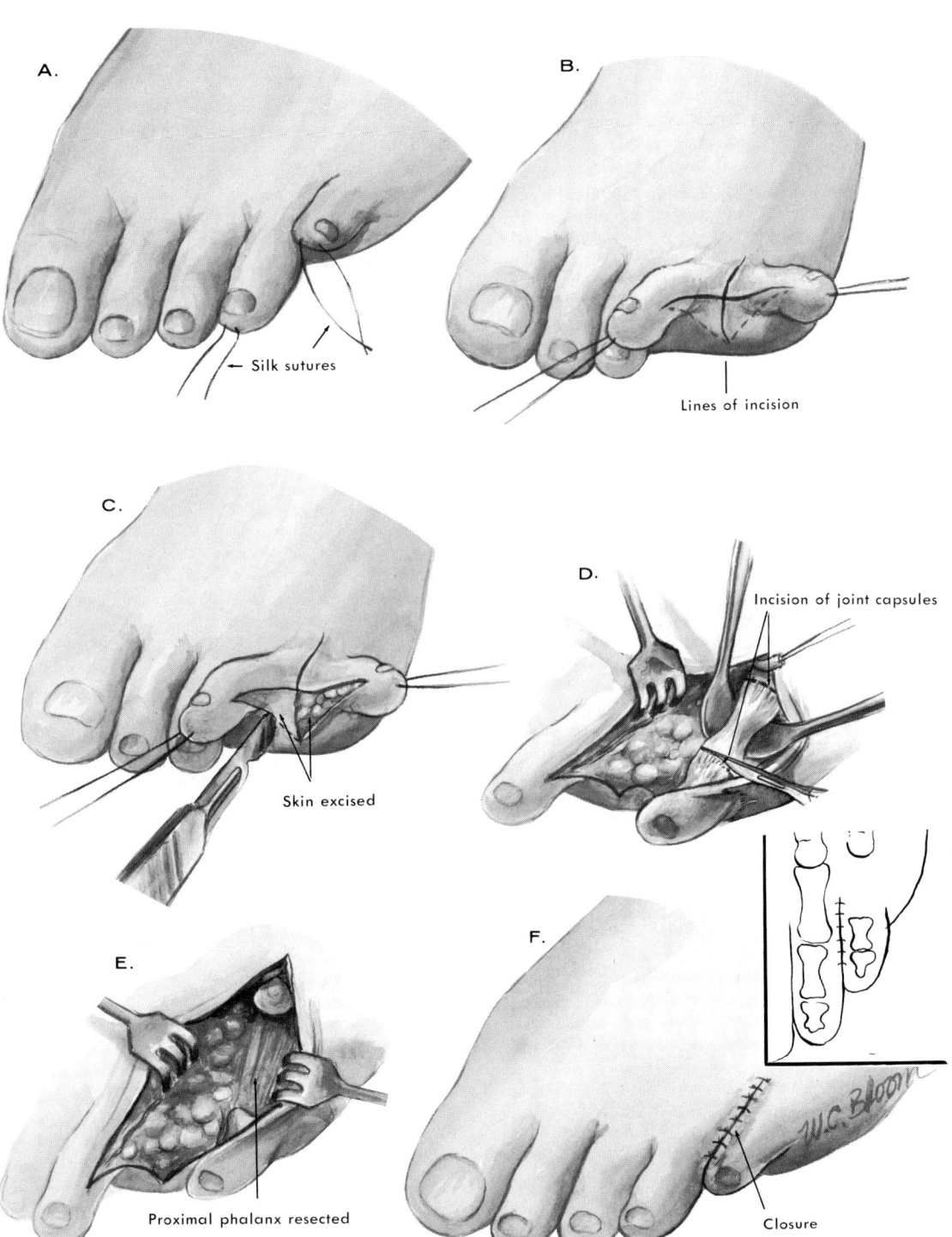

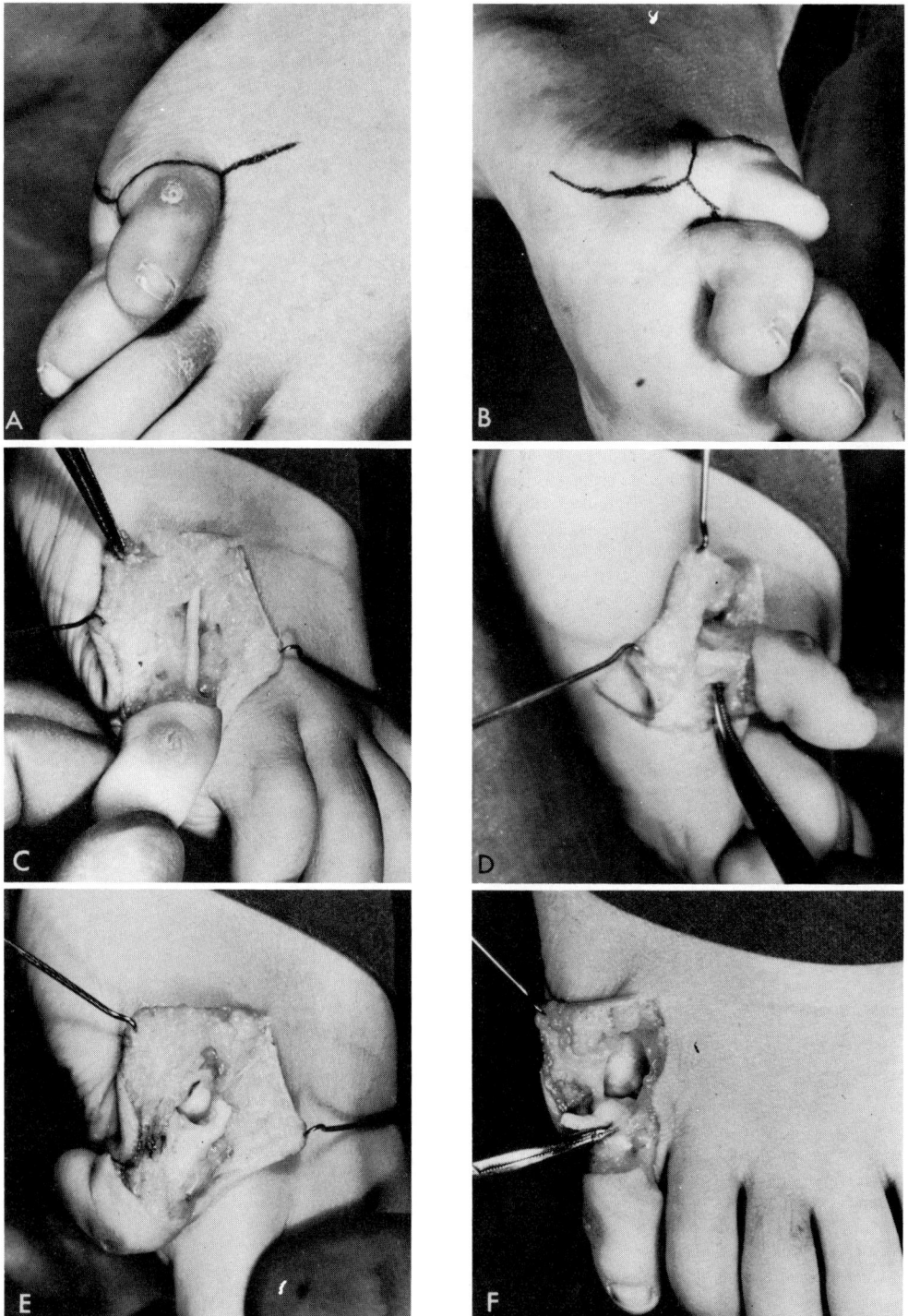

FIGURE 2–125. Butler's operation for an overriding fifth toe.

A and **B**. A dorsal racquet incision is made with a second handle added on the plantar aspect. The plantar handle is inclined laterally and is a little longer than the dorsal handle. **C** and **D**. The contracted extensor tendon to the fifth toe is exposed by elevating the skin flaps. The neurovascular bundles should be identified and carefully preserved. **E**. Sectioning of the extensor tendon and the dorsomedial part of the capsule of the metatarsophalangeal joint. **F**. In severe deformity, the articular surfaces of the metatarsophalangeal joints may be incongruous. This is due to plantar capsular adhesions.

Illustration continued on opposite page

Congenital Deformities 343

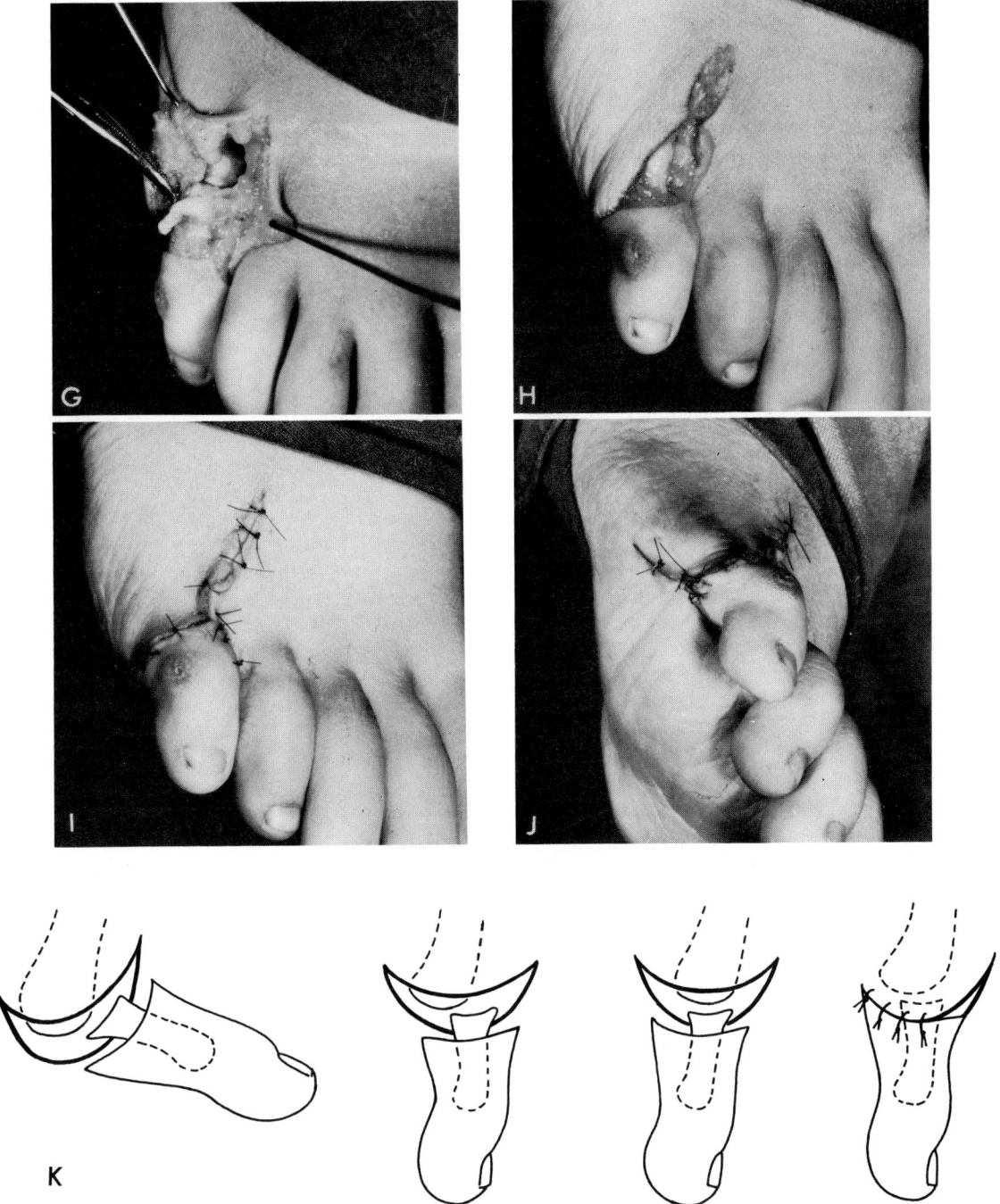

FIGURE 2–125 *Continued. Butler's operation for an overriding fifth toe.*

G. Adhesions on the plantar part of the capsule are freed by blunt dissection. Note the little toe now lies in the fully corrected position. **H.** Appearance of the toe before skin closure. It lies freely in normal alignment without tension. **I** and **J.** Closure of the wound. Skin sutures securely hold the toe in the correct position. **K.** Diagrammatic illustration of the mechanics of the operation. (From Cockin, J.: Butler's operation for an overriding fifth toe. J. Bone Joint Surg., *50-B*:78–80, 1968. Reprinted by permission.)

mobilize the toe in the corrected position are not required. The sutures are removed in 10 to 14 days, and normal activity is then allowed.

The author has utilized the Butler operation in children and has found it to be very satisfactory. In adolescents and adults, however, the potential embarrassment to circulation of the little toe is a definite drawback to the procedure.

Hallux Valgus Interphalangeus

In this congenital deformity the distal phalanx of the great toe is deviated laterally toward the second toe at the interphalangeal joint. The degree of valgus deviation varies from mild to marked (Figs. 2–126 and 2–127). In moderately severe cases the shoe pressure irritates the skin over the interphalangeal joint of the hallux, and gradually adventitious bursa and blisters develop.

In childhood treatment consists of cuneiform osteotomy through the shaft of the proximal phalanx of the hallux. The resected wedge of bone is based medially, and the bone fragments are aligned and fixed internally with a Kirschner wire (Fig. 2–128). In the skeletally mature foot, the interphalangeal joint of the great toe is fused in correct alignment following partial excision of the hypertrophied medial portion of the epiphysis.

Congenital Curly (or Varus) Toe

In this common congenital deformity one or more toes are bent plantarward, deviated medially, and rotated laterally at the distal interphalangeal joint (Fig. 2–129). The twisted terminal pulp then gradually begins to impinge upon and curl under the adjacent toe.

This affection is usually bilateral and symmetrical, and has a high familial incidence. It is most probably caused by hypoplasia of the intrinsic muscles of the affected toe. Trethowan regarded the anomaly as a congenital form of hammer toe.[28] Sweetnam coined the term *congenital curly toe*, and also observed that the deformity does not correct itself spontaneously and usually becomes exaggerated with growth.[26]

TREATMENT

If the deformity is mild and the curly toe does not impinge upon its adjacent toe, the condition can be ignored and no treatment

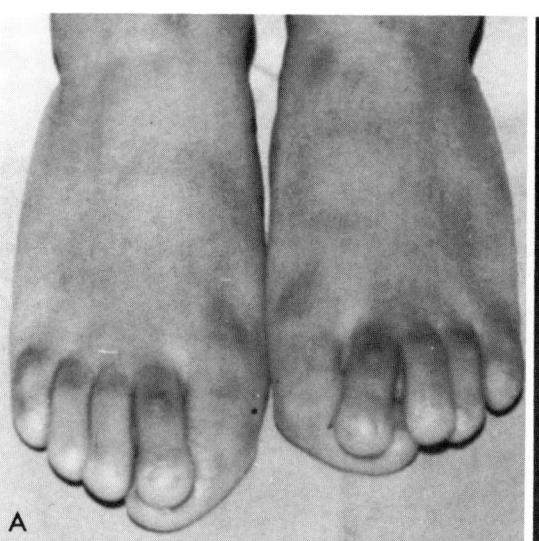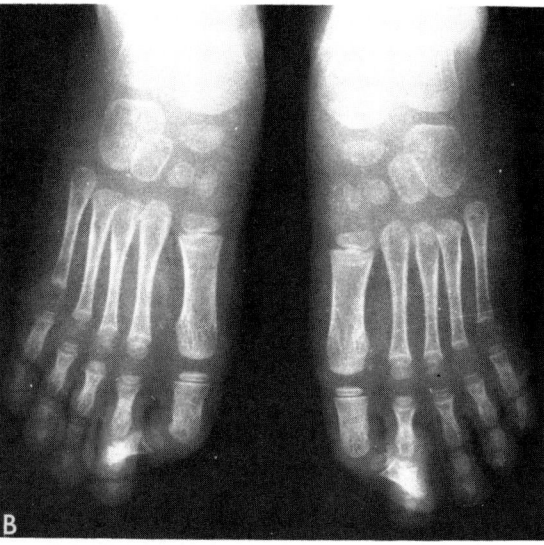

FIGURE 2–126. Bilateral hallux valgus interphalangeus.

A. Clinical appearance. Note the lateral deviation of the distal phalanx of the great toe. **B.** Anteroposterior roentgenogram of both feet showing lateral subluxation of the interphalangeal joint of the hallux.

Congenital Deformities 345

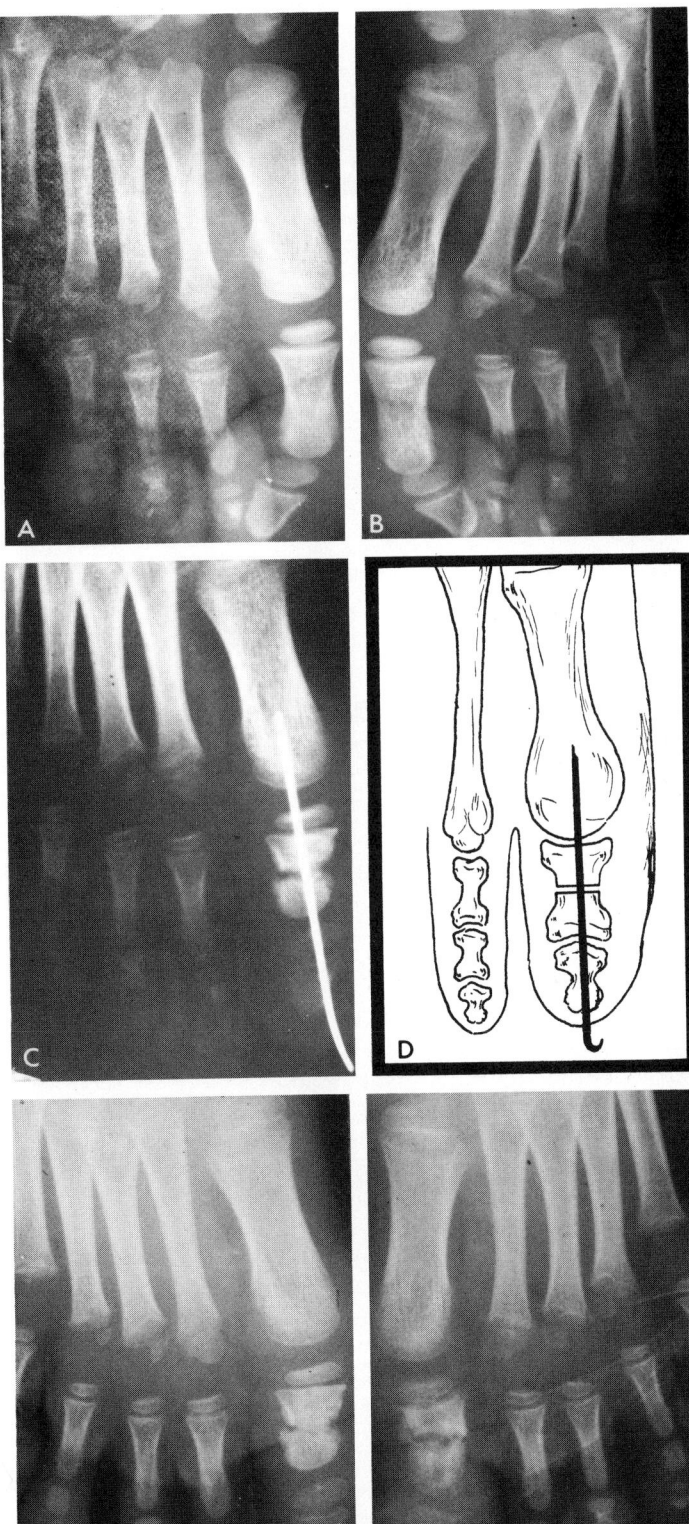

FIGURE 2–127. Congenital hallux valgus interphalangeus in a two-year-old child.

Treatment consisted of cuneiform osteotomy of the shaft of the proximal phalanx with the base of the resected wedge of bone passing medially, and internal fixation of the bone fragments with Kirschner wire. **A** and **B**. Preoperative roentgenograms. **C**. Roentgenogram showing correction maintained by Kirschner wire. **D**. Interpretive diagram. **E** and **F**. Postoperative roentgenograms of both forefeet showing excellent correction. (From Kelikian, H.: Hallux Valgus, Allied Deformities of the Forefoot and Metatarsalgia. Philadelphia, W. B. Saunders Co., 1965, p. 461. Reprinted by permission.)

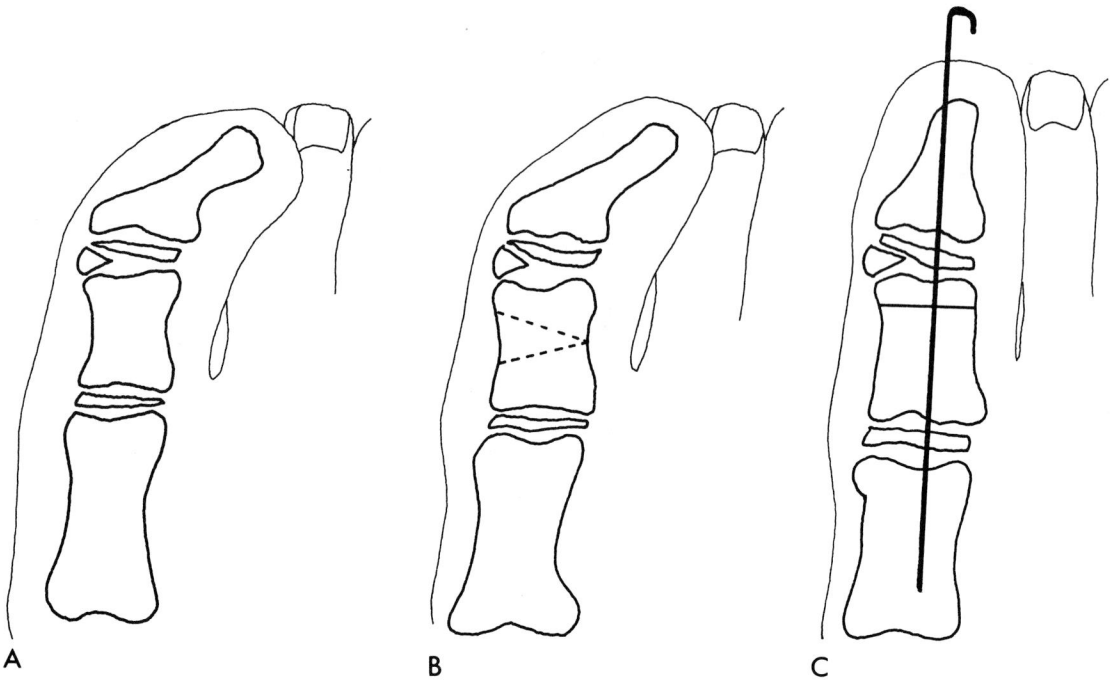

FIGURE 2–128. *Hallux valgus interphalangeus–diagram showing method of correction in childhood.*

A. Deformity. **B.** Cuneiform osteotomy of the diaphysis of the proximal phalanx of the great toe. The base of the resected bone wedge lies medially. **C.** The bone fragments are aligned and fixed internally with Kirschner wire.

is necessary. Over-and-under strapping is useless and has no permanent effect.

If the affected toe curls under the neighboring one, disabling symptoms are most likely to ensue later in life, particularly in women, in whom discomfort results from the pressure of tight shoes. Pain under the adjacent medial metatarsal head develops as the underlying toe does not permit its neighboring medial toe to touch the floor; thus more body weight is transmitted to the metatarsal head. In children, Kelikian recommends surgical syndactyly of the curly toe with its normal neighbor on the medial side.[24] Another alternative is to transfer the flexor digitorum longus tendon of the affected toe to the dorsal and lateral aspect of the extensor hood.[25, 27] This is especially indicated in children in whom the deformity is not very severe or rigid. The operative technique is as follows:

A 3-cm. longitudinal incision is made on the dorsolateral aspect of the deformed toe. The subcutaneous tissue is divided, and the digital nerve and long toe extensor tendon are pulled medially with a blunt retractor. The affected toe is acutely flexed, and on its plantar aspect the long toe flexor tendon is identified. A longitudinal incision is made in the flexor tendon sheath, and the tendon is pulled dorsally with a small hook and sectioned near its insertion. After manipulation of the distal interphalangeal joint into normal alignment, the long flexor tendon is sutured to the extensor expansion with the interphalangeal joints of the toe in full extension and with the metatarsophalangeal joint in flexion. The tourniquet is released, and the wound closed in the usual manner. Alignment of the affected toe is maintained by a smooth Kirschner wire drilled from the distal end of the toe into the base of the proximal phalanx. Adhesive strapping or a below-knee walking cast is applied. The cast and wire are removed three to four weeks after surgery. In adults, Kelikian recommends partial proximal phalangectomy with surgical syndactyly of the toes.[24]

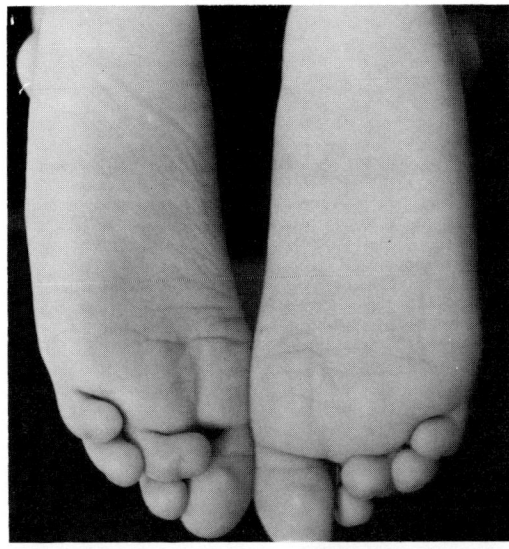

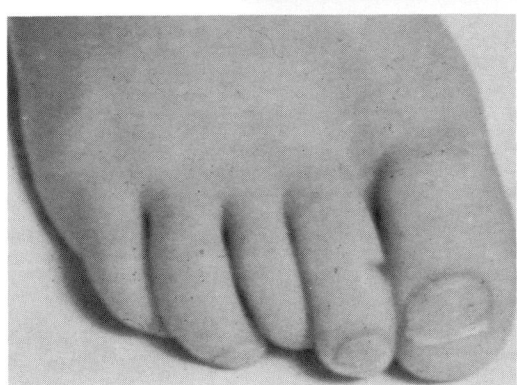
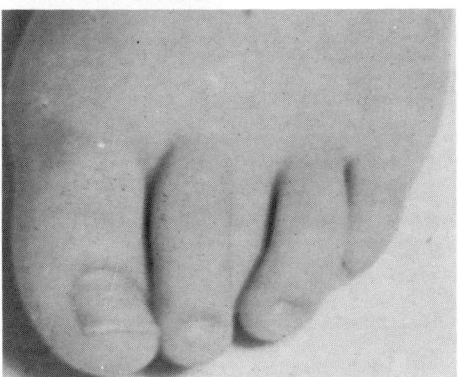

FIGURE 2–129. *Curly toes.*

References

SYNDACTYLISM

1. Blauth, W.: Congenital digital syndactylia. (Author's transl.) Z. Kinderchir. Grenzgeb., *30*:42, 1980.
2. Blauth, W., and Helbig, B.: Syndactylia recurrences and their treatment. (Author's transl.): Z. Kinderchir. Grenzgeb., *30*:53, 1980.
3. Kleiner, B. C., and Holmes, L. B.: Brief clinical report: Hallux varus and preaxial polysyndactyly in brothers. Amer. J. Med. Genet., 6:113, 1980.
4. Losch, G. M., Schrader, M., and Eckert, P.: Malformation syndrome with constriction rings, pseudoligaments, acral defects and syndactylism: Diagnosis and treatment. (Author's transl.) Z. Kinderchir. Grenzgeb., *30*:85, 1980.
5. Piza, H., and Meissl, G.: Long term results following surgical correction of syndactylia. (Author's transl.) Z. Kinderchir. Grenzgeb., *30*:57, 1980.
6. Reuter, G.: Pitfalls in surgery of syndactylism. (Author's transl.) Z. Kinderchir. Grenzgeb., *30*:61, 1980.
7. Teot, L., and Gilbert, A.: Measure of the web-space in children. (Author's transl.) Chir. Pediat., 22:31, 1981.

CONGENITAL DIGITUS MINIMUS VARUS

8. Butler, R. W.: Personal communication to J. Cockin, 1964 (see ref. 9).
9. Cockin, J.: Butler's operation for an overriding fifth toe. J. Bone Joint Surg., *50-B*:78, 1968.
10. DuVries, H. L.: Surgery of the Foot. St. Louis, C. V. Mosby Co., 1959, p. 347.
11. Gocht, H., and DeBrunner, H.: Orthopaedische Therapie. Leipzig, F. C. W. Vogel, 1925, p. 238.
12. Goodwin, F. C., and Swisher, F. M.: The treatment of congenital hyperextension of the great toe. J. Bone Joint Surg., *25*:193, 1943.
13. Kelikian, H.: Hallux Valgus, Allied Deformities of the Forefoot and Metatarsalgia. Philadelphia, W. B. Saunders Co., 1965.
14. Kelikian, H., Clayton, I., and Loseff, H.: Surgical syndactylia of the toes. Clin. Orthop., *19*:208, 1961.
15. Lantzounis, L. A.: Congenital subluxation of the fifth toe and its correction by a periosteocapsuloplasty and tendon transplantation. J. Bone Joint Surg. 22:147, 1940.
16. Lapidus, P. C.: Transplantation of the extensor tendon for correction of the overlapping fifth toe. J. Bone Joint Surg., *24*:555, 1942.
17. McFarland, B.: Congenital deformities of the spine and limbs. *In* Platt, H. (ed.): Modern Trends in Orthopedics. New York, P. B. Hoeber, Inc.; London, Butterworth & Co., 1950, p. 107.
18. Ruiz-Mora, J.: Personal communication to L. R. Straub, 1954 (see ref. 21).
19. Scrase, W. H.: The treatment of dorsal adduction deformities of the fifth toe. J. Bone Joint Surg., *36-B*:146, 1954.
20. Stamm, T. T.: Surgery of the foot. *In* British Surgical Practice. Vol. IV. London, Butterworth & Co.; St. Louis, C. V. Mosby Co., 1948, p. 160.

Correction of Hammer Toe by Resection and Arthrodesis of Proximal Interphalangeal Joint

THE PROCEDURE

A. A 3- to 4-cm. longitudinal incision is made over the dorsal aspect of the proximal interphalangeal joint parallel to and at the lateral border of the extensor digitorum longus tendon. The subcutaneous tissue is divided and the skin flaps are retracted.

B. The long extensor tendon is split and retracted to expose the capsule of the proximal interphalangeal joint. The digital vessels and nerves are protected from injury. A transverse incision is made in the capsule and the joint surfaces are widely exposed.

C and **D.** With a rongeur, wedges of bone based dorsally are resected from the head of the proximal phalanx and the base of the middle phalanx. Enough bone should be removed to allow correction of deformity.

E and **F.** The proximal and middle phalanges are held together by internal fixation with a Kirschner wire that is inserted retrograde. The Kirschner wire should not cross the metatarsophalangeal joint. The cancellous bony surfaces of the middle and proximal phalanges should be apposed, and the rotational alignment should be correct. The capsule is resutured tightly by reefing. The wound is closed in routine manner. With a pair of nose pliers, the end of the Kirschner wire is bent 90 degrees and cut, leaving 0.5 cm. protruding through the skin.

POSTOPERATIVE CARE

A below-knee walking cast is applied with a band of plaster of Paris protecting the toe. The wire and cast are removed in six weeks, when the roentgenograms show fusion of the interphalangeal joint.

Plate 10. Correction of Hammer Toe by Resection and Arthrodesis of Proximal Interphalangeal Joint

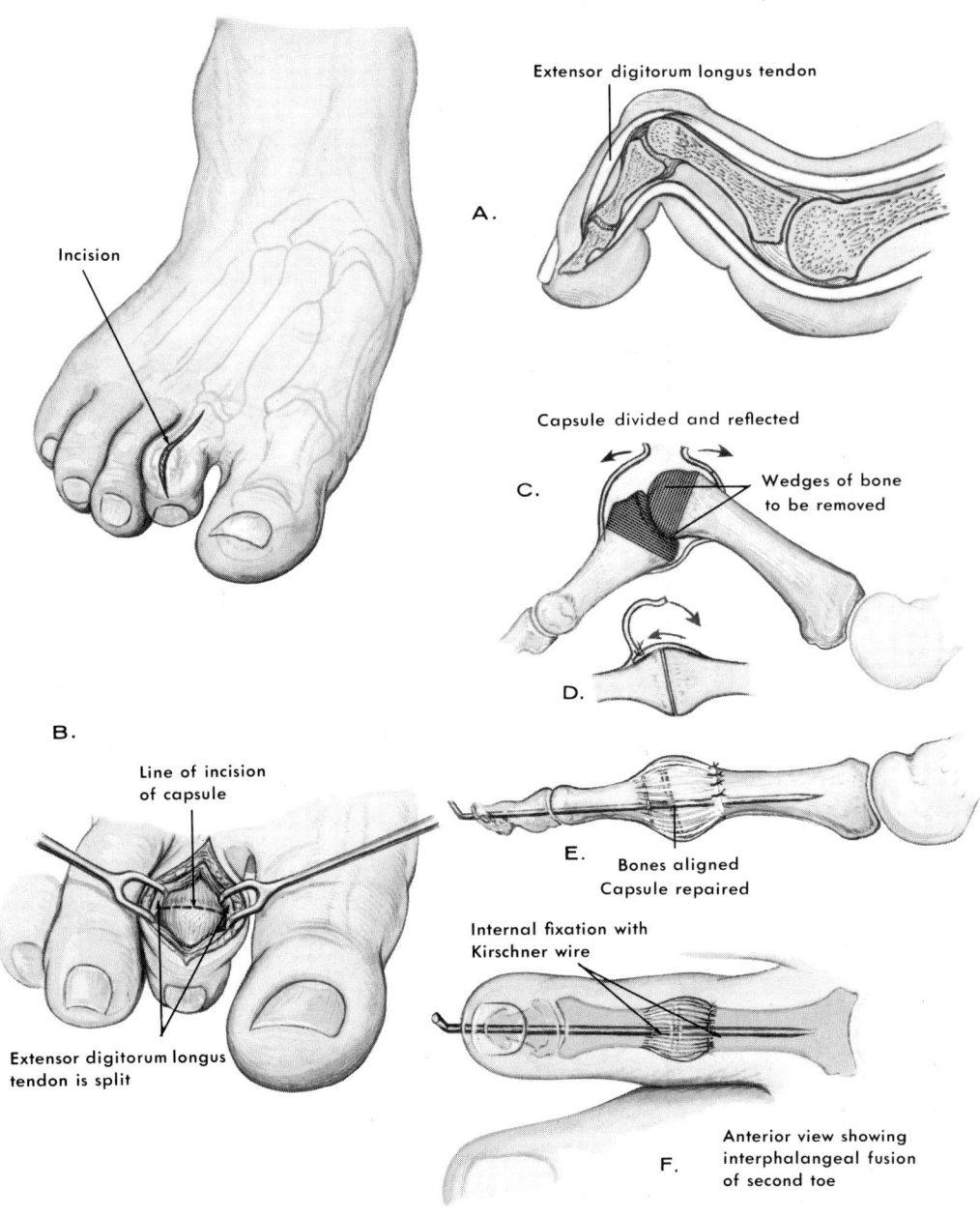

21. Straub, L. R.: Orthopedic surgery. *In* Cecil, R. L. (ed.): The Specialties in General Practice. Philadelphia, W. B. Saunders Co., 1951, p. 60.
22. Thompson, C. T.: Surgical treatment of disorders of the fore part of the foot. J. Bone Joint Surg., *46-A*:1117, 1964.
23. Wilson, J. N.: V-Y correction for varus deformity of the fifth toe. Brit. J. Surg., *41*:133, 1953.

CONGENITAL CURLY (OR VARUS) TOE

24. Kelikian, H.: Hallux Valgus, Allied Deformities of the Forefoot and Metatarsalgia. Philadelphia, W. B. Saunders Co., 1965, p. 330.
25. Sharrard, W. J. W.: The surgery of deformed toes in children. Brit. J. Clin. Pract., *17*:263, 1963.
26. Sweetnam, R.: Congenital curly toes. An investigation into the value of treatment. Lancet, *2*:398, 1958.
27. Taylor, R. G.: The treatment of claw toes by multiple transfers of flexor with extensor tendons. J. Bone Joint Surg., *33-B*:539, 1951.
28. Trethowan, W. H.: The treatment of hammertoe. Lancet, *1*:1257, 1312, 1925.

HAMMER TOE

Hammer toe is a deformity characterized by flexion contracture of the proximal interphalangeal joint. The distal interphalangeal joint may be in flexion, in neutral extension, or in slight hyperextension. Eventually, with depression of the metatarsal head, the metatarsophalangeal joint becomes hyperextended. Painful calluses develop under the metatarsal heads. The capsules and ligaments on the plantar aspect of the flexed joints and on the dorsal aspect of the hyperextended joints become contracted. The interosseus tendons become shifted dorsally. Constant irritation caused by shoe pressure may cause calluses to develop over the dorsum of the flexed interphalangeal joint and on the end of the toe. An adventitious bursa may also appear between the indurated skin and subjacent bone.

Hammer toe is often bilateral and symmetrical. There is a very high familial incidence. The second toe is most frequently affected, and less often the third and fourth toes. The deformity is usually congenital; acquired cases are ordinarily caused by mechanical pressure of a small shoe on an abnormally long toe that is forced to flex at its interphalangeal joints. Hammer toe may occur in association with hallux valgus.

Treatment

In infants and children, the deformity should be treated conservatively. Passive stretching exercises are performed by the parents. The deformity is usually not fixed; if it is marked, the interphalangeal joint is manipulated into extension and strapped with adhesive tape in the corrected position. When the child begins to walk, it is important to provide him with shoes that have adequate room. Pain from inflamed calluses over the dorsum of the flexed interphalangeal joint is alleviated by protective pads.

In the adolescent, if the deformity is severe and disabling, surgical correction is indicated. Various operative procedures are available. A simple and very satisfactory method is resection of the proximal interphalangeal joint and arthrodesis of the joint in neutral position. This was first reported by Soule, in 1910, and later was popularized by Sir Robert Jones.[6, 16] The operative correction of hammer toe by resection and fusion of the proximal interphalangeal joint is described and illustrated in Plate 10. The procedure is combined with dorsal capsulotomy of the metatarsophalangeal joint if the latter has developed fixed hyperextension contracture. In the presence of marked depression of the metatarsal head, the long toe extensor is transferred to the metatarsal head.

When the hammer toe deformity is severe with *irreducible* dorsal subluxation of the metatarsophalangeal joints, partial proxi-

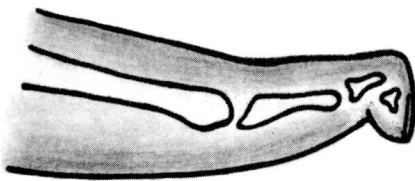

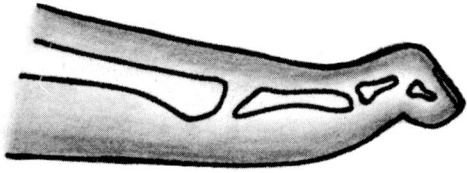

A.   **B.**

FIGURE 2–130. Mallet toe.
A. Severe. **B.** Mild.

mal phalangectomy is preferred and the adjacent digits are syndactylized surgically.

The Girdlestone operation was designed to provide active plantar flexion of the proximal phalanx by transfer of the toe flexor to the extensor hood. The author is dissatisfied with the procedure and does not recommend it because lateral deformities of the toes frequently develop following the transfer and also because it does not always correct the deformity.

References

1. Blum, A.: De l'orteil en marteau. Bull. Mem. Soc. Chir. Paris, 9:738, 1883.
2. Brahms, M. A.: Common foot problems. J. Bone Joint Surg., 49-A:1653, 1967.
3. Cahill, B. R., and Connor, D. E.: A long-term follow-up on proximal phalangectomy for hammer toes. Clin. Orthop., 86:191, 1972.
4. Ely, L. W.: Hammertoe, Surg. Clin. N. Amer., 6:433, 1926.
5. Glassman, F., Wallin, L., and Sideman, S.: Phalangectomy for toe deformities. Surg. Clin. N. Amer., 29:275, 1949.
6. Jones, R.: Notes on Military Orthopaedics. New York, P. B. Hoeber, 1917, pp. 38–57.
7. Krenz, L.: Die Hammerzchen and ihre Operation macht Bocht. Arch. Orthop. Untallchir., 21:459, 1923.
8. Lapidus, P. W.: Operation for correction of hammertoe. J. Bone Joint Sur., 21:977, 1939.
9. McConnell, B. E.: Hammer toe surgery. Southern Med. J., 68:595, 1975.
10. Margo, M. K.: Surgical treatment of conditions of the fore part of the foot. J. Bone Joint Surg., 49-A:1665, 1976.
11. Merrill, W. J.: Conservative operative treatment of hammertoe. Amer. J. Orthop. Surg., 10:262, 1912.
12. Michele, A. A., and Krueger, F. J.: Operative correction for hammertoe. Mil. Surg., 103:52, 1948.
13. Milgram, J. E.: Office measures for relief of painful foot. J. Bone Joint Surg., 46:1095, 948.
14. O'Neil, J.: An arthroplastic operation for hammertoe. J.A.M.A., 57:1207, 1911.
15. Sehig, S.: Hammertoe: A new procedure for its correction. Surg. Gynec. Obstet., 72:101, 1941.
16. Soule, R. E.: Operation for the cure of hammertoe. New York Med. J., 91:649, March 26, 1910.
17. Taylor, R. G.: An operative procedure for the treatment of hammer toe and claw toe. J. Bone Joint Surg., 22:608, 1940.
18. Trethowan, W. H.: The treatment of hammertoe. Lancet, 1:1257–1312, 1925.
19. Young, C. S.: An operation for correction of hammertoe and claw toe. J. Bone Joint Surg., 20:715, 1938.

MALLET TOE

This deformity is characterized by flexion deformity at the distal interphalangeal joint of any of the lesser toes (Fig. 2–130). Usually a single toe or two neighboring ones are affected. The condition is less common than hammer toe, in which the flexion deformity is at the proximal interphalangeal joint. Mallet toes are asymptomatic in childhood, but in adolescence or early adult life, the development of a painful corn on the tip of the toe close to the nail may be very disabling.

Conservative measures such as adhesive strapping and passive stretching exercises do not correct the deformity. Shaving the corn and padding the toe will give symptomatic relief, but surgery is often preferred. Fusion of the distal interphalangeal joint in normal alignment and section of the long toe flexor corrects the deformity. A simpler method that provides immediate relief of symptoms is amputation of the distal phalanx, but this is esthetically undesirable.

3. Neuromuscular Diseases

THE FOOT AND ANKLE IN
NEUROMUSCULAR DISEASES
    Levels of Paralysis
    Neuromuscular System as a Functional Unit
    Responses of Muscles
    Interdependence of Foot, Ankle, Knee, Hip, and Trunk
CEREBRAL PALSY
MYELOMENINGOCELE
DIASTEMATOMYELIA
POLIOMYELITIS

PERONEAL MUSCULAR ATROPHY (CHARCOT MARIE-TOOTH DISEASE)
FRIEDREICH'S ATAXIA
HYPERTROPHIC INTERSTITIAL NEURITIS
MUSCLES
    Muscular Dystrophy
    Congenital Absence of Muscles
    Accessory Muscles
    Congenital Contracture of Triceps Surae Muscle
    Achilles Tendinitis

THE FOOT AND ANKLE IN NEUROMUSCULAR DISEASES

The foot and ankle may be affected in neuromuscular diseases at various levels—the spinomuscular, the extrapyramidal, the pyramidal, the cerebellar, and the psychomotor. Disease at each level is characterized by changes in motor function peculiar to the site and extent of involvement.

Levels of Paralysis

At the *spinomuscular level* motor activity is simple; the impulses arising in the anterior horn cells of the spinal cord are transmitted through the peripheral nerves to the myoneural junctions and then to the individual muscles. In disorders at the spinomuscular level, the loss of motor power is focal and segmental, with complete paralysis of the muscles or muscle groups that are supplied by a peripheral nerve or by the anterior horn cells in the spinal cord. Muscular paralysis is flaccid or hypotonic, with reaction of degeneration, atrophy, fibrillations, and fasciculations. The deep tendon and superficial reflexes are diminished or absent. Pyramidal tract signs, abnormal involuntary movements, and ataxia are absent. There may be trophic changes in the skin, nails, and bone.

Pathologic processes at the spinomuscular level may be further classified into various sublevels. When the disease originates in the anterior horn cells, as in poliomyelitis, the *spinal level* of the motor system is affected. Other examples of diseases at the spinal level are progressive spinal muscular atrophy of the Werdnig-Hoffmann type, progressive bulbar palsy, syringomyelia, and intramedullary neoplasm. The loss of function of the anterior horn cells and the motor nuclei of the brain stem results in clinical findings of flaccid paralysis, atrophy, areflexia, reaction of degeneration, and fasciculations.

At the *neural level* of the motor system, the peripheral nerves and nerve roots are affected. Common examples of disorders at this level are obstetrical brachial plexus palsy and progressive neural muscular atrophy (Charcot-Marie-Tooth disease). In affections of nerves, sensory fibers are usually involved, with resultant sensory changes such as anesthesia or hyperesthesia. Otherwise, the clinical findings are similar to those of spinal level affections, i.e., flaccid paralysis, atrophy, reaction of degeneration, and areflexia as a result of loss of conduction of motor impulses. In the absence of sensory changes it is difficult to distinguish between diseases of the peripheral nerves and those of the anterior roots and anterior horn cells.

When the pathologic process arises at the myoneural junction, as in myasthenia gravis and familial periodic paralysis, then it is a disease at the *myoneural level*. In diseases of primarily muscular origin, the motor system is involved at the *muscular level*. The muscular dystrophies are familiar examples of disturbance of the muscular level in disease at the spinomuscular level. Paralysis is flaccid, but reflexes persist until the late stages when marked atrophy has occurred. There is loss of contractibility without loss of excitability, i.e., the muscle fibers have degenerated and have been replaced by fibroadipose tissue, but the peripheral nerves and anterior horn cells are normal.

In disorders of the motor system at the *extrapyramidal level* there is generalized involvement of the muscles of the limbs and trunk. The muscle tone is hypertonic. Atrophy, fasciculations, and reaction of degeneration are absent. Motion of the limbs is hyperkinetic, with loss of associated or automatic movements. The deep tendon and superficial reflexes are normal. There are no pyramidal tract responses and no sensory deficit. Athetoid cerebral palsy is a common example of a disease at the extrapyramidal level.

At the *pyramidal* or *corticospinal level* of involvement, motor deficit arises from affection of motor nuclei of the cerebral cortex. Paresis is usually generalized and associated with hypertonicity or spasticity of muscles. Pyramidal tract signs and pathologic reflexes are usually present. There is usually some atrophy that is not focal; it is caused by chronic paralysis and disuse. Fasciculations, trophic disturbances, reaction of degeneration, and abnormal movements are absent. The deep tendon reflexes are hyperactive, and the superficial reflexes are diminished or absent. Spastic cerebral palsy illustrates the pyramidal level of motor involvement.

Cerebellar level lesions are characterized by loss of coordination and control, or ataxia. There is no real loss of motor power. Fasciculations, reaction of degeneration, atrophy, and trophic disturbances are absent. The deep tendon reflexes may be diminished or pendular, but the superficial reflexes are normal. Pyramidal tract responses cannot be elicited.

The *psychomotor level* of motor performance is the highest level of neuromuscular activity—at which volitional movements are initiated and effected by integration, memory, and symbolization. Paralysis caused by hysteria is an example of psychomotor disturbance. Loss of motor power is bizarre, with no actual paralysis. There is no real neurologic deficit. There are no fasciculations, no atrophy, and no true ataxia.

Differential features of various levels of motor function are illustrated in Table 3–1.

Neuromuscular System as a Functional Unit

Muscles are the expressive unit of the neuromuscular system and the moving force of the body. Muscles whose contraction directly produces a specific action are classified as *agonists* or *prime movers* (protag-

Table 3-1. Differentiation of Motor Disorders at Various Levels of Neuromuscular Function*

	Spinomuscular			Extrapyramidal	Pyramidal	Cerebellar	Psychomotor
	Muscular	*Neural*	*Spinal*				
Loss of motor power	Focal-segmental Usually proximal and axial muscle groups	Focal-segmental Usually distal limb musculature	Focal-segmental Usually distal limb musculature	Generalized Entire limb and movements	Generalized Entire limb and movements	None Ataxia may simulate loss of power	No true loss Bizarre, may simulate any type
	Complete	Complete	Complete	Incomplete	Incomplete		
Tone	Flaccid	Flaccid	Flaccid	Rigid	Spastic	Hypotonic (ataxia)	Normal or variable, may be increased
Atrophy	Present	Present	Present	Absent	Minimal (due to disuse and chronic paresis)	Absent	Absent
Fasciculations	May be present	Absent	May be present	Absent	Absent	Absent	Absent
Reaction of degeneration	Present	Present	Present	Absent	Absent	Absent	Absent
EMG							
Interference pattern	Normal until late in disease	Reduced	Reduced				
Fibrillation potential	Not usually present Short duration	Present Prolonged with normal or polyphasic potentials	Usually present Prolonged with occasional giant potentials				
Action potential							

Neuromuscular Diseases

Feature	Col 1	Col 2	Col 3	Col 4	Col 5	Col 6	Col 7
Evoked sensory and mixed nerve potentials	Normal	Absent, diminished amplitude, or prolonged conduction time	Normal				
Reflexes							
Deep	Diminished and preserved until late	Absent early	Absent early	Normal or variable	Hyperactive	Diminished or pendular	Normal or increased range
Superficial	Diminished	Absent	Absent	Normal or increased	Diminished or absent	Normal	Normal or increased
Pyramidal tract response	No	No	No	No	Yes	No	No
Sensory deficit	Absent	Usually present	Absent	Absent	May be present (stereognosis or other cortical)	Absent	Absent
Trophic disturbance	Present	Present	Present	Absent	Usually absent	Absent	Absent
Ataxia	Absent	Absent	Absent	Absent	Absent	Present	Absent (may simulate ataxia)
Abnormal movements	Absent	Absent	Absent	Present	None	May be present (intention tremor and ataxia)	May be present
Associated movements	Normal	Normal	Normal	Absence of normal associated movements	Presence of pathologic associated movements	Normal	Normal

*Adapted from DeJong, R. N.: The Neurological Examination. 3rd edition. New York, Hoeber Medical Division, Harper & Row, 1967, p. 382; and Farmer, T. W.: Pediatric Neurology. New York, Hoeber Medical Division, Harper & Row, 1964, p. 612.

onists). An example is the biceps brachii in flexion of the elbow. Those muscles that oppose the agonists must be relaxed for contraction of the agonists (these are called *antagonists* or *moderators*) as, for example, the triceps brachii is in flexion of the elbow.

A motor action, even in an apparently simple motion, is quite complex. It involves the *muscles of fixation,* which stabilize the adjacent joints and afford a firm base for muscle action. The action of *synergists* is to assist the agonists and to reduce to a minimum all unnecessary motions. The execution of a motor movement requires the coordinated action of all four physiologic muscle groups—the contraction of agonists and the relaxation of antagonists as well as the associated function of the synergists and the muscles of fixation. Loss of function of any of these muscle groups will result in disturbance of motor performance.

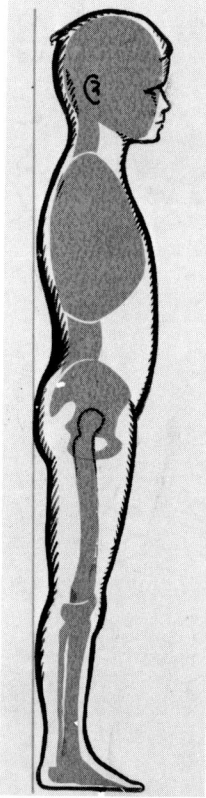

FIGURE 3–1. *Requisites for stable upright posture in stance.*

Requirements are (1) plantigrade feet and ankles, (2) slightly hyperextended knees, (3) extended hips, and (4) trunk-head-neck balanced and centered on the supporting base.

Responses of Muscles

The responses of muscles to injury and disease are predictable. Muscles that are not used atrophy. The rapidity with which such disuse atrophy develops is well illustrated by the atrophy of the quadriceps femoris that follows a painful lesion of the knee or immobilization of the knee in an above-knee cast. With progressive resistive exercises, muscles hypertrophy. Painful stimuli will cause protective spasm of a muscle, which, when maintained in its shortened position for a period of time, will tend to develop myostatic contracture. The antagonists to those muscles in spasm are weakened by being maintained in their longer stretched position and by inhibition of their function and recovery.

Muscular action affects bone growth. In the growing skeleton, muscle imbalance will cause deformity in the direction of action of the stronger muscle. Muscles are very sensitive to ischemia, as illustrated by Volkmann's ischemic contracture. Chronic systemic disease causes generalized muscle weakness and increased fatigability.

Interdependence of the Foot, Ankle, Knee, Hip, and Trunk

In the treatment of deformities of the foot and ankle in neuromuscular diseases it is imperative to assess the entire lower limb, to determine the posture and balance of the trunk, and to consider the patient as a whole.[1]

The prerequisites for a stable upright posture in stance are plantigrade feet and ankles, extended or slightly hyperextended knees and hips, and trunk, head, and neck balanced and centered on the supporting base (Fig. 3–1).

The hip and knee mark the two ends of one bone—the femur; the knee and ankle are connected by the tibia and fibula (Fig. 3–2). The ankle, knee, and hip should be treated as one functional unit. The posture of each depends upon that of the others; they reflect and affect each other. Deformity and muscle weakness at one level influence stability at the adjacent levels, requiring compensatory adaptations to achieve independent stance and gait. Each level

Figure 3–2. Interdependence of the hip, knee, and ankle.

A. The hip and knee mark the two ends of one bone—the femur. The hip, femur, and knee should be treated as a functional unit. **B.** The knee and ankle are connected by the tibia and fibula. The knee, tibia, and ankle should be treated as one functional unit.

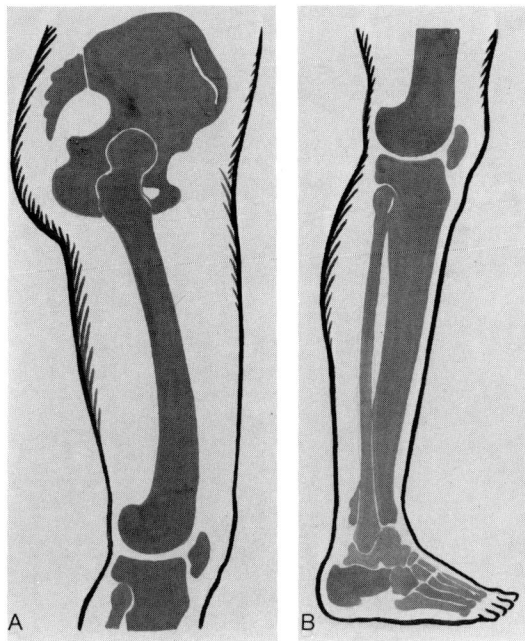

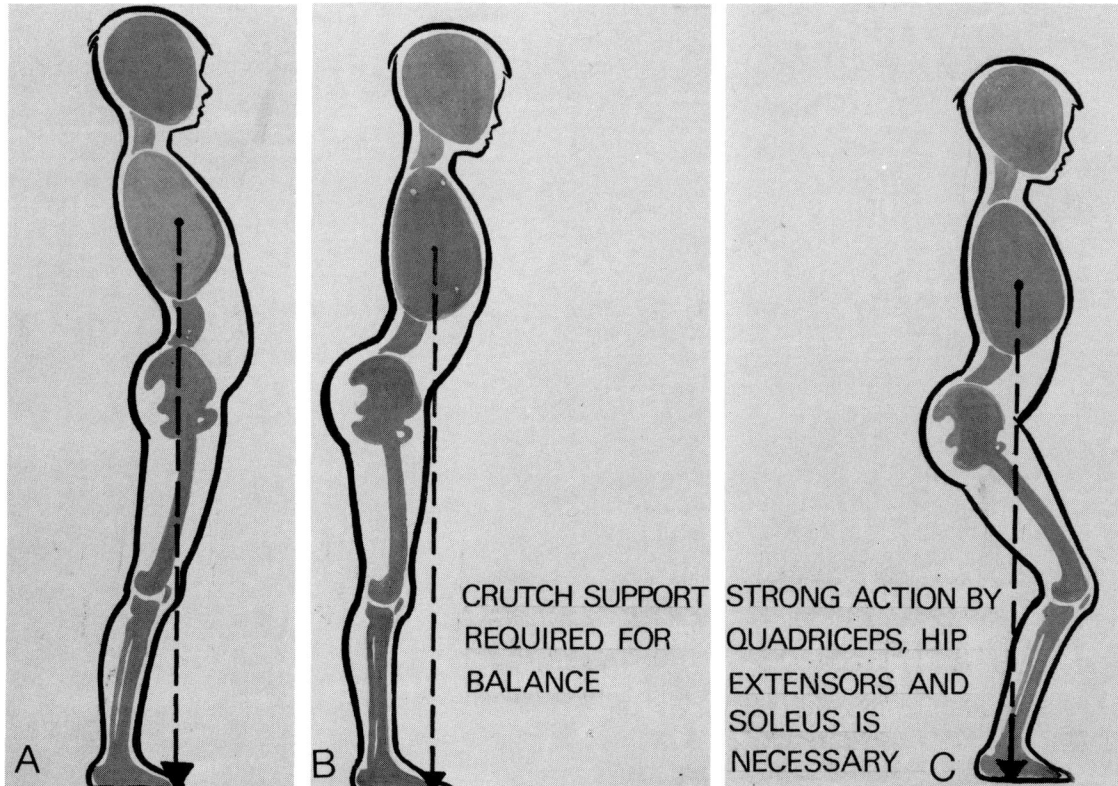

FIGURE 3–3. Hip flexion deformity; its effect on posture of the trunk, knee, and ankle.

A. Excessive lumbar lordosis is used to achieve balance. **B.** If hip flexion deformity exceeds the amount accommodated by lumbar lordosis, the trunk leans forward; with knees in extension, crutch support is required for stability of balance. **C.** With knees flexed and trunk tilted backward, balance is regained. This exerts excessive strain on the antigravity muscles—gluteus maximus, triceps surae, and quadriceps.

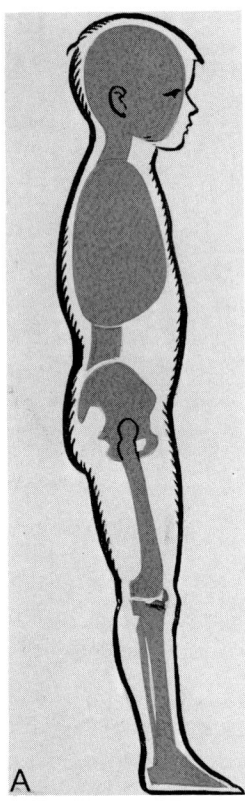
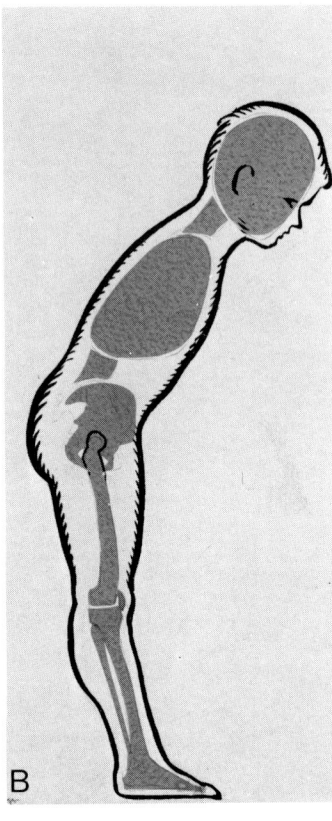

FIGURE 3–4. Compensation for fixed equinus deformity of the ankle by hip flexion.

A. When there are no compensatory accommodations at the hip and knee, the center of gravity of the body is posterior to the feet. **B**. The hips flex to bring it over them.

should be assessed both individually and in relation to adjacent levels.

Hip flexion deformity will affect the posture of the trunk, knees, and ankles. First, to achieve balance, lordosis of the lumbar spine is increased excessively (Fig. 3–3A). If the hip flexion deformity exceeds the degree that can be accommodated by lumbar lordosis, the trunk leans forward; this posture, with the knees in extension, requires support by crutches to achieve balance (Fig. 3–3B). The knees flex to restore balance and their flexed posture exerts more than normal strain on the antigravity muscles, demanding strong action on the part of the gluteus maximus, triceps surae, and quadriceps femoris (Fig. 3–3C).

When the ankles are fixed in equinus position and there are no compensatory accommodations at the hip and knee, the center of gravity of the trunk is posterior to the base of support (Fig. 3–4A). It is brought over the feet by flexion of the hips (Fig. 3–4B). Therefore, one method of compensating for fixed equinus deformity is by hip flexion. Another is by hyperextension of the knees (Fig. 3–5). In calcaneus deformity of the feet (e.g., due to overlengthening of the triceps surae), the center of body weight falls posterior to the ankle axis; this is compensated for by bringing the body weight forward by excessive knee flexion and reducing body height, the tibia tilts forward because control by the triceps surae is lacking, and as a result the posture in both stance and gait is unstable (Fig. 3–6).

Reference

1. Perry, J.: Kinesiology of lower extremity bracing. Clin. Orthop., *102*:18, 1974.

CEREBRAL PALSY

The common deformities of the foot and ankle in cerebral palsy are: talipes equinus, equinovarus, equinovalgus, calcaneus, calcaneovalgus, and calcaneovarus. Deformities of the forefoot and toes are less frequent and are of relatively minor importance. They include metatarsus varus, hallux varus, hallux valgus, and flexion deformity of the toes—mallet or hammer toes.

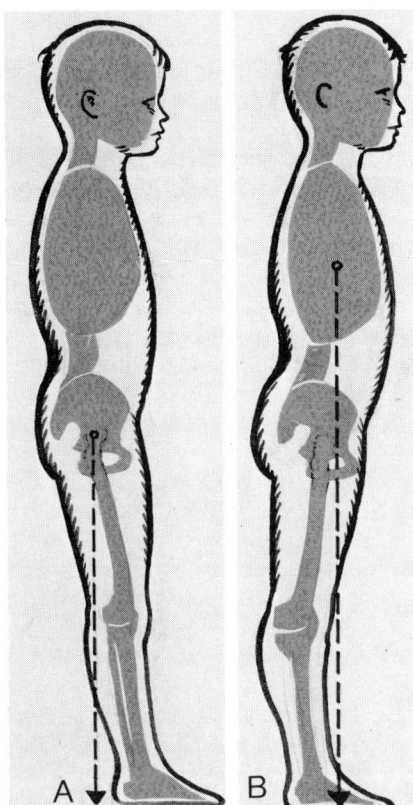

FIGURE 3–5. *Hyperextension of the knees to compensate for fixed equinus deformity of the ankle.*

A. When the equinus deformity of the ankle is fixed and there is no compensatory accommodation at the hip and knee, the center of gravity is posterior to the base of support. **B.** One method of aligning the trunk and bringing the center of gravity over the feet is by knee hyperextension. Note the hips are in neutral position or slightly hyperextended.

General Principles of Treatment and Preoperative Assessment

Prior to beginning treatment of a child with cerebral palsy and deformities of the lower limb, several vital questions have to be answered (Fig. 3–7). First, and most important, is the *diagnosis* correct? What is cerebral palsy? It is not a single disease entity but, rather, a convenient category of conditions having certain common characteristics. The generally accepted criteria of the symptom complex of cerebral palsy are:

1. It must be due to a fixed, nonprogressive brain lesion or lesions. No active disease should exist at the time of diagnosis. Thus, transient disorders or those that are the result of a progressive disease of the brain or spinal cord are excluded.

2. The original lesion must occur prenatally, at birth, or early in the postnatal period. The exact limits of this early period are not agreed upon, and it is best to avoid arbitrary age limits. The interference with the developing central nervous system by the early fixed lesion is the significant pathologic feature.

3. In certain children, the primary disorder involves the musculoskeletal system, and lack of motor control is the greater handicap; in others mental retardation, convulsions, sensory disturbance, speech impediments, or defects of hearing, language,

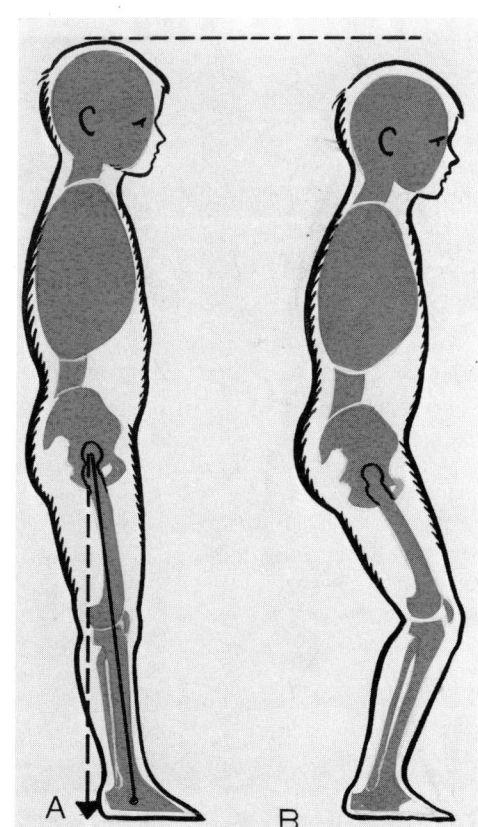

FIGURE 3–6. *The effect of calcaneus deformity of the ankle on posture of the hip and knee.*

A. In pes calcaneus (due, for example, to overlengthening of the triceps surae) the center of body weight falls behind the ankle axis. **B.** To compensate, body weight is brought anterior to the ankle axis by greater knee flexion, height is lost, and the tibia falls forward because of lack of control by the weak triceps surae. The posture in both stance and gait is unstable.

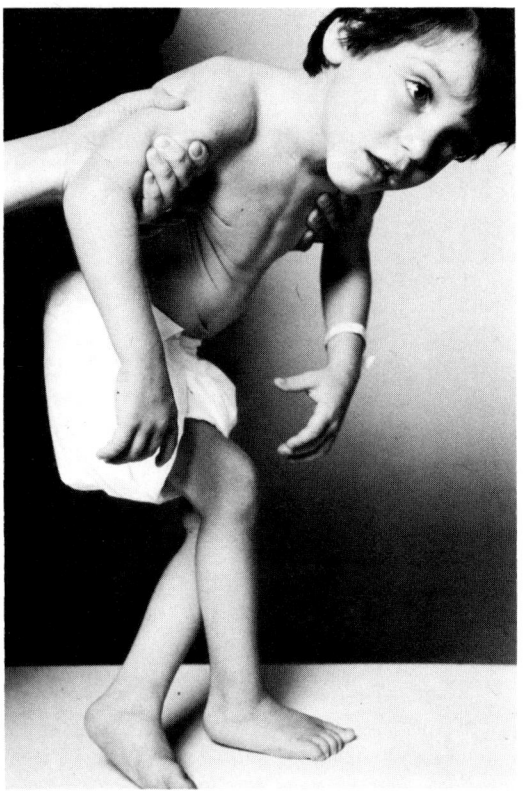

FIGURE 3–7. A child with cerebral palsy.

or eyesight may be the more important difficulty.[103]

The term *cerebral palsy* has certain administrative usefulness. The foregoing criteria of this category of disease should, however, be carefully examined. It is imperative that a neurologic consultation be obtained prior to orthopedic treatment. It is not uncommon for conditions such as neoplasms of the central nervous system, metabolic diseases such as Lesch-Nyhan syndrome, progressive hereditary paraplegia, Friedreich's ataxia, and amaurotic familial idiocy to be diagnosed erroneously as cerebral palsy.[80]

The type of cerebral palsy must be determined next. Is it pyramidal-spastic, extrapyramidal-athetoid, mixed, ataxic, rigid, or tremor? It is beyond the scope of this book to discuss the various classifications of cerebral palsy. These and the natural history and diagnosis of the disease, and assessment and principles of management of the child with cerebral palsy are discussed in the cited references.*

---

*See references 9, 10, 31, 40, 43, 44, 52, 72, 76–79, 93, 94, 103, 107, 108, 111, 117, 131, 157, 163, 164.

Operative measures are most useful in the spastic type. In the other forms of cerebral palsy—athetoid, rigid, ataxic, or tremor—soft-tissue operations on the limbs are seldom indicated. Surgery in the extrapyramidal type of cerebral palsy is limited to bony procedures such as osteotomy or fusion of joints to correct structural fixed deformities.

What is the *distribution of paralysis?* Is there monoplegia (one limb involved), hemiplegia (two limbs on same side affected), quadriplegia (all four limbs), or double hemiplegia (the arms more severely affected than the legs or the involvement asymmetrical)?

It is essential to assess carefully the symmetry of affection between two limbs. The difference between them may be slight and subtle, or marked and extreme. Completely symmetrical affection is rare; more often the involvement is asymmetrical, and the diagnosis should be double hemiplegia rather than quadriplegia or paraplegia. Recognize the asymmetry of paralysis and plan the type and extent of surgery accordingly.

Next the *neurophysiologic maturation and motor level of development* are determined.[55] There is great variation in the severity, extent of involvement, and prognosis in cerebral palsy. Are there any persistent neonatal or abnormal reflex patterns? The asymmetrical tonic neck reflex and the Moro and grasp reflexes normally disappear between four and six months of age; their presence in a two- or three-year-old child is a relative contraindication for surgery on the foot and ankle (Fig. 3–8). The protective extension of arms reflex is tested (Fig. 3–9); it should be present preoperatively. Does she have symmetrical tonic neck reflex (Fig. 3–10)? Sitting and standing balance is assessed (Fig. 3–11). Tilting reactions—in standing position preferably—should be present (Fig. 3–12). Does he crawl? Is there reciprocal motion between his upper and lower limbs? What degree of control and function does he have in his upper limbs?

In retarded children, one should note the rate of maturation of neurophysiologic and motor systems. What is his potential for further improvement with growth and development? Are his deformities interfering with his already precarious balance and hindering his stance and locomotion? It must be remembered that the nursing and perineal care of a retarded child may be

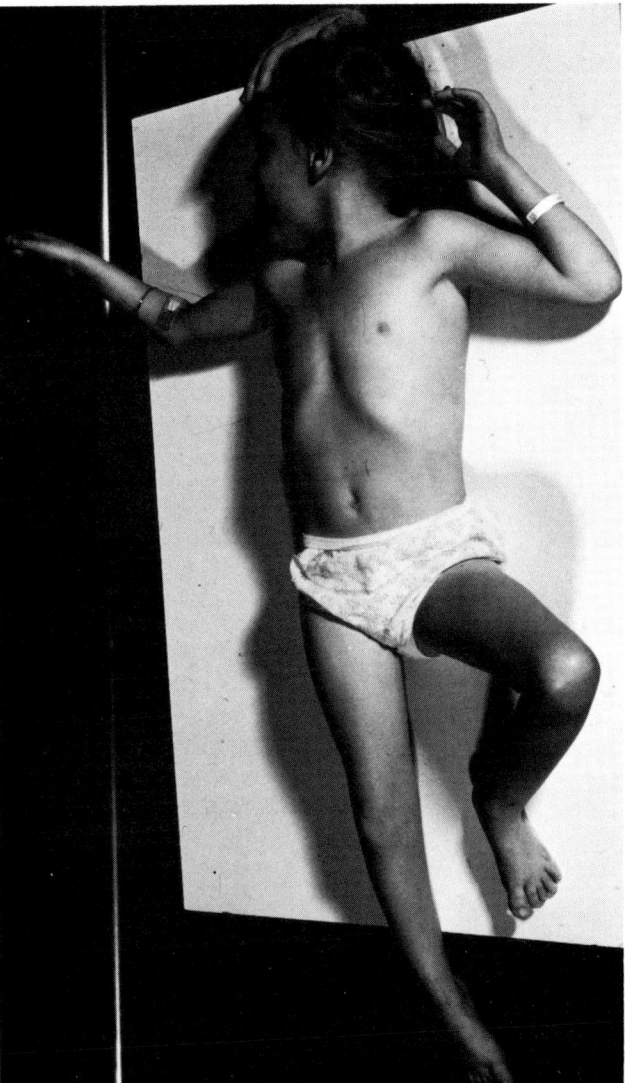

FIGURE 3–8. Asymmetrical tonic reflex in a child.

Note on the chin side, the elbow and knee are extended, whereas on the occiput side, the elbow and knee are flexed.

greatly simplified by a simple adductor myotomy of the hips. Prior to attainment of the desired level of motor and neurophysiologic maturation, surgical procedures are performed to prevent deformities, primarily hip dislocation; prevention of hip dislocation is, in fact, the principal indication for surgery before evidence of sitting balance has developed. Even though these children will never be able to walk, they will be much more comfortable, and their nursing care will be much less difficult than if their hips were dislocated. However, to perform a Grice extra-articular arthrodesis of the subtalar joint or a heel cord lengthening in a child who has no independent sitting balance and no potential for locomotion displays total lack of understanding of basic principles of management of cerebral palsy.

The whole child should be examined. Cerebral palsy is a multidisciplinary problem involving pediatrics, neurology, orthopedic surgery, physical therapy, occupational therapy, psychology, speech therapy, audiology, sociology, and vocational counseling. The care of a child with cerebral palsy extends over many years. In the course of this multidisciplinary treatment, the patient must be evaluated as an individual, as a member of the family, and as a future member of the community.

The problem is a dynamic one, changing

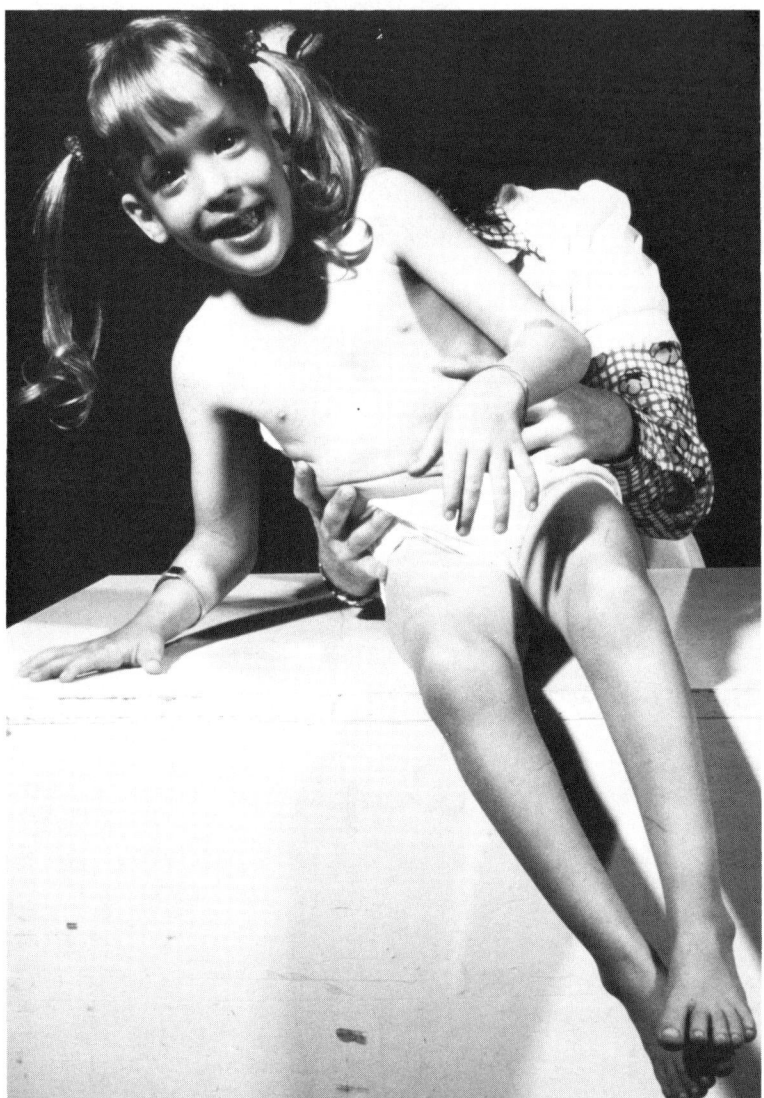

FIGURE 3–9. Protective extension of arms reflex.
The reflex is present on sitting.

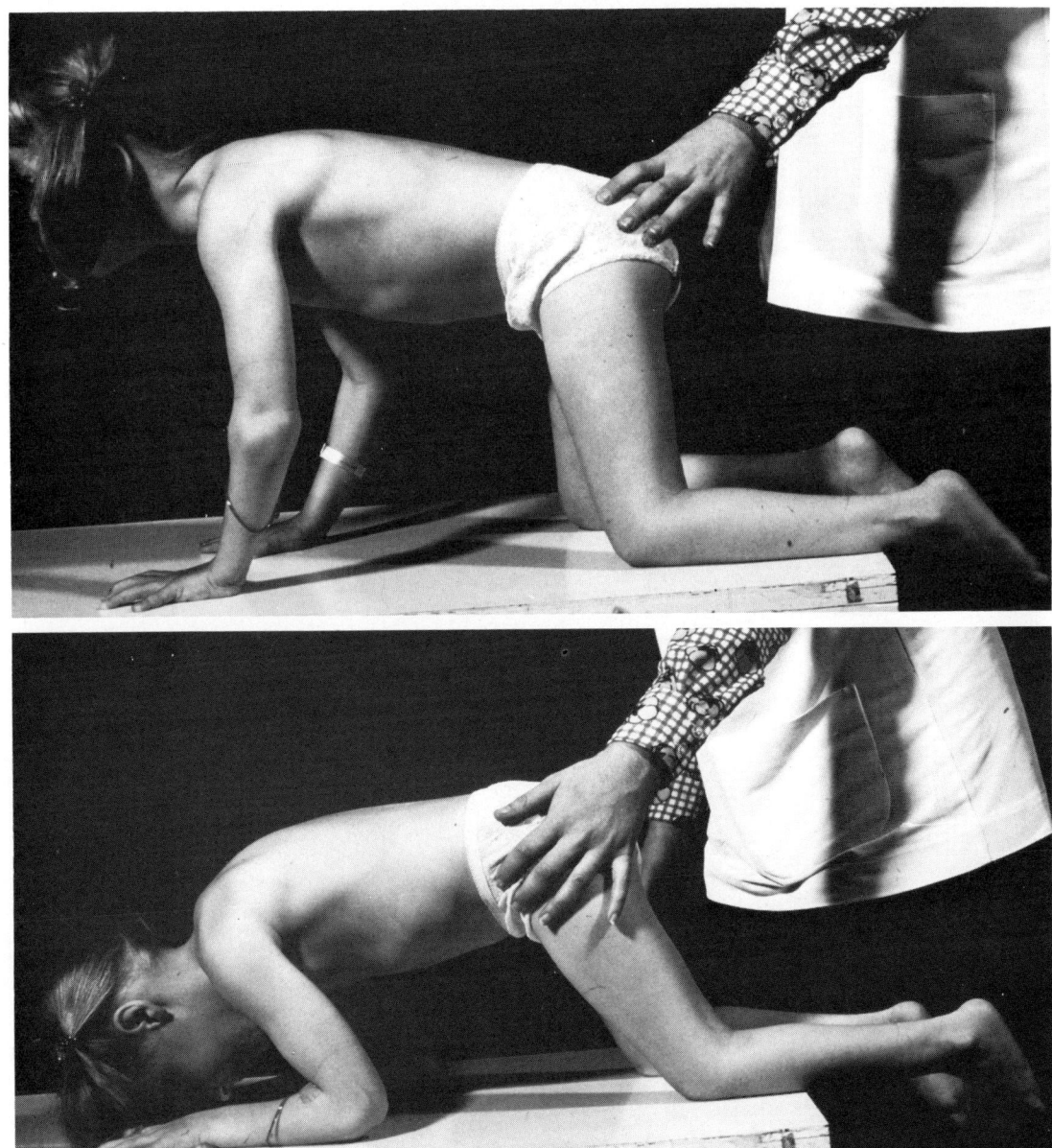

FIGURE 3–10. Symmetrical tonic neck reflex.

Note that on extension of the neck, the elbows are extended, whereas on flexion of the neck, the elbows are flexed.

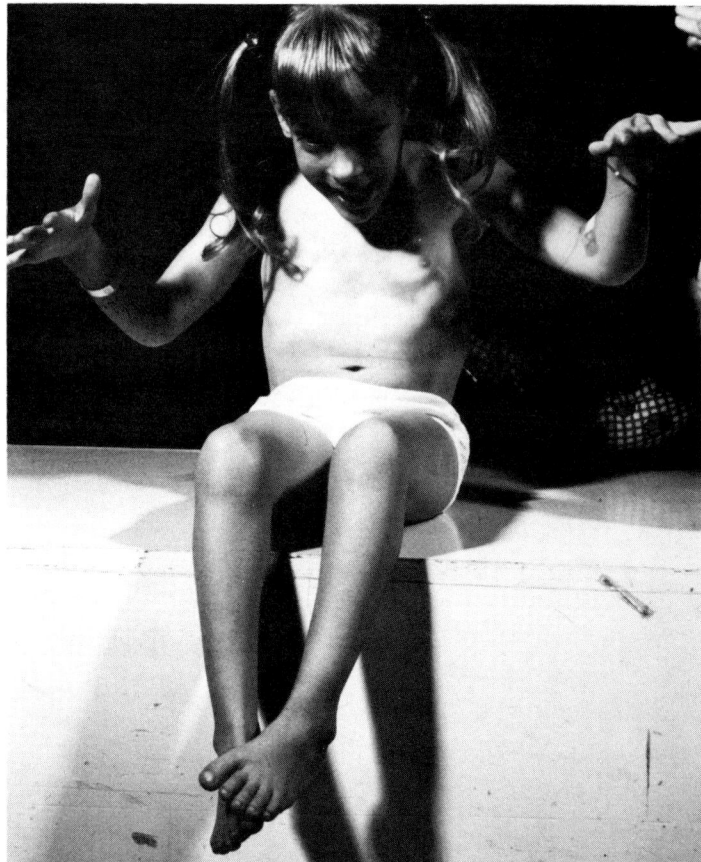

FIGURE 3–11. *Sitting balance is precarious in this child with cerebral palsy.*

FIGURE 3–12. *This child has no head tilting response.*

Note that the head does not come to the midline.

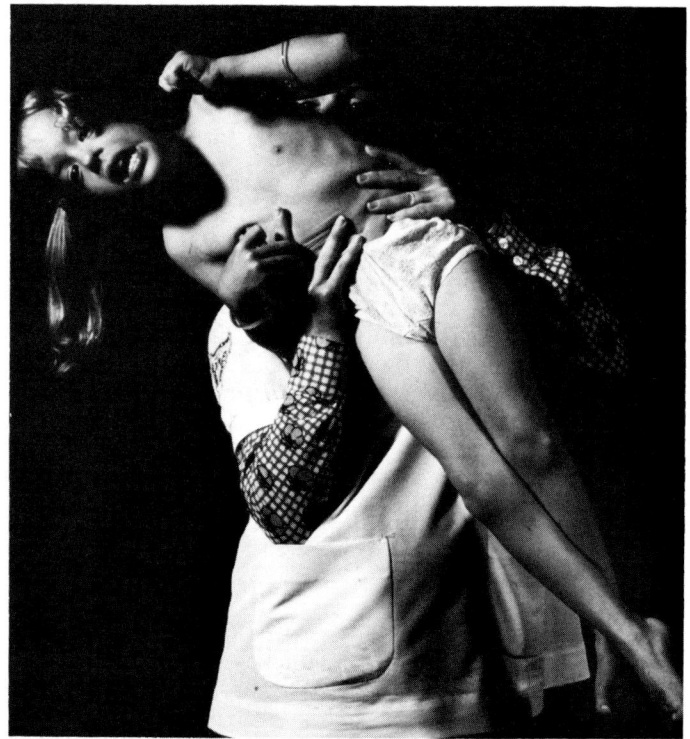

with the growth, development, and maturation of the central nervous system. As the child grows, he acquires higher levels of performance and greater skills. The objective of surgery in cerebral palsy is to improve motor function. The parents should realize that the motor handicap can be substantially improved by surgery, but that, unless other involvement is minimal, the child will never be completely normal. A child with cerebral palsy should be treated in a medical center where a team of physicians is available to provide total multidisciplinary care.

It is imperative to employ conservative measures and follow the patient for a period. Is there a changing pattern of paralysis?

Is *adequate and meticulous postoperative care* feasible? Several factors influence this, namely:

The patient's age: he should be old enough to cooperate in the postoperative period to obtain the maximum benefit from the surgery. Usually this age range is from four to six years.

The child's level of intelligence: in order to be able to cooperate with his physical therapist during the postoperative training period, he should possess a reasonable mentality. Will he be trainable after his operation? What is his span of attention? The motivational factor often determines the difference between success and failure.

Is the *home and family situation* adequate and conducive to good follow-up care? Are the parents sufficiently intelligent? How interested are they in the child? How faithfully have they kept their appointments? What has been their past performance with conservative management? In the preoperative period it is imperative to indoctrinate the patient and his family concerning exercises and night support. They should be well prepared for an aggressive postoperative training program.

The children who come for surgery on their lower limbs have had physical therapy. Details and effectiveness of previous conservative management should be determined. The physiotherapeutic methods are numerous, and their specific values are difficult to assess. Individual proponents claim their own methods are the best. In 1940, Phelps set forward the basis of conservative management of the child with brain damage. He stressed the importance of determining the type of cerebral palsy and the child's functional handicap and motor performance. The principles of Phelps's method of treatment are to strengthen hypotonic muscles, to weaken spastic muscles, to splint parts to prevent contracture, and to develop physiologic patterns of motion that proceed from individual active motions to general limb movements to balance and coordinated activity. Parents are instructed in exercises to be performed at home under periodic close supervision by the therapist. The aim of passive exercises is to maintain full range of motion and prevent myostatic contracture; they must, however, be carried out gently and should not elicit stretch reflex.[117, 118]

There are a number of schools of physical therapy that are concerned with the development of posture and reflex activity.* The most popular ones are those of Fay, Rood, and Bobath.

The problem of cerebral palsy is a dynamic one that changes with growth and development and maturation of the central nervous system. It is, therefore, difficult to assess the individual merits of all these time-consuming therapy programs.

Next, in the preoperative assessment one should study the orthotic devices worn by the child. Braces have definite disadvantages.[142] They are cumbersome and heavy, cause muscle weakness, and inhibit development of normal patterns of motion. Reciprocal hip-knee flexion and ankle dorsiflexion are essential for a normal gait pattern. A common but poor practice is to prescribe a dorsiflexion-assist ankle-foot orthosis for a child with toe-toe or toe-heel gait. The result will be to exaggerate the stretch reflex of the triceps surae muscle, cause rocker-bottom deformity of the foot, and do more harm than good. Orthoses are to be used in specific circumstances—for example, in quadriceps femoris weakness—to support the knee, to develop function in hypotonic cerebral zero anterior tibial muscles, or to control involuntary movements in athetosis.

In the past, it has been emphasized that

---

*See references 23–26, 43, 54, 59, 78, 81, 124, 126, 149.

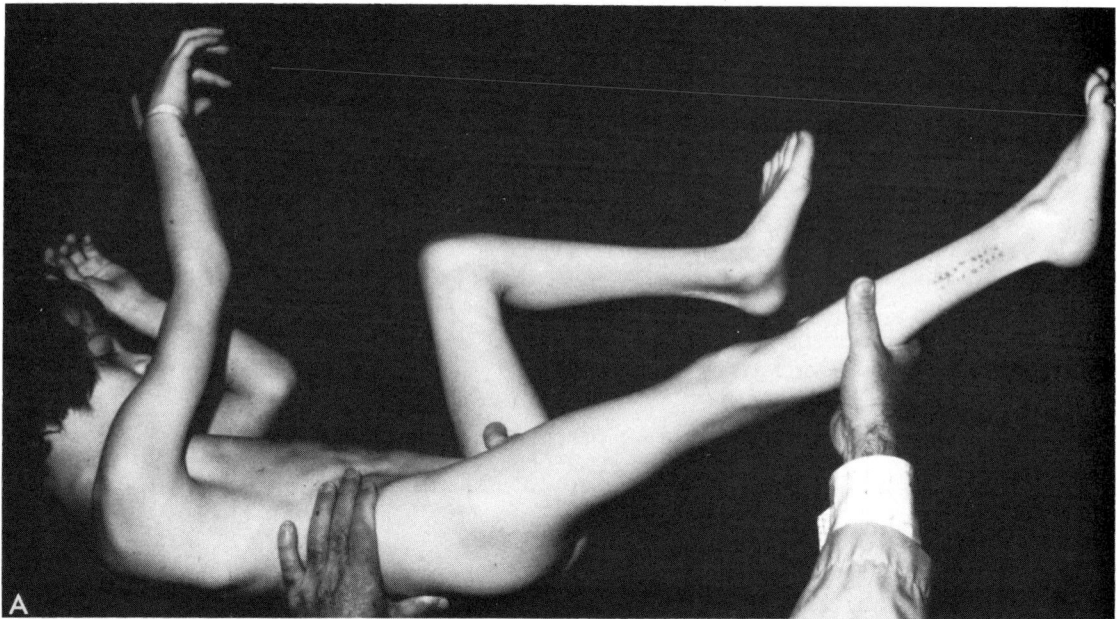

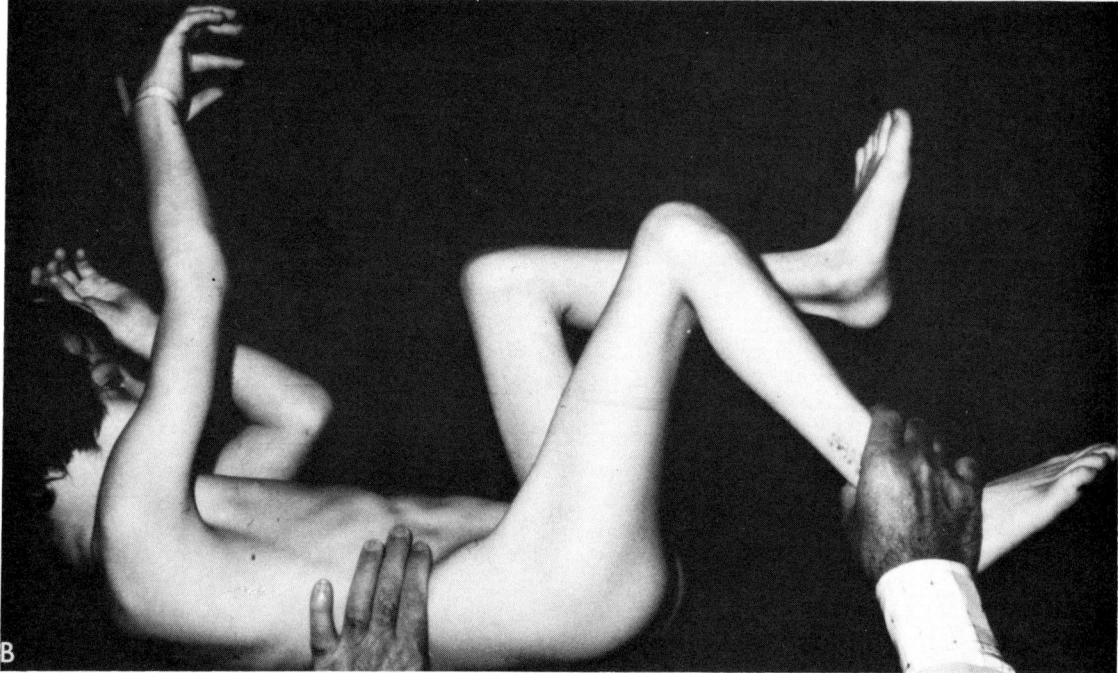

FIGURE 3–13. Side-lying Thomas test to demonstrate flexion deformity of the hip in spastic cerebral palsy.

The underlying hip is acutely flexed to obliterate lumbar lordosis. **A.** The upper hip is passively extended with the knee in full extension. **B.** Then the hip is extended with the knee in acute flexion (see text).

soft-tissue procedures should not be performed during the growth period because the deformities will recur. The results of Green and Banks and their associates have shown, however, that if the patients receive adequate postoperative care that includes a well-supervised program of exercises and night splinting, the recurrence of deformities can be prevented or markedly reduced.[7-11, 61] Unless a surgeon is willing to supervise minute details of postoperative care, he should never operate on these children. The importance of thorough preoperative assessment and detailed, meticulous postoperative care cannot be overemphasized.

The deformities of the foot and ankle are studied in relation to the lower limb and trunk as a whole. In the ambulatory patient, first the posture in stance and then the gait are analyzed. Next, the nature and the severity of deformities are determined. In cerebral palsy a deformity may be *fixed* owing to myostatic contracture, or *functional* owing to exaggerated stretch reflex with no permanent shortening of muscles; or it may be *secondary*, to compensate for a deformity at an adjacent level. The hip is examined first. Is there a flexion contracture of the hip? This is best demonstrated by the sidelying Thomas test. The underlying hip is acutely flexed on the abdomen to obliterate lumbar lordosis. Flexion deformity of the hip is primarily caused by spasticity and contracture of the iliopsoas and rectus femoris muscles. To distinguish between the two forces, the Thomas test is performed with the knee first in extension and then in flexion (Fig. 3–13). When the rectus femoris is the cause, hip flexion deformity is increased with the knee in flexion and decreased with the knee in extension; whereas when it is due to the iliopsoas muscle, the position of the knee has no effect on the degree of hip flexion contracture. Palpation for tautness of the muscle fibers of the pelvic origin of the rectus femoris muscle is also of some assistance. Often it is the iliopsoas muscle that is the principal deforming force causing hip flexion deformity. The Ely test will demonstrate spasticity and contracture of the pelvic origin of the rectus femoris muscle (Fig. 3–14). It is imperative to correct flexion deformity of the hip joint prior to heel cord lengthening.

In stance and gait a flexed attitude of the hip may be secondary to flexion deformity of the knee or equinus deformity of the ankle; also, when balance is poor, the spastic child will flex his knees and hips to lower his center of gravity and will press the knees together to support them. *Jump position* is a term referring to the posture of a spastic child who stands with his knees flexed and the ankles in equinus position (Fig. 3–15).

One of two roentgenographic methods may be used for accurate determination of the degree of hip flexion deformity in stance. In the Milch method, a line is drawn from the ischial tuberosity to the anterior superior iliac spine, and a second line is drawn parallel to the axis of the femoral shaft. The angle formed by the intersection of these two lines is the pelvifemoral angle, which normally measures 55 degrees. In the Fick method, the sacrofemoral angle is formed between lines drawn across the superior surface of the first sacral vertebra

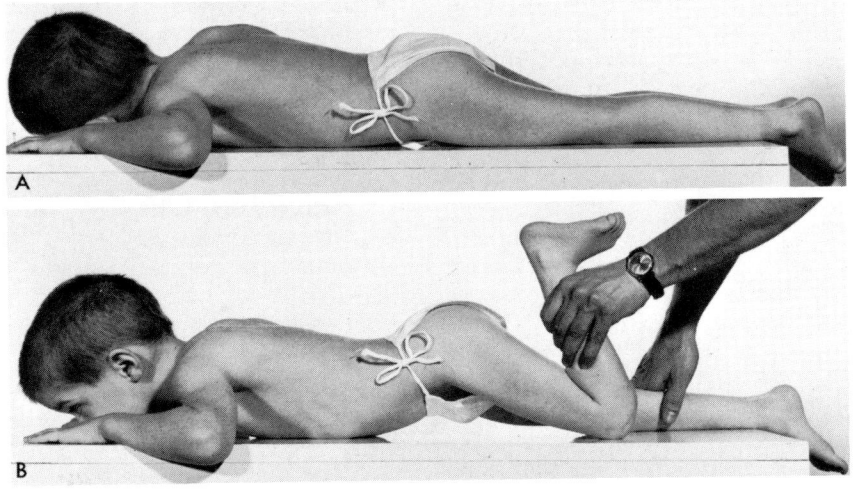

FIGURE 3–14. Positive Ely test.

A. The child is placed in prone position with the knees and hips in extension. **B.** On passive flexion of the knee the pelvis will rise off the table. The examiner records the degree of knee flexion when the pelvis begins to rise and the height of elevation of the pelvis on maximal flexion of the knee.

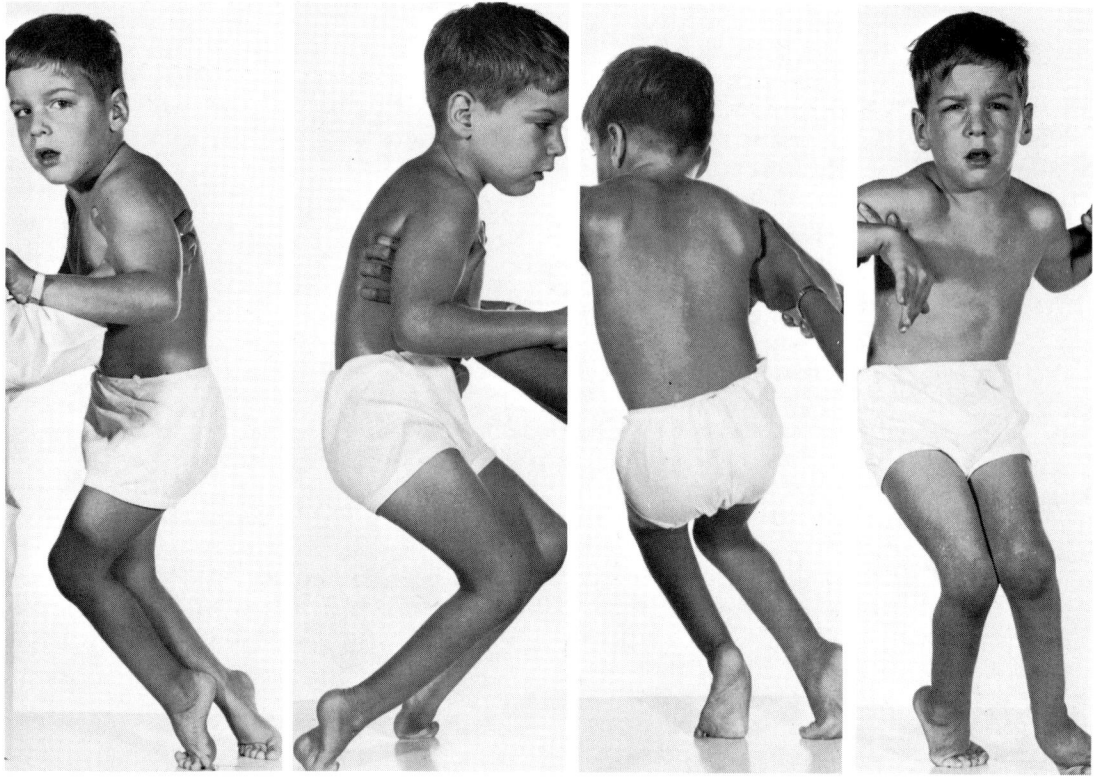

FIGURE 3–15. A five-year-old boy with spastic paraplegia with poor balance and trunk posture.

The equinus deformity of the ankles is compensatory to the hip and knee flexion contracture.

and along the axis of the femoral shaft. Normally, the sacrofemoral angle diminishes with age.[22] These roentgenographic methods of mensuration of hip flexion deformity are ordinarily impractical for routine use, as the spastic child has poor balance and often requires the support of crutches or parallel bars for standing and walking. Inspection of the standing posture of the patient and the Thomas test are of more clinical value.

Adduction deformity of the hip is caused by spasticity and contracture of the hip adductors (adductor longus, adductor brevis, adductor magnus, and pectineus), the gracilis, and the medial hamstrings (semitendinosus and semimembranosus muscles). It is important to distinguish between limitation of hip abduction caused by overaction and pull of the hip adductors and that caused by the gracilis and medial hamstrings. The two deforming components are differentiated by passive hip abduction performed with the knees in 90 degrees of flexion, which relaxes the gracilis and medial hamstring muscles (Fig. 3–16). Any asymmetry of involvement between the right and left sides should be carefully noted at this time. The hips are also examined for medial and lateral rotation deformity, femoral antetorsion, and subluxation or dislocation of the hip. Roentgenograms of the hips should be made.

The position of the knee in relation to the ankle and foot, and its effect on them, is assessed next. The knee joint should not be regarded as an isolated problem in cerebral palsy, since it is affected by deformities of the hip or ankle. The mechanism of the knee joint is complex because of the pressure of "two-joint" muscles, i.e., the hamstrings, which extend the hip and flex the knee; the gastrocnemius, which plantarflexes the ankle and flexes the knee; and the quadriceps (direct head of rectus femoris), which extends the knee and flexes the hip. Is the knee flexed, neutral, or hyperextended? A flexion deformity of the knee

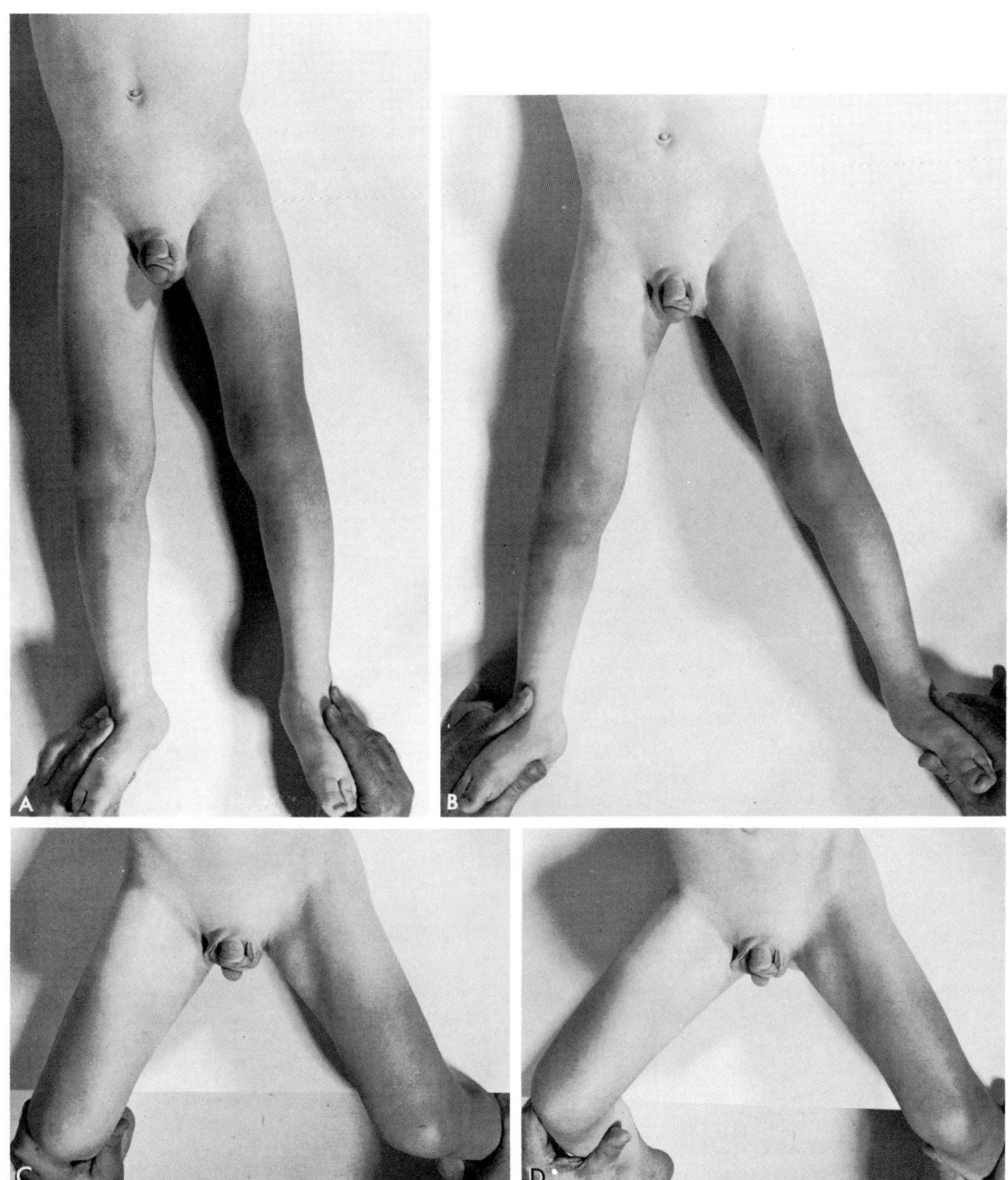

FIGURE 3–16. Determination of range of hip abduction.

The hips are in extension. **A** and **B**. The knees in extension. **C** and **D**. The knees in 90 degrees of flexion. Flexion of the knee will relax the gracilis and medial hamstring muscles, making it possible to differentiate between limitation of hip abduction due to spasticity and contracture of hip adductors and that due to the gracilis and medial hamstrings. **A** and **C** show the range of motion when the spastic muscle grabs; **B** and **D** demonstrate the maximal range of passive hip abduction.

Table 3–2. Physiologic Status Variations in Motor Strength of Muscles in Cerebral Palsy

Physiological Status	Motor Strength
Innervation normal *(IN)*	P to N
Spastic *(S)*	P to N
Hypotonic *(H)*	O to G
Cerebral zero *(OC)*	O to G

is a relative contraindication to heel cord lengthening because, postoperatively, calcaneus deformity may develop. Genu recurvatum may be caused by equinus deformity of the ankle.[139]

Muscle strength and physiologic innervation of muscles are determined next. Testing of motor power is difficult in spasticity, but it is important and an attempt should be made. It is best that muscle testing be performed by a physical therapist; the results should be recorded in the chart. Both the motor power and the physiologic status of the muscles should be designated. Motor power is graded by the standard accepted by the National Foundation for Infantile Paralysis, and the same abbreviations are used: zero, 0; trace, T; poor, P; fair, F; good, G; and normal, N. For phsyiologic status, the author uses the following notations and abbreviations: S for spastic (stretch reflex); H for hypotonic; 0C for cerebral zero (i.e., the patient has no voluntary control over the muscle); and IN for innervation normal. Table 3–2 shows various possible combinations of physiologic status and motor strength of muscles in patients with cerebral palsy.

In evaluating the motor strength of a spastic child, the following pitfalls should be borne in mind. Tension athetosis should be distinguished from spasticity. Tension athetosis is produced by the intentional effort of the athetoid patient to prevent any undesired motion of the athetoid limb. By shaking the limb, this voluntary tension can be released. The spastic extremity cannot be shaken loose because the exaggerated stretch reflex of a spastic muscle is involuntary and will occur whenever the muscle is suddenly passively elongated. It is also essential to differentiate between the voluntary resistance of a normal muscle and the exaggerated stretch reflex of a spastic muscle.

In spasticity, the deep tendon reflexes are exaggerated, and pathologic reflexes such as the Babinski and Hoffmann signs are present. Sudden dorsiflexion of the ankle or rapid distal movement of the patella may elicit clonus—alternate spasm and relaxation of the agonist and antagonist muscles.

Spastic paralysis has a certain predilection for specific groups of muscles, but there are variations that depend upon the disease syndrome. In congenital spastic paralysis, for example, the spasticity is more marked in the flexor muscles of the upper limb. The shoulder is adducted, flexed, and medially rotated; the elbow is flexed; the wrist and fingers are flexed; and the thumb is adducted in the palm. In the lower limb, the hip is adducted, flexed, and medially rotated; the knee is flexed; and the ankle is held in plantar flexion. In acquired spastic cerebral palsy, in the upper limb, the deltoid muscle may be spastic and hold the shoulder in abduction; and in the foot and ankle, the anterior tibial muscle may be spastic.

There may be specific deformities of the foot and ankle, each requiring specific treatment.

Talipes Equinus

The most common deformity of the foot and ankle in spastic cerebral palsy is talipes equinus. The triceps surae muscle comprises the gastrocnemius, a three-joint muscle (knee, ankle, and subtalar), and the soleus, a two-joint muscle (ankle and subtalar). The coordinated, harmonious action of the triceps surae with its principal antagonist, the anterior tibial, is necessary to have a normal heel-toe gait with adequate push-off. In the majority of children with spastic cerebral palsy, this normal gait pattern is lost because of equinus deformity.

Equinus deformity may be caused by contracture of both the soleus and gastrocnemius muscles or of the gastrocnemius alone. These two types of involvement may be differentiated from each other by passively dorsiflexing the ankle joint, first with the knee flexed and then with it extended (Silfverskiöld test).[136] The gastrocnemius portion of the triceps surae originates from the femoral condyles, and when the knee is passively flexed, it is, therefore, relaxed and equinus deformity that is chiefly due to contracture of the gastrocnemius disap-

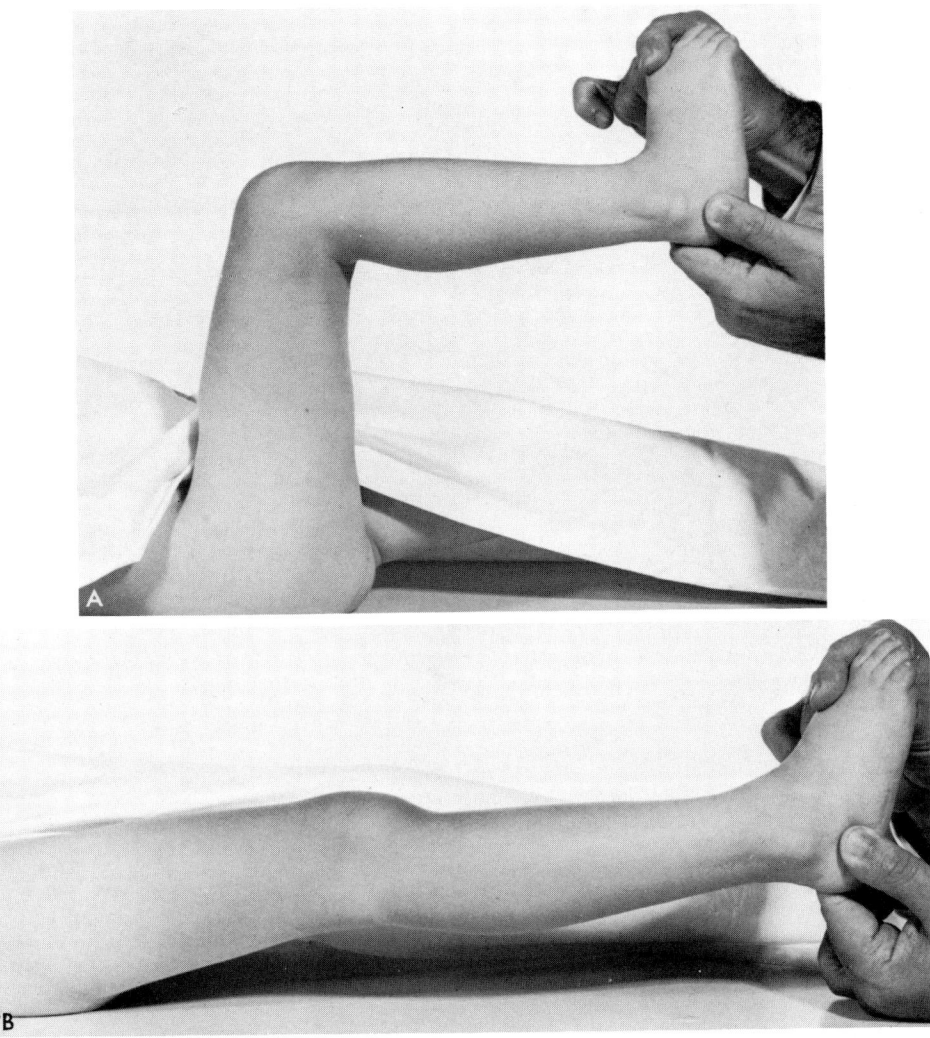

FIGURE 3–17. Testing spasticity and contracture of the triceps surae muscle by passive dorsiflexion of the ankle.

A. With the knee in flexion, the gastrocnemius muscle is relaxed and equinus deformity is caused by contracture of the soleus muscle. **B.** The part played by the gastrocnemius is tested with the knee in extension.

pears. The part played by the gastrocnemius is revealed with the knee extended (Fig. 3–17). Care should be taken to apply the dorsiflexion force to the hindfoot and not to the forefoot, as the latter maneuver brings the peroneal, tibialis posterior, and toe flexor muscles into play (Fig. 3–18). Contracture of the gastrocnemius is the primary cause of equinus deformity in spastic cerebral palsy. Electromyographic studies and gait analysis by Perry and associates have demonstrated that the Silfverskiöld test is nonselective.[114] When the ankle is passively dorsiflexed with the knee in flexion, both soleus and gastrocnemius muscles are stimulated; therefore the foregoing method of differentiation between the two types of equinus deformity is applicable only when the deformity is fixed and not functional. The gait pattern may be toe-toe if the child's body weight is insufficient to overcome the exaggerated stretch reflex of the calf muscles, as shown in Figure 3–19; or, depending upon the degree of involvement, the gait may be toe-heel or plantigrade (putting the foot down as a unit). A taut triceps surae muscle may prevent dorsiflexion of the ankle; and the tibia, acting as a lever, will thrust the knee into recurvation when the heel touches the floor.

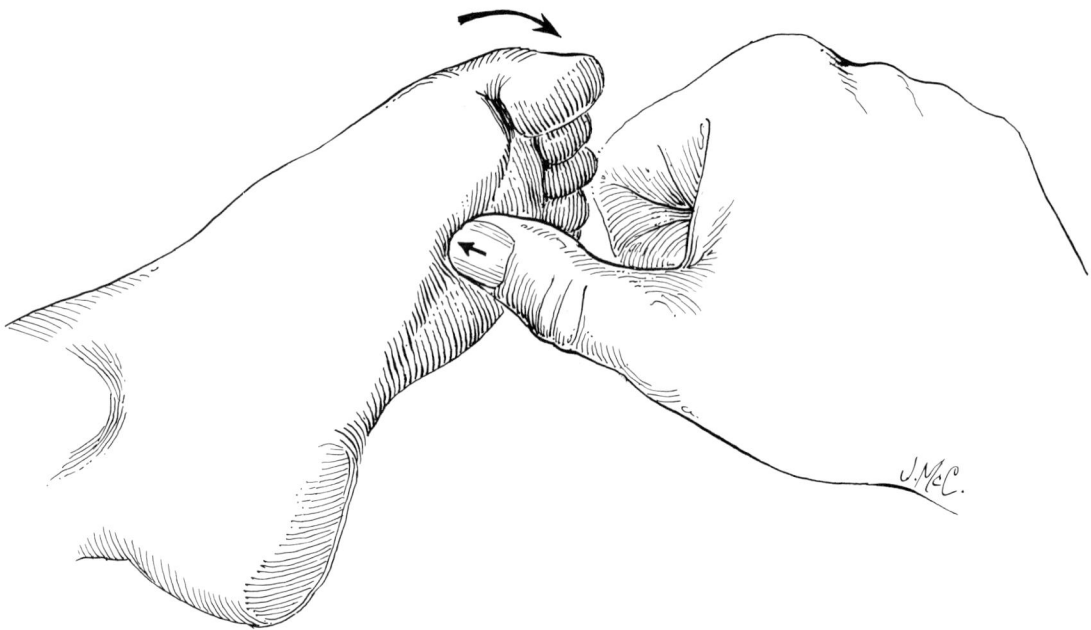

FIGURE 3–18. *Spasticity of the toe flexors is elicited by dorsiflexion of the foot by pressure over the metatarsal head.*

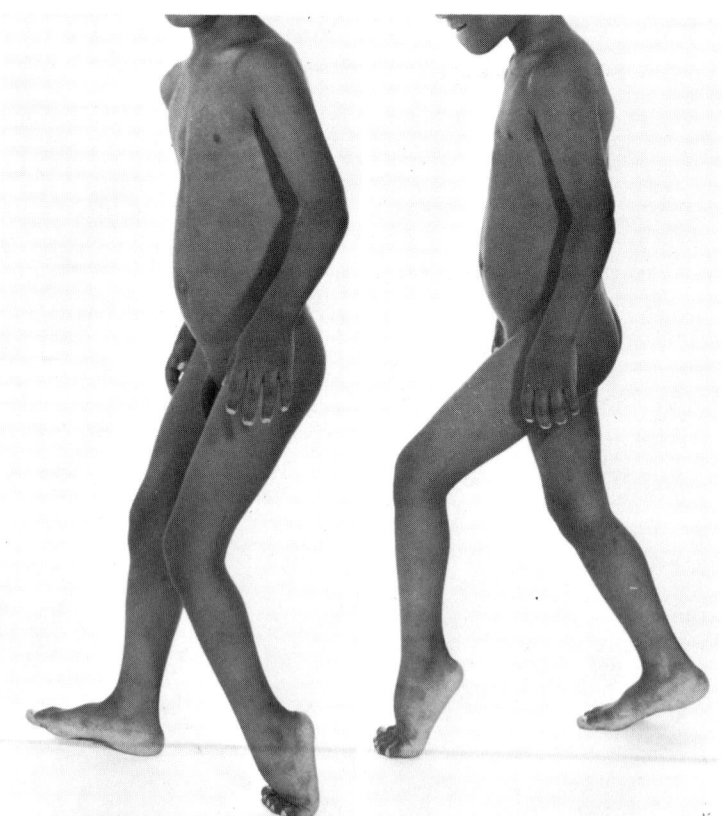

FIGURE 3–19. *Toe-toe gait in spastic hemiplegia.*

More frequently, however, the knee is held in flexion by the spastic hamstrings and a stretched-out, poorly functioning quadriceps muscle. The spastic gastrocnemius muscle plays a lesser role in producing flexion deformity of the knee. On plantar flexion of the foot, when the gastrocnemius is relaxed, any persistent knee flexion deformity is probably caused by the hamstrings.

Simon and co-workers studied the mechanisms producing genu recurvatum in 15 children with spastic cerebral palsy. The patients were aged 4 to 16 years, and all of them had genu recurvatum. The gait patterns were studied by using high-speed motion pictures, electromyography, a dynamic piezoelectric force plate, and computer data analysis. During the stance phase, recurvation began when the tibia stopped moving forward, and disappeared when the tibial movement resumed. There were two distinct patterns of genu recurvatum. In the first group (six patients), excessive activity of the triceps surae in response to the increasing dorsiflexion at the ankle produced by the foot-floor reaction stopped the forward movement of the tibia. In the second group (six patients) the contraction of the triceps surae was not strong enough to stop dorsiflexion of the ankle; the forward motion of the tibia continued until the ankle dorsiflexion was maximal and then it stopped. In both groups genu recurvatum resulted from forward motion of the femur over a stationary tibia. In no case did the activity of hamstrings prevent hyperextension of the knee. Genu recurvatum diminished and stopped as forward motion of the tibia was produced at heel-off (Group I) or as the weight on the limb was suddenly unloaded at opposite heel-strike.[139]

In equinus deformity, when the heel touches the floor, the hindfoot is often forced into valgus position as a result of the bowstring effect of the taut triceps surae on the ankle and subtalar joints. With rigid resistance to dorsiflexion of the foot, the calcaneus rotates underneath the talus and is displaced posterolaterally. Loss of support of the sustentaculum tali beneath the head of the talus causes the talus to drop into a vertical position. Dorsiflexion occurs in the midfoot, and a rocker-bottom deformity results; the calcaneus remains in equinovalgus position. The stress of weight-bearing is on the head of the talus (the midfoot) and not on the heel. This valgus deformity is increased when the peroneal muscles are spastic (Fig. 3–20).

Less often, the foot position is equinovarus, owing to spastic posterior tibial and toe flexor muscles (Fig. 3–21). On weight-bearing or passive dorsiflexion of the ankle, the posterior tibial tendon stands out as a taut band in its groove behind the medial malleolus and the toes may be flexed. In stance,

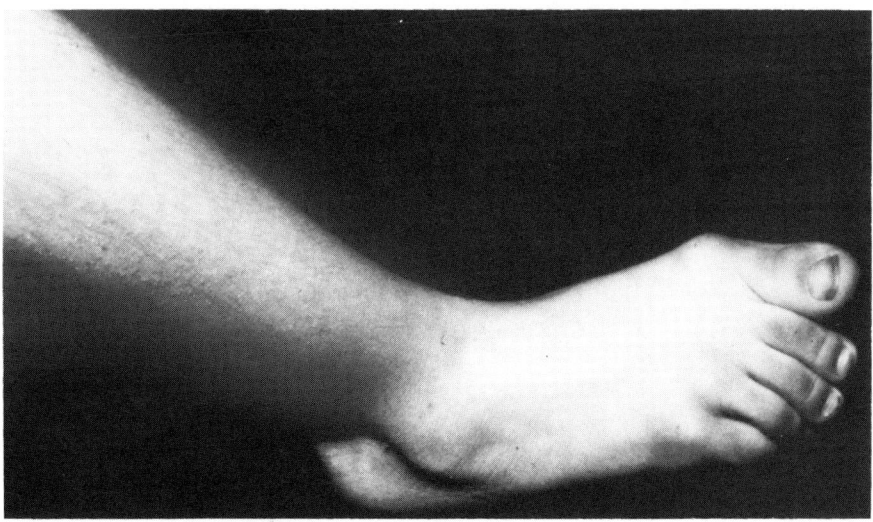

FIGURE 3–20. Pes valgus in cerebral palsy.

Spasticity of peroneal muscles increases the deformity.

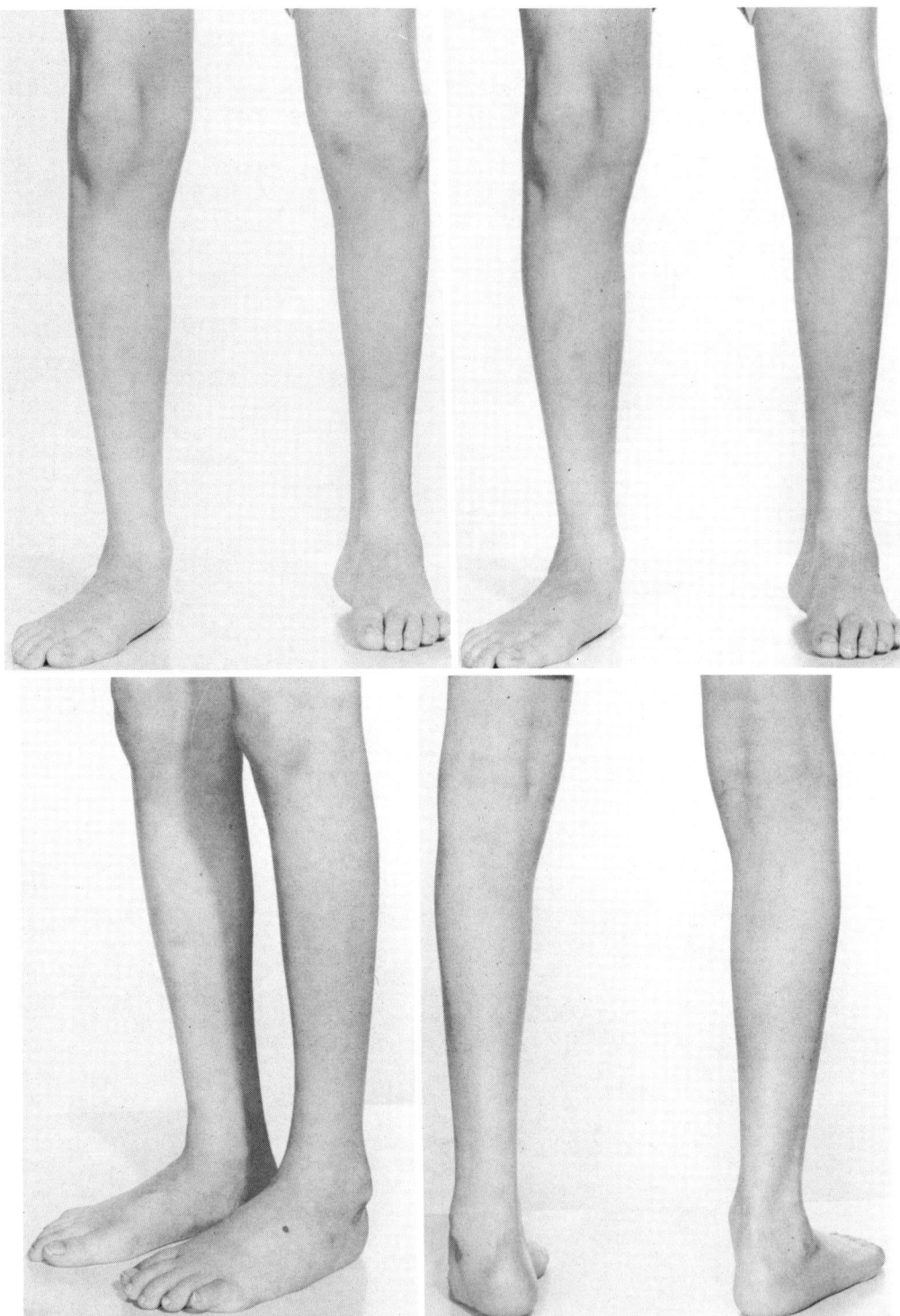

FIGURE 3-21. Spastic hemiplegia with equinovarus deformity of the left foot.
Note the taut posterior tibial tendon behind the medial malleolus.

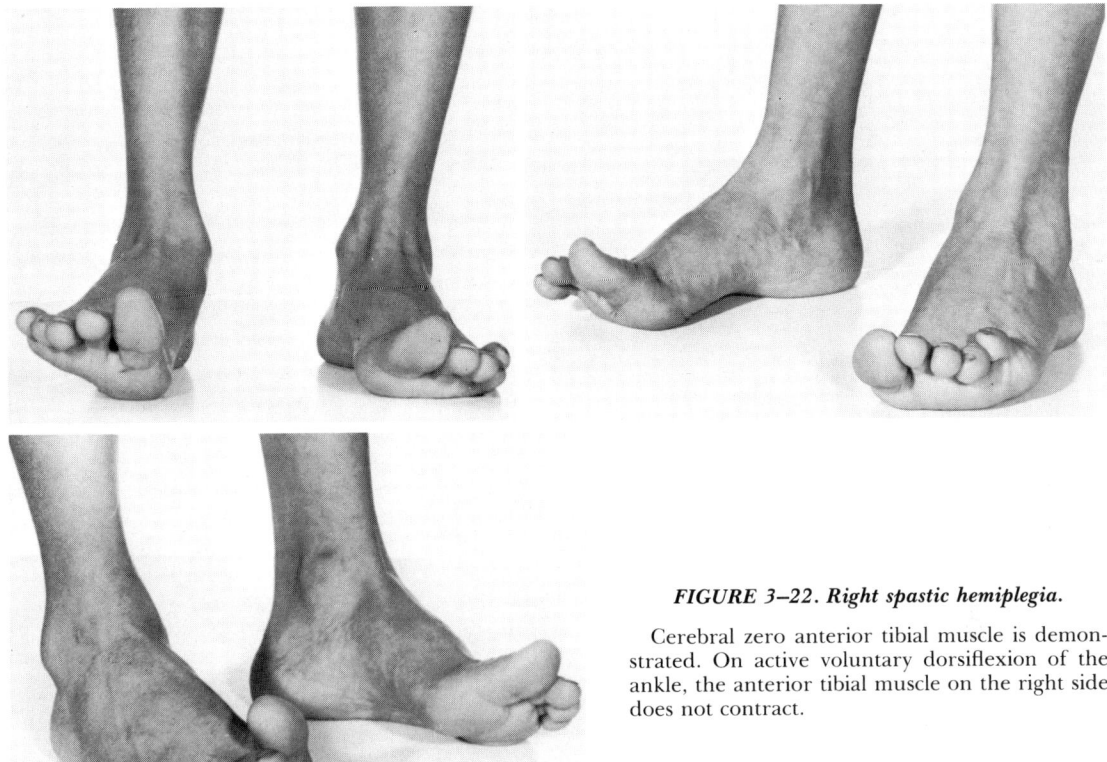

FIGURE 3–22. Right spastic hemiplegia.

Cerebral zero anterior tibial muscle is demonstrated. On active voluntary dorsiflexion of the ankle, the anterior tibial muscle on the right side does not contract.

the varus deformity is usually more marked in the forefoot, and on walking, these children toe in. Functional or fixed medial rotation deformity of the hip or excessive medial tibial torsion, or both, will aggravate the toeing in.

In acquired cerebral palsy, the anterior tibial muscle may be spastic; these children usually have varying degrees of varus deformity of both the hindfoot and the forefoot, and a plantigrade gait.

It is essential to perform a muscle test to evaluate the motor strength of the overactive muscles and their antagonists in order to determine the type and extent of surgery. Often voluntary active contraction of the anterior tibial muscle cannot be elicited with the knee in extension (Fig. 3–22). The child is asked to dorsiflex the ankle with the knee first in extension and then in flexion. The gastrocnemius portion of the triceps surae is relaxed when the knee is flexed. If the anterior tibial does not contract with the knee flexed, the child is asked to flex the hip and knee against resistance. This maneuver (called synkinesia, "confusion" or automatic reflex, or Strumpell test) will cause the anterior tibial muscle to contract, bringing the ankle and foot into dorsiflexion. In order to prevent recurrence of equinus deformity, it is essential to develop active voluntary function of the anterior tibial muscle in gait in the postoperative period.

The effect of hip and knee flexion contracture on equinus deformity of the foot should be assessed (Fig. 3–23).

CONSERVATIVE MANAGEMENT

Initially, all children should have a trial period of nonoperative treatment. The surgeon should condition the patient and his family for future care and indoctrinate them concerning exercises and night support.

Exercises. These consist of active facilitation and passive manual but gentle range of motion exercises of the ankle with the knee in extension to elongate the triceps

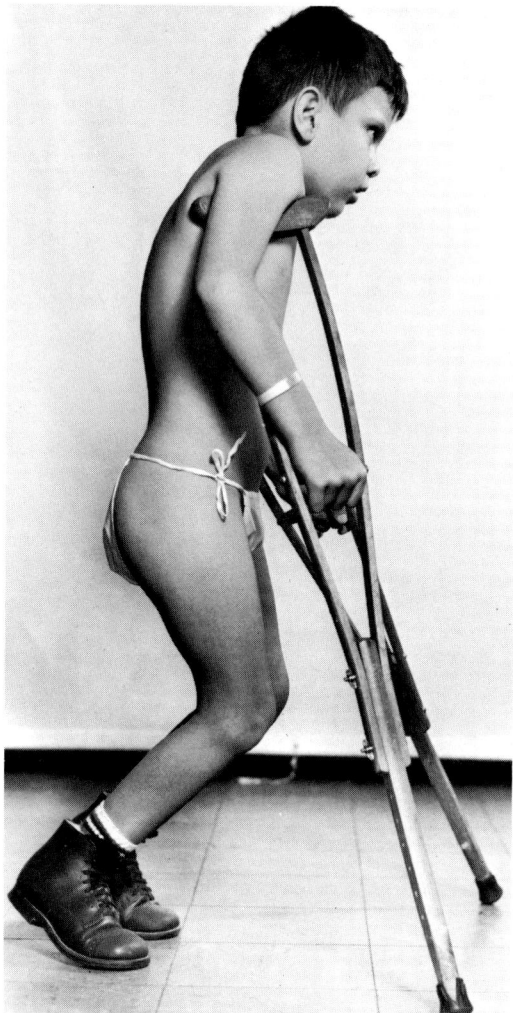

FIGURE 3–23. Equinus posture of the ankles secondary to flexion contracture of the hips and knees.

hip flexors, it is imperative that passive exercises be used and that the child sleep prone with the hips extended. During the day, part-time play activities in prone posture are also encouraged. In the presence of knee flexion deformity, hamstrings also are elongated. The parents are instructed in exercises that are to be performed at home for half an hour per day. The exercises should be pleasant for the child, and not a military drill command performance.

Night splints that hold the foot and ankle in neutral position are used to control contracture of the gastrocnemius muscle, provided they are comfortable and are well tolerated by the patient. This is especially important when the child is laid prone to maintain the hips in extension. Above-knee splints should be used, holding the knee in extension. A below-knee splint does not control the gastrocnemius and the commonly associated contracture of the hamstrings. An adjustable spreader bar between the legs will keep the hips in the desired degree of abduction and lateral rotation. The purpose of the splints is support, not correction. A common error is to make the splint in maximal dorsiflexion at the ankle; this will not be tolerated and will cause a pressure sore on the heel. Initially, it is advisable to place the knee in 5 to 10 degrees of flexion, the ankle being in neutral position or 5 to 10 degrees of plantar flexion. As equinus deformity lessens, each subsequent splint is made with the ankle in more dorsiflexion, as tolerated. There is much controversy about the indications for and the value of inhibitory casting.

Some surgeons use a below-knee night orthosis with a single caliper (rod), a right-angled stop, and a T-strap; the rod is progressively bent into increasing dorsiflexion as the triceps surae stretches out. The toe portion of the shoe may be cut out, and a large woolen sock may be worn at night until growth of the tibia is completed. The author does not recommend the use of below-knee orthoses.

Dynamic dorsiflexion-assist ankle-foot orthoses should not be used during the day because they will aggravate spasticity of the triceps surae muscle by constantly stimulating the stretch reflex and will cause an increasing equinus angulation of the ankle and a rocker-bottom deformity of the foot. The dorsiflexion-assist (Klenzak or spring)

surae muscle. They should be performed gently to avoid eliciting the stretch reflex and increasing spasticity. If the peroneal or posterior tibial muscles are contracted, they also are elongated. Active exercises are carried out to develop function and control of cerebral zero or hypotonic muscles. Gait training with the hips in extension and embodying a reciprocal pattern of ankle dorsiflexion and hip-knee flexion is essential. Use of crutches is not recommended because the child will lean forward and assume a hip flexion posture, which will inhibit function of the gluteus maximus, an important antigravity muscle. Hip flexion deformity is commonly associated with equinus deformity of the ankle. To elongate

ankle-foot orthoses do not elongate the contracted triceps surae; nor are they designed to correct fixed equinus deformity. Their primary purpose is to develop function and cerebral control over a hypotonic anterior tibial muscle, as described in the postoperative care after heel cord lengthening (see Plate 11).

The shoes should be high-topped and should fit snugly. Often, because of the smaller size of the foot in the hemiplegic, it may be necessary to obtain mismated shoes. To secure the forefoot in the shoe, an extra strap may be used over the dorsum of the foot or the shoes may be laced in the reverse direction with the bow at the base of the tongue. A sole plate is inserted between the inner and outer soles, extending to the end of the shoe and beyond the metatarsophalangeal joints in order to keep the shank from breaking. In functional equinus deformity, simple sneakers or tennis shoes are worn.

Stretching plaster casts, either wedged or the walking type with an anteriorly placed heel, to correct fixed equinus deformity are not tolerated by children with cerebral palsy. In the experience of the author they do more harm than good and should not be used. Very occasionally he employs a below-knee walking cast for an older child who has had several prior heel cord lengthenings and in whom equinus deformity has recurred because of poor postoperative care. In such a case it is imperative that the child's balance and independent gait be adequate and the cast be well padded and molded.

SURGICAL TREATMENT

Operative correction of equinus deformity is indicated if a toe-toe or toe-heel gait persists following a period of adequate conservative management. If the heel position is markedly valgus and the talus is plantarflexed in stance, because of shortening of the spastic gastrocnemius muscle, heel cord lengthening should be considered to prevent fixed valgus deformity of the foot. The development of rocker-bottom deformity of the foot is another indication. Correction of functional equinus deformity may also be indicated. If overactivity and exaggerated stretch reflex of the gastrocnemius and soleus cause equinus deformity of the foot in gait and disturb stability of balance, heel cord lengthening is indicated even though the foot can be passively dorsiflexed to neutral position.

Before surgery the child must have good sitting and standing balance and should be able to walk, at least with the assistance of appliances. The potential for independent or assisted gait is an absolute preoperative requisite. Second, the triceps surae is lengthened only when its motor strength is normal or good. Heel cord lengthening should not be performed if the triceps surae motor strength is only fair or less—calcaneus deformity is more disabling than equinus deformity. Third, hip flexion deformity should be corrected prior to correction of equinus deformity. The author does not recommend simultaneous multilevel surgery; i.e., do not lengthen the heel cord and hip flexors (iliopsoas and rectus femoris) at the same time. Spasticity and contracture of the hip flexors inhibits the action of the gluteus maximus—which is the most important antigravity muscle. The triceps surae muscle is hyperactive to compensate for hip extensor muscle weakness. Often equinus distortion is lessened following hip flexor release and acquisition of control over the gluteus maximus.

The purpose of Achilles tendon lengthening is to correct fixed myostatic contracture of the triceps surae, alter the point at which stretch reflex of the triceps surae is elicited, develop voluntary control over and motor strength in the cerebral zero anterior tibial muscle, and establish dynamic muscle balance between dorsiflexors and plantarflexors of the ankle. The key to success is the adequacy of postoperative care. It is imperative that the parents realize that surgery is only the initial stage of treatment. The child should be at least three years old; tendo Achillis lengthening should not be performed under two years of age.

During the past 150 years various techniques for elongating the triceps surae muscle have been described in the literature. The type of procedure employed is not so important; the result obtained is related to the selection of patient and the adequacy of postoperative care. The author prefers sliding lengthening of the heel cord, the White procedure, as advocated by Banks and Green.[6,8] Because anatomic continuity of the heel cord is not disturbed, one can

Sliding Lengthening of the Heel Cord

THE PROCEDURE

A. With the patient supine or in prone position, a posteromedial incision about 6 to 7.5 cm. long is made 1.5 cm. anteromedial to the medial border of the tendo Achillis. The subcutaneous tissue and tendon sheath are divided in one plane so that the latter remains attached to subcutaneous tissue and can be reconstructed effectively later on. It is not necessary to disturb the deep surface of the tendon or to dissect around the sheath.

B. The rotation of fibers of the tendo Achillis is studied next, as it varies greatly. The tendon usually rotates about 90 degrees on its longitudinal axis between its origin and insertion, so the fibers that occupy a medial position proximally twist laterally as they approach their insertion on the calcaneus and are posterior to those fibers that proximally occupied a lateral position. Straight Keith needles may be used to mark rotation of fibers.

The Achilles tendon is then transversely sectioned at two levels. The site of division must be chosen according to the degree of rotation of fibers. Usually the anteromedial half to two thirds of the tendon is divided distally near its insertion, and then the posteromedial half is divided in the proximal end of the wound.

C. The foot is then passively dorsiflexed with the knee in extension. The medial portion of the tendon will slide on the lateral portion, lengthening the tendon in continuity. (A third incision, midway between the others, is indicated at times if stretching does not occur easily; its site can be readily determined by palpation.) There is no fraying of the tendon as in the Z-plasty type of tendon lengthening. The actual amount of lengthening depends upon the degree of equinus deformity. At the end of the procedure the foot should rest comfortably in neutral position or passively dorsiflexed 5 degrees beyond neutral. Correction beyond this point should be avoided, as it may cause calcaneus deformity. The pneumatic tourniquet is released, and all bleeding vessels are clamped and coagulated.

D. The sheath, including a small portion of the subcutaneous tissues, is meticulously closed over the lengthened Achilles tendon.

E. The lower limb is immobilized in a well-padded above-knee cast with the knee in full extension or 5 degrees' flexion (but no hyperextension) and the foot-ankle in neutral position or 5 to 10 degrees of dorsiflexion. It is essential to mold the plaster cast well, particularly at the ankle, heel, and knee.

Plate 11. Sliding Lengthening of the Heel Cord

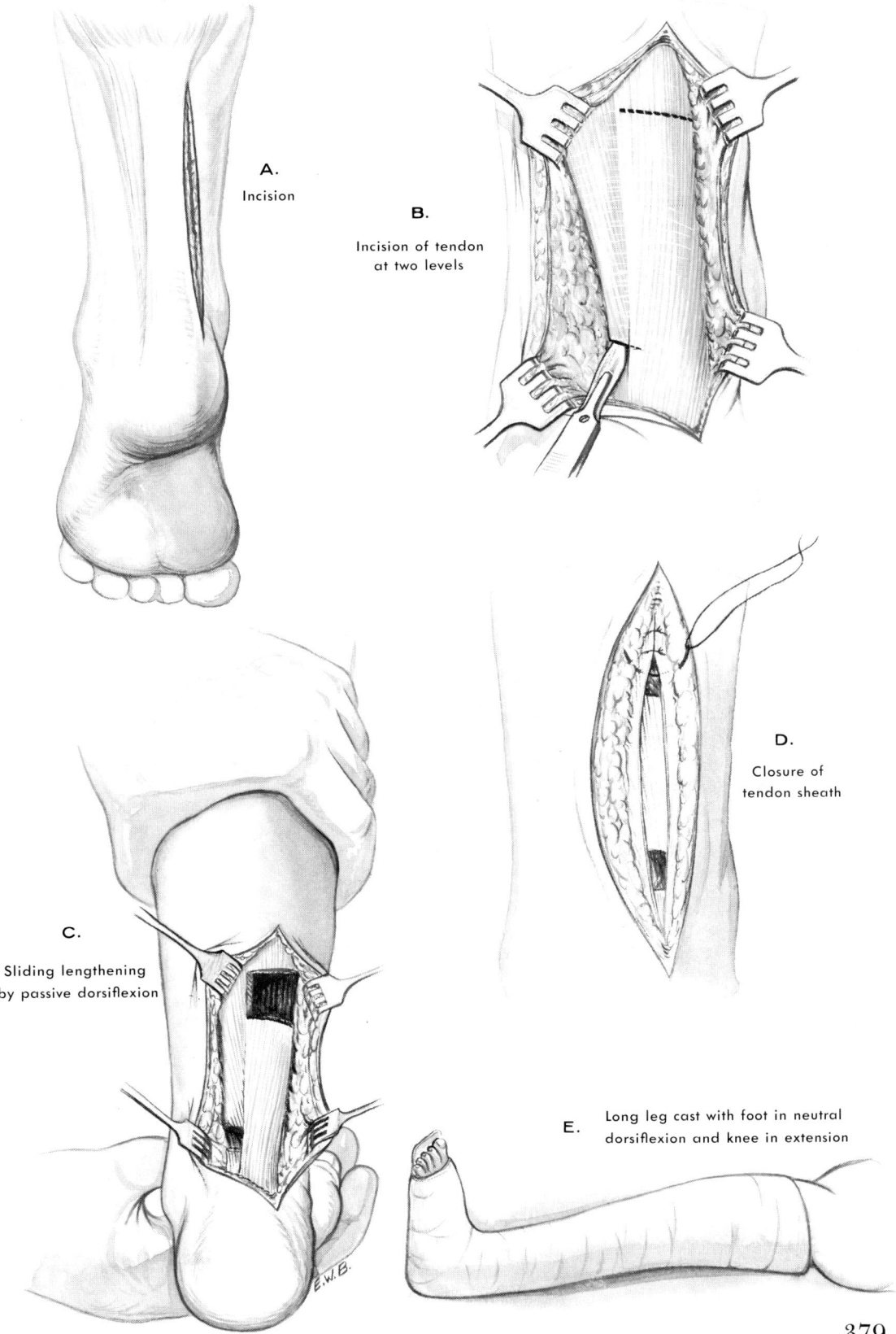

POSTOPERATIVE CARE

Meticulous execution of details of postoperative care is the key to success. The cast is bivalved and exercises are begun when the patient is comfortable, usually three to four weeks after surgery. In the immediate postoperative period, disuse atrophy is prevented by active exercises designed to develop function in both the triceps surae and anterior tibial muscles. First, with the child in supine position, the foot is dorsiflexed with the knee and hip in flexion and with manual resistance applied against the thigh to stimulate reflex function of the cerebral zero anterior tibial muscle. Gradually the position is changed from supine to upright, and the knee and hip are extended (Fig. 3–24). The range of ankle and knee motion is restored to normal by gentle passive exercises. The triceps surae muscle should not be overlengthened. To develop range of plantar flexion is as important as to develop dorsiflexion. Gastrocnemius-soleus muscle function is strengthened by plantar flexion exercises performed at first with the child lying on his side and then, against gravity, in the prone position.

An ankle-foot dorsiflexion-assist or rigid ankle orthosis should not be used in the immediate postoperative period; it will overstretch a surgically weakened triceps surae muscle and cause calcaneus deformity—more disabling than equinus deformity.

The patient is allowed to stand when the triceps surae muscle is fair in motor strength on hand testing. When he is raised to upright posture the knees are supported to prevent them from flexing, and the hips are maintained in extension (Fig. 3–25). In stance, and later during walking, a hip-knee flexion and ankle dorsiflexion pattern of locomotion is developed. The knees are always supported to prevent flexion (Figs. 3–26 and 3–27). The use of crutches (three-point gait in hemiplegics and four-point in paraplegics) to support the triceps surae under the stress of body weight has definite drawbacks. Walking or standing with crutches keeps the hips in varying degrees of flexion; this flexed posture inhibits function of the gluteus maximus—the most forceful antigravity muscle. This author does not recommend support by crutches in spastic cerebral palsy. When given, crutches should be used only under supervision and with proper instruction to maintain the hips in extension.

At night a removable bivalved cast or plastic splint is worn to maintain the foot and ankle in neutral or 5 degrees dorsiflexed position. The splint should extend to the upper thigh, holding the knee in 5 degrees of flexion, not in hyperextension. The use of night-splinting to prevent recurrence of equinus deformity cannot be overemphasized. Night-time use of splint or bivalved cast should be continued for several years, until there is dynamic balance between the muscles of ankle dorsiflexion and those of plantar flexion. It is vital that the patient sleep in prone position to maintain the hips in extension and prevent flexion posture and deformity of the hips.

If by six to nine months after tendo Achillis lengthening the anterior tibial muscle is not functioning, a dorsiflexion-assist foot-ankle orthosis may be used part time, several hours a day, to assist development of control over a cerebral zero tibialis anterior.

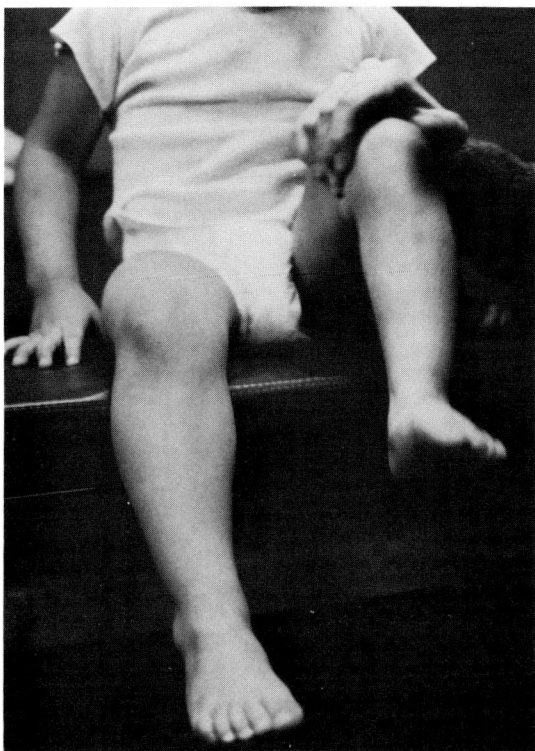

FIGURE 3–24. Active exercises to stimulate reflex function of cerebral zero anterior tibial muscle.

Ankle dorsiflexion is performed with the knee and hip in flexion and manual resistance against the thigh.

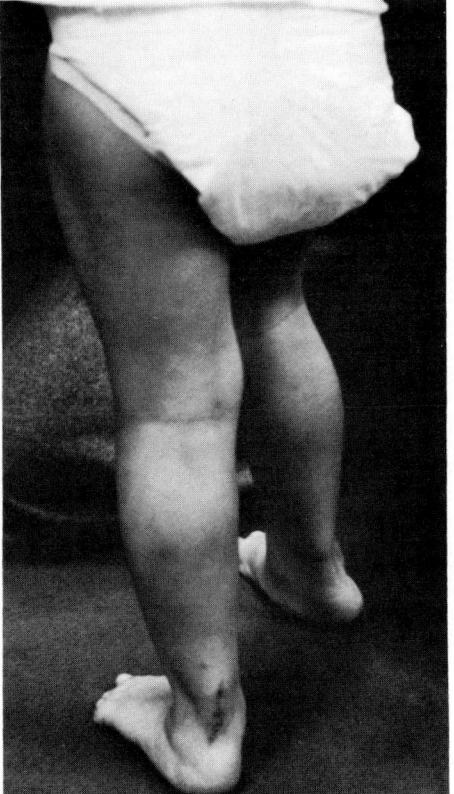

FIGURE 3–25. Following tendo Achillis lengthening the patient is raised to upright posture when the gastrocnemius-soleus muscles are fair in motor strength.

It is important to maintain the hips in extension, contracting the gluteus maximus muscle, and to prevent the knees from going into flexion. Flexion of the knee will overstretch the triceps surae muscle.

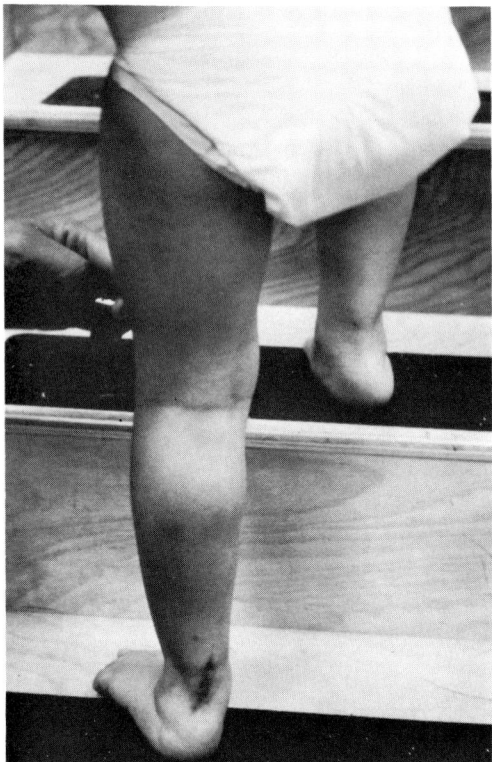

FIGURE 3–26. In the postoperative period following tendo Achillis lengthening, the triceps surae muscle should be protected from overstretching.

When the child is taught to climb up and down steps, the knees should be supported to ensure that they do not flex.

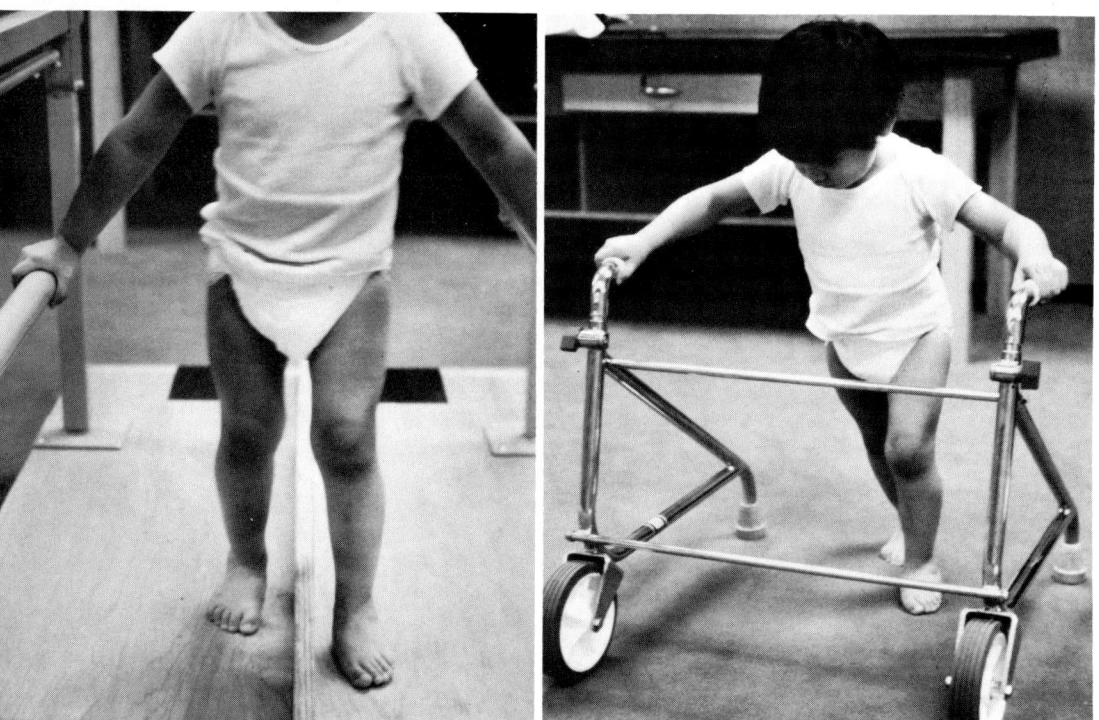

FIGURE 3–27. During gait training the triceps surae is protected by having the child hold onto parallel bars.

At home, the older child may use a walker for support. The hips should be in extension, as shown in this patient.

control the amount of lengthening, allowing relatively early mobilization. The operative procedure of sliding heel cord lengthening is described and illustrated in Plate 11 and the postoperative care is shown in Figures 3–24 through 3–27.

Subcutaneous tenotomy of the tendo Achillis was performed by Delpech in 1816 and popularized by Stromeyer (Fig. 3–28).[42, 147] The initial results in cerebral palsy were excellent; however, because of poor postoperative care the long-term results were discouraging. This author does not recommend subcutaneous lengthening of the heel cord because it is difficult to control the degree of lengthening. The same is true for Z-lengthening; it should not be performed to correct equinus deformity in spastic cerebral palsy (Fig. 3–29).

Vulpius and Stöffel, in 1913, described an operation to correct spastic equinus deformity. In their procedure the aponeurotic tendon of the gastrocnemius and soleus was divided transversely just below the middle of the leg, leaving the underlying muscle fibers intact. By forceful dorsiflexion of the ankle, the segments of the aponeurotic tendon were separated, but continuity of the soleus muscle fibers was not disturbed.[158]

Later, one or two V-shaped incisions were made instead of transverse incisions (Fig. 3–30). Compere and Schnute popularized the Vulpius procedure in the United States, and Baker further modified it, using a tongue-in-groove lengthening (Fig. 3–31).[1] In both the Vulpius and Baker operations, aponeurotic lengthening of the soleus is often performed also.

When equinus deformity is primarily caused by contracture of the gastrocnemius muscle, Silfverskiöld recommends lowering or recession of the gastrocnemius muscle heads below the level of the knee joint and partial neurectomy of the tibial motor nerves to the gastrocnemius muscle to further decrease its motor power (Fig. 3–32). This procedure does not disturb the soleus muscle, which retains its function for effective push-off in gait.[136]

In 1950, Strayer described recession of the gastrocnemius muscle in its distal portion. The gastrocnemius tendon is divided transversely at its junction with the conjoined gastrocnemius-soleus tendon. The foot is dorsiflexed to neutral position, and the retracted proximal part of the gastrocnemius tendon is resutured to the underlying soleus (Fig. 3–33).[145] In 1958, Strayer

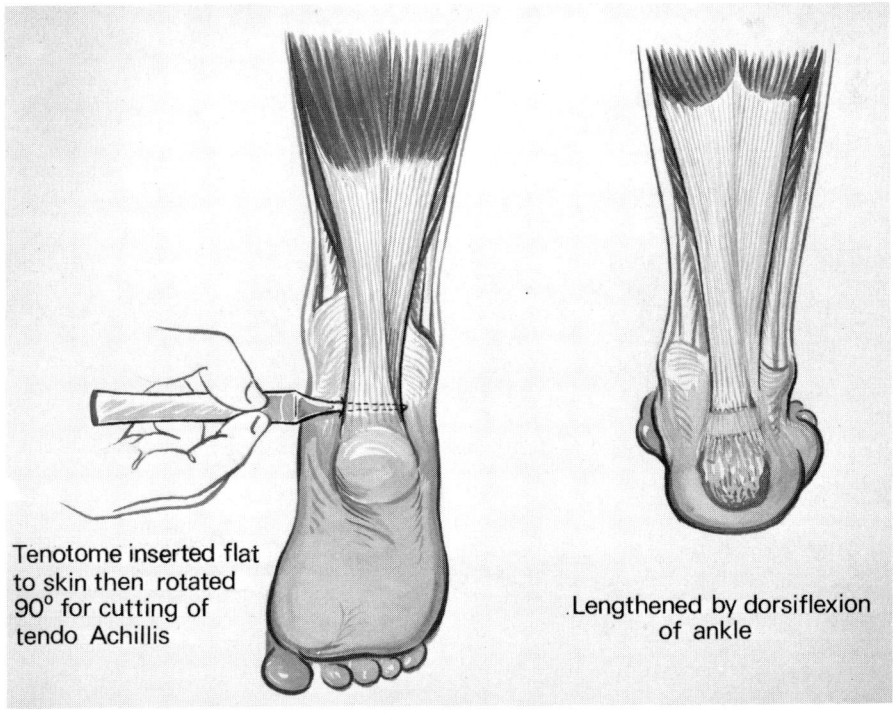

FIGURE 3–28. Subcutaneous lengthening of tendo Achillis.

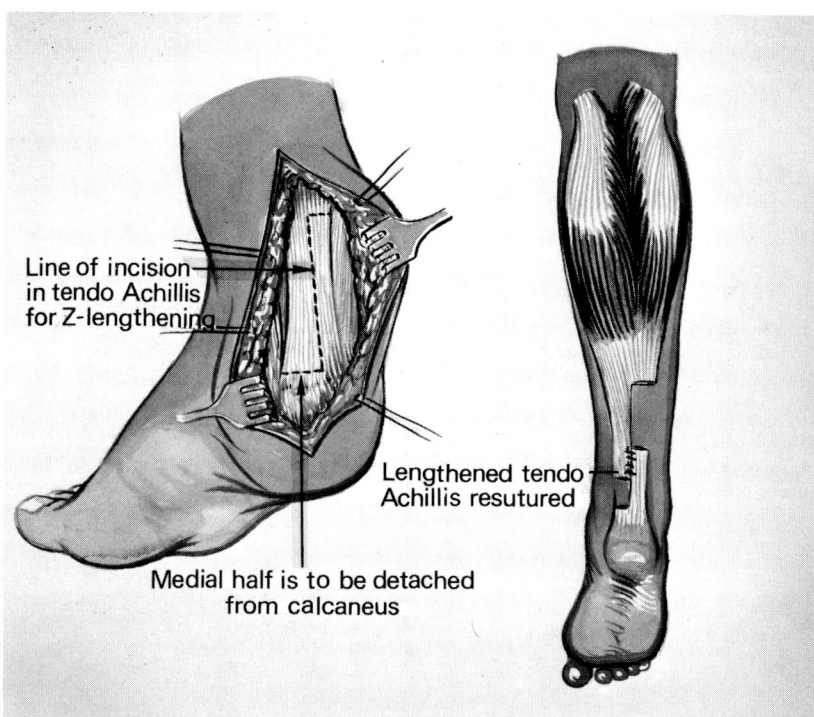

FIGURE 3–29. Z-lengthening of tendo Achillis.
This procedure should not be performed to correct equinus deformity in spastic cerebral palsy.

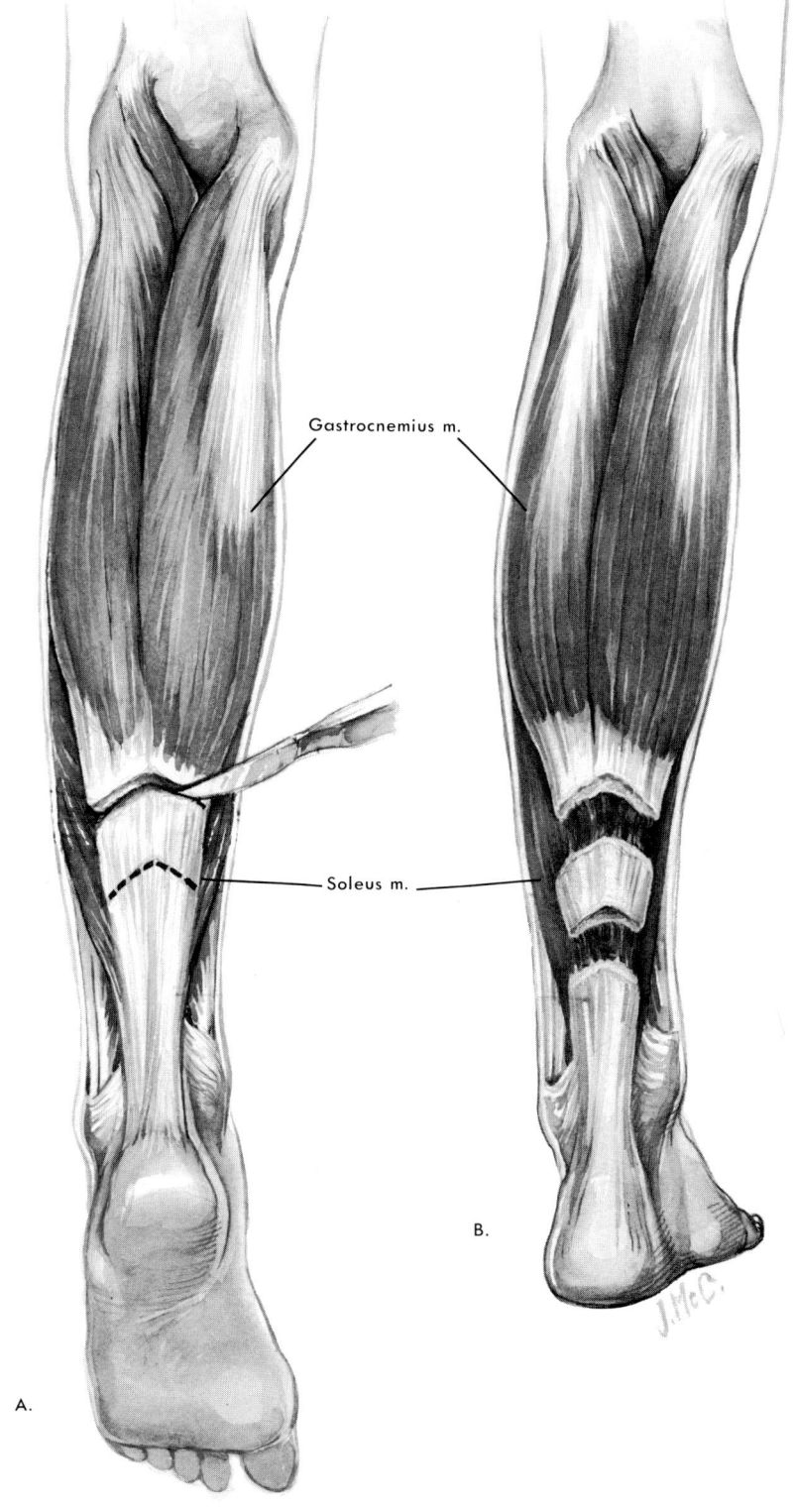

FIGURE 3–30. Lengthening of the gastrocnemius by the Vulpius technique.

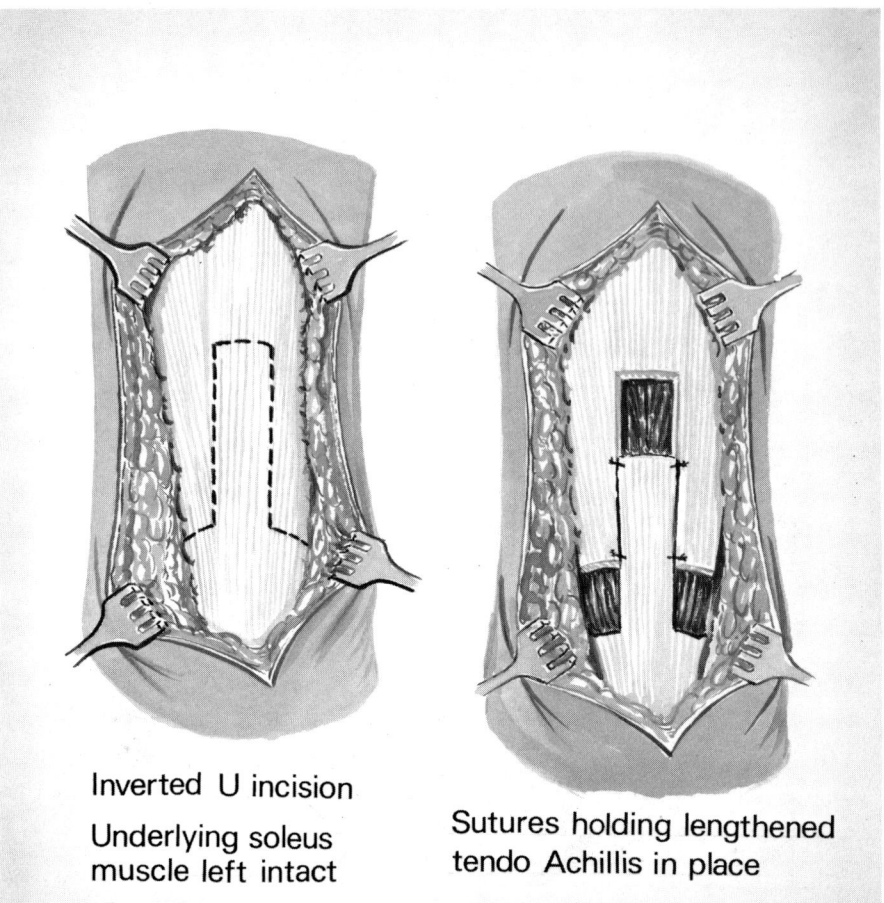

FIGURE 3–31. *"Tongue-in-groove" lengthening of gastrocnemius aponeurosis in its middle third, the Baker technique.*

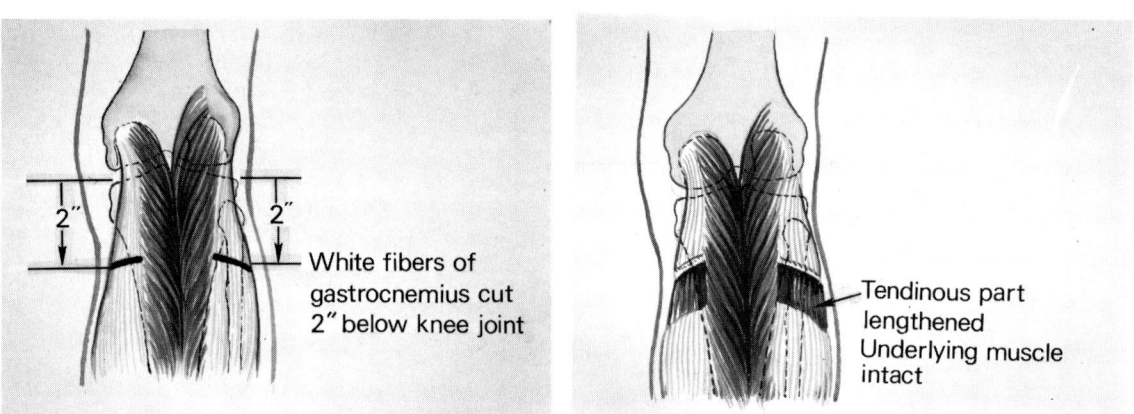

FIGURE 3–32. *Proximal (below-knee) recession of gastrocnemius, the Silfverskiöld technique.*

Silfverskiöld combined this procedure with neurectomy of the motor branch of the tibial nerve to the gastrocnemius.

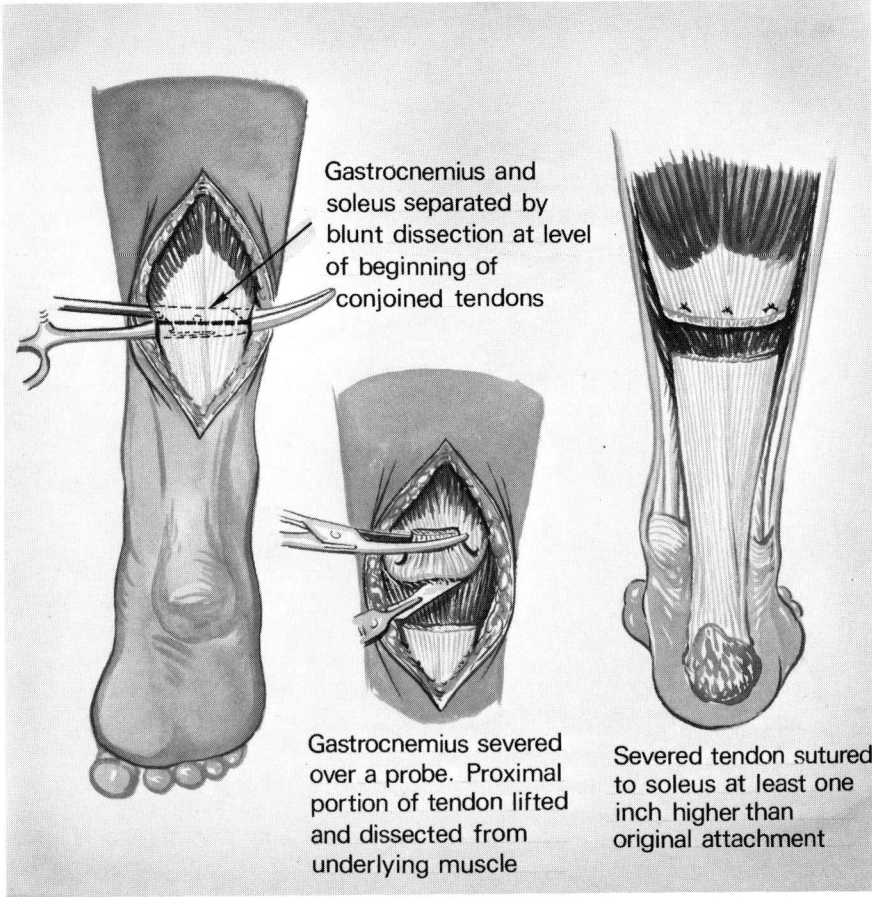

FIGURE 3-33. *Distal recession of the gastrocnemius, the Strayer technique.*

reported on distal gastrocnemius recession in 23 patients, in 16 of whom the results were good or excellent.[146]

Silver and Simon, in 1959, reported their experience with the proximal gastrocnemius recession of Silfverskiöld in 66 children on whom 110 operations were performed. In addition, they performed neurectomy of one head of the gastrocnemius. The equinus deformity recurred in five cases; on their evaluation, the failures were attributed to muscle imbalance and weakness of the dorsiflexor muscles of the foot.[137]

The advantage of the Strayer and Silfverskiöld procedures is that they preserve soleus function for push-off in gait; there are however, definite disadvantages to each. The Silfverskiöld operation removes the posterior dynamic support to the knee provided by the gastrocnemius, with the result that genu recurvatum is a potential complication. This procedure should not be performed when the hamstrings need to be lengthened at a later date or when, in gait, the knee goes into hyperextension when the heel touches the floor. Following the Strayer procedure, in which it is completely freed from the soleus, the gastrocnemius muscle may retract proximally as a small functionless knot in the upper calf. For these reasons, the Strayer procedure is not advocated.

Fractional lengthening of the gastrocnemius above the knee was described by Green and McDermott in 1942, and later by Baker in 1954 and 1956 (Fig. 3-34).[1,2,61] Its only indication is for a mild equinus deformity with fixed flexion contracture of the knee when the hamstrings are being lengthened.[61] It should not be employed as a primary procedure.

In 1913, Stöffel described neurectomy of the motor branches of peripheral nerves for

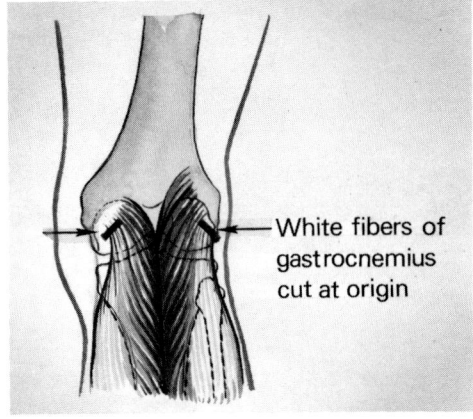

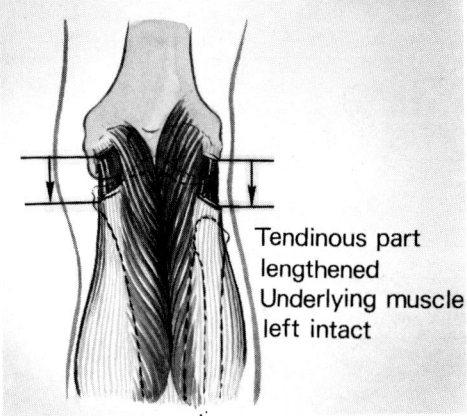

FIGURE 3–34. *Proximal (above-knee) recession of gastrocnemius, technique of Green (1942) and Baker (1954).*

the correction of spastic contractures.[144] Since then, division of motor nerves to one or both heads of the gastrocnemius to correct equinus deformity has been advocated by numerous surgeons. This author does not recommend neurectomy of motor branches of the tibial nerve because it produces fibrosis of the triceps surae muscle with consequent myostatic contracture and recurrence of fixed equinus deformity. Tibial neurectomy should be performed only when there is severe ankle clonus on weight-bearing, which hinders walking. It is imperative that one distinguish the clonus caused by the gastrocnemius from that caused by the soleus. When it diminishes or disappears on flexion of the knee, the clonus is primarily caused by the gastrocnemius; when the clonus is unaltered by changes in the position of the knee, the soleus is its chief cause. Motor branches of the tibial nerve to the spastic muscle causing the clonus are the ones to be resected. This author recommends that after the motor nerve is sectioned it be reimplanted in the muscle to prevent fibrosis. The tendo Achillis is usually not lengthened at the same time, although, on occasion, it may have to be done later. The operative technique of neurectomy of motor branches of the tibial nerve is described and illustrated in Plate 12.

Anterior advancement of the heel cord was originally described by Estève of Paris in 1936.[51] Murphy of Lexington, Kentucky, independently introduced the procedure in the United States in 1959.[120] The principle of anterior advancement of the tendo Achillis from the posterior tuberosity to the dorsum of the calcaneus immediately posterior to the subtalar joint is to shorten the lever arm and weaken the triceps surae without changing the resting length of the muscle. Murphy proposed that skeletal growth would not affect the end result and permanent correction could be achieved without the use of splints and orthotic devices. The principle of the operation is illustrated in Figure 3–35. The axis of ankle motion is the midportion of the body of the talus. The triceps surae muscle acts on the ankle joint and foot through a lever system, the fulcrum of which is located at point B in the midportion of the body of the talus. On anterior advancement of the heel cord from point C (the posterior tuberosity of the calcaneus) to point D (the upper surface of the calcaneus immediately behind the subtalar joint) the power of the triceps surae is diminished by 48 per cent according to the calculations of Pierrot and Murphy.[120] On push-off the fulcrum in the foot moves distally to the first metatarsal head (point A), weakening the push-off power by the ratio of $\frac{C + D}{AC} = 0.15 \pm 0.02$. Therefore, the advantage of anterior advancement of the heel cord is that it decreases resistance to ankle dorsiflexion by 48 per cent. This author recommends anterior advancement of the tendo Achillis to correct equinus deformity in spastic paralysis when the triceps surae muscle is of fair motor strength. The operative technique is described in Plate 13.

Throop and associates reported the results of 79 anterior advancements of the tendo calcaneus; in 17.7 per cent they were

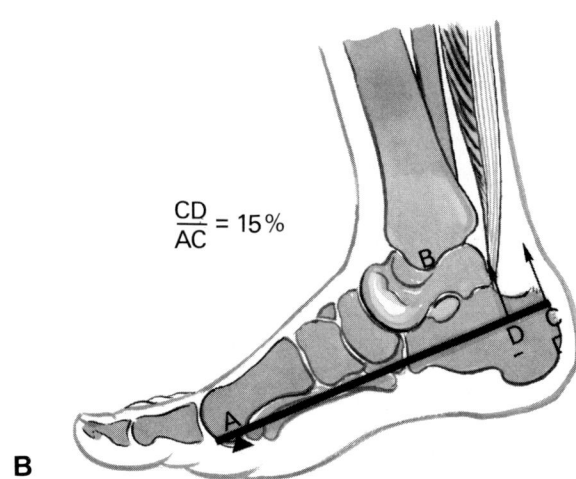

FIGURE 3–35. *The principle of anterior advancement of the heel cord for correction of pes equinus due to spastic cerebral palsy.*

A. The power of the triceps surae is reduced to 48 per cent when the Achilles tendon is transferred from C to D. B. The power of push-off of the triceps surae is reduced to only 15 per cent with transfer of the heel cord from C to D. (Redrawn from Pierrot, A. H., and Murphy, O. B.: Heel cord advancement—a new approach to the spastic equinus deformity. Orthop. Clin. N. Amer., 5:118, 1974.)

excellent (heel-toe gait, good push-off, no hyperextension of the knee); in 72.2 per cent, good (flat foot-strike with or without push-off, no hyperextension of the knee), and in 10.1 per cent, poor (toe-heel gait, recurrence of equinus deformity, calcaneus gait). Added, the percentages of excellent and good results show the operation was satisfactory in 89.9 per cent. The indication for the Murphy procedure was given as the presence of dynamic equinus angulation with no more than 15 per cent of fixed equinus deformity.[153]

If by 6 to 12 months following heel cord lengthening the patient is unable to develop voluntary control over a cerebral zero anterior tibial muscle, this author recommends shortening the stretched-out and elongated muscle by plication or excision of a segment at its distal attachment and transferring a neurophysiologically normal and strong extensor hallucis longus to the base of the first metatarsal, rerouting it through the anterior tibial muscle to promote reflex stimulation of and voluntary control over it. This procedure is a modification of that of Alfonso Tohen.[154] If any equinus deformity is present, it should be corrected by a stretching below-knee walking cast. It should be possible to passively dorsiflex the ankle joint to at least 20 degrees beyond neutral prior to surgery. The details of operative technique are illustrated in Plate 14.

Valgus or varus deformity associated with the equinus foot is usually caused by an imbalance of the muscles of inversion and eversion—the tibialis posterior and the peroneal muscles. Treatment of these deform-

Text continued on page 398

Neurectomy of Motor Branches of Tibial Nerve to Gastrocnemius

A. The patient is placed in prone position with a pneumatic tourniquet on the proximal thigh. A transverse incision 5 to 7 cm. long is made immediately proximal to the popliteal crease in line with the flexion creases of the skin.

B. The deep fascia is divided and the tibial nerve, lying superficial to the vessels, is exposed. The first branch is cutaneous; it is not disturbed. The next two branches are the motor nerves to the gastrocnemius. One branch emerges from the medial side and enters the medial head close to its origin; just prior to disappearing into the muscle, it divides into three branches. The other branch emerges from the lateral side and similarly enters the lateral head close to its origin, but it divides into only two branches. The motor branch to the soleus muscle emerges distal to that of the gastrocnemius. It is best to stimulate each branch to determine which is the principal cause of clonus.

C. The motor branches are sectioned distally at their entrance into the muscle; then a slit 1.5 cm. long is made in the muscle belly and the sectioned nerve is reimplanted into the muscle and secured with 000 plain catgut sutures. The wound is closed in layers in the usual manner. The limb is immobilized in an above-knee cast with the foot at 5 to 10 degrees of dorsiflexion at the ankle and with the knee in full extension. The cast is removed in three weeks; the postoperative care is similar to that after heel cord lengthening. (Some surgeons apply only a pressure dressing and allow the patient to walk when he is comfortable and when the wound is healed.)

Plate 12. Neurectomy of Motor Branches of Tibial Nerve to Gastrocnemius

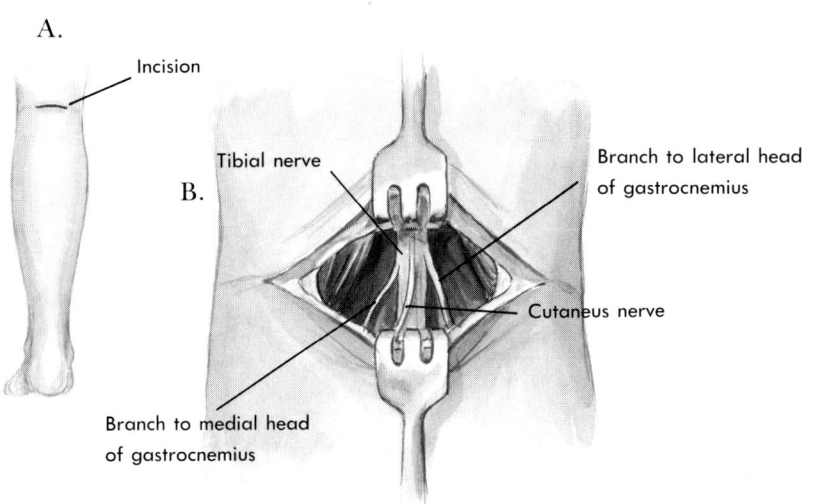

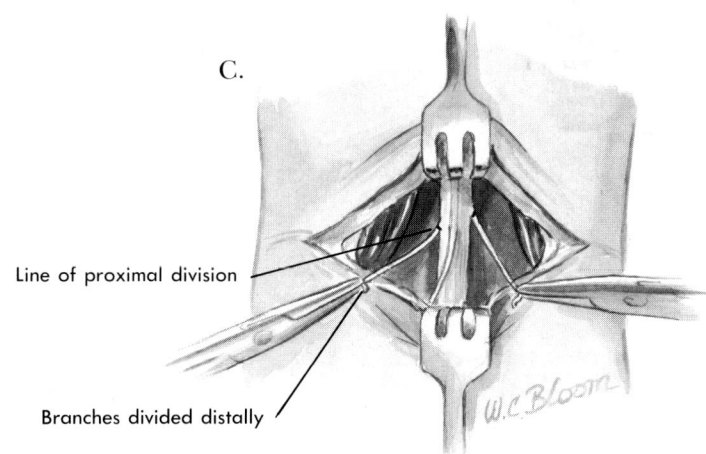

Anterior Advancement of Tendo Achillis for Correction of Spastic Equinus Deformity (Murphy Technique)

THE PROCEDURE

A. With the patient in prone position, a posteromedial incision is made about 1 cm. medial to the tendo Achillis; it begins at the os calcis and extends proximally for a length of 7.5 to 10 cm. The subcutaneous tissue and tendon sheath are divided in one plane in line with the skin incision.

B. The Achilles tendon is identified and isolated by sharp and blunt dissection to its insertion. It is detached from the calcaneal tuberosity as far distally as possible to preserve length. Caution is exercised to avoid injury to the calcaneal apophysis.

C. Next, a Bunnell pull-out wire suture is placed on the distal end of the tendo Achillis. The flexor hallucis longus tendon is identified, mobilized, and retracted medially. The upper surface of the calcaneus is exposed. A 0.6-cm. drill hole is made from the superior part of the calcaneus immediately posterior to the subtalar joint to exit on the plantar aspect of the non-weight-bearing area of the calcaneus. With a curet the drill hole is enlarged, if necessary.

D. The pull-out wire and Achilles tendon are passed through the drill hole and are tied over a sterile, thick felt pad and a button on the plantar aspect of the foot with the ankle in 15 degrees of plantar flexion. It is vital that the heel cord be routed anterior to the flexor hallucis longus. If attention is not paid to this important detail the Achilles tendon will reattach itself to its original insertion. The tourniquet is released, and after complete hemostasis the wound is closed. An above-knee cast is applied with the ankle joint in 15 degrees of plantar flexion and the knee in 10 degrees of flexion.

POSTOPERATIVE CARE

The cast and pull-out wire are removed in four to six weeks. Physical therapy is begun to restore ankle motion and develop strength of the anterior tibial and triceps surae muscles. Other details of postoperative care follow the same principles outlined for tendo Achillis lengthening.

Plate 13. Anterior Advancement of Tendo Achillis for Correction of Spastic Equinus Deformity (Murphy Technique)

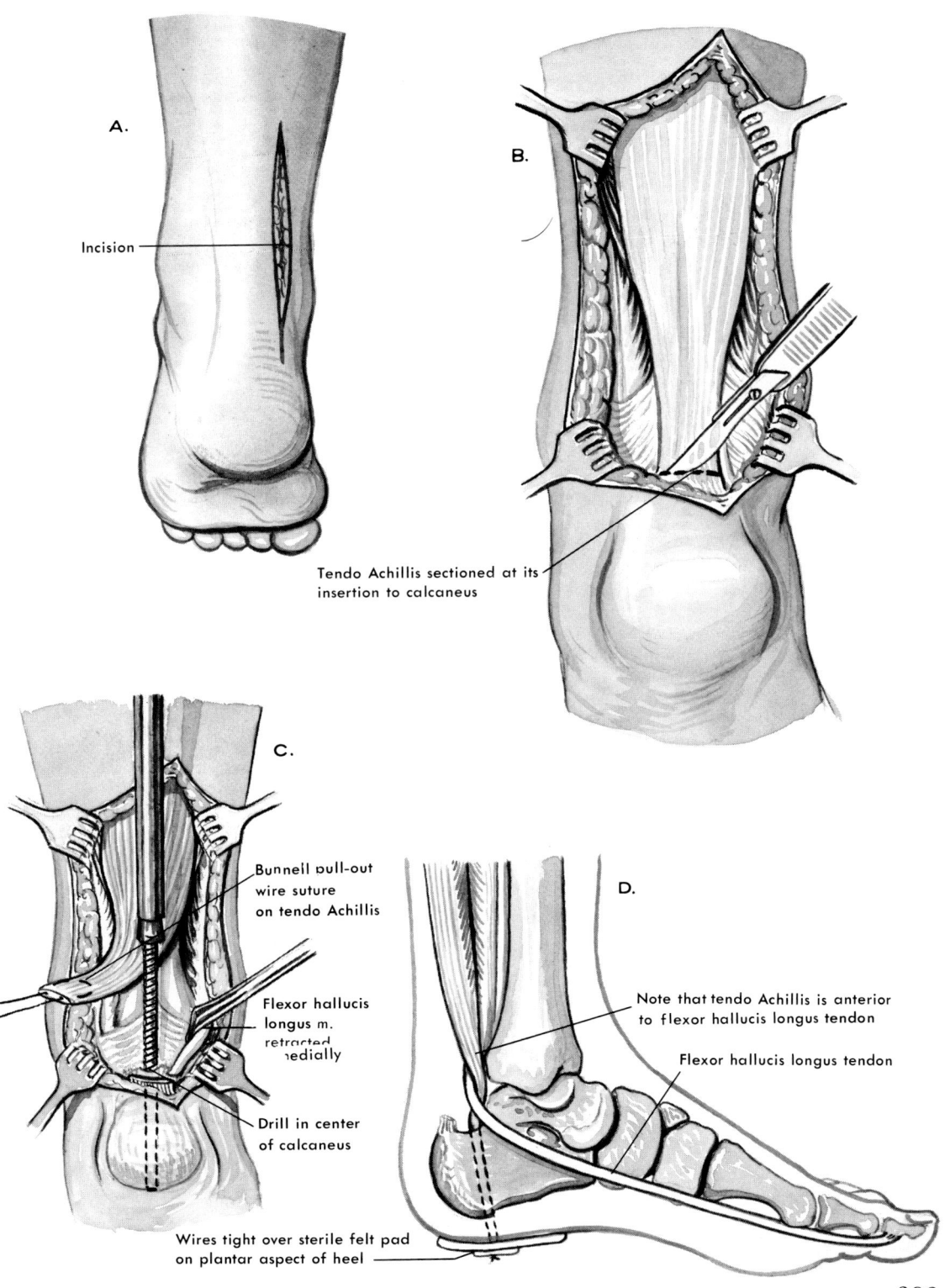

Extensor Hallucis Longus Rerouting Through Anterior Tibial Tendon and Shortening of Anterior Tibial Muscle

THE PROCEDURE

A. A longitudinal incision about 7 cm. long is made over the dorsum of the foot. It starts at the base of the proximal phalanx of the big toe and extends proximally to the first cuneiform bone. Subcutaneous tissue is divided in line with the skin incision; wound margins are undermined and gently retracted. Injury to the superficial vessels and sensory nerves is avoided.

B. The extensor hallucis longus tendon is identified and detached from its insertion as far distally as possible. The stump is sutured to the tendon of the extensor hallucis brevis with the big toe held in marked dorsiflexion to prevent plantar drop of the hallux postoperatively. (It is described in Plate 24). The tendon of the extensor hallucis longus is dissected free of its sheath as high as possible. Then a second incision is made over the course of the anterior tibial tendon in the distal third of the leg. The tendons of the extensor hallucis longus and the anterior tibial are identified. The extensor hallucis longus is pulled into the proximal wound by gentle traction.

C. With a scalpel, three slits of appropriate size are made in the anterior tibial tendon. The extensor hallucis longus tendon is rewound by passing through these slits and then delivered into the distal wound with an Ober tendon passer.

Plate 14. Extensor Hallucis Longus Rerouting Through Anterior Tibial Tendon and Shortening of Anterior Tibial Muscle

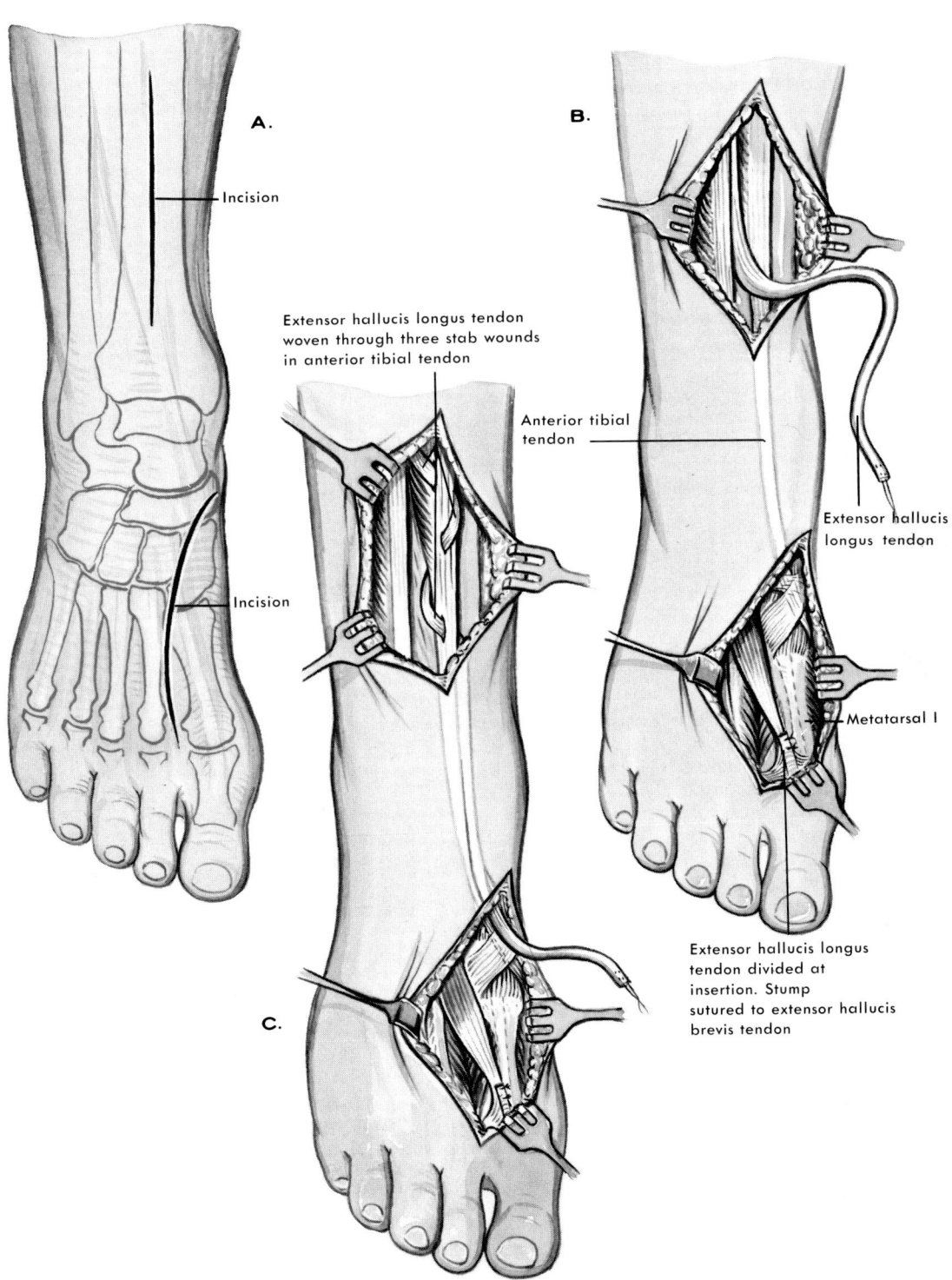

Extensor Hallucis Longus Rerouting Through Anterior Tibial Tendon and Shortening of Anterior Tibial Muscle *(Continued)*

D. The extensor hallucis longus tendon is sutured to the insertion of the anterior tibial muscle with the ankle in neutral position or 10 degrees of dorsiflexion. Any excess of the extensor hallucis longus tendon is either excised (as illustrated) or, if it is long enough, reattached to its insertion. Next, the lax anterior tibial tendon is shortened by plication and suturing to the capsule of the first metatarsal-cuneiform joint.

E. Another way of shortening the anterior tibial tendon is by excising an appropriate segment distally and suturing the cut ends together. The tourniquet is released and after complete hemostasis the wound is closed in layers in the usual fashion. The foot and ankle are immobilized in a below-knee walking cast.

POSTOPERATIVE CARE

Three weeks after surgery the cast is removed and an above-knee splint is made that maintains the ankle at 5 to 10 degrees of dorsiflexion and the knee in neutral extension; the splint is worn at night. During the day a dorsiflexion-assist below-knee orthosis is used. Active assisted exercises are performed to develop function in and cerebral control over the cerebral zero anterior tibial muscle. Gentle passive exercises are carried out to maintain range of ankle motion. During the day periods of gait training without orthosis are carried out to activate the anterior tibial muscle function. The dorsiflexion-assist orthosis is gradually discontinued over a period of three to six months. Persistent and meticulous physical therapy and night splinting is vital.

Plate 14. Extensor Hallucis Longus Rerouting Through Anterior Tibial Tendon and Shortening of Anterior Tibial Muscle

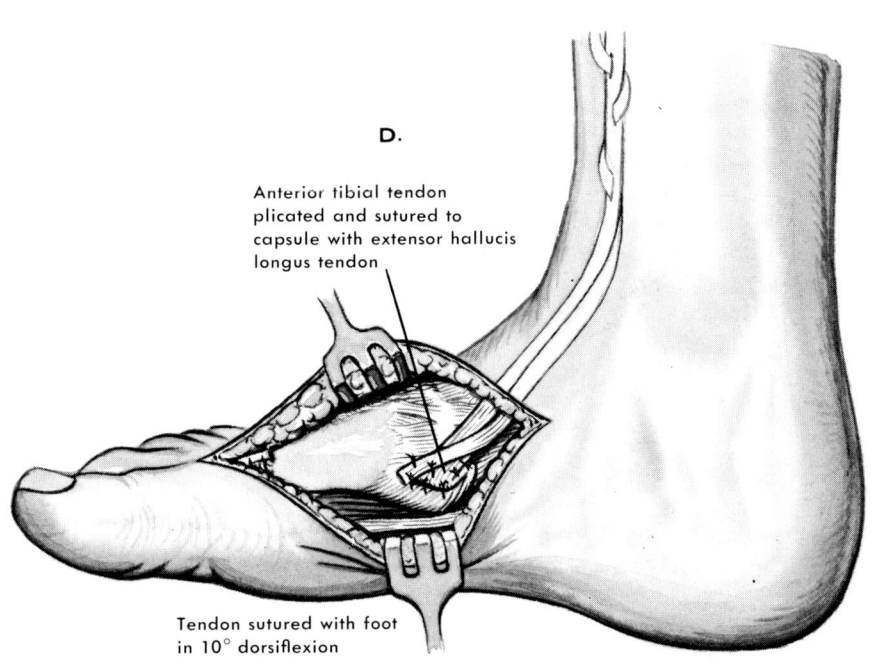

D.

Anterior tibial tendon plicated and sutured to capsule with extensor hallucis longus tendon

Tendon sutured with foot in 10° dorsiflexion

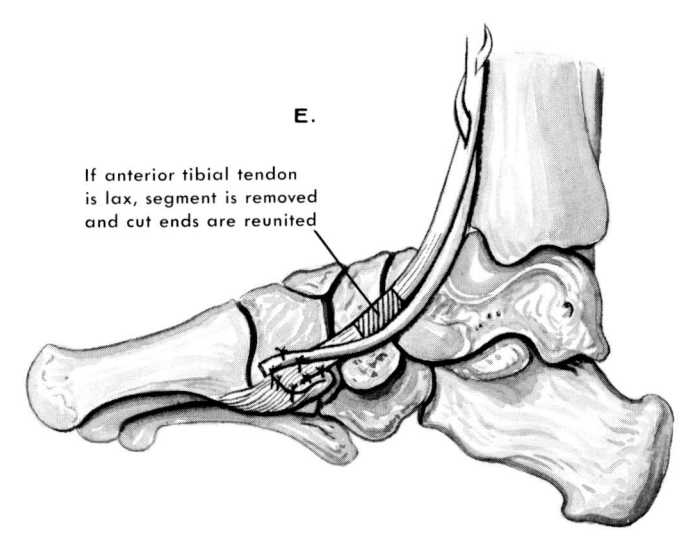

E.

If anterior tibial tendon is lax, segment is removed and cut ends are reunited

ing spastic muscles may be carried out at the same time as correction of equinus deformity.

Pes Varus

When the spastic posterior tibial muscle is causing pes varus, it may be lengthened at the same time as the heel cord. It is not necessary to make a separate incision. Through the posteromedial incision for heel cord lengthening, the posterior tibial muscle and tendon can be exposed above the medial malleolus in the distal third of the leg immediately posterior to the tibia. At two levels, 5 cm. apart and well above the site where muscle fibers terminate on the tendon, two incisions are made over the tendinous portion of the posterior tibial muscle but not into the muscle fibers themselves. The proximal incision is transverse, and the distal one oblique. The sliding lengthening of the tendon is obtained by forcing the foot into valgus position and by gentle stretching between two moist sponges (Fig. 3–36). Total section and release of the posterior tibial tendon should be avoided, as it will cause marked valgus deformity in the growing foot. Baker recommends freeing the sheath of the posterior tibial tendon behind the medial malleolus and allowing it to be displaced anterior to the malleolus.[2] The author does not advise this procedure because, in its new transposed position, the posterior tibial muscle still acts as an invertor of the foot, causing calcaneovarus deformity.

Anterior transfer of the posterior tibial tendon through the interosseous route for the correction of nonstructural varus deformity of the hindfoot in spastic paralysis has been described by several authors. Williams reported the results in 53 feet in 42 patients as follows: (1) of 28 patients who had required below-knee orthoses, 23 were able to discard them postoperatively; (2) 38 patients had improved gait with plantigrade

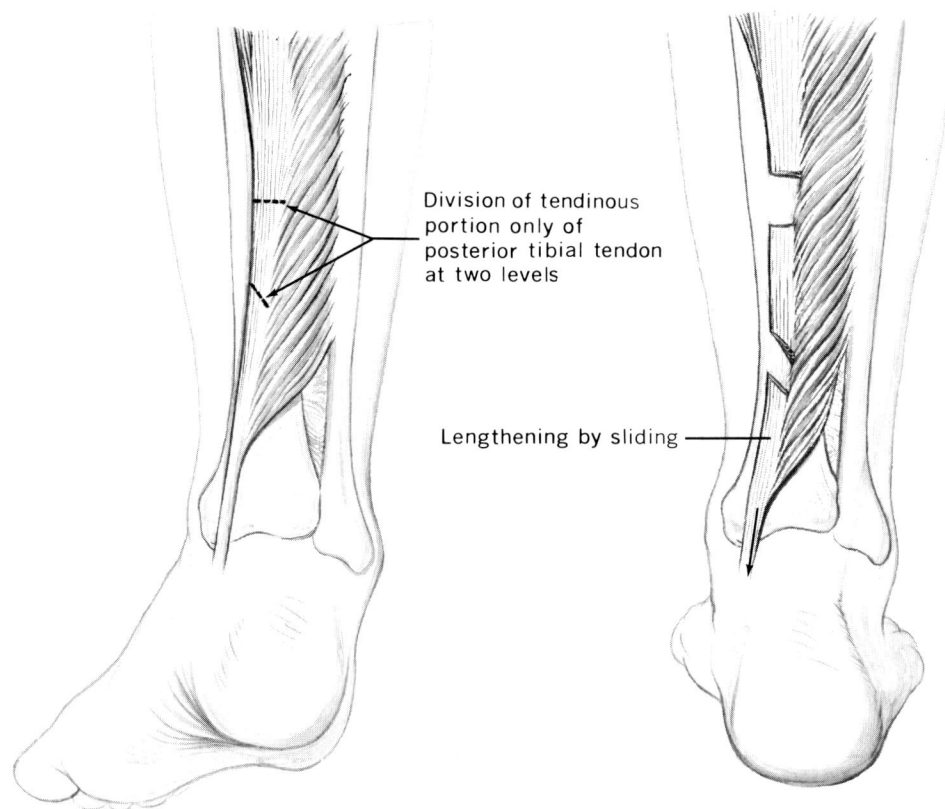

FIGURE 3–36. Sliding lengthening of the posterior tibial muscle.

position of the foot and decrease in toeing-in; (3) 24 feet showed improved shoe wear; (4) 27 feet demonstrated voluntary control over the transferred tibialis posterior; and (5) 23 feet had active contraction of the transfer in gait. (6) In seven feet all the muscles of the lower leg were in spasm, including the transferred tibialis posterior; in these patients the feet were frozen at right angles to the leg, but function was remarkably good. (7) Of the 53 feet, 5 needed further surgical procedures to obtain an acceptable result—these consisted of triple arthrodesis in 3, lengthening of the transfer to correct spastic calcaneus deformity in 1, and shortening of the transfer to overcome a drop foot in 1. The overall rating of the transfers in the 42 patients was good in 22, fair in 14, and poor in 6. Williams regarded anterior transfer of the tibialis posterior as "one of the most reliable and successful operations in cerebral palsy."[162]

This author does not share the enthusiasm of Mr. Williams. It is very difficult to train an out-of-phase transfer in a child with brain damage. The results are unpredictable, and not infrequently, a reverse deformity may develop. When the procedure is combined with heel cord lengthening, calcaneovalgus or calcaneus deformity is a common complication.

More definitive preoperative assessment by kinetic electromyography synchronized with three-plane motion pictures in gait and with force plate measurements is available in special centers. Perry and Hoffer have utilized preoperative and postoperative dynamic electromyography as an aid in planning tendon transfers in children with cerebral palsy.[113]

In the gait of a normal person, there is habitual phasic activity of groups of muscles working automatically during portions of the stance and swing phases. In cerebral palsy this selective and habitual phasic mus-

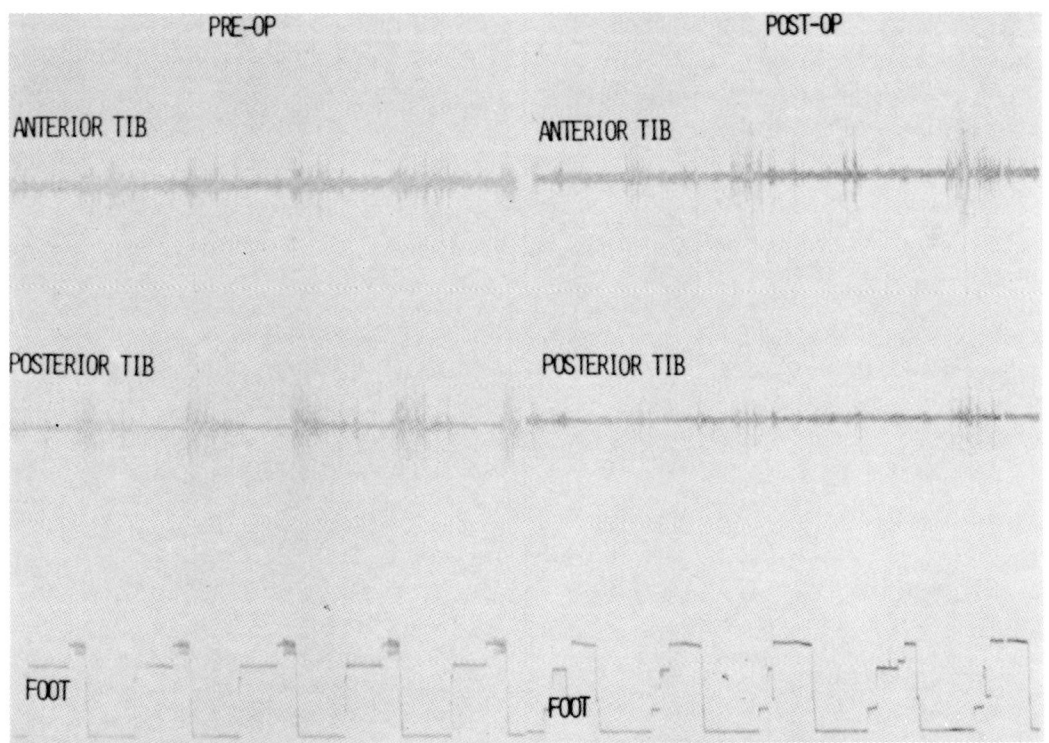

FIGURE 3–37. Preoperative and postoperative dynamic electromyographic studies of anterior transfer of posterior tibial tendon in spastic cerebral palsy.

Note that the muscle is active during the swing phase of gait both before and after anterior transfer. (From Perry, J., and Hoffer, M. M.: Preoperative and postoperative dynamic electromyography as an aid in planning tendon transfers in children with cerebral palsy. J. Bone Joint Surg., 59-A:532, 1978. Reprinted by permission.)

cle control is disturbed because primitive modes of muscle action persist in the form of patterns of activity that respond to posturing of the trunk and limbs, to different rates of stretch, and to residual perinatal reflexes. Muscle grading in cerebral palsy is difficult because of the "patterning" or stretch activation of the muscles, but electromyography will show their activity during different phases of gait. By applying this information in addition to the basic principles of tendon transfer learned in poliomyelitis—a muscle of normal or good motor strength, ample tendon excursion, a direct line of pull, normal range of joint motion, and meticulous postoperative training—one can achieve the desired function in cerebral palsy.

Perry and associates recommend anterior transfer of the posterior tibial tendon for pes varus when the muscle is active only in the swing phase preoperatively; it is prerequisite that there be full range of passive motion of the ankle and hind part of the foot. (When there is equinus deformity, anterior transfer of the posterior tibial tendon should be preceded by heel cord lengthening.) On the other hand, if the tibialis posterior is active continuously in both swing and stance phases of gait, they recommend lengthening and not transfer because the transfer frequently becomes a tenodesis. In three children the phase action of the posterior tibial muscle was reversed (i.e., it was active during the swing phase); the tendon was transferred anteriorly and all three transfers functioned automatically (Fig. 3–37). Two children had continuous activity of the posterior tibial muscle, which was lengthened at its musculotendinous junction (Fig. 3–38).[114]

As a general rule this author does *not recommend* anterior transfer of the posterior tibial tendon in spastic paralysis unless the facilities of a gait analysis laboratory are available and dynamic electromyography demonstrates that the muscle is active only during the swing phase of gait. He employs it then only if the ankle and hind part of the foot have full passive range of motion, i.e., the varus posture of the foot is not fixed. The child should be intelligent and of an age to be motivated to cooperate during the postoperative training period. The indication for transfer is drop foot due to ankle dorsiflexor insufficiency, provided the aforementioned requisites are met. Otherwise, it is safer and much simpler to lengthen the tibialis posterior.

Split posterior tibial tendon transfer is

FIGURE 3–38. Dynamic electromyograph of the posterior tibial muscle showing continuous activity in both phases of gait.

A preoperative study. This muscle is lengthened at its musculotendinous junction; it should not be transferred anteriorly. (From Perry, J., and Hoffer, M. M.: Preoperative and postoperative dynamic electromyography as an aid in planning tendon transfers in children with cerebral palsy. J. Bone Joint Surg., 59-A:532, 1978. Reprinted by permission.)

recommended by Green and Griffin when the posterior tibial muscle is diphasic, the anterior tibial muscle weak, and the peroneals weak or absent. Through a posteromedial incision, the posterior tibial tendon is split longitudinally into halves, leaving the anteromedial half attached to the navicular. The posterolateral half is passed laterally, anterior to the neurovascular bundle and the long flexors, into the sheath of the peroneus brevis tendon and sutured as far distally as possible. In 14 of the 15 feet the varus deformity of the hindfoot was corrected with no recurrence of valgus or calcaneus deformity at a two-year or more follow-up. In one foot the result was poor owing to fixed varus deformity of the hindfoot requiring calcaneal osteotomy for correction.[62a]

In the adolescent patient the hindfoot varus deformity may be severe and fixed; in such cases soft-tissue procedures will not correct it and a bony procedure is required. The author recommends a Dwyer lateral calcaneal close-up wedge osteotomy (see Plate 4) or preferably lateral displacement osteotomy of the calcaneus. It is wise to precede or combine it with soft-tissue release, such as lengthening of the posterior tibial tendon, in order to prevent recurrence of deformity.

TRANSFER OF TIBIALIS ANTERIOR

In acquired spastic paralysis the anterior tibial muscle may be hyperactive, pulling the foot into varus posture. The anterior tibial tendon may be transferred laterally to the base of the second or third metatarsal—never more laterally—to change the action of the muscle from varus dorsiflexion to pure dorsiflexion. There should be no equinus deformity. In perinatal spastic cerebral palsy, calcaneovarus deformity of the foot may develop as a complication of overlengthening of the tendo Achillis with consequent poor function of the triceps surae and overactivity of the tibialis anterior; these cases present another indication for lateral transfer of the tibialis anterior.

Split anterior tibial tendon transfer has been performed extensively at Rancho Los Amigos Hospital, Downey, California—on adults with cerebrovascular accidents and also on spastic children. Hoffer and associates presented the results of 21 split anterior tibial tendon transfers in 16 children. Gait improved in all patients; all 16 had required braces before surgery, and only 7 required them postoperatively. The fixed deformities were released in 15 feet (12 patients). Twenty of the twenty-one transfers functioned with force equal to that noted in their spastic patterns preoperatively. Deformities recurred in two feet.[71]

Later, Perry and Hoffer reported the results of four split anterior tibial tendon transfers for treatment of varus posture of the foot. All four patients required braces preoperatively, and after surgery they all became brace-free and had balanced foot posture. Preoperative dynamic electromyography had shown continuous activity of the anterior tibial during gait, and the postoperative electromyograms did not show any change. The feet improved because the force of the anterior tibial tendon was balanced.[113]

The technique of split anterior tibial ten-

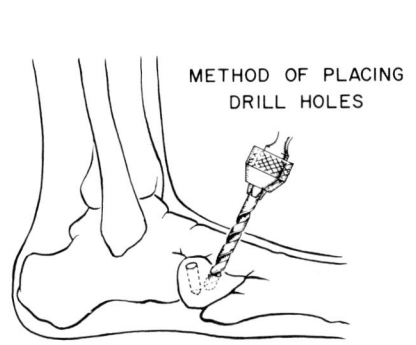
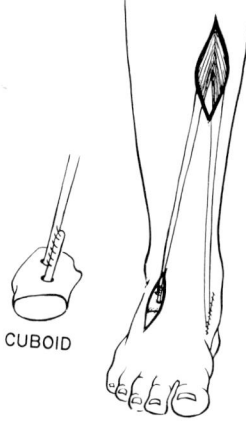

FIGURE 3–39. Split anterior tibial tendon transfer in the treatment of spastic varus hindfoot.

(From Hoffer, M. M., Reiswig, J. A., Garrett, M. M., and Perry, J.: The split anterior tibial tendon transfer in the treatment of spastic varus hindfoot in childhood. Orthop. Clin. N. Amer., 5:32, 1974. Reprinted by permission.)

don transfer is relatively simple (Fig. 3–39). A 5- to 7-cm.-long incision is made over the dorsomedial aspect of the foot, centered over the medial cuneiform. The anterior tibial tendon is identified and split into halves; the medial half is left anchored to the base of the first metatarsal. The lateral half of the tendon is sectioned, dissected free, and tagged with a whip suture. A second longitudinal incision, 7 cm. long, is made over the anterior aspect of the distal third of the leg, lateral to the crest of the tibia. With an Ober tendon passer the lateral half of the tendon is delivered to the proximal wound. A third longitudinal incision is made on the dorsolateral aspect of the foot, 5 cm. long and centered over the cuboid. The lateral half of the anterior tibial tendon is delivered into the third wound subcutaneously with an Ober tendon passer. With a 7/64-inch drill, two holes are made in the cuboid at converging angles. The holes are joined at their depth with a small curet. The dorsal roof of the cuboid should be preserved. The lateral half of the split anterior tibial tendon is passed through the hole and sutured to itself with the ankle in 5 to 10 degrees of dorsiflexion. The wounds are closed in the usual fashion and a below-knee cast is applied. Weight-bearing with the cast is permitted at two weeks; the cast is removed at six weeks. Immediately the patient is fitted with a dorsiflexion-assist ankle-foot orthosis, with the ankle joint at 5 degrees of dorsiflexion. Plastic splints are worn at night to hold the ankle in slight dorsiflexion. Active and passive exercises are performed to develop anterior tibial muscle function and to maintain range of ankle motion. Use of the ankle-foot orthosis during the daytime is usually discontinued at six months.

The split anterior tibial tendon transfer acts as a balanced yoke, and leaving its medial half attached to the base of the first metatarsal preserves its action as dorsiflexor of the first metatarsal. This author recommends split anterior tibial tendon transfer when the peroneus longus is functioning, as the action of the medial half of the anterior tibial tendon will counterbalance the plantar-flexing action of the peroneus longus and prevent the development of forefoot equinus (anterior cavus) deformity. The posterior tibial muscle, if contracted, can be fractionally lengthened at the same time. The procedure should not, however, be combined with simultaneous heel cord lengthening. It is best to stage the two operations to ensure success of the outcome.

Talipes Equinovalgus

Varying degrees of valgus deformity of the foot are commonly associated with contracture of the triceps surae because the height of the foot is reduced when the hindfoot is everted, and the tendo Achillis is relatively lengthened. The valgus deformity is severe when there is a dynamic muscle imbalance between the evertors and invertors of the foot, i.e., the peroneal muscles are spastic and strong, and the anterior and posterior tibial muscles are cerebral zero or weak.

In early childhood, management of valgus foot is approached conservatively. Supportive shoes with a Thomas heel, a 1/8- to 3/16-inch medial heel wedge, an extended medial heel counter, and a 3/8-inch longitudinal arch support are given. Gentle passive exercises to elongate the contracted triceps surae and peroneal muscles are performed several times a day. The hypotonic posterior tibial and anterior tibial muscles are strengthened by active exercise. Splints are worn at night to hold the ankle and foot in neutral position. In severe pes valgus UCBL (University of California Biomechanics Laboratory) shoe inserts are prescribed. If a dynamic orthosis is worn, a valgus corrective T-strap is added to it.

Surgical correction of equinus deformity, however, should not be long delayed, as fixed pes valgus may develop that may require extensive bony procedures for correction. A sliding heel cord lengthening is performed at the appropriate time. The distal portion of the tendo Achillis is sectioned in its lateral half to decrease the eversion pull of the triceps surae. This is combined with fractional lengthening of the peroneal muscles at their musculotendinous junction through a separate incision over the middle third of the fibula. In the postoperative period, a UCBL shoe insert is used to support the foot. Passive and active exercises are performed as already described.

Perry and Hoffer recommend lengthening of the peroneus longus or brevis when the muscles are active continuously throughout both the stance and swing phases of the gait cycle. On the other hand, if the peroneus brevis or longus is active only during the stance phase, they transfer the tendon of the hyperactive muscle posteromedially through the sheath of the tibialis posterior to the navicular. In two such transfers the muscle activity of the transferred peroneus brevis remained unchanged postoperatively.[113] This author has had no personal experience with posteromedial transfer of the peroneus longus or brevis in cerebral palsy.

By the time the child is eight to ten years of age, if the pes valgus persists and its severity is of such a degree that it interferes with shoe wear, balance, and locomotion, a subtalar extra-articular arthrodesis is performed. This will control the alignment of the foot and will help to avoid a triple arthrodesis later when growth is complete. The operative technique of extra-articular subtalar arthrodesis (Grice procedure) is described in Plate 15.

In the experience of this author, with early, preventive soft-tissue surgery, the alignment of the foot can be controlled in most cases, obviating the need for a Grice procedure.

Several end-result studies of the Grice extra-articular arthrodesis in cerebral palsy have appeared in the literature.* Banks and his colleagues reported long-term results of Grice subtalar arthrodesis in 72 valgus feet in 44 patients with cerebral palsy; the results were excellent in 43 feet, as shown in Figure 3-40, good in 15, fair in 8, and poor in 6 feet. Overcorrection and hindfoot varus deviation was the most significant complication; the heel varus deformity was minor in five feet and marked in three feet.[11] It is vital to determine the degree of correction by intraoperative roentgenograms before closure of the wound. Threaded Steinmann pins or cancellous bone screws should be used for internal fixation; they give the graft greater stability and allow immobilization of the limb with the foot in neutral position and the knee in extension to prevent hamstring contracture postoperatively. Similar results of Grice subtalar arthrodesis have been reported by the cited authors. It is well documented that the Grice procedure corrects valgus deformity of the hindfoot and restores the height of the longitudinal arch. When the graft is extra-articular it will interfere minimally with the growth of the foot. On the other hand, the Grice procedure does not correct fixed valgus or varus deformity of the mid- or forepart of the foot; it does not improve pes planus due to ligamentous relaxation and sagging of the talonavicular or naviculocuneiform joints. There are, also, drawbacks of which one should beware: the Grice arthrodesis does cause loss of lateral mobility of the hindfoot and may cause difficulty in walking on rough terrain; it also exerts excessive ligamentous strain on the ankle joint.

When performing a Grice extra-articular subtalar arthrodesis one should follow certain basic dicta rigidly:

1. Equinus deformity should be corrected first; failure to do this will result in fusion of the calcaneus to the talus with the heel in fixed equinus position and the foot in abduction and eversion. Upon weightbearing the talus will tilt into valgus position in the ankle mortise. Imperatively, one should determine preoperatively whether the calcaneus can be restored to its normal position beneath the talus; this is done by making lateral roentgenograms of the foot after it has been passively manipulated into an equinus position and inversion. When there is contracture of the triceps surae muscle, it is essential to make a lateral roentgenogram of the foot and ankle with the foot in inversion and the ankle in maximal forced dorsiflexion. Equinus deformity is corrected by heel cord lengthening, but the procedure should *not be combined* with the Grice procedure. Prolonged immobilization in a cast will cause marked atrophy of the triceps surae and result in calcaneus deformity. Stage the two operations. If it is impossible to place the calcaneus in a normal position beneath the talus, the Grice procedure should not be performed.

2. Always determine the stability of the body of the talus in the ankle mortise preoperatively by making weight-bearing stress roentgenograms of the ankle. Determine the level of the lateral malleolus in relation to the medial malleolus. Is there valgus deviation of the ankle? The distal fibular

Text continued on page 408

---

*See references 3, 11, 27–29, 36, 45, 62–64, 82, 86, 97, 109, 110, 122, 123, 134, 141.

Extra-Articular Arthrodesis of the Subtalar Joint (Grice Procedure)

THE PROCEDURE

A. A 2½-inch-long and slightly curved incision is made over the subtalar joint, centering over the sinus tarsi.

B. The incision is carried down to the sinus tarsi. The capsules of the posterior and anterior subtalar articulations are identified and left intact. The operation is extra-articular. If the capsule is opened inadvertently, it should be closed by interrupted sutures.

The periosteum on the talus corresponding to the lateral margin of the roof of the sinus tarsi is divided and reflected proximally. The fibrofatty tissue in the sinus tarsi with the periosteum of the calcaneus corresponding to the floor of the sinus tarsi and the tendinous origin of the short toe extensors from the calcaneus are elevated and reflected distally in one mass.

C. The remaining fatty and ligamentous tissue from the sinus tarsi is thoroughly removed with a sharp scalpel and curet.

Plate 15. Extra-Articular Arthrodesis of the Subtalar Joint (Grice Procedure)

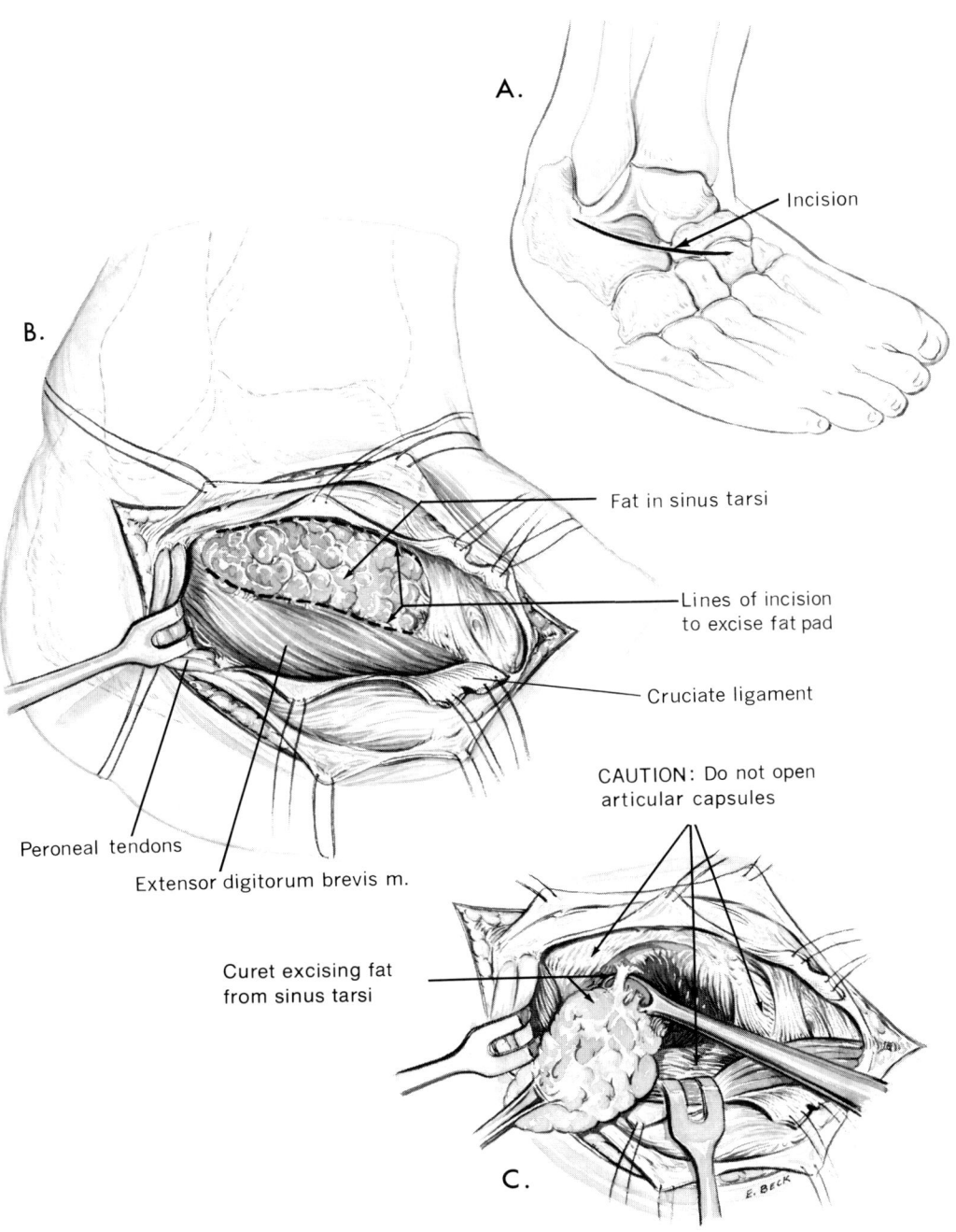

Extra-Articular Arthrodesis of the Subtalar Joint (Grice Procedure) (Continued)

D. Next the foot is manipulated into equinus position and inversion, rotating the calcaneus into its normal position beneath the talus and correcting the valgus deformity. Broad straight osteotomes of various sizes (¾ to 1¼ inches or more) are inserted into the sinus tarsi, blocking the subtalar joint and determining the length and optimum position of the bone graft and the stability that it will provide. The long axis of the graft should be parallel with that of the leg when the ankle is dorsiflexed into neutral position, and the hindfoot should be 5 degrees valgus or neutral, but never varus. Even a slight degree of varus deformity of the heel seems to increase with growth.

E. The optimum site of the bone graft bed is marked with the broad osteotome. With a dental osteotome, a thin layer of cortical bone (⅛ to 3/16 inch) is removed from the inferior surface of the talus (the roof of the sinus tarsi) and the superior surface of the calcaneus (the floor of the sinus tarsi) at the site marked for the bone graft. It is best to preserve the most lateral cortical margin of the graft bed to support the bone block and to prevent it from sinking into soft cancellous bone.

F. A bone graft of appropriate size can be taken from the anteromedial surface of the proximal tibial metaphysis as a single cortical graft that is then cut into two trapezoidal bone grafts with their cancellous surfaces facing each other. Lately the author prefers to use fibular bone grafts with the cortices intact. The corners of the base of the graft are removed with a rongeur so that it is trapezoidal in shape and can be countersunk into cancellous bone, preventing lateral displacement after operation.

The bone graft is placed in the prepared graft bed in the sinus tarsi while the foot is held in varus position. An impacter may be used to fix the cortices of the graft in place. The longitudinal axis of the graft should be parallel with the shaft of the tibia when the ankle is in neutral position.

With the foot held in the desired position, the distal soft-tissue pedicle of fibrofatty tissue of the sinus tarsi, the calcaneal periosteum, and the tendinous origin of the short toe extensors are sutured to the reflected periosteum from the talus. The subcutaneous tissue and skin are closed with interrupted sutures, and an above-knee cast is applied.

POSTOPERATIVE CARE

The cast is removed eight to ten weeks after operation. Roentgenograms are taken; if there is solid healing of the graft, gradual weight-bearing is allowed with the protection of crutches. Active and passive exercises are performed to strengthen the muscles and to increase the range of motion of the ankle and of the knee.

Plate 15. Extra-Articular Arthrodesis of the Subtalar Joint (Grice Procedure)

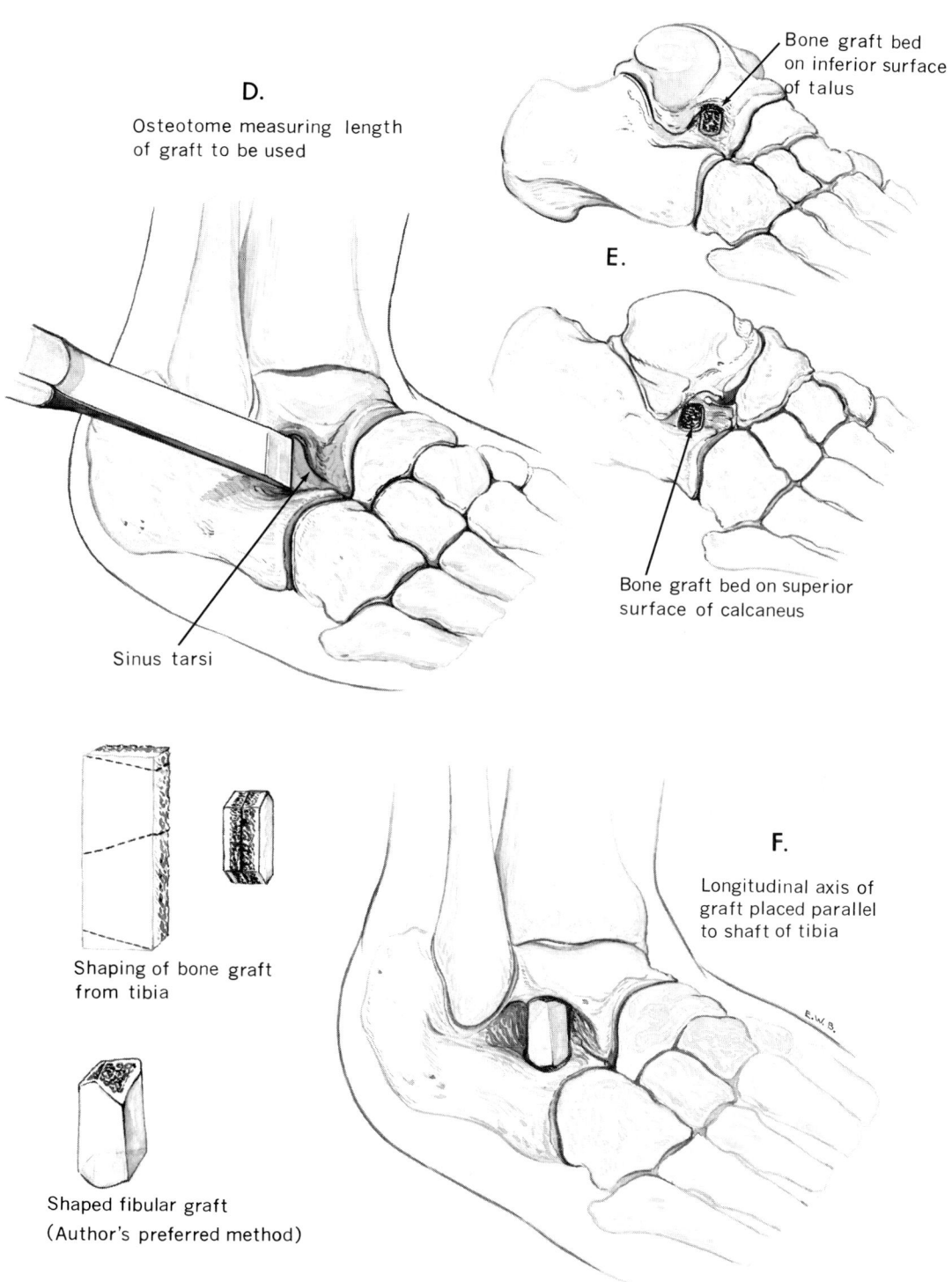

growth plate should be level with the ankle joint. In paralyzed limbs the fibula is frequently underdeveloped, the distal fibular epiphyseal plate being at the same level or at a more proximal one than that of the tibia.[99] Removal of a bone graft from the ipsilateral tibia will definitely accelerate growth of that bone and further increase the disparity in length between the fibula and tibia.[74, 109] It is better to use a fibular bone graft from the involved limb or an iliac bone graft if there is already a valgus deformity of the ankle.[36] The fibular bone graft should, however, be taken at the junction of the proximal and middle thirds of the shaft. The excised segment of the fibula should not be too long, and the periosteum should be meticulously closed to ensure union. When bilateral extra-articular subtalar arthrodesis is performed, an autogenous fibular bone graft should be taken from each leg. A common tendency is to take a long segment of the fibula from one leg to use for both feet; this, however, will result in nonunion of the fibula, a high-riding lateral malleolus, and valgus deformity of the ankle. When there is marked valgus deformity of the ankle it is corrected by calcaneofibular tenodesis in the child under eight years of age, and by supramalleolar osteotomy of the tibia in the older patient, as described in the section on myelomeningocele.

3. Avoid overcorrection and varus de-

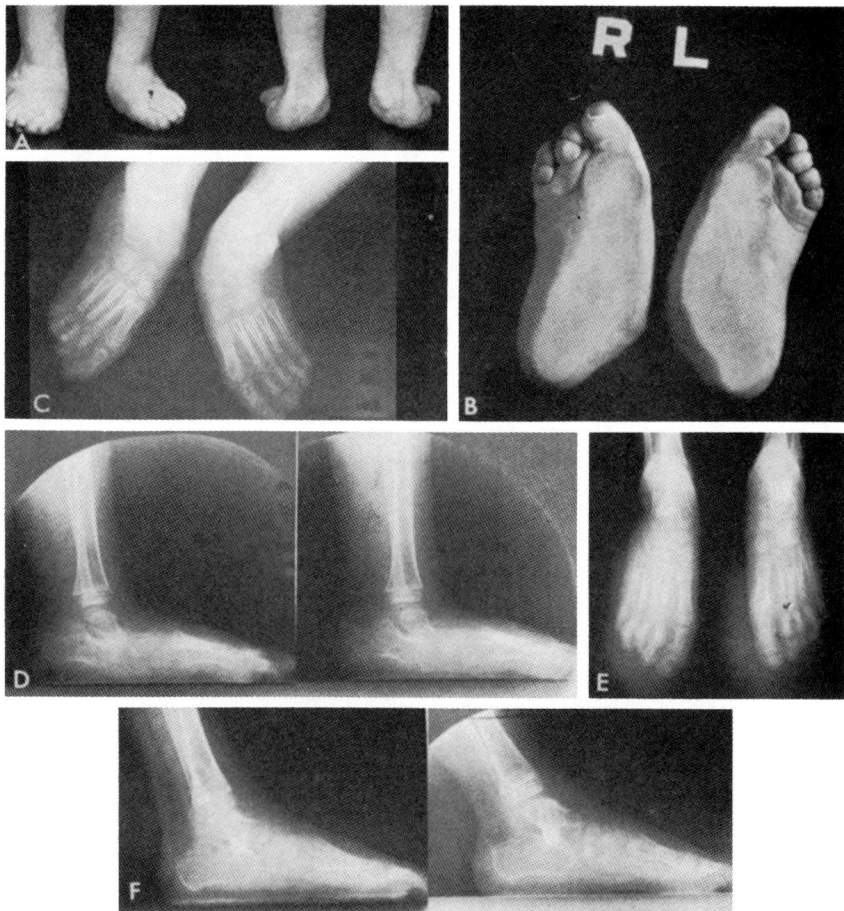

FIGURE 3–40. Equinovalgus deformity of the feet in spastic cerebral palsy.

A. Severe valgus foot deformities at age three years and three months. **B.** Plantar view of feet. **C** and **D.** Weight-bearing roentgenograms of feet preoperatively. **E** and **F.** Weight-bearing roentgenograms of feet eight months after bilateral heel cord lengthening and subtalar bone block arthrodesis. Note incorporation of talocalcaneal bone graft.

Illustration continued on opposite page

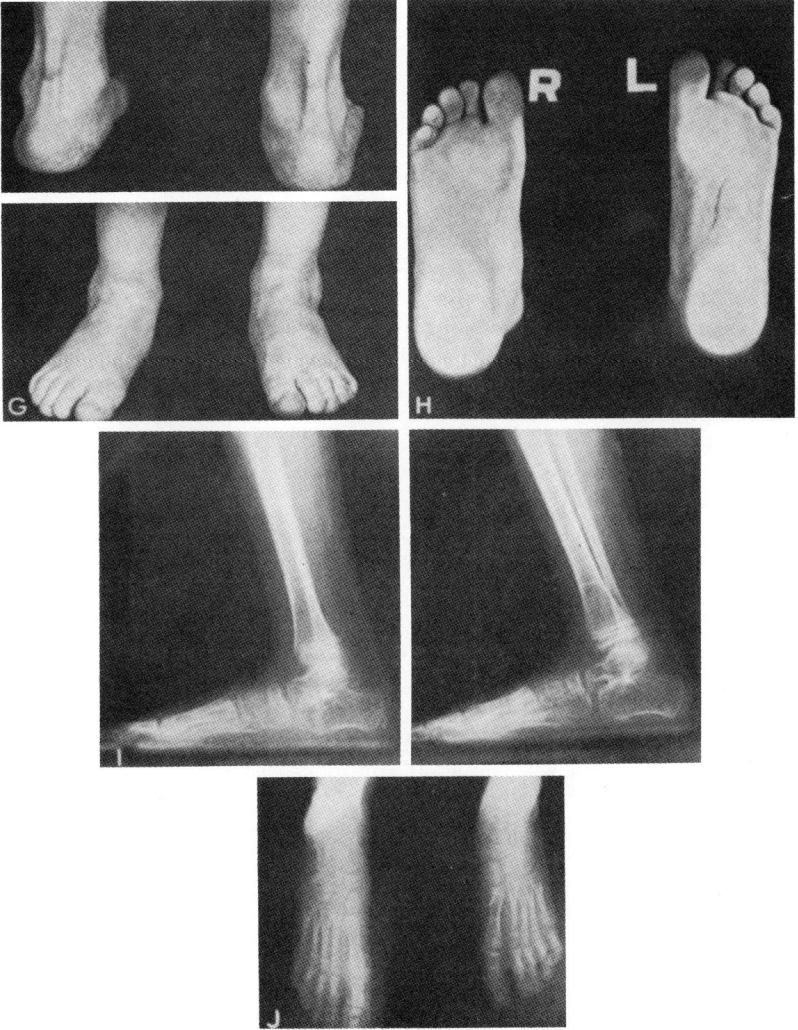

FIGURE 3–40 Continued. *Equinovalgus deformity of the feet in spastic cerebral palsy.*

G. Weight-bearing photographs of feet three years and six months postoperatively. H. Plantar weight-bearing views of feet three years and six months postoperatively. I and J. Weight-bearing roentgenograms three years and six months postoperatively. (From Banks, H., and Panagakos, P.: The role of the orthopedic surgeon in cerebral palsy. Pediat. Clin. N. Amer., *14*:495, 1967. Reprinted by permission.)

formity by taking intraoperative x-rays. After the graft is placed in the sinus tarsi, the position of the heel is carefully inspected clinically and on roentgenographic views. The hindfoot should never be fused in varus position.

4. Malposition or shifting of the bone graft in the sinus tarsi should be recognized and corrected in the operating room.

5. The dynamic balance of muscles that act on the foot should be restored, and contractural deformities should be corrected by appropriate musculotendinous lengthenings. Invertor-evertor muscle imbalance may cause recurrence of deformity in the growing foot. Overzealous correction should, however, be avoided.

6. Detect pseudarthrosis early. The bone graft may fail to unite to the talus or calcaneus, or pseudarthrosis may occur in the middle, or the entire bone graft may be resorbed. The incidence of pseudarthrosis has been greatly reduced by the use of autogenous fibular or iliac bone graft, rather than homologous bone bank bone; it will still develop in a certain percentage of

cases, however, and it is important that it be detected and revised or corrected—by insertion of another graft if necessary. Otherwise the correction will be lost and the os calcis will be united to the talus with the foot in fixed planovalgus position.

Batchelor modified the Grice extra-articular subtalar arthrodesis by inserting an autogenous fibular graft from the neck of the talus across the sinus tarsi into the calcaneus with the hind part of the foot held in neutral position. The subtalar joint is not exposed.[18, 134]

The technique of the operation is as follows: Under tourniquet hemostasis a 4-cm-long longitudinal incision is made over the dorsomedial aspect of the foot in line with and centered over the neck of the talus. (The tendency is to place the incision too far anteriorly.) The neck of the talus is exposed after it has been identified under image intensification. The calcaneus is inverted into neutral position or 5 degrees of valgus, but not varus, deviation. A smooth Steinmann pin is drilled through the body of the talus into the calcaneus, transfixing the subtalar joint. The pin also serves as a guide for the drill. Under image intensification control, a 9-mm drill is driven through the neck of the talus plantarward, posteriorly, and slightly laterally. As the electric drill passes through the inferior cortex of the talus one can feel the ease with which it traverses the sinus tarsi until it meets the resistance of the cortex of the superior surface of the calcaneus. Its position is checked under an image intensifier and, if it is correct, the drill is advanced for an additional 2 or 3 cm and then is withdrawn. Larger burrs are used if necessary, until the hole is large enough for the fibular graft. The fibular bone graft of desired length is taken from the junction of the proximal and middle thirds of the fibula. One end of the graft is trimmed to a point and is gently tapped through the hole made in the talus and calcaneus. The position of the graft is double-checked with anteroposterior and lateral roentgenograms of the foot. Inferiorly it should be well down into the calcaneus. Its superior surface should be flush with the superior surface of the neck of the talus; any excess bone is resected from the graft (Fig. 3–41). The Steinmann pin is removed, and the tourniquet is released. After complete hemostasis the wound is closed. A below-knee cast is applied and then is exchanged for a walking cast in two weeks. The total period of cast immobilization is eight weeks. Brown reported the results of the Batchelor extra-articular subtalar arthrodesis in 23 feet in 20 patients (9 of whom had cerebral palsy). Stability with survival of the graft was maintained in 17 patients for at least four years. Fracture of the graft occurred in two patients, both heavy boys 15 years old and over (Fig. 3–42). Brown does not advocate

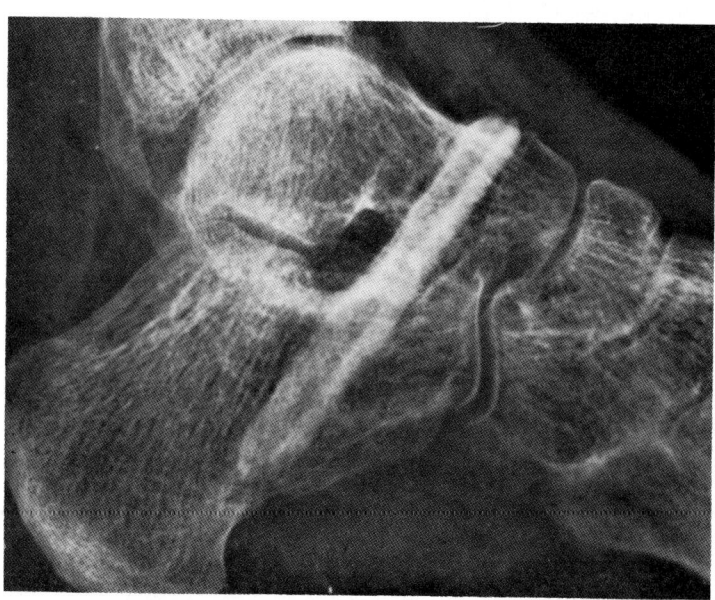

FIGURE 3–41. Batchelor subtalar extra-articular arthrodesis.

Note a fibular bone graft is inserted from the neck of the talus across the sinus tarsi into the calcaneus with the hindpart of the foot held in neutral position. The sinus tarsi is not opened. (From Brown, A.: A simple method of fusion of the subtalar joint in children. J. Bone Joint Surg., *50-B*:370, 1968. Reprinted by permission.)

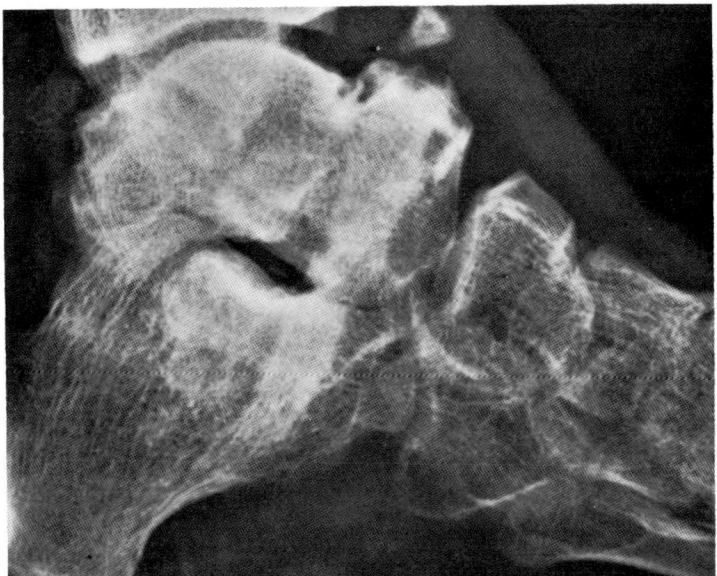

FIGURE 3–42. *Fracture of the fibular bone graft in Batchelor extra-articular subtalar arthrodesis.*

(From Brown, A.: A simple method of fusion of the subtalar joint in children. J. Bone Joint Surg., 50-B:370, 1968. Reprinted by permission.)

the procedure for patients over the age of 11 or 12 years.[29]

Seymour and Evans presented the results in 27 feet in 16 patients (5 had cerebral palsy and 10 had myelomeningocele). Follow-up periods ranged from 9 to 20 months. Avascular necrosis of the talus did not develop in any case. In two of the five cerebral palsy patients the pes valgus persisted. In the myelomeningocele group there were three failures. In one patient both grafts broke down. Seymour and Evans accord the Batchelor procedure two advantages over the Grice operation. First is the simplicity of insertion and retention of the graft with the Batchelor technique. In the Grice procedure insertion and retention of the graft in the sinus tarsi may be difficult, necessitating its placement under some compression, which may lead to overcorrection. Second, the fixation of the foot after insertion of the graft is stable and firm, permitting tendon transfers without fear of loss of alignment of the subtalar joint.[134]

Hsu, Yau, O'Brien and Hodgson studied valgus deformity of the ankle resulting from fibular resection for a graft in Batchelor-type subtalar fusion in children, of whom 30 had poliomyelitis, and 2 had cerebral palsy. They divided the patients into two groups: Group A, whose grafts were taken from the lower third of the fibula (28 legs in 25 patients), and Group B, whose grafts were taken from the middle third of the fibula (9 legs in 7 patients). In Group A, 20 of the 28 fibulae failed to regenerate fully, and fibular pseudarthrosis resulted; in 16 of these cases there was definite upward migration of the distal epiphysis of the fibula in relation to the tibia. In group B, eight of the nine legs showed regeneration of the fibula, and seven of these had no disturbance of the ankle mortise. It appears the blood supply of the fibula and its periosteum is an important consideration. Because of the subcutaneous location of the lower third of the fibula, blood supply of the periosteum comes primarily from the nutrient artery and not from the adjacent muscle arteries. When a segment of the fibula is resected from its lower third, the main blood supply of the periosteum is disrupted; hence the bone fails to regenerate to fill the defect. On the other hand, the middle third of the fibula is surrounded by muscle origins and is richly endowed with muscular and periosteal vascular anastomoses, making its regeneration more likely after removal of the fibular segment and interruption of the nutrient arterial blood supply.[74]

The experience of this author with the Batchelor technique of subtalar fusion is limited. Problems with fractures of the graft with its potential for causing upward migration of the distal fibular epiphysis and development of a valgus ankle outweigh the "simplicity" of the operation. The Grice operation is, therefore, recommended over the Batchelor technique for extra-articular arthrodesis of the subtalar joints in children. Dennyson and Fulford modified the Batchelor operation by using a metal screw instead of a bone peg for internal fixation of the subtalar joint and a cancellous graft instead of cortical bone to stimulate union.[45]

CALCANEAL OSTEOTOMY TO CORRECT HINDFOOT VALGUS DEFORMITY

Dwyer's open-up lateral osteotomy of the calcaneus with insertion of a tibial bone graft has been used by Silver and Simon for correction of hindfoot valgus deviation. They reported the results in 73 feet in 42 patients (bilateral deformities in 31 and unilateral deformity in 11). In 61 operations homogenous autoclaved tibial bone was used for the graft; the homogenous bone appeared to be as satisfactory as autogenous bone. The results in 56 feet were good (neutral position of hindfoot), in 7 fair (mild residual valgus deformity), and in 6 poor. In the poor category there were four feet in which overcorrection produced varus deformity requiring subsequent calcaneal wedge osteotomies, and in two feet there was recurrence of marked valgus deformity requiring repeat calcaneal osteotomy with homogenous bone grafts and Achilles tendon lengthening; "in retrospect the Achilles tendon lengthenings should have been done during the first operation." According to Silver, Simon, and Litchman, the advantage of calcaneal osteotomy is that it improves the weight-bearing alignment of the foot and retains approximately 50 per cent of subtalar motion. The flexibility imparted by the subtalar motion decreases the stress on the midtarsal joints and the foot, making possible better locomotion on uneven terrain.[138]

It appears to this author that Dwyer's calcaneal osteotomy creates a compensatory deformity to mask the primary site of the deformity above, i.e., at the talocalcaneonavicular joint. He strongly recommends that soft-tissue procedures (tendo Achillis and peroneal lengthening) be performed first, that postoperatively the feet be supported by UCBL shoe inserts, and that a meticulous exercise program be carried out to restore function and dynamic balance of muscles controlling the foot and ankle. Then weight-bearing roentgenograms of the feet are carefully studied; if the anteroposterior talocalcaneal angle is markedly divergent (i.e., greater than 25 degrees) and the *talus is plantar-flexed,* Dwyer's calcaneal osteotomy should not be performed. The site of deformity is the subtalar joint, and it should be stabilized by Grice subtalar extra-articular arthrodesis.

Horizontal osteotomy through the base of the posterior articular process of the calcaneus with lateral wedge grafts was used by Baker to correct hindfoot valgus deviation (Fig. 3–43). It provides normal contact between the talar and calcaneal articular surfaces, restores normal talocalcaneal alignment, and places the sustentaculum tali under the talus to provide support for the talus. The hindfoot pronation is corrected without interfering with subtalar motion. It does not create a bone block. The results in 31 feet treated by this osteotomy with an average follow-up observation of two years were as follows: in 21 feet the alignment was satisfactory, in 8 feet there was persistent mild valgus deformity, and in 2 feet there was moderate varus deformity.[4]

The operation is performed through a 5- to 7-cm. longitudinal incision over the sinus tarsi. The subcutaneous tissues are divided in line with the skin incision. The contents of the sinus tarsi are not cleaned out. The peroneal tendons and fibular collateral ligaments are identified and retracted posteriorly with a blunt dissector. Adequate exposure is provided thereby. The calcaneus is supported during the osteotomy. The line and depth of osteotomy is determined by lateral roentgenograms of the foot with two Kirschner wires inserted parallel to the posterior talocalcaneal joint. With a sharp, thin osteotome or oscillating saw an osteotomy through the base of the posterior articular process of the calcaneus is performed through the *horizontal plane*. Do not enter the subtalar joint! The osteotomy extends to, but not through, the medial cortex, which should be preserved as a hinge. Next, osteotomes of different width (1 to 2 cm.) are inserted into the osteotomy site to determine the width of the bone graft. Anteroposterior roentgenograms of the foot are made with the osteotome in place to check

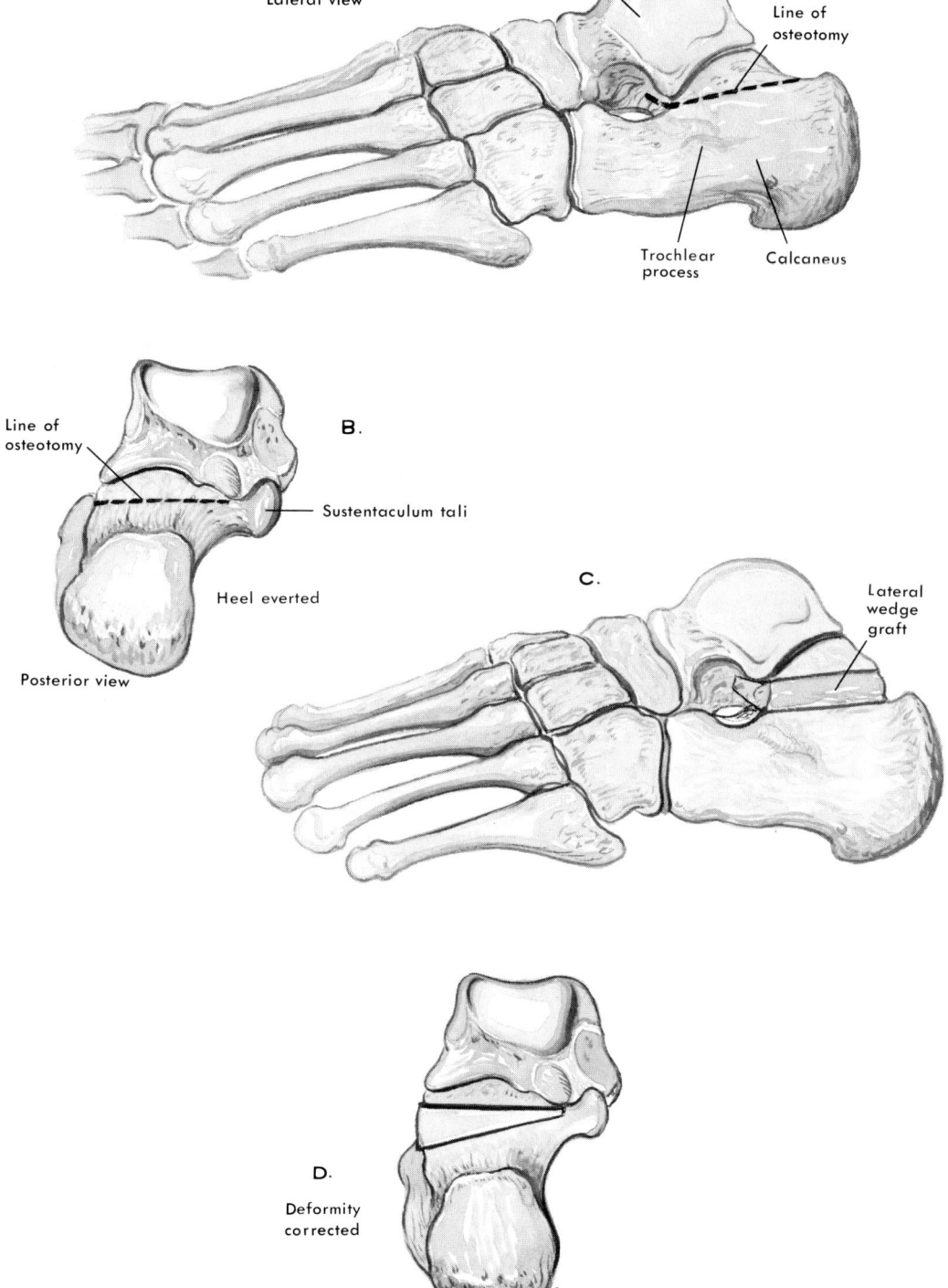

FIGURE 3–43. Horizontal osteotomy through the base of the posterior articular process of the calcaneus with lateral wedge graft.

the restoration of normal alignment between the talus and calcaneus. The anteroposterior talocalcaneal angle should be 15 degrees. Autogenous bone wedges of correct width are then taken from the ilium and inserted into the osteotomy site. The wedges are based laterally. The osteotomized segments are fixed internally with a threaded Steinmann pin. Overcorrection should be avoided. The dorsoplantar roentgenogram of the foot is repeated, and the anteroposterior talocalcaneal angle is measured; it should be 15 degrees. The wounds are closed, and an above-knee cast is applied. The Steinmann pin is removed at six weeks, and the total period of immobilization is two months. This author recommends medial displacement osteotomy of the os calcis instead of Baker's horizontal osteotomy; it is as effective and is simpler, and bone grafting is not required.

Triple arthrodesis is indicated to relieve symptoms and to correct the deformity of severe valgus deviation in the skeletally mature foot that is painful, fixed by osseous deformation, and causing serious problems in shoe wear and fitting.

Pes Calcaneus

Overlengthening of the tendo Achillis will result in calcaneus deformity of the foot and ankle (Fig. 3–44). Another cause is lengthening of a triceps surae muscle whose motor strength is fair or less. When the hips and knees have significant flexion deformity, the feet are forced into dorsiflexion,

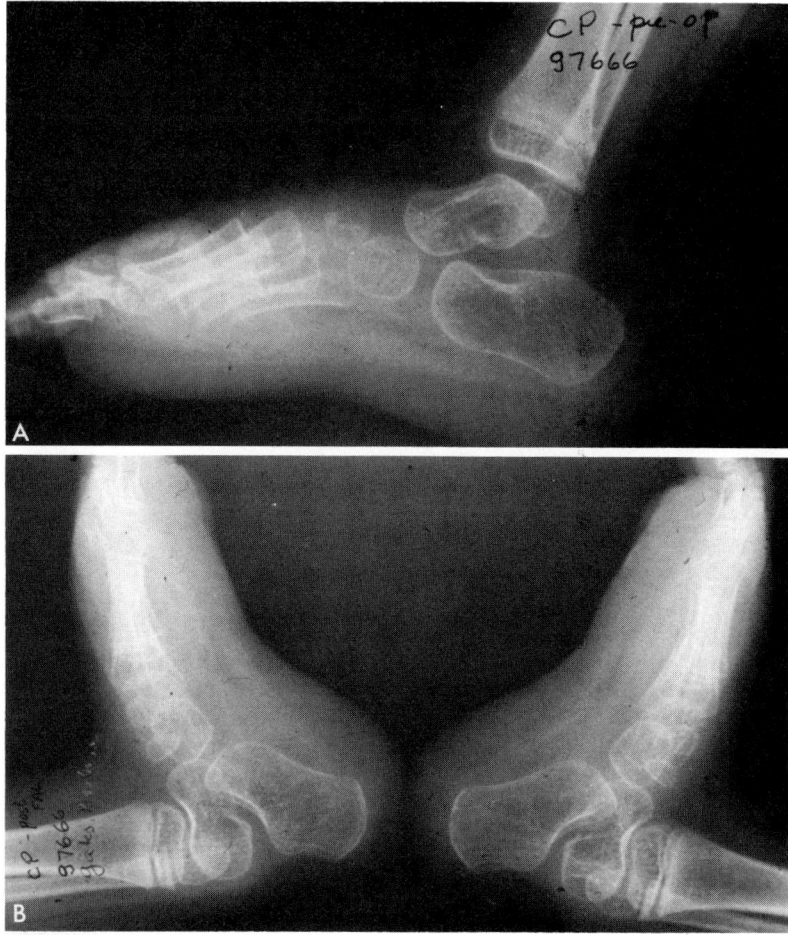

FIGURE 3–44. Calcaneus deformity of ankle and foot caused by overlengthening of heel cord in spastic cerebral palsy.

A. Preoperative lateral roentgenogram. **B**. Lateral roentgenogram of the ankles and feet two years after excessive heel cord lengthening.

and calcaneus deformity will develop. With weakness of the triceps surae the fibula will fail to develop and will be short in relation to the tibia; the lateral malleolus will be elevated, and the ankle mortise will assume a valgus tilt. Functionally, calcaneus deformity of the ankle is more disabling than equinus deformity.

Pes calcaneus can be prevented if certain basic dicta are followed: (1) Correct hip flexion deformity first, and then at a later stage lengthen the Achilles tendon; (2) lengthen the triceps surae *only* when its motor strength is normal or good; (3) do not overlengthen the tendo Achillis; and (4) provide meticulous postoperative care as outlined in the section on Achilles tendon lengthening.

Initially, treatment of calcaneus deformity is conservative: splinting at night with the ankles in plantar flexion, passive and active exercises to elongate shortened ankle dorsiflexors and strengthen weak plantarflexors, and protection of the ankles with orthoses that prevent dorsiflexion beyond neutral position. The knees should be supported so that they do not flex in stance and gait. The hip flexors should be elongated by passive exercises. The gluteus maximus should be strengthened by active exercises and pelvic tilt. Sleeping prone is of great help.

Surgical correction is indicated in the severe, persistent case. The author recommends splitting the tendo Achillis and suturing the lateral half or two thirds of it to the distal fibular metaphysis. Additional Mersilene strips are used to reinforce the tenodesis.

Deformities of the Forefoot and Toes

Metatarsus varus may be congenital, postural, or spastic in type. The congenital type is treated by manipulation and cast, whereas the postural type will correct itself spontaneously or respond to passive manipulation alone. The spastic metatarsus varus is usually associated with hallux varus and is caused by hyperactivity of the abductor hallucis. It is treated conservatively by manipulation and splinting; if conservative measures fail the abductor hallucis is lengthened fractionally at its musculotendinous junction. When the hallux is in normal position or slightly valgus, it is best to release the abductor hallucis muscle at its origin.

Hallux valgus is caused by spasticity and contracture of the adductor hallucis. This is treated by sectioning of the adductor hallucis tendon near its insertion on the lateral side of the base of the proximal phalanx of the great toe. If it is associated with significant metatarsus primus varus, osteotomy of the base of the first metatarsal may be indicated.

Hammer or mallet toe in spastic cerebral palsy is usually caused by hyperactivity of either the long or short toe flexors or both. If it does not respond to passive elongation exercises, proper shoes, and metatarsal support, it is treated by fractional lengthening of the long toe flexors in the distal part of the leg or sectioning of the short toe flexors. Severe fixed hammer toes require transfer of the long toe extensors to the metatarsal necks and fusion of the proximal interphalangeal joints. Neurectomy of the motor branches of the plantar nerves to intrinsic muscles of the foot is not recommended.

References

1. Baker, L. D.: Triceps surae syndrome in cerebral palsy. Surgery, 68:216, 1954.
2. Baker, L. D.: A rational approach to the surgical needs of the cerebral palsy patient. J. Bone Joint Surg., 38A:313, 1956.
3. Baker, L. D., and Dodelin, R. A.: Extra-articular arthrodesis of the subtalar joint (Grice procedure): Results in seventeen patients with cerebral palsy. J.A.M.A., 168:1005, 1958.
4. Baker, L. D., and Hill, L. M.: Foot alignment in the cerebral palsy patient. J. Bone Joint Surg., 46-A:1, 1964.
5. Balf, C. L., and Ingram, T. T. S.: Problems in the classification of cerebral palsy. Brit. Med. J., 2:163, 1955.
6. Banks, H. H.: The foot and ankle in cerebral palsy. In Samilson, R. L. (ed.): Orthopedic Aspects of Cerebral Palsy. Spastics International Medical Publication. Philadelphia, J. B. Lippincott Co., 1975, p. 195.
7. Banks, H. H.: The management of spastic deformities of the foot and ankle. Clin. Orthop., 122:70, 1977.
8. Banks, H. H., and Green, W. T.: The correction of equinus deformity in cerebral palsy. J. Bone Joint Surg., 40-A:1359, 1958.
9. Banks, H. H., and Panagakos, P.: Orthopaedic evaluation of the lower extremity in cerebral palsy. Clin. Orthop., 47:117, 1966.
10. Banks, H., and Panagakos, P.: The role of the orthopedic surgeon in cerebral palsy. Pediat. Clin. N. Amer. 14:495, 1967.
11. Banks, H. H., Panagakos, P., and Green, W. T.: The correction of severe foot valgus in cerebral palsy. J. Bone Joint Surg., 50-A:1479, 1968.
12. Barbieri, E., and Garcia, M.: Osservazioni sulla terapia chirurgica del piede spastico. Minerva Orthop., 21:639, 1970.
13. Barnett, H. E.: Orthopedic surgery in cerebral palsy. J.A.M.A., 150:1396, 1952.

14. Baron, M.: La chirurgie de l'infirmité motrice cérébrale chez l'enfant. Le pied. Rev. Chir. Orthop., 53:739, 1967.
15. Bassett, F. H.: The foot in cerebral palsy. In Giannestras, N. J.: Foot Disorders. Medical and Surgical Management. Philadelphia, Lea & Febiger, 1967, pp. 247–265.
16. Bassett, F. H., III: Cerebral palsy. Part II: Deformities of the feet due to cerebral palsy. A.A.O.S. Instr. Course Lect., 20:35, 1971.
17. Bassett, F. H., III, and Baker, D.: Equinus deformity in cerebral palsy. In Adams, J. P. (ed.): Current Practice in Orthopedic Surgery. Vol. 3. St. Louis, C. V. Mosby Co., 1966, p. 59.
18. Batchelor, J. S.: Personal communication to Seymour, R.
19. Berman, A., and Gartland, J. J.: Metatarsal osteotomy for the correction of adduction of the forepart of the foot in children. J. Bone Joint Surg., 53-A:498, 1971.
20. Bisla, R. S., Louis, H. J., and Albano, P. S.: Transfer of tibialis posterior tendon in cerebral palsy. J. Bone Joint Surg., 58-A:497, 1976.
21. Bleck, E. E.: Spastic abductor hallucis. Develop. Med. Child Neurol., 9:602, 1967.
22. Bleck, E. E.: Postural and gait abnormalities caused by hip flexion deformity in spastic cerebral palsy. J. Bone Joint Surg., 53-A:1468, 1971.
22a. Bleck, E. E.: Orthopedic Management of Cerebral Palsy. Philadelphia, W. B. Saunders Co., 1979.
23. Bobath, K., and Bobath, B.: Control of motor function in the treatment of cerebral palsy. Physiotherapy, 43:295, 1957.
24. Bobath, K., and Bobath, B.: The facilitation of normal postural reactions and movements in the treatment of cerebral palsy. Physiotherapy, 50:246, 1964.
25. Bobath, K., and Bobath, B.: The treatment of spastic paralysis by the use of reflex inhibition. Brit. J. Phys. Med., 13:1, 1965.
26. Bobath, B., and Finnie, N.: Re-education of movement patterns in everyday life in the treatment of cerebral palsy. Occup. Ther., 21:23, 1958.
27. Bratberg, J. J., and Scheer, G. E.: Extra-articular arthrodesis of the subtalar joint. A clinical study and review. Clin. Orthop., 126:220, 1977.
28. Broms, J. D.: Sub-talar extra-articular arthrodesis-follow-up study. Clin. Orthop., 42:139, 1965.
29. Brown, A.: A simple method of fusion of the subtalar joint in children. J. Bone Joint Surg., 50-B:2, 369, 1968.
30. Burman, M. S.: Spastic intrinsic-muscle imbalance of the foot. J. Bone Joint Surg., 20:145, 1938.
31. Cahuzac, M.: L'enfant infirme moteur d'origine cérébrale. Paris, New York, Masson & Cie, 1977.
32. Cahuzac, M., Nichil, J., and Ousset, A.: Principes d'examen d'un infirme moteur cérébral. Rev. Chir. Orthop., 52:375, 1966.
33. Cahuzac, M., Claverie, P., Ollé, R., Mansat, C., Nichil, J., and Delpech, R.: Notre expérience de la chirurgie du pied chez l'enfant infirme moteur cérébral. Chirurgie, 98:680, 1972.
34. Campbell, J., and Ball, J.: Energetics of walking in cerebral palsy. Orthop. Clin. N. Amer., 9:374, 1978.
35. Chambers, E. F. S.: An operation for correction of flexible flat feet of adolescents. Western J Surg., 54:77, 1946.
36. Chigot, P. L., and Sananes, P.: Arthrodese de Grice: Indications nouvelles et variante technique. Rev. Chir. Orthop., 51:53, 1965.
37. Conrad, L., and Bleck, E. E.: Augmented auditory feed back in the treatment of equinus gait in children. Develop. Med. Child Neurol., 22:713, 1980.
38. Cozen, L.: Effect of lengthening the Achilles tendon on the strength of gastrocnemius-soleus musculature. Clin. Orthop., 49:179, 1966.
39. Craig, J. J., and Van Vuren, J.: The importance of gastrocnemius recession in the correction of equinus deformity in cerebral palsy. J. Bone Joint Surg., 58-B:84, 1976.
40. Crothers, B., and Paine, R. S.: The Natural History of Cerebral Palsy. Cambridge, Mass., Harvard University Press, 1959.
41. Dekel, S., and Weissman, S. L.: Osteotomy of the calcaneus and concomitant plantar stripping in children with talipes cavo-varus. J. Bone Joint Surg., 55-B:802, 1973.
42. Delpech, J. M.: Tenotomie du tendon d'Achille, Chirurgie Clinique de Montpellier, ou Observations et Reféxions Tirées des Travaux de Chirurgie Clinique de Cette École. Paris, Gabon, 1823.
43. Denhoff, E., and Robinault, I. P.: Cerebral Palsy and Related Disorders. A Developmental Approach to Dysfunction. New York, McGraw-Hill Book Co., 1960.
44. Denny-Brown, E.: The Basal Ganglia and Their Relation to Disorders of Movement. London, Oxford University Press, 1962.
45. Dennyson, W. G., and Fulford, G. E.: Subtalar arthrodesis by cancellous grafts and metallic internal fixation. J. Bone Joint Surg., 58-B:507, 1976.
46. Desbrosses, J., and Stagnara, P.: Grice's operation. Rev. Chir. Orthop., 54:791, 1968.
47. Dimeglio, A., Pous, J. G., and Florensa, G.: La chirurgie du membre inférieur de l'infirme moteur cérébral. Du rééducateur au chirurgien. In Simon, L. (ed.): Actualités en Rééducation Fonctionelle et Réadaptation. Paris, New York, Masson & Cie, 1976, pp. 120–127.
48. Duncan, W. R.: Tonic reflexes of the foot. J. Bone Joint Surg., 42-A:859, 1960.
49. Dwyer, F. C.: Osteotomy of the calcaneum in the treatment of grossly everted feet with special reference to cerebral palsy. Proceedings of the 8th Congress of Orthopedic Surgeons and Trauma, New York, September, 1960. Brussels, Imprimerie Médicale et Scientifique, 1960.
50. Dwyer, F. C.: The treatment of relapsed club foot by the insertion of a wedge into the calcaneum. J. Bone Joint Surg., 45-B:67, 1963.
51. Estève, R.: Un procédé d' équilibration des pieds spastique. La Vie Medicale 1: Janvier: 51, 1970.
52. Evans, E. B.: The status of surgery of the lower extremities in cerebral palsy. Clin. Orthop., 47:127, 1966.
53. Eyring, E. J., Earl, W. C., and Brockmeyer, J. F.: Posterior tibial tendon transfers in neuromuscular conditions other than anterior poliomyelitis. Arch. Phys. Med., 55:124, 1974.
54. Fay, T.: The use of pathological and unlocking reflexes in rehabilitation of spastics. Amer. J. Phys. Med., 33:347, 1954.
55. Fiorentino, M. R.: Reflex Testing Methods for Evaluating C.N.S. Development. Springfield, Ill., Charles C Thomas, 1973.
56. Fisher, R. L., and Shaffer, S. R.: An evaluation of calcaneal osteotomy in congenital clubfoot and other disorders. Clin. Orthop., 70:141, 1970.
57. Frost, H. M.: Surgical treatment of spastic equinus in cerebral palsy. Arch. Phys. Med., 52:270, 1971.
58. Galal, Z., and Said, M.: Anterior transposition of the tibialis posterior tendon in spastic equinus. A preliminary report. Egypt. Orthop. J., 6:209, 1971.
59. Gillette, H. E.: Kinesiology of cerebral palsy. Clin. Orthop., 47:31, 1966.
60. Goldner, J. L.: Cerebral palsy. Part I: General principle. A.A.O.S. Instr. Course Lect., 20:20, 1971.
61. Green, W. T., and McDermott, L. J.: Operative treatment of cerebral palsy of spastic type. J.A.M.A., 118:424, 1942.
62. Green, W. T., and Grice, D. S.: The surgical correction of the paralytic foot. A.A.O.S. Instr. Course Lect., 10:343, 1953.
62a. Green, N. E., Griffin, P. P., and Shiair, R.: Split posterior tibial tendon transfer in cerebral palsy. J. Bone Joint Surg., 65-A:748, 1983.
63. Grice, D. S.: Extra-articular arthrodesis of the subastragalar joint for correction of paralytic flat feet in children. J. Bone Joint Surg., 34-A:927, 1952.
64. Grice, D. S.: Further experience with extra-articular arthrodesis of the subtalar joint. J. Bone Joint Surg., 37-A:246, 1955.
65. Gritzka, T. L., Staheli, L. T., and Duncan, W. R.: Posterior tibial tendon transfer through the interosseous membrane to correct equinovarus deformity in cerebral palsy. Clin. Orthop., 89:201, 1972.
66. Gunsolus, P., Welsh, C., and Houser, C.: Equilibrium reactions in the feet of children with spastic cerebral palsy and of normal children. Develop. Med. Child. Neurol., 17:580, 1975.
67. Hagberg, B., Lemperg, R., and Lundberg, A.: Transposition av gastrocnemius-muskulaturen vid spastiska former av cerebral pares hos barn. Nord. Med., 79:685, 1968.
68. Hagberg, B., Sanner, G., and Steen, M.: The dysequilibrium syndrome in cerebral palsy. Clinical aspects and treatment. Acta Paediat. Scand., Suppl., 226:1, 1972.

69. Hodgen, J. T., and Frantz, C. H.: Subcutaneous tenotomy of the Achilles tendon. J. Bone Joint Surg., 20:419, 1938.
70. Hoffer, M. M.: Basic considerations and classifications of cerebral palsy. A.A.O.S. Instr. Course Lect., 25:96, 1976.
71. Hoffer, M. M., Reiswig, J. A., Garrett, M. M., and Perry, J.: The split anterior tibial tendon transfer in the treatment of spastic varus hindfoot in childhood. Orthop. Clin. N. Amer., 5:31, 1974.
72. Holt, K. S.: Assessment of Cerebral Palsy. London, Lloyd-Luke, 1965.
73. Hoover, G. H., and Frost, H. M.: Dynamic correction of spastic rocker-bottom foot. Clin. Orthop., 65:175, 1969.
74. Hsu, L. C., Yau, A. C., O'Brien, J. P., and Hodgson, A. R.: Valgus deformity in the ankle resulting from fibular resection for a graft in subtalar fusion in children. J. Bone Joint Surg., 54-A:585, 1972.
75. Hunt, J. C., and Brooks, A. L.: Subtalar extra-articular arthrodesis for correction of paralytic valgus deformity of the foot. J. Bone Joint Surg., 47-A:1310, 1965.
76. Illingworth, R.: Recent Advances in Cerebral Palsy. London, J. & A. Churchill, 1958.
77. Illingworth, R. S.: The Development of Infants and Young Children, Normal and Abnormal. 3rd Ed. Edinburgh, E. & S. Livingstone, Ltd., 1964.
78. Ingram, T. T. S.: Pediatric Aspects of Cerebral Palsy. Baltimore, Williams & Wilkins Co., 1964.
79. Jones, A. R.: William John Little. J. Bone Joint Surg., 31-B:123, 1949.
80. Jones, M. H.: Differential diagnosis and natural history of the cerebral palsied child. In Samilson, R. L. (ed.): Orthopaedic Aspects of Cerebral Palsy. Clinics in Developmental Medicine Vols. 52/53. Philadelphia, J. B. Lippincott Co., 1975, p. 5.
81. Kabat, H., and Knott, M.: Principles of neuromuscular reeducation. Phys. Ther. Rev., 28:197, 1948.
82. Keats, S.: Cerebral Palsy. Springfield, Ill., Charles C Thomas, 1965.
83. Keats, S.: Operative Orthopedics in Cerebral Palsy. Springfield, Ill., Charles C Thomas, 1970.
84. Keats, S.: Warning: Serious complications caused by the routine rerouting of the peroneus longus and brevis tendons in performing the Grice procedure in cerebral palsy (Abstract). J. Bone Joint Surg., 56-A:1304, 1974.
85. Keats, S.: Early preventive surgery in the modern management of the preschool child. Need a cerebral palsied child be a crippled child. Int. Surg., 57:398, 1977.
86. Keats, S., and Kouten, J.: Early surgical correction of the planovalgus foot in cerebral palsy. Extra-articular arthrodesis of the subtalar joint. Clin. Orthop., 61:223, 1968.
87. Kendall, P. H., and Robson, P.: Lower limb bracing in cerebral palsy. Clin. Orthop., 47:73, 1966.
88. Khalili, A. A., and Benton, J. G.: A physiologic approach to the evaluation and management of spasticity with procaine and phenol nerve block. Clin. Orthop., 47:97, 1966.
89. Knott, M., and Voss, E. E.: Proprioceptive Neuromuscular Facilitation. New York, Paul B. Hoeber (Harper Bros.), 1956.
90. Lemperg, R., Hagberg, B., and Lundberg, A.: Achilles tendoplasty for correction of equinus deformity in spastic syndromes of cerebral palsy. Acta Orthop. Scand., 40:507, 1969.
91. Levitt, S.: Physiotherapy in Cerebral Palsy. Springfield, Ill., Charles C Thomas, 1962.
92. Lindsley, D. B., Schreiner, L. H., and Magoun, H. W.: An electromyographic study of spasticity. In Payton, O. D., Hirst, S., and Newton, R. A. (eds.): Scientific Bases for Neurophysiologic Approaches to Therapeutic Exercise. Philadelphia, F. A. Davis Co., 1977, pp. 119–123.
93. Little, W. J.: The deformities of the human frame. Lancet, 1:5, 1843.
94. Little, W. J.: On the Nature and Treatment of Deformities of the Human Frame (with Notes and Additions). London, Longmans, 1853.
95. Little, W. J.: On the influence of abnormal parturition, difficult labours, premature birth and asphyxia neonatorum on the mental and physical condition of the child, especially in relation to deformities. Trans. Obstet. Soc. Lond., 3:293, 1862.
96. McCarroll, H. R., and Schwartzman, J. P.: Spastic paralysis and allied disorders. J. Bone Joint Surg., 25:747, 1943.
97. McElroy, D. K.: Stabilization of the foot in cerebral palsy. Clin. Orthop., 34:19, 1964.
98. Majestro, T. C., Ruda, R., and Frost, H. M.: Intramuscular lengthening of the posterior tibialis muscle. Clin. Orthop., 79:59, 1971.
99. Makin, M.: Tibiofibular relationship in paralyzed limbs. J. Bone Joint Surg., 47-B:500, 1965.
100. Martz, C. D.: Talipes equinus correction in cerebral palsy. J. Bone Joint Surg., 42-A:769, 1960.
101. Masse, P., Baron, P., Cahuzac, M., Lacheretz, M., Martin, C. H., Queneau, P., and Roullet, J.: La chirurgie de l'infirmité motrice cérébrale chez l'enfant. Rev. Chir. Orthop., 53:729, 1967.
102. Mimran, R.: Transplantation du jambier postérieur sur le dos du pied. Rev. Chir. Orthop., 52:681, 1966.
103. Minear, W. L.: A classification of cerebral palsy. Pediatrics, 18:841, 1956.
104. Mortens, J., Moller, H., and Salmonsen, L.: Early stabilizing operation for spastic talipes equino-valgus by Grice's extra-articular osteoplastic subtalar arthrodesis. Acta Orthop. Scand., 32:485, 1962.
105. Mullaferoze, P., and Vora, P. H.: Surgery in lower limbs in cerebral palsy. Develop. Med. Child Neurol., 14:45, 1972.
106. Ober, F. R.: Tendon transplantation in the lower extremity. New Eng. J. Med., 209:52, 1933.
107. Paine, R. S.: Neurological examination of infants and children. Pediat. Clin. N. Amer., 7:471, 1960.
108. Paine, R. S.: Cerebral palsy: Symptoms and signs of diagnostic and prognostic significance. In Adams, J. P. (ed.): Current Practice in Orthopedic Surgery. Vol. 3. St. Louis, C. V. Mosby Co., 1966, p. 39.
109. Paluska, D. J., and Blount, W. P.: Ankle valgus after the Grice subtalar stabilization. Clin. Orthop., 59:137, 1968.
110. Parsch, K.: Grice extra-articular arthrodesis (results, extensions in the range of indication). Z. Orthop., 111:457, 1973.
111. Perlstein, M. A., and Barnett, H. E.: Nature and recognition of cerebral palsy in infants. J.A.M.A., 148:1389, 1952.
112. Perry, J.: Kinesiology of lower extremity bracing. Clin. Orthop., 102:18, 1974.
113. Perry, J., and Hoffer, M. M.: Preoperative and postoperative dynamic electromyography as an aid in planning tendon transfers in children with cerebral palsy. J. Bone Joint Surg., 59-A:531, 1977.
114. Perry, J., Hoffer, M. M., Antonelli, D., Giovan, P., and Greenberg, R.: Gait analysis of the triceps surae in cerebral palsy. A preoperative and postoperative clinical and electromyographic study. J. Bone Joint Surg., 56-A:511, 1974.
115. Phelps, W. M.: Care and treatment of cerebral palsies. J.A.M.A., 111:4, 1938.
116. Phelps, W. M.: Treatment of cerebral palsies. Clinics, 2:981, 1943.
117. Phelps, W. M.: Classification of athetosis with special reference to the motor classification. Amer. J. Phys. Med., 35:24, 1956.
118. Phelps, W. M.: Complications of orthopedic surgery in the treatment of cerebral palsy. J. Bone Joint Surg., 41-A:440, 1959.
119. Phelps, W. M.: Complications of orthopedic surgery in the treatment of cerebral palsy. Clin. Orthop., 53:39, 1967.
120. Pierrot, A. H., and Murphy, O. B.: Heel cord advancement. A new approach to the spastic equinus deformity. Orthop. Clin. N. Amer., 5:117, 1974.
121. Pollock, G. A.: Surgical treatment of cerebral palsy. J. Bone Joint Surg., 44-B:68, 1962.
122. Pollock, J. H., and Carrell, B.: Subtalar extra-articular arthrodesis in the treatment of paralytic valgus deformities. A review of 112 procedures in 100 patients. J. Bone Joint Surg., 46-A:533, 1964.
123. Rogtveit, A.: Extra-articular subtalar arthrodesis. According to Green-Grice in flat feet. Acta Orthop. Scand., 34:367, 1964.
124. Rood, M. S.: Neurophysiologic reactions as a basis for physical therapy. Physiol. Rev., 34:444, 1954.
125. Root, L.: Functional testing of the posterior tibial muscle

in spastic paralysis. Develop. Med. Child Neurol., 12:592, 1970.
126. Root, L.: Tendon surgery on the feet of children with cerebral palsy. Develop. Med. Child Neurol., 18:671, 1976.
127. Root, L., and Wise, D.: Posterior tibial tendon transfers in cerebral palsy. Presented at the Annual Meeting of the American Academy of Cerebral Palsy. New York, N.Y., Nov. 29, 1971.
128. Rosenthal, R. K., Deutsch, S. D., Miller, W., Schumann, W., and Hall, J. E.: A fixed-ankle below-the-knee orthosis for the management of genu recurvatum in spastic cerebral palsy. J. Bone Joint Surg., 57-A:545, 1975.
129. Ruda, R., and Frost, H. M.: Cerebral palsy. Spastic varus and forefoot adductus, treated by intra-muscular posterior tibial tendon lengthening. Clin. Orthop., 79:61, 1971.
130. Samilson, R. L.: Tendon transfers in cerebral palsy. Editorial. J. Bone Joint Surg., 58-B:153, 1978.
131. Samilson, R. L., and Hoffer, M. M.: Problems and complications in orthopaedic management of cerebral palsy. In Samilson, R. L. (ed.): Orthopedic Aspects of Cerebral Palsy. Philadelphia, J. B. Lippincott Co., 1975, pp. 258–274.
132. Samilson, R. L., and Perry, J.: The orthopaedic assessment in cerebral palsy. In Samilson, R. L. (ed.): Orthopaedic Aspects of Cerebral Palsy. Philadelphia, J. B. Lippincott Co., 1975, pp. 35–70.
133. Schneider, M., and Balon, K.: Deformity of the foot following anterior transfer of the posterior tibial tendon and lengthening of the Achilles tendon for spastic equinovarus. Clin. Orthop., 125:133, 1977.
134. Seymour, N., and Evans, D. K.: A modification of the Grice subtalar arthrodesis. J. Bone Joint Surg., 50-B:372, 1958.
135. Sharrard, W. J. W., and Bernstein, S.: Equinus deformity in cerebral palsy. J. Bone Joint Surg., 54-B:272, 1972.
136. Silfverskiöld, N.: Reduction of the uncrossed two-joint muscles of the leg to one-joint muscles in spastic conditions. Acta Chir. Scand., 56:315, 1923–1924.
137. Silver, C. M., and Simon, S. D.: Gastrocnemius-muscle recession (Silfverskiöld operation) for spastic equinus deformity in cerebral palsy. J. Bone Joint Surg., 41-A:1021, 1959.
138. Silver, C. M., Simon, S. D., and Litchman, H. M.: Calcaneal osteotomy for valgus and varus deformities of the foot. Int. Surg., 58:24, 1973.
139. Simon, S. R., Deutsch, S. D., Nuzzo, R. M., Mansour, M. J., Jackson, J. L., Koskinen, M., and Rosenthal, R. K.: Genu recurvatum in spastic cerebral palsy. J. Bone Joint Surg., 60-A:882, 1978.
140. Smith, J. B., and Westin, G. W.: Subtalar extra-articular arthrodesis. J. Bone Joint Surg., 50-A:1027, 1968.
141. Stahl, F.: Gastrocnemius recession. Acta. Orthop. Scand., 32:466, 1962.
142. Stamp, W. G.: Bracing in cerebral palsy. J. Bone Joint Surg., 44-A:1457, 1962.
143. Steindler, A.: Pathokinetics of cerebral palsy. A.A.O.S. Instr. Course Lect., 9:118, 1952.
144. Stöffel, A.: The treatment of spastic contractures. Amer. J. Orthop. Surg., 10:611, 1913.
145. Strayer, L. M., Jr.: Recession of the gastrocnemius, an operation to relieve spastic contracture of the calf muscles. J. Bone Joint Surg., 32-A:674, 1950.
146. Strayer, L. M., Jr.: Gastrocnemius recession. Five year report of cases. J. Bone Joint Surg., 40-A:1019, 1958.
147. Stromeyer, G. F.: Beiträgge zur operativen Orthopädik oder Erfahrungen über die subcutane Durchschneidung verkürzter Muskeln und deren Sehnen. Hanover, Helwing, 1838.
148. Sutherland, D. H., Schottstaedt, E. R., Larsen, L. J., Ashley, R. K., Callander, J. N., and James, P. M.: Clinical and electromyographic study of seven spastic children with internal rotation gait. J. Bone Joint Surg., 51-A:1070, 1969.
149. Swinyard, C. A.: Reflections about reflex therapy in cerebral palsy. Phys. Ther. Rev., 39:103, 1959.
150. Tardieu, G., Lespargot, A., and Tardieu, C.: To what extent is the tibia-calcaneum angle a reliable measurement of the triceps surae length? Radiological correction of the torque-angle curve (III). Eur. J. Appl. Physiol., 37:163, 1977.
151. Tardieu, C., Bret, M. D., Colbeau-Justin, P., and Huet de la Tour, E.: Relationship of triceps surae torques to photographed tibia-calcaneus angles in man. (II). Eur. J. Appl. Physiol., 37:153, 1977.
152. Tardieu, C., Colbeau-Justin, P., Bret, M. D.: Lespargot, A., Huet de la Tour, E., and Tardieu, G.: An apparatus and a method for measuring the relationship of triceps surae torques to tibio-tarsal angles in man. Eur. J. Appl. Physiol., 35:11, 1976.
153. Throop, F. B., DeRosa, G. P., Reeck, C., and Waterman, S.: Correction of equinus in cerebral palsy by the Murphy procedure of tendon calcaneus advancement: A preliminary communication. Develop. Med. Child Neurol., 17:182, 1975.
154. Tohen, A. Z., Carmona, J. P., and Barrera, J. R.: The utilization of abnormal reflexes in the treatment of spastic foot deformities. Clin. Orthop., 47:77, 1966.
155. Tönnis, D., and Rauterberg, E.: Ergebnisse der orthopädisch-chirurgischen Behandlung infantiler Cerebralparesen und die Indikation zur Operation. Arch. Orthop. Unfallchir., 62:29, 1967.
156. Turner, J. W., and Cooper, R. R.: Anterior transfer of the tibialis posterior through the interosseous membrane. Clin. Orthop., 83:241, 1972.
157. Twitchell, T. E.: The neurologic examination in infantile cerebral palsy. Develop. Med. Child Neurol., 5:271, 1963.
158. Vulpius, O., and Stöffel, A.: Orthopaedische Operationslehre. 2nd Ed. Stuttgart, Ferdinand Enke, 1920.
159. Watkins, M. B., Jones, R. B., Ryder, C. T., and Brown, T. H., Jr.: Transplantation of the posterior tibial tendon. J. Bone Joint Surg., 36-A:1181, 1954.
160. Wesely, M. S., and Barenfeld, P. A.: Mechanism of the Dwyer calcaneal osteotomy. Clin. Orthop., 70:137, 1970.
161. White, J. W.: Torsion of the Achilles tendon: Its surgical significance. Arch. Surg. (Chicago), 46:784, 1943.
162. Williams, P. F.: Restoration of muscle balance of the foot by transfer of the tibialis posterior. J. Bone Joint Surg., 58-B:217, 1976.
163. Woods, G.: Cerebral Palsy in Childhood. Bristol, John Wright & Sons, Ltd., 1957.
164. Zausmer, E.: Locomotion in cerebral palsy. Clin. Orthop., 47:49, 1966.

MYELOMENINGOCELE

Myelomeningocele is a developmental defect of the spinal column characterized by a failure of fusion between the vertebral arches, dysplasia of the spinal cord, and cystic distention and protrusion of the meninges. Nerve tissue is present within or adherent to the sac, and there is clinically demonstrable neurologic deficit caudal to the level of the lesion.

The incidence of myelomeningocele varies in different parts of the world. The regional and national differences are possibly due to the different genetic composition of the population and prevention of the deformity by antenatal diagnosis and genetic counseling.

Lorber reports that in Great Britain, where every year about one million babies are born, some 3,000 newborns are afflicted with myelomeningocele (3 per 1,000), and of these, 2,000 could be expected to survive if the best total surgical and medical care were available.[80]

The mortality rate is getting progressively lower with improvement of neurosurgical total care of these children, and an increasing number of them are surviving.

The incidence of myelomeningocele in the United States appears to be less. O'Hare, in a survey of nearly a million and a half births at teaching centers in the United States, reported an incidence of 1.22 per thousand.[103] In community surveys, Alter reports a rate of 1.05 per 1,000 live births in Charleston, South Carolina; and a similar rate is given by Wallace and associates in New York.[162] In Sweden, the incidence is 0.72 per 1,000 live births, and in Australia 0.95 per 1,000 births.[141a, 162]

Myelomeningocele is slightly more common in females than in males. The sex ratio of male to female is reported as 1:1.15 by Doran and Guthkelch, and as 1:1.17 by Record and McKeown.[22, 115]

The exact cause of myelomeningocele is unknown. The incidence, however, is significantly greater in the siblings of affected children than in the general population.[80]

In families already having one child with myelomeningocele, the chance of another afflicted child being born rises to 4 to 5 per cent, the risk of recurrence varying according to geographic area and genetic disposition of the population; in families with two affected children, it becomes much greater, the risk rising to 10 per cent, and after three children to 25 per cent. These figures stress the desirability of genetic counseling. Inheritance of myelomeningocele follows a multifactorial pattern with a threshold effect.[14a] It is not within the scope of this book to discuss its pathogenesis, pathology, and neurosurgical aspects. For these the reader is referred to the cited literature.*

Clinical Features

The external appearance of the meningeal sac and the local lesion is characteristic (Fig. 3–45). Assessment of the neurologic deficit and the adequacy of cerebrospinal circulation is carried out by the neurosurgeon; the genitourinary system is examined by the urologist. An intravenous pyelogram is imperative. The pediatrician will rule out the possibility of congenital heart disease, malformations of the gastrointestinal tract,

---

*See references 5, 6–9, 14, 40, 60, 65, 86, 140, 142, 166.

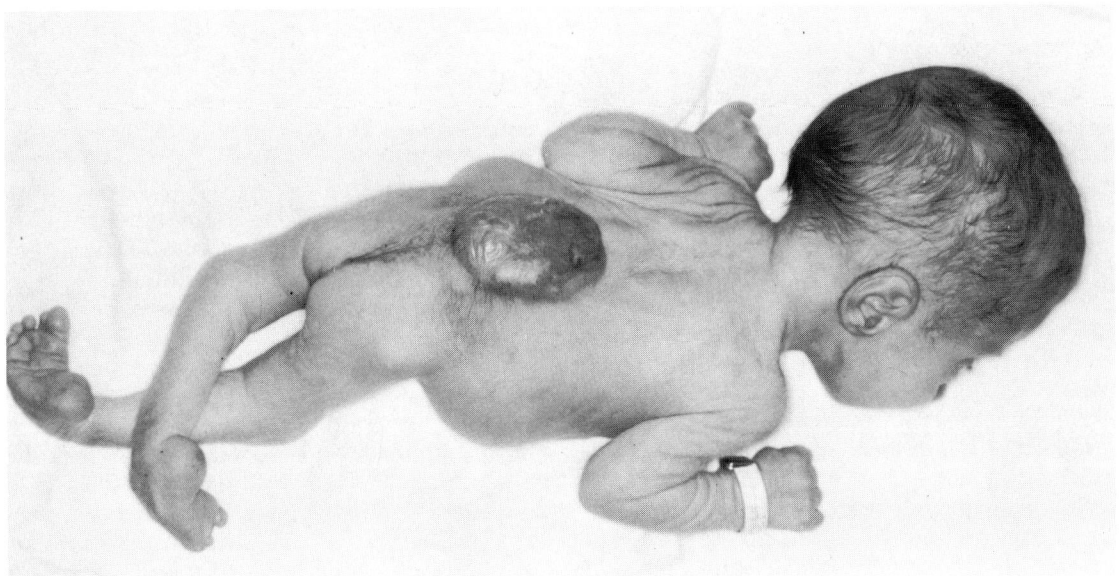

FIGURE 3–45. *Newborn infant with lumbosacral myelomeningocele.*

Note the severe equinovarus deformity of both feet.

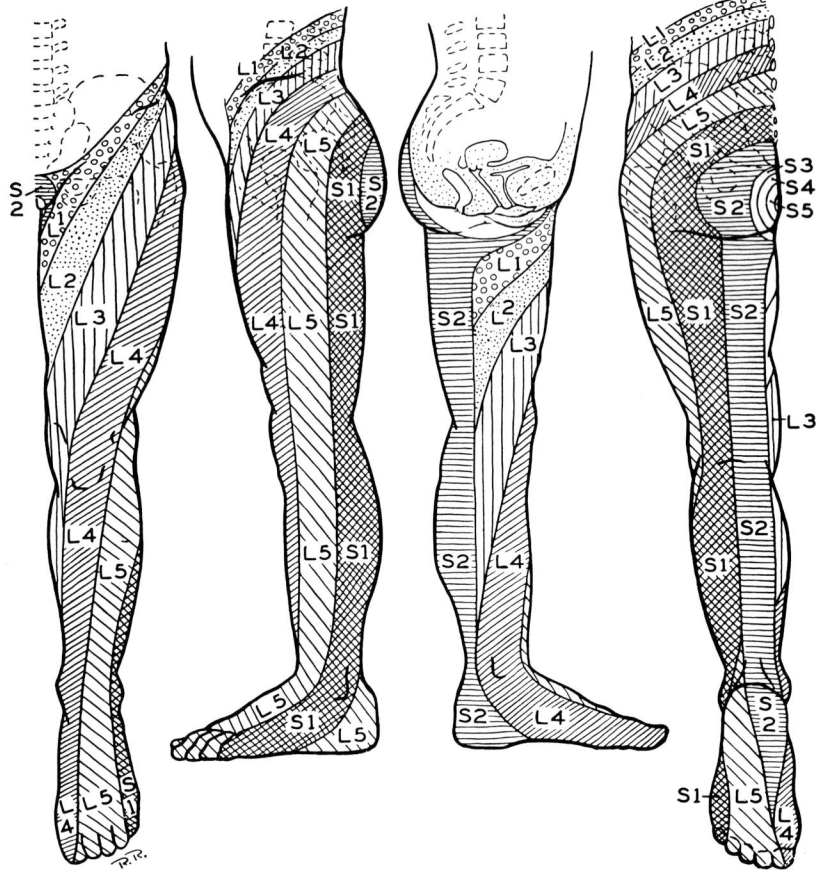

FIGURE 3–46. *The segmental innervation of cutaneous sensation of the lower limb.*

(From Keegan, J. J., and Garrett, F. D.: Segmental distribution of nerves in man. Anat. Rec., *102*:409, 1948. Reprinted by permission.)

cleft palate, and other general systemic affections. In the older child, the level of intelligence should be evaluated by a psychologist.

The orthopedic surgeon's role is to evaluate the musculoskeletal system.

The degree and distribution of paralysis should be noted. Repeated and careful muscle reflex and sensory examination will detect the segmental level of neurologic deficit.

In lumbosacral lesions, paralysis of the lower limbs is flaccid, whereas in cervicothoracic lesions, it is of the spastic type because of partial cord involvement. Paralysis may be partial or complete below a certain neurosegmental level, and function above that level may be normal. Asymmetry of involvement between the two lower limbs is noted. The upper limbs are examined for involvement.

The presence or absence of deep tendon reflexes and superficial skin reflexes is determined. In flaccid paralysis, there is total areflexia, whereas in spastic paralysis there are hyperactive deep tendon reflexes, ankle clonus, and extensor plantar response. Sensory function cannot be adequately evaluated in a newborn, but the examination should be attempted. The segmental innervation of cutaneous sensation in the lower limb is shown in Figure 3–46.

Motor strength of muscles is evaluated, both by observing active motions of the limbs and by using reflex stimulation techniques. Electromyographic studies may reveal muscle activity. Faradic current may be applied over nerve trunks and at motor points of muscles to stimulate muscle groups. The neurosegmental level of innervation of muscle groups is given in Figure 3–47; correlation between segmental inner-

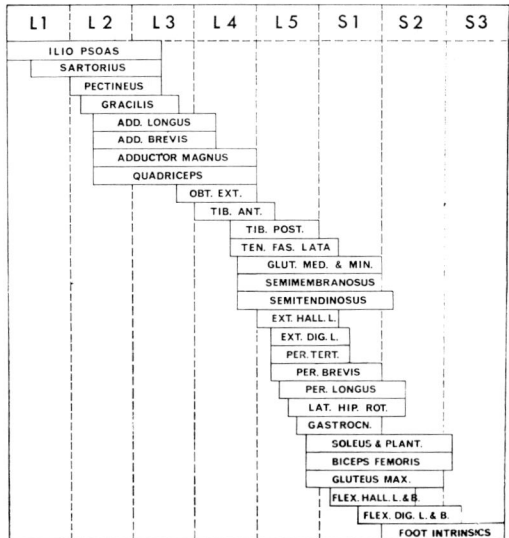

FIGURE 3–47. *Neurosegmental innervation of muscles of lower limb.*

(From Sharrard, W. J. W.: Posterior iliopsoas transplantation in the treatment of paralytic dislocation of the hip. J. Bone Joint Surg., *46-B*:427, 1964. Reprinted by permission.)

vation of reflexes, joint movement, and consequent deformities is shown in Figure 3–48.

General Principles of Treatment

The birth of an infant with myelomeningocele raises a serious ethical question, i.e., whether or not the child is to be treated. In the past there have been two possible avenues of approach: the child was treated and given every opportunity to live, or treatment was neglected and he was encouraged to die. Early closure of the sac with modern techniques of neonatal surgery has decreased the mortality rate, diminished the incidence of meningitis, and improved preservation of neurological function of the lower limbs. The newer methods of shunting for hydrocephalus have improved not only the number of survivors but the quality of their survival. These advances, however, have created tremendous problems for the family, for society, and for the child later in life.

In certain parts of the world the passport for life for the child with myelomeningocele is quadriceps function.[90] Lorber has proposed five adverse prognostic criteria that form a basis for selection; these are thoracolumbar lesions with severe paraplegia; gross enlargement of the head (at least 2 cm. above the ninetieth percentile, corrected for birth weight); severe kyphosis; major deformities of the musculoskeletal system; and associated gross congenital anomalies such as cardiac or urinary malformations. Lorber contends that selection is essential for the benefit of those affected—whether they are to receive treatment or no treatment—and in the interest of their families and the community.[82, 83] The ethical dilemma of whether to treat or not to treat the newborn infant with myelomeningocele has not yet been resolved in North America.[36, 39, 150]

In families with a history of previous

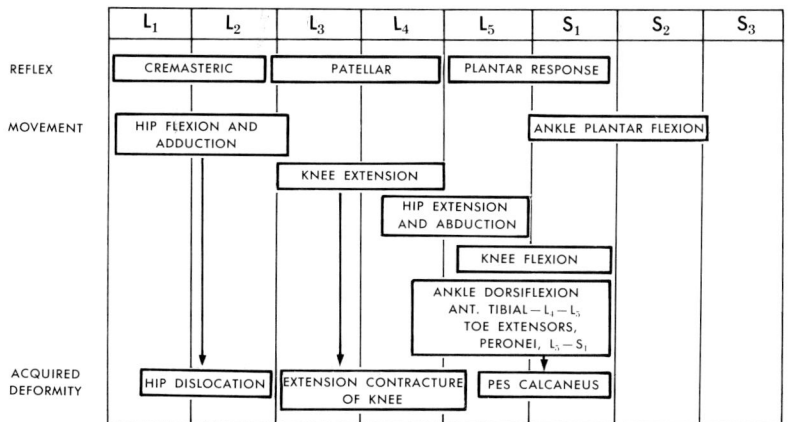

FIGURE 3–48. *Segmental innervation of reflexes, joint movement, and consequent deformities.*

congenital defects, especially myelomeningocele, antenatal diagnosis is advised. Sonar scanning of the fetal spine in longitudinal and transverse planes may detect, but cannot exclude, the presence of neural tube defects; however, anencephaly can be definitely demonstrated. Amniocentesis may reveal either the presence of sloughed epithelial cells (indicating an open ectodermal defect such as myelodysplasia) or the presence of an elevated level of alpha-fetoprotein, which suggests communication between the amniotic fluid and the cerebrospinal fluid spaces of the embryo. By combining ultrasound and amniocentesis, one can expect to detect open neural tube defects in 80 to 90 per cent of the fetuses.[118a] Fiberoptic uteroscopy will visualize the embryo and confirm or rule out the presence of a central nervous system defect. Therapeutic abortion, if acceptable to the family and the treating physician, may be performed as prophylactic therapy.[31, 34, 99, 121]

The infant with myelomeningocele has many handicaps, each dysfunction and deformity requiring the frequent attention of many medical and surgical specialists. For the average family, such care, when it involves visits to separate clinics, is prohibitively costly in time as well as money. On the other hand, the vision of a single physician can be myopic, his attention being directed to only one phase of therapy. Furthermore, frequent interdisciplinary consultation is essential to adequate comprehensive care of the child with myelomeningocele. For these reasons, it is best to care for the child in a special multidisciplinary clinic in a children's hospital, where the specialized services of the neurosurgeon, urologic surgeon, pediatric surgeon, orthopedic surgeon, neurologist, pediatrician, and physical and occupational therapists are available.[67, 155]

Social and psychologic factors also have a tremendous impact on the lives of these multiply handicapped children for whom the prognosis is pessimistic and the motivation to adjust to life and the community may be lacking. The roles of the special educator, vocational counselor, psychologist, and social worker are extremely important. By providing him with specialized education and vocational guidance, these workers enable the child with myelomeningocele to compensate for his extreme physical disability. Finally, the total care of these children should be coordinated and supervised by an interested pediatrician who functions as director of the team.

Parents' associations are extremely valuable for educating the parents of children with spina bifida, giving them the continued moral support so necessary for the adequate and proper care of these children. A stable and cooperative family is the most important part of the team in the total care of the child with myelomeningocele.

It is beyond the scope of this book to present neurosurgical, urologic, and other aspects of medical treatment of the child with myelomeningocele. These aspects are dealt with in the cited literature.[5, 6–9, 65, 86, 140]

The care of the musculoskeletal system of the infant with myelomeningocele begins on the day of birth. The orthopedist should be called in consultation at the same time as the neurosurgeon so that he may have an opportunity to examine the patient prior to closure of the lesion and to determine the neurosegmental level of the lesion and the presence or absence of deformities of the limbs and spine.

The goal of orthopedic treatment is to have these children able to walk with appropriate orthotic support by the age of 18 months. Upright posture opens new vistas with a promise of a useful and satisfying life (Fig. 3–49).

Ambulation is defined as the process by which an individual moves from one area to another by his own volition and motor power. Hoffer and associates have divided these patients into four groups according to their functional levels of ambulation.[55]

Community ambulators are those who walk indoors and outdoors for most of their activities, with or without the support of orthoses or crutches. Wheelchairs are used only for long trips out of the community.

Household ambulators are able to walk only indoors and for limited distances with the help of orthotic support. At home they are independent for their activities of daily living, getting in and out of chair and bed; but when going out into the community they need a wheelchair.

Nonfunctional ambulators walk only for ex-

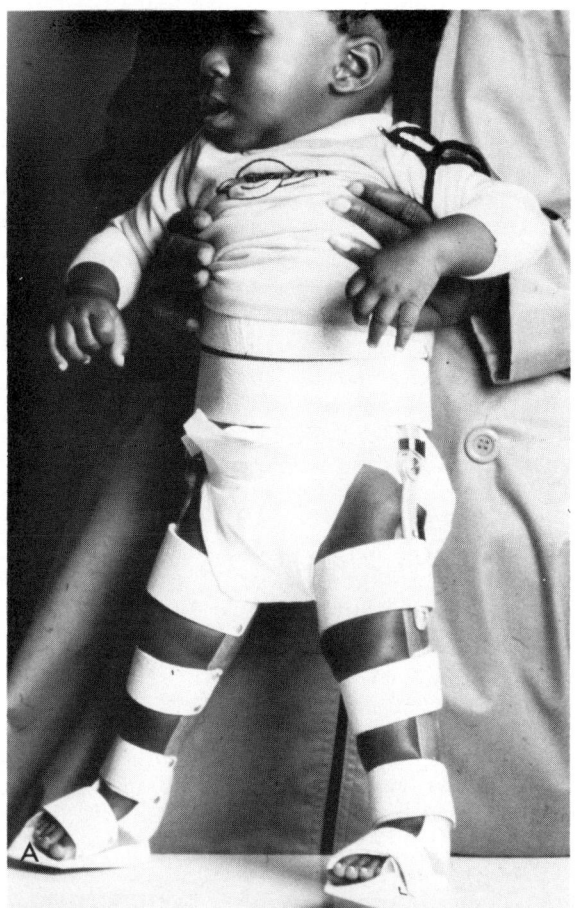

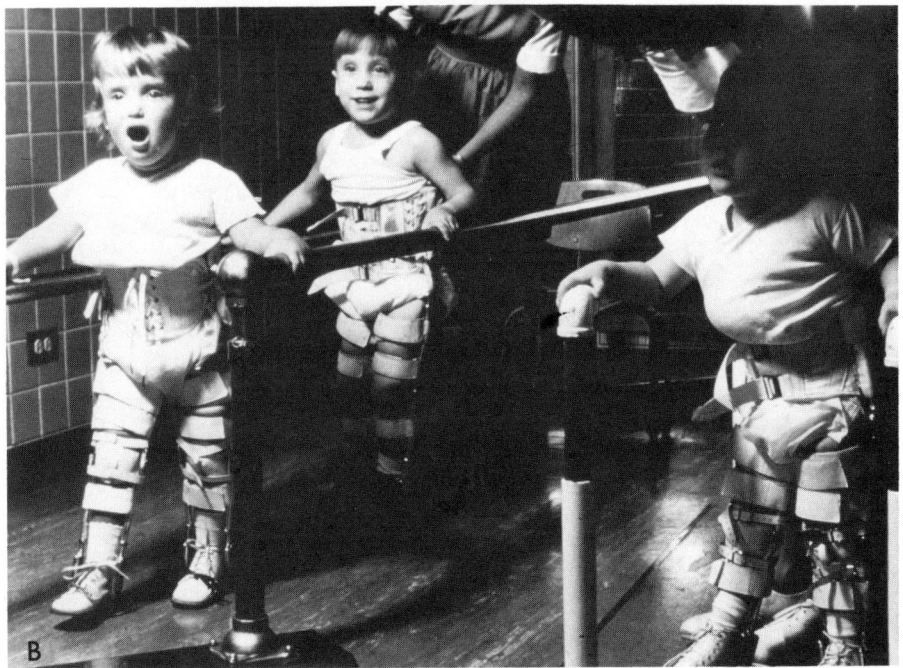

FIGURE 3–49. The goal of orthopedic management is ambulation at 16 to 18 months with the help of orthoses and crutches.

A. A 14-month-old infant with myelomeningocele held upright in braces. **B**. Gait training in parallel bars.

ercise, not for function. For all transportation they use the wheelchair. At a physical therapy session in school, in the hospital, or at home, they walk short distances with a swing-to-swing-through gait with crutches and above-knee orthoses with pelvic band.

Nonambulators are wheelchair bound but are usually able to transfer from chair to bed.

Factors that determine the functional level of ambulation are (1) the neurologic level of the lesion; (2) the presence or absence of hydrocephalus and spasticity; (3) the stability of the spine and the motor strength of the trunk; (4) the function of the upper limbs; (5) the presence of contracture and other deformities of the lower limbs; (6) associated brain damage and mental retardation; and (7) motivation, home environment, and social factors. Behavioral aberrations and an unsatisfactory family situation are detrimental to functional achievement.[55, 65]

Hoffer and associates reviewed the ambulatory status of 56 patients with myelomeningocele who were in their teens and were followed for over five years. None of those with lesions at the thoracic neurologic level functioned above the wheelchair level. All the patients with lesions at the sacral level were community ambulators. Of the 40 patients whose lesions were at the lumbar neurologic level (21 lower and 19 upper), 14 were community ambulators, 5 were household ambulators, 2 were nonfunctional ambulators, and 19 were wheelchair bound. Hoffer and his co-workers could not find any significant difference between higher and lower lumbar lesion levels with regard to ambulation. Lesions at the lumbar level present a variable picture, and factors other than the level of paraplegia are operative in determining the ultimate ambulatory status.[55]

Age is an important factor in considering the upward or downward transition of functional level of ambulation. In Hoffer's series all the patients who achieved community ambulatory status did so by nine years of age, and most of these children were at least nonfunctional ambulators by the age of five years. The household and nonfunctional ambulators are the transient group. Few of the very young nonfunctional ambulators rose in functional level; the majority of nonfunctional ambulators became wheelchair bound in their teens. About 50 per cent of household ambulators become community ambulators, and the remainder end up in wheelchairs. The transition to wheelchair usually takes place during early adolescence when the increase in height and weight overburden their capacity for energy expenditure.

It is obvious that reconstructive surgery of the lower limbs should be reserved for the functional ambulators; in the nonambulatory patients surgical efforts should be directed toward stabilization of the trunk by spinal fusion, and therapy for the lower limbs be confined to stretching exercises and splinting. It is vital to have realistic goals in the management of the child with myelomeningocele and to individualize the care of each child, depending upon his unique problems.

Deformities of the foot and ankle are very common in myelomeningocele. Some of them are congenital and others acquired postnatally. The causative factors are muscle imbalance, spasticity, fibrotic contracture of denervated muscles, intrauterine malposition assumed by a paralyzed foot, and habitual malposition of the limb adopted after birth; some deformities, however, may be of teratogenic origin.

Sharrard and Grosfield, in a study of 296 feet (148 patients with myelomeningocele), found 27 normal feet and 28 flail feet that were, however, not deformed.[135] At Children's Memorial Hospital in Chicago, 90 per cent of the patients with myelomeningocele had deformed feet; the distribution of deformities in 256 limbs in 128 children was as follows: (1) pes calcaneus—89 feet; (2) talipes equinovarus—83 feet; (3) pes equinus—30 feet; (4) congenital convex pes valgus—10 feet; and (5) miscellaneous—18 feet. There was no deformity in 26 feet. In analyzing the lower limbs of 350 patients with myelomeningocele, Lindseth found 233 (or 63 per cent) had deformities of the feet (Table 3–3).

Paralytic involvement of the lower limbs in myelomeningocele may be of two types; in the first, there is complete *flaccid* paralysis of the muscles below a certain segmental level with total loss of spinal cord function; in the second type, there is reflex *spasticity* in isolated segments distal to the cord lesion.[149] Spastic and partial flaccid paralysis can cause muscle imbalance and result in

*Table 3–3. Deformities of the Feet in 350 Children with Myelomeningocele**

Level	Clubfoot	Calcaneo-valgus Deformity	Vertical Talus	No Deformity
Thoracic	40	8	0	38
L1, L2	22	4	1	13
L3	24	2	1	9
L4	50	4	0	14
L5	11	38	5	20
Sacral	19	4	0	41
Total	166	60	7	135

*In patients with asymmetric paralysis each foot was counted separately. (From Lindseth, R. E.: Treatment of the lower extremity in children paralyzed by myelomeningocele (birth to 18 months). A.A.O.S. Instr. Course Lect., 25:79, 1976. Reprinted by permission.)

deformities with skeletal growth. Sharrard and Grosfield often observed no correlation between spontaneous motor activity and the type of deformity, but a strong correlation was noted between the deformity and the response of the lower limb muscles to faradic stimulation.[135]

The type of paralytic foot deformity may be correlated with the neurosegmental level of the lesion. When it is at or above the third lumbar segment, there is flail foot and ankle; they may be in calcaneus, equinovarus, or valgus position as a result of intrauterine or postnatal malposture (Fig. 3–50). When these children are upright and begin to walk, valgus deformity will develop in response to the static force of body weight.

When the lesion is at the fourth lumbar segment, the anterior tibial muscle will be active and strong, pulling the forefoot into dorsiflexion and inversion. The posture of the hindfoot is usually calcaneovalgus but occasionally may be equinus, and the talus is plantar-flexed with dorsolateral subluxation or dislocation of the talocalcaneonavicular joint (paralytic vertical talus).

When involvement is at the fifth lumbar level, the long toe extensors and peroneal and anterior tibial muscles are strong, whereas the triceps surae and long toe flexor muscles are paralyzed. A progressive calcaneus deformity will result if dynamic imbalance is not corrected (Fig. 3–51).

When the lesion is within the first two sacral neurosegments there is complete or partial paralysis of the long toe flexor and intrinsic muscles of the foot, with the long and short toe extensor muscles active; the resultant deformity is pes cavus with clawing of the toes. Equinovarus deformity may result from a teratologic process at any level. Dias reports an equal distribution of talipes equinovarus (82 feet in 51 patients) between the thoracic, high lumbar, and low lumbar levels.[20a]

The object of treatment is to obtain a flexible, normally aligned plantigrade foot that can bear weight safely. Deformed feet will develop pressure sores, cellulitis, and osteomyelitis, which will eventually necessitate amputation. One cannot overemphasize the importance of diligent and persistent care of the feet of children with myelomeningocele. Management, however, does present certain difficult problems due to fibrosis of denervated muscles, sensory loss, and associated paralysis of the muscles controlling the hip and knee.

Treatment should begin at birth. There is no excuse for delay. A flexible deformity will become rigid with skeletal growth. The general tendency is to postpone the treatment of foot deformities because of the fear that it may interfere with the nursing and surgical management of the spinal defect and hydrocephalus. The neurosurgeon should be requested to place the needles for intravenous administration of fluids in the upper limb when there is a deformity of the lower limb. Early soft-tissue surgery will prevent development of rigid structural bony deformities. Incomplete correction, muscle imbalance, and spasticity and fibrosis will cause a high rate of recurrence of foot deformity. It is vital to use night splints and day orthoses, to carry out an adequate physical therapy program, and to balance muscle forces surgically to prevent recurrence of deformity.

The specific deformities of the foot are discussed next.

Pes Calcaneus

Pes calcaneus is very common in myelomeningocele (Figs. 3–50 and 3–51). On gross anatomic inspection the problem appears to be benign, but functionally it is very disturbing. In calcaneus deformity the weight-bearing surface is shortened, and the stability of the base upon which the

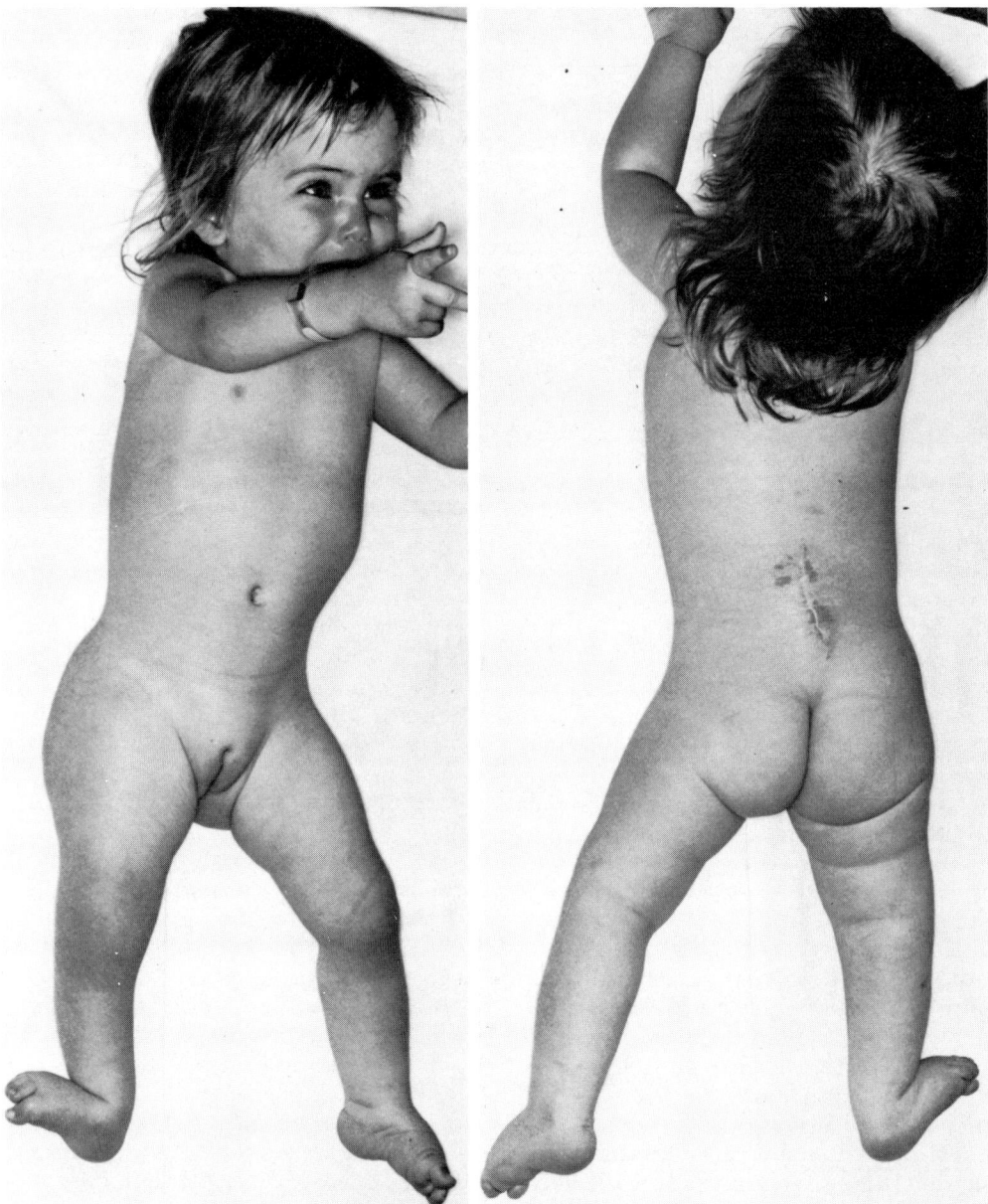

FIGURE 3–50. A one-year-old infant with myelomeningocele.

The severe calcaneovalgus deformity of the right foot is due to fibrosis of the long toe extensor and peroneal muscles.

body is supported is diminished. In addition excessive pressure is exerted on the posterior tuberosity of the dorsiflexed calcaneus and the plantar-flexed metatarsal heads. Pressure will lead to callosities and trophic ulcerations, which cause severe problems in insensitive feet.[33] Children with myelomeningocele have smaller feet than normal, and many of them put on excess weight as they get older. Hay and Walker found plantar pressures in children with myelomeningocele to be substantially higher than those in normal children of the same age.[49] This relative increase in perpendicular static pressure is partly due to the smaller feet in the child with spina bifida and, thereby, the

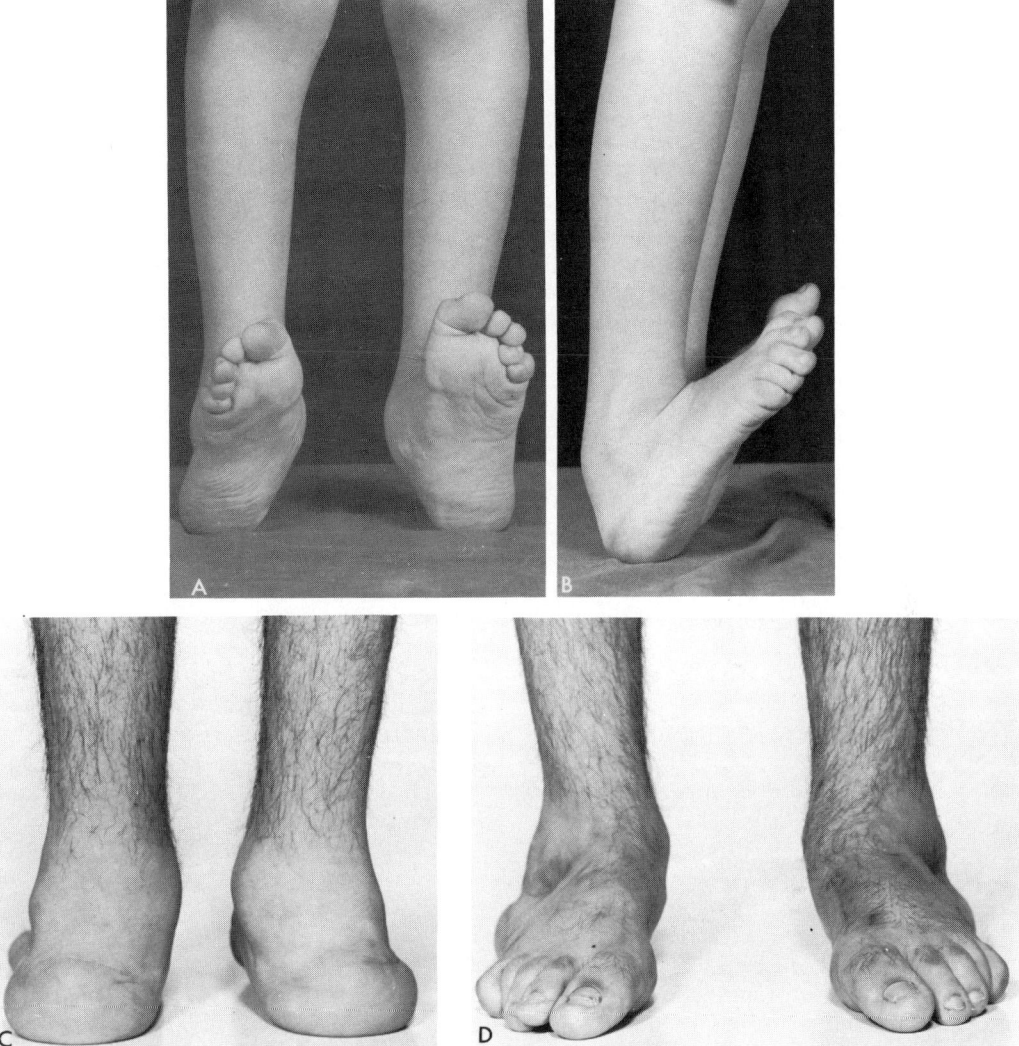

FIGURE 3–51. Severe calcaneus deformity of both feet in a child with myelomeningocele with paralytic involvement at the fifth lumbar level.

The long toe extensor, peroneal, and anterior tibial muscles are normal in motor strength, whereas the triceps surae and long toe flexors are paralyzed. Severe calcaneus deformity of both feet has developed as a result of dynamic imbalance of muscles acting on the foot and ankle. A posterior transfer of the anterior tibial and peroneal muscles was performed to restore dynamic balance. **A** and **B**. Preoperative photographs at five years of age. **C** and **D**. Postoperative photographs when 14 years old.

greater pressure per unit of surface. Greater pressure is exerted on the hindfoot because of the vertical position of the os calcis in calcaneus deformity. In the normal limb, motions at the knee and ankle reduce the impact on foot-strike and in the stance phase in ambulation. In the braced, rigid knee and ankle of the child with myelomeningocele this compensatory mechanism is lacking, and the weight borne on the plantar aspect of the foot is increased.

The deformed calcaneus foot is difficult to fit with shoes. The prominent dorsum of the midfoot and interphalangeal joints of the clawed toes are rubbed and irritated by the shoe, and ulceration results. Because the posterior part of the heel is shortened or almost absent, it is difficult to keep the shoe on. Biomechanically, calcaneus posture of the ankle and poor posterior stability in gait causes knee and hip flexion and increases the instability of an already precarious balance.[33]

The primary cause of calcaneus deformity is muscle imbalance between the active dorsiflexors of the ankle and the paralyzed plantar-flexors. Being at the highest level of innervation, the tibialis anterior will function in fourth lumbar level lesions. The long toe extensors and peroneals will be strong in lesions at the fifth lumbar level.[135] Other deforming factors are fibrosis of the denervated muscles, spasticity, and malposture—intrauterine and postnatal. Greater motor strength of the lateral extensors (peroneus tertius, extensor digitorum communis, and peroneus brevis) over the tibialis anterior will cause calcaneovalgus deformity. Underdevelopment of the fibula in relation to the tibia will result in a high-riding lateral malleolus and lateral tilting of the ankle mortise.[20] Lateral tibial torsion is often associated with valgus foot and ankle. Calcaneovarus deformity is caused by the unbalanced action of the tibialis anterior; it is much less common than calcaneovalgus deformity.

In the newborn, treatment consists of passive manipulative exercises to elongate contracted soft-tissue structures on the dorsum of the ankle and leg. The rigid and severe calcaneus deformity may require the use of a plaster of Paris cast to retain the correction achieved by manipulation. As soon as the foot is brought into 10 to 20 degrees of plantar flexion, splints are used at night to maintain correction, and passive stretching exercises are continued.

If the calcaneus deformity cannot be prevented from progressing or recurring and the anterior tibial muscle is the deforming force, it is transferred posteriorly through the interosseous route. This procedure was originally described by Peabody for treatment of calcaneus deformity secondary to poliomyelitis.[110] Green and Grice have reported their methods and experience in the management of pes calcaneus.[45] The operative technique is described and illustrated in Plate 16.

This author recommends posterior transfer of the anterior tibial through the interosseous route, transfer of the peroneus longus to the os calcis, and suture of the distal stump of the peroneus longus to the peroneus brevis if the transferred muscles are good or normal in motor strength and the long toe extensors are strong. Additional important requisites are that the patient should have good hip flexors (and preferably knee flexors also) to clear the foot, and quadriceps femoris function. The patient should be between three and four years old at the time of surgery. With adequate postoperative care, the posterior transfer will be fair or good on manual testing but poor when the patient rises on his toes. The objective of the posterior transfer is to check progression of calcaneus deformity and to provide a plantigrade foot (Fig. 3–52). If only the anterior tibial muscle is functioning and the long toe extensors are paralyzed, it is best to lengthen or simply section the anterior tibial tendon.

As reported in the literature, the results of posterior transfer of the tibialis anterior to the calcaneus have not been very encouraging; there were three failures in eight cases (37.5 per cent) reported by Hayes and colleagues, and 20 per cent of the series of 20 feet reported by Sharrard and Grosfield were failures.[51, 135] Menelaus recommends transfer of the anterior tibial tendon alone. When the toe extensors are functioning, Menelaus advises tenotomy of the extensor hallucis longus, extensor digitorum longus and peroneus tertius.[90] Smith and Duckworth reported six poor results in nine feet in which the extensor tendons were transferred to the heel, whereas in four calcaneus feet treated by extensor tenotomy there were no poor results.[144]

Posterior transfer of the anterior tibial tendon to the os calcis may be combined with tenodesis of the Achilles tendon to the tibia. Banta and co-workers reported the results in seven patients (14 feet). Postoperative gait analysis demonstrated improvement of the hindfoot and midfoot support, and better control over ankle-knee motion and walking velocity. The progression of the calcaneus deformity was checked in all cases.[2] This author recommends a combination of Achilles tendon tenodesis to the tibia with posterior transfer of the anterior tibial tendon when the deformity is calcaneovarus. Often, however, the presenting deformity is a calcaneovalgus foot with an associated valgus ankle. In such a case the author recommends a combination of posterior transfer of the anterior tibial tendon with calcaneofibular Achilles tendon tenodesis; this will stimulate distal growth of the fibula and prevent progression of the valgus inclination of the ankle.[20, 20a]

Fibrosis and contracture of the dener-

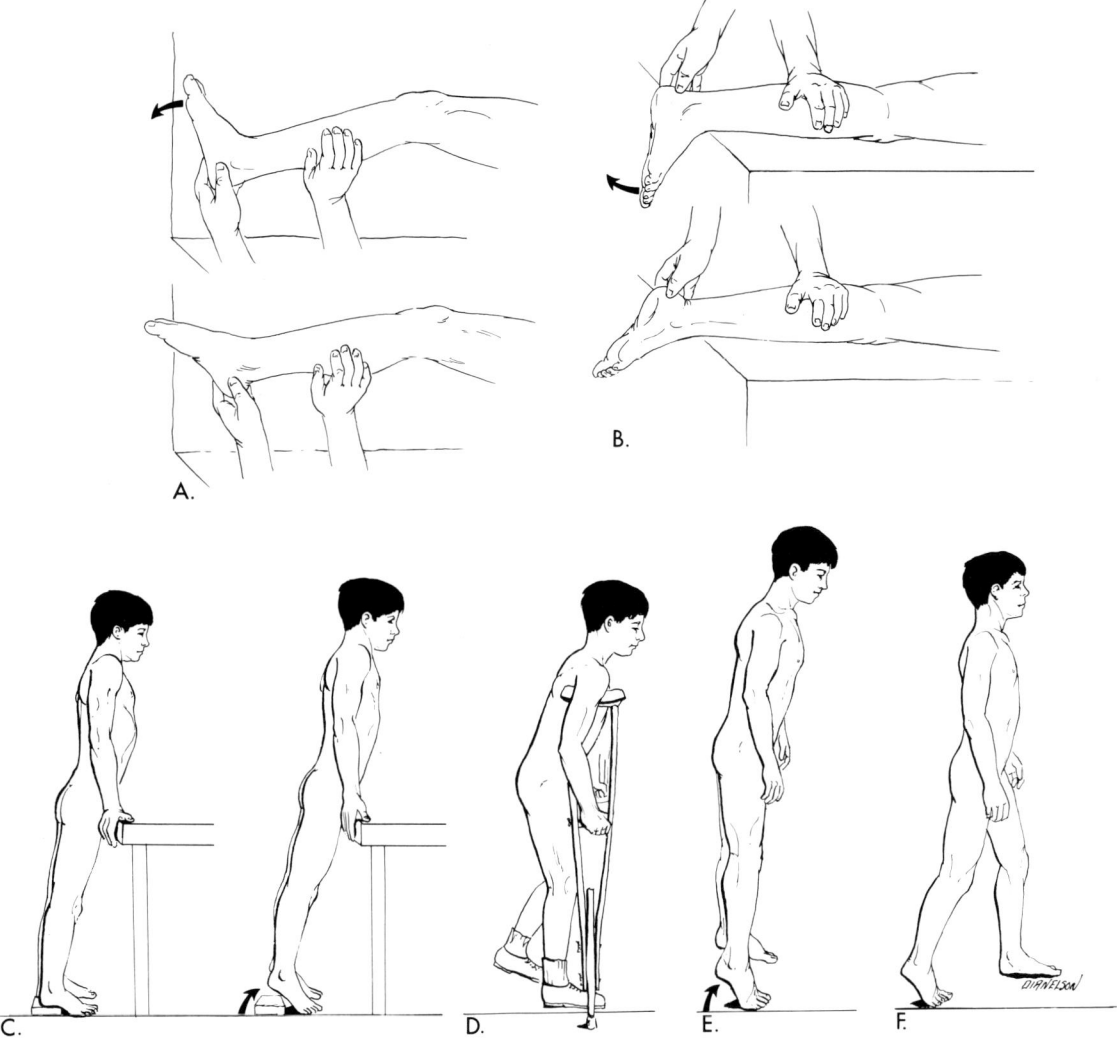

FIGURE 3–52. Postoperative exercises following posterior tendon transfer to the os calcis.

vated anterior crural muscles will cause calcaneus deformity. In severe cases there will be rigid contracture of the anterior capsule of the ankle joint. This type of pes calcaneus is treated by early radical excision of the tendons and tendon sheaths of the ankle dorsiflexors and anterior ankle capsulectomy. The skin may be very taut, preventing plantar flexion of the foot; in such a case Z-plasty lengthening of the skin is performed.

Another type of calcaneus deformity is caused by spasticity of the ankle dorsiflexors and flaccid paralysis of the triceps surae. This type is treated by excision of the spastic tendons and their tendon sheaths.

In the older child with bony deformity, the calcaneocavus foot is corrected by posterior displacement osteotomy of the os calcis, by either Mitchell's oblique or Samilson's crescentic technique; it should be combined with plantar release as described in the section of this chapter on pes cavus.[94, 119]

Valgus Ankle

Relative shortening of the fibula in relation to the tibia is common in the ankles of children with myelomeningocele. Makin described delay in ossification and shortening of the fibula in ten such patients.[85] Hol-

Text continued on page 434

Posterior Tendon Transfer to Os Calcis for Correction of Calcaneus Deformity (Green and Grice)

THE PROCEDURE

It is best to place the patient in the prone position to facilitate the surgical exposure of the heel. The posterior tibial and the peroneus longus and brevis tendons are divided distally at their insertion and delivered into the proximal wound following the technique and steps described in Plate 18, page 460. When the flexor hallucis longus tendon is to be transferred, its distal portion is sutured to the flexor hallucis brevis muscle. The anterior tibial tendon is delivered into the calf and heel through the interosseous route.

A. A 5-cm.-long posterior transverse incision is made around the heel along one of the skin creases in the part that neither presses the shoe nor touches the ground.

B. The skin and subcutaneous flaps are undercut and reflected, exposing the os calcis and the insertion of the tendo calcaneus. An L-shaped cut is made in the lateral two thirds of the insertion of the tendo calcaneus. The divided portion is reflected proximally, exposing the apophysis of the os calcis.

C. Next, with a 9/64-inch drill, a hole is made through the calcaneus, beginning in the center of the apophysis and coming out laterally at its plantar aspect. With a diamond head hand drill and curet, the hole is enlarged to receive all the transferred tendons.

Plate 16. Posterior Tendon Transfer to Os Calcis for Correction of Calcaneus Deformity (Green and Grice)

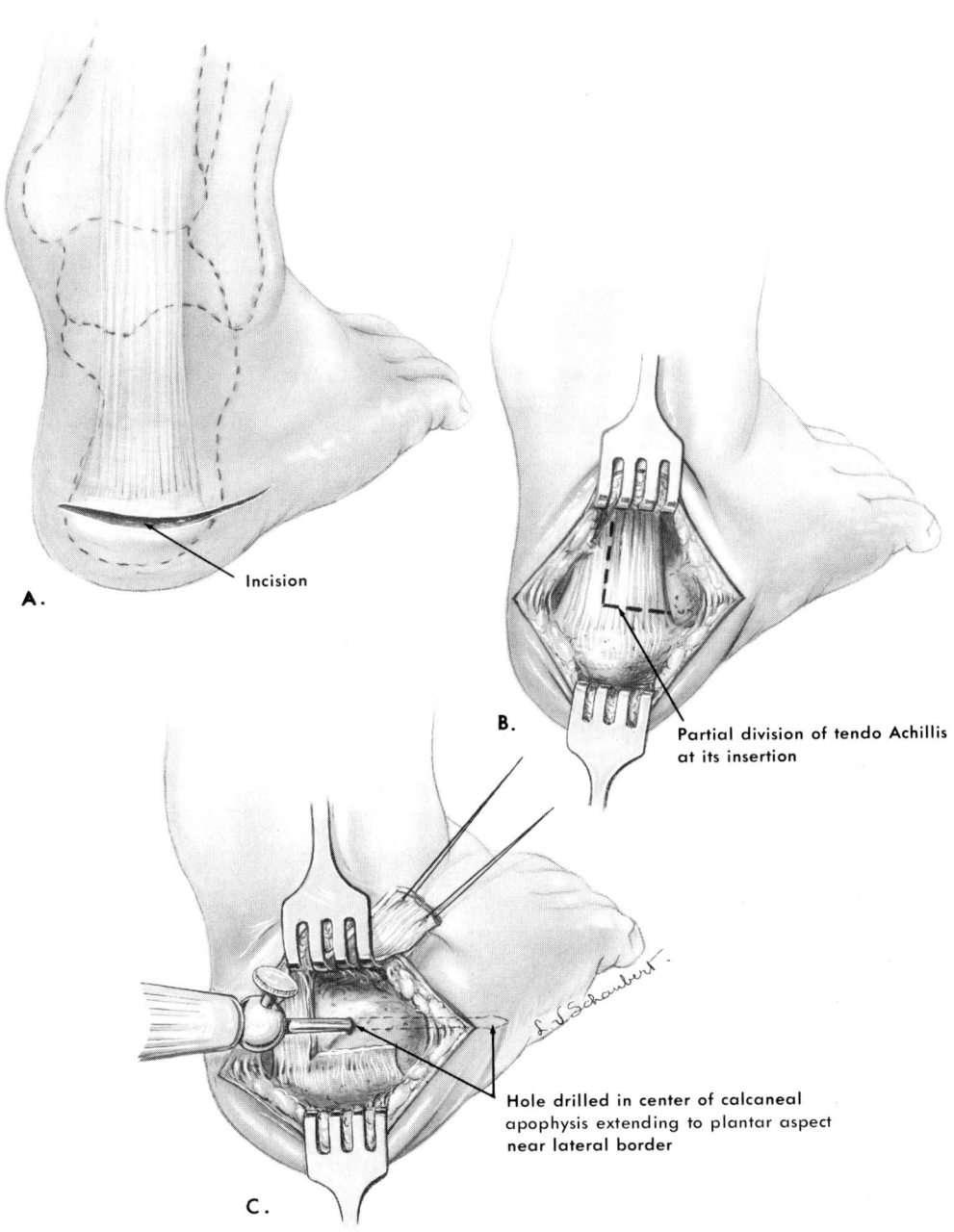

Posterior Tendon Transfer to Os Calcis for Correction of Calcaneus Deformity (Green and Grice) (Continued)

D. Through a lateral incision, the intermuscular septum is widely divided between the lateral and posterior compartments. An Ober tendon passer is inserted through the wound and directed anterior to the tendo calcaneus into the transverse incision over the os calcis. The threads of the whip sutures at the ends of the peroneal tendons are passed through the hole in the tendon passer and the tendons are delivered at the heel. The posterior tibial tendon is delivered at the heel by a similar route, through an incision in the intermuscular septum between the medial and posterior compartments and anterior to the tendo calcaneus. Next, with a twisted wire probe, the tendons are inserted in the hole and pulled through the tunnel in the calcaneus.

E. At their point of exit on the lateral aspect of the calcaneus the tendons are sutured to the periosteum and ligamentous tissues under enough tension to hold the foot at a 15-degree equinus angle when the remaining ankle dorsiflexors are fair in motor strength, and at 30 degrees if they are good or normal. The tendons are sutured to each other and to the periosteum of the apophysis of the calcaneus at the posterior end of the tunnel.

F and G. The divided portion of the tendo calcaneus is resutured in its original position posterior to the transferred tendons.

The wounds are closed and an above-knee cast is applied, the knee in 45 to 60 degrees of flexion, the hindfoot 15 to 30 degrees equinus, but the forefoot neutral. Cavus deformity of the forefoot should be avoided.

POSTOPERATIVE CARE

Three to four weeks following surgery the solid cast is removed and a new above-knee bivalved cast is made to protect the limb at all times when exercises are not being performed. It is imperative to prevent forced dorsiflexion of the ankle and stretching of the transferred tendons.

Exercises are first performed with the patient lying on his side and with gravity eliminated, and then in prone position against gravity (see Fig. 3–52 A and B). In order to teach the patient the new action of the transferred muscle, he is asked to move the foot in the direction of a component of the original action of the muscle and then to plantar-flex the foot. For example, when the peroneals are transferred, he is asked to evert and plantar-flex the foot; or when the anterior tibial is transferred, to invert and plantar-flex the foot. Soon, under supervision, guided dorsiflexion of the foot is performed along with plantar flexion. It is important to develop reciprocal motion and motor strength of agonist and antagonist muscles. Weight-bearing is not allowed. Ambulation with crutches is permitted in the above-knee bivalved cast or a plastic splint.

In about four to six weeks when the transferred tendons are fair in motor strength the patient is allowed to stand on both feet. The heel of the foot that was operated on rests on a 3-cm.-thick block to prevent stretching of the transferred tendons. Bearing partial weight on his foot, the patient should rise up on his tiptoes while holding on to a table with his hands or using two crutches.

When the transplant functions effectively on tiptoe standing, walking with crutches is begun with three-point gait and partial weight-bearing on the affected limb (Fig. 3–52D). The heel of the shoe is elevated with a 1- to 1.5-cm. lift that tapers in front (toward the toes). Walking periods are gradually increased. When the transplant works effectively in gait and take-off has been developed in walking, standing tiptoe rising exercises are started without the support of crutches (Fig. 3–52E). The knee should not be flexed and the patient should not lean forward while rising up on his toes at least three times (Fig. 3–52F). This may take a long time (as much as a year or more), but it is a very important phase of postoperative management.

A plantar-flexion-assist spring brace or a brace with a posterior elastic is worn when the patient is uncooperative in the use of crutches or when muscular control of the knee and hip is poor because of extensive paralysis. A stop at the ankle prevents dorsiflexion of the ankle beyond neutral position.

Plate 16. Posterior Tendon Transfer to Os Calcis for Correction of Calcaneus Deformity (Green and Grice)

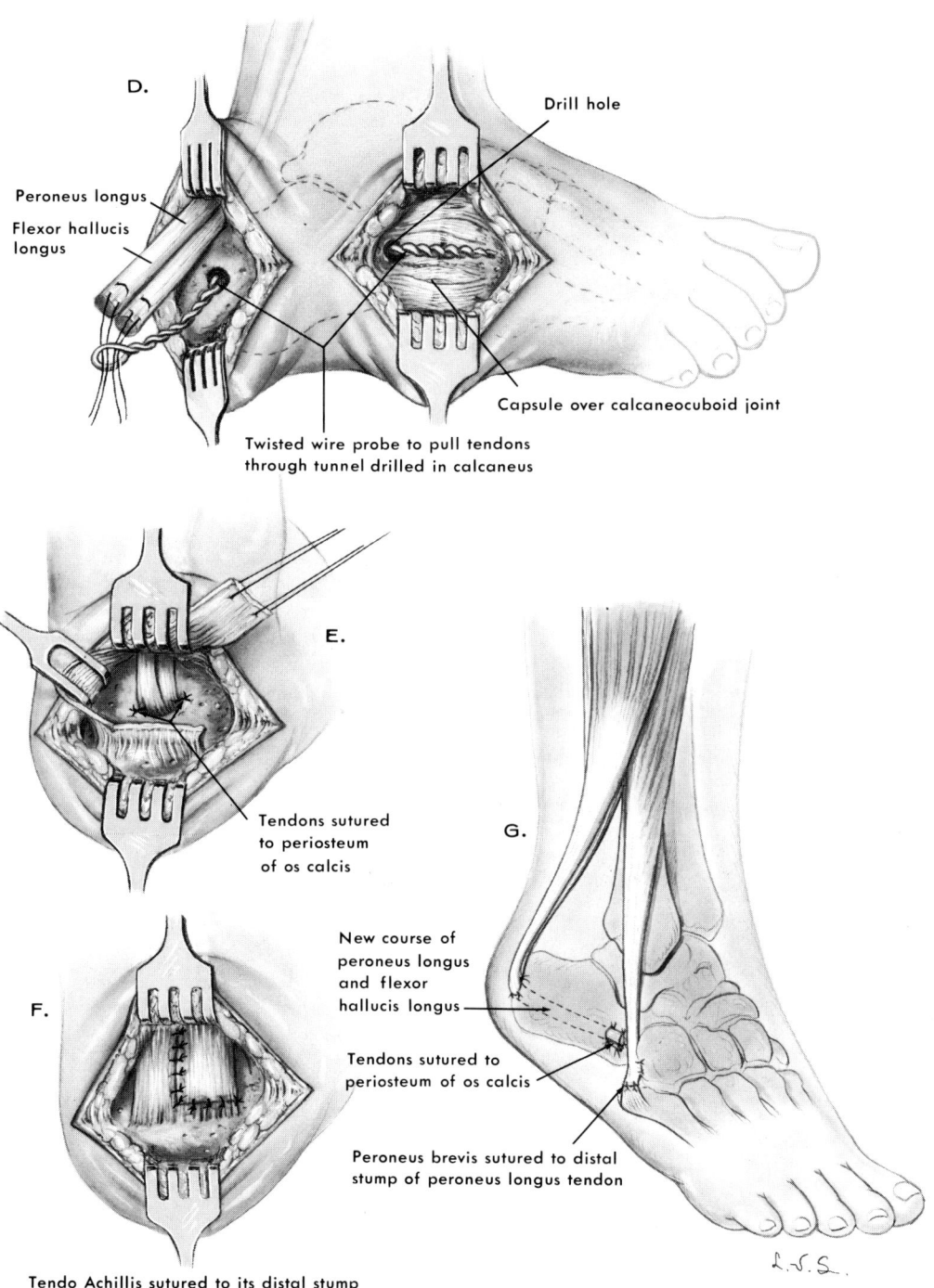

lingsworth analyzed the roentgenograms of 39 children with myelomeningocele, of whom 32 showed slight to marked shortening of the fibula and a valgus ankle.[56] Dias studied the growth of the fibula and ankle mortise in 86 children with myelomeningocele who were between the ages of 18 months and 15 years.[20] The degree of fibular shortening was determined by comparing their roentgenograms with those showing the relationship between the distal fibular growth plate and the dome of the talus in 100 normal persons. During the first four years of life the normal distal physis of the fibula is slightly superior to the dome of the talus; at five years of age it is level with the talar dome; thereafter it gradually migrates inferiorly. At skeletal maturity it is situated approximately 3 mm. distal to the dome of the talus.

The degree of fibular shortening is determined by two factors: the severity of paralysis of the triceps surae and the age of the patient. The fibula bears one sixth of the total body weight during stance and gait. Its longitudinal growth appears to be related to the strength of the posterior calf musculature, particularly of the soleus muscle. Weinert and associates have demonstrated with telephoto motion pictures and cineroentgenograms of weight-bearing and non-weight-bearing ankles that the fibula moves downward during the weight-bearing phase of the gait; this serves to deepen the mortise and adds to the stability of the ankle.[163] The muscles taking origin from the fibula are the lateral head of the soleus and the flexor hallucis longus (both having innervations from the first and second sacral segments), and the tibialis posterior (innervated from the fifth lumbar segment). Growth of the fibula is stimulated by the dynamic force of muscle action and the static loading from body weight. When the soleus muscle is paralyzed, progressive shortening of the fibula takes place (Fig. 3–53). The age of the patient is another factor to consider; the older the patient, the greater the degree of shortening. According to Dias the mean yearly increment of shortening is 1.3 mm.[20]

Relative shortening of the fibula and elevation of the lateral malleolus result in instability of the ankle mortise and increasing lateral wedging of the distal tibial epiphysis (Fig. 3–54). The medial malleolus is prominent; irritation from the shoe and the medial upright of the orthosis will cause adventitious bursitis, which may become infected. The short fibula will exert a teth-

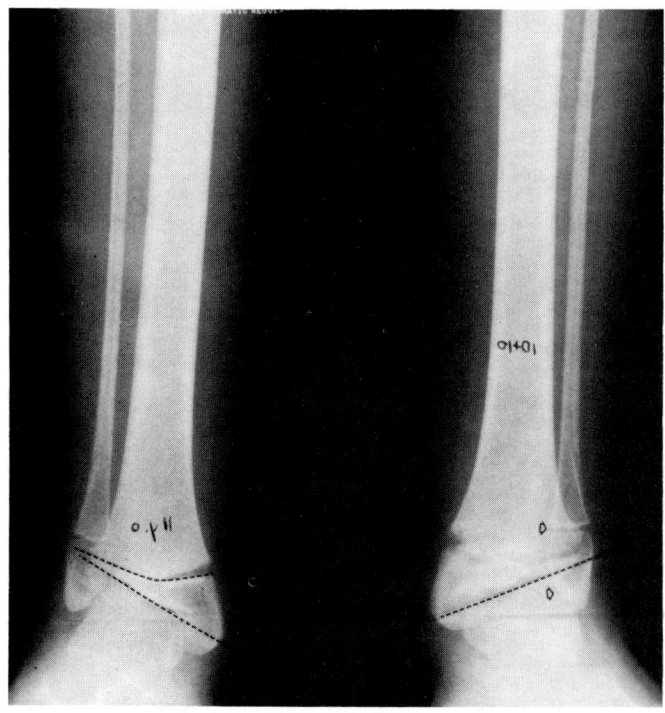

FIGURE 3–53. Anteroposterior roentgenogram of both ankles in an eight-year-old child with myelomeningocele at the fourth lumbar level.

Note the high-riding physis of the distal fibula and the valgus deformity of the ankle.

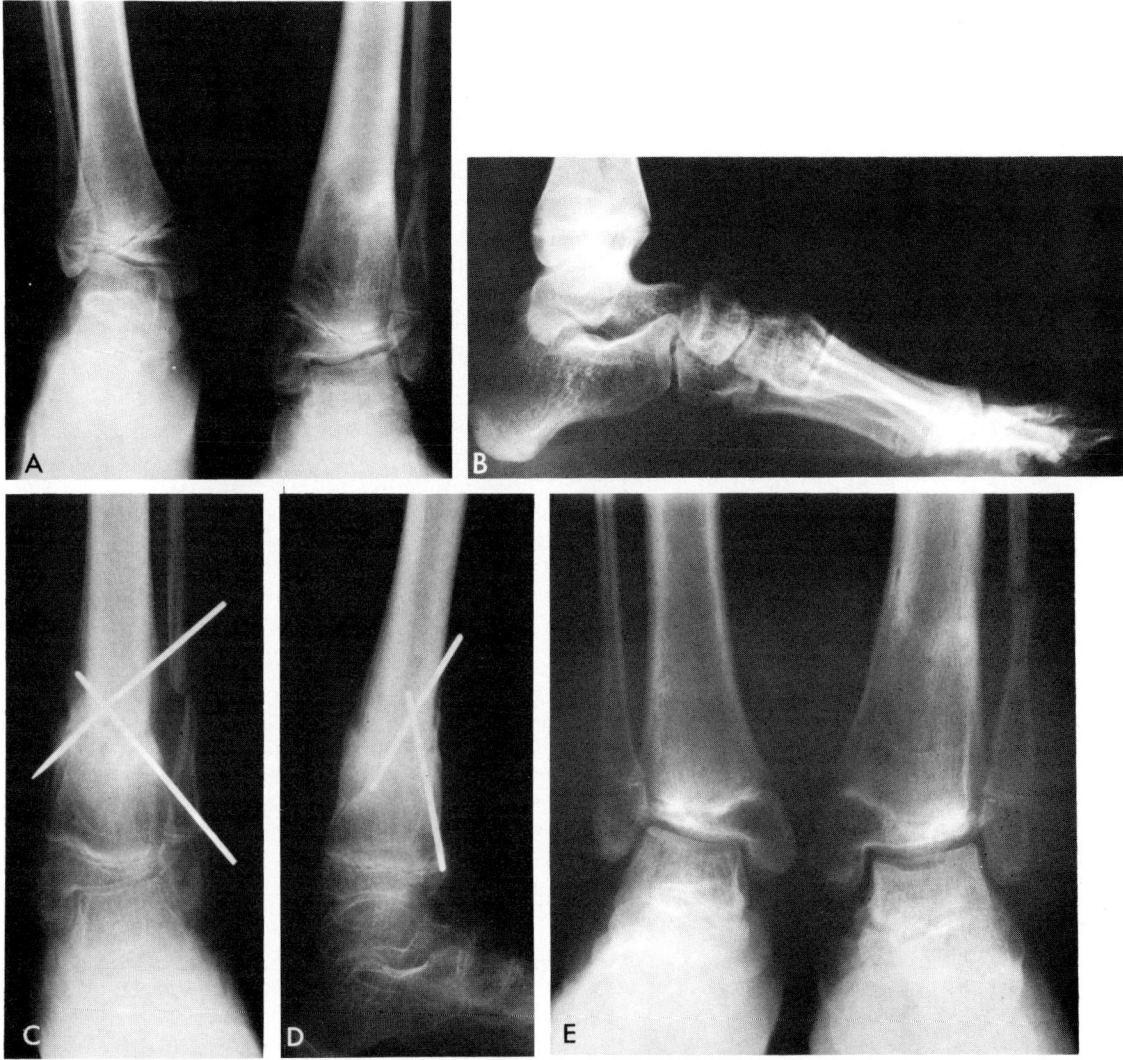

FIGURE 3–54. *The left ankle of a child with myelomeningocele at the fourth lumbar level.*

There are valgus ankle, high-riding fibular malleolus, and severe lateral wedging of the distal tibial epiphysis. **A.** Anteroposterior roentgenograms at six years old. Note the valgus ankle, especially on the left. **B.** Lateral view of the left foot, showing severe calcaneus deformity. **C** and **D.** Two-months-postoperative roentgenograms. The tendo Achillis is split and sutured to the distal fibular metaphyseal-diaphyseal junction. **E.** Two years postoperatively, roentgenograms of the left ankle show control and some correction of the valgus deviation of the ankle.

ering effect on the tibia and knee, causing progressively exaggerated lateral tibial torsion, genu valgum, and impairment of gait.

Treatment in the young child consists of calcaneofibular tenodesis. The technique is described and illustrated in Plate 17. The procedure was developed by Westin for correction of valgus ankle in poliomyelitis. Although not as effective in myelomeningocele, it does stimulate the growth of the fibula and prevents further progression of the valgus deviation of the ankle. In the active ambulatory patient, when performed at four or five years of age, it may to some degree correct the shortening of the fibula. This author strongly recommends the procedure in children between four and six years of age. In selected cases it may be combined with posterior transfer of the anterior tibial tendon to the os calcis.

In the child over eight years of age a supramalleolar tibial and fibular osteotomy

Calcaneofibular Tenodesis

THE PROCEDURE

The patient is placed in lateral position to facilitate the surgical exposure of the heel and lateral aspect of the ankle.

A. A longitudinal incision is made immediately posterior to the fibula; it begins at the tip of the lateral malleolus and extends proximally for a distance of 7 to 10 cm.

B. The subcutaneous tissue is divided, and the wound flaps are undercut and reflected, exposing the tendo calcaneus and the lateral surface of the fibula. The Achilles tendon is sectioned transversely at its musculotendinous junction, as proximally as possible. Obtain adequate length of the tendon.

C. Next, the distal physis of the fibula is identified and marked with a Keith needle. Roentgenograms are made with the Keith needle in place to verify the site of the growth plate, which should not be disturbed. With a dental drill a longitudinal slot about 3 cm. long and 0.5 to 0.75 cm. wide is made in the metaphyseal-diaphyseal area of the fibula. Its lower end should be 1 to 1.5 cm. proximal to the growth plate. The slot should be directed anteroposteriorly; do not break the lateral or medial cortex of the fibula.

D. The Achilles tendon is passed through the slot posteroanteriorly and sutured to itself under enough tension to hold the foot at an equinus angle of 15 to 20 degrees. The tendon is anchored to the periosteum of the fibula with additional sutures. Sometimes in the ankle of the child with myelomeningocele the fibula is so small and atrophied that it is safer to make a smaller slot, section the heel cord into halves, and pass only one half of the tendon through the slot and suture the other half to the fibular shaft through holes made with an electric drill. A calcaneofibular tenodesis may be combined with posterior transfer of the anterior tibial tendon to the os calcis through the interosseous route.

In calcaneus deformity secondary to overlengthening of the triceps surae in cerebral palsy, only the lateral half of the tendo calcaneus is attached to the fibula; its medial half is left continuous with the gastrocnemius-soleus muscle.

The tourniquet is released and, after complete hemostasis, an above-knee cast is applied with the ankle in 20 degrees of plantar flexion, but the forefoot in neutral position. Avoid cavus deformity of the forefoot.

POSTOPERATIVE CARE

Four weeks following surgery the solid cast is removed and a new above-knee plastic splint is made to protect the limb, preventing forced dorsiflexion of the ankle and stretching of the tenodesis.

As soon as possible the child is fitted with an ankle-foot orthosis, in which a plantar flexion assist and stop at the ankle prevent dorsiflexion beyond minus 10 to 15 degrees. He is allowed to ambulate and bear weight with the support of crutches. The splint is worn at night. With the pull of the Achilles tendon the distal fibular epiphysis will grow, and gradually the lateral tilting of the ankle mortise will be corrected.

Plate 17. Calcaneofibular Tenodesis

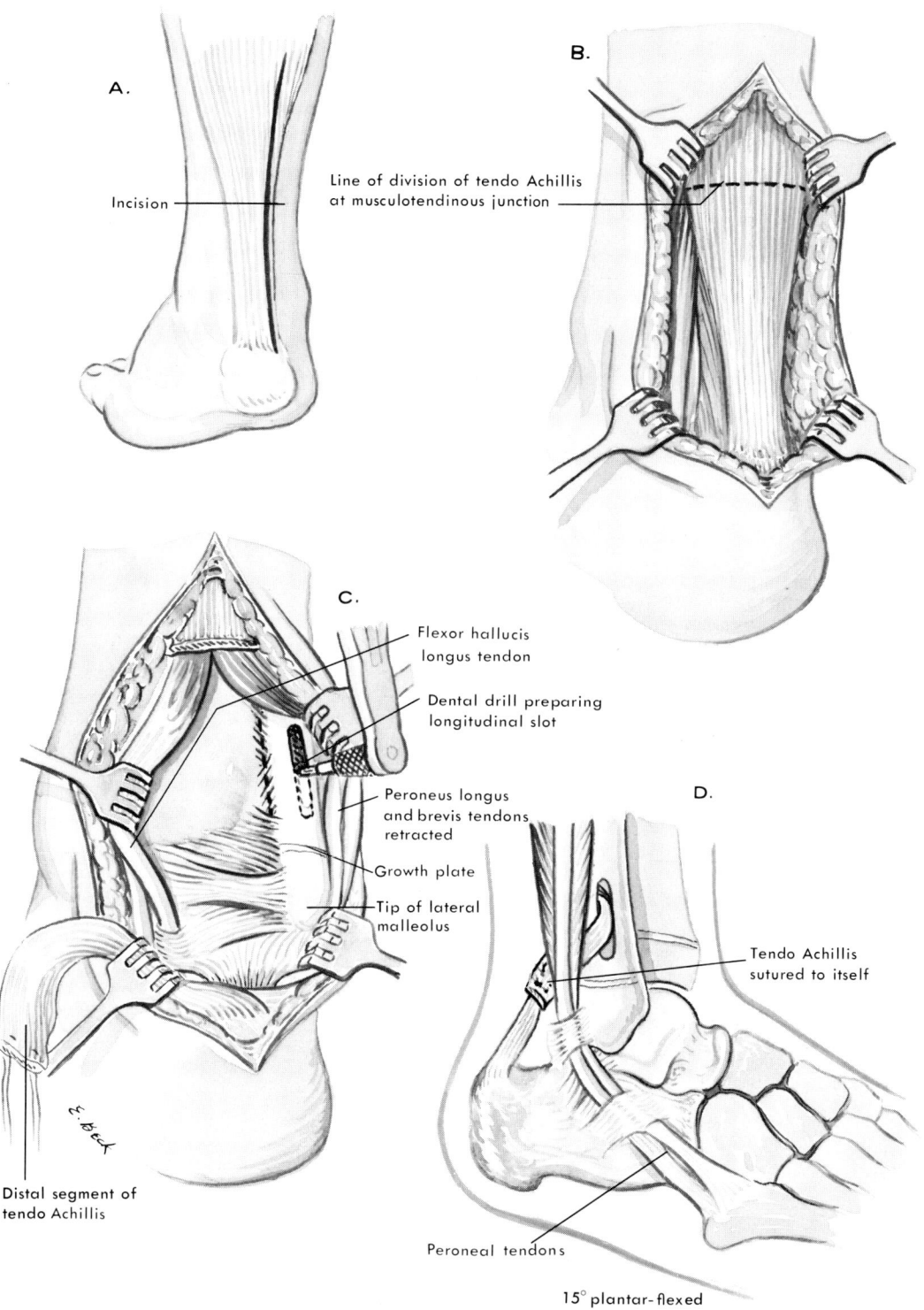

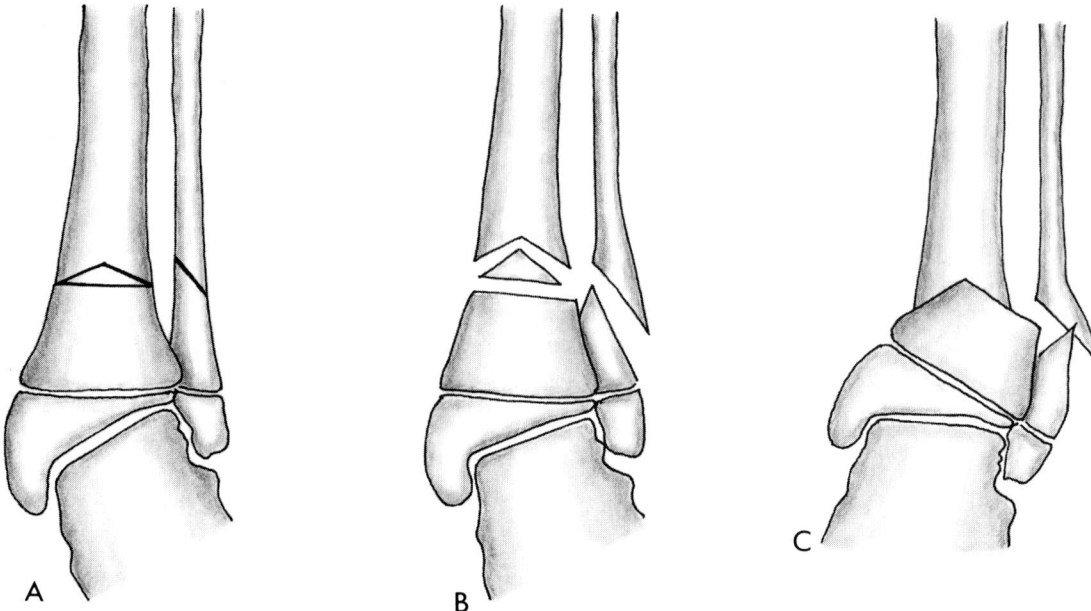

FIGURE 3–55. *Wiltse technique of triangular osteotomy of distal tibial diaphysis to correct valgus ankle.*

A. The lines of osteotomy. **B**. Triangular fragment of tibia excised. **C**. Medial rotation and lateral shift of the distal fragment will correct the valgus deformity without undesirable prominence of the medial malleolus; the shortening of the limb will be less than with a simple close-up osteotomy.

is required to correct the valgus ankle. Sharrard and Webb perform a wedge resection osteotomy of the tibia.[137] This author, however, recommends a medial displacement and tilting osteotomy, which corrects the valgus ankle, elevates the medial malleolus, and lowers the fibular malleolus.[167] The technique of supramalleolar osteotomy of the tibia and fibula is described and illustrated in Figure 3–55.

Supramalleolar osteotomy may be combined with calcaneofibular tenodesis in the child between eight and ten years of age.

Talipes Equinovarus

This is a common and most difficult deformity of the feet in myelomeningocele (Figs. 3–56 and 3–57). In the majority of

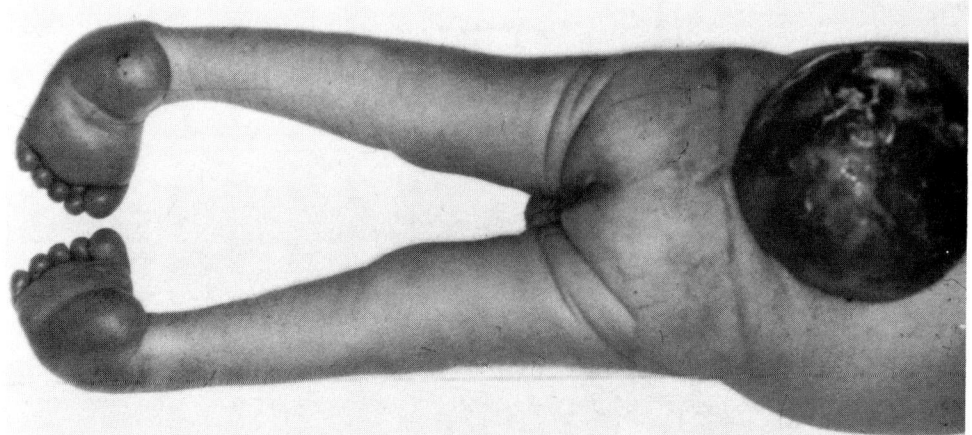

FIGURE 3–56. *Bilateral talipes equinovarus in a newborn infant with myelomeningocele.*

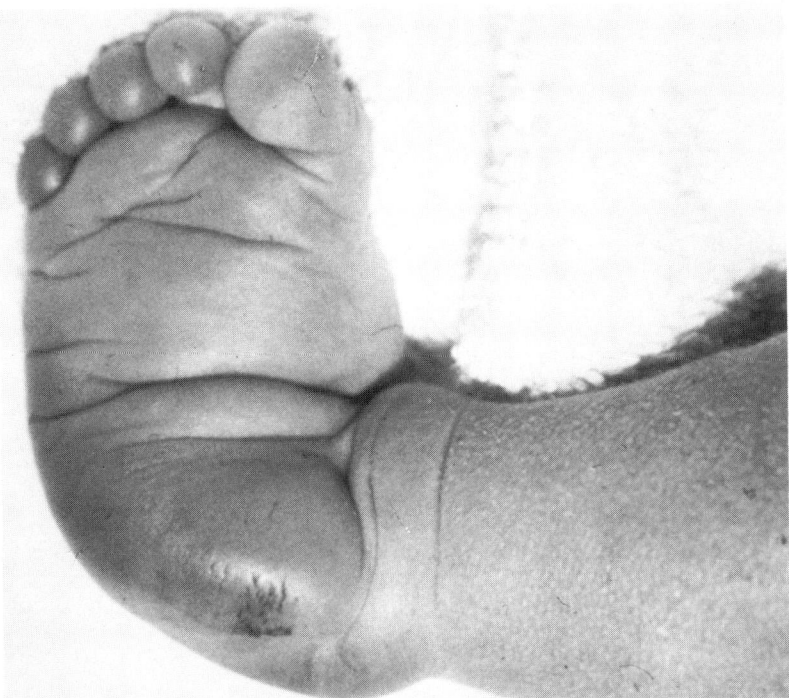

FIGURE 3–57. Pressure sore on the heel of a child with myelomeningocele and talipes equinovarus.

The cast should be applied not as a stretching device but as a retention apparatus to maintain the correction obtained by gentle manipulation.

the cases the deformity is very rigid and severe and has a high rate of recurrence despite adequate initial correction, behaving more like the clubfoot seen in arthrogryposis multiplex congenita. Talipes equinovarus in myelomeningocele is paralytic, caused by lack of normal muscle forces in utero and arrest of development of the foot beyond the fetal stage of equinovarus posture. Often there is no muscle function of the limb below the knee. In about 10 per cent of the cases the equinovarus deformity is acquired and due to muscle imbalance, spasticity, and fibrosis; the toe extensors, peroneals, and anterior tibial are paralyzed (sometimes the anterior tibial may be functioning); there is reflex activity and spasticity of the posterior tibial muscle, and fibrosis of the triceps surae, long toe flexors, and flexor hallucis longus.

Principles and details of management of talipes equinovarus are described in Chapter 2. Manipulative elongation of contracted soft tissues should be very gently performed to avoid fracture. Adhesive strapping or plaster of Paris casts should be properly padded and well molded. Sharrard reports disastrous results from attempted conservative treatment of equinus and equinovarus deformities in children with myelomeningocele.[135] The same experience has *not* been shared by the author. It is strongly advocated that contractural deformities be corrected as much as possible by conservative methods. Partial correction of soft-tissue contractures will diminish the incidence of postoperative wound dehiscence. In the flail limb it is recommended that soft-tissue release (tenotomy of anterior tibial, posterior tibial, and Achilles tendons) be performed during the neonatal period at the time of sac closure or first shunt procedure. The mildly deformed foot can be corrected by nonsurgical means; in the great majority of the cases, however, surgical correction is required. By three to six months of age, depending upon the size of the foot and general medical and neurosurgical status of the infant, an open reduction of the subluxated talocalcaneonavicular joint is performed. The Cincinnati transverse incision is ideal as it will allow complete subtalar release and correction of medial plantar subluxation of the talocalcaneonavicular joint.

In the experience of Walker, V-Y-plastic incision has been unsatisfactory. He recommends the rotation flap incision, as used by Holdsworth. The incision begins at the midpoint of the posterior aspect of the calf, extends distally to behind the medial malleolus, and then runs forward along the medial border of the foot. Then it runs laterally across the dorsum at or just behind the metatarsal heads and turns proximally along the lateral border of the foot (Fig. 3–58A). The subcutaneous tissue is divided in line with the skin incision. The wound flap is raised, staying superficial to the venous arch (Fig. 3–58 B and C). Posteromedial and plantar releases are performed to obtain full correction of the foot. The tourniquet is released, and after complete hemostasis, the flap is rotated to close the defect

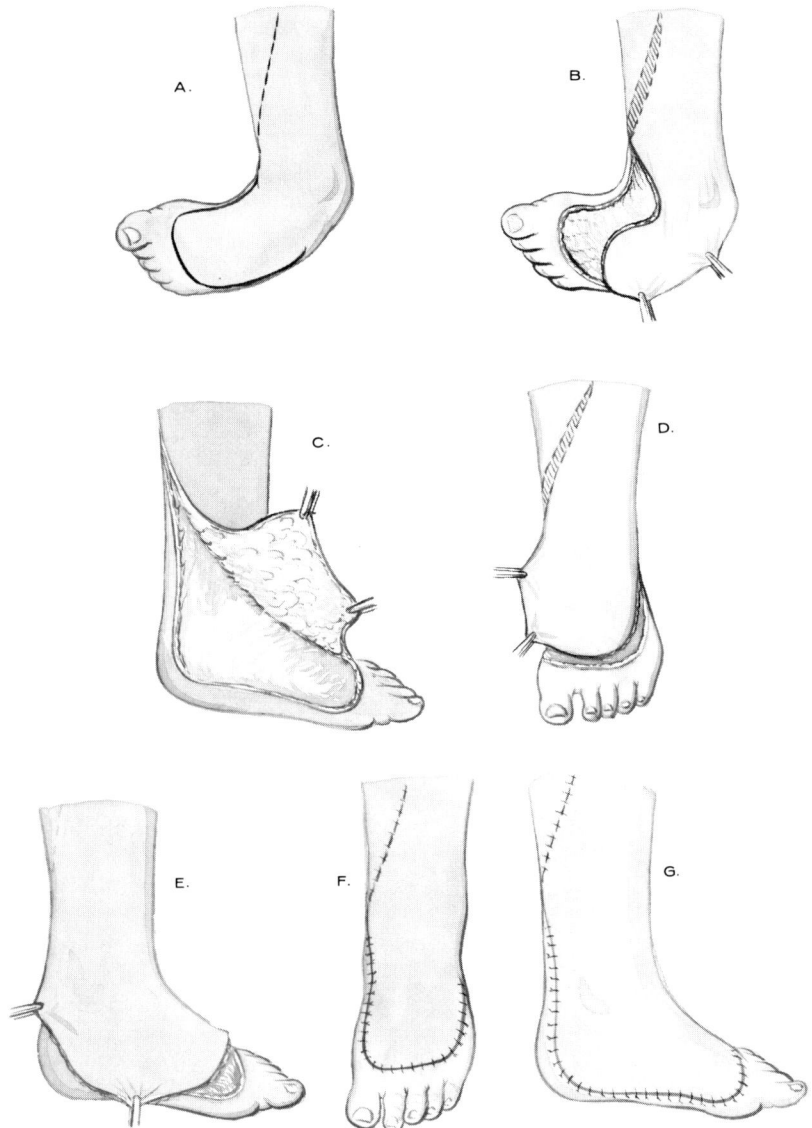

FIGURE 3–58. Rotation flap incision for correction of rigid equinovarus deformity in myelomeningocele.

A. The incision. **B** and **C.** Raising of the flap. **D.** Rotation of the flap. **E** to **G.** Resuturing of the flap with the foot in plantigrade position. (Redrawn after Walker, C.: The early management of varus feet in myelomeningocele. J. Bone Joint Surg., 53-B:465, 1977.)

on the medial aspect of the foot and ankle (Fig. 3–58D). Usually the return of circulation is adequate; occasionally there may be distal skin ischemia, which usually settles down during the period of cast immobilization. According to Walker, the rotation flap incision provides adequate skin cover at operation with the foot in plantigrade position, and scar contracture is not a problem.[160] During surgery one should excise the tendons of fibrosed muscles, the tendon sheaths, and the contracted joint capsules to prevent recurrence of deformity. It is crucial to provide meticulous postoperative care to prevent recurrence of deformity. Despite all efforts, recurrence of deformity is still high.[20, 90] Talectomy may be indicated between the ages of one and five years for the recurrent and rigid deformity.[139] Menelaus analyzed the outcome of talectomy in 41 feet (25 in patients with arthrogryposis multiplex congenita and 16 in those with spina bifida—among them, 14 with equinovarus deformity and 2 with vertical talus); the results were good in 32 feet (79 per cent); there was residual equinus deformity in 14 feet (14 per cent) and residual equinovarus deformity in 3 feet (7 per cent).[89] The technique of talectomy is described in Chapter 2. It should be combined with soft-tissue release and partial or complete resection of the cuboid bone. Menelaus states that during the past eight years the need for talectomy has been obviated by early soft-tissue release. Decancellation of the head and neck of the talus and cuboid bone (Verebelyi-Ogston procedure) is not recommended by this author.[39a, 103]

Pes Equinus

Varying degrees of pes equinus are quite common in myelomeningocele. It is caused by fibrosis and contracture of the triceps surae; if it is associated with contracture of the peronei the foot will be in equinovalgus position. Equinus deformity is very disabling, making it very difficult to fit shoes and braces. Pressure sores on the heel become a chronic problem. In the flail limb, equinus deformity can be prevented by passive range of motion exercises and splinting the foot and ankle in neutral position at night. Moderate equinus deformity is corrected by section and excision of a segment of the Achilles tendon. Severe equinus deformity, as shown in Figure 3–59, requires radical excision of tendons and tendon sheaths, posterior capsulectomy of the ankle and subtalar joints, and sometimes sectioning of the inferior syndesmosis of the tibiofibular articulation to widen the ankle mortise. Postoperatively it is essential to maintain the ankles and feet in corrected neutral position by splints at night and plastic orthoses in the shoes during the day.

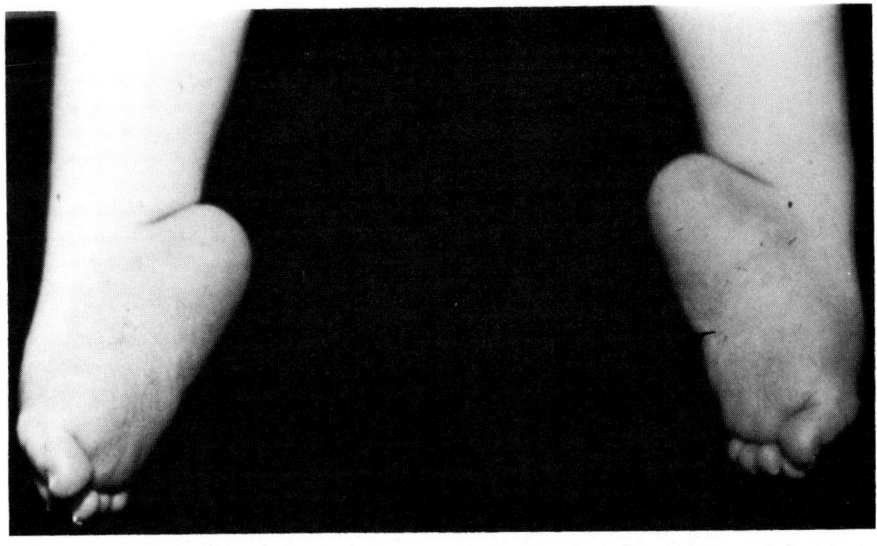

FIGURE 3–59. Severe equinus deformity of both feet due to fibrosis and contracture of the triceps surae.

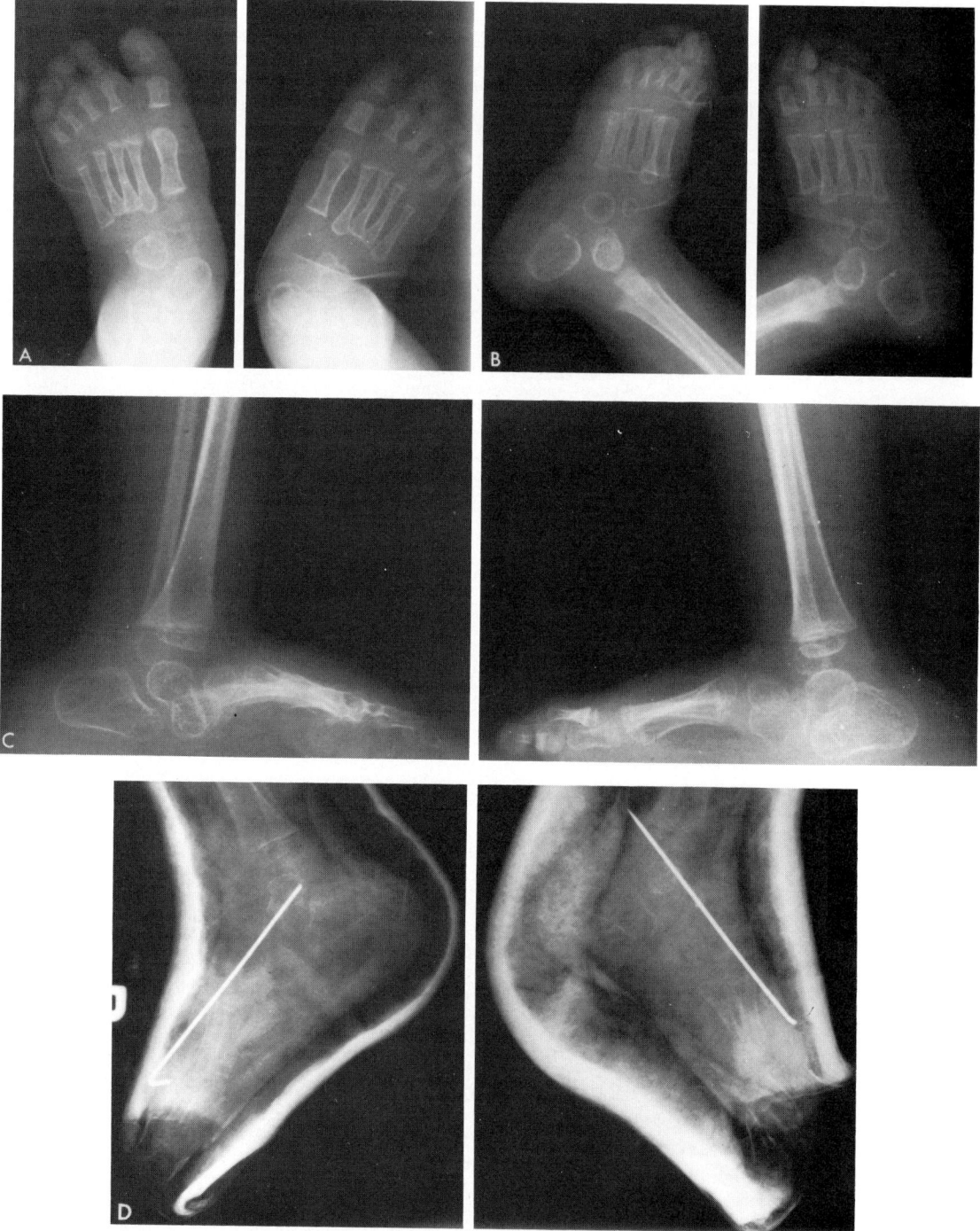

FIGURE 3–60. Paralytic congenital convex pes valgus of both feet in a child with myelomeningocele.

A and **B**. Roentgenograms of both feet at age of ten months. **C**. Lateral roentgenograms of the feet at two and one half years of age. Note the plantar-flexed talus with dislocation of the talonavicular joint. The os calcis is everted and shows some equinus deviation. The forefoot is abducted and slightly dorsiflexed. **D**. Postoperative lateral roentgenograms of both feet in cast. Open reduction of the talonavicular joint was performed. The Kirschner wire was introduced retrograde to maintain the reduction. The anterior tibial and peroneal muscles were transferred posteriorly to the os calcis.

Illustration continued on opposite page

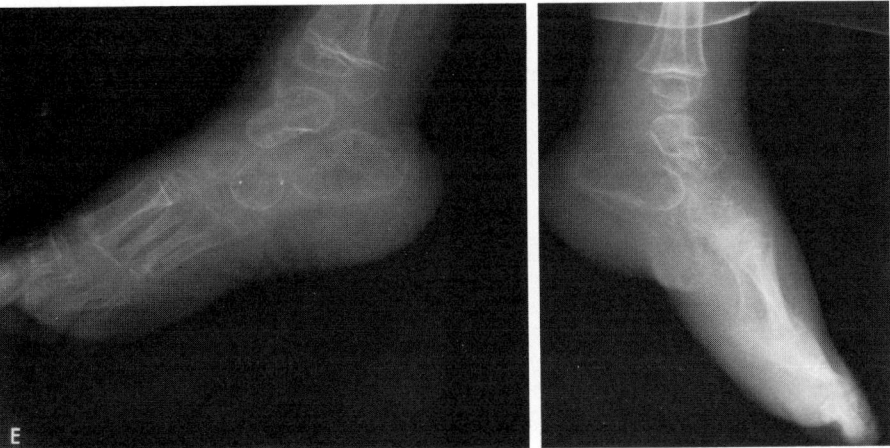

FIGURE 3–60 Continued. *Paralytic congenital convex pes valgus of both feet in a child with myelomeningocele.*

E. Six months after surgery. The roentgenograms of both feet show maintenance of reduction. The foot has normal alignment.

Paralytic Congenital Convex Pes Valgus

This is a rare congenital deformity, occurring in the feet of 5 to 10 per cent of children born with myelomeningocele. The talus is plantar-flexed, and the talocalcaneonavicular joint is subluxated or dislocated dorsally and laterally. In clinical appearance, the paralytic and nonparalytic types are quite similar. The sole of the foot is convex with the head of the talus prominent on its plantar and medial aspect; the hindfoot is everted and in equinus posture, and the forepart of the foot is abducted and dorsiflexed (Fig. 3–60).

The usual pattern of muscle imbalance found in association with paralytic vertical talus is normal strength in the anterior tibial, long toe extensor, and peroneal muscles, and paralysis of the triceps surae, tibialis posterior, long and short toe flexors, and intrinsic muscles of the foot, i.e., intact innervation down to the muscles supplied by the first sacral segment with paralysis of the muscles supplied by the second and third sacral segments. Occasionally, congenital convex pes valgus is associated with complete paralysis of all muscles of the lower limb. The pathologic anatomy and roentgenographic features are discussed in the section on congenital convex pes valgus in Chapter 2. Usually the deformity is present at birth; occasionally it develops postnatally.[25]

The deformity is very rigid and does not respond to conservative therapy. It is strongly recommended that open reduction of the talocalcaneonavicular joint be performed at three to six months of age, depending upon the general medical and neurosurgical status of the infant. The capsule of the talonavicular joint is repaired, and the joint is fixed internally with a threaded pin.

The details of the author's operative technique are illustrated in Plate 5. The muscular forces acting on the foot are balanced by appropriate tendon transfers; commonly the anterior tibial tendon is transferred to the head-neck of the talus, and the peroneus brevis posteriorly to the os calcis. The peroneus longus is left to act as plantar-flexor of the first metatarsal.

Duckworth and Smith, and Sharrard recommend the following procedure: The operation is performed through three incisions, the first of which is made over the dorsum of the foot to the lateral aspect of the subtalar joint. A segment of the taut long toe extensors and peroneus tertius is excised. (Sharrard recommends lengthening rather than sectioning of the toe extensors.) The subtalar joint is opened laterally, and the interosseous talocalcaneal ligament is divided. The peroneus longus is lengthened by Z-plasty. The peroneus brevis is detached from the base of the fifth metatarsal. By this degree of soft-tissue release, a great deal of the dorsiflexion-abduction deformity of the forefoot and the valgus deformity of the hindfoot can be corrected. A separate longitudinal incision is made on the lateral side of the Achilles tendon. The peroneus brevis is delivered into the back of the ankle, and the tendo calcaneus is lengthened by Z-plasty. A third incision is made on the medial aspect of the foot, beginning below and behind the medial malleolus and extending distally to the base of the first metatarsal. The dorsal capsule of the talonavicular joint and the tibionavicular ligament are sectioned, and the talonavicular joint is reduced. The tibialis posterior tendon is identified and isolated. The tibialis anterior tendon is detached from its insertion to the base of the first metatarsal. Next, the peroneus brevis tendon is passed across the back of the ankle joint deep to the neurovascular bundle, threaded down the tendon sheath of the tibialis posterior, and attached to the navicular bone. In case the peroneus brevis tendon is short and does not reach the navicular, it is sutured to the tibialis posterior proximal to the level of the tendon sheath. The talonavicular joint is reduced and transfixed with a Kirschner wire, and the anterior tibial tendon is transferred to the neck of the talus (Fig. 3–61). The tourniquet is released, and after complete hemostasis, the wounds are closed, and a below-knee cast is applied. The cast and Kirschner wire are removed in six weeks, at which time the limb is mobilized and walking with appropriate orthotic support is permitted.[25] Sharrard recommends simple division of the tendons in the flail limb with paralytic convex pes valgus.[133]

This author advocates preservation of muscle function, i.e., do not section the tendons of the long toe extensors and peroneous tertius; if necessary, lengthen them. The peroneus brevis is transferred posteromedially to the navicular if the tibialis posterior is paralyzed; if the posterior tibial tendon and plantar calcaneonavicular ligament are functioning, they are advanced distally to increase the support on the plantar aspect of the head of the talus. It is vital to plicate and tauten the capsule of the talonavicular joint on its medial and plantar aspects.

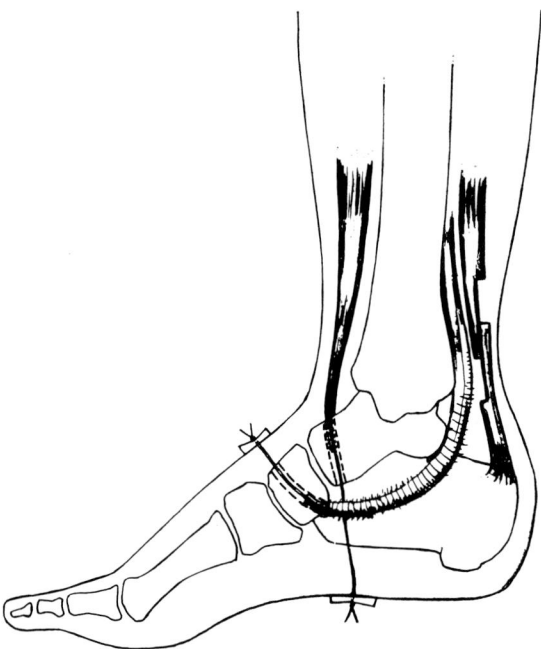

FIGURE 3–61. Composite diagram showing tendons transferred in operative correction of paralytic congenital convex pes valgus in myelomeningocele.

The tendo calcaneus is lengthened by Z-plasty. The anterior tibial tendon is transferred to the neck of the talus, and the peroneus brevis is detached from the base of the fifth metatarsal, passed behind the ankle joint deep to the neurovascular bundle, threaded down the sheath of the tibialis posterior tendon and attached to the navicular. (From Duckworth, T., and Smith, T. W. D.: The treatment of paralytic convex pes valgus. J. Bone Joint Surg., 56-B:305, 1974. Reprinted by permission.)

Pes Cavus and Claw Toes

With intact innervation down to the second sacral segment, there will be paralysis of the intrinsic muscles of the foot, but motor strength of the remaining muscles of the lower limb will be normal. The dynamic muscle imbalance between the long toe extensors and flexors and the intrinsic muscles of the foot will gradually cause pes cavus and clawing of the toes (Figs. 3–62 and 3–63). Most of these children have quite adequate motor function in their lower limbs and are very active on their feet. Meticulous care should be given to the toe and forefoot deformities, however, to prevent development of pressure sores on the toes or the plantar surface of the metatarsal heads. The type of treatment varies with the severity of deformity. In mild to moderate cases, treat-

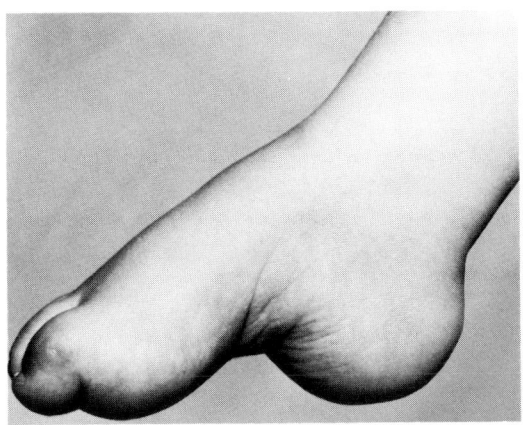

FIGURE 3–62. *Clawing of the hallux in myelomeningocele.*

ment is by passive stretching exercises and a metatarsal pad. More severe deformity may require plantar fasciotomy and transfer of long toe extensors to the metatarsal heads. In the older child, fusion of the proximal interphalangeal joint is indicated.

For clawing of the great toe in the young child, Sharrard recommends tenodesis of the flexor hallucis longus. The hallux should be flexible; rigid deformity is a contraindication to the procedure.[136]

The operation is performed under general anesthesia and tourniquet hemostasis. If cavus deformity is present, it is corrected by plantar release. A longitudinal incision is made over the medial aspect of the great toe and the distal third of the first metatarsal. The subcutaneous tissue is divided; the neurovascular bundle is identified and retracted dorsally. The flexor hallucis longus tendon is dissected free. If there is any contracture of the dorsal capsule of the metatarsophalangeal joint, it is released. In the middle half of the plantar surface of the proximal phalanx of the great toe, the periosteum and cortex are excised. Two stainless steel sutures are passed through the tendon of the flexor hallucis longus, and the tendon is secured to cancellous bone. The tension on the proximal part of the tendon maintains the metatarsophalangeal joint of the hallux in neutral extension. There should be no tension on the distal part of the tendon. A Kirschner wire is passed through both phalanges of the great toe at the first metatarsal. After closure of the wound, a below-knee walking cast is applied. The cast and pull-out wire are removed in six weeks. Sharrard has performed this operation in 17 feet and achieved good results in 15.[136] This author has had no experience with this operation. The treatment of pes cavus and pes calcaneocavus is discussed in Chapter 4; the same principles apply for treatment of pes cavus in myelomeningocele.

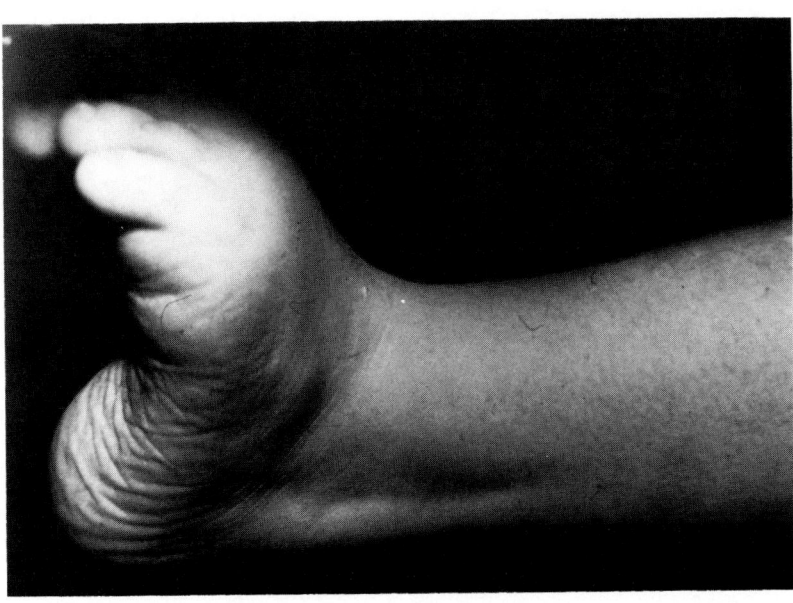

FIGURE 3–63. *Clawing of the hallux and the lesser toes in spina bifida.*

Flail Ankle

When the foot is plantigrade and free of deformity it may be stabilized by appropriate fusion, enabling the patient to discard orthotic support and use only crutches for walking. In the past, if the hip flexors and quadriceps femoris muscles were satisfactory, this author has performed a Chuinard type of ankle fusion when the child was eight or ten years old. Delayed healing and development of Charcot-like changes were a problem, however, and therefore, at present, he does not recommend ankle fusion in myelomeningocele. It should never be combined with either a Green-Grice extra-articular subtalar arthrodesis or a triple arthrodesis (i.e., pantalar fusion) because of consequent trophic skin problems under the metatarsal heads. This is contrary to the report of Ruderman and associates.[118b]

References

1. Abraham, E., Verinder, D. G., and Sharrard, W. J.: The treatment of flexion contracture of the knee in myelomeningocele. J. Bone Joint Surg., 59-B:433, 1977.
2. Banta, J. V., Sutherland, D. H., and Wyatt, M.: Anterior tibial transfer to the os calcis with Achilles tendon for calcaneus deformity in myelomeningocele. J. Pediat. Orthop., 1:125, 1981.
3. Bratberg, J. J., and Scheer, G. E.: Extra-articular arthrodesis of the subtalar joint: A clinical study and review. Clin. Orthop., 126:220, 1977.
4. Brereton, R. J., Cudmore, R. E., Irving, I. M., Lister, J., and Buyukpanukcu, N.: Screening for neural-tube defects. Lancet, 1:879, 1978.
5. Brocklehurst, G.: Spina Bifida for the Clinician. Clinics in Developmental Medicine, Vol. 57. Philadelphia, J. B. Lippincott Co., 1976.
6. Brocklehurst, G., Gleave, J. R. W., and Lewin, W. S.: Early closure of myelomeningocele with especial reference to leg movement. Develop. Med. Child Neurol. Suppl., 13:51, 1967.
7. Bunch, W. H.: General concepts. Myelomeningocele. Part I. A.A.O.S. Instr. Course Lect., 25:61–65, 1976.
8. Bunch, W. H., Cass, A. S., Bensman, A. S., and Long, D. M.: Orthopedic approaches. In Modern Management of Myelomeningocele. St. Louis, Warren H. Green, Inc., 1972, pp. 121–180.
9. Cameron, A. H.: The spinal cord lesion in spina bifida cystica. Lancet, 2:171, 1956.
10. Carroll, N.: The orthotic management of the spina bifida child. Clin. Orthop., 102:108, 1974.
11. Carroll, N.: An orthopedist's view of bracing. In McLaurin, R. L. (ed.): Myelomeningocele. New York, Grune & Stratton, Inc., 1977, pp. 411–419.
12. Carroll, N.: Hindfoot and forefoot varus. In McLaurin, R. L. (ed.): Myelomeningocele. New York, Grune & Stratton, Inc., 1977, pp. 441–445.
13. Cartaya, R. A.: A modified standing orthosis. Orthot. Prosthet., 30:25, 1976.
14. Carter, C. O.: The management of spina bifida cystica. Birth Defects, 1974.
14a. Carter, C. O.: Genetics of common simple malformations. Brit. Med. Bull., 32:21, 1976.
14b. Carter, C. O., and Evans, K.: Children of adult survivors with spina bifida cystica. Lancet, 2:924, 1973.
14c. Carter, C. O., and Evans, K.: Spina bifida and anencephalus in Greater London. J. Med. Genet., 10:209, 1973.
14d. Carter, C. O., and Fraser Roberts, J. A.: The risk of recurrence after two children with central nervous system malformation. Lancet, 1:306, 1967.
15. Chakour, K.: Deformities of the lower extremities and prosthetic devices in children with myelodysplasia. Arch. Orthop. Unfallchir., 70:101, 1971.
16. Childs, V.: Physiotherapy for spina bifida. Physiotherapy. 63:218, 1977.
17. Chrystal, M., and Hershey, L. S.: Total rehabilitation in relation to spina bifida. Phys. Ther. Rev., 31:357, 1951.
18. Davidson, B. G., and Sheffield, L. J.: Hazards of prenatal detection of neural tube defects by screening maternal serum for alpha fetoprotein. Canad. Med. Assoc. J., 118:1186, 1978.
19. DeSouza, L. J., and Carroll, N.: Ambulation of the braced myelomeningocele patient. J. Bone Joint Surg., 58-A:1112, 1976.
20. Dias, L. S.: Ankle valgus in children with myelomeningocele. Develop. Med. Child Neurol., 20:627, 1978.
20a. Dias, L.: The foot. In Schafer, M. F., and Dias, L. S.: Myelomeningocele: Orthopaedic treatment. Baltimore, Williams & Wilkins Co., 1983.
21. Dimeglio, A., Pous, J. G., Montoya, P., and Cahuaz, M.: Le membre supérieur des myéloméningocèles. Elément négligé du diagnostic fonctionnel. Rev. Chir. Orthop., 62 Suppl.:51, 1976.
22. Doran, P. A., and Guthkelch, A. N.: Studies in spina bifida cystica. I. General survey and reassessment of the problem. J. Neurol. Neurosurg. Psychiat., 24:331, 1961.
23. Drennan, J. C.: Management of myelomeningocele foot deformities in infancy and early childhood. Myelomeningocele. Part V. A.A.O.S. Instr. Course Lect., 25:82–90, 1976.
24. Drennan, J. C., and Sharrard, W. J.: The pathological anatomy of convex pes valgus. J. Bone Joint Surg., 53-B:455, 1971.
25. Duckworth, T., and Smith, T. W. D.: The treatment of paralytic convex pes valgus. J. Bone Joint Surg., 56-B:305, 1974.
26. Duncan, J. W., and Lovell, W. W.: Hoke triple arthrodesis. J. Bone Joint Surg., 60-A:795, 1978.
27. Dunn, N.: Calcaneocavus and its treatment. J. Orthop. Surg., 1:711, 1919.
28. Edvardsen, P.: Physeo-epiphyseal injuries of lower extremities in myelomeningocele. Acta Orthop. Scand., 43:550, 1972.
29. Edwards, J. H.: Congenital malformations of the central nervous system in Scotland. Brit. J. Prev. Soc. Med., 12:115, 1958.
30. Eskelund, V., and Bartels, E. D.: Spina bifida umbalis in uniovular twins. Nord. Med., (Hospitalstid), 11:2075, 1941.
31. Faber, L. A., and Ericksen, L. G.: Prenatal diagnosis of spina bifida. J. Iowa Med. Soc., 26:359, 1936.
32. Fawcitt, J.: Some radiological aspects of congenital anomalies of the spine in childhood and infancy. Proc. Roy. Soc. Med., 52:331, 1959.
33. Feiwell, E.: Paralytic calcaneus in myelomeningocele. In McLaurin, R. L. (ed.): Myelomeningocele. New York, Grune & Stratton, Inc., 1977, pp. 447–460.
34. Ferguson-Smith, M. A., Rawlinson, H. A., May, H. A., Vince, J. D., Gibson, A. A., Robinson, H. P., and Ratcliffe, J. G.: Avoidance of anencephalic and spina bifida births by maternal serum-alphafetoprotein screening. Lancet, 1:1330, 1978.
35. Floyd, W., Lovell, W., and King, R. E.: The neuropathic joint. Southern Med. J., 52:563, 1959.
36. Foltz, E. L., Kronmal, R., and Shurtleff, D. B.: To treat or not to treat: A neurosurgeon's perspective of myelomeningocele. Clin. Neurosurg., 20:147, 1973.
37. Ford, F. R.: Diseases of the Nervous System in Infancy, Childhood, and Adolescence. 5th Ed. Springfield, Ill., Charles C Thomas, 1966, pp. 84–88, 159–166.
38. Fraser, F. C.: Genetic counselling. Amer. J. Hum. Genet., 26:636, 1974.
39. Freeman, J. M.: To treat or not to treat: Ethical dilemmas of treating the infant with a myelomeningocele. Clin. Neurosurg., 20:134, 1973.
39a. Freeman, J. M.: Practical Management of Meningomyelocele. Baltimore, University Park Press, 1974.
40. Gardner, W. J.: Etiology and pathogenesis of the development of myelomeningocele. In McLaurin, R. L. (ed.): Myelomeningocele. New York, Grune & Stratton, Inc., 1977, pp. 3–30.

41. Gillies, C. L., and Hartung, W.: Fracture of tibia in spina bifida vera. Radiology, *31*:621, 1938.
42. Glancy, J.: A dynamic orthotic system for young myelomeningoceles: A preliminary report. Orthot. Prosthet., *30*:3, 1976.
43. Golding, C.: Spina bifida and epiphyseal displacement. J. Bone Joint Surg., *42-B*:387, 1960.
44. Golski, A., and Menelaus, M. B.: The treatment of intoed gait in spina bifida patients by lateral transfer of the medial hamstrings. Aust. New Zeal. J. Surg., *46*:157, 1976.
45. Green, W. T., and Grice, D. S.: The management of calcaneus deformity. A.A.O.S. Instr. Course Lect., *13*:135–149, 1956.
46. Grimm, R. A.: Hand function and tactile perception in a sample of children with myelomeningocele. Amer. J. Occup. Ther., *30*:234, 1976.
47. Gross, H. P.: Myelomeningocele in one identical twin. J. Neurosurg., *20*:439, 1963.
48. Gyepes, M. T., Newbern, D. H., and Neuhauser, E. B. D.: Metaphyseal and physeal injuries in children with spina bifida and meningomyelocele. Amer. J. Roentgen., *95*:168, 1965.
49. Hay, M. C., and Walker, G.: Plantar pressures in healthy children and in children with myelomeningocele. J. Bone Joint Surg., *55-B*:828, 1973.
50. Hayes, J. T., and Gross, H. P.: Orthopedic implications of myelodysplasia. J.A.M.A., *184*:762, 1963.
51. Hayes, J. T., Gross, H. P., and Dow, S.: Surgery for paralytic defects secondary to myelomeningocele and myelodysplasia. J. Bone Joint Surg., *46-A*:1577, 1964.
52. Hayes-Allen, M. C.: Obesity and short stature in children with myelomeningocele. Develop. Med. Child Neurol. Suppl. *27*:59, 1972.
53. Herskowitz, J., and Marks, A. N.: The spina bifida patient as a person. Develop. Med. Child Neurol., *19*:413, 1977.
54. Hewson, J. E.: Basic physiotherapy of spina bifida. Devel. Med. Child Neurol., Suppl. *37*:117, 1976.
55. Hoffer, M. M., Feiwell, E., Perry, R., Perry, J., and Bonnett, C.: Functional ambulation in patients with myelomeningocele. J. Bone Joint Surg., *55-A*:137, 1973.
56. Hollingsworth, R. P.: An x-ray study of the valgus ankles in spina bifida children with valgus flat foot. Proc. Roy. Soc. Med., *68*:481, 1975.
57. Hostler, S. L.: Development of the infant with myelomeningocele. Myelomeningocele. Part III. A.A.O.S. Instr. Course Lect., *25*:70–75, 1976.
58. Hostler, S. L.: The adolescent with myelomeningocele. Myelomeningocele. Part VI. A.A.O.S. Instr. Course Lect., *25*:90–93, 1976.
59. Ingalls, T. H., Pugh, T. F., and MacMahon, B.: Incidence of anencephalus, spina bifida, and hydrocephalus related to birth rank and maternal age. Brit. J. Prev. Soc. Med., *8*:17, 1954.
60. Ingraham, F. D., and Matson, D. D.: Neurosurgery in Infancy and Childhood. Springfield, Ill., Charles C Thomas, 1954.
61. Jolson, R. A.: Split triceps transfer for recurrent equinus. *In* McLaurin, R. L. (ed.): Myelomeningocele. New York, Grune & Stratton, Inc., 1977, pp. 427–436.
62. Judet, H., and Judet, J.: La réorientation de l'articulation tibio-tarsienne. Chirurgie, *97*:638, 1971.
63. Katz, J. F.: Spontaneous fractures in paraplegic children. J. Bone Joint Surg., *35-A*:220, 1953.
64. Kilfoyle, R. M., Foley, J. J., and Norton, P. L.: The spine and pelvic deformity in childhood and adolescent paraplegia. J. Bone Joint Surg., *47-A*:659, 1965.
65. Kopits, S. E.: Orthopedic aspects in meningomyeloceles. *In* Freeman, J. M. (ed.): Practical Management of Meningomyelocele. Baltimore, University Park Press, 1974, pp. 106–165.
66. Kowalski, M.: The place of orthopedic surgery in early rehabilitation of children with spina bifida. Acta Orthop. Belg., *43*:297, 1977.
67. Kupka, J., Geddes, N., and Carroll, N. C.: Comprehensive management in the child with spina bifida. Orthop. Clin. N. Amer., *9*:97, 1978.
68. Lambert, K. L.: The weight-bearing function of the fibula. A strain gauge study. J. Bone Joint Surg., *53-A*:507, 1971.
68a. Langenskiöld, A.: Supination deformity of the forefoot. Acta Orthop. Scand., *48*:325, 1977.
69. Laurence, K. M.: The natural history of spina bifida cystica: Detailed analysis of 407 cases. Arch Dis. Child., *59*:41, 1964.
70. Lenzi, L., and Manzoni, A.: Piede cavo essenziale e piede cavo mielodisplasico. Chir. Organi Mov., *54*:123, 1965.
71. Laurence, K. M.: The survival of untreated spina bifida cystica. Develop. Med. Child. Neurol., *8*:Suppl. 11:10, 1966.
72. Laurence, K. M., and Tew, B. J.: Follow-up of 65 survivors from the 425 cases of spina bifida born in South Wales between 1956 and 1962. Develop. Med. Child Neurol., Suppl. 13:1, 1967.
73. Levitt, R. L., Canale, S. T., and Gartland, J. J.: Surgical correction of foot deformity in the older patient with myelomeningocele. Orthop. Clin. N. Amer., *5*:19, 1974.
74. Lindseth, R. E.: Treatment of the lower extremity in children paralyzed by myelomeningocele (birth to 18 months). Myelomeningocele. Part IV. A.A.O.S. Instr. Course Lect., *25*:76–82, 1976.
75. Lindseth, R. E.: Valgus and rotational deformities of the knee, ankle and foot in myelomeningocele. *In* McLaurin, R. L. (ed.): Myelomeningocele. New York, Grune & Stratton, Inc., 1977, pp. 475–488.
76. Lodge, T.: Bone, joint, and soft tissue changes following paraplegia. Acta Radiol., *46*:435, 1956.
77. Long, C. H., and Lawton, E. B.: Functional significance of spinal cord lesion level. Arch. Phys. Med., *36*:249, 1955.
78. Lonton, A. P.: Hand preference in children with myelomeningocele and hydrocephalus. Develop. Med. Child Neurol., Suppl. 37:143, 1976.
79. Lorber, J.: The family history of spina bifida cystica. Pediatrics, *35*:589, 1965.
80. Lorber, J.: Incidence and epidemiology of myelomeningocele. Clin. Orthop., *45*:81, 1966.
81. Lorber, J.: Neurologic assessment of neonates with spina bifida. Clin. Pediat., *7*:676, 1968.
82. Lorber, J.: Results of treatment of myelomeningocele. An analysis of 524 unselected cases, with special references to possible selection for treatment. Develop. Med. Child Neurol., *13*:279, 1971.
83. Lorber, J.: Spina bifida cystica: Results of treatment of 270 consecutive cases. Arch. Dis. Child., *47*:854, 1972.
84. Lorber, J., and Levick, K.: Spina bifida cystica: Incidence of spina bifida occulta in parents and in controls. Arch. Dis. Child., *42*:171, 1967.
85. Makin, M.: Tibio-fibular relationship in paralyzed limbs. J. Bone Joint Surg., *47-B*:500, 1965.
86. Matson, D. D.: Surgical repair of myelomeningocele. J. Neurosurg., *27*:180, 1967.
87. Melton, J.: Life with spina bifida. Brit. Med. J., *1*:47, 1978.
88. Menelaus, M. B.: Dislocation and deformity of the hip in children with spina bifida cystica. J. Bone Joint Surg., *51-B*:238, 1969.
89. Menelaus, M. B.: Talectomy for equinovarus deformity in arthrogryposis and spina bifida. J. Bone Joint Surg., *53*:468, 1971.
90. Menelaus, M. B.: The Orthopedic Management of Spina Bifida Cystica. 2nd Ed. Edinburgh, E. & S. Livingstone, 1980.
91. Menelaus, M. B.: Orthopaedic management of children with myelomeningocele: A plea for realistic goals. Develop. Med. Child Neurol., Suppl. 37:31, 1976.
92. Menelaus, M. B., and Burrows, H. J.: Conditions affecting the hip—paralytic dislocation of the hip. *In* The Orthopaedic Management of Spina Bifida Cystica. Edinburgh, E. & S. Livingstone, 1977, pp. 51–65.
93. Milunsky, A., and Alpert, E.: Maternal serum AFP screening. New Eng. J. Med., *298*:738, 1978.
94. Mitchell, G. P.: Posterior displacement osteotomy of the calcaneus. J. Bone Joint Surg., *59-B*:233, 1977.
95. Montagnani, C. A.: Traitement chirurgical des malformations osseuses multiples en cas de myelomeningocele. Ann. Chir. Infant. (Paris), *10*:115, 1969.
96. Morris, J., and Laurence, K. M.: The effectiveness of genetic counselling for neural-tube malformations. Develop. Med. Child Neurol., Suppl. 37:157, 1976.
97. Morris, J. V.: Familial spina bifida. J. Irish Med. Assoc., *40*:154, 1957.
98. Morrissy, R. T.: Spina bifida: A new rehabilitation problem. Orthop. Clin. N. Amer., *9*:379, 1978.
98a. Murphy, E. A., and Chase, G. A.: Principles of Genetic

Counselling. Chicago, Year Book Medical Publishers, 1975.
99. Nadler, H. L.: Present status of the prevention of neural tube defects. Pediatrics, 55:751, 1975.
100. Naglo, A. S., and Hellstrom, B.: Results of treatment in myelomeningocele. Acta Paediat. Scand., 65:565, 1976.
101. Nöh, E., and Kienzler, G.: Ein Beitrag zum Problem der Analgesie beim Kind. Arch. Orthop. Unfallchir., 73:263, 1972.
102. Norton, P. L., and Foley, J. J.: Paraplegia in children. J. Bone Joint Surg., 41-A:1291, 1959.
103. Ogston, A.: A new principle of curing clubfoot in severe cases in children a few years old. Brit. Med. J., 1524, 1902.
104. Padovani, J. P., Rigault, P., Pouliquen, J. C., Guyonvarch, G., and Durand, Y.: L'astragalectomie chez l'enfant. Résultats, technique, indications, d'après notre expérience de 33 cas. Rev. Chir. Orthop., 62:475, 1976.
105. Parsch, K.: Early orthopedic treatment of children with myelomeningocele. Acta Orthop. Belg., 38:204, 1972.
106. Parsch, K., and Rossak, K.: Die pathologischen Frakturen bei Spina bifida. Arch. Orthop. Unfallchir., 68:165, 1970.
107. Parsch, K., and Schulitz, K. P.: Rehabilitation of the spina bifida child. Z. Orthop., 110:997, 1972.
108. Parsch, K., and Manner, G.: Prevention and treatment of knee problems in children with spina bifida. Develop. Med. Child Neurol., Suppl. 37:114, 1976.
109. Passo, S. D.: Positioning infants with myelomeningocele. Amer. J. Nurs., 74:1658, 1974.
110. Peabody, C. W.: Tendon transplantation in the lower extremities. A.A.O.S. Instr. Course Lect., 6:178, 1949.
111. Quilis, A. N.: Fractures in children with myelomeningocele. Acta. Orthop. Scand., 45:883, 1974.
112. Rali, S. Z. A., Rali, S. H. M., Randall, M., Watkins, G., and Blake, P. D.: Changes in shape, ossification and quality of bones in children with spina bifida. Develop. Med. Child Neurol., Suppl. 37:29, 1976.
113. Raycroft, J. F.: Care of the flexible foot in infants and younger children with myelodysplasia. In McLaurin, R. L. (ed.): Myelomeningocele. New York, Grune & Stratton, Inc., 1977, pp. 421–425.
114. Raycroft, J. F.: Talectomy: Application in children with myelodysplasia. In McLaurin, R. L. (ed.): Myelomeningocele. New York, Grune & Stratton, Inc., 1977, pp. 437–440.
115. Record, R. G., and McKeown, T.: Congenital malformations of the central nervous system. I. A survey of 930 cases. Brit. J. Soc. Med., 3:183, 1949.
116. Renoirte, P., and Bellen, P.: Place of orthoses in the treatment of sequelae of meningomyelocele. Acta Orthop. Belg., 43:345, 1977.
117. Rickham, P. P.: The swing of the pendulum: The indications for operating on myelomeningoceles. Med. J. Aust., 2:743, 1976.
118. Rodeck, C. H., and Campbell, S.: Early prenatal diagnosis of neural-tube defects by ultrasound-guided fetoscopy. Lancet, 1:1128, 1978.
118a. Rogers, J. C.: Genetic counselling and antenatal diagnosis. In Menelaus, M. B.: The Orthopedic Management of Spina Bifida Cystica. Edinburgh, London, New York, Churchill Livingstone, 1980, pp. 20–22.
118b. Ruderman, R. J., Goldner, J. L., and Hardaker, W. T.: Pantalar fusion in myelodysplasia: a procedure too hastily rejected? Orthop. Trans., 4:152, 1980.
119. Samilson, R. L.: Crescentic osteotomy of the os calcis for calcaneocavus feet. In Bateman, J. E. (ed.): Foot Science, Philadelphia, W. B. Saunders Co., 1976, p. 18.
119a. Schafer, M. F., and Dias, L. S.: Myelomeningocele: Orthopaedic Treatment. Baltimore, Williams & Wilkins Co., 1983.
120. Schulitz, K. P., Schumacher, G., and Parsch, K.: Congenital rocker-bottom foot. Z. Orthop., 115:55, 1977.
121. Scrimgeour, J. B.: Antenatal diagnosis: Present and future. Practitioner, 220:612, 1978.
122. Seeligmüller, K.: V-osteotomy for the correction of popliteal fossa contractures in spina bifida children. Z. Orthop., 113:776, 1975.
123. Sharrard, W. J. W.: Congenital paralytic dislocation of the hip in children with myelo-meningocele. J. Bone Joint Surg., 41-B:622, 1959.
124. Sharrard, W. J. W.: The mechanism of paralytic deformity in spina bifida. Develop. Med. Child Neurol., 4:310, 1962.
125. Sharrard, W. J. W.: Posterior iliopsoas transplantation in the treatment of paralytic dislocation of the hip. J. Bone Joint Surg., 46-B:426, 1964.
126. Sharrard, W. J. W.: Spina bifida. Physiotherapy, 50:44, 1964.
127. Sharrard, W. J. W.: Paralytic deformity in the lower limb. J. Bone Joint Surg., 49-B:731, 1967.
128. Sharrard, W. J. W.: The orthopaedic surgery of spina bifida. Clin. Orthop., 92:195, 1973.
129. Sharrard, W. J. W.: The orthopaedic management of spina bifida. Acta Orthop. Scand., 46:356, 1975.
130. Sharrard, W. J. W.: General orthopaedic management and operative treatment. In Brocklehurst, G. (ed.): Spina Bifida and the Clinician. Clinics in Developmental Medicine, Vol. 57. Philadelphia. J. B. Lippincott Co., 1976, pp. 84–100.
131. Sharrard, W. J. W.: Specific orthopaedic problems. In Brocklehurst, G. (ed.): Spina Bifida for the Clinician. Clinics in Developmental Medicine. Vol. 57. Philadelphia, J. B. Lippincott Co., 1976, pp. 101–121.
132. Sharrard, W. J. W.: Assessment of the myelomeningocele child. In McLaurin, R. L. (ed.): Myelomeningocele. New York, Grune & Stratton, Inc., 1977, pp. 389–410.
133. Sharrard, W. J. W.: Paralytic convex pes valgus. (Paralytic vertical talus.) In McLaurin, R. L. (ed.): Myelomeningocele. New York, Grune & Stratton, Inc., 1977, pp. 461–467.
134. Sharrard, W. J. W.: Paralytic pes cavus and claw toes. In McLaurin, R. L. (ed.): Myelomeningocele. New York, Grune & Stratton, Inc., 1977, pp. 469–474.
135. Sharrard, W. J. W., and Grosfeld, I.: The management of deformity and paralysis of the foot in myelomeningocele. J. Bone Joint Surg., 50-B:456, 1968.
136. Sharrard, W. J. W., and Smith, T. W. D.: Tenodesis of flexor hallucis longus for paralytic clawing of the hallux in childhood. J. Bone Joint Surg., 58-B:224, 1976.
137. Sharrard, W. J. W., and Webb, J.: Supramalleolar wedge osteotomy of the tibia in children with myelomeningocele. J. Bone Joint Surg., 56-B:458, 1974.
138. Sharrard, W. J. W., Zachary, R. B., Lorber, J., and Bruce, A. M.: A controlled trial of immediate and delayed closure of spina bifida cystica. Arch. Dis. Child., 38:18, 1963.
139. Sherk, H. H., and Ames, M. D.: Talectomy in the treatment of the myelomeningocele patient. Clin. Orthop., 110:218, 1975.
140. Shillito, J. Jr.: Surgical approaches to spina bifida and myelomeningocele. Clin. Neurosurg., 20:114, 1973.
141. Shulman, K., and Ames, M.: Intensive treatment of fifty children born with myelomeningocele. New York J. Med., 68:265, 1969.
141a. Simpson, D.: Congenital malformations of the nervous system. Med. J. Aust., 1:700, 1976.
142. Smith, E. D.: Spina Bifida and the Total Care of Spinal Myelomeningocele. Springfield, Ill., Charles C Thomas, 1965.
143. Smith, R. S.: Orthopedic considerations in the treatment of spina bifida. Surg. Gynec. Obstet., 62:218, 1936.
144. Smith, T. W. D., and Duckworth, T.: The management of deformity of the foot in children with spina bifida. Develop. Med. Child Neurol., Suppl. 37:104, 1976.
145. Solovay, J., and Solovay, H. U.: Paraplegic neuroarthropathy. Amer. J. Roentgen., 61:475, 1949.
146. Soutter, F. E.: Spina bifida and epiphyseal displacement.: Report of two cases. J. Bone Joint Surg., 44-B:106, 1962.
147. Specht, E. E.: Congenital paralytic vertical talus. An anatomical study. J. Bone Joint Surg., 57-A:842, 1975.
148. Stark, G. D.: Spina bifida. Problems and management. London, Oxford Blackwell Scientific Publications, 1977.
149. Stark, G. D., and Baker, G. C. W.: The neurological involvement of the lower limbs in myelomeningocele. Develop. Med. Child Neurol., 9:732, 1967.
150. Stein, S. C., Schut, L., and Ames, M. D.: Selection of early treatment of myelomeningocele: A retrospective analysis of selection procedures. Develop. Med. Child Neurol., 17:311, 1975.
151. Stills, M.: Clinical experience with the "solid-ankle" orthosis. Orthot. Prosthet., 30:13, 1976.
152. Stoyle, T. F.: Prognosis for paralysis in myelomeningocele. Develop. Med. Child Neurol., 8:755, 1966.
153. Strach, E. H.: The spring implant operation: a preliminary report. Develop. Med. Child Neurol., Suppl. 27:121, 1972.

154. Sugar, M., and Kennedy, C. M.: The use of electrodiagnostic techniques in the evaluation of the neurological deficit in infants with meningomyelocele. Neurology (Minneap.), 15:787, 1965.
155. Swinyard, C. A.: Comprehensive Care of the Child with Spina Bifida Manifesta. Rehabilitation Monograph No. 31. New York, Institute of Rehabilitation Medicine, 1966.
156. Taillard, W., Compère, J., Vasey, H., and Berney, J.: L'orthopédie des spina bifida. Ann. Chir. Infant. (Paris), 10:87, 1969.
157. Tzimas, N., and Badell-Ribera, A.: Orthopedic and habilitation management of patients with spina bifida and myelomeningocele. Med. Clin. N. Amer., 53:502, 1969.
158. Vanderick, L. P.: Pathology and treatment of feet and knees in myelomeningocele. Acta Orthop. Belg., 43:306, 1977.
158a. Wald, N. J., and Cuckle, H.: Maternal serum alpha fetoprotein measurement in antenatal screening for anencephaly and spina bifida in early pregnancy. Reports of a collaborative study of alpha fetoprotein in relation to neural tube defect. Lancet, 1:1323, 1977.
159. Wald, N., Cuckle, H., and Polani, P. E.: Alpha-fetoprotein in antenatal diagnosis of neural tube defects. Brit. Med. J., 1:238, 1978.
160. Walker, G.: The early management of varus feet in myelomeningocele. J. Bone Joint Surg., 53-B:462, 1977.
161. Walker, G., and Cheong-Leon, P.: The surgical management of paralytic vertical talus in myelomeningocele. J. Bone Joint Surg., 55-B:876, 1973.
162. Wallace, H. M., and Baumgartner, L., and Rich, H.: Congenital malformations and birth injuries in New York City. Pediatrics, 12:525, 1953.
163. Warkany, J.: Morphogenesis of spina bifida. In McLaurin, R. L. (ed.): Myelomeningocele. New York, Grune & Stratton, Inc., 1977, pp. 31–39.
164. Westin, W.: Calcaneofibular tenodesis. Personal communication and Pediatric Orthopedic International Seminar. San Francisco, Cal., 1978.
165. Weinert, C. R., McMaster, J. H., Scranton, P. E., Jr., and Ferguson, R. J.: Human fibular dynamics. In Bateman, J. E. (ed.): Foot Science, Philadelphia, W. B. Saunders Co., 1976, p. 1.
166. Wilson, M. A.: Multidisciplinary problems of myelomeningocele and hydrocephalus. J. Amer. Phys. Ther. Assoc., 45:1139, 1965.
167. Wiltse, L. L.: Valgus deformity of the ankle. J. Bone Joint Surg., 54-A:595, 1972.
168. Yen, S., and McMahon, B.: Genetics of anencephaly and spina bifida. Lancet, 2:623, 1968.
169. Young, B. H.: The orthopaedic surgeon takes a closer look at congenital paraplegia. Bull. Tulane Med. Fac., 20:33, 1960.
170. Zerbi, E.: Il piede cavo essenziale a la spina bifida occulta. Arch. Ortop., 72:615, 1959.

DIASTEMATOMYELIA*

Diastematomyelia is a congenital malformation of the neural axis in which there is a sagittal division of the spinal cord or its intraspinal derivatives by a projecting osseous or fibrocartilaginous mass that is attached anteriorly to one or more vertebral bodies and posteriorly to the dura. This entity should be distinguished from diplomyelia, a very rare anomaly in which the spinal cord is duplicated, that usually occurs in association with excessive spina bifida.

The pathogenesis of diastematomyelia is unknown. It appears that during the organization of the neural tube from the primitive neuroectoderm, aberrant mesodermal cells protrude into the neural tissue on its anterior surface instead of becoming arranged entirely around its periphery. They persist in this location, developing into a bony and dural septum. Associated multiple congenital anomalies of the vertebrae with some degree of incomplete spinal fusion are often present.

The bony spicule is usually located in the lumbar region, though it may be seen at a segmental level as high as the fifth thoracic vertebra. The osseous septum transfixes the spinal cord or cauda equina at a low anatomic level, checking its normal ascent during growth of the vertebral column. Progressive neurologic deficit distal to the level of the lesion develops as a result of traction on the cord.

The condition is more common in the female, with about 75 per cent of the cases occurring in girls.

Clinical Picture

Abnormalities of motor function in the lower limbs are not ordinarily detected at birth. Hallmarks of the condition are the various skin defects that are found near the midline at the level of the lesion. The cutaneous abnormalities include tufts of hair, dimpling of the skin, ill-defined subcutaneous fatty tumors, and cutaneous vascular malformations. Localized scoliosis due to congenital anomalies of the vertebrae is not uncommon.

During the first two years of life increasing disturbance of function of the lower limbs develops. The child may fail to walk at the expected time, or some abnormality of gait may develop after the child has learned to walk properly. Muscle paralysis is often present and may be spastic or flaccid, depending upon the level of the lesion. The anterior tibial and peroneal muscles are often paralyzed. The type of limp depends upon the muscles involved. Atrophy of one or both lower limbs is common, and frequently there is a varus, valgus, or cavus deformity of the foot. In thoracic lesions, the deep tendon reflexes are hyperactive with a positive ankle clonus and dorsiflexion response to the Babinski stimulus. In lum-

---
*See references 1–15.

bar lesions the deep tendon reflexes may be diminished or absent. Rectal sphincter tone is poor, and urinary incontinence is frequent. Sensory examination may demonstrate a definite deficit, particularly in the saddle area. Diastematomyelia is a common finding in congenital scoliosis and other deformities of the spine.[6, 15]

Roentgenographic Findings

Roentgenograms of the spine disclose widening of the spinal canal and interpedicular distance that is maximal at the level of the lesion, but that may extend over several adjacent segments (Fig. 3–64). The absence of thinning of the pedicles and erosion of

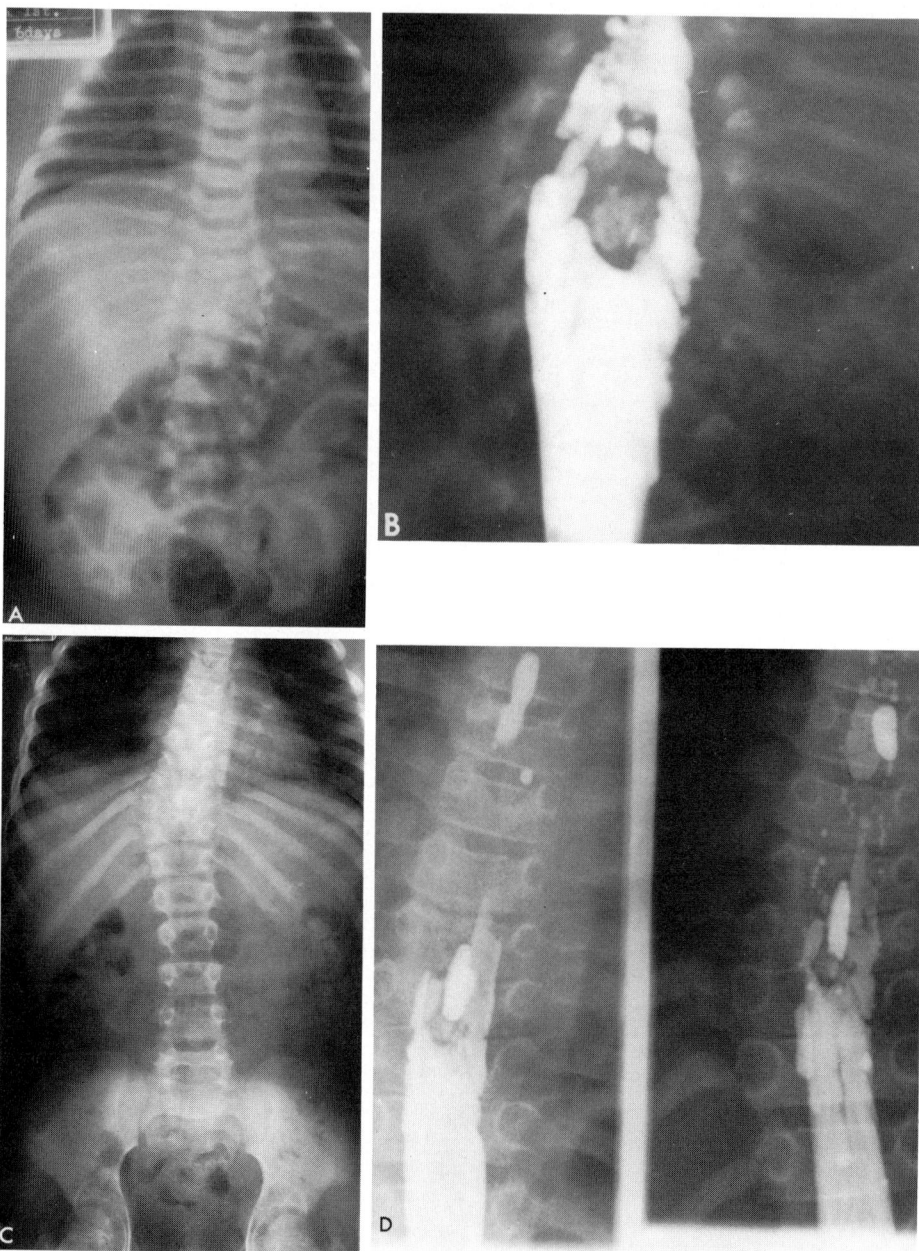

FIGURE 3–64. Diastematomyelia.

A and **B**. Diastematomyelia in a six-day-old infant. In the plain roentgenogram of the spine, note the widening of the interpediculate distance and hemivertebra, and in the myelogram the midline bony spicule around which the opaque medium is divided into two columns. **C** and **D**. Diastematomyelia in an eight-year-old boy. Note the bony spicule and widening of the intraspinal canal.

the posterior aspect of the vertebral bodies suggests a congenital origin for the widening of the spinal canal rather than an expanding intraspinal mass, which would cause pressure erosion.

The bony spicule is best visualized in the anteroposterior projection as an irregular fragment of increased density, lying in the midline of the spinal canal. It is approximately 1 cm. in length. In the lateral projection, the bony spicule may be seen as a radiopaque septum arising from the posterior surface of the vertebral body.

Various other anomalies of the vertebrae are also present. These include decrease in the anteroposterior diameter of the vertebral bodies, hemivertebrae, failure of segmentation of vertebrae, and incomplete fusion or lack of fusion of laminae, resulting in spina bifida.

Myelography with or without CT scan will usually visualize the pathologic changes and help to determine the exact level and extent of diastematomyelia. A characteristic finding is the division of the opaque medium into two columns that flow readily around the midline bony spicule and dural septum. Myelography is of significant help in surgery, but is not always essential for diagnosis, as plain roentgenograms are often satisfactory.

Treatment

The purpose of surgery in diastematomyelia is to prevent the progression of neurologic deficit. It is prophylactic rather than curative. In diastematomyelia, the spinal cord and cauda equina are transfixed by the midline bony spicule, and the normal migration of the cord is obstructed, producing progressive neurologic deficit. The aim of surgery is not so much to attempt to reverse changes that are already present as to prevent further neurologic deficit by allowing the spinal cord to ascend and mature normally.

The operation is a neurosurgical procedure.[7] A local laminectomy is performed, and most of the bony spicule is resected subperiosteally. Next, the dura is incised, arachnoidal adhesions to the medial dural reflections are divided, and the remaining portion of the bony spicule and dural septa are excised. Thus the separate halves of the cord are freely movable and approximate each other. The dura is not closed anteriorly; posteriorly, however, it is approximated in a linear manner. Hydrocephalus or other clinical evidence of the Arnold-Chiari malformation are not postoperative complications.

The role of the orthopedic surgeon is the care of muscle paralysis and deformities affecting the lower limbs. Treatment of foot deformities follows the same principles discussed in the section on poliomyelitis.

References

1. Bligh, A. S.: Diastematomyelia. Clin. Radiol., *12*:158, 1961.
2. Bremer, J. L.: Dorsal intestinal fistula: Accessory neurueteric canal; diastematomyelia. Arch. Path. (Chicago), *54*:132, 1952.
3. Cohen, J., and Sledge, C. B.: Diastematomyelia. Embryologic interpretation. Amer. J. Dis. Child., *100*:257, 1960.
4. Cowie, T. N.: Diastematomyelia with vertebral column defects. Brit. J. Radiol., *24*:156, 1951.
5. Cowie, T. N.: Diastematomyelia: Tomography in diagnosis. Brit. J. Radiol., *25*:263, 1952.
5a. Guthkelch, A. N.: Diastematomyelia with median septum. Brain, *97*:729, 1974.
5b. Hilal, S. K., Marton, D., and Pollack, E.: Diastematomyelia in children. Radiology, *112*:609, 1974.
5c. Hood, R. W., Riseborough, E. J., Nehme, A.-M., Micheli, L. J., Strand, R. D., and Neuhauser, E. B. D.: Diastematomyelia and structural spinal deformities. J. Bone Joint Surg., *62-A*:520, 1980.
6. Keim, H. A., and Greene, A. F.: Diastematomyelia and scoliosis. J. Bone Joint Surg., *55-A*:1425, 1973.
7. Matson, D. D., Woods, R., Campbell, J., and Ingraham, F. D.: Diastematomyelia (congenital clefts of the spinal cord): Diagnosis and surgical treatment. Pediatrics, *6*:98, 1950.
8. Maxwell, H., and Bucy, P.: Diastematomyelia. J. Neuropath. Exp. Neurol., *5*:165, 1946.
9. Neuhauser, E. B. D., Wittenborg, M. H., and Dehlinger, K.: Diastematomyelia. Radiology, *54*:659, 1950.
10. Perret, G.: Diagnosis and treatment of diastematomyelia. Surg. Gynec. Obstet., *105*:69, 1957.
11. Perret, G.: Symptoms and diagnosis of diastematomyelia. Neurology (Minneap.), *10*:51, 1960.
12. Sands, W. W., and Clark, W. K.: Diastematomyelia. Amer. J. Roentgen., *72*:64, 1954.
12a. Shaw, J. F.: Diastematomyelia. (Editorial.) Dev. Med. Child Neurol., *17*:361, 1975.
13. Sheptak, P. E., and Susen, A. F.: Diastematomyelia. Amer. J. Dis. Child., *113*:210, 1967.
14. Walker, R. E.: Dilation of the vertebral canal associated with congenital anomalies of the spinal cord. Amer. J. Roentgen., *52*:571, 1944.
15. Winter, R. B., Haven, J. J., Moe, J. H., and Lagaard, S. M.: Diastematomyelia and congenital spinal deformities. J. Bone Joint Surg., *56-A*:27, 1974.

POLIOMYELITIS

Poliomyelitis is an acute infectious disease caused by a group of neurotropic viruses that initially invade the gastrointestinal and respiratory tracts and subsequently spread to the central nervous system through the hematogenous route. The poliomyelitis virus has a special affinity for the anterior horn cells of the spinal cord and for certain motor nuclei of the brain stem. These cells undergo necrosis with loss of innervation of the motor units that they supply.

The course of the disease is subdivided into acute, convalescent, and chronic (or residual) stages.[65, 66]

The acute phase (lasting from five to ten days) is the period of acute illness during which paralysis may occur. It is further subdivided into the preparalytic phase and the paralytic phase. The acute phase is ordinarily considered as terminating 48 hours following the return to normal temperature.

The convalescent phase encompasses the 16-month period following the acute phase; during this time a varying degree of spontaneous recovery in muscle power takes place. This phase is also further subdivided into the sensitive phase (lasting from two weeks to several months) characterized by hypersensitivity of muscles, which are tender and "in spasm," and the insensitive phase, in which the muscles are no longer sensitive but are still in the period of recovery.

The chronic or residual phase is the final stage of the disease after the recovery of muscle power has taken place. It encompasses the rest of the patient's life span following termination of the convalescent period.[110]

This book deals with the general principles of management of paralytic deformities of the foot and ankle resulting from poliomyelitis. These principles are not only applicable to the treatment of poliomyelitis but are fundamental to the management of similar problems of flaccid paralysis due to other causes.

Tendon Transfer

The fundamentals of tendon transfer were established in the treatment of poliomyelitis.[64, 120–123, 134, 138, 139]

Tendon transfer is the shifting of the insertion of a muscle from its normal attachment to another site to replace active muscular action that was lost by paralysis and to restore dynamic muscle balance. The procedure was originally described by Nicoladoni in 1882. Many surgeons have devised various types of tendon transfers and established their usefulness. Lange, Velpeau, Vulpius, Codivilla, Mayer, Biesalski, Goldthwait, Ober, Steindler, Bunnell, and Green are some who may be mentioned.* The term *tendon transplantation* should not be used interchangeably with the term *tendon transfer,* as the two are not synonymous. Tendon transplantation refers to the procedure of excision of a tendon and its use as a free graft. In *muscle transplantation,* both the origin and insertion of a muscle are detached, and the entire muscle with its intact neurovascular supply is transplanted to a completely new site.

PRINCIPLES OF TENDON TRANSFER

Basic principles of tendon transfers have been outlined by Green:[64]

1. The muscle to be transferred must have adequate motor strength to carry out the new function. As a rule, the motor rating of the muscle should be good or normal to warrant transfer. The function that the transferred muscle is intended to perform is another consideration. In the lower limb, for example, in the presence of drop foot, anterior transfer of the peroneus longus is adequate to produce effective ankle dorsiflexion, whereas in calcaneus limp, posterior transfer of the peroneus longus alone to the os calcis is not sufficient to substitute for the gastrocnemius-soleus action, and the additional action of two or three motors such as the flexor digitorum communis and anterior tibial muscles is required. Ordinarily one grade of motor power is lost after a muscle is transferred.

2. The range of motion of muscles on contraction is an important consideration. This range must be similar to that of the muscles for which they are being substituted; also, whenever muscles are transferred in combination, their range of contraction should not differ significantly. The transfer of antagonistic muscles ordinarily is not as effective as that of muscles having similar function or corollary activity. With meticulous postoperative care, however, antagonistic muscles may be transferred effectively with good results; the posterior trans-

---

*See references 14, 19, 34, 62–68, 122, 123, 131, 133, 134, 163, 164.

fer of the anterior tibial to the os calcis and of the hamstring muscles to the patella are common examples of such antagonistic transfers.

3. In choosing the muscles for transfer, the loss of original function that will result from the tendon transfer must be balanced against the gains to be obtained. For example, in the presence of hip flexor weakness, the hamstring muscles should not be transferred to the patella for quadriceps paralysis, as loss of active knee flexion added to lack of hip flexion will be a greater disability. Whenever possible, muscle balance must be restored. Ideally, a deforming muscle force must be shifted so as to substitute for an essential weakness. In the foot and ankle, for example, the muscles of inversion and eversion and those of plantar flexion and dorsiflexion should be balanced. A common pitfall is transfer of the peroneus longus muscle posteriorly to the os calcis in the presence of a strong anterior tibial muscle. Normally, the anterior tibial muscle dorsiflexes the first metatarsal and the peroneus longus opposes this action. With posterior transfer of the peroneus longus, the unopposed anterior tibial gradually causes the first metatarsal to ride up, producing a dorsal bunion. Thus the peroneus longus should not be transferred to the os calcis unless the anterior tibial is shifted from its insertion on the first metatarsal to the midline of the foot.

4. The joints upon which the transferred muscle is to act should have functional range of motion. All contractural deformity should be corrected by wedging casts or soft-tissue release prior to tendon transfer. An anterior transfer for drop foot, for example, should not be performed in the presence of equinus deformity of the ankle.

5. A smooth gliding channel with adequate space must be provided for excursion of the tendon in its new location. The paratenon and synovial sheath are preserved over the tendon surface during dissection. It is preferable to pass the tendon beneath the deep fascia through tissues that permit free gliding rather than subcutaneously. A wide portion of the intermuscular septum is excised whenever muscles are passed from one muscle compartment to another. Sufficient space should be provided for the tendon so that adhesions will not form. An Ober tendon passer of appropriate size should be used to redirect the tendon to its new insertion; it spreads the tissues and prevents binding.

6. The neurovascular supply of the transferred muscle must not be damaged while the tendon is being transferred. One must be careful not to denervate the muscle while freeing it for redirection. When the tendon is pulled up from the distal wound into the proximal incision, traction should not be applied on the origin of the muscle. Stretching of the motor nerve is prevented by use of the double hand technique, i.e., with a moist sponge, the proximal segment of the tendon is held steady while, with another sponge, traction is applied on its distal segment. Acute angulation or torsion of the neurovascular bundle is another cause of injury. Gentle handling is imperative for preservation of innervation and function of the transferred muscle.

7. In the rerouting of the tendon a *straight line* of contraction must be provided between the origin of the muscle and its new insertion. Angular courses and passages over pulley systems should be avoided. In order to allow adequate freeing of the muscle toward its origin, the incision over the belly of the muscle must be long and proximally located.

8. The tendon should be reattached to its new site under sufficient tension so that the transferred muscle will have a maximal range of contraction. The transferred muscle should be tested at surgery to ensure that it will hold the part in optimal position. Ordinarily, in the lower limb, where weight-bearing forces are involved, the tendon is attached to bone, whereas in the upper limb, it is sutured to the tendon. An important technical detail is scarification of the distal segment of the tendon that is to be anchored to a bone or tendon; this is achieved by excision of the sheath and paratenon and "roughening" of the tendon by scraping and crosshatching it with a knife. The position of immobilization in a plaster cast should allow the transferred tendon to be relaxed in order to diminish any tension on the tendon while it is healing. For example, when the flexor carpi ulnaris is transferred to the extensor carpi radialis longus, the tension on the tendon should be sufficient to hold the wrist in 20 degrees of dorsiflexion. Yet when the cast is applied, the wrist is immobilized in the overcorrected

position of 35 to 45 degrees of dorsiflexion.[64]

POSTOPERATIVE CARE AND TRAINING

The following fundamental principles as stated by Green are prerequisite to obtaining a good result and should be followed meticulously.

First, the age of the patient at the time of tendon transfer is an important preoperative consideration. The child should be old enough, preferably over four years of age, to cooperate in the training of the transfer. A delay in tendon transfer in the presence of muscle imbalance will lead to progressive deformity. Usually, conservative measures should be undertaken to control deforming factors, but in certain instances, early surgery is indicated when such a delay of tendon transfer will result in increasing structural deformity. A common example is the rapid development of progressive calcaneus deformity of the foot with paralysis of the gastrocnemius-soleus muscles while ankle dorsiflexors remain strong. An early posterior transfer will prevent the development of a deformed foot.

Support of the part in overcorrected position should be continued until the muscle has assumed full function and until there is no tendency for the deformity to recur. Use of a bivalved cast will serve to hold the transferred tendon in a relaxed position.

It is best to teach the patient preoperatively to localize contracture in the muscle to be transferred. Active exercises are resumed postoperatively as soon as the reaction to surgery and pain has subsided. The surgeon should assist the physical therapist during the initial exercises. When tendon transfer is combined with arthrodesis, muscle re-education is delayed until adequate bony union has taken place.

The patient is instructed to contract the transferred muscle voluntarily, moving the part through the arc of motion that was the original normal action of the muscle, while the therapist manually guides the part to move in the direction that is intended to be provided by the transfer. For example, when the peroneus longus muscle is transferred anteriorly to the base of the second metatarsal, the active motion called upon is eversion in combination with guided dorsiflexion, or if the anterior tibial muscle has been transferred posteriorly to the os calcis, active inversion is combined with guided plantar flexion of the ankle; in anterior transfer of the hamstrings to the patella for quadriceps femoris paralysis, the patient is placed in side-lying position and is asked to extend the hip actively (using the hamstrings) as the knee is guided into extension; or when the flexor carpi ulnaris is transferred to the extensor carpi radialis longus, the wrist is gently guided into extension as the patient deviates it ulnarward. With one hand, the therapist should palpate the belly and tendon of the transferred muscle to ensure its contraction. In the beginning, the exercises are performed in the bivalved cast. Motion of the concerned joint is executed slowly, steadily, and smoothly through as full a range as possible. Soon the limb is taken out of the plaster cast and is properly positioned, and at this time measures are taken to prevent stretching of the tendon out of its resting position.

Occasionally the patient is unable to contract the transferred muscle actively and has difficulty in "finding" it. To enable him to use the transfer actively and to assist him in acquiring the feeling desired, one may exert gentle mild tension on the transferred tendon, shift positions while actively contracting it, or use corollary motions. If, after two weeks, such difficulty in "finding" the transfer persists, electrical stimulation may be employed to initiate contraction as the patient himself attempts to use the muscle. After a few sessions, the patient begins to "feel" the transfer and to contract it voluntarily.

As soon as the patient is able to contract the transferred muscle actively, exercises in the direction of the original action of the muscle are discontinued and only those motions in the new function provided by the transfer are performed.

When the transferred muscle develops poor motor strength, i.e., can carry the part through the full range of motion with gravity eliminated, the physical therapist teaches one of the parents to perform the exercises with the patient. The exercise regimen is supervised by the physical therapist and the surgeon, who check it at weekly or biweekly intervals.

In the beginning, the limb should be

retained in the bivalved cast for support except during the exercise periods. As soon as the motor strength of the transfer becomes fair, the use of a bivalved cast during the day is gradually discontinued. Controlled activities are permitted to develop function. These are permitted sooner in the upper limb than in the lower one. The age and dependability of the patient are other considerations. Resistive exercises to develop power are begun whenever the transfer has a normal range of action and is fair in strength. It is also important to exercise the antagonistic muscles to prevent disuse atrophy.

The next stage of training is the incorporation of the transfer into the new functional pattern. This is particularly important in the lower limb, in which the muscles are concerned with gait. For example, the action of the peroneus transfer may be good, dorsiflexing the ankle through full range and taking moderate resistance; yet, during locomotion, voluntary control over the transfer is "lost" and the patient walks with a drop-foot gait. The transition to walking requires diligent supervision. Of particular importance is the use of crutches—they serve to protect the limb from undue strain and at the same time allow the patient to be taught the use of the transfer and to become accustomed to it. First the patient is asked to take a single step, ensuring that the muscle contracts and dorsiflexes the ankle. As soon as the transfer functions throughout all the phases of a single step, the walking periods are gradually increased until the normal gait pattern becomes a conditioned reflex.

The use of orthoses in the postoperative period should be judicious and for specific reasons. Orthotic support protects the part and allows early activity. This is indicated particularly when paralysis is extensive, as in myelomeningocele. In a posterior transfer to the os calcis, for example, a plantar flexion–assist orthosis with a dorsiflexion stop at right angles with crutches may be used to aid developing function in the transfers and prevent stretching. However, standing and walking exercises are also performed without the brace to stimulate function in the transfer.

Prolonged use of night splinting is very important to prevent the development of contractural deformity that will oppose the action of the transfer, as for example, in the instance of anterior transfer for dorsiflexion, equinus deformity of the ankle. From the beginning, daily stretching exercises should be a part of the exercise regimen. Stretching and night support are continued over a long period of time, until the muscle has developed full strength and there is balanced function between the agonist and antagonist muscles with no tendency for recurrence of the original deformity. In fact, stretching and active exercises should be a simple rule of daily living.

Arthrodesis to provide stability and correct osseus deformity may be indicated, particularly in the foot. If dynamic balance is established prior to development of structural deformity, however, arthrodesis may be unnecessary. When it is necessary to combine arthrodesis with tendon transfer, muscle re-education must be delayed until adequate bony union has taken place.

SPECIFIC DEFORMITIES OF THE FOOT AND ANKLE

Paralysis of the muscles acting on the foot may result in various deformities and functional disability of the foot, depending upon the particular muscle or muscles involved and the strength of the remaining musculature.

The stability of the foot is dependent on several factors: the contour of the bones and the articular surfaces, the integrity of the ligamentous and capsular support, and the motor strength of the muscles.

The combined mobility of the foot and ankle is equal to that of a universal joint. Motions of the ankle, subtalar, and midtarsal joints are related to each other. In inversion of the hindfoot, for example, the os calcis is displaced forward, producing adduction and inversion of the forefoot; when the hindfoot is everted, the os calcis moves backward and the forefoot is abducted and everted. When the ankle joint is plantar flexed, the hindfoot inverts, whereas, in dorsiflexion of the ankle, the hindfoot everts. The foot is most stable in eversion and dorsiflexion and least stable in equinus position and inversion.

The muscles that produce *plantar flexion*

Table 3-4. Tendon Transfers for Paralytic Deformities of the Foot and Ankle

Dynamic Imbalance Paralyzed or Weak	Dynamic Imbalance Normal or Strong	Deformity of Foot	Tendon Transfer	Remarks
Peroneus longus Peroneus brevis	*Anterior tibial* Extensor hallucis longus Extensor digit. communis Posterior tibial Gastrocnemius-soleus Flexor hallucis longus Flexor digit. longus	Varus Dorsal bunion (first metatarsal dorsiflexed because of unopposed action of anterior tibial)	Lateral transfer of anterior tibial to base of second metatarsal	Perform transfer before fixed deformity develops Lateral stability will be retained Do not transfer more lateral than second metatarsal in presence of strong extensor digit. communis (will cause pes valgus)
Peroneus longus Peroneus brevis Extensor digit. communis Extensor hallucis longus	*Anterior tibial* Posterior tibial Gastrocnemius-soleus Flexor hallucis longus Flexor digit. longus	Varus, some equinus	Lateral transfer of anterior tibial to base of third metatarsal	Do not transfer further lateral than base of third metatarsal (will cause pes valgus)
Peroneus longus Peroneus brevis Extensor digit. communis Extensor hallucis longus Anterior tibial	*Posterior tibial* Gastrocnemius-soleus Flexor hallucis longus Flexor digit. longus	Equinovarus	Anterior transfer of posterior tibial tendon through interosseous space to base of third metatarsal	Preoperatively, equinovarus deformity should be fully corrected by stretching cast or soft-tissue surgery May consider reinforcing posterior tibial transfer by adding flexor hallucis longus or flexor digit. longus to anterior transfer through interosseous space; anterior tenodesis to prevent dropping down of foot is another choice Postoperatively, support transfer by dorsiflexion assist below-knee orthosis
Anterior tibial	*Peroneus longus* Peroneus brevis Extensor hallucis longus Extensor digit. communis Gastrocnemius-soleus Posterior tibial Flexor hallucis longus Flexor digit. longus	Equinovalgus Cock-up deformity of toes (overactivity of toe extensors displaces proximal phalanges of toes into hyperextension and depresses metatarsal heads Occasionally cavovarus deformity of foot results (unopposed peroneus longus acts as depressor of first metatarsal)	Anterior transfer of peroneus longus to base of second metatarsal (suture peroneus brevis to distal stump of peroneus longus)	Do not attach peroneus longus to first metatarsal (will displace it upward and cause dorsal bunion) Transfer long toe extensors to heads of metatarsals if cock-up deformity of toes is present If both peroneals are transferred, lateral instability of foot will develop, necessitating stabilization by subtalar extraarticular or triple arthrodesis
Gastrocnemius-soleus (motor strength zero or trace)	*Peroneus longus* Peroneus brevis *Flexor hallucis longus* *Posterior tibial* Flexor digit. longus *Anterior tibial* Extensor hallucis longus Extensor digit. communis	Calcaneus or Calcaneocavus	Posterior transfer (to os calcis) of both peroneals, posterior tibial, and flexor hallucis longus	*Caution*—Prevent development of dorsal bunion by lateral transfer of anterior tibial to base of second metatarsal within a year In adolescent patient with fixed calcaneus deformity, before tendon transfers, perform triple arthrodesis with posterior shift of os calcis to correct bony deformity In young child, calcaneus deformity will correct with subsequent growth; however, subtalar extra-articular arthrodesis may be required for lateral stability

Table 3-4. Tendon Transfers for Paralytic Deformities of the Foot and Ankle (Continued)

Dynamic Imbalance Paralyzed or Weak	Normal or Strong	Deformity of Foot	Tendon Transfer	Remarks
Gastrocnemius-soleus (motor strength poor)	As already described	Calcaneus or Calcaneocavus	Posterior transfer (to os calcis) of posterior tibial and peroneus longus	Suture distal stump of peroneus longus to peroneus brevis Watch closely for possible development of dorsal bunion; lateral transfer of anterior tibial to base of second metatarsal may be indicated
Gastrocnemius-soleus Posterior tibial Peroneus longus Peroneus brevis	*Anterior tibial* *Flexor hallucis longus* Extensor hallucis longus Extensor digit. communis Flexor digit. longus	Calcaneovarus	Posterior transfer (to os calcis) of anterior tibial and flexor hallucis longus	Suture distal stump of flexor hallucis longus to flexor hallucis brevis Interphalangeal joint fusion of great toe may be necessary
Anterior tibial Gastrocnemius-soleus	*Peroneus longus* *Peroneus brevis* *Posterior tibial* Flexor hallucis longus Flexor digitorum longus Extensor hallucis longus Extensor digitorum longus	Calcaneovarus	Posterior transfer (to os calcis) of both peroneals and posterior tibial	Perform triple arthrodesis in adolescence to provide lateral stability to hindfoot.
Gastrocnemius-soleus Posterior tibial Peroneus longus Peroneus brevis Flexor hallucis longus Flexor digit. longus	*Anterior tibial* Extensor hallucis longus Extensor digit. communis	Calcaneovarus	Posterior transfer (to os calcis) of anterior tibial	Protect transfer with plantar flexion assist orthosis until skeletal maturity Consider tendo Achillis tenodesis In adolescence, if adequate function exists in transferred anterior tibial, foot is stabilized by triple arthrodesis If anterior tibial function is inadequate, Chuinard type ankle fusion is performed (will provide stability and gait will improve considerably)
Gastrocnemius-soleus Posterior tibial Peroneus longus Peroneus brevis Flexor hallucis longus Flexor digit. longus Anterior tibial	Extensor hallucis longus Extensor digit. communis	Calcaneovalgus (minimal)	Ankle fusion (Chuinard type)	Stability and muscle control of knee should be adequate Full knee extension and functioning hamstrings are prerequisite
Flail ankle and foot (all muscles paralyzed)	None except short toe flexors and intrinsic muscles of foot	Flexion of toes and metatarsus varus Hindfoot neutral or valgus (may be in inversion due to contracture of plantar fascia)	Pantalar arthrodesis Resect motor branches of plantar nerves	As above
Anterior tibial Extensor hallucis longus Extensor digit. communis Peroneus longus Peroneus brevis Posterior tibial	Gastrocnemius-soleus Flexor digit. longus Flexor hallucis longus	Equinus	Anterior transfer of flexor digit. longus and flexor hallucis through interosseous space Anterior tenodesis	Do not lengthen tendo Achillis (will produce calcaneus deformity) Disability is little (patient must lift leg to clear toes) Stretch triceps surae, use night support to prevent fixed equinus deformity

are the gastrocnemius-soleus, flexor hallucis longus, flexor digitorum longus, peroneus longus, peroneus brevis, and posterior tibial. *Dorsiflexor muscles* are the anterior tibial, extensor hallucis longus, extensor digitorum communis, and peroneus tertius. The muscles that produce *inversion* are the posterior tibial, flexor hallucis longus, and anterior tibial; the *evertors* of the foot are the peroneus brevis, peroneus tertius, extensor digitorum communis, and extensor hallucis longus. The muscles that plantar flex the ankle and foot provide the force for forward propulsion of the body during locomotion. The dorsiflexor muscle group clears the foot during the swing phase of gait.

About two thirds of the total musculature of the leg is constituted by the triceps surae—one of the strongest muscles in the body. It acts on the foot as a first-class lever with the ankle joint as a fulcrum. The working capacity of the triceps surae is 6.5 kg.-m., whereas that of the dorsiflexors of the ankle joint is only 1.4 kg.-m., or a relative ratio of 4:1. This gross discrepancy of muscle mass between the plantar flexors and dorsiflexors of the ankle is the result of developmental and mechanical factors. The strength of the calf muscles is a necessary antigravitational force against the elevated center of gravity of the body in the upright posture. Also, since the center of gravity of the human body falls anterior to the ankle joint, there is a strong rotatory component in ankle dorsiflexion that the triceps surae must counteract. The muscles that provide lateral stability to the foot in plantar flexion are the posterior tibial and peroneals, whereas in dorsiflexion it is provided by the action of the anterior tibial and extensor digitorum communis.

Muscle imbalance will produce progressive deformity. This is flexible in the beginning, but with skeletal growth, fixed soft-tissue and structural osseous deformity will develop. The deformities of the foot and loss of function produced by muscle imbalance are predictable. The *dynamic imbalance* from paralysis of the major muscle groups, the resultant deformity, and its treatment are presented in Table 3–4.

Paralysis of Peroneal Muscles. When the peroneus longus and brevis muscles are paralyzed, the os calcis is pulled into inversion by the strong posterior tibial muscle. The forefoot adducts following inversion of the hindfoot and also because of the unopposed action of the anterior tibial muscle. Gradually, a varus deformity of the foot is produced (Fig. 3–65). Normally, the peroneus longus depresses the first metatarsal and the anterior tibial raises it. When the peroneus longus muscle is paralyzed, the first metatarsal becomes dorsiflexed by the unopposed action of the anterior tibial, and a dorsal bunion will result. The opposing actions of the peroneus longus and anterior tibial muscles on the first metatarsal should always be considered whenever there is a dynamic imbalance between the two.

Treatment consists of lateral transfer of

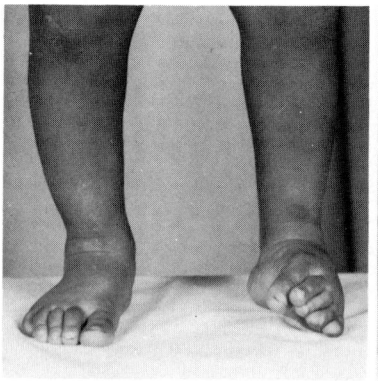 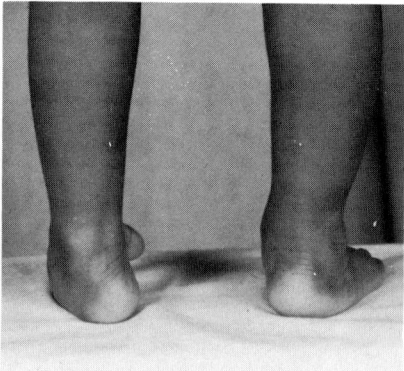 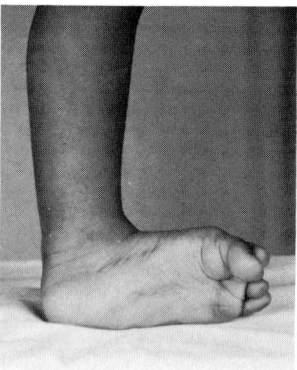

FIGURE 3–65. Paralytic pes varus.

The deformity is the result of paralysis of the peroneus longus and brevis muscles. The hindfoot is inverted by the pull of the strong posterior tibial muscle, and the forefoot is adducted and inverted by the unopposed action of the anterior tibial muscle. Note that the first metatarsal is dorsiflexed and a dorsal bunion is produced.

the anterior tibial to the base of the second metatarsal bone. Lateral stability of the foot will then be adequate, and arthrodesis is not required.

Paralysis of Peroneals, Extensor Digitorum Longus, and Extensor Hallucis Longus. The deformity resulting from paralysis of these muscles will be moderately varus and somewhat equinus. Dynamic balance of the foot is restored by lateral transfer of the anterior tibial muscle to the base of the third metatarsal bone. Pes valgus may result if the anterior tibial is transferred to the fourth or fifth metatarsal bone. The operative technique of lateral transfer of the anterior tibial tendon is as follows:

A longitudinal incision is made over the medial aspect of the foot; it begins at the base of the first metatarsal bone and extends proximally parallel to the course of the anterior tibial tendon for a distance of 3 cm. The anterior tibial tendon is detached from its insertion into the base of the first metatarsal bone and the medial and under surface of the first cuneiform bone. A Mersilene or Dacron whip suture is inserted into the distal end of the tendon. By sharp dissection, the tendon is mobilized over the dorsum of the foot. The dorsalis pedis artery, lying between the tendon of the extensor hallucis longus and the first tendon of the extensor digitorum longus, should not be divided.

Then a second 8- to 10-cm. longitudinal incision is made over the anterior tibial compartment in the distal third of the leg beginning at the upper border of the transverse crural ligament. The subcutaneous tissue and deep fascia are divided. The anterior tibial tendon is located immediately on the tibia. The anterior tibial vessels lie between the anterior tibial and extensor hallucis longus muscles in the middle third of the leg. At the ankle, the extensor hallucis longus tendon crosses the anterior tibial vessels from the lateral to the medial side. The deep peroneal nerve is located on the lateral side of the anterior tibial vessels in the upper third of the leg, in front of the artery in the middle third, and then again lateral in the distal third. Caution should be exercised in order not to injure the deep peroneal nerve and the anterior tibial vessels. The anterior tibial sheath is divided and by gentle traction, using the two-hand technique, the tendon is delivered into the proximal wound. Transfer of the anterior tibial tendon on the dorsum of the foot distal to the transverse crural ligament from the medial to the lateral side will not correct the varus action of the muscle.

Next, an incision 3 cm. long is made over the dorsum of the foot with its center over the base of the third metatarsal bone. With an Ober tendon passer, the anterior tibial tendon is delivered into the dorsum of the foot, passing deep to the transverse crural ligament to produce straight dorsiflexion. It is securely fixed to the base of the third metatarsal bone with the ankle joint in neutral position or dorsiflexed 5 degrees. The muscle should be under physiologic tension. The wounds are closed in routine fashion and a long leg cast is applied, with the ankle in 5 degrees of dorsiflexion and the knee in 45 degrees of flexion.

Paralysis of Anterior Tibial Muscle. Dorsiflexor and inversion power of the foot is lost when the anterior tibial muscle is paralyzed, and equinovalgus deformity of the foot will develop (Fig. 3–66). The toe extensors are overactive in an attempt to substitute for the action of the anterior tibial in dorsiflexion of the ankle. The proximal phalanges of the toes become hyperextended and depress the metatarsal heads, causing cock-up deformity of the toes. Equinus deformity of the ankle gradually results from contracture of the triceps surae. Occasionally cavovarus deformity of the foot may result because of the action of the peroneus longus muscle, which acts as a depressor of the first metatarsal. On active dorsiflexion of the ankle, the forefoot is everted, but on weight-bearing it goes into inversion to permit horizontal contact of all metatarsal heads with the ground. The heel will invert following the forefoot inversion.

During the convalescent phase of poliomyelitis, aggressive measures should be taken to retain passive range of dorsiflexion of the ankle joint. Passive heel cord stretching exercises are performed every day. At night, a bivalved cast or a plastic splint is used to hold the ankle in neutral position, and during the day an ankle-foot dorsiflexion-assist orthosis supports the ankle and foot.

If proper treatment is neglected, fixed

Text continued on page 464

Anterior Transfer of Peroneus Longus Tendon to Base of Second Metatarsal

The patient is placed in semilateral position with a sandbag under the hip on the affected side.

A. A 3- to 4-cm.-long incision is made over the lateral aspect of the foot, extending from the base of the fifth metatarsal to a point 1 cm. distal to the tip of the lateral malleolus. Subcutaneous tissue is divided and the tendons of the peroneus longus and brevis are exposed. Then a second incision is made over the fibular aspect of the leg; it begins 3 cm. above the lateral malleolus and extends proximally for a distance of 7 cm. Subcutaneous tissue and deep fascia are incised, and the peroneal tendons are exposed by dividing their sheath. The peroneus longus tendon lies superficial to that of the peroneus brevis. The muscle is inspected to ensure that it is of normal gross appearance.

B. Next, the peroneus brevis muscle is detached from the base of the fifth metatarsal and a whip suture is inserted into its distal end.

C and **D.** The peroneus longus tendon is divided as far distally as possible. The peroneus brevis is sutured to the distal stump of the peroneus longus to preserve the longitudinal arch and depression of the first metatarsal.

Plate 18. Anterior Transfer of Peroneus Longus Tendon to Base of Second Metatarsal

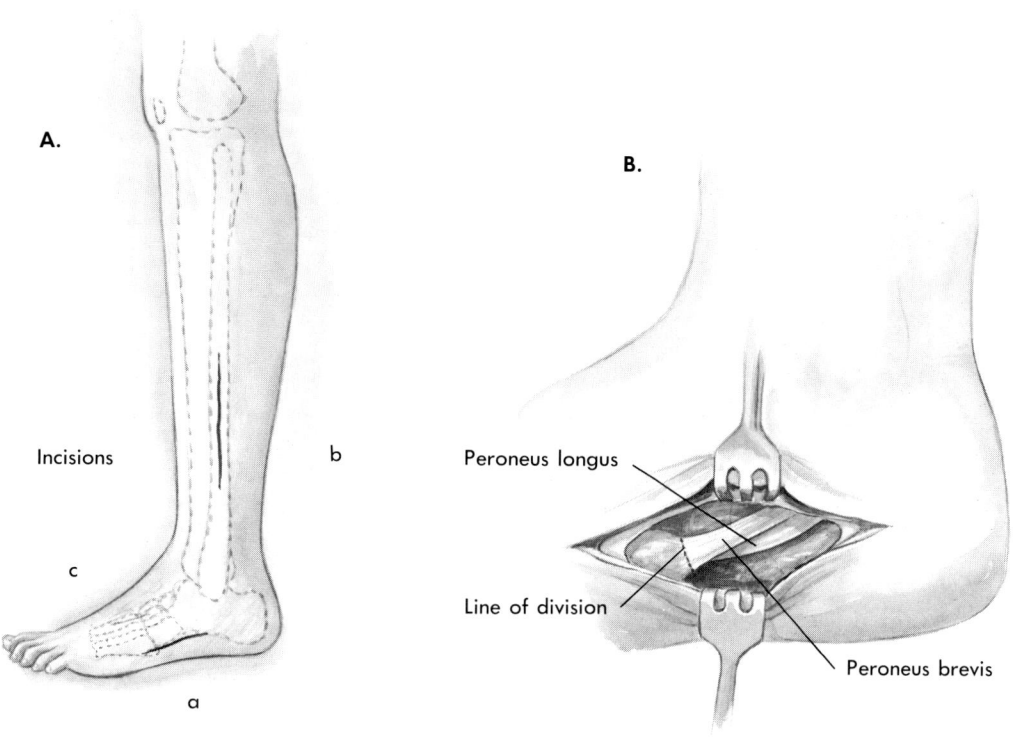

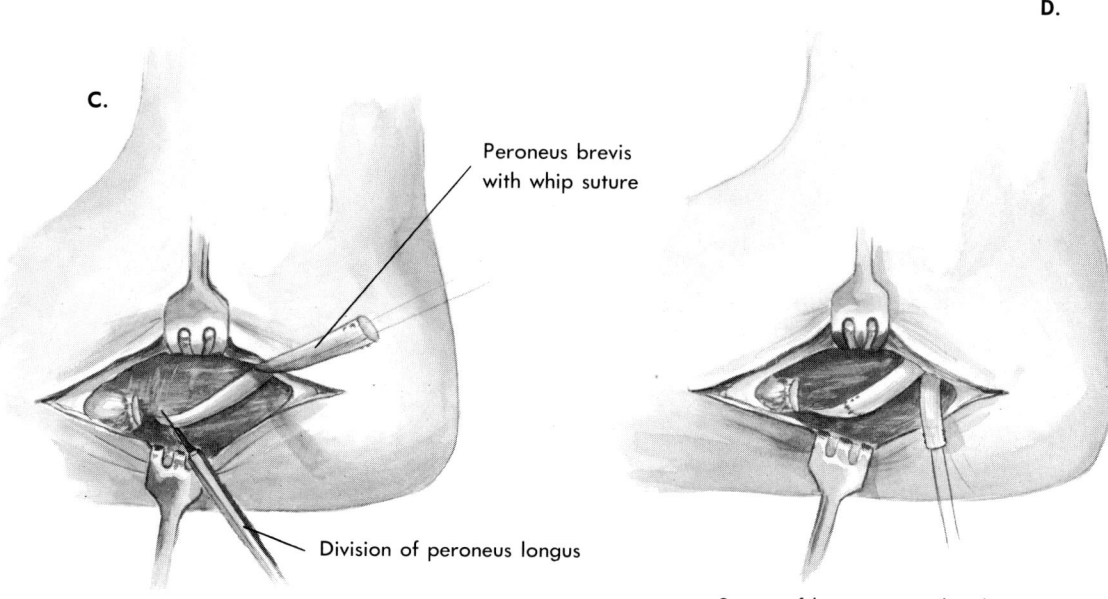

461

Anterior Transfer of Peroneus Longus Tendon to Base of Second Metatarsal (Continued)

E and **F.** The peroneus longus tendon is mobilized, and with the two-hand technique, it is gently pulled into the proximal wound in the leg. The origin of the peroneus brevis from the fibula should not be disrupted.

An adequate opening is made in the intermuscular septum, taking care not to injure neurovascular structures.

G and **H.** A 2- to 3-cm. longitudinal incision is made over the dorsum of the foot, centering over the base of the second metatarsal bone. The deep fascia is divided and the extensor tendons are retracted to expose the proximal one fourth of the second metatarsal bone. The periosteum is divided longitudinally and the cortex of the recipient bone is exposed.

With an Ober tendon passer, the peroneus longus tendon along with its sheath is passed into the anterior tibial compartment, deep to the cruciate crural and tarsal ligaments, and delivered into the incision on the dorsum of the foot. The author does not recommend a subcutaneous route. It should be ensured that there is a direct line of pull of the peroneus longus tendon from its origin to its insertion.

I and **J.** A drill hole is made in the base of the second metatarsal. A star-head hand drill is used to enlarge the hole to receive the tendon adequately. The peroneus longus tendon is passed through the recipient hole and sutured on itself under correct tension. If the peroneus longus tendon is not of adequate length, two small holes are made 1.5 cm. distal to the large hole at each side of the metatarsal shaft. The silk sutures at the end of the tendon are passed from the large central hole to the lateral distal small holes and the tendon is securely sutured to the bone. The ankle tourniquet is released and hemostasis is obtained. The wounds are closed in routine manner. A long leg cast is applied with the ankle in 5 degrees of dorsiflexion and the knee in 45 degrees of flexion. Postoperative care follows the guidelines outlined in the section on principles of tendon transfer.

Plate 18. Anterior Transfer of Peroneus Longus Tendon to Base of Second Metatarsal

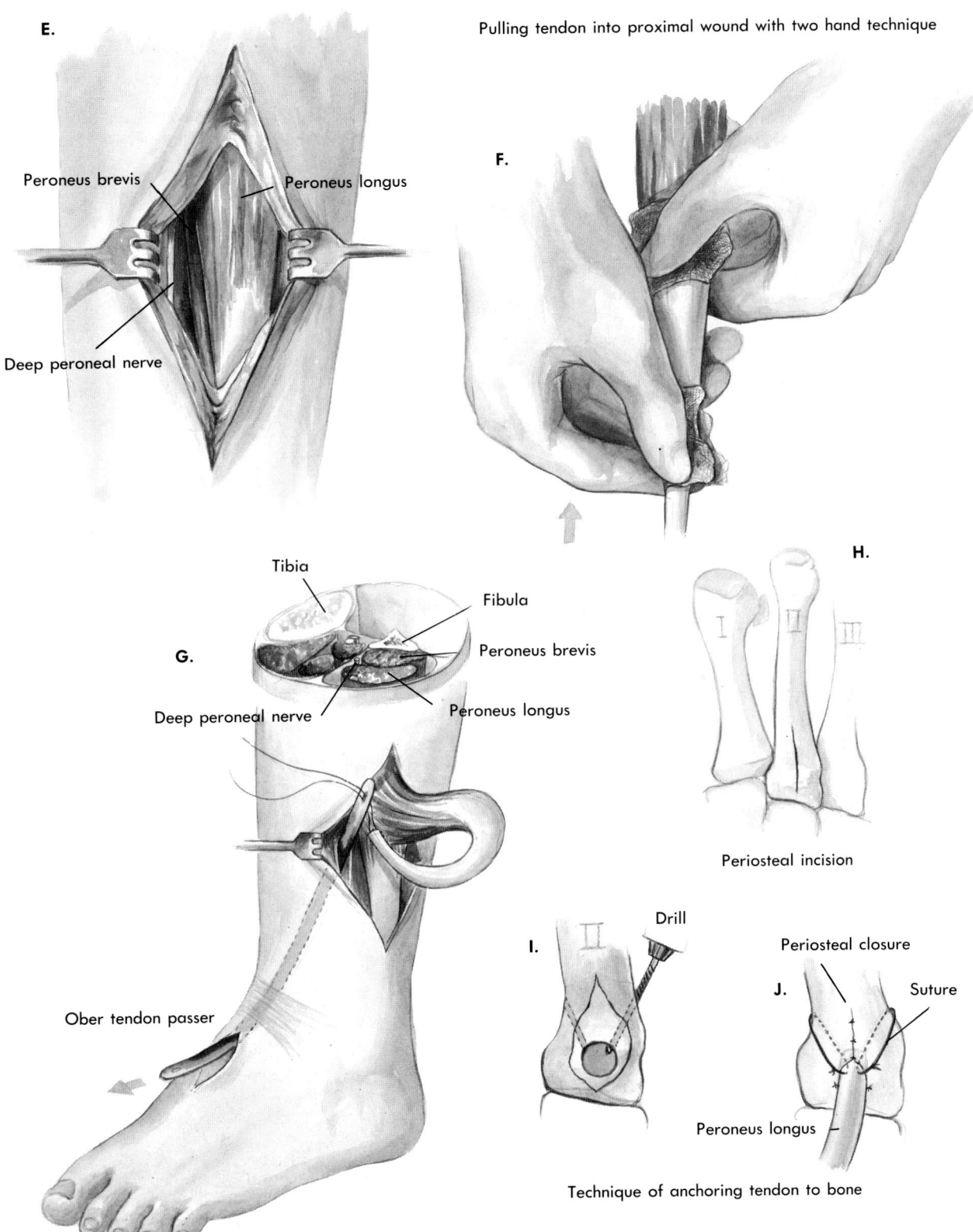

463

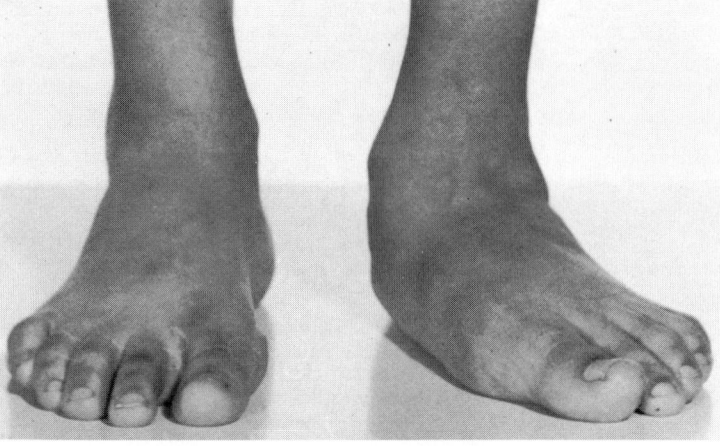

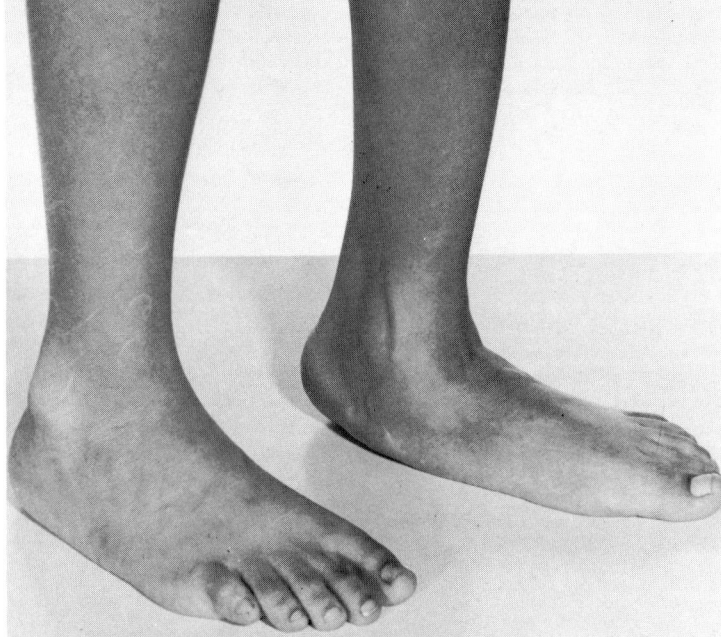

FIGURE 3–66. *Equinovalgus deformity of the foot as a result of paralysis of the anterior tibial muscle.*

equinus deformity may develop. In that event, the heel cord should not be lengthened, and every effort should be made to retain full function of the triceps surae muscle. Range of dorsiflexion of the ankle may be obtained with a wedging cast or a below-knee walking cast with an anterior heel. In severe fixed equinus deformity, posterior capsulotomy of the ankle and subtalar joints is performed and the heel cord is stretched with skeletal traction through a threaded Steinmann pin in the os calcis. Functional disability is great following loss of plantar flexion power.

Dorsiflexion power of the ankle is restored by anterior transfer of the peroneus longus tendon to the base of the second metatarsal bone. The peroneus brevis is sutured to the distal stump of the peroneus longus. The operative technique and postoperative care of anterior transfer of the peroneus longus are described and illustrated in Plate 18. The peroneus longus tendon should not be attached to the base of the first metatarsal, since it will displace the bone upward and cause a dorsal bunion. If there is a cock-up deformity of the toes, the long toe extensors are transferred to the heads of the metatarsals. If both peroneals are transferred, lateral instability of the foot will develop, necessitating stabilization of the hindfoot by extra-articular subtalar arthrodesis or triple arthrodesis.

Paralysis of Anterior Tibial, Toe Extensors, and Peroneals. Equinovarus deformity of the foot will develop from the unopposed action of the posterior tibial and triceps surae muscles (Fig. 3–67). Treatment consists of anterior transfer of the posterior tibial tendon through the interosseous space to the base of the third metatarsal or second cuneiform (Plate 19). Preoperatively, equinovarus deformity should be fully corrected by a stretching cast. Soft-tissue release may be indicated for correction of the fixed pes varus.

The flexor digitorum longus or flexor hallucis longus may be transferred anteriorly through the interosseous route to reinforce the strength of dorsiflexion power of the posterior tibial transfer. Anterior tenodesis is another method of preventing the foot from dropping down in plantar flexion. In the postoperative period, the anterior transfer and tenodesis should be supported in an ankle-foot dynamic dorsiflexion-assist orthosis during the day and a bivalved cast or plastic splint at night.

Paralysis of Triceps Surae Muscle. When the gastrocnemius and soleus muscles are weak or paralyzed, the patient walks with a calcaneus limp, i.e., there is weakness or lack of push-off. The tibia is displaced posteriorly on the talus by the forward thrust of the trunk, and the foot is forced into excessive dorsiflexion at the ankle joint.

The tendo Achillis inserts into the posterior aspect of the apophysis of the os calcis. Normally, the force exerted by the triceps surae muscle elevates the heel, depresses the anterior end of the os calcis, and pushes the body forward. The longitudinal arch is flattened as the head of the talus plantarflexes with the anterior end of the os calcis. In paralysis of the gastrocnemius and soleus muscles, the head of the talus and anterior end of the os calcis are displaced upward to a more vertical position. This results in the disappearance of the normal prominence of the heel and an increase in the range of dorsiflexion of the ankle (Fig. 3–68). When the accessory plantar flexor muscles (i.e.,

Text continued on page 470

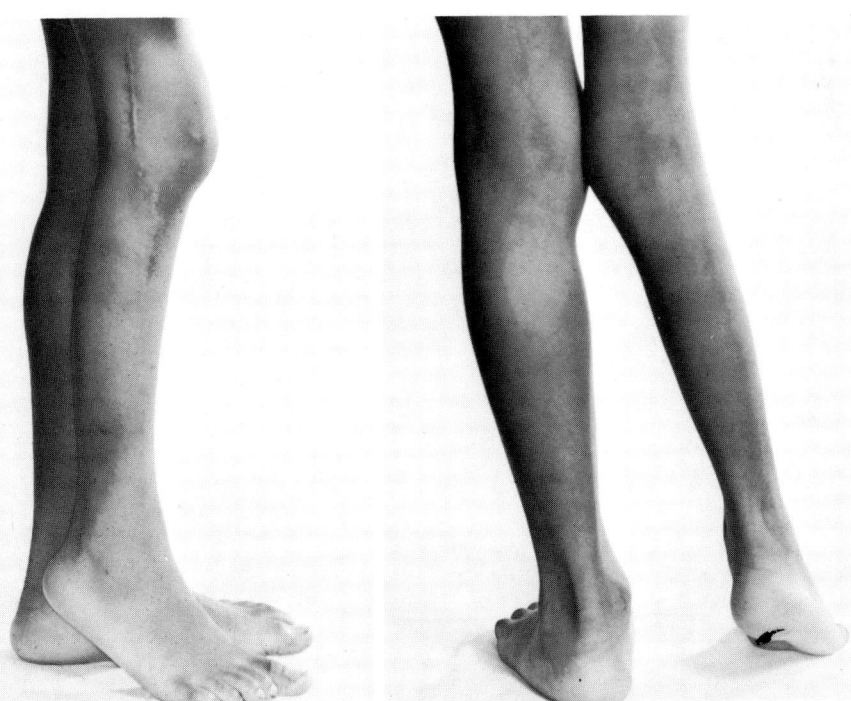

FIGURE 3–67. *Equinovarus deformity of right ankle and foot caused by unopposed action of the triceps surae and posterior tibial muscles.*

Anterior Transfer of Posterior Tibial Tendon Through Interosseous Membrane

A. A 4-cm.-long incision is made over the medial aspect of the foot, beginning posterior and immediately distal to the tip of the medial malleolus and extending to the base of the first cuneiform bone. A second longitudinal incision is made 1.5 cm. posterior to the subcutaneous medial border of the tibia, beginning at the center of the middle third of the leg and ending 3 cm. from the tip of the medial malleolus.

B. The posterior tibial tendon is identified at its insertion, and its sheath is divided. The tendon is freed and sectioned at its attachment to the bone, preserving maximal length. The peritenon of the distal 3 cm. of the tendon is excised and a 00 silk whip suture is inserted in its distal end.

C. The posterior tibial muscle is identified in the leg incision and its sheath opened and freed. Traction on the stump in the foot incision will aid in its identification. Moist sponges and the two-hand technique are used to deliver the posterior tibial tendon into the proximal wound. The muscle belly is freed well up the tibia. One should be careful to preserve the nerve and blood supply to the posterior tibial muscle.

D. Next, a longitudinal skin incision is made anteriorly, one fingerbreadth lateral to the crest of the tibia, starting at the proximal margin of the cruciate ligament of the ankle and extending 7 cm. proximally. Then a 4-cm. longitudinal incision is made over the dorsum of the foot, centering over the base of the second metatarsal.

Plate 19. Anterior Transfer of Posterior Tibial Tendon Through Interosseous Membrane

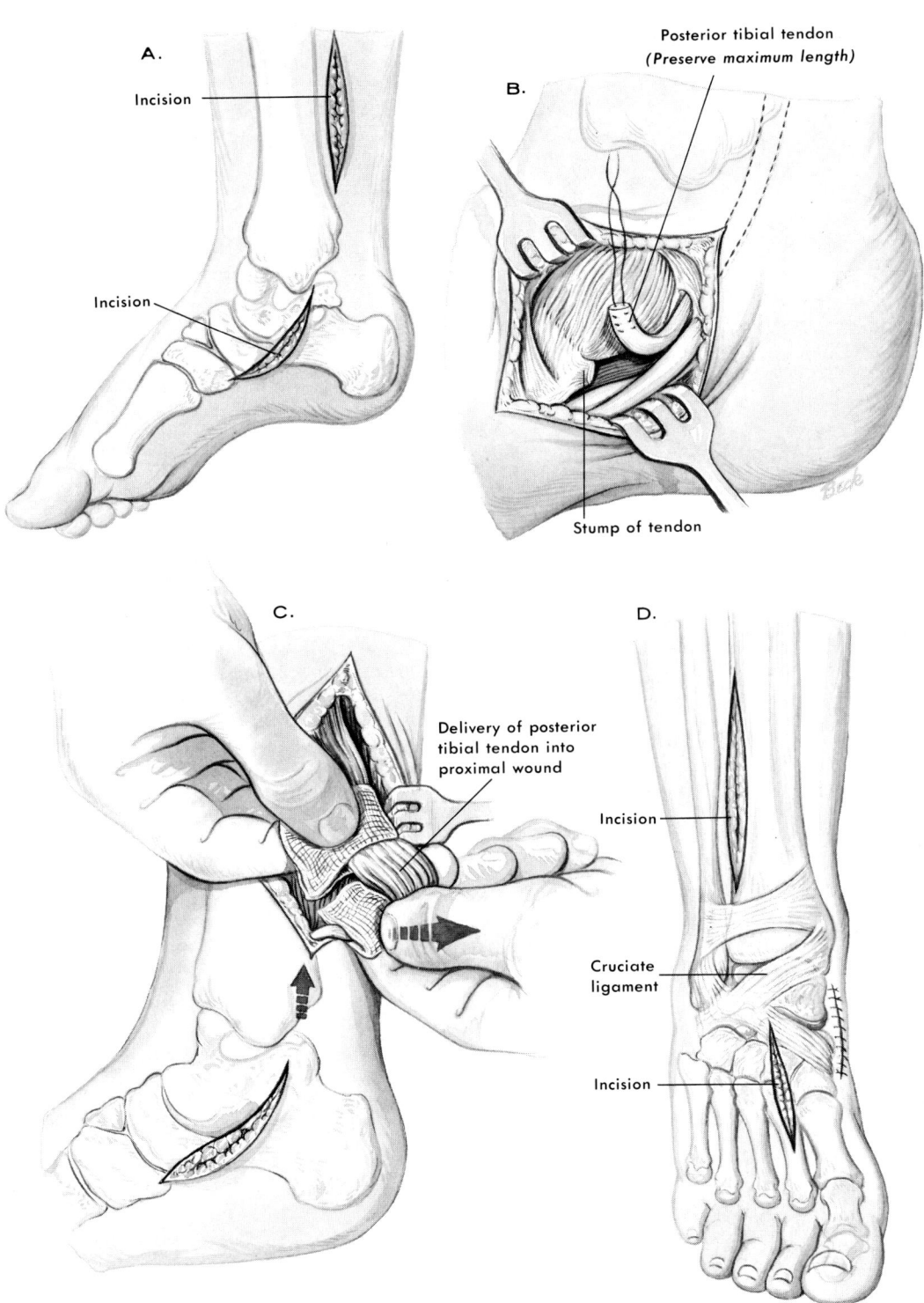

Anterior Transfer of Posterior Tibial Tendon Through Interosseous Membrane *(Continued)*

E. The anterior tibial muscle is exposed, and elevated from the anterolateral surface of the tibia together with the anterior tibial artery and extensor hallucis longus muscle. It is retracted laterally, exposing the interosseous membrane. Next, a large rectangular window is cut in the interosseous membrane. One should avoid stripping the periosteum from the tibia or fibula.

F and **G.** Then, with an Ober tendon passer, the posterior tibial tendon is passed through the window in the interosseous membrane from the posterior into the anterior tibial compartment. One should be careful not to twist the tendon or to damage its nerve or blood supply. Next, with an Ober tendon passer, the posterior tibial tendon is passed beneath the cruciate ligament and the extensors and delivered into the wound on the dorsum of the foot. It is anchored to the base of the second metatarsal bone according to the method described in anterior transfer of peroneal tendons (Plate 18). The wounds are closed in layers in the usual manner. A long leg cast is applied, holding the foot in neutral position at the ankle joint and the knee in 45 degrees of flexion.

The principles of postoperative care are the same as for any tendon transfer.

Plate 19. Anterior Transfer of Posterior Tibial Tendon Through Interosseous Membrane

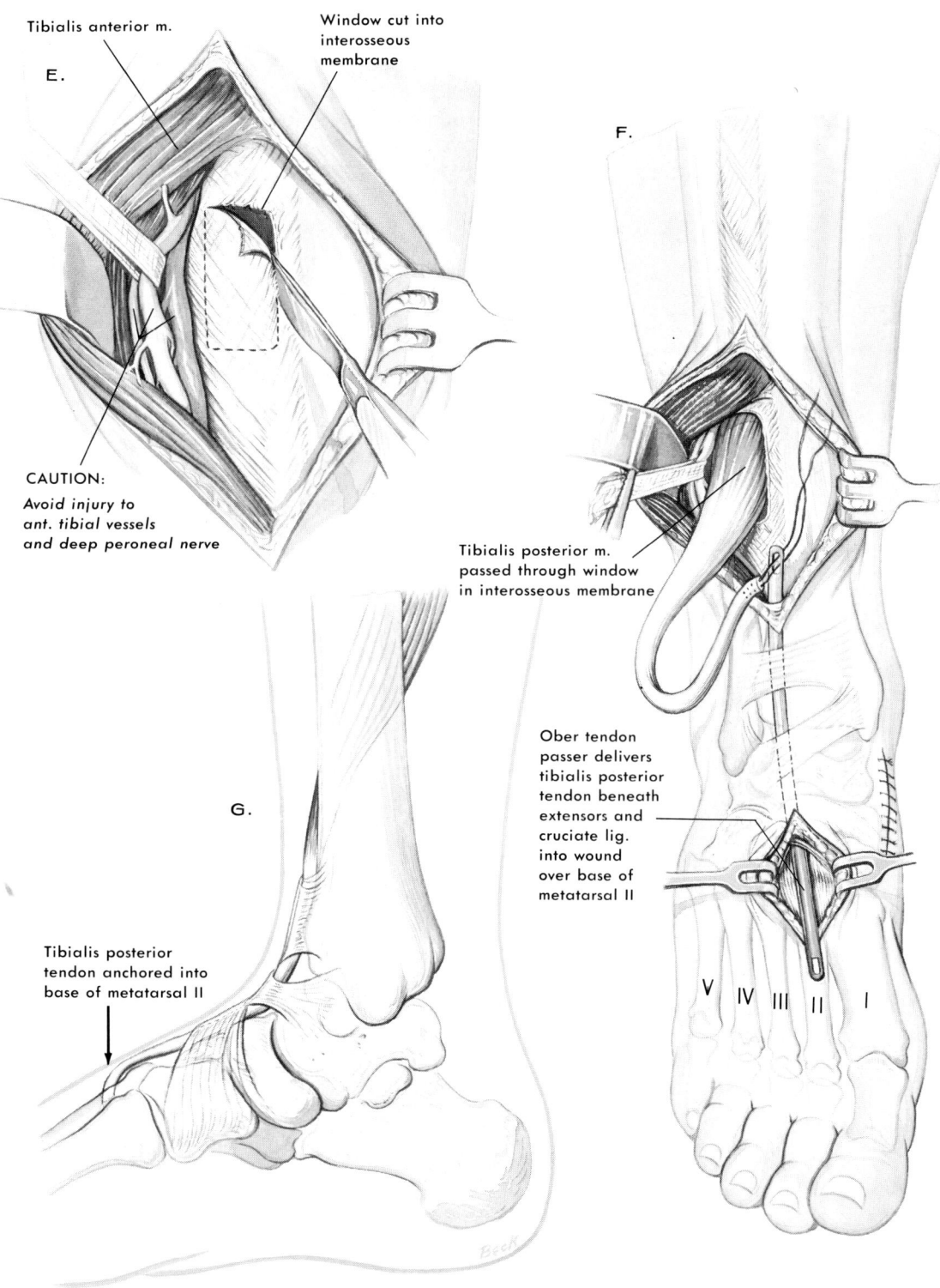

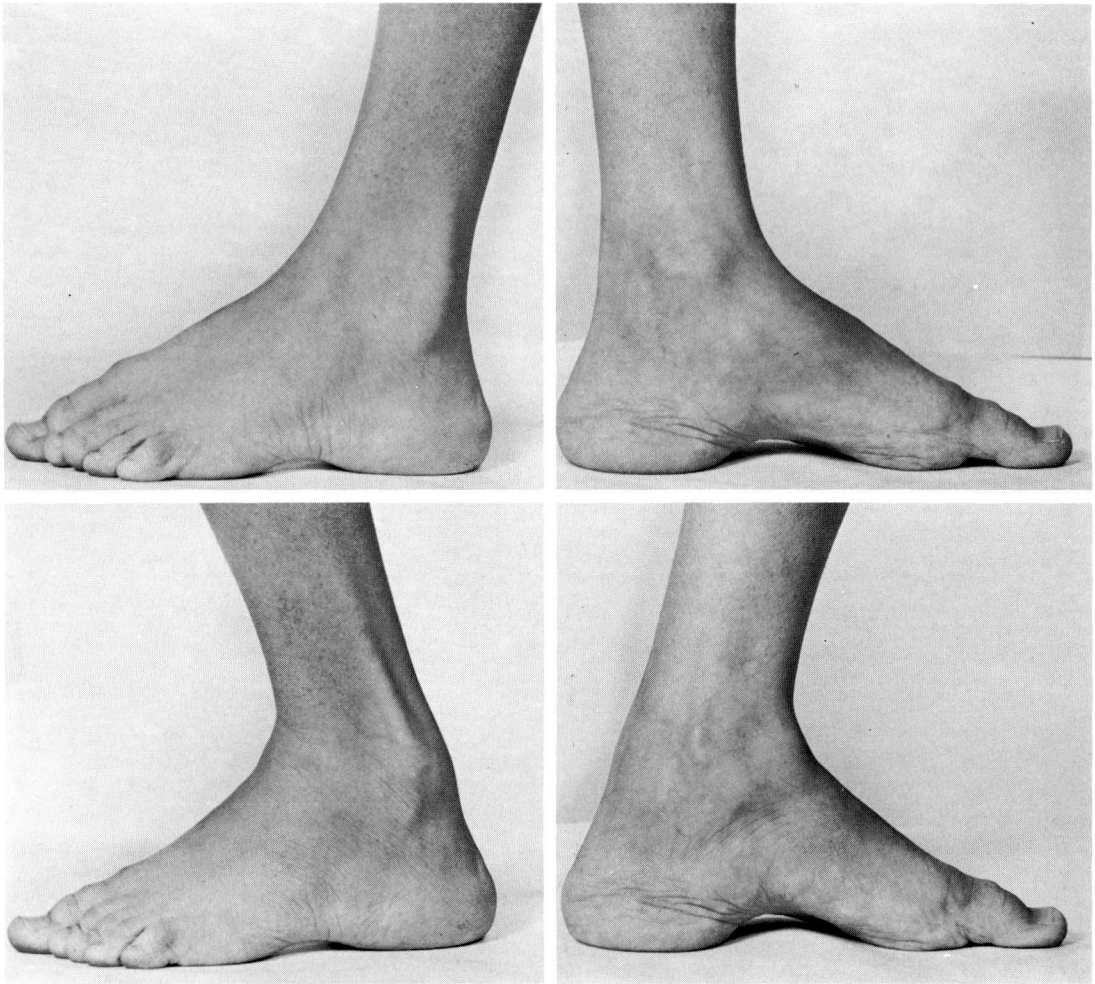

FIGURE 3–68. Calcaneus deformity of the foot and ankle.

Note the posterior shift of the tibia over the talus during push-off.

the posterior tibial, flexor hallucis longus, flexor digitorum longus, and peroneals) are strong, the forefoot is forced into equinus position, producing a calcaneocavus deformity. The foot is shortened by plantar flexion of the metatarsals and by rotation of the os calcis into a vertical position. Soon the plantar fascia and short flexors of the toes will contract and act as a bowstring, pulling together the metatarsal heads and the os calcis, and increasing the cavus deformity (Fig. 3–69). The calcaneocavus deformity progressively increases with every step. With paralysis of the triceps surae, growth of the apophysis of the os calcis is retarded. This is particularly important in a young child in whom, following an early and successful posterior tendon transfer to the os calcis, the calcaneus deformity of the heel may be restored to normal.

As stated previously, the triceps surae muscle is the strongest muscle of the foot. Therefore, it is desirable to transfer three or four muscles posteriorly to the os calcis depending upon their availability and the degree of weakness of the triceps surae. Plantar flexion at the ankle is more important functionally than dorsiflexion.

When the motor strength of the triceps surae muscle is zero, both peroneus longus and brevis, the posterior tibial, and the flexor hallucis longus are transferred to the os calcis. The anterior tibial is transferred laterally to the base of the second metatarsal

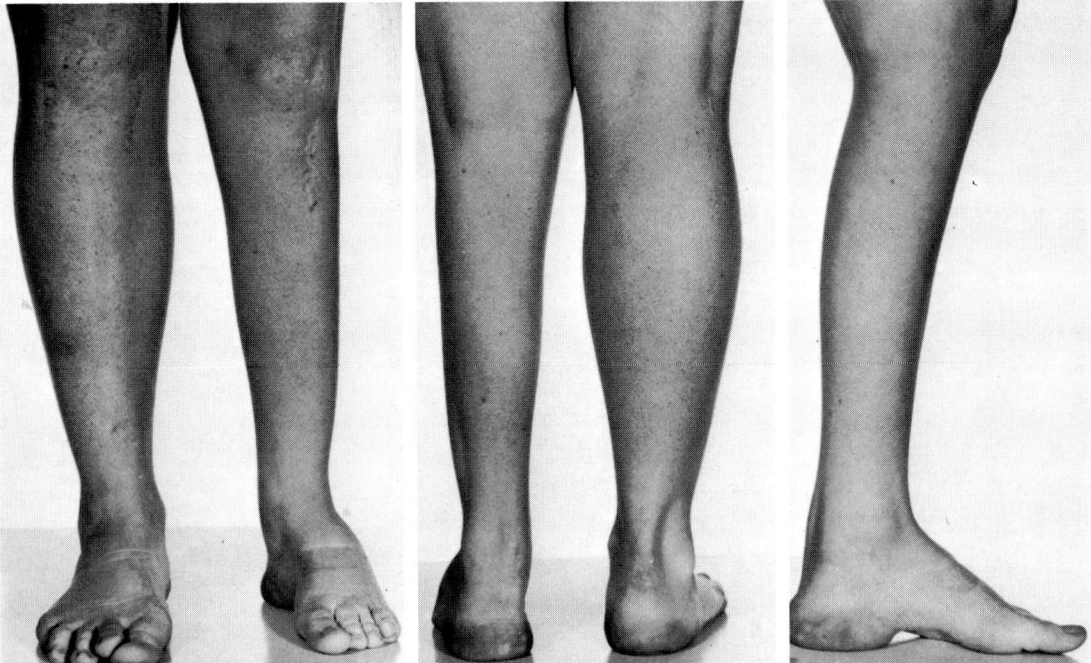

FIGURE 3–69. Calcaneocavus deformity of the left foot and ankle.

within a year to prevent formation of a dorsal bunion. In adolescents with fixed calcaneus deformity, the hindfoot is stabilized by triple arthrodesis, the bony deformity is corrected, and the os calcis is shifted posteriorly. In a young child, calcaneus deformity will be corrected by subsequent growth if the posterior transfer is successful; however, a subtalar extra-articular arthrodesis may be required later for lateral stability.

When the gastrocnemius-soleus muscles are poor in motor strength, only the peroneus longus and posterior tibial muscles are transferred. The distal stump of the peroneus longus is sutured to the peroneus brevis. If a dorsal bunion tends to develop, lateral transfer of the anterior tibial to the base of the second metatarsal may again be indicated.

When the posterior tibial and peroneal muscles are paralyzed along with the triceps surae, the muscles available for posterior transfer are the anterior tibial and flexor hallucis longus. The flexor digitorum longus may be added if necessary. The interphalangeal joints, particularly that of the great toe, are fused.

When the anterior tibial muscle is paralyzed with the triceps surae, posterior transfer of both peroneals and the posterior tibial is performed; lateral stability of the hindfoot is provided by triple arthrodesis.

When all the plantar flexor muscles are paralyzed, the anterior tibial muscle is transferred to the os calcis. The posterior transfer is protected with a plantar flexion-assist ankle-foot orthosis until skeletal maturity. Tendo Achillis tenodesis may be performed to provide posterior stability to the ankle joint. In adolescence, if plantar flexion function of the transferred anterior tibial is adequate, the hindfoot is stabilized by triple arthrodesis.

When the anterior tibial function is inadequate, Chuinard-type ankle fusion is performed. When only the toe extensors are functioning, there will be no muscles available for posterior transfer. An ankle fusion is performed, provided there is adequate stability and muscle control of the knee.

The operative technique and postoperative care of posterior tendon transfer to the os calcis are presented in Plate 16, and of Chuinard-type distraction-compression bone graft arthrodesis of the ankle in Plate 22.

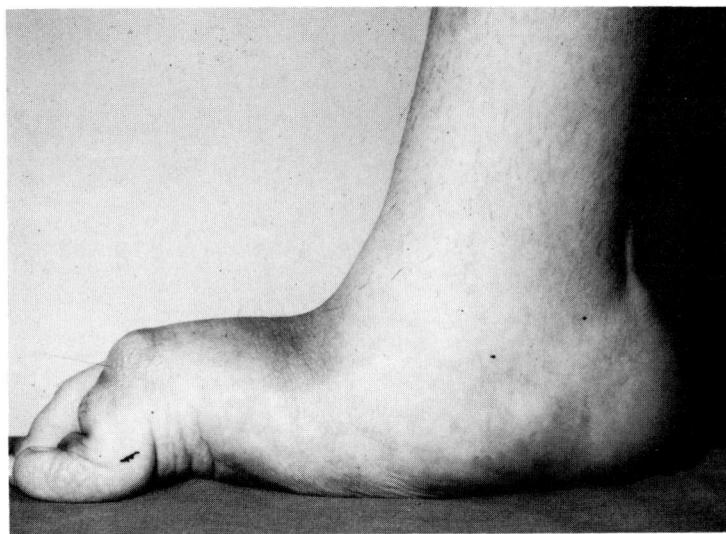

FIGURE 3–70. Dorsal bunion of left foot.

Note the dorsiflexion of the first metatarsal and plantar flexion of the great toe. (Courtesy of Dr. D. W. McKay.)

Dorsal bunion is characterized by dorsiflexion of the first metatarsal and plantar flexion of the great toe (Fig. 3–70). It is caused by muscle imbalance—weakness or absence of the peroneus longus muscle (plantar flexor of the first metatarsal) against normal strength of the anterior tibial muscle (dorsiflexor of the first metatarsal) or flexor hallucis brevis and longus. There are two types of dorsal bunion—one in which there is primary dorsiflexion of the first metatarsal and secondary plantar flexion of the hallus, and another in which there is primary plantar flexion of the hallux with resultant upward displacement of the metatarsal head. The author has treated dorsal bunion successfully by open-up wedge osteotomy of the base of the first metatarsal and transfer of the flexor hallucis longus to the head of the first metatarsal (Plate 20). McKay transfers tendinous insertions of the flexor hallucis brevis and abductor and adductor hallucis to the neck of the first metatarsal (Fig. 3–71). He believes these muscles have better mechanical advantage after transfer than the flexor hallucis longus; furthermore, the deforming action of the flexor hallucis brevis is also removed. The operative technique is as follows: a longitudinal incision is made on the medial aspect of the foot, extending from the base of the first metatarsal to the interphalangeal joint of the great toe. The abductor hallucis and medial part of the flexor hallucis brevis are identified, detached from their insertion, and dissected free; as much tendon as possible should be preserved (Fig. 3–72A). Then the lateral tendon of the flexor hallucis brevis and the tendon of the adductor hallucis are sectioned from their insertion and dissected free. The sesamoid bones in the tendinous part of the flexor hallucis brevis are carefully removed. If there is associated hallux valgus the abductor hallucis is left intact; if hallux varus is present the adductor hallucis is left attached to its insertion. Next, a circumferential incision is made in the periosteum of the first metatarsal at its neck and elevated for a distance of 1 cm. The abductor hallucis and medial part of the flexor hallucis brevis are transferred medially to the dorsal aspect of the metatarsal neck; the adductor hallucis and lateral part of the flexor hallucis brevis are transferred dorsally between the first and second metatarsals (Fig. 3–72B). All four tendons are sutured together, creating a myotendinous ring around the neck of the metatarsal (Figs. 3–71C and 3–72C). The collar of periosteum is sutured to the tendon. Next the interphalangeal joint of the great toe is stabilized by tenodesis or arthrodesis. A below-knee walking cast is applied and worn for three to four weeks. McKay reports complete correction in ten feet (Figs. 3–73 and 3–74).[14]

Arthrodesis of the Foot and Ankle

In the operative treatment of the paralyzed foot, a multitude of surgical proce-

Text continued on page 477

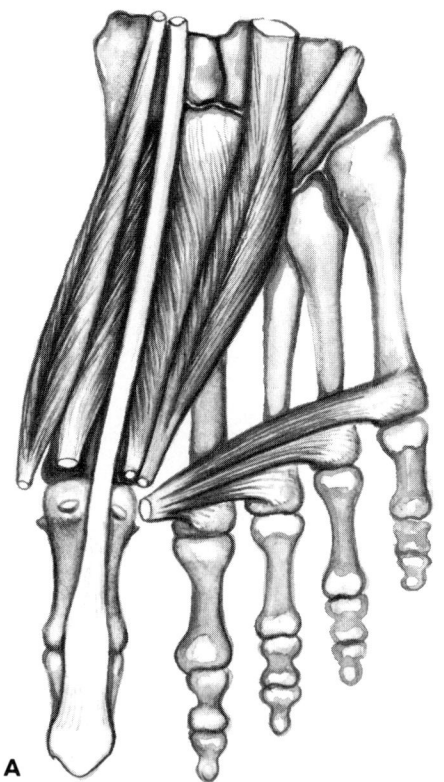
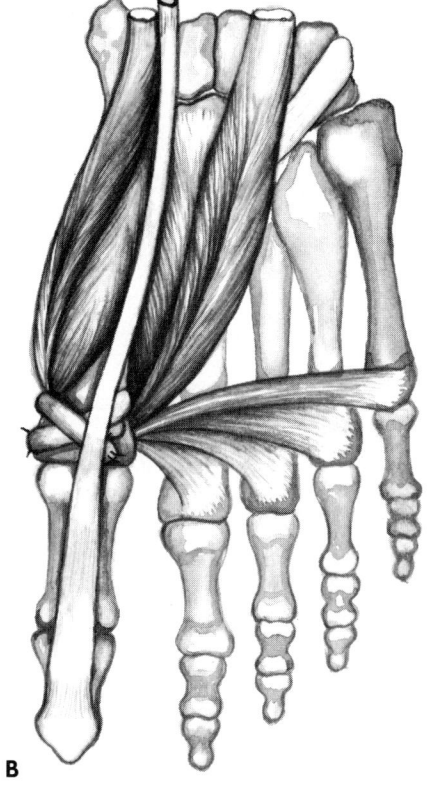
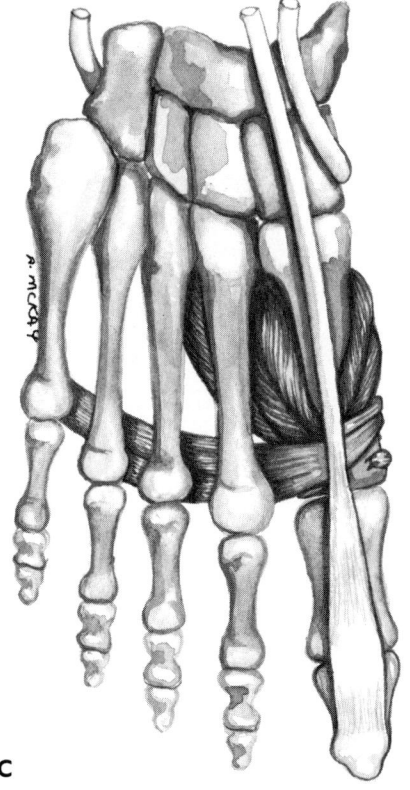

FIGURE 3–71. *McKay's technique for correction of dorsal bunion.*

A. Plantar view of right foot showing section of abductor hallucis, adductor hallucis, and flexor hallucis brevis from base of proximal phalanx. **B**. Tendinous portions of these muscles transferred to neck of first metatarsal as seen from plantar aspect. **C**. Dorsal view showing tendons transferred to the dorsum of the first metatarsal neck. (Courtesy of Dr. D. W. McKay.)

Treatment of Dorsal Bunion by Open-Up Osteotomy of Base of First Metatarsal

A. A longitudinal incision is made over the dorsomedial aspect of the foot, starting at the first cuneiform bone and extending distally to the first metatarsal head, where it is curved plantarward.

B. The base of the first metatarsal is exposed. A dorsal capsulotomy of the tarsometatarsal and navicular-cuneiform joint may be necessary to bring the first metatarsal bone into plantar flexion. With a starter and drill, the line of open-up osteotomy on the dorsal aspect of the base of the first metatarsal is marked. The plantar cortex should be left intact. Next, with a scalpel, a U-shaped flap of capsule is raised from the dorsum of the metatarsophalangeal joint with its base attached to the proximal phalanx. If necessary, any abnormally prominent bone on the metatarsal head is excised. If the flexion contracture of the great toe is not corrected by manipulation, capsulotomy of the plantar aspect of the first metatarsophalangeal joint is performed. Next the flexor hallucis longus tendon is divided near its insertion and delivered into the proximal part of the wound. A tunnel is drilled in the head of the first metatarsal from its dorsal to its plantar aspect.

C. Next the osteotomy of the dorsal, medial, and lateral parts of the base of the first metatarsal is completed. The distal part of the metatarsal is manipulated into plantar flexion, taking due care not to break the plantar cortex. A wedge of autogenous bone graft from the tibia or fibula is obtained and inserted at the osteotomy site, correcting the dorsiflexion deformity of the first metatarsal. The flexor hallucis longus tendon, with a whip suture in its distal end, is brought from plantar to dorsal aspect through the tunnel in the first metatarsal head and sutured to itself; this makes the flexor hallucis longus muscle a plantar-flexor of the first metatarsal instead of the great toe.

D. The dorsal U-flap of the capsule is sutured to the flexor hallucis longus tendon on the dorsum of the metatarsal head, holding the great toe in neutral position. The wound is closed in the usual fashion. A below-knee walking cast is applied and is worn for five to six weeks.

Plate 20. Treatment of Dorsal Bunion by Open-Up Osteotomy of Base of First Metatarsal

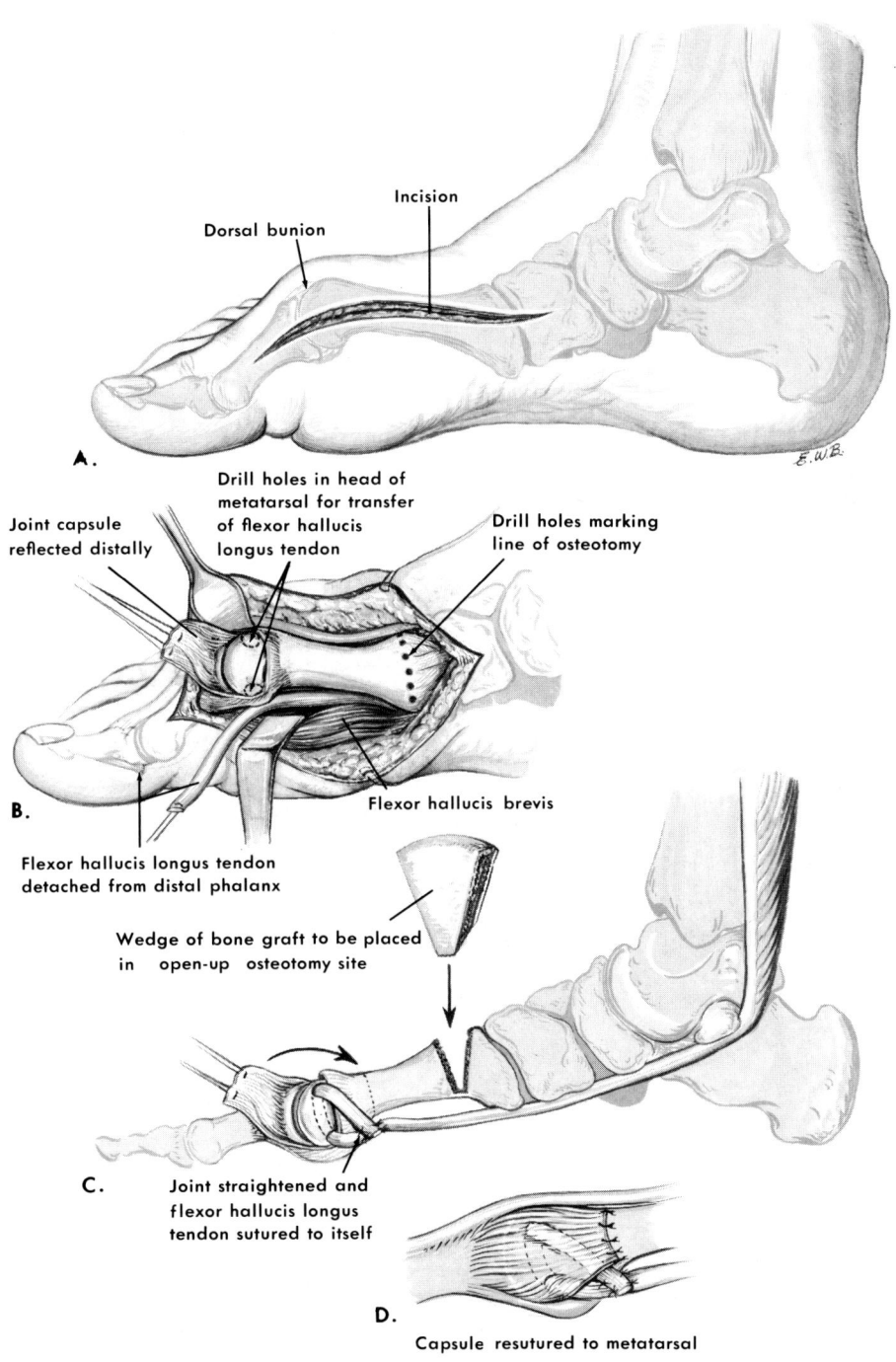

476 Neuromuscular Diseases

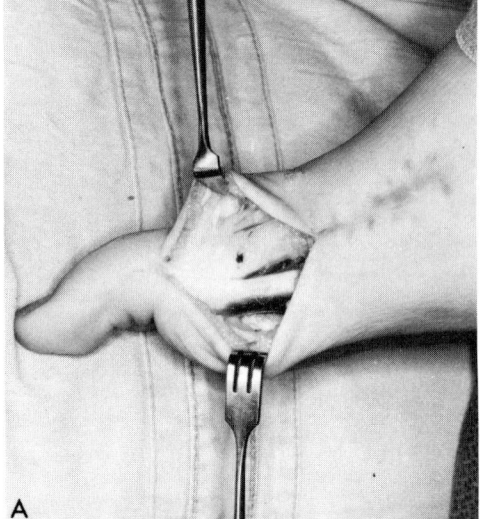

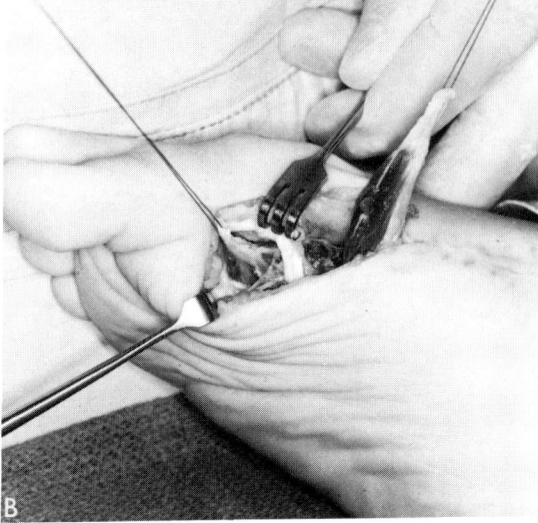

FIGURE 3–72. *McKay's technique for correction of dorsal bunion as seen during surgery.*

A. Note the abductor hallucis muscle. **B.** The suture on the right is attached to the abductor hallucis and the medial head of the flexor hallucis brevis; the other suture is attached to the adductor hallucis and the lateral head of the flexor hallucis brevis. The flexor hallucis longus tendon is in the middle of the wound. **C.** The four tendons are sutured over the dorsum of the neck of the first metatarsal and to the adjoining capsule and periosteum, providing a myotendinous ring. (Courtesy of Dr. D. W. McKay.)

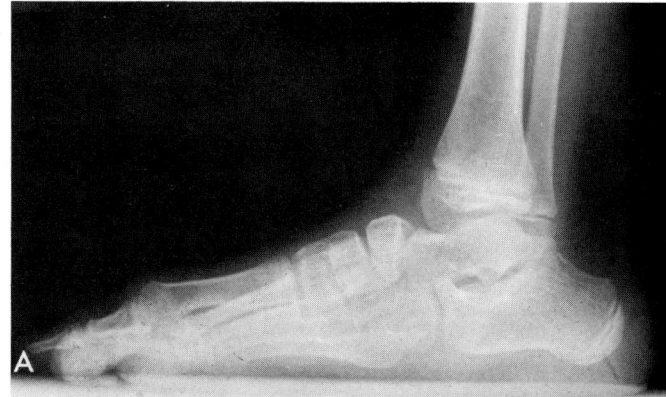

FIGURE 3–73. *McKay's technique for correction of dorsal bunion.*

A. Preoperative lateral roentgenogram of the foot, showing the deformity. **B.** Postoperative lateral x-ray of the foot. Note the excellent correction. (Courtesy of Dr. D. W. McKay.)

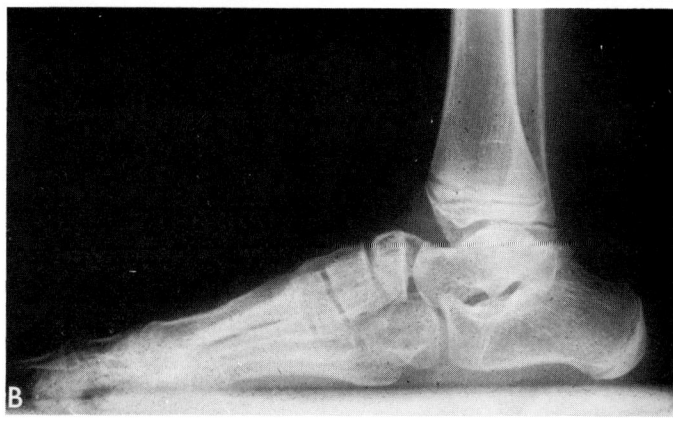

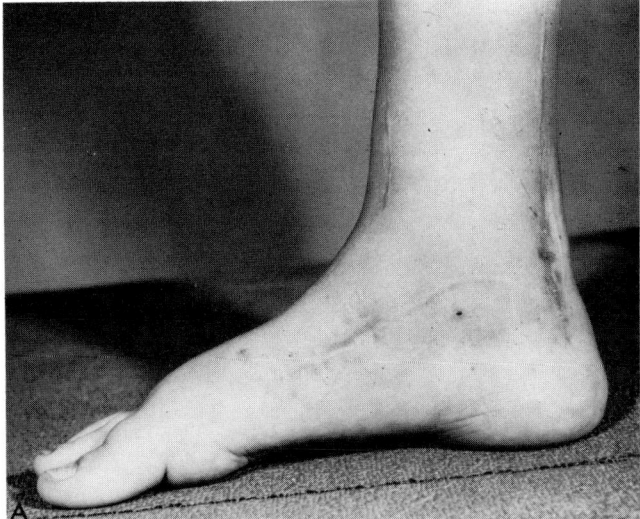
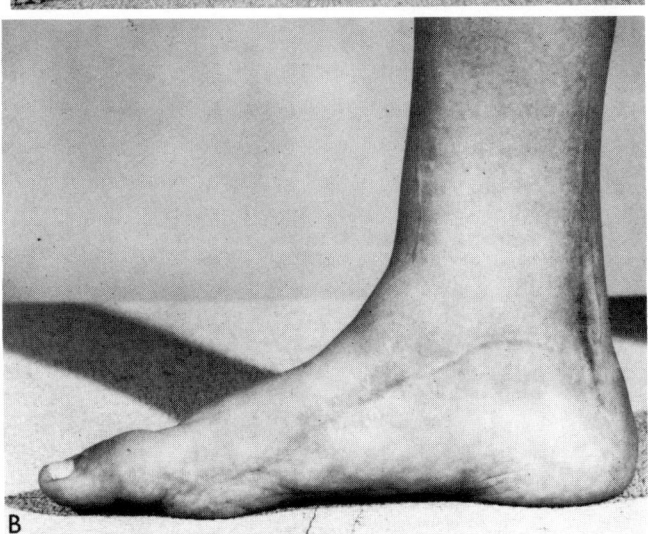

FIGURE 3–74. Dorsal bunion corrected by McKay's technique.

A. Preoperative photograph. Patient had developed dorsal bunion following cuneiform open wedge osteotomy (Fowler's procedure) for cavovarus foot. **B.** Postoperative lateral view of foot showing correction. (Courtesy of Dr. D. W. McKay.)

dures have been developed to provide stability, to correct deformity, and to improve function.

The history of the evolution of stabilizing operations of the foot and ankle is given in Table 3–5. Detailed accounts of these procedures are to be found in the original contributions and in the comprehensive historical reviews by Hart, Hallgrimson, and Schwartz.[74, 76, 150]

In general, stabilizing operations on the foot and ankle can be subdivided into the following: (1) triple arthrodesis, (2) extraarticular subtalar arthrodesis, (3) ankle fusion, and (4) anterior or posterior bone blocks to limit motion at the ankle joint. These procedures may be performed alone or in combination.

TRIPLE ARTHRODESIS

This procedure was devised by Ryerson in 1923 and consists of fusion of the subtalar, calcaneocuboid, and talonavicular joints.[148] The operation is designed to provide lateral stability, and it will also correct deformity if the articular surfaces are resected by pattern. In locomotion, the essential motions of the foot and ankle are plantar flexion and dorsiflexion. In the presence of muscle weakness, triple arthrodesis will stabilize the hindfoot and diminish the functional demand on the remaining active muscles by reducing the number of joints that they control.

The operative technique of triple arthrodesis is described and illustrated in Plate 21.

Text continued on page 482

Triple Arthrodesis

A pneumatic tourniquet is placed on the proximal thigh, and the patient is positioned semilaterally with a large sandbag under the hip on the affected side.

A. A curvilinear incision is made, centering over the sinus tarsi. It starts one fingerbreadth distal and posterior to the tip of the lateral malleolus and extends anteriorly and distally to the base of the second metatarsal bone.

B. Skin flaps should not be developed. The incision is carried to the floor of the sinus tarsi. By sharp dissection, with scalpel and periosteal elevator, the periosteum of the calcaneus, the adipose tissue contents of the sinus tarsi, and the tendinous origin of the exterior digitorum brevis are elevated in one mass from the calcaneus and lateral aspect of the neck of the talus and retracted distally. It is essential to provide a viable soft-tissue pedicle to obliterate the dead space remaining at the end of the operation.

Next, an incision is made superiorly over the periosteum of the talus, and the head and neck of the talus are carefully exposed. The upper flap of the skin, subcutaneous tissue, and periosteum should be kept as thick as possible to avoid necrosis. Traction sutures are placed on the periosteum. At no time are the skin edges to be retracted. It is not necessary to divide the peroneal tendons or their sheaths. By subperiosteal dissection, the peroneal tendons are retracted posteriorly for exposure of the subtalar joint.

C and D. The capsules of the calcaneocuboid, talonavicular, and subtalar joints are incised. These joints are opened and their cartilaginous surfaces clearly visualized by turning the foot into varus position. A laminar spreader placed in the sinus tarsi will aid in exposure of the posterior subtalar joint. Before excision of articular cartilaginous surfaces, one should review the deformity of the foot and decide on the wedges of bone to be removed to correct the deformity (Figs. 3–76 and 3–77). The blood supply of the talus and the complications of avascular necrosis of the talus and arthritis of the ankle following triple arthrodesis should always be kept in mind. The height of the foot is another consideration. A low lateral malleolus will cause difficulty with wearing shoes. At times, it is best to add a bone graft rather than resect wedges of bone. With a sharp osteotome, the cartilaginous surfaces of the calcaneocuboid joint are excised. Next, the articular cartilage surface of the talonavicular joint is exposed, the plane of osteotomy being perpendicular to the long axis of the neck of the talus and parallel to the calcaneocuboid joint. When the beak of the navicular is unduly prominent medially, or when, in a varus foot, one cannot obtain adequate exposure of the talonavicular joint without excessive retraction, a second dorsomedial incision may be used to expose the talonavicular joint.

Plate 21. Triple Arthrodesis

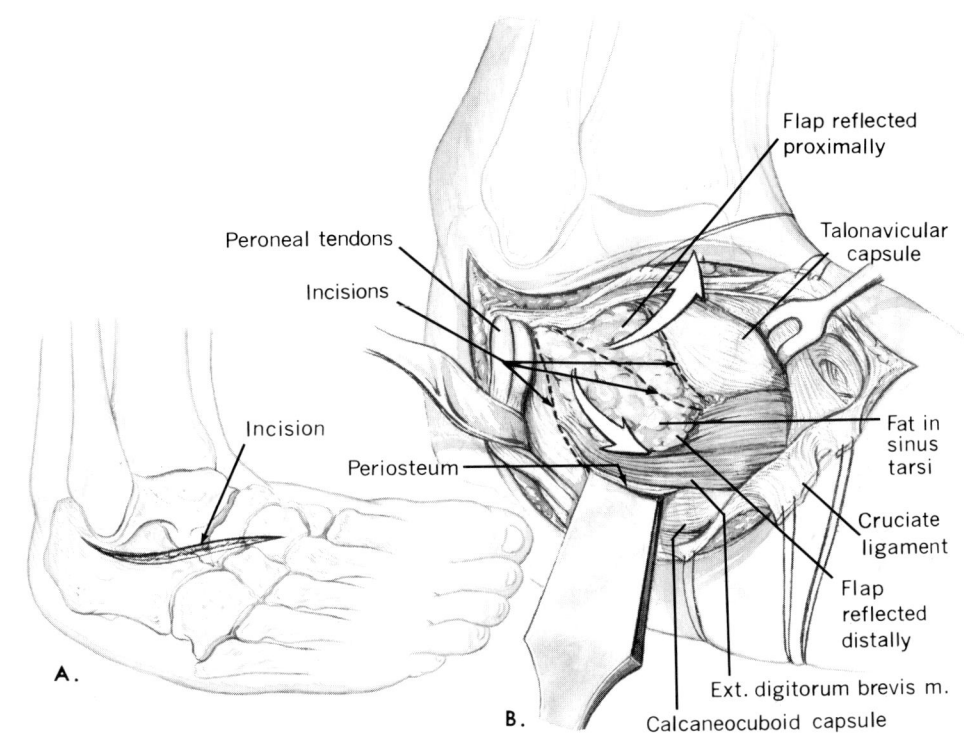

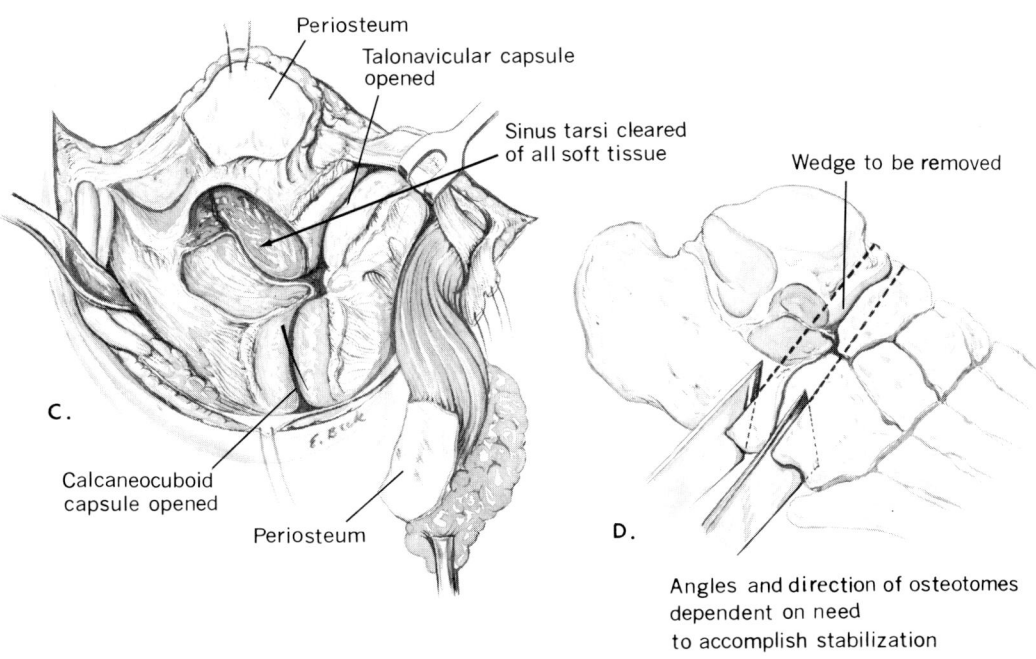

Triple Arthrodesis *(Continued)*

E to H. With a laminar spreader in the sinus tarsi, the subtalar joint is widely exposed and the cartilage of the anterior and posterior joints is excised. One should keep in mind the neurovascular structures behind the medial malleolus. The wedges of bone that must be removed to correct the deformity are excised in one mass with the articular cartilage. It is of great help to leave the osteotome used on the opposing articular surface in place and held steady by the assistant as a second osteotome or gouge is used to take contiguous cartilage and bone. The divided articular surfaces of the joints to be arthrodesed are "fish-scaled" for maximum raw cancellous bony contact.

The skin is closed with interrupted sutures. A well-molded long leg cast is applied, holding the foot in the desired position. The author has not found necessary and does not recommend fixation of the joints by staples. In foot stabilization in children with cerebral palsy, especially in the severely athetoid or spastic, secure criss-cross Kirschner wires are used to maintain position. These are removed in six to eight weeks.

Plate 21. Triple Arthrodesis

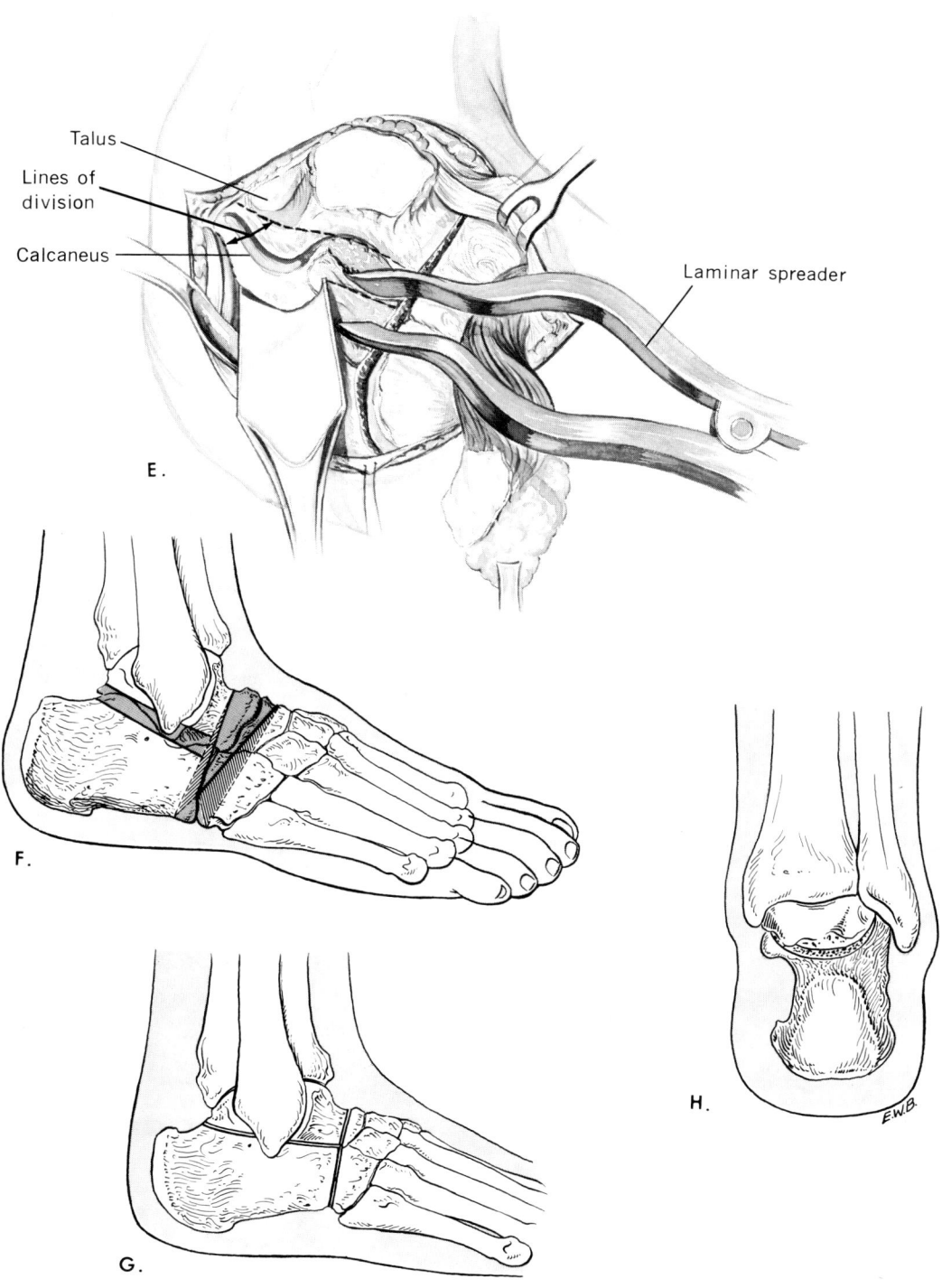

Table 3-5. *History of Stabilizing Operations of the Foot and Ankle*

1879	Albert	Tibiotarsal or ankle joint arthrodesis
1879	Von Lesser	Tibiotarsal or ankle joint arthrodesis
1884	Samster	Ankle and subtalar joint arthrodesis
1901	Whitman	Talectomy and posterior displacement of the foot
1905	Nieny	Talocalcaneal and talocalcaneonavicular or subtalar arthrodesis
1908	Jones	Talocalcaneal and talocalcaneonavicular or subtalar arthrodesis
1908	Goldthwait	Supratalar and infratalar arthrodesis
1911	Lorthioir	Pantalar arthrodesis (temporary removal of the talus)
1911	Ombredanne	Surgical approach for exposure of the subtalar and midtarsal joints
1912	Soule	Talonavicular arthrodesis
1912	Soule	Talonavicular and subtalar arthrodesis
1913	Davis	Subtalar arthrodesis (transverse horizontal section of the tarsus) with posterior displacement of the foot
1915	Albee	Talonavicular arthrodesis with bone graft peg
1916	Davis	Subtalar or calcaneotalar and calcaneotalonavicular arthrodesis
1919	Dunn	Midtarsal tarsectomy and calcaneotalar arthrodesis
1920	Toupet	Posterior bone check
1921	Hoke	Calcaneotalonavicular arthrodesis resection, reshaping and reimplantation of head and neck of the talus, and posterior displacement of the foot.
1922	Dunn	Excision of navicular bone, calcaneotalocuneiform and calcaneocuboid arthrodesis with posterior displacement of the foot
1922	Putti	Anterior bone check
1922	Steindler	Pantalar arthrodesis (talus not temporarily removed)
1923	Ryerson	Triple (subtalar and calcaneocuboid) arthrodesis
1923	Ryerson	Lateral arthrodesis (cuneonavicular, first and fifth tarsometatarsal arthrodesis)
1923	Campbell	Posterior bone block
1925	Smith and von Lackum	Calcaneotalonavicular and calcaneocuboid arthrodesis, excision of head and neck of talus with posterior displacement of the foot
1927	Lambrinudi	Resection of wedge of bone from plantar aspect of head and neck of talus to lock the talus in equinus position at the ankle while the rest of the foot is in the desired degree of dorsiflexion
1933	Brewster	Calcaneonaviculocuneiform arthrodesis, excision of head and neck of the talus, posterior displacement of the foot and countersinking of the body of the talus in the os calcis
1935	Girard	Arthrodesis of subtalar and calcaneocuboid joints; shortening of the neck of the talus; posterior displacement of foot; construction of ankle joint mortise
1952	Grice	Extra-articular arthrodesis of subtalar joint
1963	Chuinard and Peterson	Distraction-compression bone graft arthrodesis of the ankle
1966	Siffert	"Beak" triple arthrodesis for correction of severe cavus deformity
1977	Williams and Menelaus	Triple arthrodesis by lateral inlay grafting

The subtalar and midtarsal joint motions are particularly important for balance when an individual is walking upon rough or uneven terrain. The loss of lateral mobility of the hindfoot following triple arthrodesis may result in difficulty in locomotion on an irregular surface.

Triple arthrodesis may exert excessive ligamentous strain on the ankle joint. It is imperative to determine the stability of the body of the talus in the ankle mortise. This is done clinically by testing passive lateral motion of the ankle. If ankle stability is questionable, weight-bearing anteroposterior roentgenograms of the ankle with the hindfoot first in forced maximal eversion and abduction and then in forced inversion and adduction are taken. Normally, there is no lateral motion of the body of the talus in the ankle mortise except when the ankle is in marked plantar flexion; then it may be present in minimal amount. When there is marked instability of the ankle joint, varus or valgus deformity of the hindfoot may recur following triple arthrodesis, and stabilization of the ankle joint may be indicated.

Anterior subluxation of the ankle joint may be present in severe equinus deformity; this should be ruled out by making lateral roentgenograms of the ankle with the foot in maximal plantar flexion and in forced dorsiflexion.

Alignment and weight-bearing lines of the lower limb should be carefully studied. The presence of bowleg, knock-knee, or any excessive medial or lateral tibial torsion should be noted. Lateral tibial torsion and

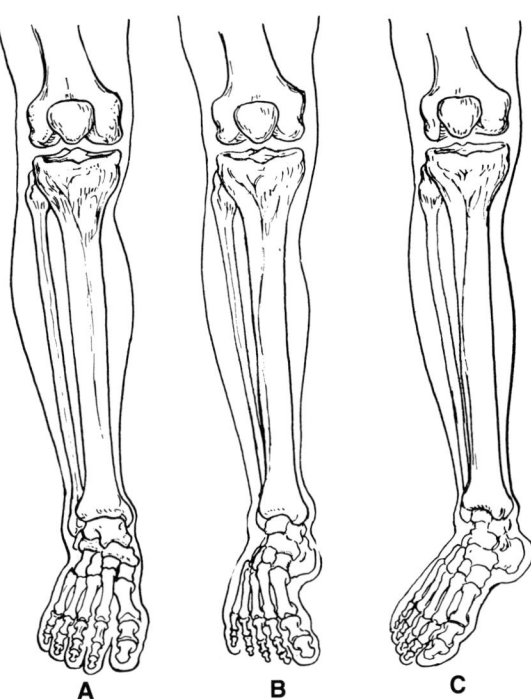

FIGURE 3–75. *Alignment of the foot.*

A. Normal foot, ankle, and knee alignment without tibial torsion. **B**. *Incorrect.* Foot is aligned with knee, not ankle, in the presence of external tibial torsion. **C**. *Correct.* Foot is aligned with ankle joint in the presence of external tibial torsion. (From Patterson, R. L., Parrish, F. F., and Hathaway, E. N.: Stabilizing operations on the foot. J. Bone Joint Surg., *32-A*:3, 1950. Reprinted by permission.)

genu valgum are common deformities in poliomyelitis. In stance, does the center of gravity of the body fall on the second metatarsal bone? Failure to recognize malalignment of the leg will result in improper positioning of the foot. During surgery, it is mandatory that the knee be draped sterile in the operative field. The foot should be aligned with the ankle mortise and not with the knee (Fig. 3–75). If there is significant torsional or angular deformity of the leg, it is corrected at a subsequent operation.

The growth of the foot in a young child should not be disturbed. The tarsal bones grow concentrically at their periphery, and resection of their articular surfaces will inhibit their growth. Triple arthrodesis should be deferred until the foot has achieved skeletal maturity, which in girls is 10 to 12 years, and in boys, 12 to 14 years.

The osseous deformity of the foot should be carefully analyzed in the preoperative roentgenograms. These should include anteroposterior and mediolateral weight-bearing views of the foot and ankle. It is important to make the roentgenograms with the foot held in the positions of maximum correction. Tracings of the foot are made on x-ray negative films. The foot and ankle are divided into three segments, according to function: (1) the talus with the tibia and ankle joint; (2) the os calcis; and (3) the tarsal bones, the joints distal to the midtarsal joint, the metatarsals and phalanges. The talus is the only tarsal bone that transmits the entire body weight; thus, the importance of double-checking the stability of the body of the talus in the ankle mortise cannot be overemphasized.

The pattern of osteotomies and the plane of resection of the articular surfaces of each joint should be carefully and precisely planned. It is best to draw these lines on tracings of the preoperative lateral roentgenograms of the foot.

In the correction of varus deformity a wedge of bone with its base facing laterally is resected from the talonavicular and calcaneocuboid joints (Fig. 3–76). Lateral displacement of the forefoot is often prevented by the "beak" of the navicular bone, which projects posteriorly along the medial side of the head of the talus. It is important to excise this "beak" flush with the main body of the navicular—through a separate incision if necessary. The planes of osteotomies of the talonavicular and calcaneocuboid joints should be parallel to each other in the vertical axis in order to have close apposition of bones. To correct varus deformity of the heel, a laterally based wedge is resected from the subtalar joint. Most of the bone should be removed from the superior surface of the calcaneus. Only a minimal amount of bone should be excised from the talus. A slight valgus position of

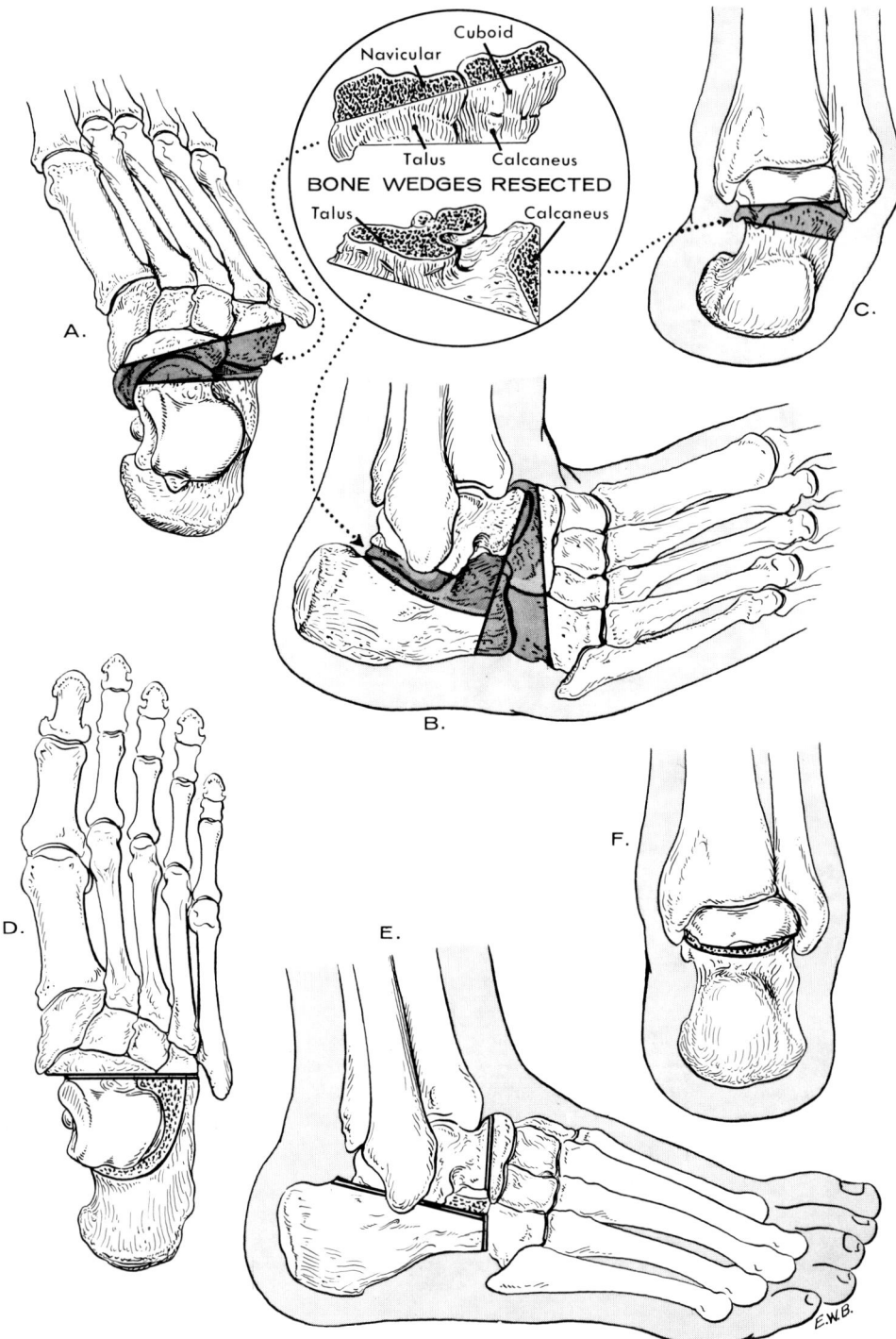

FIGURE 3–76. Wedge of bone to be removed for correction of pes varus.

A to **C**. Three views of the varus deformity. Shaded areas show amount of bone to be resected. **D** to **F**. Corrected positions of the bones postoperatively.

the heel will provide stability; however, the hindfoot should not be placed in more than 5 to 10 degrees of eversion, as it will cause difficulty in the proper wearing of shoes and is not cosmetically satisfactory. A varus position of the heel should not be accepted.

Valgus deformity of the foot is corrected by excision of a medially based wedge from the midtarsal area and another wedge, also based medially, from the subtalar region. The use of a laminectomy spreader in the subtalar joint will adequately expose the medial side of the hindfoot. Great care should be exercised not to injure the posterior tibial nerves and artery, which lie adjacent and superficial to the flexor hallucis longus tendon. In the valgus foot, the os calcis is everted and the head of the talus is plantar-flexed over the medial aspect of the foot. The common tendency is to excise a large wedge in order to reduce the calcaneus medially beneath the talus. This should be avoided, as it will reduce the height of the hindfoot and lower the malleoli, resulting in a wide ankle contour and extreme difficulty in fitting shoes. When correcting severe valgus, varus, or calcaneus deformity of the foot, it is best to add bone graft wedges rather than to excise too much bone. Resection of excessive bone from the talus and navicular may also cause avascular necrosis of these tarsal bones with subsequent degenerative arthritis of the ankle and pseudarthrosis of the talonavicular joint.

For restoration of alignment of the calcaneus foot, a wedge of bone based posteriorly is resected from the subtalar joint (Fig. 3–77). Often there is associated cavus deformity, which is corrected by excising a wedge based dorsally from the talonavicular and calcaneocuboid joints. It is imperative to displace the os calcis posteriorly to provide a longer lever arm. When contracted, the anterior capsule of the ankle joint is stretched out preoperatively by passive manipulation and corrective casts. Release of soft-tissue contracture may be indicated when the contracture is very fixed. It is imperative to obtain normal range of plantar flexion of the ankle.

In severe talipes calcaneus, the bony deformity and soft-tissue contracture are rigid, fixing the talus and os calcis in marked dorsiflexion. The associated cavus deformity will be marked, with severe contracture of the plantar fascia and osseous changes in the midtarsal bones. Correction of deformity by wedge resections will result in appreciable reduction in the height and length of the foot.

Plantar fasciotomy is performed first. The anterior capsule of the ankle joint is released through an anterolateral approach. Next, the articular surfaces of the subtalar and talonavicular and calcaneocuboid joints are minimally resected, exposing raw cancellous bone. The calcaneus deformity is corrected by inserting an anteriorly based wedge of bone graft in the subtalar joint. Forefoot equinus deformity can be corrected by excising a wedge of bone based dorsally from the talonavicular and calcaneocuboid joints. Frequently, the author postpones surgical correction of the cavus deformity until solid healing of the triple arthrodesis has taken place. During the application of the long leg cast, however, it is important to immobilize the heel in moderate plantar flexion and the forefoot in maximal dorsiflexion. The common pitfall is to hold the forefoot in equinus position, permitting the cavus deformity to increase. The metatarsal heads should be well padded to prevent skin slough. Three to four months later, the metatarsals are osteotomized at their base and elevated into dorsiflexion, correcting the forefoot equinus deformity. In this way, some degree of mobility of the naviculocuneiform and cuneiform metatarsal joints is preserved.

Talectomy will correct the severe calcaneus deformity.[81, 111, 167, 177, 178] However, it reduces the height of the foot, lowers the malleoli, and causes great difficulty in fitting shoes. This is particularly disturbing to women. Fibroarthrosis and degenerative arthritis of the ankle joint will often develop in later years. For these reasons, astragalectomy is not recommended.

In classic triple arthrodesis, it is difficult to displace the os calcis backward. Dunn described a method of excising the navicular and part of the head and neck of the talus to permit posterior displacement of the calcaneus.[48, 49] Hoke had previously resected the navicular and head and neck of the talus; after subtalar joint resection and posterior displacement of the foot, he recommended reshaping and reimplanting the head and neck of the talus.[80] The Hoke and Dunn procedures, however, shorten the foot and increase the likelihood of pseudarthrosis of the talonavicular joint. For these reasons, the author prefers correction of calcaneus deformity by bone graft wedges.

In correction of pes equinus, fixed contracture of the posterior capsule of the ankle and subtalar joints and the triceps surae muscle must be corrected preoperatively. As stated previously, function of the gastrocnemius-soleus muscles should be maintained as much as possible. Wedging casts are tried first, followed by posterior

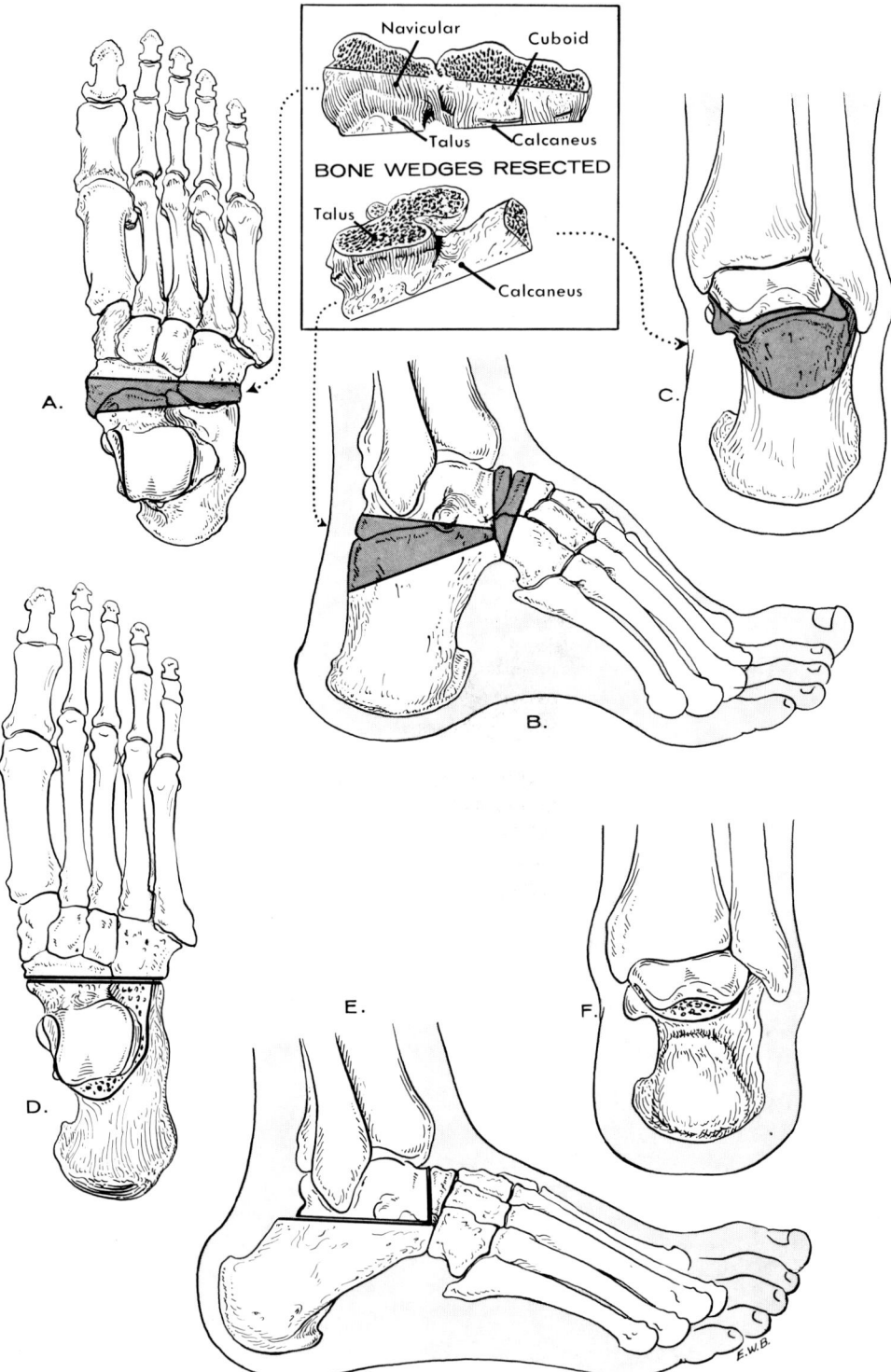

FIGURE 3–77. Wedges of bone to be removed for correction of calcaneocavus deformity.

A, B, and **C**. Dorsal, lateral, and posterior views show the deformity. Shaded areas indicate amount of bone removed. **D** to **F**. Positions of the bones after correction of deformity by triple arthrodesis. Note the posterior displacement of the hindfoot.

capsulotomy and skeletal traction through the os calcis. In severe equinus deformity, limited heel cord lengthening may have to be performed, but it is preferable to leave some tightness of the triceps surae. It is imperative that the foot be dorsiflexed to neutral position; otherwise a rocker-bottom deformity will result. In patients with cerebral palsy, the author maintains reduction with a large Kirschner wire. One pin is placed through the os calcis into the talus and across the ankle joint into the tibia, while the other transfixes the talonavicular joint. When equinus posture is due simply to drop foot and the foot can be passively dorsiflexed beyond neutral position, it is preferable to perform tendon transfer anteriorly to provide power of active dorsiflexion. If adequate muscles are not available for anterior transfer, the triple arthrodesis may be modified to prevent the foot from dropping down into plantar flexion. Lambrinudi, in 1927, described a method of triple arthrodesis in which a wedge of bone is excised from the plantar aspect of the head and neck of the talus and the distal sharp margin of the body of the talus is inserted into a prepared trough in the navicular. Thus the talus is locked in equinus position at the ankle joint, whereas the rest of the foot is maintained in the desired degree of dorsiflexion.[97]

The Lambrinudi operation is not recommended by the author, as his experience with it has been unsatisfactory. For adequate correction of equinus deformity, too much bone has to be resected from the talus, with consequent development of avascular necrosis of the talus, talonavicular pseudarthrosis, flattening of the superior surface of the talus, and painful arthritis of the ankle.[52, 77, 98, 113, 118, 136]

EXTRA-ARTICULAR SUBTALAR ARTHRODESIS

Grice, at the suggestion of William T. Green, developed a method of fusion of the subtalar joint by insertion of autogenous bone grafts in the sinus tarsi in the lateral aspect of the foot for correction of paralytic pes valgus and restoration of the height of the longitudinal arch.[69, 71] Any interference with subsequent normal growth of the foot is minimal, at most, because the procedure is extra-articular. The operative technique is described and illustrated in Plate 15. Pitfalls and complications are discussed in the section on cerebral palsy.

ANKLE FUSION AND PANTALAR ARTHRODESIS*

When surgical reconstruction is being considered for a flail foot and ankle, their relationship to the lower limb as a whole should be carefully assessed, since there is often associated paralysis of the muscles throughout the lower limb.

Pantalar arthrodesis is surgical fusion of the joints around the talus, i.e., the ankle, subtalar, and talonavicular joints; the calcaneocuboid joint (which is not an articulation of the talus) is also included in the stabilization, thus making the procedure a combination of triple arthrodesis and ankle fusion.

Lorthioir, as he originally reported the procedure in 1911, extirpated and replaced the talus as an autogenous bone graft.[109] In 1922, Steindler advised against the temporary removal of the talus from the wound because of the danger of avascular necrosis; he also included the calcaneocuboid joint in the fusion to provide stability and to maintain correction.[163]

When the muscles below the knee are paralyzed, pantalar arthrodesis will provide stability to the ankle and hindfoot, thus eliminating the need for orthotic support, provided the gluteus maximus is of adequate strength and the knee is stable. Extensor strength of the knee is desirable but not imperative. When the quadriceps muscle is paralyzed, stability of the knee joint is provided by shifting the center of gravity of the body forward anterior to the plane of the knee joint. To lock the knee in extension, the tibia should not be allowed to come forward through a dorsiflexion movement of the ankle, either by a strong triceps surae muscle or by a fixed equinus ankle joint. A good gluteus maximus muscle will transmit push-off power to the ball of the foot when the ankle is rigid and the knee is locked in extension.

Position of ankle fusion is an important consideration. In arthrodesis of the ankle, excessive plantar flexion to stabilize the knee in extension during the stance phase of gait or to compensate for a short limb will result in increased pressure on the metatarsal heads. Callosities will form and eventually the skin will ulcerate. Consequently, in later adult life, pain in the forefoot will be a constant complaint. Unequal heel

Text continued on page 492

---

*See references 4, 9, 15, 25, 27, 63, 75, 84, 92, 106, 136.

Arthrodesis of Ankle Joint Through Anterior Approach Without Disturbing Distal Tibial Growth Plate

THE PROCEDURE

A and **B.** A longitudinal skin incision is made, beginning 7 cm. proximal to the ankle joint between the extensor digitorum longus and extensor hallucis longus tendons; it extends distally across the ankle joint in line with the third metatarsal and ends 4 cm. distal to the ankle joint.

The subcutaneous tissue is divided and the skin flaps are mobilized and retracted to their respective sides. The veins crossing the field are clamped, divided, and coagulated. The intermediate and medial dorsal cutaneous branches of the superficial peroneal nerve are identified and protected by retraction to one side of the wound.

C. The deep fascia and transverse crural and cruciate crural ligaments are divided in line with the skin incision. The ligaments are marked with 00 silk suture for accurate closure later.

Plate 22. Arthrodesis of Ankle Joint Through Anterior Approach Without Disturbing Distal Tibial Growth Plate

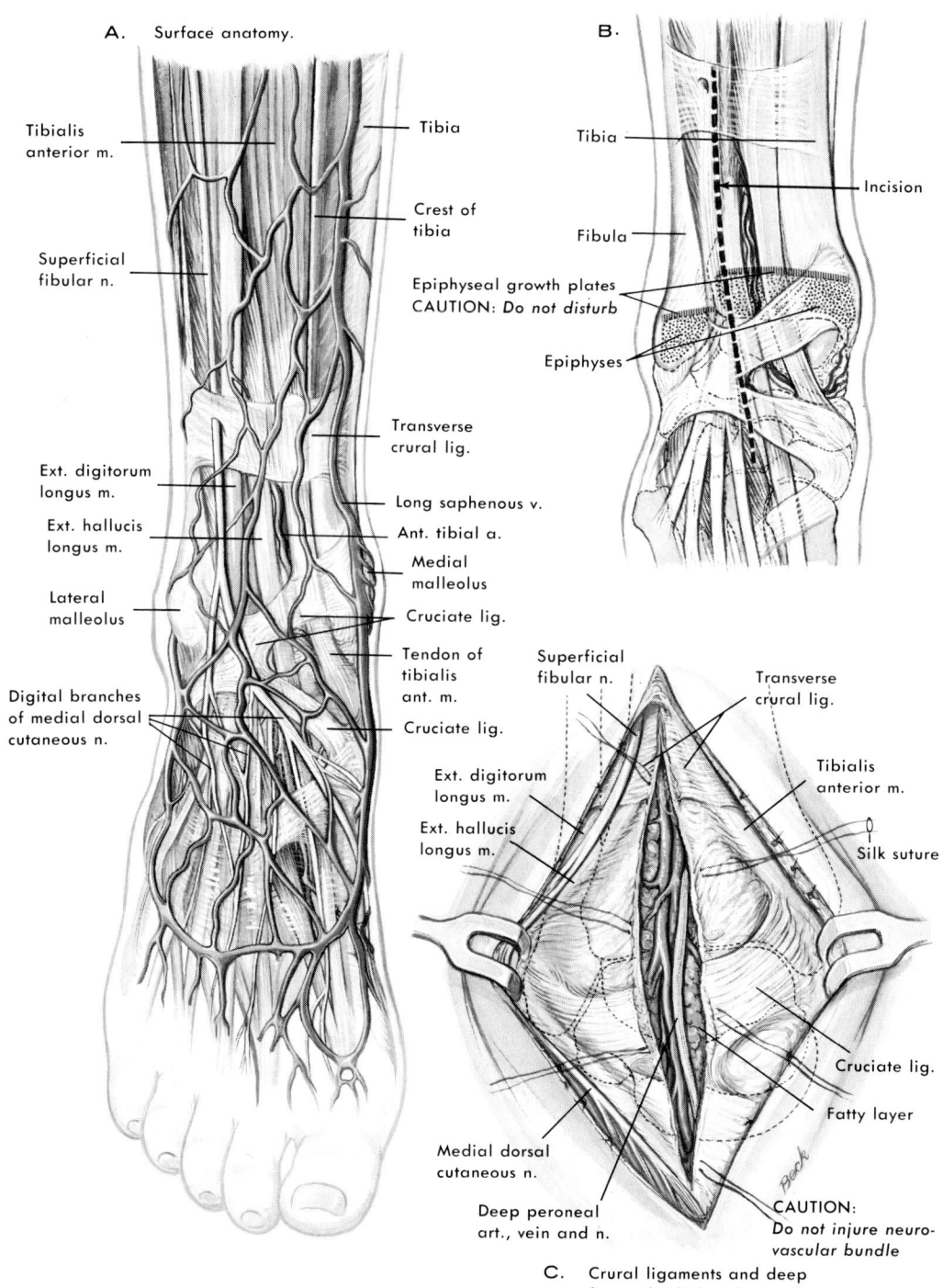

Arthrodesis of Ankle Joint Through Anterior Approach Without Disturbing Distal Tibial Growth Plate *(Continued)*

D. The neurovascular bundle (deep peroneal nerve, anterior tibial–dorsalis pedis vessels) is identified, isolated, and retracted laterally with the extensor hallucis longus, extensor digitorum longus, and peroneus tertius tendons. The anterolateral malleolar and lateral tarsal arteries are isolated, clamped, divided, and ligated. The distal tibia, ankle joint, and talus are identified. A transverse incision is made in the capsule of the talotibial joint from the posterior tip of the medial malleolus to the lateral malleolus. The edges of the capsule are marked with 00 silk suture for meticulous closure later.

E to G. The capsule is reflected and retracted distally on the talus and proximally on the tibia. The periosteum of the tibia should not be divided. The distal tibial and fibular epiphyseal plates should not be disturbed in growing children. With thin curved and straight osteotomes, the cartilage and subchondral bone are removed from the opposing articular surfaces of the distal tibia and proximal talus down to raw bleeding cancellous bone. Cartilage chips should not be left posteriorly.

H. Next, a large piece of bone for grafting is taken from the ileum and fashioned to fit snugly in the ankle joint. The graft should have both cortices intact and should be thicker at one end, wedge-shaped. The cortices of the graft are perforated with multiple tiny drill holes. The ankle joint is held in the desired position and the bone graft is firmly fitted into the joint with an impacter. If any space is left on each side of the graft, it is packed with cancellous bone from the ilium. The graft in the ankle joint gives compressional force to the arthrodesis and adds to the height of the foot and ankle. The arthrodesis may be fixed internally with a smooth Steinmann pin; it is introduced up through the calcaneus and the talus, across the ankle, and through the lower half of the tibia. The capsule of the ankle joint and the transverse crural and cruciate crural ligaments are closed carefully in layers. The deep fascia and the wound are closed in the usual manner. Roentgenograms are obtained in anteroposterior and lateral views to ensure that the ankle joint is in the desired position.

I. An above-knee cast is applied with the ankle joint in the desired position of plantar flexion (boys, 10 degrees; girls, 15 to 20 degrees) and the knee in 45 degrees of flexion.

POSTOPERATIVE CARE

Periodic roentgenograms are obtained to determine the position of the graft and the extent of healing. Eight to ten weeks after surgery, the solid cast is removed and roentgenograms are obtained with the cast off. Ordinarily, by this time, the fusion is solid and the patient is gradually allowed to be ambulatory. The Steinmann pin is extracted when the cast is removed. Full weight-bearing is begun two to three weeks later.

Plate 22. Arthrodesis of Ankle Joint Through Anterior Approach Without Disturbing Distal Tibial Growth Plate

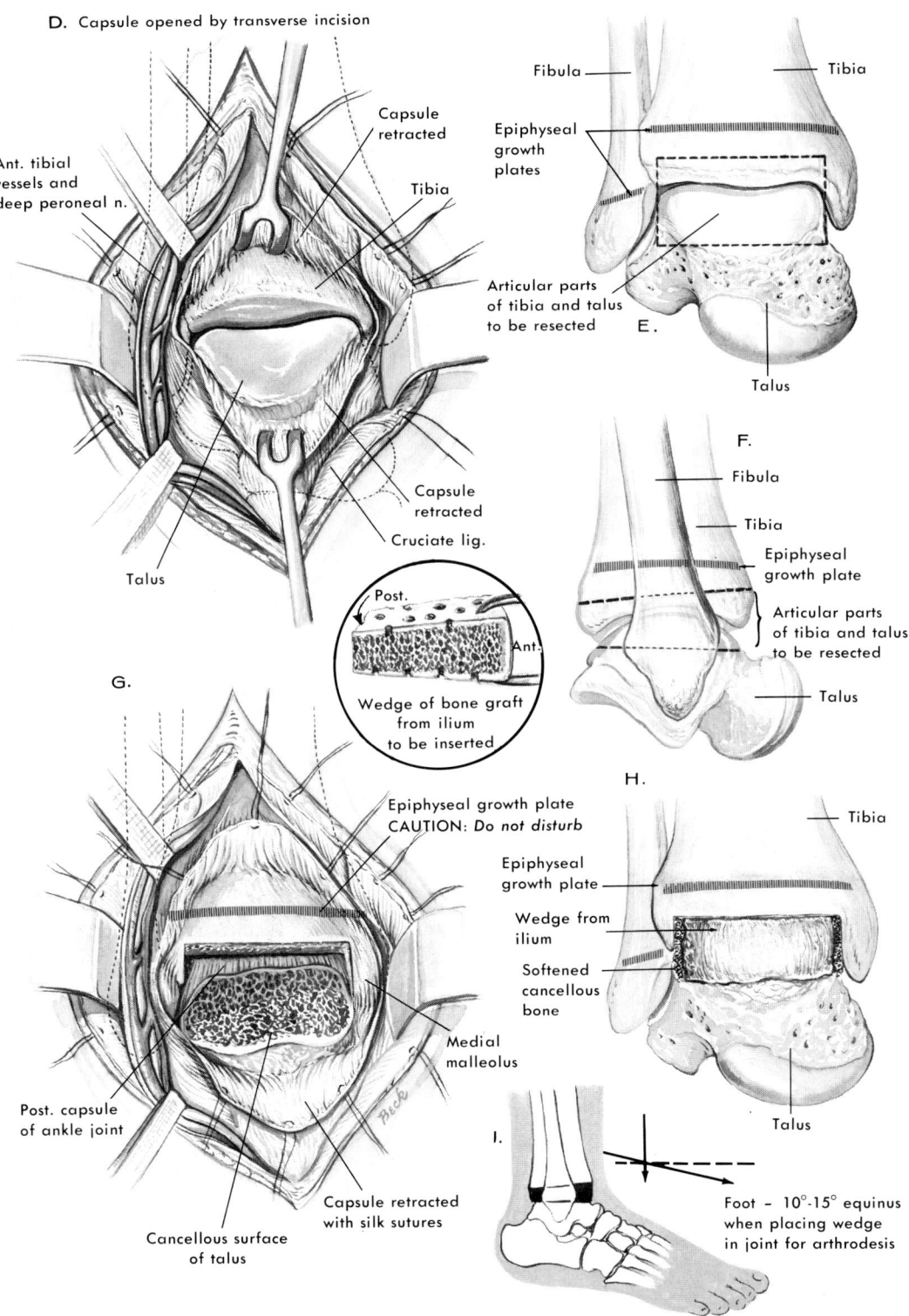

heights are another cause of dissatisfaction; often patients would rather accept shortening and a full sole build-up. It is imperative that the position of ankle fusion be 5 to 10 degrees equinus. Lateral roentgenograms of the foot and ankle should be made at the time of surgery, and the position of stabilization of the ankle accurately measured with a goniometer.

Pronation or supination of the forefoot results in unequal pressure on its sides and may also cause painful callosities and ulceration. When the forefoot is in supination, callosities develop over the fifth metatarsal head, whereas in pronation they develop over the first and second metatarsal heads; and when in excessive equinus inclination, over the first and fifth metatarsal heads.

The plantar surface of the foot should be in the normal weight-bearing position, with no pronation or supination or uneven pressure under the metatarsal heads. The lateral border of the foot should be straight, with the heel in neutral or slightly valgus position and the ankle in less than 10 degrees of plantar flexion.

Waugh, Wagner, and Stinchfield reported the results of 116 pantalar arthrodeses in 97 patients with a mean follow-up of five years and an average follow-up of 6.9 years. In general, pantalar arthrodesis was found to be an effective and satisfying procedure. About 80 per cent of the patients had no complaints referable to their pantalar arthrodesis. Adequate compensatory motion developed in the forepart of the foot, so that rigidity of the feet was not a problem, despite fusion of the ankle and hindpart of the foot. Of the 52 patients who had used an orthosis preoperatively, 47 were able to discard it following fusion. Pseudarthrosis occurred in 14.7 per cent of the cases.[173]

When the foot has normal alignment and adequate bony and ligamentous stability, the author recommends ankle fusion only, using the distraction-compression bone graft arthrodesis described by Chuinard and Peterson (Plate 22).[32] In the paralyzed limb, there are no compressional forces to maintain the tibia and talus in close apposition, and the weight of the cast pressing on the dorsum of the foot may distract them.

ANTERIOR OR POSTERIOR BONE BLOCKS TO LIMIT MOTION AT ANKLE

In pes calcaneus, construction of a bone buttress anteriorly in the talus will limit dorsiflexion of the ankle by impinging upon the anterior lip of the distal tibia, whereas in equinus deformity of the foot, plantar flexion of the ankle may be restricted by bone block construction on the posterior aspect of the talus.[22, 23, 58, 59] These procedures were developed for use in cases of paralytic calcaneus or drop foot, when there is no musculature available for transfer to provide plantar flexion or dorsiflexion power. Long-term follow-up studies of bone block operations have disclosed a high incidence of recurrence of deformity and fibrous ankylosis or painful degenerative arthritis of the ankle joint. The author does not recommend bone blocks to limit motion at the ankle, as the procedure has all the disadvantages of arthrodesis of the ankle without providing the pain-free stability of the latter.

The only indication for a posterior bone block is in a female patient who desires to wear shoes with heels of varying height and who has fair strength of the triceps surae muscle but no dorsiflexor power. Following triple arthrodesis, small subarticular grafts are placed posteriorly to lift the articular surface of the posterior aspect of the talus and limit plantar flexion. Massive bone grafts that abut the posterior aspect of the tibia should not be used. The small blocks placed beneath the articular surface of the talus are just as effective, heal rapidly, can be performed in combination with triple arthrodesis, and are less likely to cause pain.[68]

References

1. Albert, E.: Zur Resektion des Kniegelenkes. Wien. Med. Presse, *20*:705, 1879.
2. Albert, E.: Chirurgische Mittheilungen. Zbl. Chir., *8*:766, 1881.
3. Alldredge, R. H., and Riordan, D. C.: The use of staples and bone-chip grafts for internal fixation in foot-stabilization operations. J. Bone Joint Surg., *35-A*:951, 1953.
4. Ansart, M. B.: Pan-arthrodesis for paralytic flail foot. J. Bone Joint Surg., *33-B*:503, 1951.
5. d'Aubigné, R. M.: Chirurgia Orthopedique des Paralysis. Paris, Masson & Cie, 1959.
6. Auriach, A., Puig-Manera, R., and Loton, J.: Qu'en est-il

de la poliomyélite de l'enfant en centre de rééducation en 1976? *In* Simon, L. (ed.): Acualités en rééducation fonctionnelle et réadaptation. Paris, New York, Masson & Cie, 1976, pp. 147–153.
7. Axer, A.: Transposition of gluteus maximus, tensor fasciae latae and ilio-tibial band for paralysis of lateral abdominal muscles in children after poliomyelitis. A preliminary report. J. Bone Joint Surg., *40-B*:644, 1958.
8. Baker, L. D., and Dodelin, C. D.: Extra-articular arthrodesis of the subtalar joint (Grice procedure). J.A.M.A., *168*:1005, 1958.
9. Barr, J. S., and Record, E. E.: Arthrodesis of the ankle for correction of foot deformity. Surg. Clin. N. Amer., *27*:1281, 1947.
10. Beau, A., Prevot, J., and Masse, P.: Intervention de Grice dans le pied plat valgus paralytique. Rev. Chir. Orthop., *47*:233, 1961.
11. Benyi, P.: A modified Lambrinudi operation for drop foot. J. Bone Joint Surg., *42-B*:333, 1960.
12. Bertrand, P.: Transplantations tendineuses pour pied talus paralytique. A propos de 38 observations. Rev. Chir. Orthop., *47*:212, 1961.
13. Bickel, W. H., and Moe, J. H.: Translocation of the peroneus longus tendon for paralytic calcaneus deformity of the foot. Surg. Gynec. Obstet., *78*:627, 1944.
14. Biesalski, H., and Mayer, L.: Die Physiologische Sehnenverpflanzung. Vol. 14. Berlin, Julius Springer, 1916.
15. Bingold, A. C.: Ankle and subtalar fusion by a transarticular graft. J. Bone Joint Surg., *38-B*:862, 1956.
16. Bradford, E. H., and Lovett, R. W.: Treatise on Orthopedic Surgery. London, Baillière, Tindall & Cox, 1915, p. 486.
17. Brewster, A. H.: Countersinking the astragalus in paralytic feet. New Eng. J. Med., *209*:71, 1933.
18. Broms, J. D.: Subtalar extra-articular arthrodesis. Followup study. Clin. Orthop., *42*:139, 1965.
19. Bunnell, S.: Restoring flexion to the paralytic elbow. J. Bone Joint Surg., *33-A*:566, 1951.
20. Caldwell, G. D.: Correction of paralytic footdrop by hemigastrosoleus transplant. Clin. Orthop., *118*:81, 1976.
21. Camera, R.: La double tenodese des extenseurs du pied dans le traitement du pied équin paralytique. Rev. Orthop., *35*:242, 1949.
22. Campbell, W. C.: An operation for the correction of "dropfoot." J. Bone Joint Surg., *5*:815, 1923.
23. Campbell, W. C.: End results of operation for correction of drop-foot. J.A.M.A., *85*:1927, 1925.
24. Carayon, A., Bourrel, P., Bourges, M., and Touze, M.: Dual transfer of the posterior tibial and flexor digitorum longus tendons for drop foot. Report of thirty-one cases. J. Bone Joint Surg., *49-A*:144, 1967.
25. Carmack, J. C., and Hallock, H.: Tibiotarsal arthrodesis after astragalectomy, a report of eight cases. J. Bone Joint Surg., *29*:476, 1947.
26. Chambers, E. F. S.: Operation for correction of flexible flat fleet in adolescents. Western J. Surg., *54*:77, 1946.
27. Charnley, J.: Compression arthrodesis of the ankle and shoulder. J. Bone Joint Surg., *33-B*:180, 1951.
28. Charnley, J.: Compression Arthrodesis. London, E. & S. Livingstone, Ltd., 1953.
29. Chigot, P.: Transplantations tendineuses dans le paralysies des extenseurs dorsaux et lateraux du pied. Résultats et indications. Rev. Chir. Orthop., *47*:200, 1961.
30. Chigot, P. L., and Sananes, P.: Arthrodèse de Grice. Variente technique. Rev. Chir. Orthop., *51*:53, 1965.
31. Cholmeley, J. A.: Elmslie's operation for the calcaneus foot. J. Bone Joint Surg., *33-B*:228, 1951.
32. Chuinard, E. G., and Peterson, R. E.: Distraction-compression bone-graft arthrodesis of the ankle. A method especially applicable for children. J. Bone Joint Surg., *45-A*:481, 1963.
33. Close, J. R., and Todd, F. N.: The phasic activity of the muscles of the lower extremity and the effect of tendon transfer. J. Bone Joint Surg., *41-A*:189, 1959.
34. Codivilla, A.: Meine Erfahrugen über Schnenverpflanzungen. Z. Orthop. Chir., *12*:221, 1904.
35. Coonrad, R. W., Irwin, C. E., Gucker, T., III, and Wray, J. B.: The importance of plantar muscles in paralytic varus feet. The results of treatment by neurectomy and myotenotomy. J. Bone Joint Surg., *38-A*:563, 1956.
36. Crego, C. H., Jr., and McCarroll, H. R.: Recurrent deformities in stabilized paralytic feet. A report of 1100 consecutive stabilizations in poliomyelitis. J. Bone Joint Surg., *20*:609, 1938.
37. Cross, A. B.: Crawling patterns in neglected poliomyelitis in the Solomon Islands. J. Bone Joint Surg., *59-B*:428, 1977.
38. Davis, G. G.: Wedge-shaped resection of the foot for the relief of old cases of varus. New York J. Med., *56*:379, 1892.
39. Davis, G. G.: The treatment of hollow foot (pes cavus). Amer. J. Orthop. Surg., *11*:231, 1913.
40. Decoulx, P., Decoulx, R. J., and Duquennoy, A.: Le traitement du pied équin paralytique de l'adulte par l'operation de Lambrinudi associée à la transplantation du jambier posterieur. Acta Orthop. Belg., *34*:845, 1968.
41. Dennyson, W. G., and Fulford, G. E.: Subtalar arthrodesis by cancellous grafts and metallic internal fixation. J. Bone Joint Surg., *58-B*:507, 1976.
42. Der Azvazadurian, A., and Gambier, R.: Transplantations tendineuses dans le pied paralytique. Résultats de 92 observations. Rev. Chir. Orthop., *47*:228, 1961.
43. Descamps, L.: Transposition des peroniers en aviant. Rev. Chir. Orthop., *47*:227, 1961.
44. Dickson, F. D., and Diveley, R. L.: Operation for correction of mild claw foot, the result of infantile paralysis. J.A.M.A., *87*:1275, 1926.
45. Drew, A. J.: The late results of arthrodesis of the foot. J. Bone Joint Surg., *33-B*:496, 1951.
46. Ducroquet, R., Ducroquet, J., and Ducroquet, P.: Remarques sur le pied creux paralytique et le steppage. Rev. Chir. Orthop., *47*:219, 1961.
47. Duncan, J. W., and Lovell, W. W.: Hoke triple arthrodesis. J. Bone Joint Surg., *60-A*:795, 1978.
48. Dunn, N.: Stabilizing operations in the treatment of paralytic deformities of the foot. Proc. Roy. Soc. Med. (Section of Orthopaedics), *15*:15, 1922.
49. Dunn, N.: Suggestions based on ten years' experience of arthrodesis of the tarsus in the treatment of deformities of the foot. *In* Robert Jones Birthday Volume. London, Oxford University Press, 1928, p. 395.
50. Elmslie, R. L.: *In* Turner, G. G. (ed.): Modern Operative Surgery. 2nd Ed. London, Cassell & Co., Ltd., 1934.
51. Emmel, H. E., and LeCoco, J. F.: Hamstring transplant for the prevention of calcaneocavus foot in poliomyelitis. J. Bone Joint Surg., *40-A*:911, 1958.
52. Fitzgerald, F. P., and Seddon, H. J.: Lambrinudi's operation for drop-foot. Brit. J. Surg., *25*:283, 1937.
53. Flint, M. H., and MacKenzie, I. C.: Anterior laxity of the ankle. A cause of recurrent paralytic drop foot deformity. J. Bone Joint Surg., *44B*:377, 1962.
54. Francillon, M. R.: Transplantations tendineuses au niveau des extremities inférieures. Considerations physiologiques. Rev. Chir. Orthop., *47*:196, 1961.
55. Fried, A., and Hendel, C.: Paralytic valgus deformity of the ankle. Replacement of the paralyzed tibialis posterior by the peroneus longus. J. Bone Joint Surg., *39-A*:921, 1957.
56. Friedenberg, Z. B.: Arthrodesis of the tarsal bones. A study of failure of fusions. Arch. Surg. (Chicago), *57*:162, 1948.
57. Gallie, W. E.: Tendon fixation in infantile paralysis. A review of 150 operations. Amer. J. Orthop. Surg., *14*:18, 1916.
58. Gill, A. B.: An operation to make a posterior bone block at the ankle to limit foot-drop. J. Bone Joint Surg., *15*:166, 1933.
59. Girard, P. M.: Ankle joint stabilization with motion. J. Bone Joint Surg., *29*:802, 1935.
60. Goldner, J. L.: Paralytic equinovarus deformities of the foot. Southern Med. J., *42*:83, 1949.
61. Goldner, J. L., and Irwin, C. E.: Paralytic deformities of the foot. A.A.O.S. Instr. Course Lect., *5*:190, 1948.
62. Goldthwait, J. E.: Tendon transplantation in the treatment of deformities resulting from infantile paralysis. Boston Med. Surg. J., *133*:447, 1895.
63. Goldthwait, J. E.: An operation for the stiffening of the ankle joint in infantile paralysis. Amer. J. Orthop. Surg., *5*:271, 1908.
64. Green, W. T.: Tendon transplantation in rehabilitation. J.A.M.A., *163*:1235, 1957.
65. Green, W. T., and Grice, D. S.: The treatment of polio-

myelitis: Acute and convalescent stages. A.A.O.S. Instr. Course Lect., *13*:261, 1951.
66. Green, W. T., and Grice, D. S.: The management of chronic poliomyelitis. A.A.O.S. Instr. Course Lect., *9*:85, 1952.
67. Green, W. T., and Grice, D. S.: The surgical correction of the paralytic foot. A.A.O.S. Instr. Course Lect., *10*:343–363, 1953.
68. Green, W. T., and Grice, D. S.: The management of calcaneus deformity. A.A.O.S. Instr. Course Lect., *13*:135–149, 1956.
69. Grice, D. S.: An extra-articular arthrodesis of the subastragalar joint for correction of paralytic flat feet in children. J. Bone Joint Surg., *34-A*:927, 1952.
70. Grice, D. S.: Further experience with extra-articular arthrodesis of the subtalar joint. J. Bone Joint Surg., *36-A*:246, 1955.
71. Grice, D. S.: The role of subtalar fusion in the treatment of valgus deformities of the feet. A.A.O.S. Instr. Course Lect., *16*:127, 1959.
72. Guildal, P., and Sodeman, T.: Results of 256 tri-articular arthrodeses of the foot in sequelae of infantile paralysis. Acta Orthop. Scand., *1*:499, 1930–1931.
73. Gunn, D. R., and Molesworth, B. D.: The use of tibialis posterior as a dorsiflexor. J. Bone Joint Surg., *39-B*:674, 1957.
74. Hallgrimsson, S.: Studies on reconstructive and stabilizing operations on the skeleton of the foot, with special reference to subastragalar arthrodesis in treatment of foot deformities following infantile paralysis. Acta Chir. Scand., *88*:Suppl. 78:1, 1943.
75. Hamsa, W. R.: Panastragaloid arthrodesis. A study of end-results in eight-five cases. J. Bone Joint Surg., *18*:732, 1936.
76. Hart, V. L.: Arthrodesis of the foot in infantile paralysis. Surg. Gynec. Obstet., *64*:794, 1937.
77. Hart, V. L.: Lambrinudi operation for drop-foot. J. Bone Joint Surg., *22*:937, 1940.
78. Henderson, M. S.: Reconstructive surgery in paralytic deformities of the lower leg. J. Bone Joint Surg., *11*:810, 1929.
79. Herndon, C. H., Strong, J. M., and Heyman, C. H.: Transposition of the tibialis anterior in the treatment of paralytic talipes calcaneus. J. Bone Joint Surg., *38-A*:751, 1956.
80. Hoke, M.: An operation for stabilizing paralytic feet. Amer. J. Orthop. Surg., *3*:494, 1921.
81. Holmdahl, H. C.: Astragalectomy as a stabilizing operation for foot paralysis following poliomyelitis; results of a follow-up investigation of 153 cases. Acta Orthop. Scand., *25*:207, 1956.
82. Howorth, M. B.: Triple subtalar arthrodesis. Clin. Orthop., *99*:175, 1974.
83. Hunt, J. C., and Brooks, A. L.: Subtalar extra-articular arthrodesis for correction of paralytic valgus deformity of the foot. Evaluation of forty-four procedures with particular reference to associated tendon transference. J. Bone Joint Surg., *47-A*:1310, 1965.
84. Hunt, W. S., Jr., and Thompson, H. A.: Pantalar arthrodesis. A one-stage operation. J. Bone Joint Surg., *36-A*:349, 1954.
85. Inclan, A.: End results in physiological blocking of flail joints. J. Bone Joint Surg., *31-A*:748, 1949.
86. Ingersoll, R. E.: Transplantation of peroneus longus to anterior tibial insertion in poliomyelitis. Surg. Gynec. Obstet., *86*:717, 1948.
87. Ingram, A. J., and Hundley, J. M.: Posterior bone block of the ankle for paralytic equinus. An end-result study. J. Bone Joint Surg., *33-A*:679, 1951.
88. Jacobs, J.: Achilles tenodesis for paralytic calcaneocavus foot. Clin. Orthop., *47*:143, 1966.
89. Jones, B. S.: A method of posterior bone block for paralytic drop foot in children. S. Afr. Med. J., *44*:1139, 1970.
90. Judet, J., and Judet, R.: Greffe inter-astragalocalcanéenne. Rev. Chir. Orthop., *45*:350, 1959.
91. Judet, R., and Kliszowski, H.: Les transplantations tendineuses du long péronier latéral sur le jambier antérieur et du court péronier latéral sur le long dans les pieds équins poliomyélitiques. Presse Méd., *74*:7, 1966.
92. King, B. B.: Ankle fusion for the correction of paralytic drop foot and calcaneus deformity. Arch. Surg. (Chicago), *40*:90, 1940.
93. Kirk, A. A., Kunkle, H. M., and Waive, H. J.: Ledge tenodesis of the extensor hallucis longus. A substitution for the Jones operation. J. Bone Joint Surg., *53-A*:774, 1971.
94. Kramer, J., and Laturnus, H.: Arthrodesen am Fuss mit dem Cloward-Instrumentarium. Z. Orthop., *115*:112, 1977.
95. Kuhlmann, R. F., and Bell, J. F.: A clinical evaluation of tendon transplantations for poliomyelitis affecting the lower extremities. J. Bone Joint Surg., *34-A*:915, 1952.
96. Lahdenranta, U., and Pylkkanen, P.: Subtalar extraarticular fusion in the treatment of valgus and varus deformities in children. A review of 162 operations in 136 patients. Acta Orthop. Scand., *43*:438, 1972.
97. Lambrinudi, C.: New operation on drop-foot. Brit. J. Surg., *15*:193, 1927.
98. Lambrinudi, C.: A method of correcting equinus and calcaneus deformities at the sub-astragaloid joint. Proc. Roy. Soc. Med. (Section of Orthopaedics), *26*:788, 1933.
99. Lance, P.: Conclusions générales. Symposium sur le traitement du pied paralytique par les transplantations tendineuses. Rev. Chir. Orthop., *47*:239, 1961.
100. Lance, P., LeCoeur, P., and Anquex: Transplantations tendineuses pour pieds paralytiques. Considerations sur 470 cas. Rev. Chir. Orthop., *47*:235, 1961.
101. Lasserre, J.: Transplantations tendineuses dans les paralysies du triceps sural. Indications et résultats. Rev. Chir. Orthop., *47*:209, 1961.
102. Leavitt, D. G.: Subastragaloid arthrodesis for the os calcis type of flat foot. Amer. J. Surg., *59*:501, 1943.
103. LeCoeur, P.: Principes mécaniques des transplantations tendineuses. Rev. Chir. Orthop., *47*:184, 1961.
104. Legg, A. T., and Merrill, J. T.: Physical Therapy in Infantile Paralysis. Hagerstown, Md., W. F. Prior Co., Inc., 1932.
105. Leikkonen, O.: Astragalectomy as ankle-stabilizing operation in infantile paralysis sequelae. Acta Chir. Scand., Suppl. 152, 1950.
106. Liebolt, F. L.: Pantalar arthrodesis in poliomyelitis. Surgery, *6*:31, 1939.
107. Lipscomb, P. R.: Osteotomy of calcaneus, triple arthrodesis, and tendon transfer for severe paralytic calcaneocavus deformity. Report of a case. J. Bone Joint Surg., *51-A*:548, 1969.
108. Lipscomb, P. R., and Sanchez, J. J.: Anterior transplantation of the posterior tibial tendon for persistent palsy of the common peroneal nerve. J. Bone Joint Surg., *43-A*:60, 1961.
109. Lorthioir, J.: Huit cas d'arthrodèse du pied avec extirpation temporaire de l'astragale. J. Chir. Ann. Soc. Belge Chir., *11*:184, 1911.
110. Lovett, R. W.: The Treatment of Infantile Paralysis. Philadelphia, P. Blakiston's Son & Co., 1916.
111. MacAusland, W. R., and MacAusland, A. R.: Astragalectomy (the Whitman operation) in paralytic deformities of the foot. Ann. Surg., *80*:861, 1924.
112. McFarland, B.: Paralytic instability of the foot (editorial). J. Bone Joint Surg., *33-B*:493, 1951.
113. MacKenzie, I. G.: Lambrinudi's arthrodesis. J. Bone Joint Surg., *41-B*:738, 1959.
114. McKay, D. W.: A new technique for correction of dorsal bunion in children. Personal communication, 1976; Paper presented at Pediatric Orthopedic International Seminar, Chicago, Ill., 1975.
115. Makin, M.: Tibiofibular relationship in paralyzed limbs. J. Bone Joint Surg., *47-B*:500, 1965.
116. Makin, M., and Yossipovitch, Z.: Translocation of the peroneus longus in the treatment of paralytic pes calcaneus. A follow-up study of thirty-three cases. J. Bone Joint Surg., *48-A*:1541, 1966.
117. Malvarez, O.: Arthrodesis subastragalina extraarticular en el pie valgo pronado paralitico. Arthrodesis minima. Estudio de 87 casos. Rev. Ortop. Trauma., Lat. Amer., *2*:251, 1957.
118. Marek, F. M., and Schein, A. J.: Aseptic necrosis of the astragalus following arthrodesing procedures of the tarsus. J. Bone Joint Surg., *27*:587, 1945.
119. Masse, P., and Courtois, B.: Transplantations tendineuses au niveau du pied chez les enfants de moins de 5 ans. Rev. Chir. Orthop., *47*:223, 1961.
120. Mayer, L.: The physiological method of tendon transplantation. I. Historical; anatomy and physiology of tendons. Surg. Gynec. Obstet., *22*:182, 1916.
121. Mayer, L.: The physiological method of tendon transplantation. II. Operative technique. Surg. Gynec. Obstet., *22*:298, 1916.

122. Mayer, L.: The physiological method of tendon transplantation. III. Experimental and clinical experiences. Surg. Gynec. Obstet., 22:472, 1916.
123. Mayer, L.: The physiologic method of tendon transplants. Reviewed after forty years. A.A.O.S. Instr. Course Lect., 13:116, 1956.
124. Meary, M. R.: L'operation de Lambrinudi dans le traitement du pied équin paralytique. Rev. Chir. Orthop., 37:66, 1951.
125. Meary, R., Filipe, G., Aubriot, J.-H., and Tomeno, B.: Etude fonctionnelle de la double arthrodèse du pied. Rev. Chir. Orthop., 63:345, 1977.
126. Miller, O. L.: Surgical management of pes calcaneus. J. Bone Joint Surg., 18:169, 1936.
127. Mimran, R.: Transplantation du jambier postérieur sur le dos du pied. Rev. Chir. Orthop., 52:681, 1966.
128. Minguella-Sola, J.: Tratamiento del pie talus paralitico mediante transplantes tendinosos. Rev. Ortop. Trauma., 13:729, 1969.
129. Mortens, J., and Pilcher, M. F.: Tendon transplantation in the prevention of foot deformities after poliomyelitis in children. J. Bone Joint Surg., 38-B:633, 1956.
130. Mortens, J., Gregersey, P., and Zachariae, L.: Tendon transplantation in the foot after poliomyelitis in children. Acta Orthop. Scand., 27:153, 1957–1958.
131. Nicoladoni, C.: Nachtrag zum Pes calcaneus und zur Transplantation der Peronealsehnen. Arch. Klin. Chir., 27:660, 1881.
132. Nieny, K.: Zur Behandlung der Fussdeformitaten bei ausgedehnten Lahmungen. Arch. Orthop. Unfallchir., 3:60, 1905.
133. Ober, F. R.: Operative and postoperative treatment of infantile paralysis. New Eng. J. Med., 205:300, 1931.
134. Ober, F. R.: Tendon transplantation in the lower extremity. New Engl. J. Med., 209:52, 1933.
135. Paluska, D. J., and Blount, W. P.: Ankle valgus after the Grice subtalar stabilization: The late evaluation of a personal series with a modified technic. Clin. Orthop., 59:137, 1968.
136. Patterson, R. L., Parrish, F. F., and Hathaway, E. N.: Stabilizing operations on the foot. A study of the indications, techniques used, and end results. J. Bone Joint Surg., 32-A:1, 1950.
137. Pauker, E.: Correction of the outwardly rotated leg from poliomyelitis. J. Bone Joint Surg., 41-B:70, 1959.
138. Peabody, C. W.: Tendon transposition: An end-result study. J. Bone Joint Surg., 20:193, 1938.
139. Peabody, C. W.: Tendon transposition in the paralytic foot. A.A.O.S. Instr. Course Lect., 6:178, 1949.
140. Picard, J. J., and Mimran, R.: Operation de Grice et transplantation tendineuse dans le traitement des pieds valgus et talus valgus paralytiques. Rev. Chir. Orthop., 47:231, 1961.
141. Picard, J. J., and Mimran, R.: Operation de Grice. Rev. Chir. Orthop., 47:590, 1967.
142. Pollock, J. H., and Carrell, B.: Subtalar extra-articular arthrodesis in the treatment of paralytic valgus deformities. A review of 112 procedures in 100 patients. J. Bone Joint Surg., 46-A:533, 1964.
143. Putti, V.: Rapporti statici fra piede e ginocchio nell'arto paralitico. Chir. Organi. Mov., 6:125, 1922.
144. Pyka, R. A., Coventry, M. B., and Moe, J. H.: Anterior subluxation of the talus following triple arthrodesis. J. Bone Joint Surg., 46-A:16, 1964.
145. Reidy, J. A., Broderick, T. F., Jr., and Barr, J. S.: Tendon transplantations in the lower extremity. A review of end results in poliomyelitis. I. Tendon transplantations about the foot and ankle. J. Bone Joint Surg., 34-A:900, 1952.
146. Robles, E., and Blanco-Arguelles, M.: Transposicion aislada del peroneo lateral largo en las paralisis de triceps sural. Rev. Ortop. Trauma., 13:657, 1969.
147. Rugtveit, A.: Extra-articular arthrodesis, according to Green-Grice, in flat feet. Acta Orthop. Scand., 34:367, 1964.
148. Ryerson, E. W.: Arthrodesing operations on the feet. J. Bone Joint Surg., 5:453, 1923.
149. Scheer, G. E., and Crego, C. H., Jr.: A two-stage stabilization procedure for correction of calcaneocavus. J. Bone Joint Surg., 38-A:1247, 1956.
150. Schwartz, R. P.: Arthrodesis of subtalus and midtarsal joints of the foot; historical review, preoperative determinations, and operative procedure. Surgery, 20:619, 1946.
151. Seitz, D. G., and Carpenter, E. B.: Triple arthrodesis in children. A ten-year review. Southern Med. J., 67:1420, 1974.
152. Seymour, N., and Evans, D. K.: A modification of the Grice subtalar arthrodesis. J. Bone Joint Surg., 50-B:372, 1968.
153. Sharrard, W. J. W.: Muscle recovery in poliomyelitis. J. Bone Joint Surg., 37-B:63, 1955.
154. Shneider, D. A., and Smith, C. F.: Medial subtalar stabilization with posterior medial release in the treatment of varus feet: A preliminary report. Orthop. Clin. N. Amer., 7:949, 1976.
155. Sideman, S.: Surgery of poliomyelitis of the lower extremity. Surg. Clin. N. Amer., 45:175, 1965.
156. Siffert, R. S., Forster, R. I., and Nachamie, B.: "Beak" triple arthrodesis for correction of severe cavus deformity. Clin. Orthop., 45:101, 1966.
157. Smith, A. deF., and von Lackum, H. L.: Subastragaloid arthrodesis. Surg. Gynec. Obstet., 40:836, 1925.
158. Smith, J. B., and Westin, G.: Subtalar extra-articular arthrodesis. J. Bone Joint Surg., 50-A:1027, 1968.
159. Soren, A.: Complications post-opératoires et mauvais résultats dans les arthrodèses du pied. Rev. Chir. Orthop., 54:249, 1968.
160. Soule, R. E.: Further considerations of arthrodesis in the treatment of lateral deformity of the foot. Amer. J. Orthop. Surg., 12:422, 1915.
161. Stagnara, P., and Desbrosses, J.: Arthrodèse sousastragalienne et medio-tarsienne pour le traitement des pieds plats valgus paralytiques. Rev. Chir. Orthop., 47:232, 1961.
162. Staples, O. S.: Posterior arthrodesis of the ankle and subtalar joints. J. Bone Joint Surg., 38-A:50, 1956.
163. Steindler, A.: The treatment of the flail ankle; panastragaloid arthrodesis. J. Bone Joint Surg., 5:284, 1923.
164. Steindler, A.: Orthopedic Operations. Indications, Technique, and End Results. Springfield, Ill., Charles C Thomas, 1940, p. 129.
165. Straub, L. R., Harvey, J. P., Jr., and Fuerst, C. E.: A clinical evaluation of tendon transplantation in the paralytic foot. J. Bone Joint Surg., 39-A:1, 1957.
166. Takebe, K., and Hirohata, K.: EMG biofeedback in tendon transplantation for foot drop. Arch. Orthop. Trauma. Surg., 97:77, 1980.
167. Thompson, T. C.: Astragalectomy and the treatment of calcaneovalgus. J. Bone Joint Surg., 21:627, 1939.
168. Townsend, W. R.: Treatment of the paralytic clubfoot by arthrodesis. Amer. J. Orthop. Surg., 3:378, 1905.
169. Von Lesser, L.: Ueber operative Behandlung des Pes varus paralyticus. Zbl. Chir., 6:497, 1879.
170. Wagner, L. C.: Modified bone block (Campbell) of ankle for paralytic drop foot with report of twenty-seven cases. J. Bone Joint Surg., 13:142, 1931.
171. Wang, C. J.: An evaluation of ankle fusion in children. Clin. Orthop., 98:233, 1974.
172. Watkins, M. B., Jones, J. B., Ryder, C. T., Jr., and Brown, T. H., Jr.: Transplantation of the posterior tibial tendon. J. Bone Joint Surg., 36-A:11181, 1954.
173. Waugh, T. R., Wagner, J., and Stinchfield, F. E.: An evaluation of pantalar arthrodesis. A follow-up study of one hundred and sixteen operations. J. Bone Joint Surg., 47-A:1315, 1965.
174. Weissman, S. L., and Herold, H. Z.: Résultats eloignés du blocage de la sous-astragalienne dans le traitement du pied plat valgus paralytique. Rev. Chir. Orthop., 50:825, 1964.
175. Weissman, S. L., Torok, G., and Kharmosh, O.: L'arthrodèse extraarticulaire avec transplantation tendineuse concomitante dans le traitement du pied plat valgus paralytique du jeune enfant. Rev. Chir. Orthop., 43:79, 1957.
176. Westin, G. W.: Tendon transfers about the foot, ankle, and hip in the paralyzed lower extremity. J. Bone Joint Surg., 42-A:1430, 1965.
177. Whitman, A.: Astragalectomy and backward displacement of the foot. An investigation of its practical results. J. Bone Joint Surg., 4:266, 1922.
178. Whitman, R.: The operative treatment of paralytic talipes of the calcaneus type. Amer. J. Med. Sci., 122:593, 1901.
179. Willard, DeF. P.: Subastragalar arthrodesis in lateral deformities of paralytic feet. Amer. J. Orthop. Surg., 14:323, 1916.
180. Williams, P. F., and Menelaus, M. B.: Triple arthrodesis in inlay grafting—a method suitable for the undeformed or valgus foot. J. Bone Joint Surg., 59-B:333, 1977.

181. Wilson, F. C., Jr., Fay, G. F., Lamotte, P., and Williams, J. C.: Triple arthrodesis. A study of the factors affecting fusion after three hundred and one procedures. J. Bone Joint Surg., *47-A*:340, 1965.
182. Zachariae, L.: The Grice operation for paralytic flat feet in children. Acta Orthop. Scand., *33*:80, 1963.

PERONEAL MUSCULAR ATROPHY
(Charcot-Marie-Tooth Disease)

Peroneal muscular atrophy of Charcot-Marie-Tooth may be defined as a hereditary and familial degenerative disorder of the peripheral nerves, motor nerve roots, and the spinal cerebellar tracts. The process is slowly progressive; it begins in the feet and legs and spreads to the hands and forearms after a lapse of several years. It is characterized by atrophy of certain muscle groups, particularly the peroneals and the intrinsic musculature of the hands and feet.

The condition was described in 1886, almost simultaneously, by Charcot and Marie of France and Tooth of England,[10, 56] It was first considered to be a myopathy; Tooth, however, and later Hoffmann emphasized its neuritic features.[28, 56] The radicular pathologic changes were pointed out by England and Denny-Brown, who showed the pattern of sensory loss.[22] Stressing the hereditary aspects, Herringham, in 1888, reported a study of four generations of one family in which only males were affected.[27]

Incidence

The incidence of peroneal muscular atrophy is highly variable. In some geographic areas it is rare, only one or two cases being seen per year in large neurologic clinics, whereas in others it is one of the more common degenerative diseases of the peripheral nervous system. Boys are more frequently affected than girls. According to Jacobs and Carr, the Negro race appears to be exempt from Charcot-Marie-Tooth disease.[33]

Genetic Factors

The peripheral neuropathies have a variable pattern of heredity—as an autosomal dominant, an autosomal recessive, or a sex-linked recessive trait.[2, 13, 21, 23, 27, 40, 43, 50, 52] There usually is a family history of the disorder, but on occasion there may be none. The classification given by Dyck and Lambert is very useful.[17] Type I includes the hypertrophic neuropathy of Charcot-Marie-Tooth disease and the Roussy-Levy syndrome (hereditary areflexic dystaxia).[45, 46] Type I is inherited as an autosomal dominant trait, although sporadic cases do occur. Type II is the neuronal form of Charcot-Marie-Tooth disease; its inheritance is by autosomal dominant pattern. Histopathologically, Type II shows neuronal degeneration rather than the segmental demyelination and hypertrophic changes of Type I. It is characterized by the onset of distal lower limb weakness after the age of 25 to 30 years. Type III is the hypertrophic neuropathy of infancy; it is inherited as an autosomal recessive trait, as is Type IV (Refsum's disease). The symptoms of repeated attacks and remissions of distal motor and sensory loss in the hands and feet develop in childhood or at puberty. Type V is inherited as an autosomal dominant disease; its major problem is spastic paraplegia. Patients with Type VI have optic atrophy and present with the clinical picture of Type I, whereas those with Type VII have retinitis pigmentosa.

Pathology

The peripheral nerves and motor nerve roots show degenerative changes with loss of myelin and fragmentation of axis cylinders. In the spinal cord, there may be secondary loss of anterior horn cells and degeneration of posterior roots and posterior columns. There is disagreement as to whether other spinal tracts are involved. Occasionally there are degenerative changes in the lateral funiculi that cannot be considered secondary to primary nerve root or peripheral nerve degeneration. The muscle fibers show neural atrophy, with blastic proliferation and infiltration of fat cells.[25, 31]

Clinical Picture

The onset of symptoms is usually between 5 and 15 years, but may be deferred until the third decade. The presenting complaints may include difficulty in walking or in wearing shoes, muscle cramps, and paresthesia in the legs.

The muscular atrophy is symmetrical and distal in distribution. The peroneals and intrinsic muscles of the feet are affected first. As a result of muscular imbalance, pes

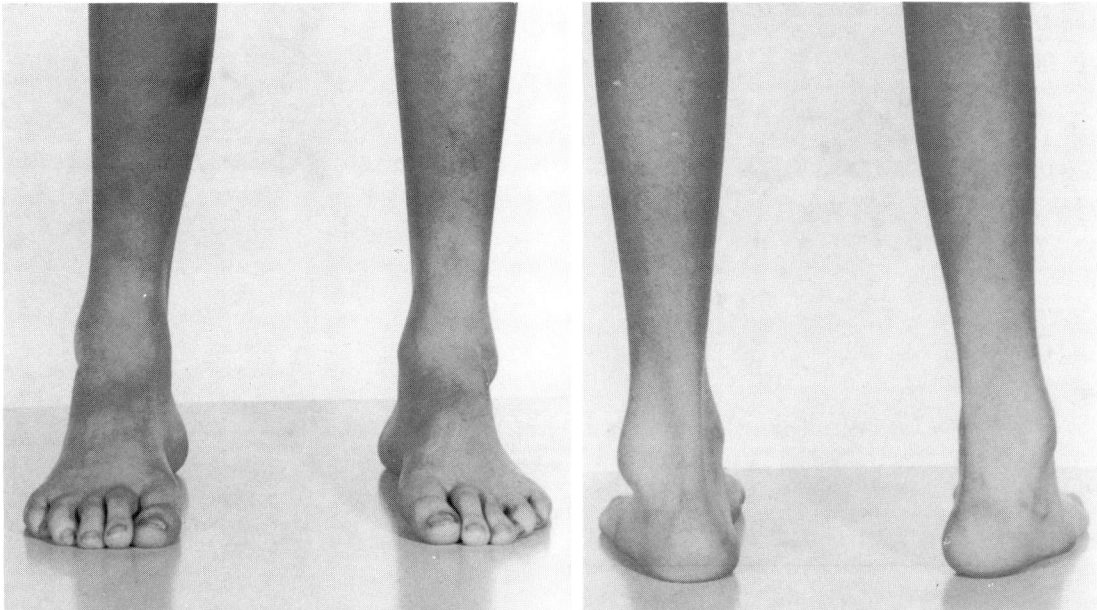

FIGURE 3–78. *Charcot-Marie-Tooth disease.*

Moderate varus and slight equinus deformity of both feet result from atrophy of peroneal, anterior tibial, and toe extensor muscles.

varus is the early deformity. Later, the atrophy spreads to the anterior compartment, involving the anterior tibial and the toe extensor muscles (Fig. 3–78). The patient walks with a toe-heel gait. Soon cavovarus deformity of the feet and claw toes develop (Fig. 3–79). With steady progression of the disease, the gastrocnemius and other calf muscles eventually atrophy.

The upper limbs are involved at a later stage. In most cases, at the time there is atrophy of the calves, the intrinsic muscles of the arms and thighs are usually not yet affected, and the face and trunk muscles are practically always spared. Therefore, in the moderately advanced case, the legs, feet, forearms, and hands are wasted and very slender, whereas the thighs and upper arms are normally developed. The contrast between the plump thighs and the slender legs with their claw toes gives the characteristic appearance of an inverted champagne bottle, which has been termed "ostrich legs."

The motor weakness is essentially a flaccid paralysis, often with fascicular twitchings in the wasting muscles. Contractural deformity, particularly equinus deformity of the ankle, may develop. The deep tendon reflexes are decreased or absent. The ankle jerk is the first to be involved, followed by the radial periosteal reflex when the upper limbs are affected. The patellar, biceps, and triceps reflexes are usually preserved.

Sensory examination may reveal diminution in vibration and position senses, and in some cases, definite areas of hypoesthesia. Ataxia is not present. Sphincter tone is normal. Intelligence is not affected. The condition progresses slowly, and life expectancy is normal. The patients are often ambulatory and, in many instances, remain remarkably free of serious disability until well past the fourth decade of life. Spinal deformity may develop.[26] Optic atrophy and visual disturbance may occur.[41, 48]

Diagnosis

Peroneal muscular atrophy, or Charcot-Marie-Tooth disease, is suggested by (1) weakness and atrophy that begin in the peroneal group of muscles and extend slowly to other muscles of the anterior tibial compartment, the intrinsic muscles of the foot, and later to the intrinsic muscles of the hand and muscles of the forearm, with relative sparing of the muscles of the thigh and upper arm; (2) the slow course of the disease; and (3) the positive family history.

The conduction velocity of the peripheral motor nerves is low in Charcot-Marie-Tooth disease.[9, 12, 20, 24, 25, 32, 42] Dyck, Lambert, and Mulder studied a total of 157 members of a family with peroneal muscular atrophy; 103 of these had neurologic examinations

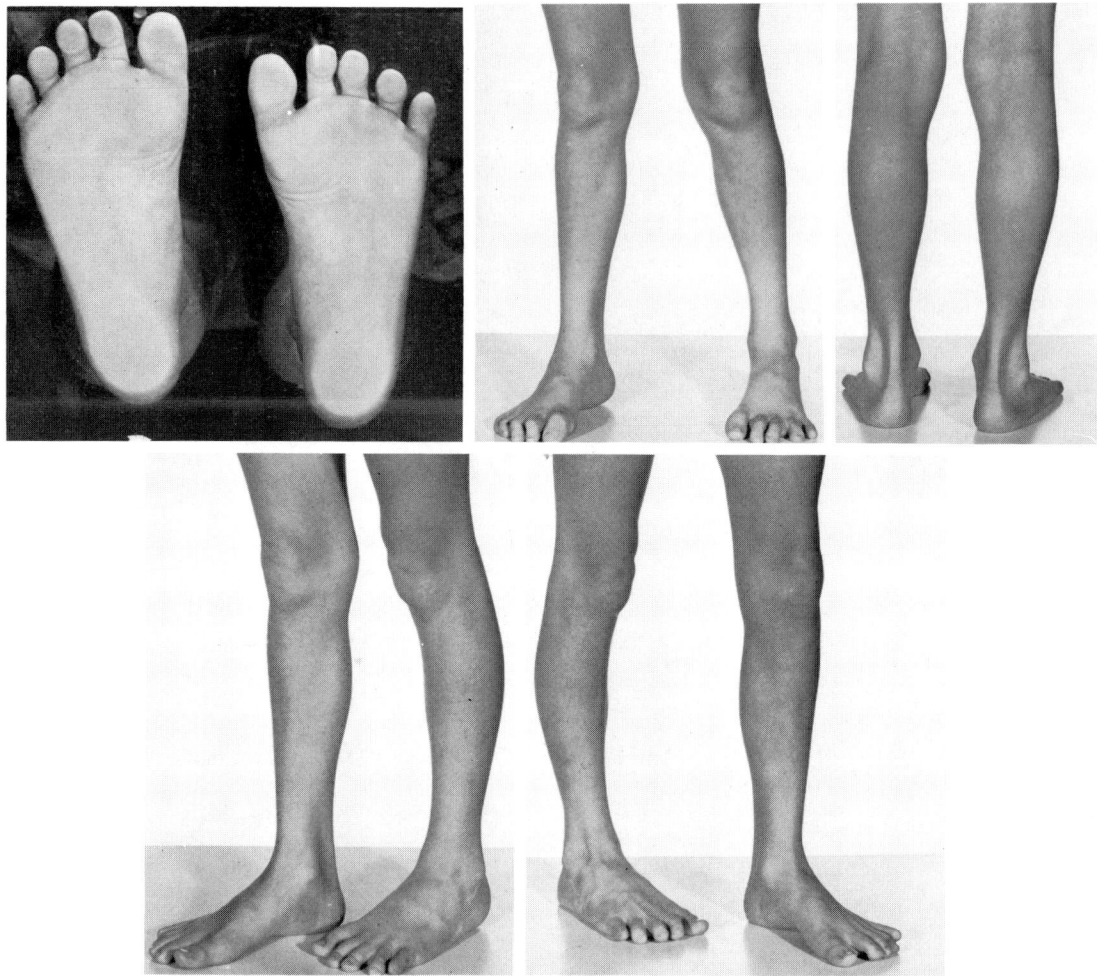

FIGURE 3–79. *Charcot-Marie-Tooth disease.*
There is moderate pes cavus. Note the beginning of development of claw toes.

and studies of nerve conduction. Each of the 16 persons who showed definite evidence of Charcot-Marie-Tooth disease on clinical examination also had low conduction velocity of the peripheral motor nerves. In addition, seven persons who showed no certain clinical evidence of the disease had low conduction velocity. Dyck and his coworkers concluded that determination of conduction velocity was a valuable method for identifying carriers of the disease trait, at least in this family.[18]

The cerebrospinal fluid findings are normal, although occasionally the protein content may be slightly elevated. The electromyogram will disclose reduction of electrical reactions.

In the differential diagnosis, one should consider distal muscular dystrophy, various forms of chronic polyneuritis, hypertrophic interstitial neuritis of Dejerine-Sottas, Roussy-Lévy syndrome, and Friedreich's ataxia.[4, 8, 44, 53, 57]

Roussy-Lévy syndrome, characterized by familial bilateral pes cavus and absence of deep tendon reflexes, is very similar to peroneal muscular atrophy.[36, 45, 46, 58] Symonds and Shaw expressed the view that it is a forme fruste of Charcot-Marie-Tooth disease.[55] Conduction velocity is low in both conditions. Static tremor of the hands is the distinguishing feature of Roussy-Lévy syndrome. Friedreich's ataxia is characterized by the presence of cerebellar signs, speech disturbance, nystagmus, and positive Babinski response.

Treatment

In the early stages, treatment consists of passive stretching exercises and splinting at night in an overcorrected position to prevent the development of fixed varus, equinovarus, or cavus deformities. Active exercises to maintain the strength of the weakened peroneals, toe extensors, and anterior tibial muscles are in order. Muscle testing at regular intervals is essential to record the progress of the disease.

In the advanced case, properly chosen surgical procedures can correct and prevent deformities. Often functional disability can be substantially diminished.[30, 33, 35, 37] The type of operation depends upon the muscle picture and the severity of foot deformity. When the peroneal muscles are of trace or zero strength, the anterior tibials are fair plus or good, and the posterior calf muscles are good or normal, the indicated procedure is anterior transfer of the posterior tibial tendon through the interosseous route to the base of the third metatarsal and lateral transfer of the anterior tibial tendon to the base of the second metatarsal. Triple arthrodesis is performed to stabilize the hindfoot and to correct the cavovarus deformity. Plantar fasciotomy is performed if the fascia is contracted. It is best to correct equinus deformity by wedging casts rather than by lengthening the tendo Achillis. If the motor strength of the anterior tibial is less than fair, the posterior tibial muscle only is transferred anteriorly through the interosseous route to the base of the third metatarsal.

References

1. Alajouanine, T., Castaigner, P., Cambier, J., and Escourolle, R.: Maladie de Charcot-Marie. Presse Méd., 75:2745, 1967.
2. Allan, W.: Relation of hereditary pattern to clinical severity as illustrated by peroneal atrophy. Arch. Intern. Med., 63:1123, 1939.
3. Amick, L. D., and Lemmi, H.: Electromyographic studies in peroneal muscular atrophy (Charcot-Marie-Tooth disease). Arch. Neurol. (Chicago), 9:273, 1963.
4. Bourguignon, G.: Association of Friedreich's disease and atrophy of Charcot-Marie type. Rev. Neurol. (Paris), 83:284, 1950.
5. Brihaye, M., Nenquin-Klaassen, E., and Berthdet, G.: Neurogenic muscular atrophy of Charcot-Marie-Tooth. Hoffman type combined with bilateral optic atrophy. Acta Neurol. Belg., 56:302, 1956.
6. Brodal, A., Böyesen, S., and Frövig, A. G.: Progressive neuropathic atrophy. (Charcot-Marie-Tooth). Arch. Neurol. Psychiat., 70:1, 1953.
7. Brody, L. A., and Wilkins, R. H.: Charcot-Marie-Tooth disease. Arch. Neurol. (Chicago), 17:552, 1967.
8. Bulgarelli, R., and Leva, R.: Are Friedreich, Charcot-Marie-Tooth and Dejerine-Sottas diseases distinct nosologic entities? Minerva Pediat., 6:497, 1954.
9. Caccia, M. R.: Study of the dispersion of motor nerve conduction in Charcot-Marie-Tooth-Hoffmann disease and in the Steinert syndrome. Electromyogr. Clin. Neurophysiol., 12:91, 1972.
10. Charcot, J. M., and Marie, P.: Sur une forme particulière d'atrophie musculaire progressive, souvent familiale, débutant par les pieds et les jambes et ateignant plus tard les mains. Rev. Méd. (Paris), 6:97, 1886.
11. Christiaens, L., Poingt, O., and Farriaux, J. P.: Charcot-Marie disease in a four-year old. Lille Méd., 8:513, 1963.
12. Christie, B. G.: Electrodiagnostic features of Charcot-Marie-Tooth disease. Proc. Roy. Soc. Med., 54:321, 1961.
13. Crank, H. H., and Reider, N.: Genetic features in the Charcot-Marie-Tooth type of muscular atrophy. Bull. Menninger Clin., 3:88, 1939.
14. Currie, R. A.: Case of the Charcot-Marie-Tooth type of muscular atrophy, with a note on the condition of the bones. Glasgow Med. J., 107:28, 1927.
15. Dawson, C. W., and Roberts, J. B.: Charcot-Marie-Tooth disease. J.A.M.A., 188:659, 1964.
16. Dejerine and Armand-Delille: Un cas d'atrophie musculaire, type Charcot-Marie, suivi d'autopsie. Rev. Neurol. (Paris), 11:1198, 1903.
17. Dyck, P. J., and Lambert, E. H.: Lower motor and primary sensory neuron disease with peroneal muscular atrophy. Part I. Neurologic, genetic and electrophysiologic findings in hereditary polyneuropathies. Part II. Neurologic, genetic, and electrophysiologic findings in various neuronal degenerations. Arch. Neurol. (Chicago), 18:603, 619, 1968.
18. Dyck, P. J., Lambert, E. H., and Mulder, D. W.: Charcot-Marie-Tooth disease. Nerve conduction and clinical studies of a large kinship. Neurology (Minneap.), 13:1, 1963.
19. Dyck, P. J., Winkelmann, R. K., and Bolton, C. F.: Quantitation of Meissner's corpuscles in hereditary neurologic disorders. Charcot-Marie-Tooth disease. Roussy-Lévy syndrome, Dejerine-Sottas disease, hereditary sensory neuropathy, spinocerebellar degeneration and hereditary spastic paraplegia. Neurology, 16:10, 1966.
20. Earl, W. C., and Johnson, E. W.: Motor nerve conduction velocity in Charcot-Marie-Tooth disease. Arch. Phys. Med., 44:247, 1963.
21. Eisenbud, A., and Grossman, M.: Peroneal form of progressive muscular atrophy. A clinical report of two families. Arch. Neurol. Psychiat., 18:766, 1927.
22. England, A. C., and Denny-Brown, D.: Severe sensory changes, and trophic disorder, in peroneal muscular atrophy (Charcot-Marie-Tooth type). Arch. Neurol. Psychiat., 67:1, 1952.
23. Erwin, W. G.: A pedigree of sex-linked recessive peroneal atrophy. J. Hered., 35:24, 1944.
24. Gilliatt, R. W., and Thomas, P. K.: Extreme slowing of nerve conduction in peroneal muscular atrophy. Ann. Phys. Med., 4:104, 1957.
25. Haase, G. R., and Shy, G. M.: Pathological changes in muscle biopsies from patients with peroneal muscular atrophy. Brain, 83:631, 1960.
26. Hensinger, R. N., and MacEwen, G. D.: Spinal deformity associated with heritable neurological conditions. Spinal muscular atrophy, Friedreich's ataxia, familial dysautonomia, and Charcot-Marie-Tooth diseases. J. Bone Joint Surg., 58-A:13, 1976.
27. Herringham, W. P.: Muscular atrophy of the peroneal type affecting many members of a family. Brain, 11:230, 1889.
28. Hoffmann, J.: Ueber progressive neurotische Muskelatrophie. Arch. Psychiat. (Berlin), 10:660, 1889.
29. Hoyt, W. F.: Charcot-Marie-Tooth disease with primary optic atrophy. Arch. Ophthal. (Chicago), 64:925, 1960.
30. Hsu, J. D., and Hoffer, M. M.: Posterior tibial tendon transfer anteriorly through the interosseous membrane: A

modification of the technique. Clin. Orthop., *131*:202, 1978.
31. Hughes, J. T., and Brownell, B.: Pathology of peroneal muscular atrophy (Charcot-Marie-Tooth disease). J. Neurol. Neurosurg. Psychiat., *35*:648, 1972.
32. Humberstone, P. M.: Nerve conduction studies in Charcot-Marie-Tooth disease. Acta Neurol. Scand., *48*:176, 1972.
33. Jacobs, J. E., and Carr, C. R.: Progressive muscular atrophy of the peroneal type (Charcot-Marie-Tooth disease). Orthopedic management and end-result study. J. Bone Joint Surg., *32-A*:27, 1950.
34. Jammes, J. L.: The autonomic nervous system in peroneal muscular atrophy. Arch. Neurol. (Chicago), *27*:213, 1972.
35. Karlholm, S., and Nilsonne, U.: Operative treatment of the foot deformity in Charcot-Marie-Tooth disease. Acta Orthop. Scand., *39*:101, 1968.
36. LaPresle, J.: Contribution à l'étude de la dystasie aréflexique héréditaire. Etat actuel de quatre des sept cas princeps de Roussy et Mlle. Lévy, trente ans après la première publication de ces auteurs. Sem. Hôp. Paris, *32*:2473, 1956.
37. Levitt, R. L., Canale, S. T., Cooke, A. T., and Gartland, J. J.: The role of foot surgery in progressive neuromuscular disorders in children. J. Bone Joint Surg., *55-A*:1396, 1973.
38. Lidge, R. T., and Chandler, F. A.: Charcot-Marie-Tooth disease. J. Pediatr., *43*:152, 1953.
39. Littler, W. A.: Heart block and peroneal muscular atrophy. A family study. Quart. J. Med., *39*:431, 1970.
40. MacKlin, M. T., and Bowman, J. T.: Inheritance of peroneal atrophy. J.A.M.A., *86*:613, 1926.
41. Milhorat, A. T.: Progressive muscular atrophy of peroneal type associated with atrophy of the optic nerves. Arch. Neurol. Psychiat., *50*:279, 1943.
42. Nielsen, V. K., and Pilgaard, S.: On the pathogenesis of Charcot-Marie-Tooth disease. A study of the sensory and motor conduction velocity in the median nerve. Acta Orthop. Scand., *43*:4, 1972.
43. Popovian, M. D., Dubinskaia, E. E., and Ageeva, T. S.: Polymorphism of Charcot-Marie-Tooth neural amyotrophy in uniovular twins. Zh. Nevropat. Psikhiat., *77*:1466, 1977.
44. Ross, A. T.: Combination of Friedreich's ataxia and Charcot-Marie-Tooth atrophy in each of two brothers. J. Nerv. Ment. Dis., *95*:680, 1942.
45. Roussy, G., and Lévy, G.: Sept cas d'une maladie familiale particulière: Troubles de la march, pieds bots et aréfléxie tendineuse généralisée, avec accessoirement, légère maladresse des mains. Rev. Neurol. (Paris), *45*:427, 1926.
46. Roussy, G., and Lévy, G.: A propos de la dystasie aréfléxique héréditaire. Rev. Neurol. (Paris), *62*:763, 1934.
47. Sachs, B.: The peroneal form or the leg-type of progressive muscular atrophy. Brain, *12*:447, 1890.
48. Schneider, D. E., and Bels, M. M.: Charcot-Marie-Tooth disease with primary optic atrophy. Report of two cases occurring in brothers. J. Nerv. Ment. Dis., *85*:541, 1937.
49. Schwartz, A. R.: Charcot-Marie-Tooth disease. A 45-year follow-up. Arch. Neurol. (Chicago), *9*:623, 1963.
50. Schwartz, L. A.: Clinical, histopathological and inheritance factors in peroneal muscular atrophy (Charcot-Marie-Tooth type.). J. Mich. Med. Soc., *43*:219, 1944.
51. Siegel, I. M.: Charcot-Marie-Tooth disease. A diagnostic problem. J.A.M.A., *228*:873, 1974.
52. Skre, H.: Genetic and clinical aspects of Charcot-Marie-Tooth's disease. Clin. Genet., *6*:98, 1974.
53. Spillane, J. D.: Familial pes cavus and absent tendon jerks. Its relationship with Friedreich's disease and peroneal muscular atrophy. Brain, *63*:275, 1940.
54. Stranak, V.: Charcot-Marie-Tooth-Hoffman syndrome. Beitr. Orthop. Trauma., *15*:564, 1968.
55. Symonds, C. P., and Shaw, M. E.: Familial claw-foot with absent tendon-jerks. A "forme fruste" of the Charcot-Marie-Tooth disease. Brain, *49*:387, 1926.
56. Tooth, H. H.: The Peroneal Type of Progressive Muscular Atrophy. London, H. K. Lewis, 1886.
57. Van Bogaert, L., and Moreau, M.: Combinaison de l'amyotrophie de Charcot-Marie-Tooth et de la maladie de Friedreich, chez plusieurs membres d'une même famille. Encephale, *34*:312, 1939–1941.
58. Yudell, A., Dyck, P. J., and Lambert, E. H.: A kinship with the Roussy-Lévy syndrome. Arch. Neurol. (Chicago), *13*:432, 1965.
59. Zellweger, H., Schochet, S. S., Jr., Pavone, L., and Bodensteiner, J.: Charcot-Marie-Tooth disease with early onset. Presentation of a family. Pediatria (Napoli), *79*:198, 1971.

FRIEDREICH'S ATAXIA
(Hereditary Spinocerebellar Ataxia)

In Friedreich's ataxia, the most common of the hereditary cerebellar ataxias, both the cerebellar and spinal cord pathways are involved.[1-31] In the spinal cord there are degenerative changes in the dorsal and ventral spinocerebellar tracts, the corticospinal tracts, and the posterior column. The anterior horn cells are usually normal. In the cerebellum there is atrophy of the Purkinje cells and the dentate nuclei. Changes may occur in the brain stem. Degeneration of the corticospinal tract may occasionally extend above the level of the medulla to involve the cerebral cortex.[15, 16]

The etiology of the disease is unknown. Males and females are affected equally. It is definitely hereditary and is usually transmitted by an autosomal recessive gene. Often it can be traced through a number of generations. Some members of a family may have it only in the mild and incomplete form.[1, 6]

Clinical Features

The onset of symptoms usually occurs in childhood between the ages of seven and ten years, but often is so insidious that it is difficult to determine when the condition was first present.

An unsteady gait is almost always the first symptom to attract attention. The child has a tendency to stagger and fall, has difficulty in making sudden turns, and is unable to keep pace with his playmates in motor activities. Over a period of years, these symptoms progress, and ataxia of the upper limbs develops. Parents notice that the child cannot handle a fork or spoon without spilling the food. He has difficulty in learning to write.[4]

On examination certain characteristic musculoskeletal deformities are observed. A slowly progressive scoliosis, usually in the thoracic region, is most common and is present in approximately 80 to 90 per cent of cases. The feet, as a rule, show symmetrical cavus deformity with marked elevation of the longitudinal arch, equinus deformity of the forefoot, and claw toes. The plantar fascia is contracted in about half the cases. Varus deformity is present with the pes cavus and increases the disability. In the early phases the cavus deformity is flexible and can be passively corrected by elevation of the metatarsal heads. Later, however, the deformity increases with skeletal growth and becomes fixed.

Muscle imbalance is an important factor in the pathogenesis of pes cavus. On muscle examination of 43 patients with Friedreich's ataxia, Makin found definite muscle weakness in 27 cases. Ten patients had normal musculature, and for six the muscle picture was unrecorded. Peroneal muscle weakness was the most common finding, either in isolated form or in combination with paresis of the anterior tibial.[19] According to Duchenne, clawfoot results from weakness of the intrinsic musculature of the foot whose action is to flex the metatarsophalangeal joint. The overactive long toe extensors, which are taut like a bowstring, hold the toes in hammer toe position. It is a combination of intrinsic and extrinsic muscle imbalance that causes pes cavus.[11, 26]

The gait is unsteady and has a wide base. Heel-to-toe walking is usually impossible. The patient sways and reels and places the feet irregularly. Stance is unsteady, and Romberg's sign may be present. The ataxia is both spinal and cerebellar in type. There is always a greater degree of ataxia in the legs than in the upper limbs. Heel-to-shin ataxia and later finger-to-nose ataxia may be demonstrated. Alternating movements of the hands are slow.

Speech is often explosive, slurred, and staccato. Head tremor may be seen. Cranial nerves are normal; eventually, however, a horizontal or rotatory nystagmus develops.

The deep tendon reflexes — the knee and ankle jerks — in the lower limbs are usually absent very early in the course of the disease. Subsequently, the biceps and triceps jerks in the arms disappear. The plantar response will in time become extensor, but this sign may be delayed for a few years.

Position and vibration sense and two-point discrimination are lost, initially in the feet, and later in the hands. Touch, pain, and temperature modalities of sensation are preserved.[9]

Later in the course of the disease, tachycardia and evidence of cardiac failure develop.[10, 13, 14, 20, 30]

Diagnosis

The diagnosis is suggested when a child has pes cavus, scoliosis, signs of involvement of tracts in the posterior half of the spinal cord, and a positive family history of similar disorders.

Cardiac manifestations will further substantiate the diagnosis of Friedreich's ataxia. In the electrocardiogram, conduction defects with bundle branch block or complete heart block resulting from myocardial fibrosis may be seen, and there may be changes consistent with acute or chronic occlusive coronary artery disease.

Roentgenograms of the spine will reveal the structural scoliosis. The cerebrospinal fluid findings are within normal limits.

Roussy-Lévy syndrome consists of familial pes cavus and absence of deep tendon reflexes, and it may be considered an abortive form of Friedreich's ataxia.[25] The differential diagnosis of chronic progressive ataxia is presented in Table 3–6.

Prognosis

The course of classic Friedreich's ataxia is steadily progressive to complete disability. An early onset is a poor prognostic sign. The history of the course of the disease in other members of the family will aid the physician in estimating the rate of progression.

Death usually results from myocardial failure due to interstitial myocarditis or from respiratory infection. The average duration of the disease from its onset until death is 16 years. Abortive cases are not uncommon; the disease may become arrested at almost any stage or may have such a slow course of progression that the patient will have a normal life span.

Treatment

There is no specific treatment for the fundamental disease process. Prevention and adequate correction of the foot deformity will help to prolong the period of ambulation and delay the day the patient will

Table 3-6. *Differential Diagnosis of Chronic Progressive Ataxia**

Clinical Disorder	Preceding History	Usual Year of Onset in Children	Examination	Usual Laboratory Examination	Usual Prognosis
Arnold-Chiari malformation	Headache, dysphagia		Palatal and tongue weakness, pyramidal signs, ataxia	May have hydrocephalus, spina bifida	Slowly progressive; stationary after surgery
Hereditary spinocerebellar ataxia	Stumbling, dizziness, familial incidence	7–10	Ataxia, loss of position sense, extensor plantar responses, kyphoscoliosis, pes cavus	Occasional associated EKG changes	Progressive with death usually by 30 years of age
Bassen-Kornzweig syndrome	Fatty diarrhea at 6 weeks to 2 years of age	2–17	Cerebellar ataxia, posterior column signs, retinitis pigmentosa, scoliosis, pes cavus	Acanthocytosis, lack of beta-lipoprotein in serum	Slowly progressive
Dentate cerebellar ataxia	Myoclonus, convulsions	7–17	Ataxia with severe intention tremor		Slowly progressive
Hereditary cerebellar ataxia	Familial incidence	3–17	Ataxia, optic atrophy, occasionally associated posterior column and pyramidal tract signs	Pneumoencephalogram: small cerebellar folia	Slowly progressive
Ataxia telangiectasia	Recurrent sinopulmonary infections in 2/3 of cases; familial incidence	1–3	Oculocutaneous telangiectasia at 4 to 6 years; ataxia, choreoathetosis, dysarthria	Chest X-ray may reveal bronchiectasis	Death before 25 years of age
Cerebellar tumors	Headache, vomiting		Papilledema, ataxia, nystagmus	Skull X-rays: separation of sutures	Progressive until operation
Multiple sclerosis	Preceding neurologic symptoms	14–17	Optic neuritis; brain stem, cerebellar, pyramidal or sensory signs	Spinal fluid may reveal increased cells, protein or gamma globulin	Exacerbations and remissions
Spinal cord tumor	May have numbness or bladder disorder		Ataxia with weakness or sensory loss	Defect on myelography	Progressive until operation

*From Farmer, T. W.: Pediatric Neurology. New York, Hoeber Medical Division, Harper & Row, 1964, p. 525. Reprinted by permission.

eventually become bedridden. Pes cavus is the most frequent deformity; its management is discussed in Chapter 4. Tendon transfers are occasionally performed on the hand to improve function.

Makin, in a review of the end results of operative procedures on 34 patients with Friedreich's ataxia with an average follow-up of 7.2 years, emphasized that structural foot deformities and instability often contribute to abnormalities of gait and stance, and that the correction of these deformities has a markedly beneficial effect on the ataxia.[19]

References

1. Andermann, E., Remillard, G. M., Goyer, C., Blitzer, L., Andermann, F., and Barbeau, A.: Genetic and family studies in Friedreich's ataxia. Can. J. Neurol. Sci., 3:287, 1976.
2. Andermann, F.: Nicolaus Friedreich and degenerative atrophy of posterior columns of the spinal cord. Can. J. Neurol. Sci., 3:275, 1976.
3. Barbeau, A.: Design of investigation. Can. J. Neurol. Sci., 3:271, 1976.
4. Barbeau, A.: Friedreich's ataxia 1976 — an overview. Can. J. Neurol. Sci., 3:389, 1976.
5. Barbeau, A., Breton, G., Lemieux, B., and Butterworth, R. F.: Bilirubin metabolism — preliminary investigation. Can. J. Neurol. Sci., 3:365, 1976.
6. Barbeau, A., Le Siege, M., Breton, R., Coallier, R., and Bouchard, J. P.: Friedreich's ataxia: Preliminary results of some genealogical research. Can. J. Neurol. Sci., 3:303, 1976.
7. Barbeau, A., Butterworth, R. F., Ngo, T., Breton, G., Helancon, S., Shapcott, D., Geoffroy, G., and Lemieux, B.: Pyruvate metabolism in Friedreich's ataxia. Can. J. Neurol. Sci., 3:379, 1976.
8. Boyer, S. H., Chisholm, A. W., and McKusick, V. A.: Cardiac aspects of Friedreich's ataxia. Circulation, 25:493, 1962.
8a. Buffoni, L., and Reboa, E.: Contributo allo studio ed all'inquadramento nosologico delle lesioni extraneurologiche del morbo de Friedreich. Minerva Pediat., 21:1540, 1969.
8b. Bureau, M. A., Ngassam, P., Lemieux, B., and Trias, A.: Pulmonary function studies in Friedreich's ataxia. Quebec cooperative study of Friedreich's ataxia. Can. J. Neurol Sci., 3:343, 1976.
8c. Cadotte, M., Barbeau, A., and Breton, G.: Friedreich's ataxia: observations with Q and G banding of human chromosomes. Quebec cooperative study of Friedreich's ataxia. Can. J. Neurol. Sci., 3:307, 1976.
9. Butterworth, R. F., Shapcott, D., Melançon, S., Breton, G., Geoffroy, G., Lemieux, B., and Barbeau, A.: Clinical laboratory findings in Friedreich's ataxia. Can. J. Neurol. Sci., 3:355, 1976.
9a. Cote, M., Elias, G., Soli, A., Geoffroy, G., Lemieux, B., and Barbeau, A.: Hemodynamic findings in Friedreich's ataxia. Quebec cooperative study of Friedreich's ataxia. Can. J. Neurol. Sci., 3:333, 1976.
10. Cote, M., Davignon, A., Pecko-Drouin, K., Solignac, A., Geoffroy, G., Lemieux, B., and Barbeau, A.: Cardiological signs and symptoms in Friedreich's ataxia. Can. J. Neurol. Sci., 3:319, 1976.
10a. Curtis, P. H.: Neurologic diseases of the foot. In Giannestras, N. J.: Foot Disorders. Medical and Surgical Management. Philadelphia, Lea & Febiger, 1967, pp. 361–378.
11. Duchenne, G. B.: Physiologie des Movements. Paris, J. B. Ballière & Fils. 1867.
12. Friedreich, N.: Über degenerative Atrophie der spinalen Hinterstränge. Virchow. Arch. Path. Anat., 26:391, and 27:1, 1863.
12a. Gattiker, H. F., Davignon, A., Bozio, A., Batlle-Diaz, J., Geoffroy, G., Lemieux, B., and Barbeau, A.: Echocardiographic findings in Friedreich's ataxia. Quebec cooperative study of Friedreich's ataxia. Can. J. Neurol. Sci., 3:329, 1976.
12b. Geoffroy, G., Barbeau, A., Breton, G., Lemieux, B., Aube, M., Leger, C., and Bouchard, J. P.: Clinical

description and roentgenologic evaluation of patients with Friedreich's ataxia. Quebec cooperative study of Friedreich's ataxia. Can. J. Neurol. Sci., 3:279, 1976.
13. Guerin, R., Elias, G., Davignon, A., Cote, M., Geoffroy, G., Lemieux, B., and Barbeau, A.: Cardiac angiographic findings in Friedreich's ataxia. Can. J. Neurol. Sci., 3:337, 1976.
14. Hartman, J. M., and Booth, R. W.: Friedreich's ataxia. A neurocardiac disease. Amer. Heart J., 60:716, 1960.
15. Heck, A. F.: A study of neural and extraneural findings in a large family with Friedreich's ataxia. J. Neurol. Sci., 1:226, 1964.
16. Hewer, R. L.: Study of fatal cases of Friedreich's ataxia. Brit. Med. J., 3:649, 1968.
17. LaPresle, J.: Contribution à l'étude de la dystasie aréfléxique héréditaire. Etat actuel de quatre des sept cas princeps de Roussy et Mlle. Lévy, trente ans après la première publication de ces auteurs. Sem. Hôp. Paris, 32:2473, 1956.
18. Levitt, R. L., Canale, S. T., Cooke, A. J., and Gartland, J. J.: The role of foot surgery in progressive neuromuscular disorders in children. J. Bone Joint Surg., 55-A:1396, 1973.
19. Makin, M.: The surgical treatment of Friedreich's ataxia. J. Bone Joint Surg., 35-A:425, 1953.
20. Malo, S., Latour, Y., Cote, M., Geoffroy, G., Lemieux, B., and Barbeau, A.: Electrocardiographic and vectocardiographic findings in Friedreich's ataxia. Can. J. Neurol. Sci., 3:323, 1976.
21. Podolsky, S., Pothier, A., Jr., and Krall, L. P.: Association of diabetes mellitus and Friedreich's ataxia. A study of two siblings. Arch. Intern. Med. (Chicago), 114:533, 1966.
22. Robinson, N.: An enzyme study of the myocardium in Friedreich's ataxia. Neurology (Minneap.), 16:1135, 1966.
23. Rombold, C. R., and Riley, H. A.: The abortive type of Friedreich's disease. Arch. Neurol. Psychiat., 16:301, 1926.
24. Roth, M.: On a possible relationship between hereditary ataxia and peroneal muscular atrophy. With a critical review of the problems of "intermediate forms" in the degenerative disorders of the central nervous system. Brain, 71:416, 1948.
25. Roussy, G., and Lévy, G.: Sept cas d'une maladie familiale particulaire: Troubles de la marche, pieds bots et aréfléxie tendineuse generalisée, avec accessoirement, légère maladresse des mains. Rev. Neurol. (Paris), 45:427, 1926.
26. Saunders, J. T.: Etiology and treatment of clawfoot. Arch. Surg. (Chicago), 30:179, 1935.
27. Spillane, J. D.: Familial pes cavus and absent tendon jerks. Its relationship with Friedreich's disease and peroneal muscular atrophy. Brain, 63:275, 1940.
28. Sylvester, P. E.: Some unusual findings in a family with Friedreich's ataxia. Arch. Dis. Child., 33:217, 1958.
29. Symonds, C. P., and Shaw, M. E.: Familial claw-foot with absent tendon jerks. Brain, 49:387, 1926.
30. Thilenius, O. G., and Grossman, B. J.: Friedreich's ataxia with heart disease in children. Pediatrics, 27:246, 1961.
31. Yudell, A., Dyck, P. J., and Lambert, E. H.: A kinship with Roussy-Lévy syndrome. Arch. Neurol. (Chicago), 13:432, 1965.

HYPERTROPHIC INTERSTITIAL NEURITIS

Dejerine and Sottas, in 1893, described a chronic familial polyneuropathy of childhood and adolescence.[9] This condition had been previously described by Gombault and Mallet, in 1889, as a pathologic variant of tabes dorsalis.[11] The original cases described by Dejerine and Sottas were in siblings with presumably unaffected parents. Later reports, however, traced the disorders through three to five generations.[1, 4, 8, 16] The disease is believed to be inherited as a dominant trait.

The etiology of the condition is unknown. Disturbance of pyruvate metabolism was proposed by Joiner and associates; subsequent studies, however, have failed to show evidence of any thiamine deficiency. Allergic factors may play a role in the pathogenesis.[6, 13]

Pathology

Peripheral nerves are enlarged as a result of the proliferation of perineurial and endoneurial connective tissue. The axis cylinders gradually decrease in size and eventually disappear. On cross section of nerve fibers, concentrically laminated structures are found about the nerve fibers—the so-called onion bulb formation. This characteristic finding is caused by proliferation of the Schwann cells. Muscles show atrophy of neural origin.

Clinical Features

Difficulty in locomotion is the usual presenting complaint. Walking is delayed. The child is unsteady, falls frequently, and has difficulty in going up and down stairs. He is unable to run and "keep up" with his playmates. His feet are weak and floppy. The abnormality of gait is similar to that of steppage gait. Subjective sensory disturbances such as paresthesias and lightning-type pains of the limbs may occur. Pes cavus and muscle weakness in the lower limbs, which is distal in distribution, develop early, antedating the more florid findings by several years. Paralysis of the intrinsic muscles of the hand appears later. Flexion contracture of the fingers and wrist is usually present toward the end of the first decade. Scoliosis develops during the rapid growth of the spine in early adolescence.

The deep tendon reflexes are diminished or absent. Superficial skin reflexes such as abdominal and cremasteric reflexes are lost later. Sensory loss involves all modalities of sensation. Anesthesia to light touch and pinprick is of the "stocking-glove" type. Proprioceptive sensory disturbance is shown by the loss of sensation of position and vibration and by the presence of a positive Romberg sign. Abnormalities of the pupil, such as the Argyll Robertson phenomenon, result from involvement of the cranial nerves. Nystagmus and slurred speech occur in some cases. Incoordination and motor deficit result from the combination of muscle weakness and sensory deficit.

Enlargement of the peripheral nerves is a late manifestation; it first develops in the proximal segments of the nerves.

Laboratory Findings

The total protein level in the cerebrospinal fluid is elevated abnormally. On manometric tests there is no block to cerebrospinal fluid circulation. Total and differential cell counts are within normal range.

Serum aldolase and creatine phosphokinase levels are not increased. The serologic test for syphilis should be performed to rule out luetic infection of the central nervous system.

Roentgenograms of the entire spine should be obtained to rule out the possibility of an intraspinal tumor. Myelography may demonstrate spinal nerve root enlargement; it should not, however, be performed routinely.

Pyruvate metabolism may be studied by determination of concentration of pyruvate in whole blood before and at intervals after the administration of glucose by mouth. Excessive accumulation of pyruvate in the blood, occurring as a response to a glucose load, is an indication that effective levels of thiamine are lacking in the body. In interstitial hypertrophic neuritis, there is no evidence of thiamine deficiency and the hydrochloric acid concentration of gastric contents is normal. Levels of blood glucose are determined to rule out diabetes. Lead or arsenic poisoning should also be ruled out.

Electromyography may disclose evidence of muscle atrophy of neural origin with reduced interference pattern, the presence of fibrillation potentials, and action potentials that are prolonged with normal or polyphasic potentials. Nerve conduction studies should be performed; evoked sensory and mixed nerve potentials will be absent or diminished in amplitude, or conduction time will be prolonged.

Muscle and nerve biopsies should be performed to confirm the diagnosis by histologic examination of the tissues.

Prognosis and Treatment

The course of the disease is one of slow progression with remissions and exacerbations. In mild cases, the diseases may reach a plateau and life expectancy may be normal.

There is no specific treatment. Adrenal steroids are reported to improve the condition and may be tried in severe cases or during acute exacerbations.[3] Orthopedic management consists of passive stretching exercises and use of night splints to prevent development of contractural deformity. In advanced cases, orthotic support of the lower limbs and spine may be indicated. Pes cavus may require surgical correction. Tendon transfers are performed to balance muscle forces acting on the foot and ankle.

References

1. Andermann, F., Lloyd-Smith, D. I., Mavor, H., and Mathieson, G.: Observations on hypertrophic neuropathy of Dejerine and Sottas. Neurology (Minneap.), *12*:712, 1962.
2. Anderson, R. M., Dennett, X., Hopkins, I. J., and Shield, L. K.: Hypertrophic interstitial polyneuropathy in infancy. Clinical and pathologic features in two cases. J. Pediat., *82*:619, 1973.
3. Austin, J. H.: Observations on the syndrome of hypertrophic neuritis (the hypertrophic interstitial radiculoneuropathies.) Medicine (Balt.), *35*:187, 1956.
4. Bedford, P. D., and James, F. E.: A family with progressive hypertrophic polyneuritis of Dejerine and Sottas. J. Neurol. Neurosurg. Psychiat., *19*:46, 1956.
5. Bradley, W. G.: Disorders of Peripheral Nerves. Oxford, Blackwell Scientific Publications, 1974.
6. Byers, R. K., and Taft, L. T.: Chronic multiple peripheral neuropathy in childhood. Pediatrics, *20*:517, 1957.
7. Cooper, E. L.: Progressive familial hypertrophic neuritis (Dejerine-Sottas). Brit. Med. J., *1*:793, 1936.
8. Craft, P. B., and Wadia, N. H.: Familial hypertrophic polyneuritis. Review of a previously reported family. Neurology (Minneap.), *7*:356, 1957.
9. Dejerine, J., and Sottas, J.: Sur la névrite interstitielle, hypertrophique et progressive de l'enfance. C. R. Soc. Bio. (Paris), *5*:63, 1893.
10. Dyck, P. J., and Lambert, E. H.: Lower motor and primary sensory neuron diseases with peroneal muscular atrophy. Part I. Neurologic, genetic and electrophysiologic findings in hereditary polyneuropathies. Part II. Neurologic, genetic, and electrophysiologic findings in various neuronal degenerations. Arch. Neurol. (Chicago), *18*:603, 1968.
11. Gombault, A., and Mallet: Un cas de tabès ayant débuté dans l'enfance. Arch. Med Exper., *1*:385, 1889.
12. Isaacs, H.: Familial chronic hypertrophic polyneuropathy with paralysis of the extremities in cold weather. S. Afr. Med. J., *34*:758, 1960.
13. Joiner, C. L., McArdle, B., and Thompson, R. H. S.: Blood pyruvate estimations in the diagnosis and treatment of polyneuritis. Brain, *73*:431, 1950.
14. Koeppen, A. H., Messmore, H., and Stehbens, W. B.: Interstitial hypertrophic neuropathy: Biochemical study of the peripheral nervous system. Arch. Neurol. (Chicago), *24*:340, 1971.
15. Krishna Rao, C. V. G., Fitz, C. R., and Harwood-Nash, D. C.: Dejerine-Sottas syndrome in children (hypertrophic interstitial polyneuritis). Amer. J. Roentgen., *122*:70, 1974.
16. Russell, W. R., and Garland, H. G.: Progressive hypertrophic polyneuritis, with case reports. Brain, *53*:376, 1930.

17. Thomas, P. K., and Lascelles, R. G.: Hypertrophic neuropathy. Quart. J. Med., 36:223, 1967.
18. Weller, R. O., and Das Gupta, T. K.: Experimental hypertrophic neuropathy: An electron microscope study. J. Neurol. Neurosurg. Psychiat., 31:34, 1968.

PROGRESSIVE MUSCULAR DYSTROPHY

Progressive muscular dystrophy, a genetically determined primary degenerative disease of skeletal muscle, is generally classified as a myopathy. The most adequate classification, from the clinical and genetic standpoints, is given in Table 3–7.

Duchenne muscular dystrophy is the most common type, occurring in 1 in 3,000 live births and constituting 80 per cent of all cases.[2] It is transmitted by sex-linked recessive inheritance and occurs only in males; females are carriers. About one third of the cases represent new mutations.[3]

The initial symptoms of the disease are usually apparent within the first three years of life and are slowness in learning to walk or run at the usual age, tendency to fall frequently, and difficulty in climbing stairs and rising from the floor. In a few cases, the disease may start between the third and sixth years or, rarely, in adolescence. Initial symmetrical involvement of the pelvic girdle musculature is followed after three to five years by affection of the muscles of the shoulder girdle.

The child stands with a protuberant abdomen and excessive lumbar lordosis. The shoulders are carried behind the pelvis. The calf muscles are enlarged. A predominant feature of the condition is pseudohypertrophy, caused by accumulation of fat. The shoulders have a sloping appearance because of the weakness of the shoulder girdle muscles.

*Table 3–7. Classification of Muscular Dystrophy**

"Pure" muscular dystrophies
  Duchenne-type muscular dystrophy
    Sex-linked recessive
    Autosomal recessive
  Limb-girdle muscular dystrophy
    Autosomal recessive or rarely dominant
  Facioscapulohumeral muscular dystrophy
    Autosomal dominant (rarely recessive)
  Distal muscular dystrophy
  Ocular myopathy
  Congenital muscular dystrophy
Cases with myotonia
  Myotonia congenita
  Dystrophia myotonica
  Paramyotonia congenita

*Adapted from Walton, J. N. (ed.): Disorders of Voluntary Muscle. Boston, Little, Brown, & Co., 1964.

The gait is waddling. Contracture of the triceps surae is due to weakness of the anterior tibial and long toe extensors. Pes planovalgus develops because the foot is forced into eversion by the limited ankle dorsiflexion. Often children in whom Duchenne muscular dystrophy is subsequently diagnosed were initially seen between the ages of two and four years because of flat feet. At this stage of the disease the affected child "climbs up on his legs" when rising from the floor (positive Gower's sign), and the diagnosis can be confirmed by elevated creatine phosphokinase serum levels and positive muscle biopsy.[1, 6, 12]

With increasing contracture of the calf muscle the child develops toe-heel and then toe-toe gait. When caught off balance he tends to fall because his knees give way. He may walk and stand by placing his feet wide apart to increase his base of support, and often utilizes trick movements to maintain equilibrium.

The course of Duchenne muscular dystrophy is steady and rapid progression, resulting in inability to walk late in the second decade. Later in the course of the disease, when the child is confined to a wheelchair or bed, contractures develop because of remaining in one position for prolonged periods; these are commonly seen in the hamstrings, the hip flexors, and the iliotibial band.

Scoliosis and kyphoscoliosis are common in the late stages; they result from weakness of the trunk and abdominal muscles. Eventually the patient is unable to sit and is confined to bed with little or no residual active movement in his limbs, except some weak grasp with his hands and flexion of his toes and feet. The muscles of the face and those of respiration and swallowing are relatively spared.

Myocardial degeneration with fatty infiltration and fibrosis eventually develops. Cardiomegaly and persistent tachycardia are frequently present in the late stages. Survival beyond the age of 30 years is a rarity. Most patients die from sudden cardiac failure or pulmonary infection. A few in whom the onset of disease was comparatively late may survive until the fourth or fifth decade.

There is no specific treatment for muscular dystrophy. Progressive muscle weakness eventually leads to inevitable wheelchair and bed confinement. Loss of independent ambulation is often prema-

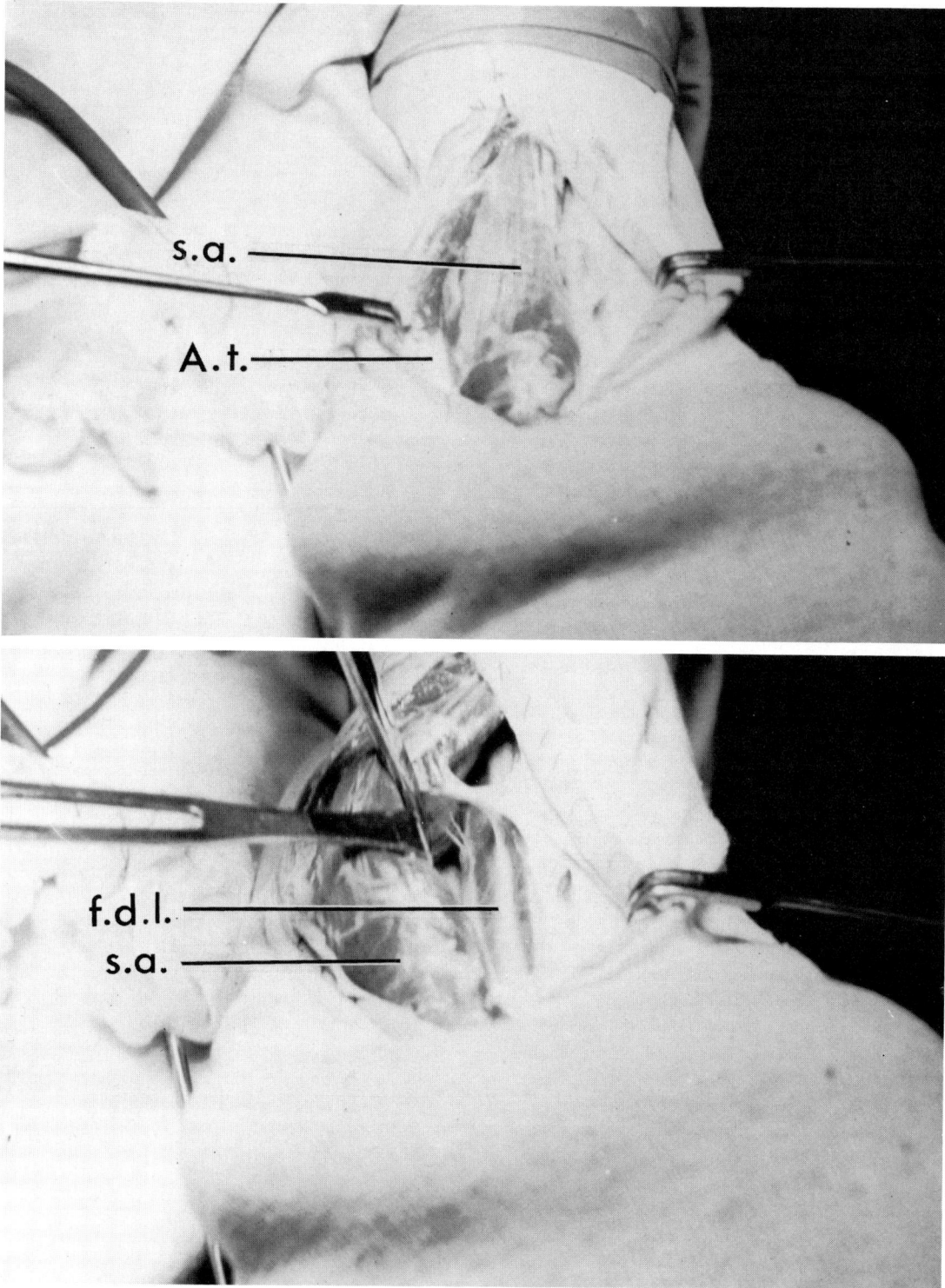

FIGURE 3–80. Soleus accessorius muscle simulating a soft-tissue tumor.

Gross appearance at surgery. s.a., Soleus accessorius muscle; A.t., Achilles tendon; f.d.l., flexor digitorum longus muscle and tendon. (From Dunn, A. W.: Anomalous muscles simulating soft tissue tumors in the lower extremities. J. Bone Joint Surg., *47-A*:1398, 1965. Reprinted by permission.)

ture; efforts should be directed to maintaining it as long as possible.[11] The factors involved are muscle weakness, contractural deformity, inactivity, and emotional problems. Contractural deformity can be prevented by passive stretching exercises and appropriate splinting. Fixed equinus deformity is corrected by heel cord lengthening and immediate external support with light plastic orthoses.[9, 10] Often these patients develop progressive varus deformity of the feet; therefore prophylactic anterolateral transfer of the posterior tibial tendon is performed at the time of heel cord lengthening. Fixed hip and knee flexion deformities are corrected by soft-tissue release. These procedures and knee-ankle-foot orthotic support will significantly prolong walking ability.

Management of scoliosis and kyphosis is beyond the scope of this book.[4, 7, 8] Muscular dystrophy patients tolerate anesthesia poorly; adequate preoperative assessment and meticulous postoperative management are crucial.[5]

References

1. Dubowitz, V., and Brooke, M. H.: Muscle Biopsy. A Modern Approach. Philadelphia, W. B. Saunders Co., 1973.
2. Duchenne, G. B.: Recherches sur le paralysie musculaire pseudo-hypertrophique ou paralysie myosclerosique. Arch. Gen. Med., *11*:5, 179, 305, 421, 552, 1868.
3. Emery, A. E. H.: Duchenne muscular dystrophy. Genetic aspects, carrier detection and antenatal diagnosis. Brit. Med. Bull., *36*:117, 1980.
4. Gibson, D. A., Koreska, J., Robertson, D., Kahn, A., III, and Albisser, A. M.: The management of spinal deformity in Duchenne's muscular dystrophy. Orthop. Clin. N. Amer., *9*:437, 1978.
5. Gronert, G. A.: Malignant hyperthermia. Anesthesiology, *53*:395, 1980.
6. Gowers, W. R.: Pseudohypertrophic Muscular Paralysis. London, Churchill, 1879.
7. Robin, G. C., and Brief, L. P.: Scoliosis in childhood muscular dystrophy. J. Bone Joint Surg., *53-A*:466, 1971.
8. Sakai, D. N., Hsu, J. D., Bonnett, C. A., and Brown, J. C.: Stabilization of the collapsing spine in Duchenne muscular dystrophy. Clin. Orthop., *128*:256, 1977.
9. Shapiro, F., and Bresnan, M. J.: Orthopedic management of childhood neuromuscular disease. Part III. Diseases of muscle. J. Bone Joint Surg., *64-A*:1102, 1982.
10. Siegel, I. M., Miller, J. E., and Ray, R. D.: Subcutaneous lower limb tenotomy in the treatment of pseudohypertrophic muscular dystrophy. Description of technique and presentation of twenty-one cases. J. Bone Joint Surg., *50-A*:1437, 1968.
11. Spencer, G. E., Jr., and Vignos, P. J., Jr.: Bracing for ambulation in childhood progressive muscular dystrophy. J. Bone Joint Surg., *44-A*:234, 1962.
12. Vignos, P. J., Jr.: Diagnosis of progressive muscular dystrophy. J. Bone Joint Surg., *49-A*:1212, 1967.

CONGENITAL ABSENCE OF MUSCLES

Developmental abnormalities in the fetus may lead to hypoplasia or aplasia of various skeletal muscles. Any of the voluntary muscles may be congenitally absent in whole or in part, but certain muscles are deficient more frequently than others. The pectoralis, particularly the sternocostal part of the pectoralis major, is most commonly involved.[3, 6] Next in order of frequency are the trapezius, quadratus femoris, serratus magnus, omohyoideus, semimembranosus, brachioradialis, abdominis, deltoid, latissimus dorsi, sternocleidomastoid, rhomboid, supraspinatus and infraspinatus, biceps brachii, thenar or hypothenar of the hand, and quadriceps femoris.[1, 5]

Usually the abnormality is discovered at birth or soon afterward. It tends to be unilateral and may involve a single muscle or a related group of muscles. The resulting functional disability remains stationary.

Congenital absence of a muscle may be combined with congenital abnormalities of other organs. Some of the best known examples of these are agenesis of the pectoral muscles in conjunction with syndactyly or microdactyly, and malformations of the genitourinary and alimentary tracts associated with congenital absence of the abdominal musculature (prune belly).[2, 4, 7, 8]

References

1. Bing, R.: Ueber angeborene Muskeldefecte. Virchow. Arch. Path. Anat., *170*:175, 1902.
2. Brown, J. B., and McDowell, I.: Syndactylism with absence of the pectoralis major. Surgery, *7*:599, 1940.
3. Christopher, F.: Congenital absence of the pectoral muscles. J. Bone Joint Surg., *10*:350, 1928.
4. Krabbe, K.: Les lésions embryonnaires à la lumière des défectuosités mammaire et pectorale de la syndactylie et de la microdactylie. Acta Psychiat.Neurol., *24*:539, 1949.
5. LeDouble, A. F.: Traité des Variations de Système Musculaire de l'Homme et Leur Signification au Point de Vue de l'Anthropologie Zoologique. Paris. Schleicher Frères, 1897.
6. Morley, E. B.: Congenital defect of pectoral muscle. Lancet, *1*:1101, 1923.
7. Resnick, E.: Congenital unilateral absence of the pectorial muscles often associated with syndactylism. J. Bone Joint Surg., *24*:925, 1942.
8. Silverman, F. N., and Huang, N.: Congenital absence of the abdominal muscles associated with malformations of the genitourinary and alimentary tracts: Report of cases and review of literature. Amer. J. Dis. Child., *80*:91, 1950.

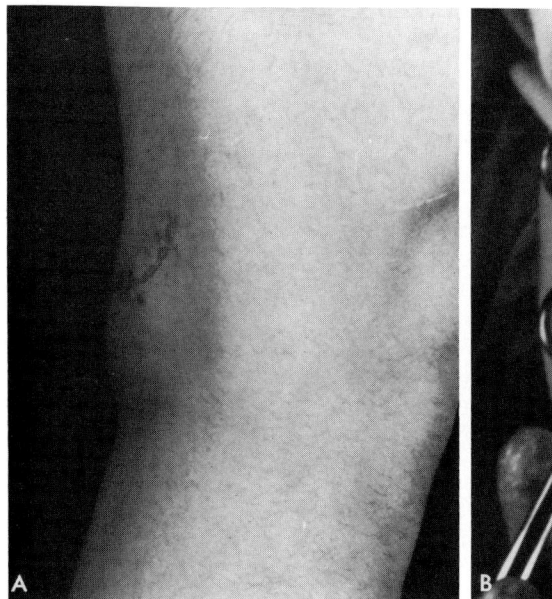 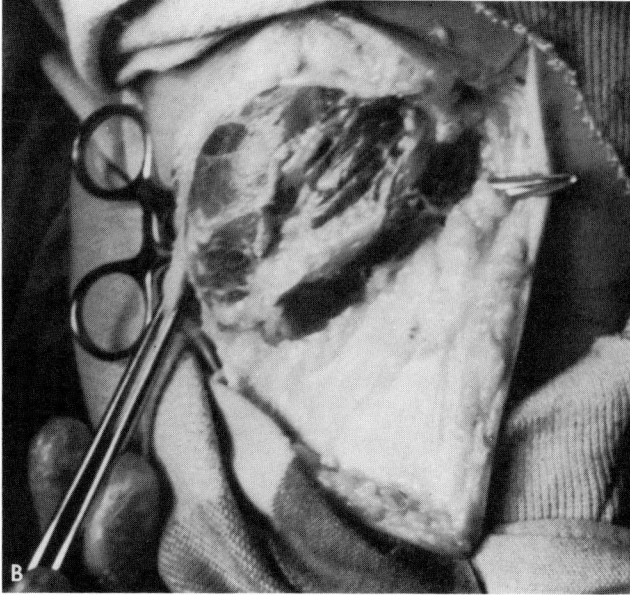

FIGURE 3–81. Anomalous hamstring muscle presenting as a popliteal cyst.

A. Clinical appearance. **B.** Findings at operation. Note that muscle crosses the popliteal fossa from the lateral to the medial side. The thumb forceps is pulling the semitendinous tendon medially. (From Dunn, A. W.: Anomalous muscles simulating soft tissue tumors in the lower extremities. J. Bone Joint Surg., 47-A:1399, 1965. Reprinted by permission.)

ACCESSORY MUSCLES

Supernumerary muscles are rare. In the limbs, they often simulate soft-tissue tumors, and because of the possibility of malignancy, surgical exploration is carried out. Dunn reports two cases of soleus accessorius muscles, both of which appeared bilaterally as a mass anteromedial to the Achilles tendon (Fig. 3–80).[3] An anomalous accessory hamstring muscle may be manifest as a popliteal swelling (Fig. 3–81). This usually originates from the linea aspera of the femur and passes medially to insert into the dorsal part of the capsule of the knee joint.[3,6]

References

1. Bardeen, C. R.: Development and variation of nerves and musculature of the inferior extremity and neighboring regions of the trunk in man. J. Anat., 6:259, 1907.
2. Bonnell, J., and Cruess, R.: Anomalous insertion of the soleus muscle as a cause of fixed equinus deformity. (Case report). J. Bone Joint Surg., 51-A:999, 1969.
3. Dunn, A. W.: Anomalous muscles simulating soft tissue tumors in the lower extremities. Report of three cases. J. Bone Joint Surg., 47-A:1397, 1965.
4. Ger, R., and Sedlin, E.: The accessory soleus muscle. Clin. Orthop., 116:200, 1976.
5. Gordon, S. L., and Matheson, D. W.: The accessory soleus. Clin. Orthop., 97:129, 1973.
6. Gray, D. J.: Some anomalous hamstring muscles. Anat. Rec., 91:33, 1945.
7. Humphrey, G. M.: Observations in Myology. London, MacMillian & Co., Ltd., 1872.
8. LeDouble, A. F.: Traité de Variations du Système Musculaire de l'Homme et de leur Signification au Point de Vue de l'Anthropologie Zoologique. Paris. Schleicher Frères, 1897.

CONGENITAL CONTRACTURE OF TRICEPS SURAE MUSCLE

Walking on tiptoes is normal when children first begin to walk. Within three to six months they "grow out" of the toe-toe or toe-heel gait pattern and learn to walk with a heel-toe gait. In some children, however, toe walking persists because of congenital short tendo calcaneus, an entity described by Hall, Salter, and Bhalla.[1] The affected children walk on their toes, though on volition, they are able to lower their heels to the ground. When they attempt heel-toe gait, their knees hyperextend and their gait is awkward; toe walking is naturally more comfortable. The range of dorsiflexion of the ankle is limited, with the degree of equinus deformity varying from case to case. On deep palpation, an abnormally low insertion of the hypertrophied soleus muscle may be felt in the region of the tendo Achillis. Neurologic examination is completely normal.

In the differential diagnosis, one should consider an abnormally large soleus or accessory soleus muscle, hyperkinesia due to minimal brain damage syndrome, delayed maturation of corticospinal tracts, spastic paraplegia, diastematomyelia, and muscular dystrophy.

In delayed maturation of the corticospinal tracts in the early stages, there is no fixed equinus deformity. The deep tendon reflexes may be hyperactive, and the Babinski sign may be equivocal. Other signs of spasticity cannot be elicited. The condition is usually familial, the toe walking normally disappearing between six and eight years of age.

Treatment

Conservative measures are indicated in the young child and consist of passive stretching exercises of the triceps surae muscle performed by the parents 15 to 20 times in several daily sessions. A splint or bivalved cast that holds the ankle in neutral position is worn at night.

If there is permanent contracture of the triceps surae muscle, a below-knee walking cast with an anterior walking heel is applied to stretch the triceps surae muscle. The cast is changed at two-week intervals, each time bringing the foot and ankle into further dorsiflexion. Uusally two or three stretching casts are required to correct the equinus deformity. Following removal of the cast, gait training, passive stretching exercises and active exercises of the triceps surae, and active exercises to strengthen the anterior tibial function are important measures that will prevent recurrence of equinus deformity and toe walking. Occasionally a dorsiflexion-assist below-knee orthosis is worn to establish the pattern of heel-toe gait.

When the child has reached the age of six to eight years, and if one or two trials of conservative management have failed, a sliding heel cord lengthening may be indicated (see Plate 11). An abnormally low insertion of the soleus muscle on the Achilles tendon or an accessory soleus is a common finding at surgery, in which instance the accessory soleus or distal one fourth of the muscle belly of the soleus is excised. Postoperative care follows the same guidelines as outlined in the section on cerebral palsy. The presence of hyperkinesia and minimal brain damage should alert the orthopedist to undertake more aggressive measures during the postoperative period.

Reference

1. Hall, J. E., Salter, R. B., and Bhalla, S. K.: Congenital short tendo calcaneus. J. Bone Joint Surg., *49-B*:695, 1967.

ACHILLES TENDINITIS

In children and adolescents, a painful heel is a common complaint that may arise from affections of any of the structures composing the heel. The most common cause, however, is nonspecific tendinitis of the heel cord. Symptoms usually develop following strenuous physical activity. The Achilles tendon is swollen and tender near its insertion. Roentgenograms demonstrate soft-tissue swelling. Fragmentation and irregular radiopacity of the calcaneal apophysis are normal findings, however, and an erroneous diagnosis of calcaneal apophysitis or Sever's disease should not be made.

In mild cases, the counter of the heel shoe is softened and a ¼- to ⅜-inch lift is added to the heel to decrease the tension of the triceps surae on the apophysis of the calcaneus. Sports, running, jumping, and prolonged walking are curtailed. These measures will usually relieve symptoms within three to four weeks. If tendinitis is severe, additional complete rest for the foot and leg is provided by immobilization for three weeks in a below-knee walking cast with the ankle joint at a 20-degree equinus angle; in the three-week period following cast removal, the patient is allowed to walk with a raised heel on the shoe.

4. Pes Cavus and Claw Toes

PES CAVUS

Pes cavus is a fixed equinus deformity of the forefoot on the hindfoot (Fig. 4–1). When associated with clawing of the toes, the term *clawfoot* is sometimes used to describe the condition.

Etiology and Pathogenesis

Cavus deformity of the foot is usually a manifestation of some underlying neuromuscular disease. The lesion may be in muscle (myopathic pes cavus), peripheral nerves or lumbosacral spinal nerve roots, anterior horn cells of the spinal cord, spinocerebellar tracts, pyramidal or extrapyramidal systems of the brain, or cerebral cortex. Examples are: at the *muscular level,* muscular dystrophy (particularly the distal type); at the *peripheral nerve or spinal nerve root level,* Dejerine-Sottas interstitial hypertrophic neuritis, Charcot-Marie-Tooth disease, polyneuritis, and traumatic lesions of the sciatic nerve; at the *spinal cord level,* poliomyelitis, myelomeningocele, diastematomyelia, and cord tumors; as heredofamilial affections of spinocerebellar tracts, Friedreich's ataxia and Roussy-Lévy syndrome; at the *pyramidal and extrapyramidal levels,* cerebral palsy (spastic hemiplegia or athetosis) and dystonia musculorum deformans; and at the *cerebral level,* hysteria in which, when the position of pes cavus is maintained constantly for prolonged periods, permanent contracture and fixed deformity may develop. Some cases of pes cavus are congenital; in others no specific cause or neurologic deficit can be demonstrated, in which case the term *idiopathic pes cavus* is used.

In the pathogenesis of pes cavus, several factors should be considered:

Muscle Imbalance Between Weak Anterior Tibial and Strong Peroneus Longus Muscles. The medial cuneiform and the base of the first metatarsal are elevated by the action of the anterior tibial muscle and depressed by the peroneus longus muscle. Bentzon advanced the theory that when the anterior tibial muscle is weak, the first metatarsal is plantar-flexed by a strong peroneus longus muscle. The forefoot is pronated by the action of the peroneus longus muscle, and the valgus deviation is further aggravated by the pull of the long toe extensors. Varying degrees of equinus deformity due to contracture of the triceps surae muscle and posterior soft tissues of the ankle are usually found. In attempting to substitute for the dorsiflexing action of the weakened anterior tibial muscle, the long toe extensors pull the proximal phalanges of the toes into hyperextension; and the tension on the long toe flexor muscle brings the distal two phalanges of the toes into plantar flexion.[10] The "windlass" mechanism pulls the metatarsals, especially the first, into plantar flexion and elevates the medial longitudinal arch. The plantar soft tissues become shortened. This hypothesis of dynamic imbalance between a weak anterior muscle and a strong peroneus longus muscle sounds very plausible and is of definite value in planning treatment. It is supported by the studies of Missirian and Mann.[89a] It fails, however, to explain the actual clinical findings. In poliomyelitis, when the anterior tibial muscle is weak and the peroneal muscles are strong, a valgus deformity results. The os calcis is everted, the head of the talus is plantar-flexed, the medial longitudinal arch is flattened, and the toes are flat on the ground. In walking, however, although the toe extensors do pull the toes into extension, a fixed claw toe deformity does not develop. Also in contradiction to the theory of Bentzon is the absence of definite anterior tibial muscle weakness in most cases of pes cavus.

Isolated Weakness of Peroneus Brevis Muscle. Another theory is that, in an attempt to compensate for the paralysis of the peroneus brevis muscle, the peroneus longus hypertrophies and overpowers the action of the anterior tibial muscle. The first metatarsal and medial cuneiform are pulled into plantar flexion, and the forefoot is pronated. The long toe extensors are hyperactive to compensate for dorsiflexion insufficiency caused by peroneus brevis muscle weakness; consequently, the proximal phalanges of the toes are pulled into hyperextension and their distal phalanges into flexion by the tension on the long toe flexors. The hindfoot inverts to compensate for eversion of the forefoot, enabling the first and fifth metatarsals to rest evenly on the ground. The dynamic imbalance between a weak peroneus brevis and a strong posterior tibial muscle may also be a factor in producing a varus heel. In support of this attractive theory, one finds an occasional patient with poliomyelitis who has isolated paralysis of the peroneus brevis muscle and a deformity of the foot quite similar to pes cavus.

Paralysis of Intrinsic Muscles of Foot. Duchenne described a cavus clawfoot with atrophy of the muscles that insert into the sesamoids of the great toe and the interossei of the foot. The proximal phalanges are hyperextended so that they are subluxated on the metatarsal heads, and the middle and distal phalanges are flexed. The result is clawing of the toes and a considerable increase in the curvature of the plantar arch. Duchenne proposed the following theory of the pathogenesis of cavus clawfoot:

> When the interossei are paralyzed or weakened, the force of the muscles which extend the proximal phalanges and the muscles which flex the middle and distal phalanges lose the moderating action of the interossei. The clawing of the toes sets in and gradually increases. The bases of the proximal phalanges progressively depress the heads of the metatarsals with increase of the degree of subluxation of the proximal phalanges; the curvature of the plantar arch increases considerably and the plantar aponeurosis contracts in time. Following this, all the joints, especially the mediotarsal joints and their ligaments, become deformed in a manner characteristic of all cavus feet.[33]

Duchenne believed the mechanism of the clawing of the foot to be similar to that of the clawhand seen following paralysis of the intrinsic muscles of the hand, i.e.,

> ... the heads of the medial four metacarpals are equally pushed by the proximal phalanges of the fingers, resulting in a form of cavus of the palm and of the hand.[33]

It should be noted, however, that the interossei in the foot insert mainly into the bases of the proximal phalanges, an anatomic fact that contradicts the theory of Duchenne of the "moderating action of the interossei" on the middle and distal phalanges in preventing flexion at the interphalangeal joints.[73]

Paralysis of the intrinsic muscles of the foot produces pes planovalgus, not pes cavus. Coonrad, Irwin, Gucker, and Wray observed that persistent function of the short toe flexors and other intrinsic muscles of the foot in an otherwise flail foot resulted in the development of cavovarus deformity of the foot.[27] Garceau and Brahms demonstrated the importance of functioning intrinsic muscles in the production of pes cavus and pes cavovarus; they recommended resection of the motor branches of both the medial and lateral plantar nerves. In their experience the results of 47 operations in 40 patients were encouraging.[47]

Electromyographic studies of the intrinsic muscles of the foot and the extrinsic muscles of the foot and leg in patients with pes cavus have been performed by Bertrand and Ingelrans. Both authors have demonstrated definite abnormality in the short toe flexors and other intrinsic muscles of the foot. Ingelrans also observed abnormal activity in the long toe extensor and peroneus longus muscles.[11, 69] The author has repeatedly observed such changes, but has found it difficult to correlate electromyographic findings in pes cavus with dynamic muscle imbalance and abnormal forces causing the cavus deformity.

Lambrinudi supported Duchenne's theory of interosseus insufficiency as the cause of clawfoot and devised an operation consisting of arthrodeses of both interphalangeal joints and sectioning of the long toe extensors. Stiffening the interphalangeal joints brings the entire action of the long toe flexor to bear on the metatarsophalangeal joint; thus, during locomotion, the toes are pressed on the ground and the metatarsal heads are supported.[77]

Triceps Surae Muscle. The triceps surae muscle has been blamed as a factor in the pathogenesis of pes cavus. When the gas-

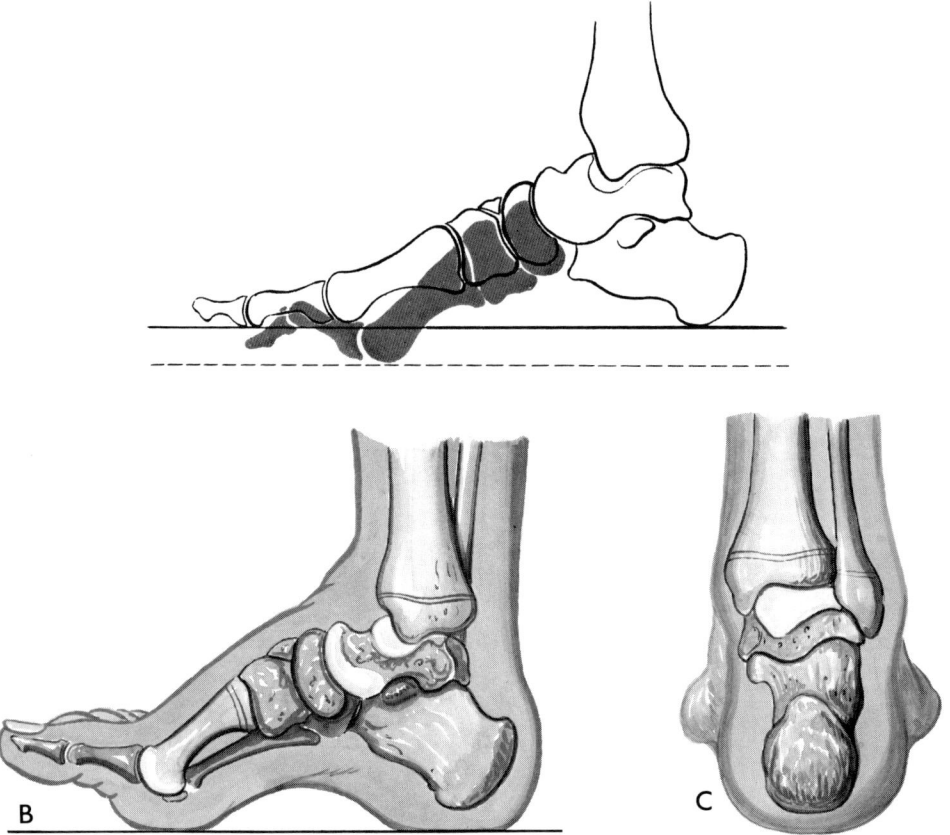

FIGURE 4–1. Cavus deformity of the foot.

A. Pes cavus. There is fixed equinus deformity of the forefoot on the hindfoot. **B** and **C.** Simple pes cavus. The plantar flexion deformity of the forefoot is equal in its medial and lateral columns and the heel is in neutral position.

Illustration continued on opposite page.

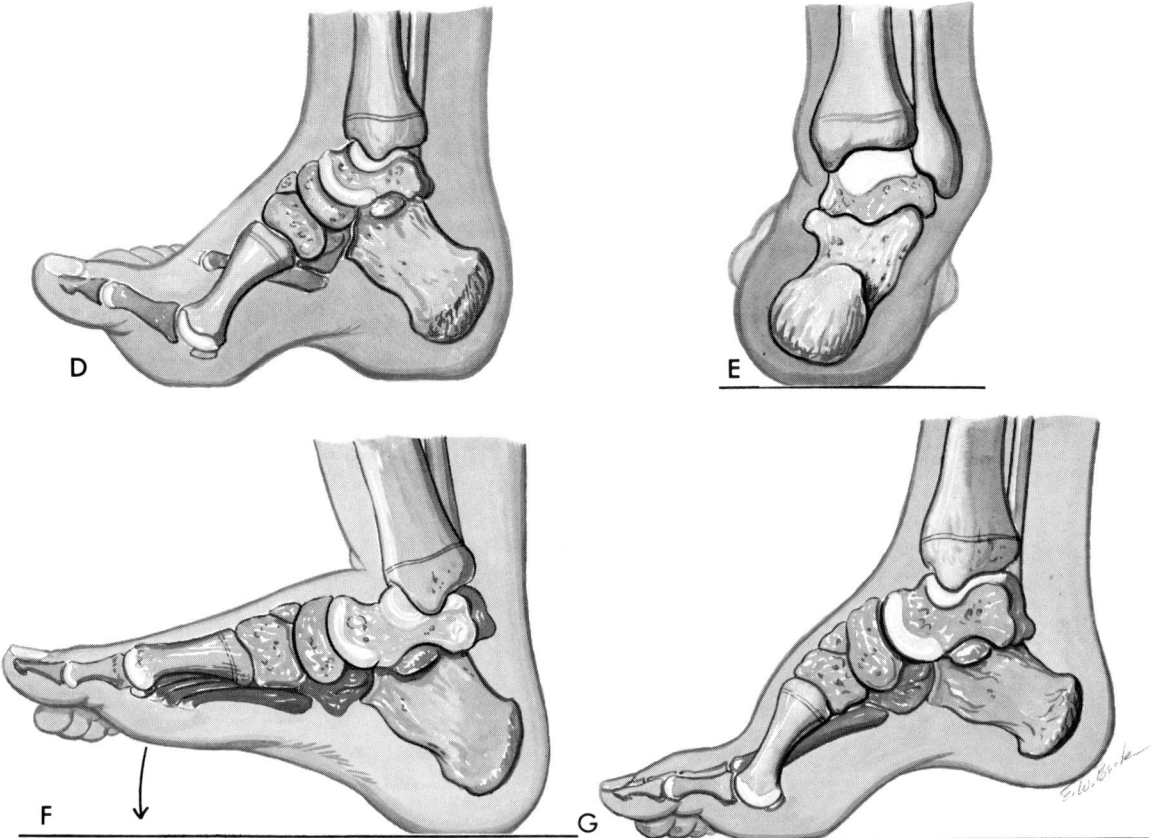

FIGURE 4–1 Continued. Cavus deformity of the foot.

D and **E.** Pes cavovarus. Note the plantar flexion of the medial column of the forefoot and the inversion of the heel. **F.** Calcaneocavus deformity. Note the calcaneus position of the hindfoot. The forefoot drops into equinus position, developing calcaneocavus deformity. **G.** Pes equinocavus. In addition to the forefoot, the hindfoot and ankle are in equinus position.

trocnemius-soleus muscles are paralyzed, the normal long toe flexor muscles substitute for the lost action of the triceps surae during the push-off phase of gait, with resultant clawing of the toes. The forefoot becomes plantar-flexed because of the depressing action of the claw toes. In paralytic neuromuscular disease, calcaneocavus deformity may result from such a mechanism.

Hyperactivity of Intrinsic Muscles of Foot. This is considered by Coonrad and associates and by Garceau and Brahms to be a cause of pes cavovarus.[27, 47] This theory fails, however, to explain the hyperextension deformity of the proximal phalanges of the toes.

Muscle Fibrosis and Contracture. Fibrosis and permanent contracture of the short toe flexors and other intrinsic muscles of the foot and plantar aponeurosis have been repeatedly demonstrated at surgery in pes cavus. As stated previously, the intrinsic muscles of the foot insert into the bases of the proximal phalanges, not into the metatarsal heads. The proximal phalanx of the toes in pes cavus is hyperextended, not flexed.

Genetic Factors. In idiopathic pes cavus there is a high rate of familial incidence; an exact method of hereditary transmission has not, however, been delineated. The genetic aspects of degenerative diseases of the spinocerebellar tracts and spina bifida are discussed in Chapter 3.

In summary, the exact pathogenesis of pes cavus is not known. Diverse factors may be operative in it. In some cases, equinus forefoot may be the primary deformity; in others, clawing of the toes; and occasionally, inversion of the hindfoot. Pes cavus is a manifestation of neuromuscular disease unless proved otherwise. It is imperative, therefore, that the following studies be performed to determine various possible etiologic factors: (1) a thorough family history (which should include foot examinations and neurologic assessments of the siblings and parents); (2) a muscle examination to rule out paralytic disease; (3) a thorough neurologic evaluation (often it is best to obtain consultation with a pediatric neurologist); (4) roentgenography of the *entire* spine; (5) nerve conduction and electromyographic studies; and (6) in selected cases when indicated, lumbar puncture, myelography, and computed tomography of the spine.

Clinical Features

There are various types of pes cavus that should be distinguished: In *simple pes cavus,* the plantar flexion deformity of the forefoot is equal in its medial and lateral columns, with even distribution of weight on the first and fifth metatarsal heads. The heel is in neutral position or a few degrees valgus, which is normal (see Fig. 4–1 B and C). In *pes cavovarus* only the medial column of the forefoot is dropped in plantar flexion; consequently, the longitudinal axes of the first metatarsal and, to a lesser degree, of the second metatarsal are at a marked equinus angle, while that of the fifth metatarsal is in normal horizontal position (Figs. 4–1 D and E and 4–2 A, B, and C). Examination of the non-weight-bearing foot (with the patient sitting and his leg hanging at the edge of the table) will reveal that the fifth metatarsal can easily be dorsiflexed into neutral position, whereas the first metatarsal is fixed in equinus position and cannot be passively manipulated into neutral extension. Closer scrutiny and analysis will disclose that the forefoot, particularly the first metatarsal, is in 20 to 30 degrees of pronation. The longitudinal arch is elevated. In the early stages the hindfoot is in neutral position, and in stance and locomotion there is excessive pressure on the pronated first metatarsal head; in order to relieve this pressure the whole foot (forefoot and hindfoot) is inverted (Fig. 4–2 D to I). Initially, the varus deformity of the hindfoot is reducible and can be expected to disappear when the fixed equinus deformity and pronation of the first metatarsal are corrected. With time, however, the hindfoot deformity becomes fixed and cannot be corrected by aligning the forefoot (Fig. 4–3). *Calcaneocavus deformity* of the foot usually occurs in flaccid paralysis, such as that seen in poliomyelitis or myelomeningocele. The triceps surae muscle is paralyzed. The hindfoot is in calcaneus position and the forefoot is fixed in equinus position (cf. Fig. 4–1F). *Pes equinocavus* is usually secondary to talipes equinovarus; in addition to the forefoot, the hindfoot and ankle are in equinus posture (cf. Fig. 4–1G). Occasionally cavus deformity of the feet is present at birth. The terms *talipes cavus* and *congenital cavus foot* are used to describe the condition.

On examination, the forefoot of the cavovarus foot (especially the first metatarsal) is plantar-flexed and pronated, whereas the hindfoot is in varus supination. The hindfoot and forefoot are interdependent; i.e., the forefoot pronation supinates the flexible

---

Figure 4–2. Pes cavovarus.

A to C. Diagrams of mediolateral view of the foot demonstrating that only the medial column of the forefoot is dropped in plantar flexion. Note the longitudinal axis of the first metatarsal is markedly equinus, whereas that of the fifth metatarsal is in normal alignment. On push-up test, the first metatarsal cannot be passively manipulated into neutral extension. **D to F.** Diagrams of the mechanism of inversion of the hindfoot in pes cavovarus. In the normal foot, the weight-bearing forces are equally distributed on the first and fifth metatarsal heads (D). In pes cavovarus the first metatarsal is fixed in equinus position and the forefoot is in 20 to 30 degrees of pronation. In stance and locomotion, there is excessive pressure on the pronated first metatarsal head (E). Excessive pressure on the first metatarsal head is relieved by inverting the whole foot (both forefoot and hindfoot) (F) **G to I.** Posterior views of the ankle and foot, showing the normal, pronated, and inverted hindfoot. The hindfoot assumes a varus inclination as the forefoot is inverted.

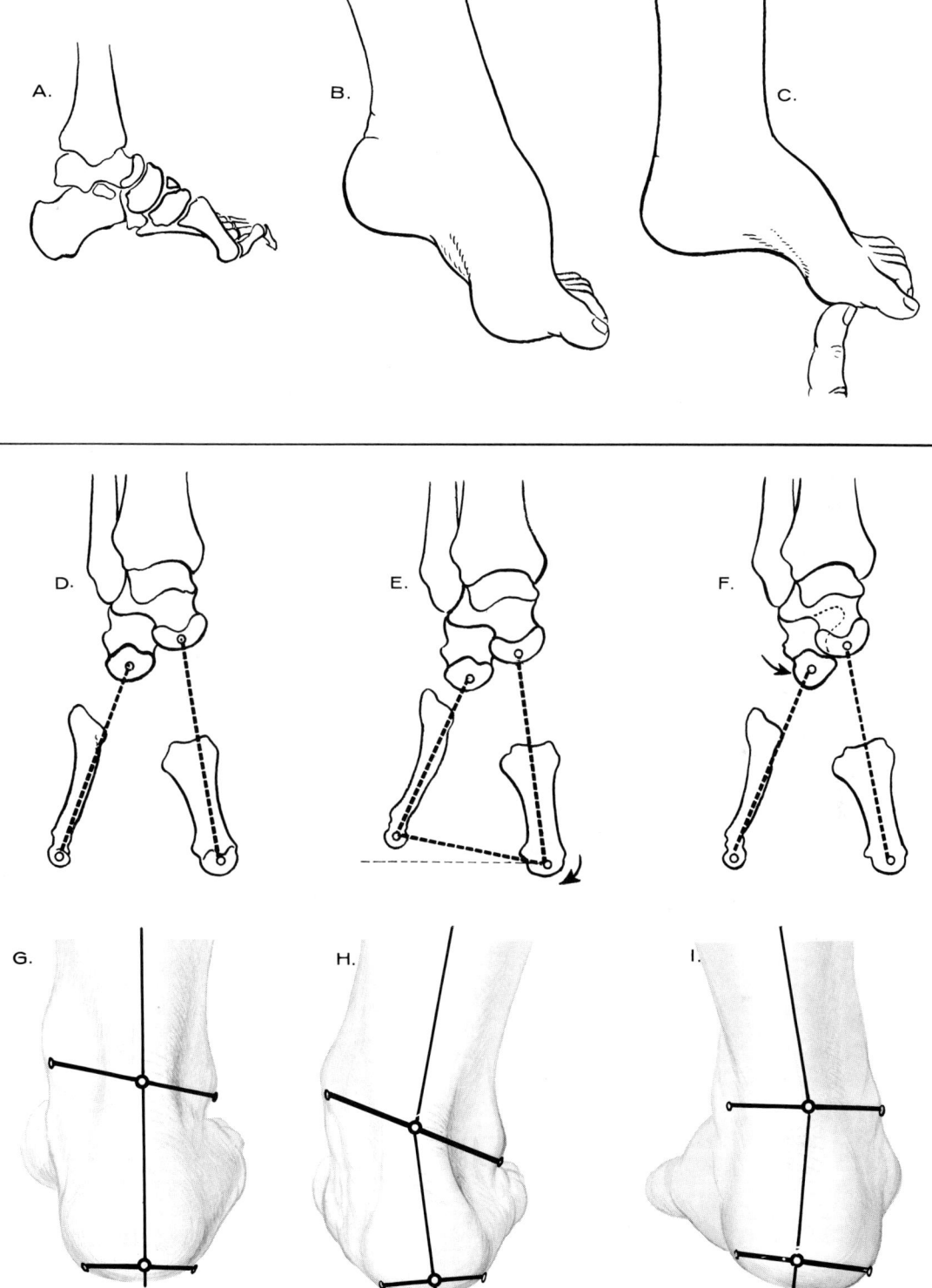

Figure 4–2. See legend on opposite page

hindfoot owing to the "tripod" effect. The medial longitudinal arch is elevated and the soft tissues in the plantar aspect of the foot are taut, fixing the forefoot in plantar flexion. The contracted structures are the plantar aponeurosis, the abductor hallucis, the flexor hallucis brevis, the flexor digitorum brevis, the abductor digiti quinti, the interossei, the tendinous insertions of the posterior tibial tendon on the plantar aspect of the cuneiform and the base of the metatarsals, the Y-ligament (calcaneocuboid and calcaneonavicular), and the capsule on the plantar aspect of the naviculocuneiform and the cuneiform-metatarsal joints. Bony and articular deformities gradually follow the soft-tissue contracture. The head of the first metatarsal is prominent beneath the sole of the foot.

In pes cavus the toes may be normal, but usually they become progressively retracted and clawed, with hyperextension of the metatarsophalangeal joints and flexion of the interphalangeal joints. The great toe and the fifth toe are ordinarily the most severely deformed (Fig. 4–3D). A painful

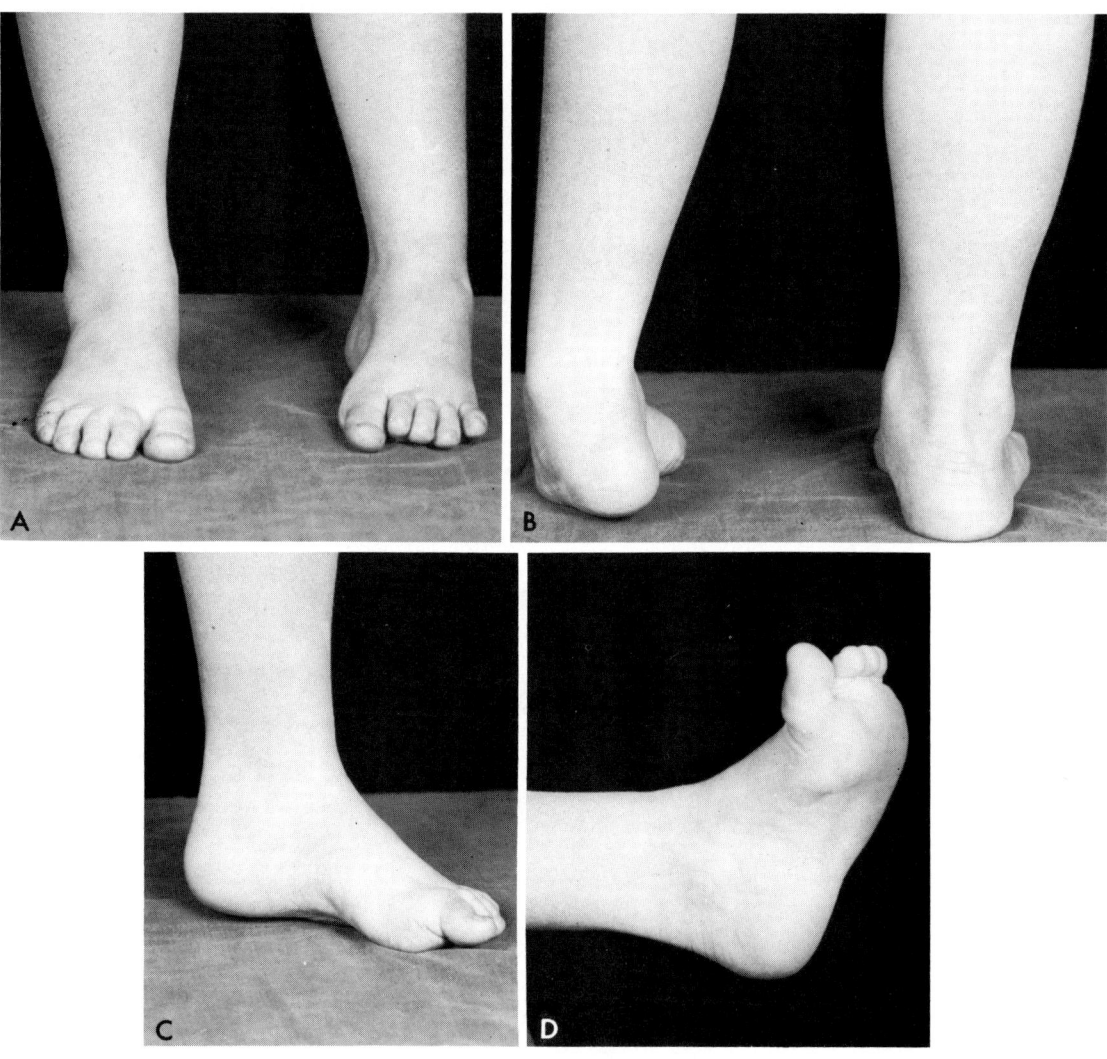

Figure 4–3. Cavovarus deformity of left foot.

A and **B.** Anterior and posterior views showing varus deformity of both forefoot and hindfoot. **C.** Medial view of left foot showing the equinus forefoot. Note also that the heel is not touching the floor, indicating associated contracture of the triceps surae muscle. **D.** Range of active dorsiflexion of ankle and foot. Note the clawing of the great toe.

Illustration continued on opposite page

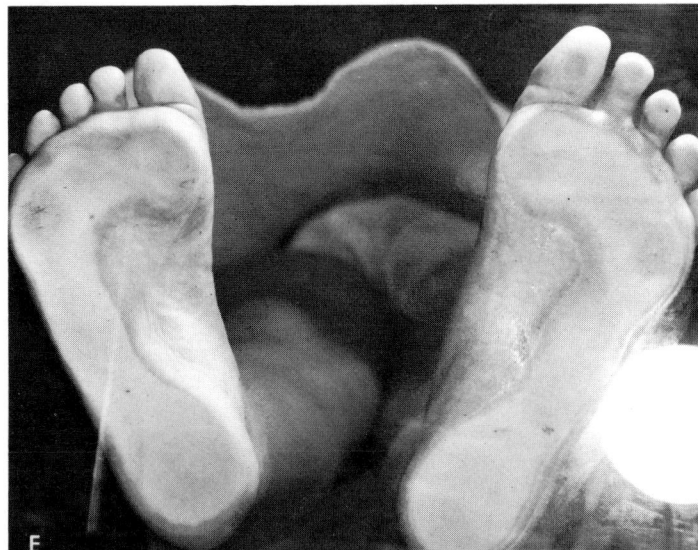
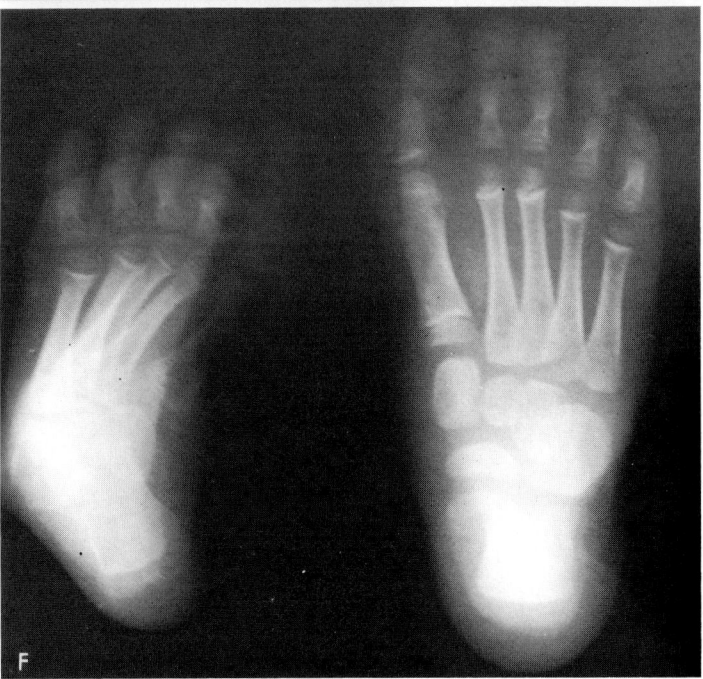

Figure 4–3 Continued. Cavovarus deformity of left foot.

E. Plantar standing view. **F.** Weight-bearing anteroposterior roentgenogram of both feet, depicting the varus deformity of forefoot and hindfoot on the left.

adventitious bursa may develop over the dorsum of the interphalangeal joint as a result of irritation by the shoe; with dorsal subluxation of the metatarsophalangeal joints, the bases of the proximal phalanges press against the metatarsal heads and exaggerate the forefoot equinus deformity. In severe claw toe deformity, the toes do not touch the ground at all and lose their function of propulsion in gait; consequently, most of the body weight as transmitted to the metatarsal heads, and plantar keratosis develops.

Depending upon the type of pes cavus, the position of the hindfoot may be neutral, inverted, equinus, or calcaneus. In pes cavovarus, the heel is inverted and the talocalcaneal angle is decreased in the roentgenogram. In pes equinocavus, contracture of the triceps surae muscle causes the hindfoot to be fixed in plantar flexion, and in stance the heel does not touch the floor (Fig. 4–3C). Most of the body weight is borne on the metatarsal heads. If the equinus deformity is not corrected, painful callosities develop on the plantar aspect of the metatarsal heads. The keratotic skin eventually ulcerates and secondary infection sets in.

Roentgenographic Findings

Weight-bearing anteroposterior and lateral roentgenograms of the feet are made. Lateral projections of the foot in maximal dorsiflexion demonstrate the apex of the cavus deformity. In the normal foot, the distal and proximal articular surfaces of the first cuneiform bone are almost parallel to each other. In pes cavus the forefoot equinus inclination is usually maximal at the first cuneiform bone, and the articular surfaces of the bone converge in the plantar aspect of the foot. Less often the tarsal navicular is at the apex of the cavus deformity. Occasionally the forefoot will drop into equinus posture more distally at the tarsometatarsal joints.

Different methods may be used to gauge the degree of pes cavus. Hibbs measures the angle formed between two lines drawn through the centers of the longitudinal axes

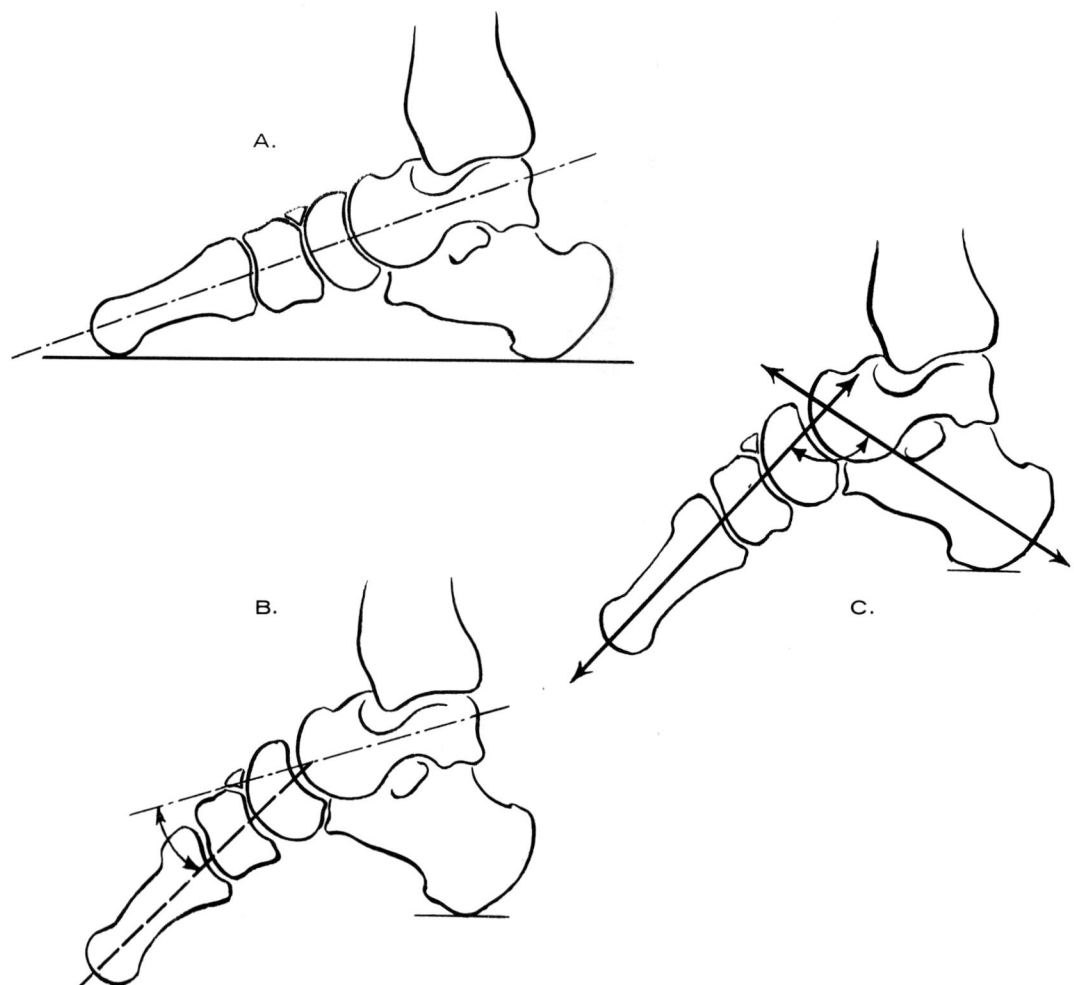

FIGURE 4–4. Methods of measuring the degree of pes cavus in the standing lateral roentgenogram of the foot.

A. In the normal foot, the longitudinal axis of the talus is parallel with that of the first metatarsal. **B.** *Méary* measures the angle formed between lines drawn through the centers of the longitudinal axes of the talus and the first metatarsal. **C.** *Hibbs* measures the angle formed between two lines drawn through the centers of the longitudinal axes of the calcaneus and the first metatarsal.

of the calcaneus and the first metatarsal (Fig. 4–4C).[64] Méary measures the angle formed between two lines drawn through the centers of the longitudinal axes of the talus and the first metatarsal (Fig. 4–4B).[87]

The talocalcaneal angle is measured in the anteroposterior roentgenogram; in pes cavovarus it will be decreased. Routine standing roentgenograms of the ankle should be made also to detect any medial tilting of the ankle mortise, which may be the cause of varus deformity of the hindfoot.

Treatment

Conservative measures are indicated in early and mild cases. Passive stretching exercises of the contracted plantar fascia and the short plantar muscles are performed several times a day. For comfort, a supportive insole with a 1-cm. pad just behind the metatarsals is placed in the shoe to relieve pressure from the metatarsal heads and redistribute the weight (Fig. 4–5). A Plastizote shoe insert of medium density is usually used. The toe portion of the shoes should be wide enough not to press on the toes. A 1/8- to 3/16-inch wedge on the lateral side of the heel is given if the hindfoot tends to go into inversion. Thin padding on the tongue of the shoe will relieve pressure on the dorsum of the foot. The objective of these measures is to provide symptomatic relief. Special shoes, shoe inserts, and ankle-foot orthoses neither correct cavovarus deformity of the foot nor prevent it from increasing in severity.

Surgical measures are indicated when the deformity is severe and disabling. Preoperative assessment should be thorough. The factors that determine the type of operation are as follows: (1) The *location of the apex of cavus deformity*. Is it anterior at the naviculocuneiform or tarsometatarsal joints or more posterior at the talonavicular and calcaneocuboid articulations? (2) The *type of*

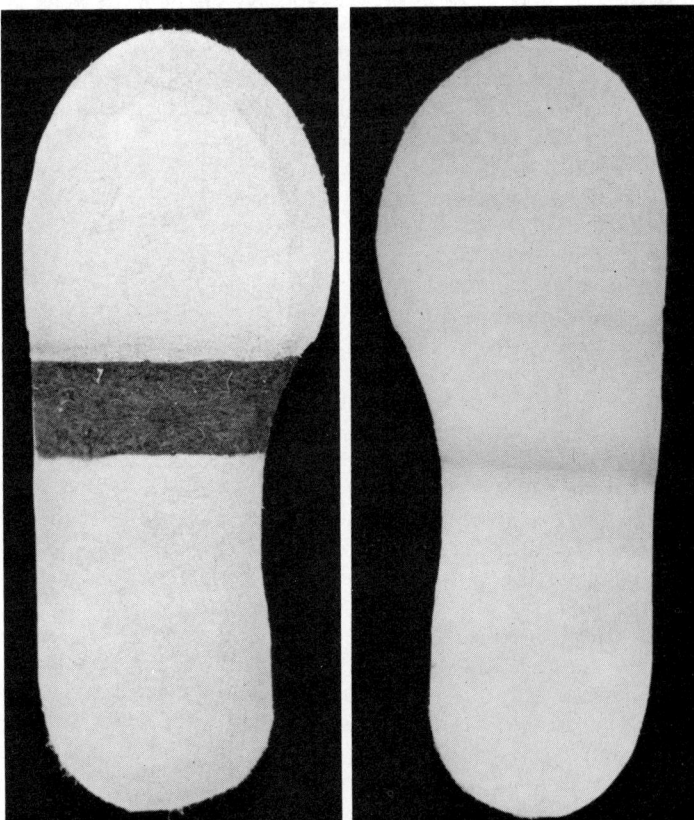

FIGURE 4–5. Insole with a 3/8-inch pad placed just behind metatarsal heads.

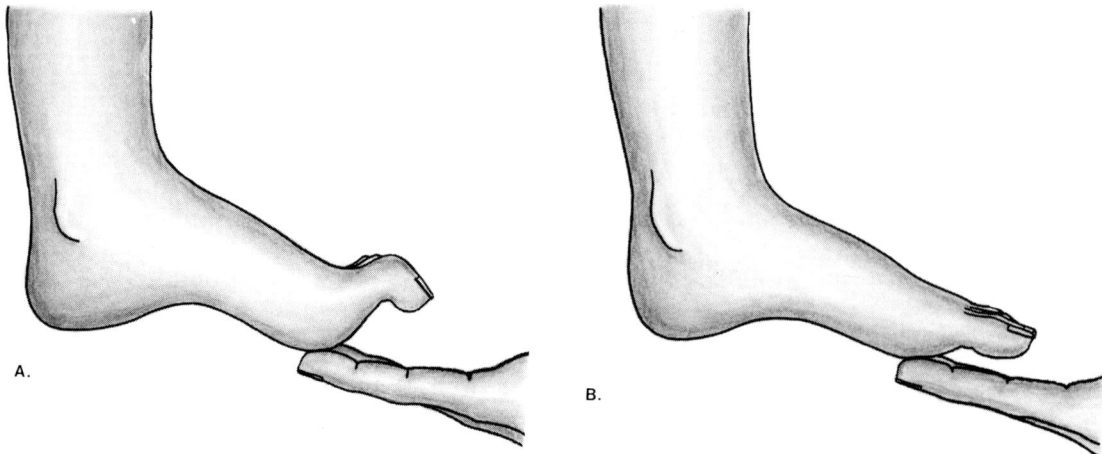

FIGURE 4–6. *Kelikian's "push-up" test for flexibility of the metatarsophalangeal and interphalangeal joints in clawfoot.*

On passive dorsiflexion of the metatarsal heads the hyperextended metatarsophalangeal joints extend to neutral position and the interphalangeal joints extend fully.

pes cavus. Is it a simple cavus or a cavovarus deformity? Is there pronation of the forefoot, particularly of the first metatarsal? (3) The *position of the hindfoot.* Is it inverted, neutral, or everted? Is there calcaneus or equinus deformity of the heel? (4) The *deformity of the toes.* Are they clawed? Do the tips of the toes touch the ground? Is there painful adventitious bursitis over the dorsum of the interphalangeal joints? How flexible is the deformity of the toes? On passive dorsiflexion of the metatarsal heads do the metatarsophalangeal joints flex from hyperextension to neutral position and do the flexed toes extend fully (Fig. 4–6)? The passive range of motion of the proximal and distal interphalangeal joints is noted. On weight-bearing, do the tips of the toes touch the floor? (5) The *condition of the sole* on the plantar aspect of the metatarsal heads. Are there painful callosities? Is the skin ulcerated? (6) The *shoe wear.* Is it abnormal? (7) The *rigidity of the deformities* and their severity. How taut are the plantar soft tissues: How far can the forefoot be dorsiflexed out of equinus posture? Is there contracture of the triceps surae muscle? Does the hindfoot evert beyond neutral on passive manipulation?

Coleman and Chestnut have described a simple test for hindfoot flexibility in the cavovarus foot (Fig. 4–7). The "cavovarus test," or standing lateral block test, is performed as follows: Place the patient's foot on a 2.5- to 4-cm.-thick wooden block with the heel and the lateral border of the foot on the block and bearing full weight while the first through third metatarsals are allowed to hang freely into plantar flexion and full pronation; this maneuver neutralizes the tripod mechanism and negates any effect that the forefoot may have on the hindfoot in stance (Fig. 4–7 A to C). A flexible hindfoot will assume a normal valgus position. The degree of correction of hindfoot varus deviation is recorded by photographs and roentgenograms. An anteroposterior roentgenogram is made of the foot with the tube directed 30 degrees cephalad toward the dome of the talus; then, with the patient still standing on the block (but without increasing the height of the block), normal weight-bearing and lateral anteroposterior roentgenograms of the foot are also made. The talocalcaneal angle is measured. If the decreased talocalcaneal angle is restored to normal value by this maneuver, the hindfoot is flexible and therapeutic efforts should be directed toward the forefoot. If, however, the talocalcaneal angle remains decreased it means the varus deformity of the hindfoot is fixed and surgical measures should be employed to correct both the forefoot and hindfoot deformations (Fig. 4–7 D to F).[26] This author finds the test to be reliable in assessing and documenting whether or not the hindfoot is flexible during stance phase. (8) *Strength of muscles* controlling foot and ankle. Is there any dynamic imbalance between the anterior tibial (dorsiflexor of the first metatarsal bone) and the peroneus longus (plantar flexor of the first metatarsal bone), and between the evertors and invertors of the foot and dorsiflexors and plantar flexors of the ankle? Is it necessary to provide stability to the foot by arthodesis? (9) *Stability of the neurologic picture.* Is there any progressive neuromuscular deficit? Can the primary neurologic affection be corrected by appropriate neurosurgical treatment? Determination of the nature of the disease process is vital. What is the rate and pattern of progression of paralysis? For example, in Charcot-Marie-Tooth disease, the posterior tibial muscle may be the only muscle left functioning for effective anterior transfer. (10) The *age of the patient* and the skeletal maturity of the foot.

In general, operative measures should be delayed until several periodic examinations have ruled out progressive neuromuscular deficit. As a rule surgical correction of pes cavus should be executed in stages in a systematic, progressive approach. First, a plantar release is always carried out. Sectioning of the taut plantar fascia, short plantar muscles, and plantar ligaments will allow

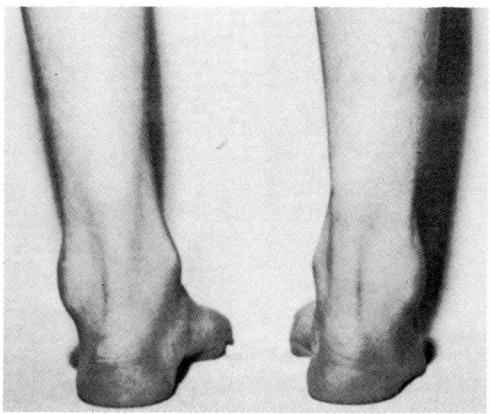

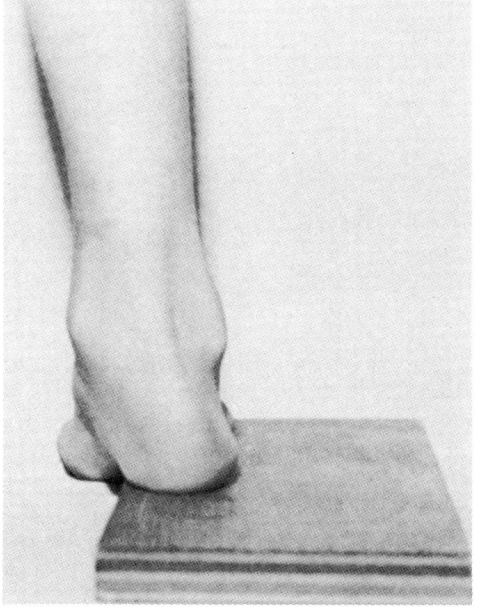

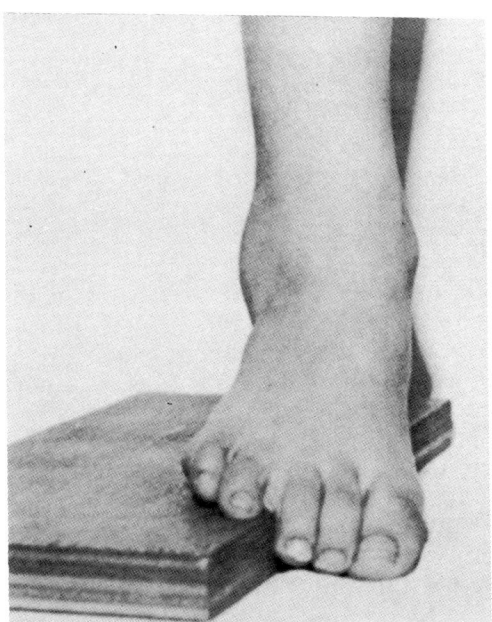

FIGURE 4–7. Test to determine hindfoot flexibility in cavovarus foot (Coleman's cavovarus test).

A. Posterior view of both feet, standing. Note the varus deformity of the right heel. **B** and **C.** Posterior and anterior views of the right foot, standing. The heel and the lateral border of the foot are bearing full weight on a block 2.5 cm. thick, whereas the first through third metatarsals are plantar-flexed into pronation.

Illustration continued on following page

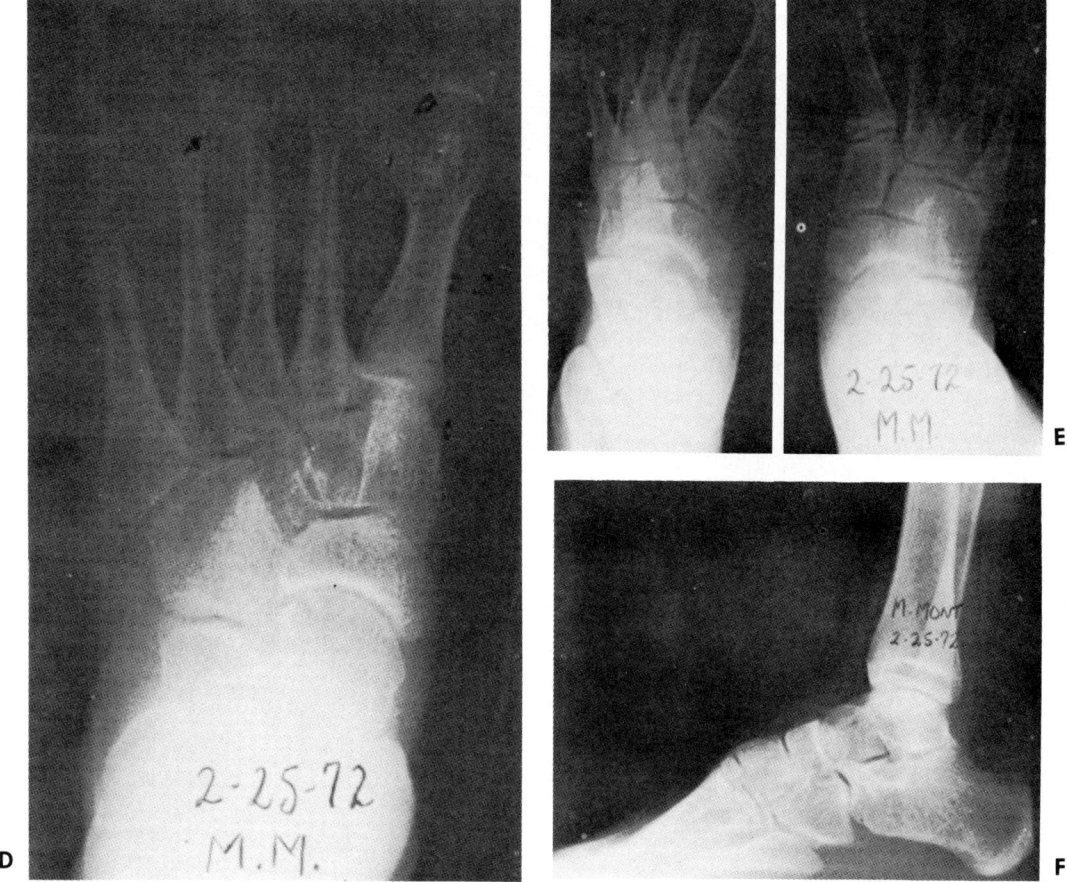

FIGURE 4–7 Continued. *Test to determine flexibility in cavovarus foot (Coleman's cavovarus test).*

D. Anteroposterior roentgenogram of the right foot with the patient standing on the block. Note the restoration of normal articulation between the talus and calcaneus; the talocalcaneal angle is normal. **E.** Standing anteroposterior roentgenogram of both feet. Note the decreased talocalcaneal angle of the cavovarus foot (on the left of the photograph). **F.** Standing lateral roentgenogram of the same right foot. Note the forefoot equinus deformity, the high arch, and the "through-and-through" visualization of the subtalar joint. (From Coleman, S. S., and Chesnut, W. J.: A simple test for hindfoot flexibility in the cavovarus foot. Clin. Orthop., *123*:60, 1977. Reprinted by permission.)

the forefoot to be elevated from equinus posture into neutral dorsiflexion. This basic dictum should never be violated. Second, the correction obtained is assessed clinically and radiologically to determine the degree of rigidity of the osseous changes. If the hindfoot varus deformity is flexible, the long toe extensor tendons are transferred to the metatarsal heads, and any invertor-evertor dynamic muscle imbalance is corrected by appropriate muscle and tendon transfers. If the varus hindfoot is rigid on the lateral block test and the forefoot cannot be elevated to neutral position, the fixed osseous changes are corrected by appropriate bony procedures prior to tendon transfers. Pes cavus is a dynamic deformity during the period of skeletal growth. Success or failure in correcting it is often determined by the diligence of detailed postoperative care.

SOFT-TISSUE PROCEDURES

Release of Contractures on Plantar Aspect of Foot

SUBCUTANEOUS SECTION OF PLANTAR APONEUROSIS. In the past, in paralytic pes cavus due to poliomyelitis, this procedure was performed when the contracture of the plantar fascia was moderate and that of the short plantar muscles was minimal. It was followed by a series of stretching casts to obtain full correction. The technique is illustrated in Plate 23A. Fibrositis of the plantar fascia is an occasional but bothersome complication of this simple procedure. This author recommends that the contracted plantar fascia be excised by open surgery rather than released by percutaneous section.

SECTION OF PLANTAR APONEUROSIS AND SHORT PLANTAR MUSCLES NEAR THEIR ORIGIN FROM TUBEROSITY OF CALCANEUS. In 1920, Steindler described a stripping operation for pes cavus in which a longitudinal incision was made on the medial side of the calcaneus, and the long plantar ligament was transversely sectioned. The flexor digitorum brevis, abductor digiti quinti, and abductor hallucis brevis were also subperiosteally stripped and released from the calcaneus.[115–117] The Steindler procedure should not be performed because the operative scar in the instep contracts, hypertrophies because of irritation from the shoe, and acts as a deforming force. Other drawbacks of the Steindler plantar fascial stripping are the potential injury to neurovascular structures and the inadequate correction of forefoot equinus deformity.

The author prefers a midline incision on the sole of the foot when contracture of plantar soft tissues is moderate. The resultant scar is minimal and not bothersome, and the exposure is adequate for the complete release of moderately contracted plantar soft tissues. The operative technique is described in Plate 23B.[109a, 128] Westin, after Lucas, performs the plantar release through a lateral incision.[128] Inadvertent injury to neurovascular structures should be avoided. It is imperative postoperatively to apply a series of stretching casts with an anterior heel for a total period of at least eight weeks.

If more extensive soft-tissue release is indicated, the procedure described by Bost, Schottstaedt, and Larsen is carried out.[15]

A curvilinear incision is made over the medial aspect of the foot; it begins over the posterior tuberosity of the calcaneus in line with skin creases, extends dorsally and anteriorly to a point 1 cm. inferior to the medial malleolus, and then extends distally to terminate at the base of the first metatarsal. Subcutaneous tissues are elevated in line with the skin incision. The wound edges are undermined, elevated, and retracted. The abductor hallucis muscle is released entirely at its origin and retracted distally. In severe cavovarus deformity this author will excise the abductor hallucis muscle; it will facilitate surgical exposure and closure of the wound.

Next, the neurovascular bundle is identified, isolated, and traced to its bifurcation into medial and lateral plantar branches. The flexor digitorum longus and flexor hallucis longus tendons are identified, and the master knot of Henry is sectioned. A generous portion of the plantar aponeurosis is excised. Next, the short flexors and plantar muscles are sectioned extraperiosteally from their calcaneal origin and dissected distally up to the talonavicular and calcaneocuboid joints. The contracted tendinous expansions of the posterior tibial tendon should be sectioned at their metatarsal and cuneiform attachments because they fix the first metatarsal in equinus posture. The Y-ligament (the calcaneocuboid and calcaneonavicular ligaments) and the plantar portion of the capsules of the cuneiforms and the first three metatarsals are sectioned. The tourniquet is released, and after complete hemostasis the wound is closed with closed suction Hemovac tubes. A below-knee cast is applied. The postoperative care is similar to that after plantar release through a midline incision.

Transfer of Long Toe Extensors to Heads of Metatarsals.[23, 44, 71, 110] This procedure is indicated when, on active dorsiflexion of the foot, the toes hyperextend but the metatarsal heads do not elevate and remain in equinus posture. The tendon transfer will increase the power of dorsiflexion of the foot and elevate the metatarsal heads, providing a dynamic force against forefoot equinus deformity. By routing the tendons from the medial to the lateral side, the transfer will also be given some inversion power, which acts against the pronation deformity of the forefoot in pes cavovarus.

For the tendon transfers to function effectively, the foot should be flexible. First, a release of contracted soft tissues on the plantar aspect of the foot is carried out. In cases of mild deformity the two procedures can be combined at the same operation; however, in moderate and severe deformities, the use of stretching casts for a period of two to three months is essential to correct

Plantar Fasciotomy and Release of Contracted Soft Tissues on Plantar Aspect of Cavus Foot

SUBCUTANEOUS SECTION OF PLANTAR APONEUROSIS

A. This procedure is performed when contracture of the plantar fascia is moderate, but that of the short plantar muscles is minimal. It is not recommended by this author.

A sharp Ryerson knife is inserted deep to the plantar fascia with the blade flat to the skin. Then the sharp edge of the blade is rotated 90 degrees, bringing its sharp edge toward the plantar fascia. By pushing it against the knife with the index finger of the opposite hand, the plantar fascia is completely divided. It is sectioned at two levels about 2.5 cm. apart, and stretched by holding the heel steady and bringing the forefoot into dorsiflexion. A below-knee walking cast is applied. The cast is changed every two to three weeks, and each time the forefoot is manipulated into further dorsiflexion. The metatarsal heads and the heel should be adequately padded and the cast well molded to prevent pressure sores.

The total period for which stretching casts should be used is about eight weeks, depending upon the severity and fixity of deformity. At night, following removal of the solid cast, the forefoot is held out of equinus and in neutral position in a posterior ankle-foot polypropylene splint; the metatarsal heads can be elevated into further dorsiflexion by a Plastizote metatarsal insert glued to the insole of the splint. The night splints are worn for several years, depending upon the cause of pes cavus and the severity of deformity. Metatarsal pads are worn in the shoes during the day. Passive stretching exercises of the plantar fascia are performed several times a day.

SECTION OF PLANTAR APONEUROSIS AND SHORT PLANTAR MUSCLES THROUGH MIDLINE INCISION

B. The Steindler stripping operation for pes cavus should not be performed because of its possible inherent complications of contracture of the scar in the instep, injury to neurovascular structures, and inadequate correction of equinus forefoot. The author recommends the following technique when contracture of plantar soft tissues is moderate.

A midline incision is made on the sole of the foot, extending from 1 cm. distal to the tuberosity of the calcaneus to the base of the metatarsals. The subcutaneous tissue is divided and the wound flaps are undermined and elevated. The central, medial, and lateral portions of the plantar aponeurosis are widely excised. The abductor hallucis is sectioned at its origin from the medial process of the tuberosity of the calcaneus and the laciniate ligament. The flexor digitorum brevis, abductor digiti quinti, and quadratus plantae muscles and the long plantar ligaments are detached from their origin on the tuberosity of the calcaneus. By keeping the dissection immediately adjacent to bone, injury to neurovascular structures is avoided. The pneumatic tourniquet is released and after complete hemostasis the skin is approximated by interrupted sutures. A below-knee walking cast is applied with the heel held in valgus posture and the forefoot in some degree of supination. This position of the foot in the cast tends to correct the cavovarus deformity by flattening the longitudinal arch. Weight-bearing is not allowed during the first postoperative week. Ten to fourteen days after surgery the cast is removed; the wound is inspected for healing, but the sutures are not removed. A new below-knee walking cast is applied. This author uses plaster of Paris cast for the first two layers and then reinforces it with several layers of plastic adhesive tape. This allows better molding of the cast and makes it much stronger. An anterior heel is applied to the cast. If the wound edges are healthy the heel is manipulated and held into a greater valgus inclination and the forefoot into further supination, obtaining additional correction of the cavovarus deformity. The patient is allowed and encouraged to walk on the cast. The casts are changed biweekly, for a total period of cast immobilization of eight weeks.

Plate 23. Plantar Fasciotomy and Release of Contracted Soft Tissues on Plantar Aspect of Cavus Foot

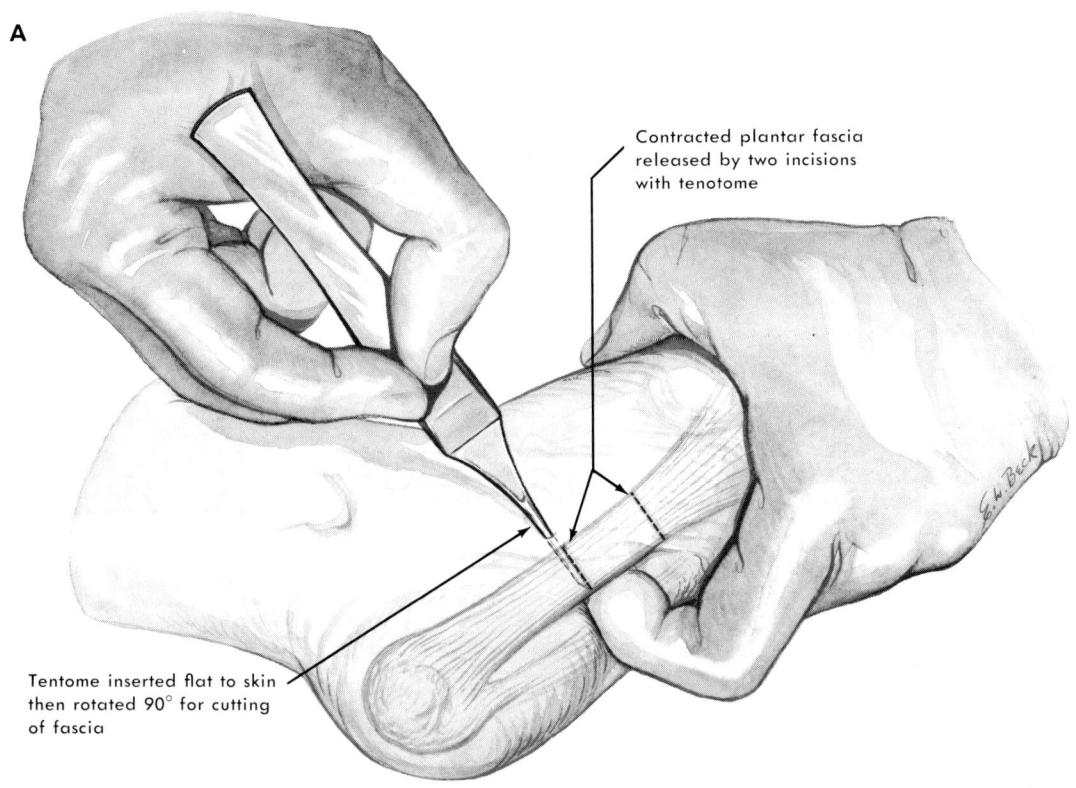

A

Contracted plantar fascia released by two incisions with tenotome

Tentome inserted flat to skin then rotated 90° for cutting of fascia

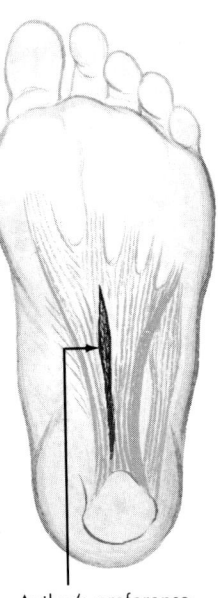

B

Author's preference: Skin incision centered on sole of foot if an open fasciotomy is necessary

the position of the forefoot. Tendon transfers are performed only when fixed cavus deformity has been fully corrected—the importance of this prerequisite cannot be overemphasized.

In 1919, Hibbs described an operation for correction of clawing of the lesser toes. The tendons of the extensor digitorum longus were divided as far distally as possible and anchored en masse into the third cuneiform bone.[64] The Hibbs operation should not be performed for pes cavus, as it fails to provide a dynamic force to elevate the metatarsal heads.

The operative technique of transfer of the long toe extensors to the metatarsal heads is described and illustrated in Plate 24. When there is associated clawing of the toes, it is combined with fusion of the proximal interphalangeal joints.

Transfer of Anterior Tibial Tendon to Dorsum of Base of First Metatarsal. This procedure, described by Fowler and associates, is combined with an opening-wedge vertical extension osteotomy of the medial cuneiform.[43] The osteotomy site is opened up on its plantar aspect and held by a triangular wedge of autogenous bone based plantarward. The osteotomized fragments are transfixed by a threaded Steinmann pin. Plantar release is always performed first. The transferred anterior tibial tendon acts as a dorsiflexor of the first metatarsal. The opening-wedge dorsiflexion osteotomy of the medial cuneiform bone elevates and elongates the medial ray of the foot. In Fowler's experience, when the hindfoot is flexible and there is satisfactory extrinsic muscle balance, the procedure will correct the cavovarus deformity. When there is fixed plantar flexion deformity of the first ray, this author recommends combination of Fowler's procedure with transfer of the extensor hallucis longus to the first metatarsal head, as shown in Figure 4–8, and of the long toe extensors to the second, third, and fourth metatarsal necks.

The anterior tibial tendon should not be transferred laterally to decrease the inversion deformity in pes cavovarus because it will enhance the action of the peroneus longus as plantar-flexor of the first metatarsal, nor should the posterior tibial tendons be lengthened in an attempt to correct hindfoot varus deformity. In paralytic pes cavovarus, as in Charcot-Marie-Tooth disease, function of the posterior tibial muscle must be preserved because it will have to be transferred anteriorly to provide dorsiflexion of the ankle and foot (see Chapter 3).

In idiopathic flexible pes cavovarus, fractional lengthening at the musculotendinous junction of the peroneus longus may be indicated to weaken its action as plantarflexor and pronator of the first metatarsal when the anterior tibial tendon is transferred to the dorsum of the base of the first metatarsal.

Selective neurectomy of the motor nerves to plantar muscles in pes cavus is not recommended by the author, as, in his experience, the results have been poor. The procedure was described by Garceau and Brahms for the treatment of paralytic cavovarus deformity of the feet following poliomyelitis; they reported encouraging results.[47] Coonrad and co-workers recommend neurectomy of the motor branches of the lateral plantar nerve and partial excision of the short toe flexors and plantar fascia in paralytic pes cavovarus.[27] Such a procedure is indicated only when the short toe flexors and other intrinsic muscles of the foot are functioning in an otherwise flail foot.

PROCEDURES ON BONE

In the adolescent or adult patient with a skeletally mature foot, osseous structural changes may fix the forefoot in marked equinus position and pronation and the hindfoot in rigid varus position. Such rigid cavovarus feet require bony procedures to correct the deformity. A number of operations have been described in the literature. In general they can be subdivided into those to correct the equinus deformity of the forefoot and those to correct the varus deformity of the hindfoot. As mentioned previously, prior to performing operations on bone, one should release the contracted soft tissues on the plantar aspect of the foot. These two procedures should be performed in separate stages.

Bony Procedures to Correct Forefoot Equinus Deformity

DORSAL TARSAL WEDGE OSTEOTOMY. Dorsal wedge resection at the level of the cuneiform and cuboid bones was devised by

Text continued on page 532

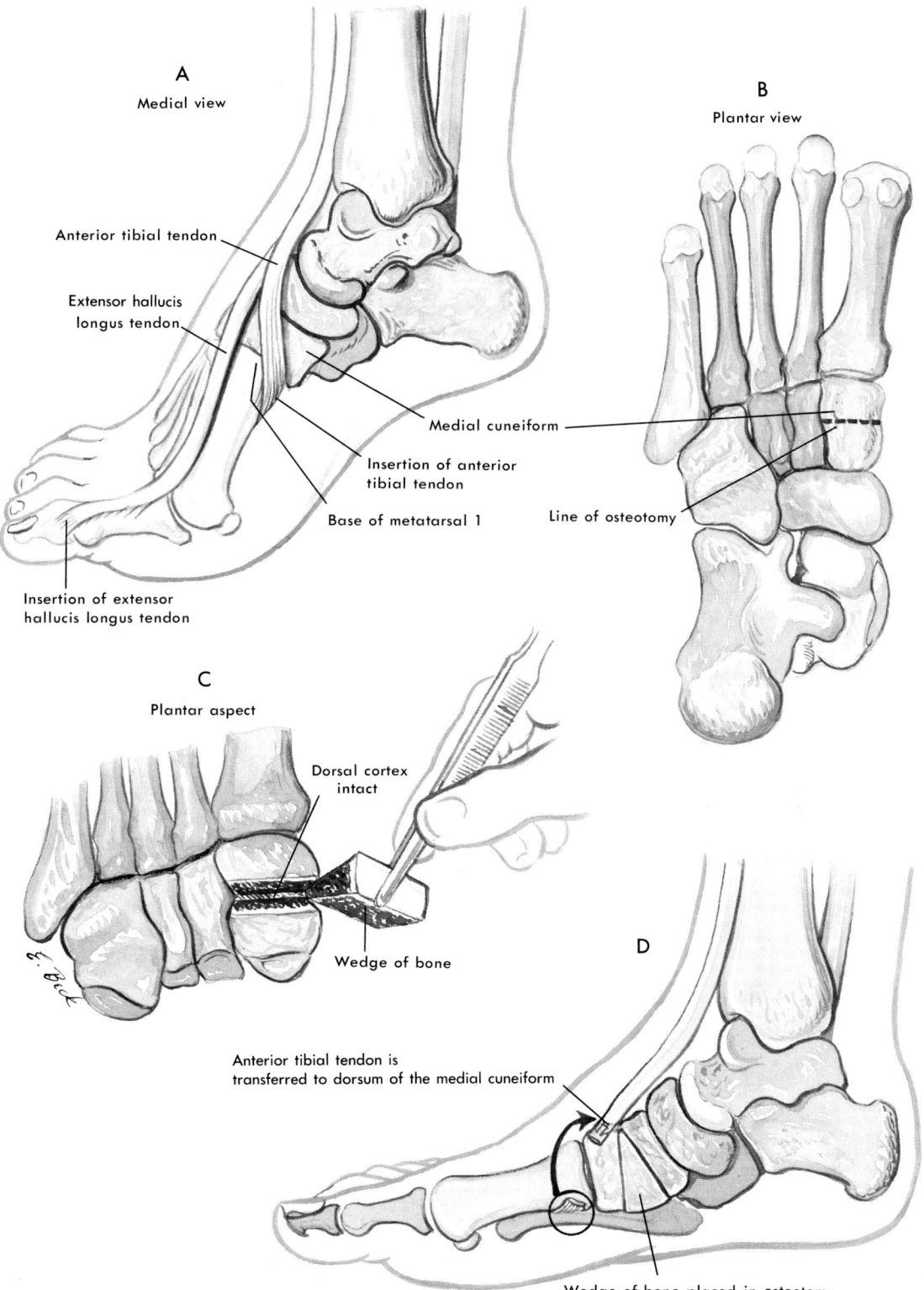

FIGURE 4–8. *Vertical osteotomy of the medial cuneiform with a wedge of bone graft based on the plantar aspect.*

This is usually combined with transfer of the anterior tibial tendon to increase action as a dorsiflexor of the first metatarsal. The extensor hallucis longus is transferred to the head of the first metatarsal.

Transfer of Long Toe Extensors to Heads of Metatarsals

A. A longitudinal incision is made on the dorsomedial aspect of the first metatarsal, extending from the base of the proximal phalanx to the proximal one fourth of the metatarsal shaft. The incision should be placed medial to the extensor hallucis longus tendon, toward the second metatarsal. The subcutaneous tissue is divided and the wound flaps are retracted with 0 silk sutures. The digital nerves and vessels should not be injured.

B. The extensor hallucis longus and brevis tendons are identified and sectioned at the base of the proximal phalanx. An alternate technique is to leave the insertion of the extensor hallucis brevis tendon intact; the stump of the extensor hallucis longus tendon is sutured to the intact brevis tendon. (This latter method is faster and is utilized by the author when the long toe extensors of all five toes are to be transferred to the heads of the metatarsals.)

C. Silk whip sutures (00) are inserted in the ends of the long and short toe extensors. The long toe extensor is dissected free, and with a sharp scalpel its sheath is thoroughly excised as far proximally as possible.

D. The epiphyseal plate of the first metatarsal is proximal, whereas that of the lateral four metatarsals is distal in location. The extensor hallucis longus tendon is transferred to the head of the first metatarsal. The long toe extensors of the lesser toes are transferred to the distal one third of the metatarsal shafts, with care taken not to disturb the growth plate. When the patient is over the age of 10 to 12 years, the tendons are transferred to the heads of the metatarsals, as by then, growth of the foot is almost complete.

With small Chandler elevator retractors, the soft tissues are retracted. The periosteum is not stripped. Through a stab wound in the periosteum, a hole is drilled in the center of the first metatarsal head and is enlarged to receive the tendon. The extensor hallucis longus tendon is passed through the hole in the first metatarsal in a medial to lateral direction and sutured to itself, with the forefoot in maximal dorsiflexion.

E. The extensor hallucis brevis tendon is then sutured to the stump of the long toe extensor, holding the toe in neutral extension or in 10 degrees of dorsiflexion.

A similar technique is employed to transfer the long extensor tendons of the lesser toes. Longitudinal incisions are made between the second and third metatarsals, and between the fourth and fifth metatarsals. The extensor brevis tendon of the little toe is either absent or not of adequate size to transfer to the stump of the longus.

The tourniquet is released and complete hemostasis is obtained. The wounds are closed with interrupted sutures. A below-knee walking cast is applied, to be worn for four to six weeks. A sturdy well-padded toe plate is made in the cast. The plantar aspect of the metatarsals should be well padded.

Special muscle training for the transferred tendons is not required, as the transfer is in phase.

Plate 24. Transfer of Long Toe Extensors to Heads of Metatarsals

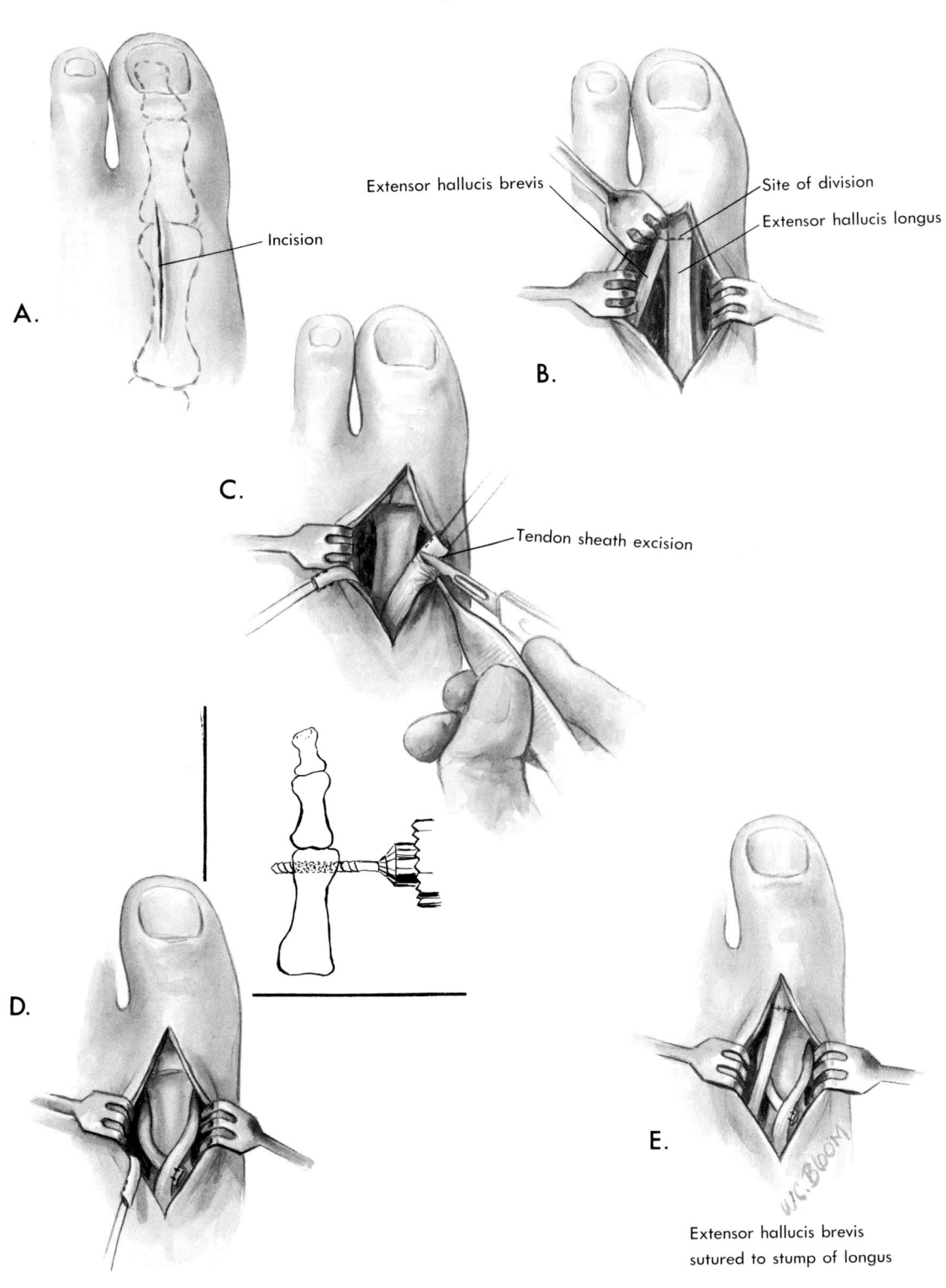

A. Incision

B. Extensor hallucis brevis — Site of division — Extensor hallucis longus

C. Tendon sheath excision

D. Extensor hallucis longus passed through hole in metatarsal head and sutured to itself

E. Extensor hallucis brevis sutured to stump of longus

Dorsal Wedge Resection for Pes Cavus

The dorsal aspect of the tarsal bones may be exposed by several means. Cole and Japas make a single dorsal longitudinal incision approximately 6 to 8 cm. long in the midline of the foot, centering over the midtarsal arch (naviculocuneiform junction). Subcutaneous tissue is divided, and the long toe extensors are identified and separated. The plane between the long extensor tendons of the second and third toes is developed, and the extensor digitorum brevis muscle is identified, elevated, and retracted laterally with the peroneus brevis tendon. The anterior tibial tendon and the long extensor tendons of the second and big toes are retracted medially. The periosteum is incised, longitudinally elevated, and retracted medially and laterally.[25, 70]

Méary makes two longitudinal incisions, each about 5 to 6 cm. in length on the dorsum of the foot. The medial incision is parallel to the longitudinal axis of the second metatarsal and is centered over the intermediate cuneiform bone. The extensor hallucis longus tendon, dorsalis pedis vessels, and the anterior tibial tendon are identified, dissected free, and retracted medially. The lateral incision is about 3 cm. long, and is centered over the cuboid bone. The peroneus brevis is identified and retracted laterally.

This author uses two longitudinal incisions, one dorsolateral and the other medial.

THE PROCEDURE

A and **B.** Two longitudinal skin incisions are made. The medial incision, about 5 cm. long, is over the medial aspect of the navicular and first cuneiform bones in the interval between the anterior tibial and posterior tibial tendons. The subcutaneous tissue is divided. The anterior tibial tendon is retracted dorsally; the posterior tibial tendon is partially detached from the tuberosity of the navicular and is retracted plantarward to expose the medial and dorsal aspects of the navicular and first cuneiform bones. The dorsolateral incision, about 4 cm. long, is centered over the cuboid bone. The extensor brevis muscle is identified, elevated, and retracted distally and laterally with the peroneus brevis tendon. The long toe extensors are retracted medially.

C. Next, through the medial wound, the capsule and periosteum of the navicular and first cuneiform bones are incised and elevated. The soft tissues are retracted dorsally and plantarward with Chandler elevator retractors. The capsule of the talonavicular joint should not be disturbed. If in doubt, one should take roentgenograms to identify the tarsal bones with certainty.

D and **E.** With osteotomes, a wedge of bone is excised, including the naviculocuneiform articulation. The base of the wedge is dorsal, its width depending upon the severity of the forefoot equinus deformity to be corrected. Through the dorsolateral incision, the wedge osteotomy of the cuboid is completed.

F. The forefoot is then manipulated into dorsiflexion. If the plantar fascia is contracted, a plantar fasciotomy is performed. In severe cases the short plantar muscles are also sectioned. The first cuneiform bone should be dorsally displaced over the navicular bone. Two Steinmann pins are inserted to transfix the tarsal osteotomy. The medial pin is inserted into the shaft of the first metatarsal, directed posteriorly through the first cuneiform, across the osteotomy site into the navicular and the head of the talus. The lateral pin is started posteriorly along the longitudinal axis of the calcaneus, across the calcaneocuboid joint, into the cuboid and the base of the fifth metatarsal. (Méary uses staples to maintain position of the osteotomy.) Roentgenograms are taken to verify the position of the pins and the maintenance of correction of forefoot equinus deformity. The tourniquet is released and complete hemostasis is obtained. The incisions are closed. The pins are cut subcutaneously and a below-knee cast is applied.

POSTOPERATIVE CARE

The foot and leg are immobilized for six weeks, at which time the cast, pins, and sutures are removed. A new below-knee walking cast is given—to be worn for another two to four weeks.

Plate 25. Dorsal Wedge Resection for Pes Cavus

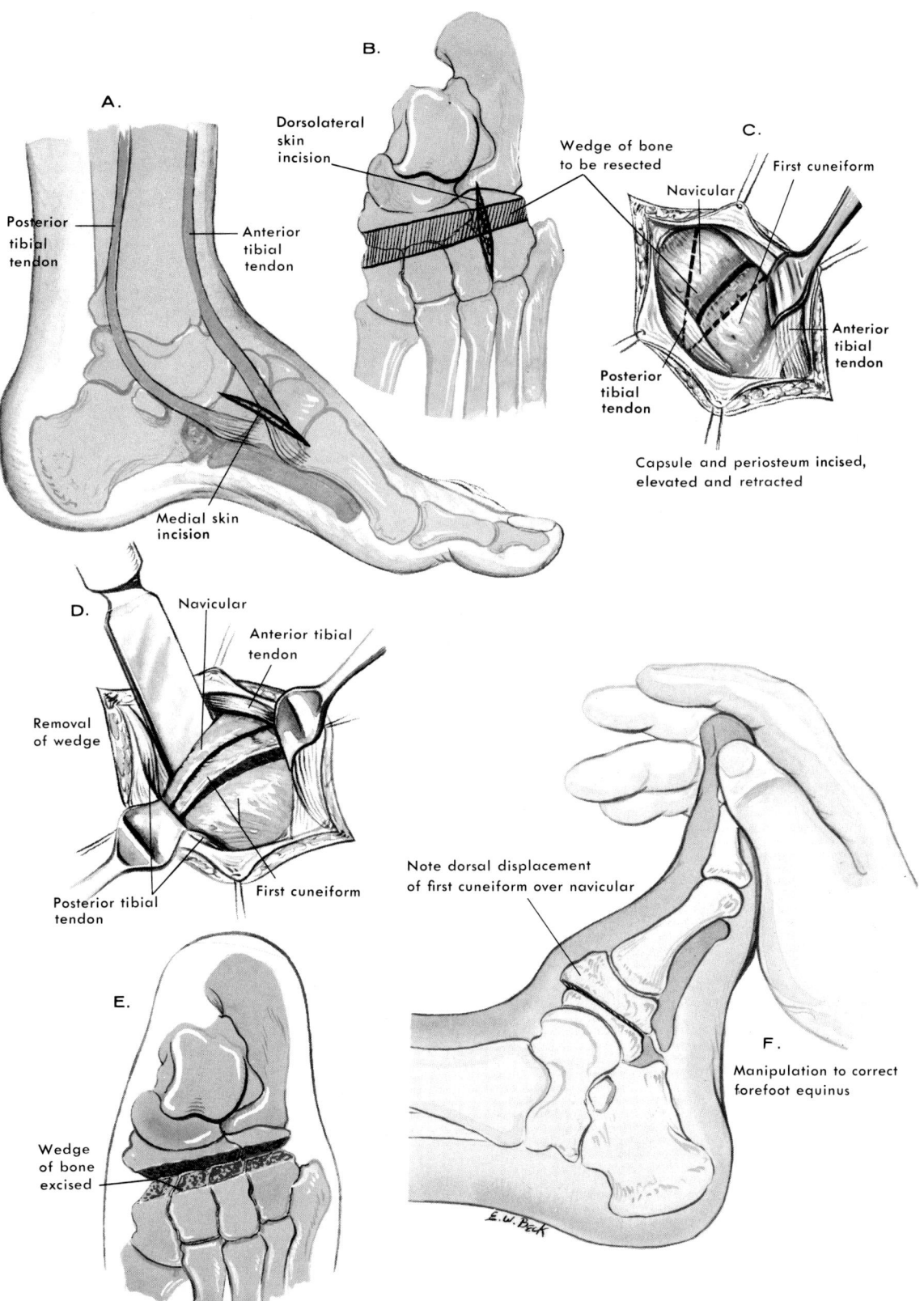

Saunders and popularized by Cole.[25, 102] It is described and illustrated in Plate 25. While preserving motion at the metatarsotarsal, midtarsal, and subtalar joints, the operation corrects the cavus deformity, provided the apex of the arch is at the midfoot. It should always be preceded by release of the contracted plantar soft tissues. Often equinus deformity of the first metatarsal will persist, necessitating a dorsiflexion osteotomy of the first metatarsal at its base or first metatarsocuneiform fusion for correction at a later stage. Wedge resection of the tarsus will shorten the foot—it should therefore never be performed in a skeletally immature foot. Circulatory insufficiency of the toes is a definite hazard. The procedure should not be combined with Dwyer osteotomy of the os calcis for correction of varus heel, since gangrene of the toes is a probable complication.

V-Osteotomy of the Tarsus. This procedure for pes cavus, originally described by Japas, is shown in Plate 26.[70] The foot is not shortened by resection of a bone wedge. The forefoot is elevated by depressing the base of the distal fragment plantarward. The procedure lengthens the concave plantar surface of the foot. Japas recommends the operation in children over six years of age. The author's personal experience with the procedure is limited; at present it is utilized in the skeletally mature foot in cases of unilateral involvement when length of the foot and shoe size are important considerations.

First Metatarsotarsal Dorsal Wedge Resection with Fusion and Dorsal Wedge Osteotomy of Lateral Four Metatarsals at Their Bases. This procedure is indicated in the skeletally immature foot when the apex of the cavus deformity is located anteriorly in the metatarsotarsal area, especially when painful keratoses develop on the plantar aspect of the foot under the metatarsal heads. The physes of the lateral four metatarsals are distal, and osteotomy at their bases will not disturb growth. The growth plate of the first metatarsal is proximal; therefore, to prevent physeal injury, dorsal wedge resection and fusion of the first metatarsocuneiform joint is performed (Fig. 4–9). The lateral four tarsometatarsal joints are left intact. The base of the wedge is dorsal, measuring 8 to 15 mm. The osteotomy is performed with an oscillating saw and finished with an osteotome. Care is exercised to avoid rotational malalignment. The joint of the first metatarsal and the cuneiform is fixed internally with a Steinmann pin.

In the skeletally mature foot in which previous dorsal tarsal wedge resection has failed to correct fixed equinus deformity of the metatarsals, and when the apex of the deformity is at the tarsometatarsal joints, dorsal wedge osteotomy of all five metatarsals is performed at their bases, leaving the tarsometatarsal articulation intact (Fig. 4–10). The slight remaining mobility of the Lisfranc joint will be of definite functional help. The bases of all five metatarsals and the tarsometatarsal joints are exposed through a transverse or longitudinal incision. The shape of the osteotomy is cuneiform, with a buttress based plantarward. In order to avoid sloughing of the skin edges, the wound flaps should be retracted gently and the cast should be padded on the dorsum of the foot. Excessive correction will result in painful bony prominences at the bases of the metatarsals. Rotational malalignment or adduction or abduction of the distal fragments will produce deformities of the forefoot.

Fusion of the First Metatarsocuneiform Joint. McElvenny and Caldwell proposed that varus distortion of the hindfoot in pes cavovarus is caused by pronation of the first metatarsal. They recommended elevation and supination of the first metatarsal and fusion of the first metatarsocuneiform joint in this position. If the forefoot dropped into equinus position in this area, they also fused the naviculocuneiform joint. They stressed that only the first metatarsal should be supinated, not the entire forefoot. If the cavovarus deformity was fixed, they recommended plantar fasciotomy and a series of stretching casts to correct the hindfoot varus deformity and to provide flexibility to the forefoot.[83]

Vertical Opening-Wedge Osteotomy of Medial Cuneiform. The vertical osteotomy with a wedge of bone graft based on the plantar aspect was recommended by Fowler and associates to elevate the first metatarsal into dorsiflexion as described earlier.[43]

Dorsal Wedge Resection and Fusion of Talonavicular and Calcaneocuboid Joints. This is carried out when the

Text continued on page 538

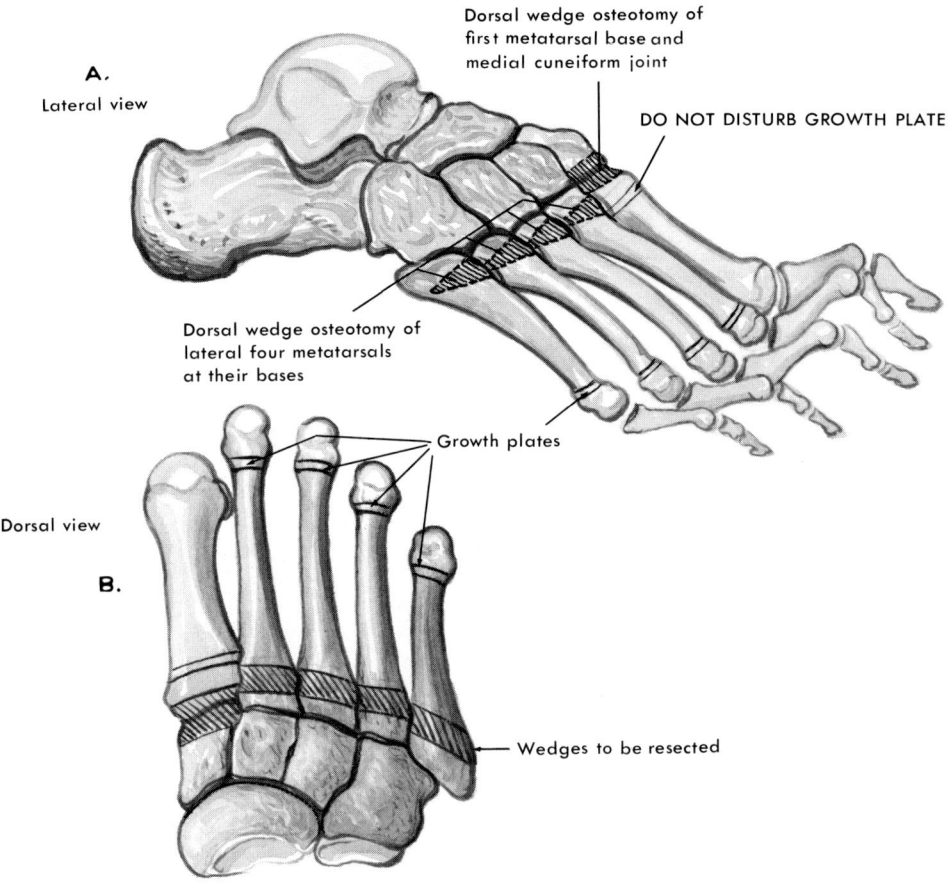
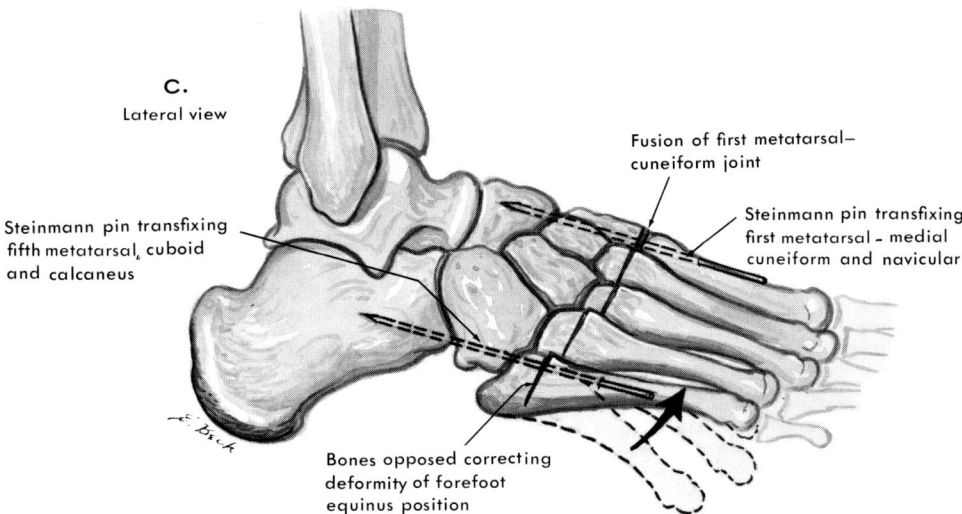

FIGURE 4–9. *Dorsal wedge osteotomy of the lateral four metatarsals at their bases with dorsal wedge osteotomy and fusion of the first metatarsal–cuneiform joint.*

Japas V-Osteotomy of the Tarsus

THE PROCEDURE

A. The dorsal aspect of the tarsal bones is exposed by a longitudinal incision 6 to 8 cm. long in the midline of the foot, i.e., between the second and third rays; it is centered over the midtarsal area at the naviculocuneiform junction.

B and **C.** The subcutaneous tissue is divided. The superficial nerves are isolated and protected. The long toe extensor tendons are identified and separated, and the plane between those of the second and third toes is developed. The extensor digitorum brevis muscle is identified, extraperiosteally elevated, and retracted laterally with the peroneal tendons. The extensor hallucis longus tendon, dorsalis pedis vessels, and anterior tibial tendon are identified, dissected free, and retracted medially. The osteotomy site is exposed extraperiosteally.

The talonavicular joint is identified next. Caution! Do not injure the midtarsal joint and compromise its function. If bony landmarks are distorted, roentgenograms are made for proper orientation. Inadvertent partial ostectomy of the head of the talus will result in aseptic necrosis and traumatic arthritis. The V line of the osteotomy is marked; its apex is located in the midline of the foot at the height of the arch of the cavus deformity; its medial limb extends to the middle of the medial cuneiform, exiting proximal to the cuneiform–first metatarsal joint, and its lateral limb extends to the middle of the cuboid, emerging proximal to the cuboid–fifth metatarsal joint. Often the V is shallow, shaped more like a dome.

Plate 26. Japas V-Osteotomy of the Tarsus

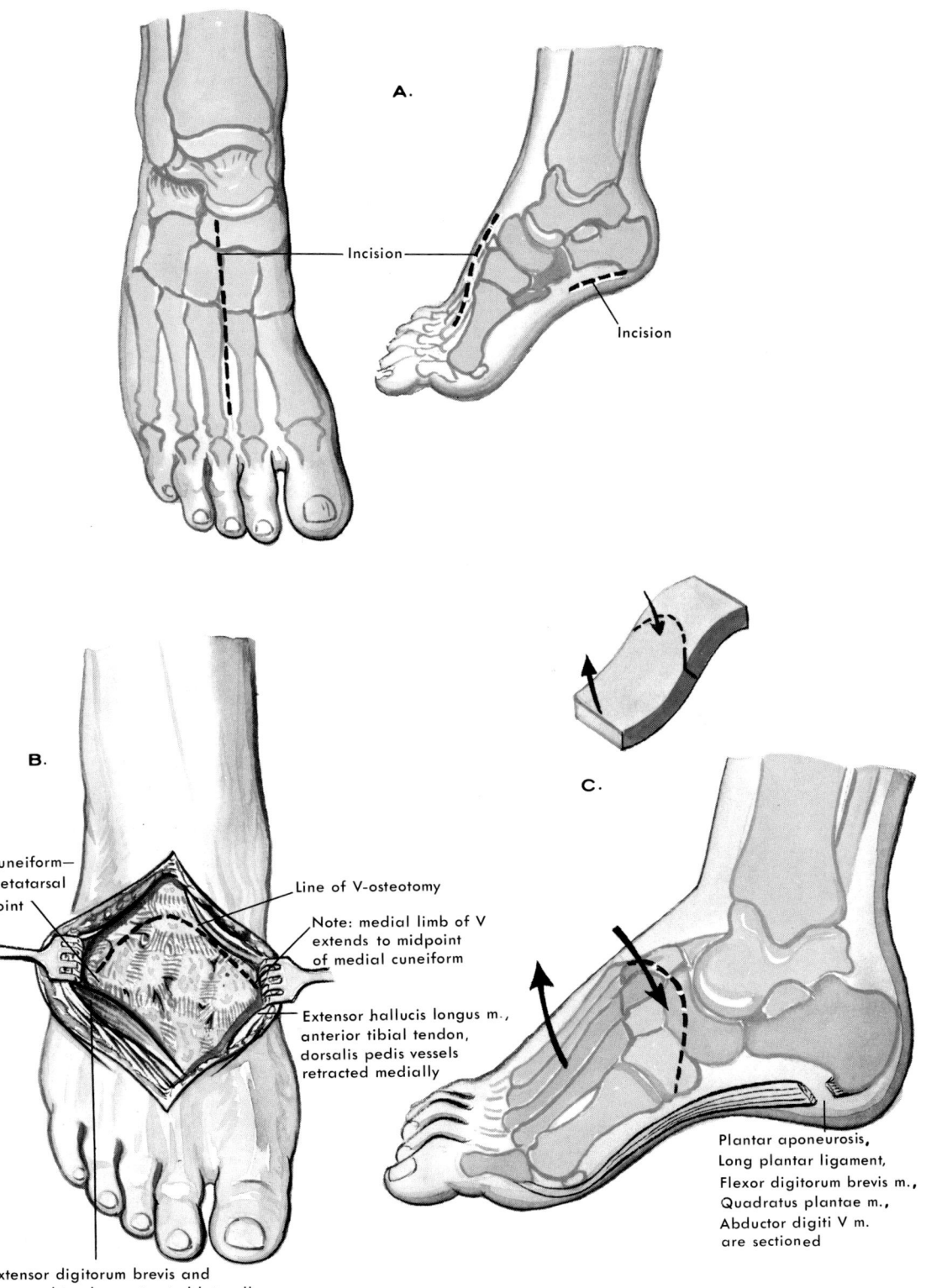

Japas V-Osteotomy of the Tarsus (Continued)

D and **E.** The osteotomy is begun with an oscillating bone saw and completed with an osteotome. Splintering of the ends of the medial and lateral limbs should be avoided. Next, a curved periosteal elevator is inserted into the osteotomy site, manual traction is applied on the forefoot, and with the elevator used as a lever, the base of the distal fragment is depressed plantarward. This maneuver corrects the cavus deformity and lengthens the concave plantar surface of the foot. The foot is not shortened, as it would be by resection of a bone wedge, and any abduction or adduction deformity can be corrected if necessary.

F. Once desired alignment is achieved, a single Steinmann pin is inserted through the distal part of the first metatarsal and directed posteriorly and laterally to terminate in the lateral part of the calcaneus or the cuboid. Roentgenograms are made to verify the completeness of correction. Then the tourniquet is removed, hemostasis obtained, and the wound closed with interrupted sutures. The pin is cut subcutaneously, and a below-knee cast is applied.

POSTOPERATIVE CARE

Two weeks after surgery a walking heel is placed posteriorly—under the long axis of the tibia—and gradual partial weight-bearing is permitted with crutches. In six weeks the cast, sutures, and Steinmann pin are removed. Roentgenograms are made. If healing is not adequate, another below-knee cast is applied for an additional two to four weeks.

Plate 26. Japas V-Osteotomy of the Tarsus

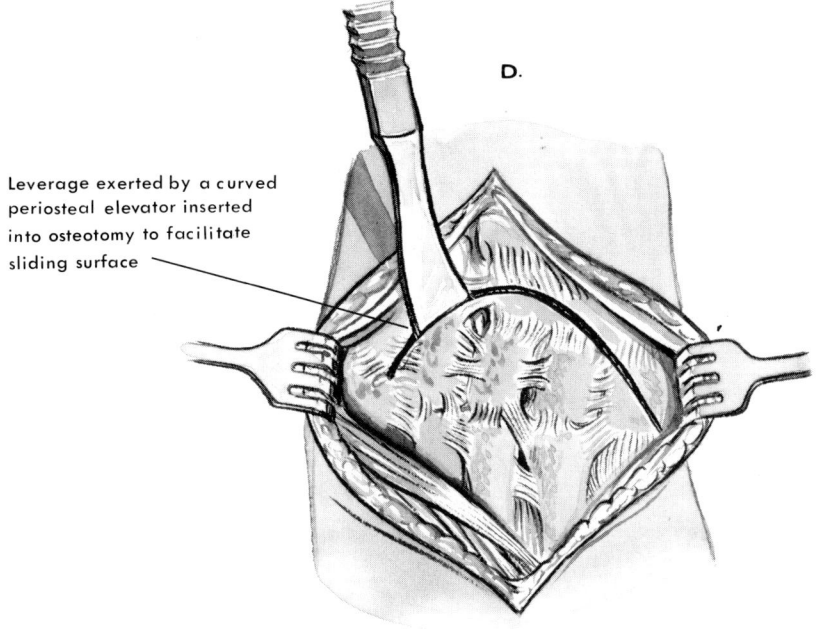

D.

Leverage exerted by a curved periosteal elevator inserted into osteotomy to facilitate sliding surface

E.

Forefoot elevated by depressing base of distal fragment plantarward

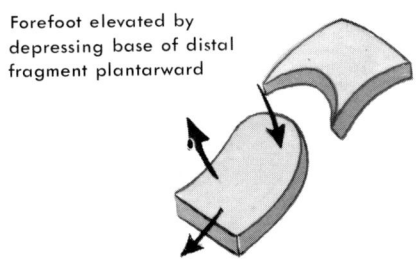

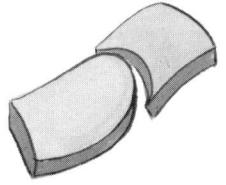

Distal traction applied on forefoot

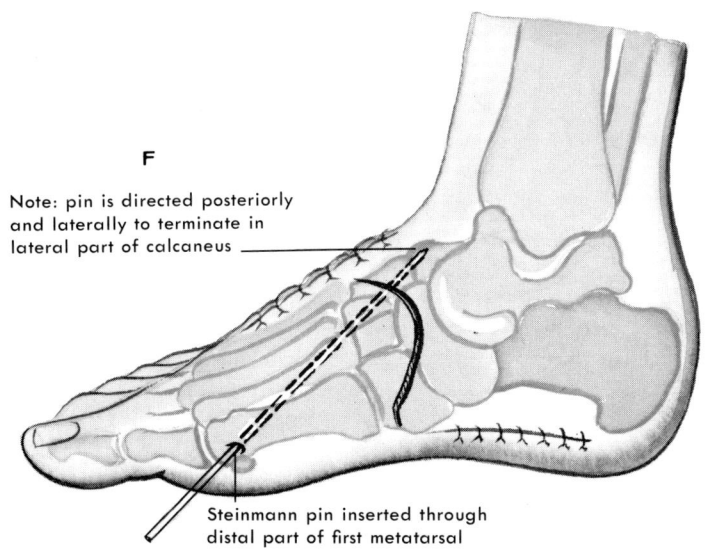

F

Note: pin is directed posteriorly and laterally to terminate in lateral part of calcaneus

Steinmann pin inserted through distal part of first metatarsal

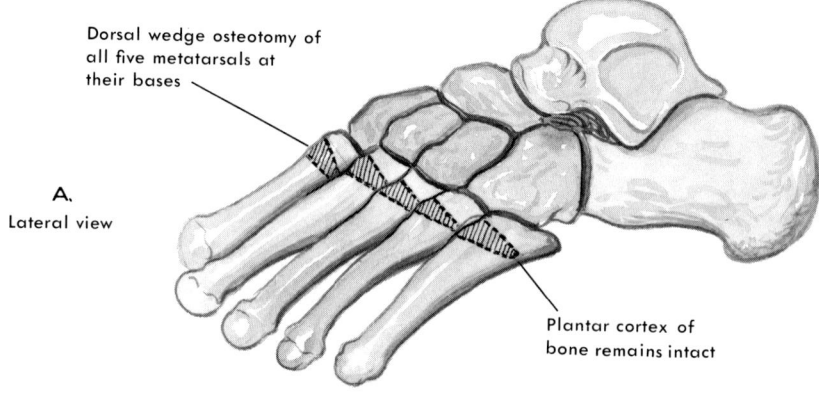

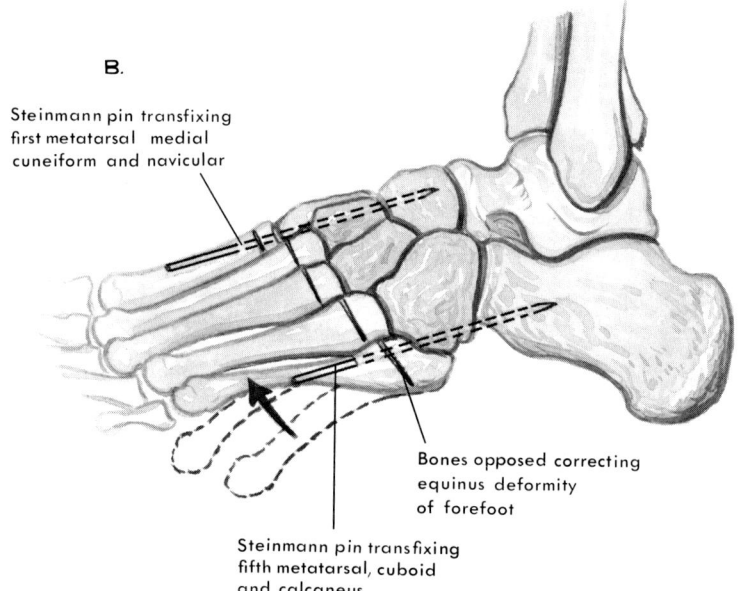

FIGURE 4–10. *Dorsal wedge osteotomy of all five metatarsals at their base.*

apex of pes cavus is more posterior in the midtarsal area. It is usually combined with subtalar fusion to correct any hindfoot varus distortion that is present. In paralytic pes cavovarus, triple arthrodesis will provide stability and at the same time correct the deformity.

"BEAK" TRIPLE ARTHRODESIS. In this technique, described by Siffert, correction of severe pes cavus and flattening of the arch is obtained by downward displacement and depression of the proximal end of the forefoot segment under the head and neck of the talus (Figs. 4–11, 4–12, and 4–13). The operation is performed through medial and lateral incisions. The subtalar and calcaneocuboid joints are denuded of hyaline articular cartilage as in an ordinary triple arthrodesis. The cartilage on the proximal surface and the cortex on the dorsal surface of the navicular bone are resected. Appropriate wedges are resected from the calcaneocuboid joint. The soft tissues on the dorsum of the talus and anterior part of

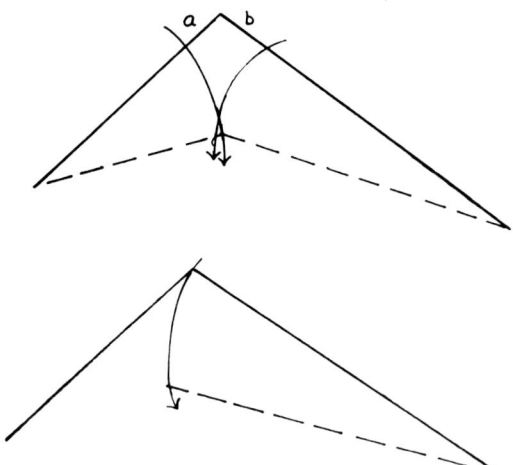

FIGURE 4–11. *The principle of "beak" triple arthrodesis for correction of severe posterior cavus deformity.*

Top. In order to obtain adequate flattening of the arch, an extensive amount of bone has to be resected from the talar head (a) and the navicular and cuneiform bones (b). This may compromise circulation to the talus. *Bottom.* The same degree of flattening of the arch is achieved by plantar displacement and depression of the proximal end of the forefoot segment under the head and neck of the talus. (From Siffert, R. S., Forster, R. I., and Nachamie, B.: "Beak" triple arthrodesis for correction of severe cavus deformity. Clin. Orthop., 45:102, 1966. Reprinted by permission.)

the talus should not be disturbed. In severe deformity the navicular may have to be excised; in such an instance the proximal and dorsal surfaces of the medial cuneiform are denuded. Then the inferior one half or one third of the talar head and neck are undercut to form a "beak" (a dorsal buttress). Next, the proximal end of the forefoot is pushed downward, and the navicular is locked under the talar beak. The bone segments are usually stable in their corrected position, and a plaster cast is adequate to maintain it. Occasionally one or two staples or threaded Steinmann pins (across the talocalcaneal and calcaneocuboid joints) are inserted for secure internal fixation.[111] This author finds the procedure effective in correcting posterior cavus deformity. It has the definite advantages of preserving circulation to the neck of the talus and maintaining the integrity of the anterior capsular and ligamentous structures of the ankle joint.

CLOSE-UP LATERAL WEDGE OSTEOTOMY OF CALCANEUS (DWYER). This procedure is combined with a release of contracted soft tissues on the plantar aspect of the foot for correction of varus hindfoot.[34] The operation should only be performed in children over eight years of age; the operative tech-

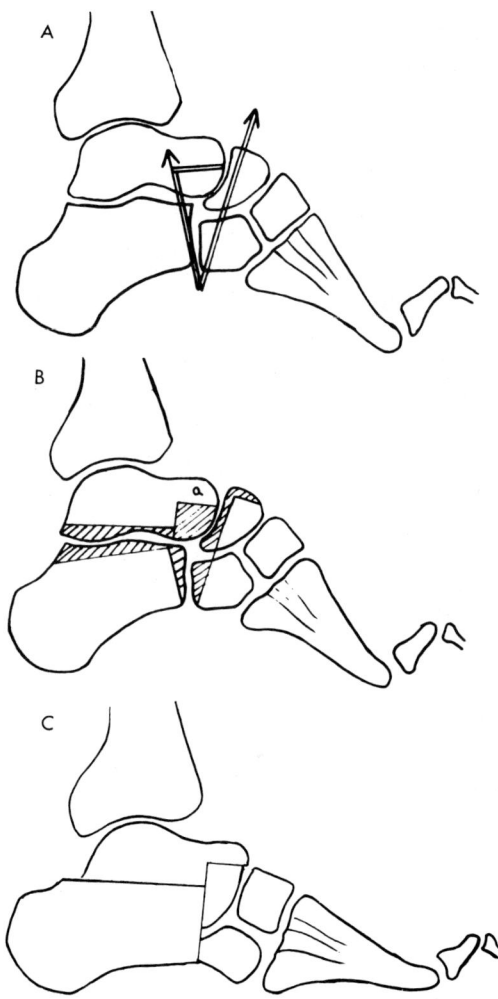

FIGURE 4–12. *Technique of "beak" triple arthrodesis for correction of severe pes cavus deformity.*

Medial and lateral incisions are employed for exposure of the subtalar, talonavicular, and calcaneocuboid joints. With the exception of the head of the talus, all joint surfaces are denuded of hyaline cartilage as in an ordinary triple arthrodesis. A dorsal-based wedge is removed from the calcaneocuboid joint and navicular bone. The plantar half or one third of the talar head-neck is resected to form a beak. Care is taken not to disturb the soft tissues in the superior aspect of the talus and anterior part of the ankle joint. **A.** The lines of osteotomy are indicated. **B.** The area of bone resected is shown by hatched areas. **C.** The final result demonstrating correction of the cavus deformity. Note that the forefoot is displaced plantarward and locked under the talar beak. (From Siffert, R. S., Forster, R. I., and Nachamie, B.: "Beak" triple arthrodesis for correction of severe cavus deformity. Clin. Orthop., 45:102, 1966. Reprinted by permission.)

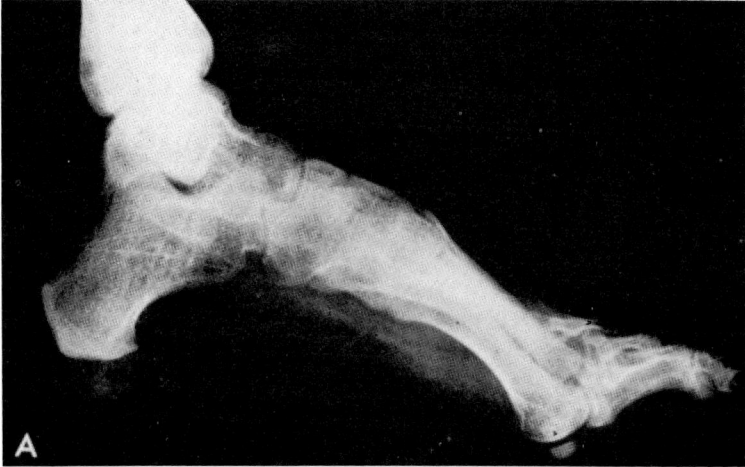
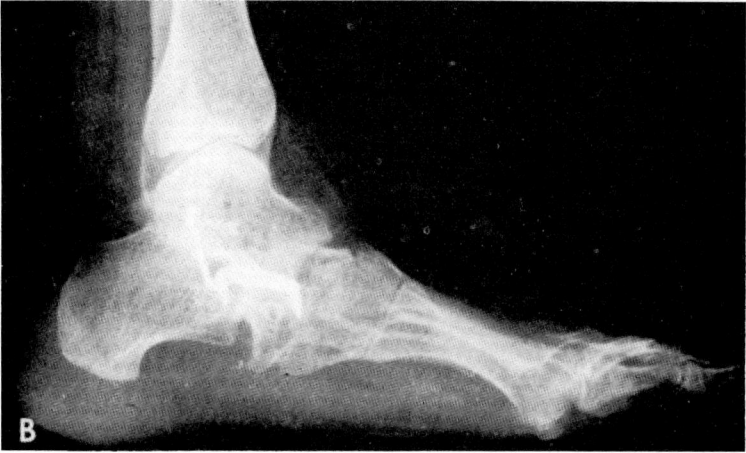

FIGURE 4–13. *Roentgenograms of the left foot showing the correction obtained by "beak" triple arthrodesis in a postpoliomyelitic cavus foot.*

A. Preoperative roentgenogram. **B.** Postoperative roentgenogram. Note the displacement of the forefoot under the talar beak and the excellent degree of correction obtained. (From Siffert, R. S., Forster, R. I., and Nachamie, B.: "Beak" triple arthrodesis for correction of severe cavus deformity. Clin. Orthop., 45:104, 1966. Reprinted by permission.)

nique is described and illustrated in Plate 27.

Bony Procedures to Correct Hindfoot Varus Deformity

In the skeletally mature foot the varus deformity of the hindfoot may be so rigid that soft-tissue releases alone are ineffective and bony procedures are required for correction. In the orthopedic arsenal, procedures available are Dwyer's osteotomy of the calcaneus (either medial opening- or lateral closing-wedge), lateral displacement osteotomy of the calcaneus, and triple arthrodesis. An axial (or Harris) view of the calcaneus is made. If there is true varus deformity of the calcaneus, Dwyer's closeup lateral wedge osteotomy of the calcaneus is indicated; the operative technique is described and illustrated in Plate 27.[34] This author does not recommend openingwedge osteotomy of the calcaneus, as the vertical height of the hindfoot is not a consideration in pes cavus and wound healing problems are greater in opening-wedge than in closing-wedge osteotomy. The operation should be performed only in children over eight years of age and it should be preceded by or combined with a plantar release.

Lateral displacement osteotomy of the calcaneus is indicated when the hindfoot varus deformity is fixed but the calcaneus is not derotated medially. Triple arthrodesis is indicated in paralytic pes cavovarus when provision of stability is desirable or when the fixed varus deformity is at the subtalar or talocalcaneonavicular joints. This author recommends that in general it is best not to combine forefoot and hindfoot operations at one stage.

OSTEOTOMY OF THE CALCANEUS FOR CORRECTION OF PES CALCANEOCAVUS. In the past pes calcaneus was corrected by an

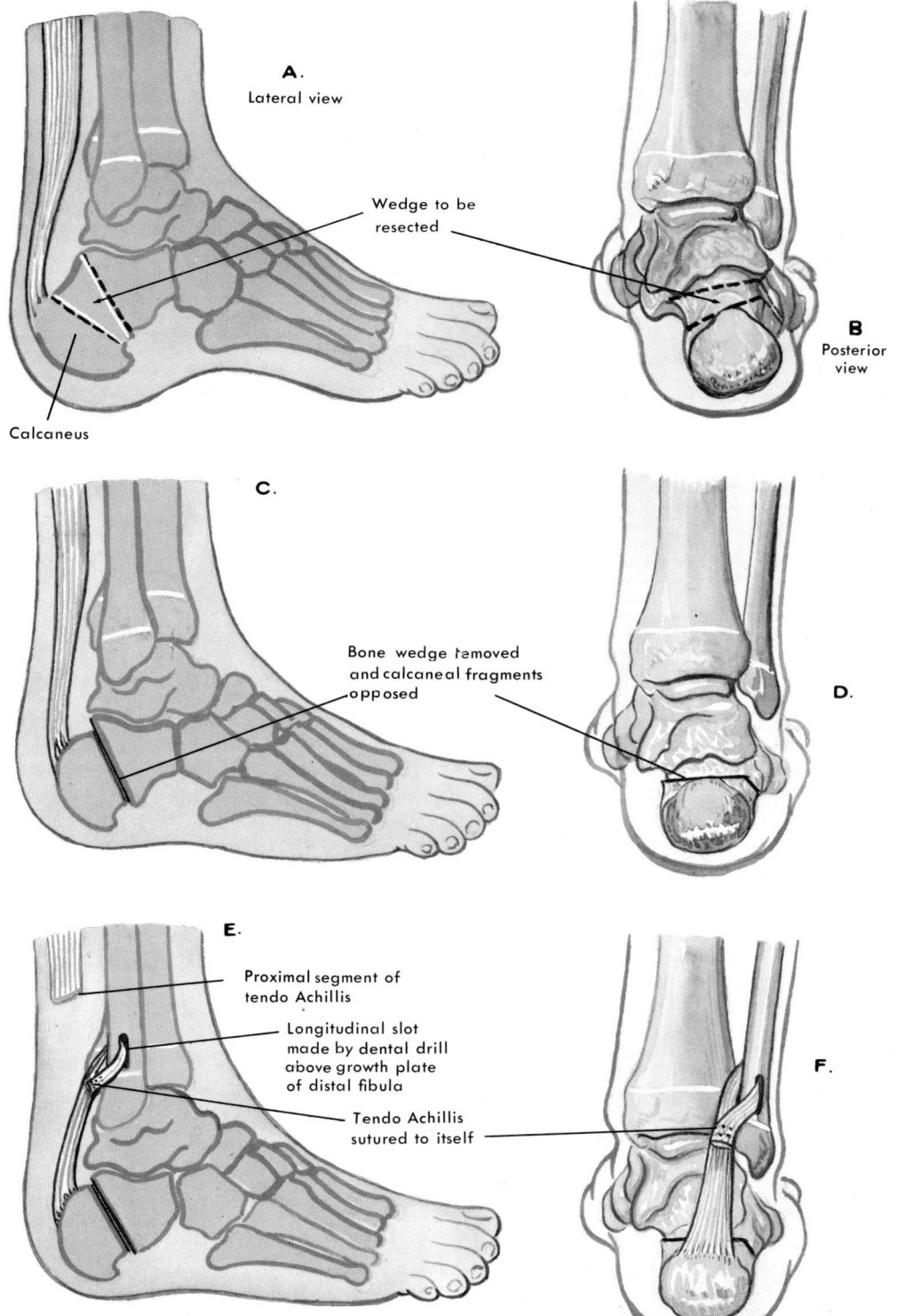

FIGURE 4–14. Correction of calcaneus deformity of the hindfoot by resection of a dorsal wedge from the os calcis.

A and **C.** A wedge, based superiorly and as wide as possible, is excised from the dorsal surface of the calcaneus. The height of the os calcis is reduced and the heel is brought closer to the plane of the forefoot. **B** and **D.** By taking the bone wedge wider on its medial or lateral side, valgus or varus deformity of the hindfoot can be corrected. In this drawing the base of the wedge is medial to correct the valgus heel. **E** and **F.** Tenodesis of the Achilles tendon to the distal fibular metaphysis is performed when the triceps surae is zero in motor strength and there is associated valgus deformity of the ankle.

Dwyer Lateral Wedge Resection of Calcaneus for Pes Cavus

Forefoot equinus deformity is corrected first, either by plantar soft-tissue release or by dorsal wedge tarsal resection, depending upon the age of the patient and the severity of the deformity. Close-up lateral wedge resection of the os calcis is designed to correct the varus deformity of the hindfoot in which the heel is of adequate height and size.

THE PROCEDURE

A. A 5-cm.-long oblique incision is made on the lateral aspect of the calcaneus parallel to, but 1.5 cm. posterior and inferior to, the peroneus longus tendon. The subcutaneous tissue is divided and the wound flaps are retracted.

B and **C.** The peroneal tendons are identified and retracted dorsally and distally. The calcaneofibular ligament is sectioned, and the periosteum is incised. The lateral surface of the calcaneus is subperiosteally exposed; with Chandler elevator retractors, the superior and inferior aspects of the calcaneus are partially exposed. With a pair of osteotomes of adequate width, a wedge of the os calcis with its base directed laterally is excised. The site of osteotomy is immediately inferior and posterior to the peroneus longus tendon. The medial cortex should be left intact. The width of the base of the wedge depends upon the severity of the varus deformity of the heel.

D. Next, a Steinmann pin is inserted transversely across the posterior segment of the calcaneus. The forefoot is dorsiflexed, putting tension on the Achilles tendon, and, the Steinmann pin serving as a lever, the bone gap is closed. The heel should be 5 degrees valgus. The wound is closed and an above-knee cast is applied, the pin being incorporated in the cast. The knee is in 45 degrees of flexion.

POSTOPERATIVE CARE

The cast, pin, and sutures are removed in four weeks. Then a below-knee walking cast is applied for an additional two weeks, by which time the osteotomy should be healed.

Plate 27. Dwyer Lateral Wedge Resection of Calcaneus for Pes Cavus

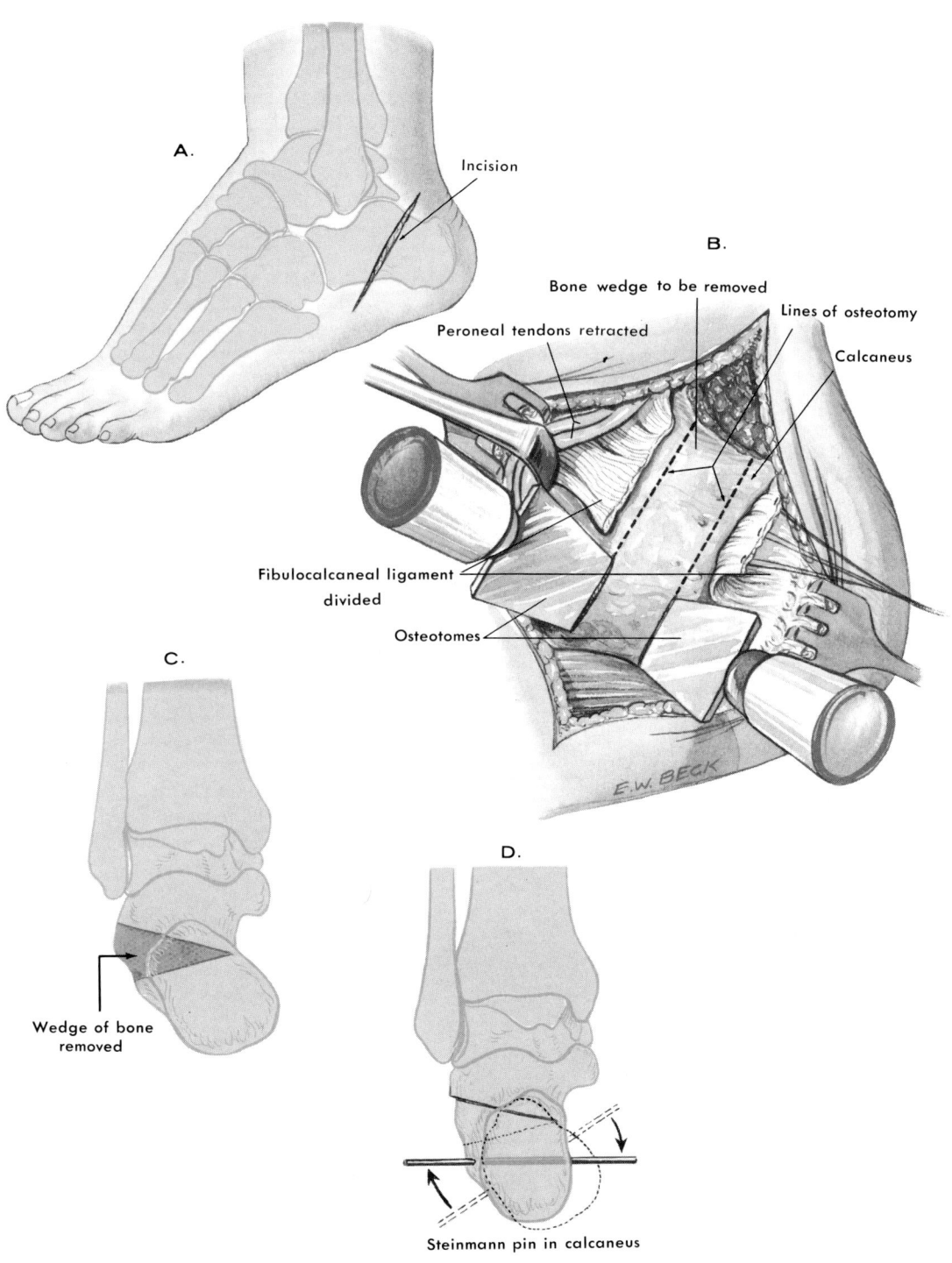

Elmsie type of triple arthrodesis in which a posteriorly based wedge was resected from the subtalar joint. The operation is difficult and complicated.

Dwyer, in 1964, reported on dorsal wedge osteotomy of the calcaneus for correction of calcaneus deformity.[35] The objective of surgery was to reduce the height of the calcaneus so that the heel would be brought closer to the plane of the forefoot. By taking the wedge wider on its medial or lateral aspect any valgus or varus deformity of the hindfoot could be corrected at the same time. In addition, leveling of the forefoot with the hindfoot allowed weight-bearing on the metatarsal heads (Fig. 4–14). Dwyer recommended preserving the wedge taken from the calcaneus; it was trimmed and inserted into a V-shaped cut in the neck of the talus to act as a permanent bone block, preventing excessive dorsiflexion of the ankle. Dwyer gave credit to Professor Bryan McFarland as the originator of the operation. This author does not recommend bone block; a more functional result is achieved with a tenodesis of the Achilles tendon to the distal fibular metaphysis (see Fig. 4–14 E and F and Plate 17). The McFarland-Dwyer dorsal wedge resection of the calcaneus has the definite drawback of shortening the os calcis.

Since 1956, Mr. George P. Mitchell of Edinburgh, Scotland, has performed a posterior and upward displacement osteotomy of the calcaneus; it is combined with an extensive plantar release. The calcaneocavus deformity is corrected without resection of bone (Fig. 4–15). The procedure is simple and has the advantage of lengthening the posterior lever arm of the calcaneus.[90] The technique of the Mitchell operation is depicted in Plate 28 L and M.

It is imperative to perform an extensive plantar release. Mr. Mitchell carries it out through a short horizontal medial incision. This author is concerned with the potential contracture and hypertrophy of the operative scar in the instep, because it may act as a deforming force in the calcaneocavovarus foot. In pes calcaneocavovalgus, however, it does not cause any difficulty. In moderate cases this author performs plantar release through a lateral or a midline incision; in severe contractures the surgical approach advocated by Bost, Schottstaedt, and Larsen is carried out.

Mr. Mitchell reviewed the long-term results in 15 feet. In five patients the triceps surae was weak and was reinforced by posterior tendon transfers. Eight feet required triple arthrodesis at a later stage.[90]

Samilson described a crescentic osteotomy of the os calcis for calcaneocavus feet.[101] The operative technique is described in Plate 28. Samilson uses staples or Kirschner wires for internal fixation. The results in 11 feet were excellent at follow-up between 5 and 12 years later. The indications for surgery were symptoms related to the calcaneocavus deformity of the feet; seven of the patients were spastics and four had idiopathic pes calcaneocavus. Before surgery

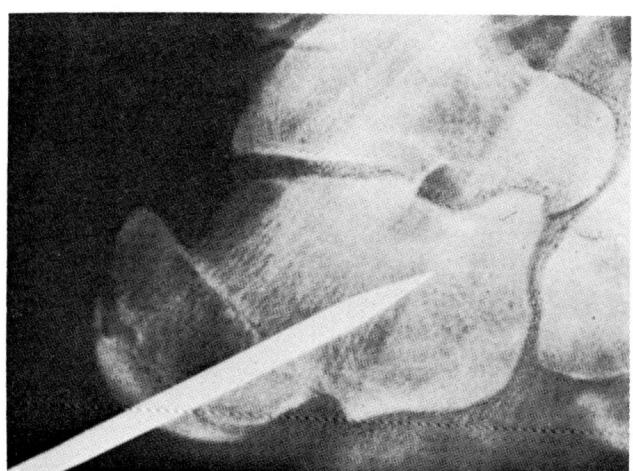

FIGURE 4–15. *A lateral roentgenogram of the hindfoot made at operation.*

Note the typical displacement of the osteotomy transfixed by a Steinmann pin. (From Mitchell, G. P.: Posterior displacement osteotomy of the calcaneus. J. Bone Joint Surg., 59-B:233, 1977. Reprinted by permission.)

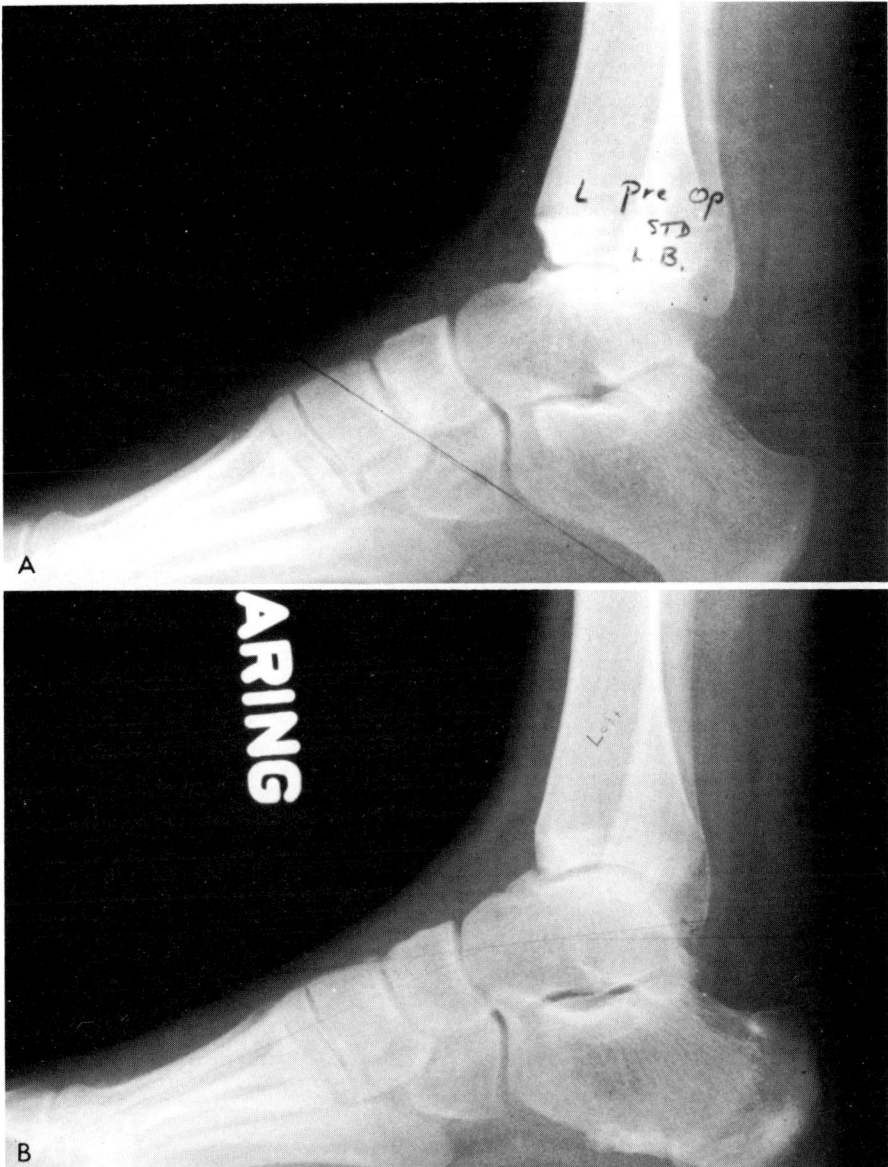

FIGURE 4–16. *Correction of a calcaneocavus foot by posterior and superior displacement crescentic osteotomy of the os calcis.*

Standing lateral roentgenograms of the foot. **A.** Preoperatively. **B.** Five years postoperatively. (From Samilson, R. L.: Crescentic osteotomy of the os calcis for calcaneocavus feet. *In* Bateman, J. E. (ed.): Foot Science. Philadelphia, W. B. Saunders Co., 1976. pp. 18–25. Reprinted by permission.)

the calcaneal pitch was 41 degrees, and postoperatively it was 19.5 degrees (Fig. 4–16). There were no infections, and all osteotomies healed. The motor strength of the triceps surae muscle did not change after surgery. Samilson found the procedure to be simple and effective in correcting calcaneocavus deformity; it does not, however, correct cavus deformity when the apex is located at the midtarsal or tarsometatarsal area.[101]

SESAMOIDECTOMY. In the adult patient, irritation of the sesamoids under the first metatarsal head causes them to hypertrophy and become inflamed. Axial views demonstrate enlargement of the sesamoids and

Text continued on page 552

Posterior and Superior Displacement Osteotomy of Os Calcis for Correction of Pes Calcaneocavus

THE PROCEDURE

A. The entire lower limb is prepared and draped in the usual manner, and the operation is performed under tourniquet ischemia. An oblique lateral incision is made over the body of the calcaneus, behind the peroneal tendons and the subtalar joint. The upper end of the incision is 3 cm. posterior to its plantar end.

B. The subcutaneous tissue is divided in line with the skin incision. First, an extensive plantar release is performed. This is vital; otherwise an adequate backward and upward displacement of the posterior segment of the calcaneus is not feasible. Mitchell uses a medial horizontal incision, as described in the text. This author carries out the plantar release as follows: the plantar fascia, abductor digiti quinti, and lateral part of the short plantar muscles are divided with scissors through the lateral incision. If one stays close to bone, this maneuver is safe and neurovascular injury is avoided.

C. An alternative approach for plantar release is through a midline plantar incision. Next, a longitudinal incision, 5 cm. long, is made on the plantar aspect of the foot, in line with the second ray.

D and **E.** With a periosteal elevator the plantar fascia and short plantar muscles are stripped from the tuberosity of the calcaneus and elevated forward.

The short and long plantar ligaments, the plantar calcaneonavicular ligament, and the capsule of the calcaneocuboid joint are divided. The foot is manipulated to correct the cavus deformity as much as possible.

At this time the lateral and plantar wounds are packed with hot moist sponges and the tourniquet is released. In a few minutes the packing is removed and the wounds are thoroughly inspected for bleeding. After complete hemostasis the tourniquet is reinflated.

Plate 28. Posterior and Superior Displacement Osteotomy of Os Calcis for Correction of Pes Calcaneocavus

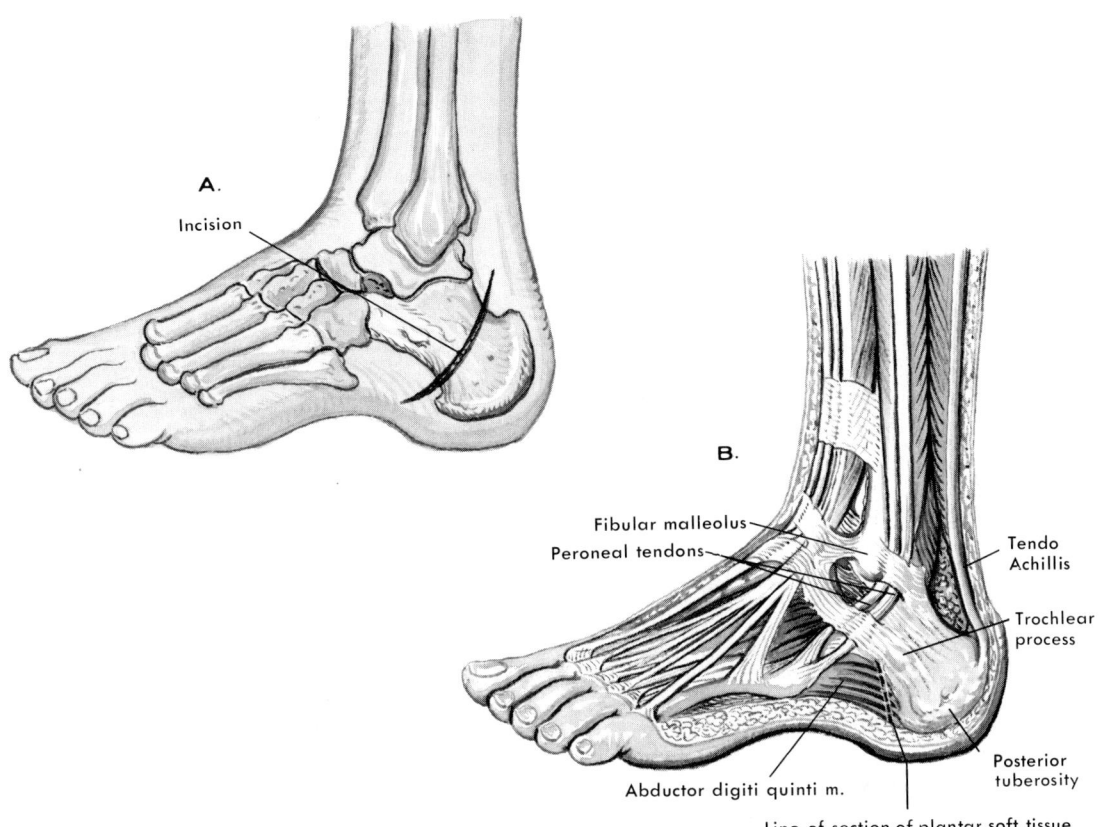
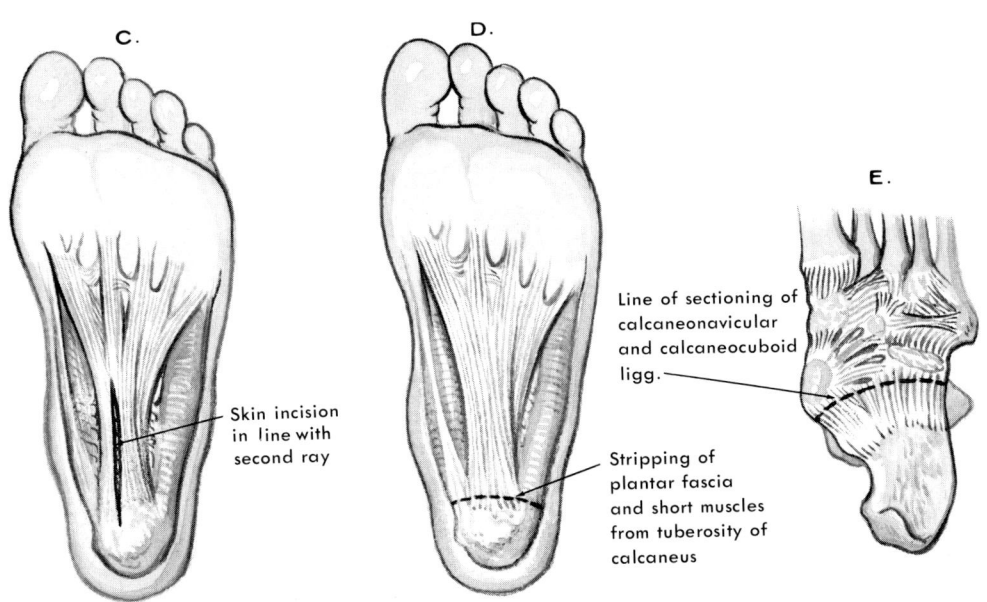

Posterior and Superior Displacement Osteotomy of Os Calcis for Correction of Pes Calcaneocavus *(Continued)*

F to J. Then, the lateral surface of the body of the calcaneus is exposed. The calcaneofibular ligament is sectioned and retracted. The peroneal tendons are pulled forward as far as possible, but there is no need to elevate them from their groove. Chandler elevators are placed on the superior and plantar surfaces of the calcaneus. The line of osteotomy is marked with multiple drill holes. Samilson makes a crescentic osteotomy (**I, J,** and **K**); whereas Mitchell's osteotomy is oblique transverse, inclining forward and plantarward (see **L** and **M**).

With an electric bone saw or a large curved sharp osteotome, the osteotomy is made.

K. A threaded Steinmann pin is inserted through the skin into the center of the apophysis of the calcaneus and the posterior bone segment. By manipulation and using the Steinmann pin as a lever, the posterior fragment is displaced backward and upward, reducing the calcaneocavus deformity. The degree of correction obtained is checked by stress-lateral roentgenograms of the foot. The calcaneal pitch should be 10 to 20 degrees. (The calcaneal pitch is the angle formed between the sole line—joining the plantar aspects of the metatarsal heads and the calcaneal tuberosity—and the plantar calcaneal line—drawn between the posterior and anterior calcaneal tuberosities (see Fig. 5–9). If correction is satisfactory the Steinmann pin is drilled into the anterior part of the os calcis, transfixing the osteotomized bones securely. This author prefers that the threaded Steinmann pin exit through the skin over the dorsolateral aspect of the midfoot and remain subcutaneous or flush with the calcaneus posteriorly.

Plate 28. Posterior and Superior Displacement Osteotomy of Os Calcis for Correction of Pes Calcaneocavus

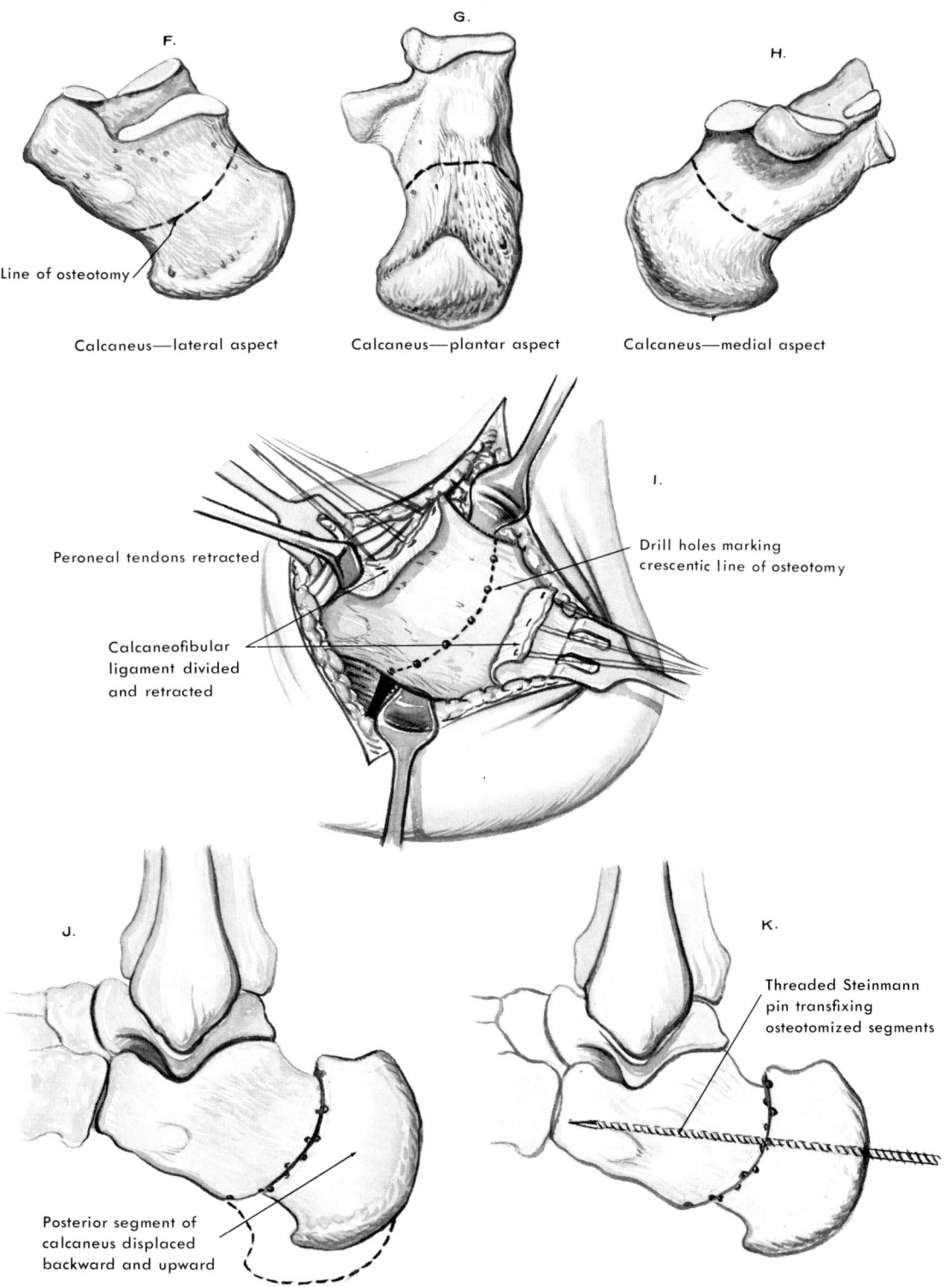

549

Posterior and Superior Displacement Osteotomy of Os Calcis for Correction of Pes Calcaneocavus *(Continued)*

L, M, and **N.** Oblique transverse osteotomy according to the technique of Mitchell. The line of osteotomy from the superior part inclines downward and forward. Drill holes are not made in the soft cancellous bone. The osteotomy is performed with a wide straight osteotome. The foot is manipulated, and with the leverage of the Steinmann pin, the posterior fragment is displaced backward and upward. This is easily done if all plantar soft tissues attached to the posterior tuberosity of the calcaneus are divided.

The wound is closed in the usual manner. A below-knee plaster of Paris cast is applied, incorporating the pin in the cast. This author prefers an above-knee cast with the knee flexed 45 degrees.

POSTOPERATIVE CARE

Weight-bearing is not allowed for three to four weeks, at which time the first cast and pin are removed. A new below-knee walking cast is applied for another two to three weeks. Then weight-bearing is permitted.

Plate 28. Posterior and Superior Displacement Osteotomy of Os Calcis for Correction of Pes Calcaneocavus

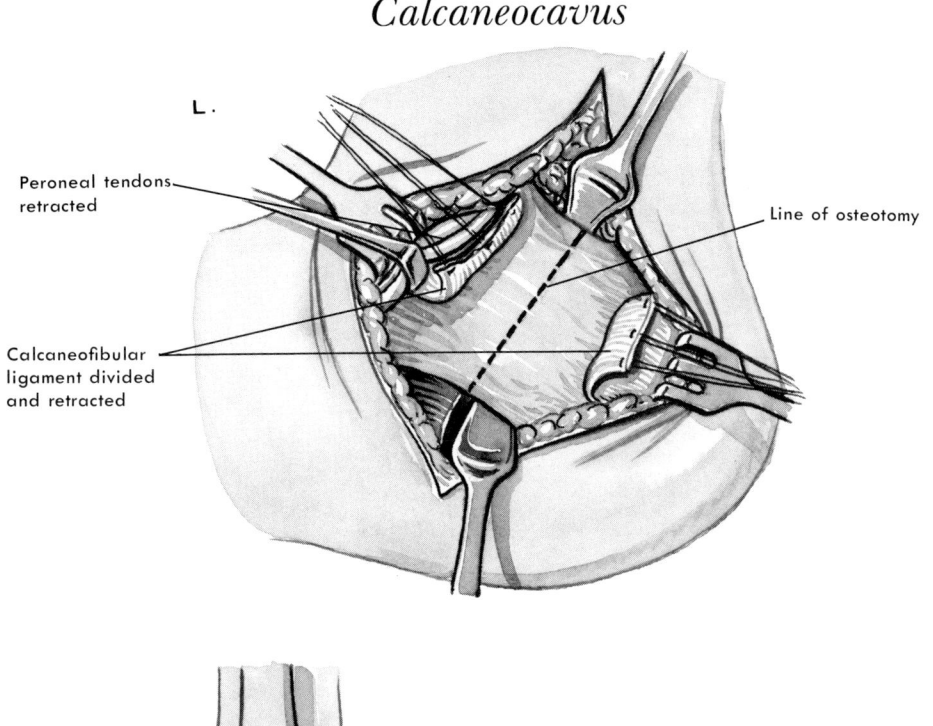

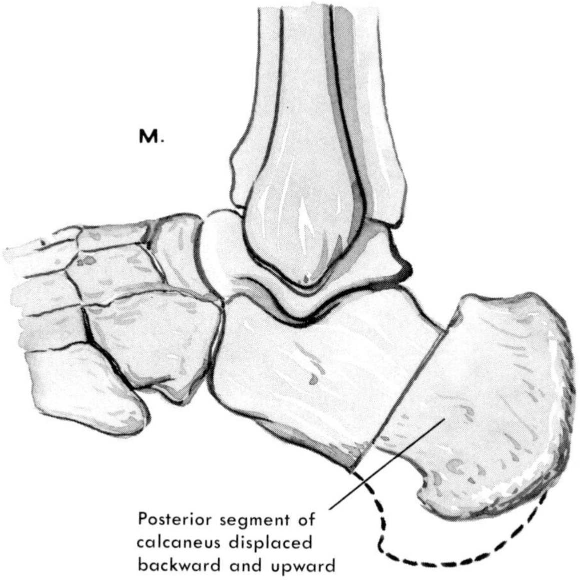

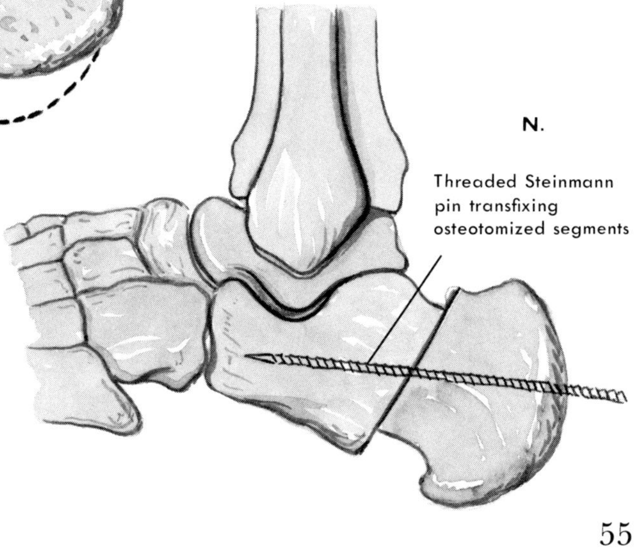

irregularity on their plantar surfaces. In such an instance, excision of one or both sesamoid bones affords complete symptomatic relief.

SUBTOTAL EXCISION OF THE TALUS. This may be indicated in a paralyzed cavovarus foot. Occasionally amputation of the toes is carried out if they are so deformed and inflamed that fitting shoes poses a formidable problem.

References

1. Alvik, I.: Operative treatment of pes cavus. Acta Orthop. Scand., 23:137, 1953.
2. Anzoletti, A.: Annotazioni intorno al piede equino cavo acquisito ed all'equinocavismo quale sintomo di affenzione nervosa non ancora descritta. Arch. Ortop., 22:356–377, 1905.
3. Arandes, Adan, R., Viladot Perice, A., and Vilanova Montiu, X.: Pie cavo. In Clinica y tratamiento de las enfermedades del pie (podologia). Barcelona, Editorial Cientifico Medical, 1956, pp. 149–159.
4. Barenfeld, P. A., Weseley, M. S., and Munter, M.: Dwyer calcaneal osteotomy. Clin. Orthop., 53:147, 1967.
5. Barenfeld, P. A., Weseley, M. S., and Shea, J. M.: The congenital cavus foot. Clin. Orthop., 79:119, 1971.
6. Bargellini, D.: Sul piede cavo con spina bifida occulta. Arch. Ortop., 32:65, 1915.
7. Bartolini, G.: Il trattamento chirurgico del piede cavo arteriore: La metatarsectomia (Note di tecnica). Arch. Ortop., 73:650, 1960.
8. Barwell, R.: Pes planus and pes cavus: An anatomical and clinical study. Edinburgh Med. J., 3:113, 1898.
9. Benages, A.: Chirurgie du pied creux. Revista espanola orthopedia et traumatologia. Rev. Esp. Cir. Osteoart., 1:115, 1966.
10. Bentzon, P. G. K.: Pes cavus and the m. peroneus longus. Acta Orthop. Scand., 4:50, 1933.
11. Bertrand, P.: Discussion. Symposium—le pied creux essentiel. Rev. Chir. Orthop., 53:423, 1967.
12. Beykirch, A.: Ein Beitrag zur Ätiologie und Therapie des Klanenhohlfusses. Z. Orthop. Chir., 52:41, 1929.
13. Boppe, M., and Janvier: A propos du pied creux essentiel de la second enfance. Rev. Med. Franc., 19:519, 1938.
14. Bosch, J.: Die Osteotomie nach Dwyer beim Ballenhohlfuss. Z. Orthop., 94:325, 1961.
15. Bost, F. C., Schottstaedt, E. R., and Larsen, L. J.: Plantar dissection. An operation to release the soft tissues in recurrent or recalcitrant talipes equinovarus. J. Bone Joint Surg., 42-A:151, 1960.
16. Brewerton, D. A., Sandifer, P. H., and Sweetman, D. R.: "Idiopathic" pes cavus, an investigation of its etiology. Brit. Med. J., 5358:659, 1963.
17. Brewster, A. H., and Larson, C. B.: Cavus feet. J. Bone Joint Surg., 22:361, 1940.
18. Brockway, A.: Surgical correction of talipes cavus deformities. J. Bone Joint Surg., 22:81, 1940.
19. Busatti, R.: Cura del piede cavo. Atti del XVI Congr. Soc. Ital. di Ortop., 1925.
20. Camera, U.: Il mio indirizzo sul trattamento delle deformita neurogene sul piede in equinismo e cavismo con particolare riguardo al piede cavo anteriore dell'adoelscenza. Boll. Mem. Soc. Piemontese Chir., 9:216, 1939.
21. Catalano, V.: Sul trattamento chirurgico del piede cavo. Arch. Putti, 5:431, 1954.
22. Chawap, A. R.: Rôle et chirurgie de l'aponévrose plantaire dans la déformation en pied creux. Thèse médecine, Paris, 1956.
23. Chuinard, E. G., and Baskin, M.: Claw-foot deformity. Treatment by transferring the long extensors into the metatarsals and fusion of the interphalangeal joints. J. Bone Joint Surg., 55-A:351, 1973.
24. Ciaccia, S.: Sul trattamento del piede cavo. Chir. Organi. Mov., 11:483, 1926.
25. Cole, W. H.: The treatment of claw-foot. J. Bone Joint Surg., 22:895, 1940.
26. Coleman, S. S., and Chesnut, W. J.: A simple test for hindfoot flexibility in the cavovarus foot. Clin. Orthop., 123:60, 1977.
27. Coonrad, R. W., Irwin, C. E., Gucker, T., III, and Wray, J. B.: The importance of plantar muscles in paralytic varus feet: results of treatment by neurectomy and myoneurectomy. J. Bone Joint Surg., 38-A:563, 1956.
28. Cralley, J., Fitch, K., and McGonagle, W.: Lumbrical muscles and contracted toes. Anat. Anz., 138:348, 1975.
29. Davis, G. G.: The treatment of hollow foot (pes cavus). Amer. J. Orthop. Surg., 11:231, 1913.
30. Daw, S. W.: Claw-foot. Clin. J., 61:13, 1932.
31. Debrunner, W.: Ueber die Wirkung Einiger Fussmuskeln insbesondere im Hinblick auf den Hohlfuss. Z. Orthop., 45:111, 1924.
32. Dekel, S., and Weissman, S. L.: Osteotomy of the calcaneus and concomitant plantar stripping in children with talipes cavo-varus. J. Bone Joint Surg., 55-B:802, 1973.
33. Duchenne, B. G.: Physiology of Motion. (Translated and edited by E. B. Kaplan.) Philadelphia, W. B. Saunders Co., 1959, p. 384.
34. Dwyer, F. C.: Osteotomy of the calcaneum for pes cavus. J. Bone Joint Surg., 41-B:80, 1959.
35. Dwyer, F. C.: Relationship of variations in the size and inclination of the calcaneum to the shape and function of the whole foot. Ann. Roy. Col. Surg. Eng., 34:120, 1964.
36. Dwyer, F. C.: The present status of the problem of pes cavus. Clin. Orthop., 106:254, 1975.
37. Faye, C. L.: A propos de 50 observations de pied creux. Étude étiologique et thérapeutique (traitement chirurgical). Thèse médecine, Paris, 1961.
38. Farill, J., A tendon transfer for the treatment of certain cases of cavus deformity of the foot. J. Bone Joint Surg., 45-A:1779, 1963.
39. Filipe, G., and Queneau, P.: Osteotomy of the calcaneus for pes cavus in childhood. Rev. Chir. Orthop., 63:563, 1977.
40. Fixsen, J. A.: Pes cavus. In Klenerman, L. (ed.): The Foot and Its Disorders. The Foot in Childhood. Oxford, Blackwell Scientific Publications, 1976, pp. 69–72.
41. Flint, M., and Sweetnam, R.: Amputation of all toes. A review of forty-seven amputations. J. Bone Joint Surg., 42-B:90, 1960.
42. Forrester-Brown, M. F.: Tendon transplantation for clawing of great toe. J. Bone Joint Surg., 20:57, 1938.
43. Fowler, B., Brooks, A. L., and Parrish, T. F.: The cavovarus foot. J. Bone Joint Surg., 41-A:757, 1959.
44. Frank, G. R., and Johnson, W. M.: The extensor shift procedure in the correction of clawtoe deformities in children. Southern Med. J., 59:889, 1966.
45. Galeazzi, R.: Pes cavus and principles for effectual treatment. Arch. Ital. Chir., 13:697, 1925.
46. Garceau, G. J.: Pes cavus. A.A.O.S. Inst. Course Lect., 18:184, 1961.
47. Garceau, G. J., and Brahms, M. A.: A preliminary study of selective plantar-muscle denervation for pes cavus. J. Bone Joint Surg., 38-A:553, 1956.
48. Gaunel, C., Louyot, P., and Tréheux, A.: Étude radiologique de la cavitation plantaire. Rev. Rhum., 28:581, 1971.
49. Gaunel, C., Louyot, P., and Tréheux, A.: Étude radiologique des désaxations en pronation ou supination du pied. Rev. Rhum., 28:591, 1971.
50. Geiges, F.: Ein Beitrag zur Aetiologie des Klauenhohlfusses. Bruns Beitr. Klin. Chir., 1:78, 1912.
51. Giaccai, L., and Simonetti, E.: Caratteristiche patogenetiche del piede cavo cosidetto essenziale e suo trattamento conla resezione-artrodesimodellante della mediotarsica. Arch. Putti Chir. Organi. Mov., 25:303, 1970.
52. Gilroy, E.: Pes cavus: A clinical study with special reference to its etiology. Edinburgh Med. J., 36:749, 1929.
53. Girardi, V. C.: Pie cavo. Semana Méd., 2:776 and 851, 1942.
54. Giriat, A., Taussig, G., and Masse, P.: Plantar release in the treatment of pes cavus in childhood. Technique and indications. (Author's transl.) Rev. Chir. Orthop., 65:77, 1979.
55. Giuntini, L.: Modalita e risultati della cura chirurgica nel piede cavo. Arch. Ortop., 54:459, 1938.

56. Goff, C. W.: The pes cavus of congenital syphilis. J.A.M.A., *86*:392, 1926.
57. Gudas, C. J.: Mechanism and reconstruction of pes cavus. J. Foot Surg., *16*:1, 1977.
58. Guradze: Operative Behandlung des Klauenhohlfusses mit Exstirpation des Os naviculare. Ver. Deutsch. Orthop. Ges., *15*:348, 1921.
59. Hackenbrock, M.: Der Hohlfuss. Ergebn. Chir. Orthop., *17*:457, 1924.
60. Halgrimssen, S.: Pes cavus, seine Behandlung und einige Bemerkungen "uber seine" Ätiologie. Acta Orthop. Scand., *10*:73, 1939.
61. Hammond, G.: Elevation of the first metatarsal bone with hallux equinus. Surgery, *13*:240, 1943.
62. Heron, J. R.: Neurological syndromes associated with pes cavus. Proc. Roy. Soc. Med., *62*:270, 1969.
63. Heyman, C. H.: The operative treatment of clawfoot. J. Bone Joint Surg., *14*:335, 1932.
64. Hibbs, R. A.: An operation for "claw-foot." J.A.M.A., *73*:1583, 1919.
65. Hoffmann-Kuhnt, H.: Der Tibialis Auticus beim Plattfuss und beim Hohlfuss. Z. Orthop., *79*:519, 1950.
66. Howard, R. J.: Operative treatment of early cavus feet. Southern Med. J., *4*:558, 1971.
67. Hughes, W. K.: Talipes cavus. Brit. Med. J., *2*:902, 1940.
68. Imhauser, G.: Surgical treatment of pes cavus with or without claw toes. Z. Orthop., *106*:488, 1969.
69. Ingelrans, P.: Discussion. Symposium—le pied creux essentiel (Méary, R., Ed.). Rev. Chir. Orthop., *53*:422, 1967.
70. Japas, L. M.: Surgical treatment of pes cavus by tarsal V-osteotomy. Preliminary report. J. Bone Joint Surg., *50-A*:927, 1968.
71. Jones, R.: The soldier's foot and the treatment of common deformities of the foot. Part II: Claw-foot. Brit. Med. J., *1*:749, 1916.
72. Karlstrom, G., Lonnerholm, T., and Olerud, S.: Cavus deformity of the foot after fracture of the tibial shaft. J. Bone Joint Surg., *57-A*:893, 1975.
73. Kelikian, H.: Hallux Valgus, Allied Deformities of the Forefoot, and Metatarsalgia. Philadelphia, W. B. Saunders Co., 1965, p. 305.
74. Kleinberg, S., Horwitz, T., and Sobel, R.: Pes cavus. Bull. Hosp. Joint Dis., *10*:252, 1949.
75. Kollicker: Der Hohlfuss. Z. Orthop., *45*:106, 1924.
76. Lake, N. C.: Pes cavus. *In* The Foot. 3rd Ed. Baltimore, The Williams & Wilkins Co., 1948, p. 284–287.
77. Lambrinudi, C.: An operation for claw-toes. Proc. Roy. Soc. Med., *21*:239, 1927.
78. Lelievre, J.: Le pied creux anterieur. *In* Pathologie du Pied. Paris, Masson & Cie, 1970, p. 405.
79. Lenzi, L., and Manzoni, A.: Piede cavo essenziale e piede cavo mielodisplasico. Chir. Organi Mov., *54*:123, 1965.
80. Little, N. J.: Claw foot. Med. J. Aust., *2*:495, 1938.
81. Lorenz, A.: Zum Redressement des Hohlfuss. Z. Orthop., *62*:149, 1934.
82. Lumsden, R. M., Schottstaedt, E. F., and Tsou, P. M.: Pes cavus. *In* Samilson, R. L. (ed.): Children's foot, ankle and leg problems. Course Syllabus, September, 1971. San Francisco, American Academy of Orthopaedic Surgeons, 1971, pp. 197–214.
83. McElvenny, R. T., and Caldwell, G. D.: A new operation for correction of clavus foot. Fusion of first metatarsocuneiform-navicular joints. Clin. Orthop., *11*:85, 1958.
84. Mann, R., and Inman, V. T.: Phasic activity of intrinsic muscles of the foot. J. Bone Joint Surg., *46-A*:469, 1964.
85. Mattéi, C. R.: La tarsectomie antérieure dans la correction du pied creux. Thèse médecine, Paris, 1974.
86. Mau, C.: Die Calcaneusosteotomie beim Hohlfuss. Verh. Deutsch. Orthop. Ges., *21*:488, 1927.
87. Méary, R.: Le pied creux essentiel. Symposium. Rev. Chir. Orthop., *53*:389, 1967.
88. Méary, R., Mattéi, C. R., and Toméno, B.: Tarsectomie antérieure pour pied creux. Indications et résultats lointains. Rev. Chir. Orthop., *62*:231, 1976.
89. Mills, G. P.: The etiology and treatment of claw foot. J. Bone Joint Surg., *6*:142, 1924.
89a. Missirian, J., and Mann, R. A.: Pathophysiology of Charcot-Marie-Tooth disease. Presented at Foot Society, Anaheim, California, March, 1983.
90. Mitchell, G. P.: Posterior displacement osteotomy of the calcaneus. J. Bone Joint Surg., *59-B*:233, 1977.
91. Mitroszewska, H., and Szulc, W.: Idiopathic pes cavus and its surgical treatment. Chir. Narzad. Ruchu Ortop. Pol., *42*:543, 1977.
92. Ollerenshaw, R.: The treatment of pes cavus. Proc. Roy. Soc. Med. (Section of Orthopedics), *20*:1126, 1927.
93. Parkin, A.: Causation and mode of production of pes cavus. Brit. Med. J., *1*:1285, 1891.
93a. Paulos, C. E., Coleman, S. S., and Samuelson, K. M.: Pes cavovarus: Review of a surgical approach using soft tissue procedures. J. Bone Joint Surg., *62-A*:942, 1980.
94. Pitzen, P.: Development of medial arch in newborn. Z. Orthop., *84*:44, 1953.
95. Pizziolo, I.: Sul trattamento del piede cavo. Arch. Ortop., *56*:157, 1940.
96. Rocher, H. L., and Dupin, J.: Aplasie musculaire jambière presque totale dans un double pied bot "varus cavus" congenital. Tarsectomie. Guérison, J. Med. Bordeaux, *130*:920, 1953.
97. Rosati, G., Granieri, E., Aiello, I., Pinna, L., De Bastiani, P., and Tola, R.: Ataxia telangiectasia: Apropos of a case with pes cavus and distal neural amyotrophy. Acta Neurol. (Napoli), *32*:764, 1977.
98. Rosenzweig, A.: Die operative Behandlung des Hohlfusses. Zbl. Chir., *61*:2037, 1934.
99. Rugh, J. T.: An operation for the correction of plantar and adduction contraction of the foot arch. J. Bone Joint Surg., *6*:664, 1924.
100. Rutt, A.: Der Hohlfuss (Pes cavus). *In* Hohmann, G. (ed.): Handbuch der Orthopädie. Stuttgart, Georg Thiem Verlag, 1961, Vol. IV, Part II, pp. 1068–1095.
101. Samilson, R. L.: Crescentic osteotomy of the os calcis for calcaneocavus feet. *In* Bateman, J. E. (ed.): Foot Science. Philadelphia, W. B. Saunders Co., 1976. pp. 18–25.
102. Saunders, J. T.: Etiology and treatment of clawfoot. Arch. Surg. (Chicago), *30*:179, 1935.
103. Scalone, I.: Sul tratamento operativo ded piede cavo. Chir. Organi Mov., *6*:83, 1922.
104. Scheer, G. E., and Crego, C. H., Jr.: A two-stage stabilization procedure for correction of calcaneocavus. J. Bone Joint Surg., *38-A*:1247, 1956.
105. Scherb, R.: Bemerkungen zur Aetiologie des Klauenhohlfusses. Z. Orthop., *44*:564, 1924.
106. Schlegel, K. F.: Spina bifida occulta and pes cavus with marked hammertoes. On the pathogenesis and causal treatment of so-called idiopathic talipes cavus. Ergebn. Chir. Orthop., *45*:268, 1964.
107. Schnepp, K. H.: Hammer-toe and claw-foot. Amer. J. Surg., *36*:351, 1937.
108. Sell, L. S.: Pes cavus. Spectator Correspondence Club Letter. Dec. 11, 1961.
109. Sharrard, W. J. W.: Congenital pes cavus (arcuatus). *In* Paediatric Orthopaedics and Fractures. Congenital and Developmental Abnormalities of Foot and Toes. Oxford, Blackwell Scientific Publications, pp. 283–286.
109a. Sherman, F. C., and Westin, G. W.: Plantar release in the correction of deformities of the foot in childhood. J. Bone Joint Surg., *63-A*:1382, 1981.
110. Sherman, H. M.: The operative treatment of pes cavus. Amer. J. Orthop. Surg., *2*:374, 1904–1905.
111. Siffert, R. S., Forster, R. I., and Nachamie, B.: "Beak" triple arthrodesis for correction of severe cavus deformity. Clin. Orthop., *45*:101, 1966.
112. Spillane, J. D.: Familial pes cavus and absent tendon-jerks: Its relationship with Friedreich's disease and peroneal muscular atrophy. Brain, *63*:275, 1940.
113. Spitzy, H.: Operative correction of claw foot. Surg. Gynec. Obstet., *45*:813, 1927.
114. Stauffer, R. N., Nelson, G. E., and Bianco, A. J.: Calcaneal osteotomy in treatment of cavovarus foot. Mayo Clin. Proc., *45*:624, 1970.
115. Steindler, A.: Operative treatment of pes cavus. Surg. Gynec. Obstet., *24*:612, 1917.
116. Steindler, A.: Stripping of the os calcis. J. Orthop. Surg., *2*:8, 1920.
117. Steindler, A.: The treatment of pes cavus. Arch. Surg. (Chicago), *2*:325, 1921.
118. Swanson, A. B., Browne, H. S., and Coleman, J. D.: The cavus foot concept of production and treatment by metatarsal osteotomy. J. Bone Joint Surg., *48-A*:1019, 1966.
119. Taylor, T. G.: The treatment of claw toes by multiple

transfer of flexors into extensor tendons. J. Bone Joint Surg., 33-B:539, 1951.
120. Thomas, W.: Treatment talipes cavus. Birmingham Med. Rev., 34:1, 1893.
121. Todd, A.: Treatment of pes cavus. Lancet, 2:758, 1934.
122. Tomeno, B.: Essential pes cavus. Rev. Prat., 31:1019, 1981.
123. Turner, M.: Pathogenesis of pes cavus, chronaximetric study. Arch. Argent. Pediat., 38:38, 1952.
124. Walsham, W. J., and Hughes, W. K.: Talipes cavus. In The Deformities of the Human Foot. London, Baillière, Tindall & Co., 1895, Chap. XIII, pp. 490–495.
125. Wang, G., and Shaffer, L. W.: Osteotomy of the metatarsals for pes cavus. Southern Med. J., 70:77, 1977.
126. Weseley, M. S.: Calcaneal osteotomy for the treatment of the cavus deformity. Bull. Hosp. Joint Dis., 31:93, 1970.
127. Weseley, M. S., and Barenfield, P. A.: Mechanism of the Dwyers calcaneal osteotomy. Clin. Orthop., 70:137, 1970.
128. Westin, G. W.: Personal communication, 1978.
129. Whitman, R.: Orthopaedic Surgery. Philadelphia, Lea & Febiger, 1930. pp. 853, 896.
130. Williams, M., and Lissner, H. R.: Parallel forces in one plane. In Biomechanics of Human Motion. Philadelphia, W. B. Saunders Co., 1962. pp. 34–68.
131. Williams, P. F., and Menelaus, M. B.: Triple arthrodesis by inlay grafting—a method suitable for the undeformed or valgus foot. J. Bone Joint Surg., 59-B:333, 1977.

CLAW TOES

Clawing of the toes is characterized by hyperextension of the metatarsophalangeal joint and flexion of both the proximal and distal interphalangeal joints (Figs. 4–17 and 4–18). The deformity may be secondary to pes cavus, or it may be paralytic in its pathogenesis. During the push-off phase of gait, when the long toe flexors contract to substitute for the paralyzed triceps surae muscle, the interphalangeal joints of the toes are flexed, and the metatarsophalangeal joints are hyperextended. A reverse mechanism by which clawing of the toes may also occur acts when the anterior tibialis muscle is weakened or zero in motor strength, and the extensor hallucis longus and extensor digitorum longus muscles are used to substitute for its action. In this latter type, clawing of the toes is produced during the swing phase of the gait. The great toe is usually more severely affected than the lesser toes. Painful callosities gradually develop over the dorsum of the interphalangeal joints, which become fixed in flexion. Pressure keratoses under the metatarsal heads aggravate the disability.

Treatment

Treatment is dependent upon the type of claw toes, the degree of flexibility of the interphalangeal and metatarsophalangeal joints, and the age of the patient. The Girdlestone-Taylor operation (in which the long toe flexor is transferred to the dorsal expansion of the long toe extensors) should *not* be performed for clawing of the toes, as it causes rotational malalignment of the toes.[4, 11] The experience of Taylor, who obtained good results in 27 of 38 patients, is not shared by others. Pyper, reviewing the results of the Girdlestone-Taylor operation in 45 feet with clawing of the toes, found that in approximately 20 per cent of cases, the extensor tendons regenerated and the deformity recurred. The interphalangeal joints were stiff in 60 per cent, and in no case was there significant improvement in metatarsal pain and callosities. Worthwhile improvement was achieved in about 50 per cent of the cases, with the best results in those with only the mildest symptoms. The advantages observed by Pyper were: improvement in the shape of the toes with consequent easier fitting of shoes, disappearance of corns over the interphalangeal joints, and general improvement in walking.[9]

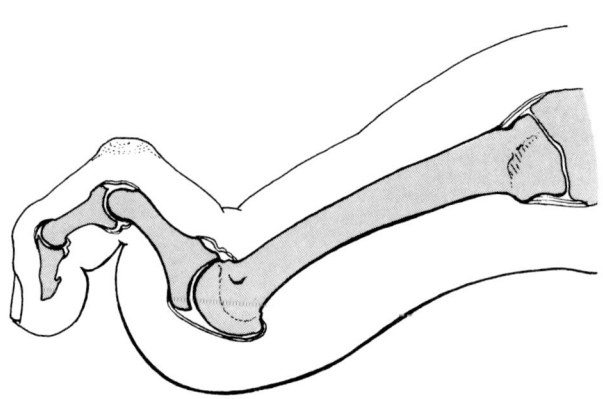

FIGURE 4–17. Claw toe.

The deformity is characterized by hyperextension of the metatarsophalangeal joint and flexion of both proximal and distal interphalangeal joints.

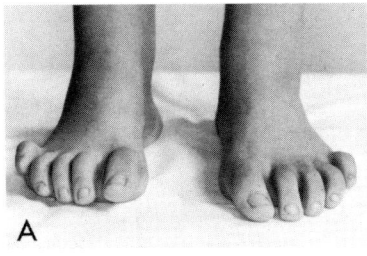 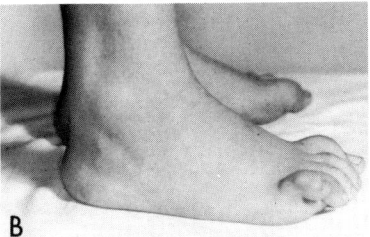 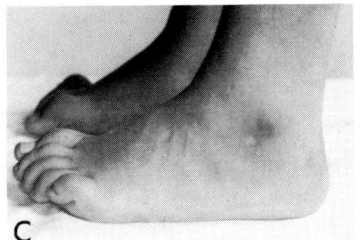

FIGURE 4–18. Bilateral clawing of the toes.

For clawing of the great toe, Dickson and Dively advise transfer of the extensor hallucis longus tendon to the flexor hallucis longus tendon, and resection and arthrodesis of the interphalangeal joint in normal alignment.[1] This author has had no experience with this operation.

In paralytic claw toes, the dynamic imbalance causing the deformity should be corrected whenever feasible. In the presence of anterior tibial muscle weakness, the motor power of ankle dorsiflexion should be restored by appropriate tendon transfer. First, associated equinus deformity is corrected by stretching casts; then the peroneal muscles are transferred to the base of the second metatarsal, or in the presence of peroneal muscle weakness, the long toe extensors are transferred to the metatarsal heads. The fixed flexion deformity of the interphalangeal joints is corrected by wedge resections and arthrodesis. If the primary cause of claw toes is triceps surae muscle weakness and hyperactive long toe flexors, posterior transfer of the appropriate muscles to the os calcis is performed to restore active power of plantar flexion. If the claw toes represent triceps surae muscle weakness and hyperactive long toe flexors, posterior transfer of the appropriate muscles to the os calcis is performed to restore active power of plantar flexion. If the claw toes are secondary to pes cavus, equinus deformity of the forefoot is corrected. Fixed claw toes are treated by dorsal capsulotomy of the metatarsophalangeal joints and transfer of the long toe extensors to the metatarsal heads and fusion of the interphalangeal joints as described in Plate 10 for correction of hammer toes.

References

1. Dickson, F. D., and Dively, R. L.: Operation for correction of mild claw foot, the result of infantile paralysis. J.A.M.A., 87:1275, 1926.
2. Forrester-Brown, M. F.: Tendon transplantation for clawing of the great toe. J. Bone Joint Surg., 20:57, 1938.
3. Frank, G. R., and Johnson, W. M.: The extensor shift procedure in the correction of clawtoe deformities in children. Southern Med. J., 59:889, 1966.
4. Girdlestone, G. R.: Physiotherapy for hand and foot. Journal of Chartered Society of Physiotherapy, 32:176, 1947.
5. Heyman, C. H.: Operative treatment of claw foot. J. Bone Joint Surg., 14:335, 1932.
6. Hibbs, R. A.: An operation for "claw foot." J.A.M.A., 73:1583, 1919.
7. Lambrinudi, C.: An operation for claw-toes. Proc. Roy. Soc. Med., 21:239, 1927.
8. Parrish, T. F.: Dynamic correction of clawtoes. Orthop. Clin. N. Amer. 4:97, 1973.
9. Pyper, J. B.: The flexor-extensor transplant operation for claw toes. J. Bone Joint Surg., 40-B:528, 1958.
10. Sharrard, W. J. W., and Smith, T. W. D.: Tenodesis of the flexor hallucis longus for paralytic clawing of the hallux in childhood. J. Bone Joint Surg., 58-B:224, 1976.
11. Taylor, T. G.: The treatment of claw toes by multiple transfers of flexor into extensor tendons. J. Bone Joint Surg., 33-B:539, 1951.

5. Flexible Pes Planovalgus (Flat Foot)

Flat foot is a loose generic term used to describe any condition of the foot in which the longitudinal arch is abnormally low or absent. It covers a multitude of conditions that differ in their etiology, pathology, degree of severity, prognosis, and treatment. The term *pes planus* is more esoteric. In the literature *pes planus* is often modified by adjectives such as *rigid* or *flexible*, *static* or *paralytic*, *congenital* or *acquired* and is sometimes denoted by more complex combinations of terms such as *congenital rigid pes planus with vertical talus* or *congenital convex pes valgus*.

The simplicity of the term *flat foot*, or *pes planus*, is deceptive, resulting in faulty diagnosis in a large number of children with normal feet that appear flat. It is vital to avoid vagaries and to be more exact in terminology. A classification of flat foot is given in Table 5–1. The disorder includes both congenital and acquired forms, with the deformity either rigid or flexible. In the acquired type the defect may be ligamentous, muscular, articular, bony, or contractural. This chapter deals with flat foot due to excessive ligamentous laxity; the other entities are described in other sections of this book.

The integrity of the longitudinal and transverse arches of the foot is dependent upon the configuration of tarsal bones and joints and the strength of the ligaments that bind them together. The longitudinal arch of the foot is *not* maintained by the active contraction of muscles. Electromyographic studies by Basmajian and associates demonstrated minimal or no electrical activity in the intrinsic and extrinsic muscles of the foot and leg of the person standing at rest. The main concerns of the primary muscles of the lower limb are to maintain balance, to propel the body forward, and to protect the ligaments from abnormal stress such as in walking on rough terrain.[4, 5]

The exact cause of hyperlaxity of ligaments in flexible pes planovalgus is unknown; the condition is, however, familial.

Table 5–1. *Classification of Flat Foot*

Congenital
  Rigid
    Congenital convex pes valgus
    Tarsal coalition
  Flexible
    Talipes calcaneovalgus
    Talipes valgus due to contracture of triceps surae muscle (calcaneal equinus deformity)
    Hypoplasia of sustentaculum tali

Acquired
  Due to *ligamentous hyperlaxity*
    Familial
    Part of a generalized syndrome (e.g., Ehlers-Danlos, Marfan's, Down's, osteogenesis imperfecta)
  Due to *muscle weakness and imbalance*
    Accessory tarsal navicular with insufficiency of tibialis posterior muscle
    Myopathic (e.g., muscular dystrophy)
    Peripheral nerve injuries
    Spinal cord affections (e.g., poliomyelitis, myelodysplasia)
    Cerebral palsy (spastic or hypotonic)
  Arthritic
    Inflammatory conditions involving subtalar and midtarsal joints (e.g., rheumatoid arthritis)
    Traumatic arthritis (in children usually in rare conditions such as congenital insensitivity to pain)
  Contractural
    Due to myostatic contracture of peroneal muscles
    Due to acquired contracture of triceps surae

Analysis of Deformity and Roentgenographic Features

In flat foot the basic deformity is depression of the longitudinal arch. The sag in the arch may result from plantar deviation of any one or all three of the components that constitute the arch—namely, the talocalcaneal, talonavicular, and naviculocuneiform joints. The cuneiform-metatarsal articulation does not sag because it is a stable joint with very limited range of motion.

When the hypermobile foot is loaded under the static force of body weight the calcaneus pronates under the talus. The anterior end of the calcaneus moves laterally and dorsally, whereas the head of the talus moves medially and plantarward (Fig. 5–1). The plantar calcaneonavicular ligament is elongated because of ligamentous hyperlaxity and does not support the head of the talus. The talocalcaneal interosseous ligament is lax, allowing the heel to evert. Horizontal movement takes place at the talonavicular joint; the navicular abducts in relation to the talar head, moving in unison with the anterior end of the calcaneus. The forepart of the foot follows the navicular, and the center of gravity of the body is shifted over or medial to the first metatarsal bone (Fig. 5–2A). Normally the weight falls

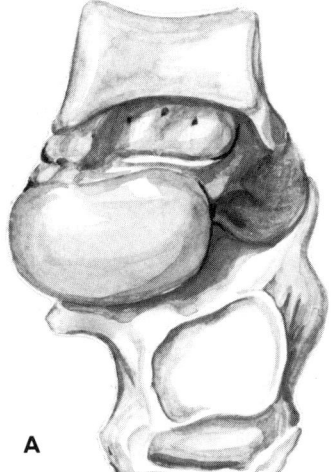
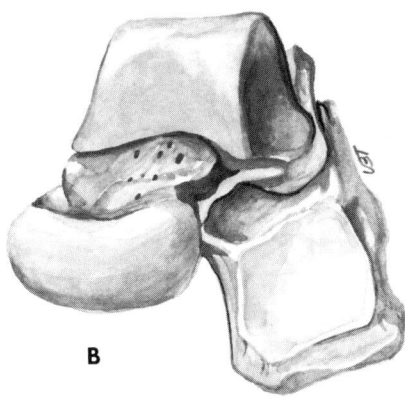

FIGURE 5–1. *Hypermobile flat foot.*

A. Non-weight-bearing. **B.** Weight-bearing. Note that the anterior end of the calcaneus moves laterally and dorsally, whereas the head of the talus moves medially and plantarward.

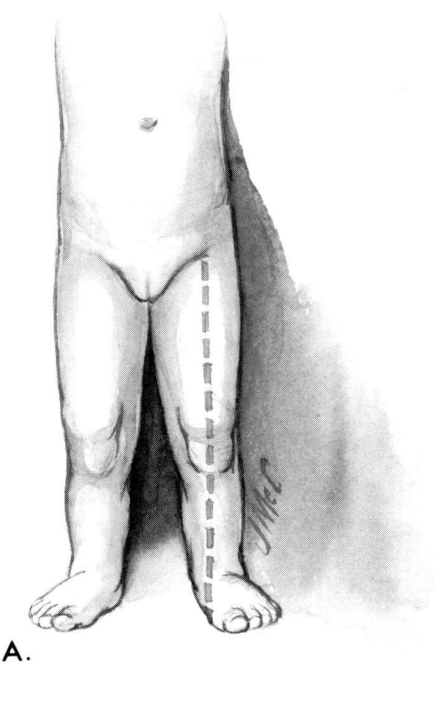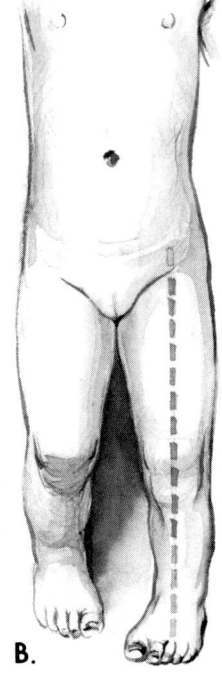

FIGURE 5–2. Flexible flat foot.

A. In stance, the center of gravity of the body is over or medial to the first metatarsal bone. **B.** Protective toeing-in so that the body weight is shifted laterally toward the center of the foot.

between the second and third rays, which is the center of the foot. A foot that on weight-bearing assumes a valgus posture because of extreme laxity of the ligaments with medial displacement of the static load of body weight produces excessive stress and strain on the foot. It is not the flatness of the longitudinal arch but rather the medial shift in weight-bearing that makes the pronated foot mechanically weak. Nature makes the child toe-in actively so that the center of gravity of the body is shifted laterally toward the center of the foot (Fig. 5–2B). With toeing-in the forepart of the foot is adducted. In the literature there is some controversy over whether the active supi-

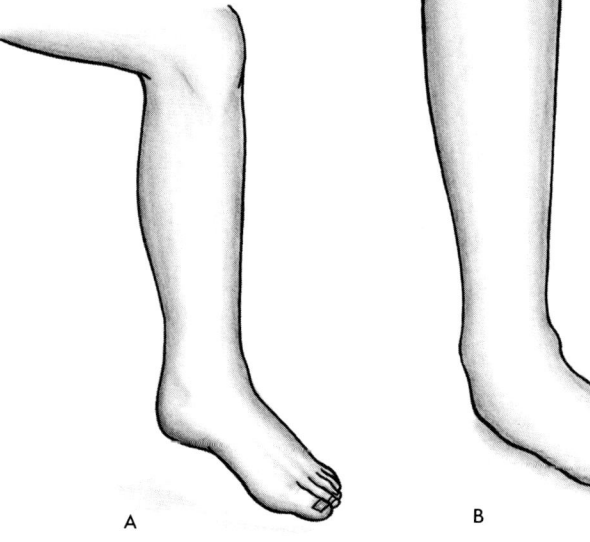

FIGURE 5–3. Flexible flat foot.

A. When not weight-bearing, the suspended foot has normal contour and longitudinal arch. **B.** On weight-bearing the longitudinal arch is flattened.

nation and adduction of the forefoot are part of the complex deformity of flexible pes planovalgus. This author proposes that toeing-in in gait and supination of the medial rays of the forefoot in stance are secondary compensatory mechanisms and not the primary deformity.

In the flexible flat foot caused by excessive ligamentous laxity there is no fixed deformity—in stance the foot assumes valgus posture, but when not bearing weight it has a normal contour and longitudinal arch (Fig. 5–3).

When there is associated myostatic contracture of the triceps surae muscle, the calcaneus is tilted into plantar flexion, losing its normal pitch, the valgus posture of the foot in stance is exaggerated, and the child is unable to protect his feet by compensatory toeing-in.

Roentgenographic examination of the feet will demonstrate the malalignment of the joints and the anatomic site of the break in the longitudinal arch, whether at the talonavicular joint, the naviculocuneiform joint, or at both joints. The roentgenograms should be made with the patient standing with the muscles relaxed. If the feet are flexible clinically, non-weight-bearing roentgenograms are not usually required.

In the lateral projection of a normal weight-bearing foot, lines drawn through the center of the longitudinal axes of the talus, navicular, medial cuneiform, and first metatarsal form a straight line (Fig. 5–4A). A vertical line is drawn through the center of the navicular parallel to its proximal articular surface. In the normal foot the longitudinal axis of the talus crosses the navicular vertical line at a right angle (Figs. 5–4A and 5–5).

When the break occurs *at the talonavicular joint alone,* the long axis of the talus points plantarward, exiting on the lower quarter of the navicular, posterior to the medial cuneiform. The long axes of the first met-

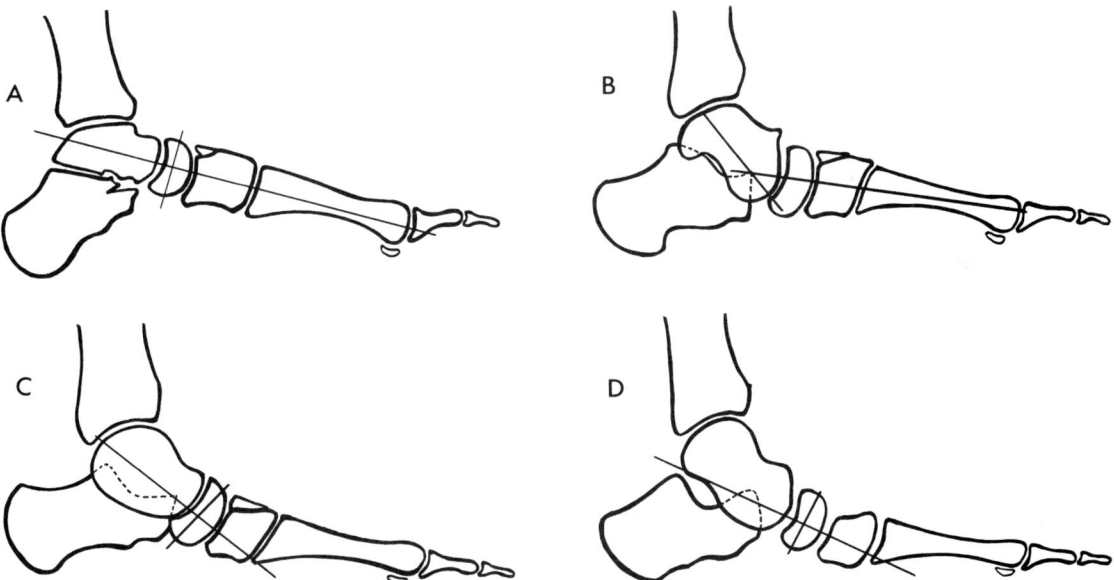

FIGURE 5–4. Line drawing of the lateral roentgenogram of weight-bearing feet.

Lines are drawn through the center of the longitudinal axes of the talus, navicular, medial cuneiform, and first metatarsal. A vertical line is drawn through the center of the navicular parallel to its proximal articular surface. **A.** *Normal foot.* The longitudinal axes of the talus, navicular, medial cuneiform, and first metatarsal form a straight line; the longitudinal axis of the talus crosses the navicular vertical line at a right angle. **B.** Flexible flat foot due to *talonavicular sag.* The longitudinal axis of the talus points plantarward, exiting on the inferior quadrant of the navicular, behind the medial cuneiform. The long axes of the first metatarsal, medial cuneiform, and navicular are in a straight line and cross the long axis of the talus at an angle. **C.** Flexible flat foot due to *naviculocuneiform sag.* The longitudinal axes of the talus and navicular make a straight line and bisect the navicular vertical line at right angles, but they exit on the plantar aspect of the medial cuneiform proximal to the base of the first metatarsal. **D.** Flexible flat foot due to sag at both the talonavicular and naviculocuneiform joints. The line drawn through the longitudinal axis of the navicular when extended proximally and distally lies plantar to the center of the talar and first metatarsal segments.

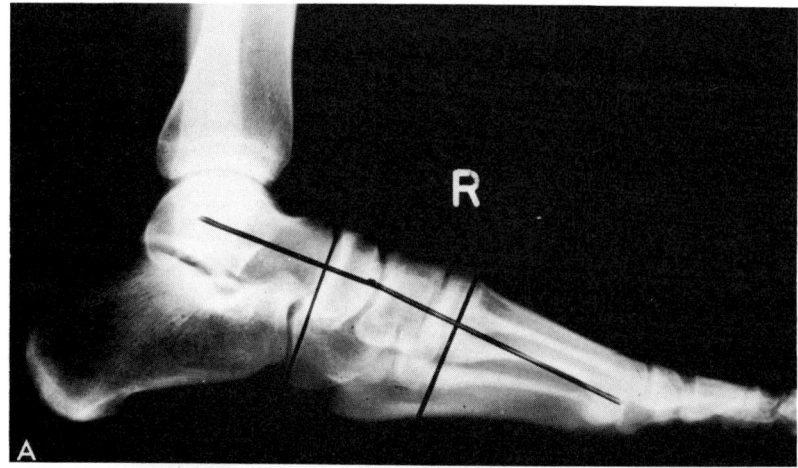
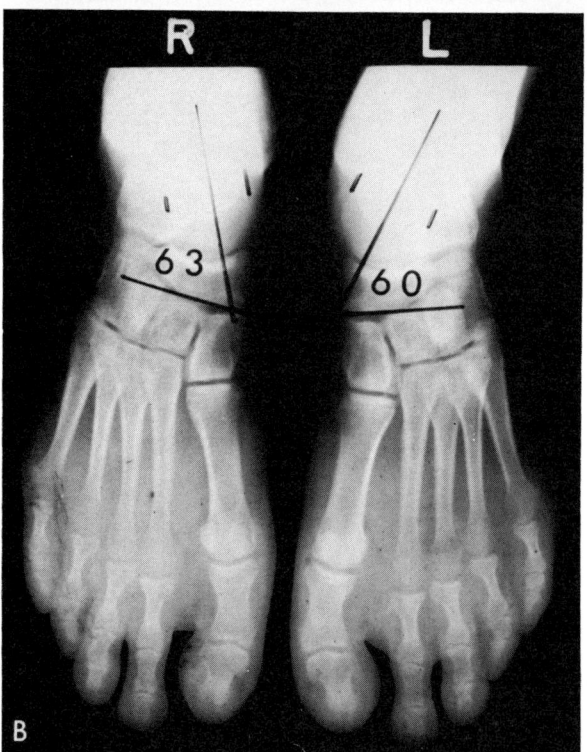

FIGURE 5–5. Roentgenograms of a normal foot, weight-bearing in stance.

A. Lateral view. Lines are drawn parallel to the proximal articular surface of the navicular and the distal articular surface of the medial cunieform. The line drawn through the center of the longitudinal axis of the talus bisects the navicular line at a right angle. On forward projection the long axis of the talus crosses the medial cuneiform line at a right angle and extends to the plantar aspect of the first metatarsal head. Note the line is slightly angulated dorsally at the naviculocuneiform joint. A straight line is considered the lower limit of normal.
B. Anteroposterior view. The dorsoplantar talonavicular angle is that formed between the longitudinal axis of the talus (bisecting the talar head-neck) and a line drawn parallel to the distal articular surface of the navicular. The normal value is between 60 and 80 degrees. Note that in the right foot it is 63 degrees and in the left foot 60 degrees. An angle less than 60 degrees is considered abnormal. (From Giannestras, N.: Flexible valgus flatfoot resulting from naviculocuneiform and talonavicular sag. Surgical correction in the adolescent. *In* Bateman, J. E. (ed.): Foot Science. Philadelphia, W. B. Saunders Co., 1976, pp. 67–105. Reprinted by permission.)

atarsal, medial cuneiform, and navicular, however, remain in a straight line and intersect the long axis of the talus at an angle (Fig. 5–4B).

The *plantar-flexion angle of the talus* is defined as the angle formed between the horizontal plantar line and a line drawn through the center of the longitudinal axis of the talus (bisecting the talar neck and head) on a weight-bearing lateral projection. The normal plantar-flexion angle of the talus measures 26.5 degrees (S.D., 5.3 degrees).[11]

The talus, in addition to being plantarflexed, deviates medially. In the anteroposterior roentgenogram, with the medial deviation of the talus and the lateral tilting of the anterior end of the calcaneus, the anteroposterior talocalcaneal angle is widened, usually to more than 35 degrees. The navicular is displaced laterally in relation to the head of the talus. Giannestras assesses the degree of medial deviation of the talar head in relation to the navicular by the dorsoplantar talonavicular angle. One line is drawn parallel to the distal articular surface of the navicular; another line is drawn through the longitudinal axis of the talus (bisecting the talar head-neck). The two lines form an angle of between 60 and 80 degrees. An angle of less than 60 degrees is abnormal and indicates medial deviation of the talus (Figs. 5–5 and 5–6).[38]

When the break takes place *at the naviculocuneiform joint alone*, in the lateral roentgenogram of the foot the longitudinal axes of the talus and the navicular make a straight line and bisect the navicular vertical line perpendicularly, but they exit on the plantar aspect of the medial cuneiform proximal to the base of the first metatarsal (see Fig. 5–4C). In the lateral view of the standing roentgenogram of the foot, Giannestras draws lines over the proximal articular surface of the navicular and over the distal articular surface of the medial cuneiform. In a normal foot the longitudinal axis of the talus (bisecting the talar head) crosses the navicular articular line at a right angle. A line drawn from the plantar aspect of the first metatarsal head is perpendicular to the medial cuneiform articular line. The line running through the long axis of the talus to the plantar aspect of the first metatarsal head in the normal foot is slightly angulated dorsally at the naviculocuneiform joint as shown in Figure 5–5A; when the line is straight it is considered to be the lower limit of the normal. When there is a sag at the naviculocuneiform joint the line is angulated plantarward (Fig. 5–7.)[38]

When the break occurs *at both the talonavicular and naviculocuneiform joints*, Jack recommends drawing a line through the longitudinal axis of the navicular, which when extended proximally and distally, lies plantar to the talar and first metatarsal segments (see Fig. 5–4D).[65]

An example of severe flexible flat foot due to breaks in all three components that make up the longitudinal arch—talocalcaneal, talonavicular, and naviculocuneiform joints—is illustrated in Figure 5–8.

The angle formed between the horizontal and a line drawn along the plantar border of the calcaneus extending between its posterior and anterior tuberosities on the lateral projection of the weight-bearing roentgenogram of the foot is called the calcaneal pitch; its normal value is 15 to 20 degrees. In flat foot with contracture of the triceps surae muscle, the calcaneal pitch is low (less than 15 degrees); in pes calcaneus it is high (30 degrees or more) (Fig. 5–9).

Clinical Features

In children, flexible flat foot is asymptomatic. It is the parents who are concerned about the appearance of the feet; or it may be a problem of abnormal shoe wear. In the obese older child or the adolescent, prolonged standing may give rise to foot strain, with pain in the longitudinal arch, abnormal fatigue, and discomfort extending upward on the legs. If there is associated myostatic contracture of the triceps surae muscle, the presenting complaint may be pain in the calf. The permanent shortening of the gastrocnemius-soleus muscle is demonstrated by testing the range of passive dorsiflexion of the ankle with the hindfoot in slight inversion or neutral (never valgus) position and the knee in neutral extension. The angle that the plantar aspect of the foot makes with the longitudinal axis of the leg is observed from the fibular side. During

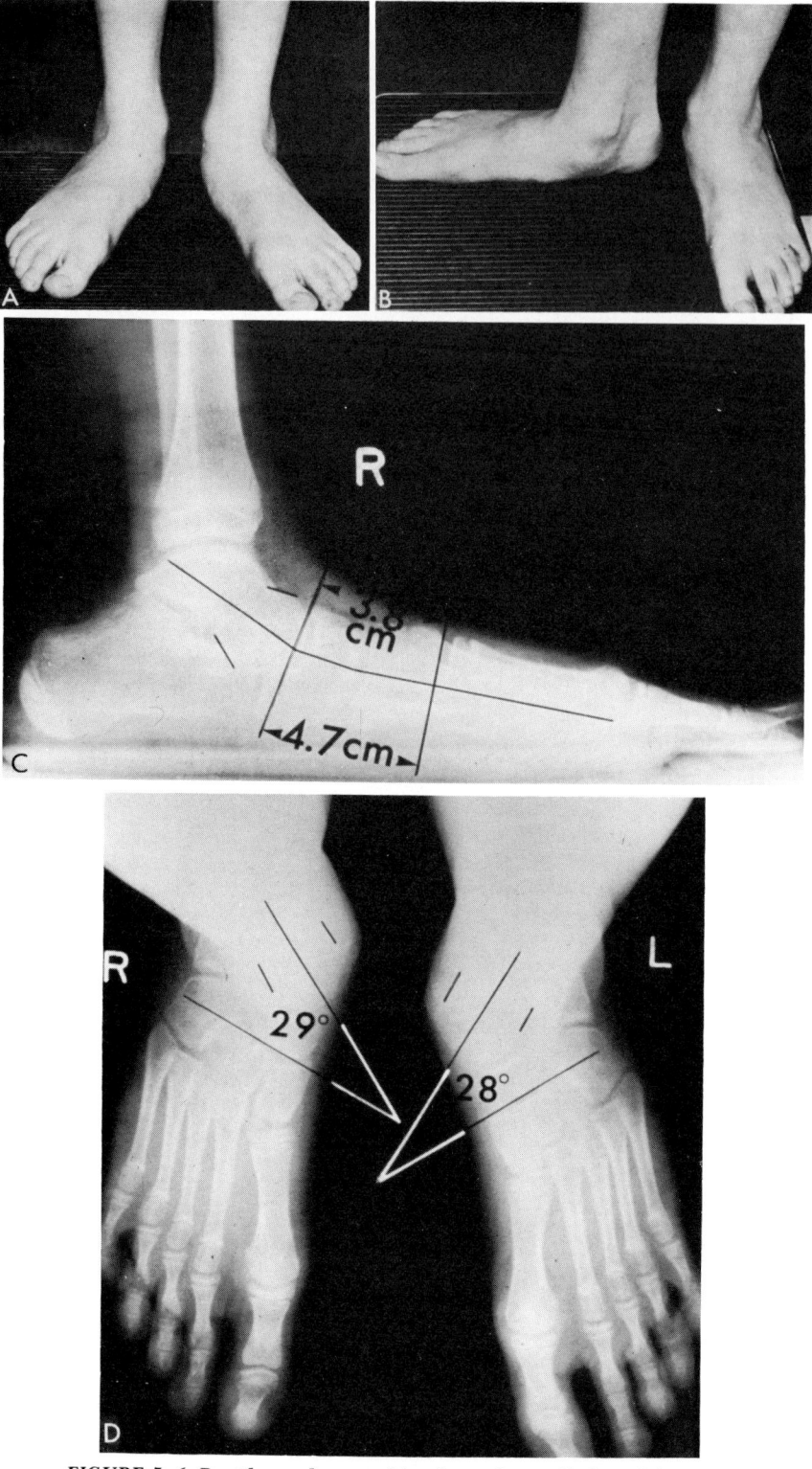

FIGURE 5–6. Pes planovalgus resulting from plantar flexion of the talus.

A and **B.** Clinical appearance showing complete absence of the longitudinal arch and the prominent plantar-flexed head of the talus just below the medial malleolus. The heels are in valgus position. **C.** Standing lateral roentgenogram of the right foot. The talus is plantar-flexed. The sag at the naviculocuneiform joint is minimal. **D.** Anteroposterior standing roentgenogram of both feet. The head of the talus is deviated medially, and the dorsoplantar talonavicular angle is markedly diminished. (From Giannestras, N.: Flexible valgus flatfoot resulting from naviculocuneiform and talonavicular sag. Surgical correction in the adolescent. *In* Bateman, J. E. (ed.): Foot Science. Philadelphia, W. B. Saunders Co., 1976, pp. 67–105. Reprinted by permission.)

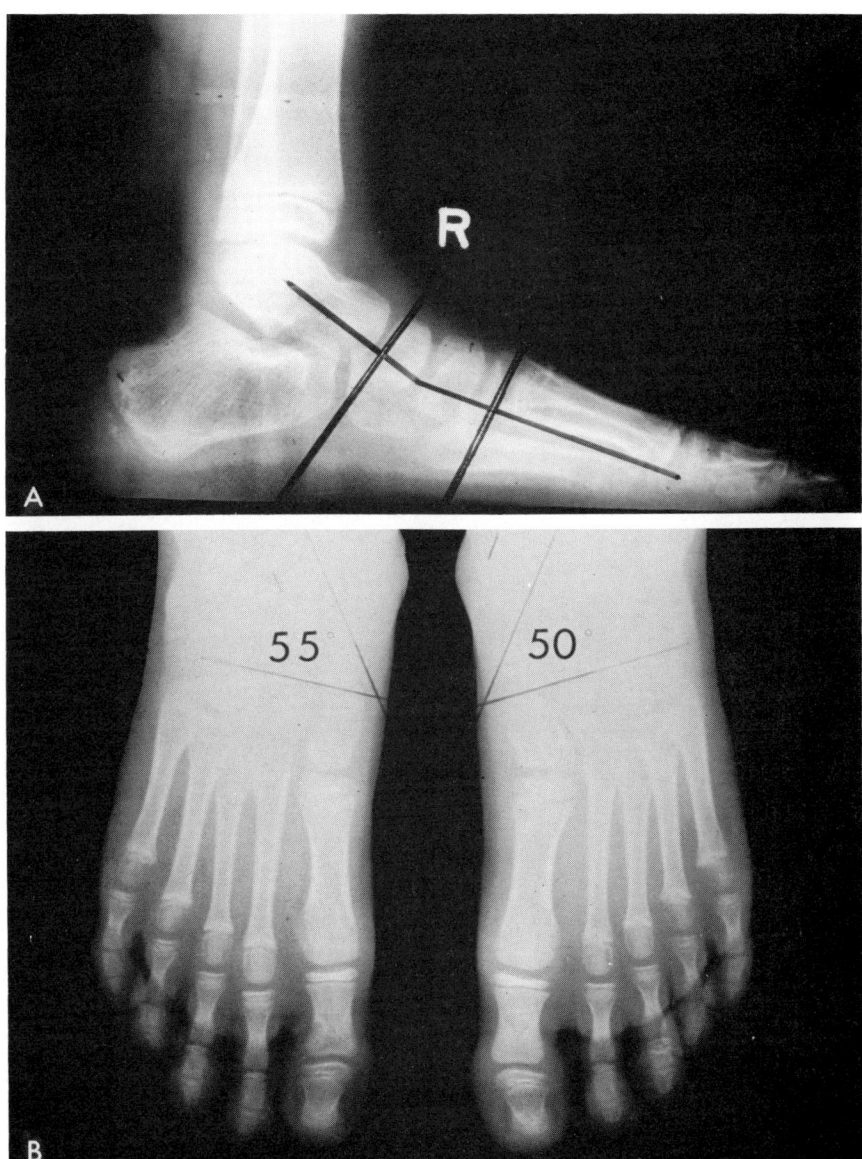

FIGURE 5–7. *Flexible flat foot due to sag at the naviculocuneiform joint.*

A. In the standing lateral roentgenogram the lines drawn through the long axes of the talus and the first metatarsal are angulated plantarward at the naviculocuneiform joint. **B.** The standing anteroposterior roentgenogram of both feet shows the decrease in the dorsoplantar talonavicular angles (the lower limit of normal is 60 degrees). (From Giannestras, N.: Flexible valgus flatfoot resulting from naviculocuneiform and talonavicular sag. Surgical correction in the adolescent. *In* Bateman, J. E., (ed.): Foot Science. Philadelphia, W. B. Saunders Co., 1976, pp. 67–105. Reprinted by permission.)

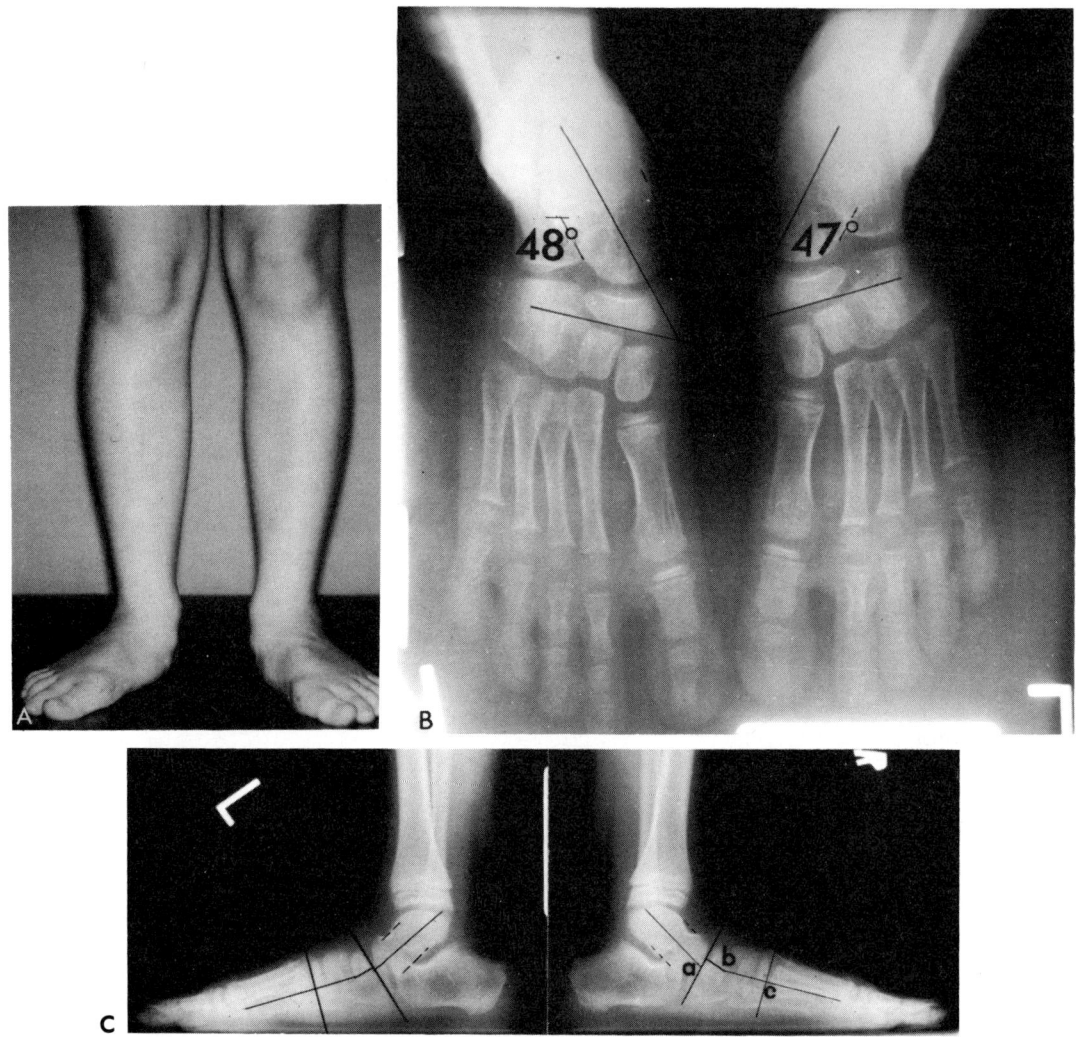

FIGURE 5–8. Severe pes planovalgus resulting from malalignment of the talocalcaneal, talonavicular, and naviculocuneiform joints.

A. Clinical appearance. **B.** Anteroposterior standing roentgenograms of both feet show decrease in the dorsoplantar talonavicular angle, 48 degrees on the right and 47 degrees on the left. **C.** In the lateral view note that the talus is plantar-flexed (a) with a plantar sag at the talonavicular joint (b). The longitudinal line drawn perpendicular to the distal articular surface of the cuneiform extends to the plantar aspect of the first metatarsal head, indicating a normal tarsometatarsal joint (c). (From Giannestras, N.: Flexible valgus flatfoot resulting from naviculocuneiform and talonavicular sag. Surgical correction in the adolescent. *In* Bateman, J. E. (ed.): Foot Science. Philadelphia, W. B. Saunders Co., 1976, pp. 67–105. Reprinted by permission.)

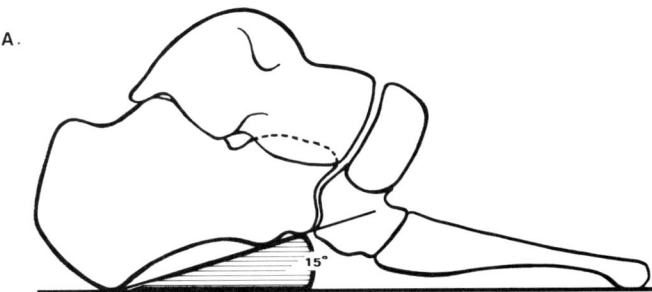

FIGURE 5–9. Calcaneal pitch.

Calcaneal pitch is determined in the standing lateral roentgenogram of the foot. It is the angle formed between the horizontal and a line drawn along the plantar border of the calcaneus extending between its posterior and anterior tuberosities. **A.** In flat foot it is decreased to less than 15 degrees. **B.** Its normal value is 20 to 25 degrees. **C.** In calcaneus feet the calcaneal pitch is high—over 30 degrees. (Redrawn from Gamble, F. O., and Yale, I.: Clinical Foot Roentgenology. 2nd Ed. New York, Robert E. Krieger Publishing Co., Inc., 1975, p. 194.)

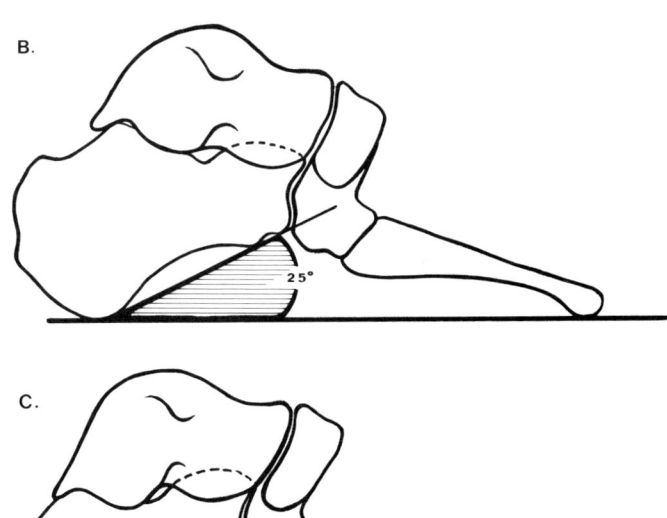

this test, the dorsiflexors of the ankle should not contract actively, as their contraction will cause reciprocal relaxation of the triceps surae muscles.

Faulty shoes or abusive use of the feet will aggravate the symptoms. Prolonged bed rest due to ill health will increase the ligamentous laxity and consequently exaggerate pronation of the feet.

Flexible flat foot is divided into three categories of severity: *Mild* or *first degree*—in which on weight-bearing the longitudinal arch is depressed but still visible; *moderate* or *second degree*—in which the longitudinal arch is not visible in stance; and *severe* or *third degree*—in which the longitudinal arch is absent and the medial border of the foot is convex with the head of the talus presenting on the plantar aspect of the foot immediately below and anterior to the medial malleolus (Fig. 5–10).

When not bearing weight, as when the patient is sitting on the examining table with the legs dangling, the feet have normal longitudinal arch and contour; under the weight of the body, however, the longitudinal arch becomes obliterated and the foot appears flat. There may be varying degrees

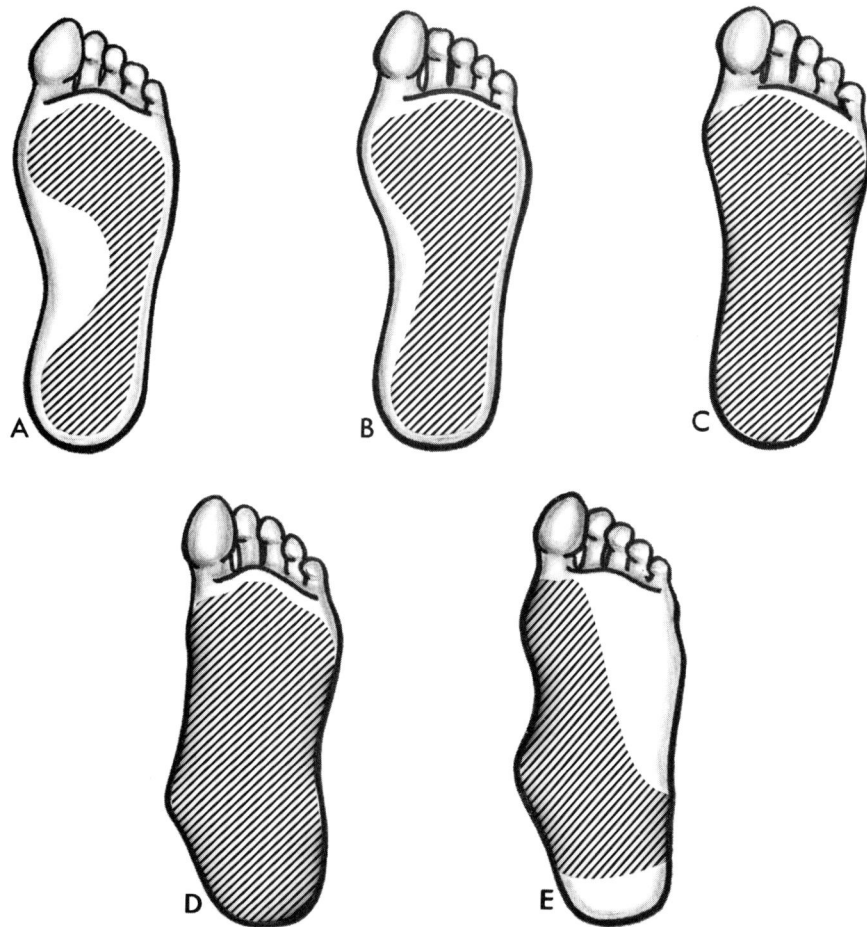

FIGURE 5–10. Foot prints of varying degrees of flat foot.

A. Normal. **B.** Mild or first-degree. The longitudinal arch is low but still visible. **C.** Moderate or second degree—the longitudinal arch is absent. **D.** Severe or third degree—the longitudinal arch is absent and the medial border of the foot is convex with the head of the talus pressing on the plantar aspect of the foot. **E.** Rocker-bottom deformity in congenital convex pes valgus. The heel is in equinus position, the forefoot is dorsiflexed and everted, and the head of the talus is prominent on the sole. The deformity is rigid; it does not disappear when not weight-bearing.

of valgus deviation of the hindfoot and plantar flexion and medial deviation of the talus.

On clinical examination it is difficult to detect the site of the sag, whether it is at the naviculocuneiform joint, at the talonavicular joint, or combined in both joints. The "toe-raising test" described by Jack will give an indication but is not infallible.[65] The patient stands bearing weight on both feet. On passive hyperextension of the big toe the longitudinal arch is elevated in all cases of naviculocuneiform sag and in most cases of combined (naviculocuneiform and talonavicular) breaks; this maneuver, however, does not restore the arch when the talus is plantar-flexed and the sag is at only the talonavicular joint (Fig. 5–11). It seems the flexor hallucis longus does not have sufficient leverage to force the navicular under the head of the talus. When the triceps surae is contracted, the toe-raising test cannot be performed because the flexor hallucis is inefficient.

Examination of the child often reveals that the excessive ligamentous laxity is generalized, as shown by the hyperextensibility of the elbows, wrists, thumbs, and knees. Muscle testing is performed to rule out muscle weakness and imbalance. A neurologic examination is carried out to detect neurologic defect.

In adult life, structural changes may gradually develop in the tarsal bones, and the planovalgus deformity may become progressively rigid. Eventually foot strain may cause disabling pain. Adult women tend to have more discomfort in the forepart of the foot (the so-called anterior or transverse arch) because of wearing shoes with high heels, which causes the weight to be transmitted to the metatarsal heads.

Treatment

In the infant and the young child up to three years of age the plantar surface of the foot appears to be flat. The portion of the foot that subsequently becomes the longitudinal arch is filled with a pad of fat. These feet are normal. As the child gets older this fat pad shrinks, the ligaments become taut, and a normal longitudinal arch develops. These normal feet should be left alone.

The mild or first-degree flat foot requires no treatment. A proportion of the human race has low longitudinal arches; such "flat feet" are normal provided they are flexible, have good muscle control, the hindfoot is not pronated more than 10 to 15 degrees, and there is no associated myostatic contracture of the triceps surae muscle. They will stand as much hard usage without producing pain or disability as do feet with so-called "normal arches." As stated earlier, the child with moderately flat feet toes-in actively so that the center of gravity of the body is shifted laterally toward the center of the foot (see Fig. 5–2B). That such toeing-in is Nature's way of protecting a child's foot and is therefore good for him should be explained to the parents, who may find it difficult to comprehend, especially when they have sought medical advice because their child is toeing-in. The toeing-

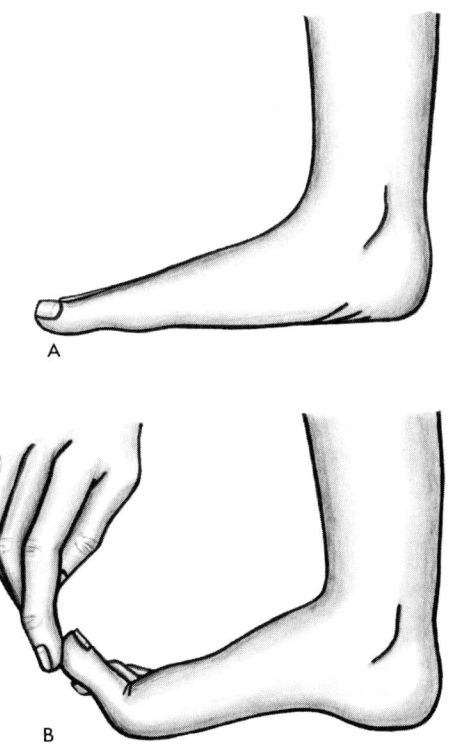

FIGURE 5–11. The "toe-raising test" of Jack.

A. Pes planus due to sag at the naviculocuneiform joint. **B.** On passive dorsiflexion of the great toe the longitudinal arch is elevated. When the talus is plantar-flexed and the sag is only at the talonavicular joint, hyperextension of the big toe does not restore the longitudinal arch. The test is not reliable in the presence of triceps surae contracture.

in calls into action the tibialis anterior and posterior muscles, the long and short toe flexors, and the adductors of the foot; using them gives additional muscular support to the longitudinal arch. Toeing-in should *not* be discouraged nor should any effort be made to prevent it by reversing shoes, putting lateral wedges on the soles of the shoes, or using Denis Browne splints or other orthoses. The more the child toes-in and shifts the center of the body weight to the center of the foot, the sooner he will correct the associated physiologic genu valgum. The parents are assured of satisfactory foot function later on in life. Nature should be left alone.

Flexible flat foot in children does not cause pain. Pain is indicative of the presence of some other pathologic condition. Commonly it is the result of contracture of the triceps surae muscle, and occasionally it is due to tarsal coalition or an inflammatory process such as rheumatoid arthritis involving the subtalar and midtarsal joints. Roentgenograms of the foot are made and, if indicated, bone imaging with ^{99m}technetium is performed to rule out rare lesions such as osteoid osteoma or stress fracture. If there is restriction of motion of the tarsal joints, a CT scan of the foot may be indicated to detect obscure tarsal coalition.

Foot strain may occur in children with normal arches as well as in those with flat feet. It is not the flatness of the longitudinal arch, but rather the medial shift in weight-bearing that is the important factor in producing foot strain. It occurs more commonly in children who are overweight and physically sluggish. A foot with a high arch is more susceptible to pain and disability than is the flexible flat foot.

CONSERVATIVE MANAGEMENT

Children with mild or moderate flexible flat foot should be allowed to go without shoes on sand at the beach, on grass in a yard or park, or on a thick rug at home. The bare foot will respond to contact with natural terrain by dynamic action of all the muscles controlling the foot and normal motion of the joints. There is absolutely no scientific evidence that encasing the foot in stiff leather above-ankle shoes and shoe modifications such as built in longitudinal arch supports, scaphoid pads, Thomas heels, medial heel wedges, or extended medial heel counters are of any therapeutic value for correcting flexible flat foot.[10, 112, 113] Unfortunately, in urban living, a child may have to spend hours walking on hard floors and pavements. Nature did not plan the human foot for such hard terrain. In such circumstances the feet are supported in a pair of good Oxford shoes.

Various exercise programs to strengthen the muscles of the foot and leg have been advocated in the literature.[7, 19, 62, 127] This author does not, however, believe that muscle weakness causes flexible pes planovalgus. Active exercises such as toe curling or picking up objects with the toes or tip-toe walking or walking with the feet inverted have no therapeutic value. It is archaic to force these children to perform exercises for 15 to 30 minutes each day. Such "toe twiddling" should be abandoned. Instead of being forced to stay in his room and pick up marbles with his toes, the poor child should be allowed to go out in the yard and play with his friends. The overanxious parents should be soothed through some other outlet, such as jogging or swimming and exercising themselves. Often the parents require more reassurance than the children with flat feet need treatment.

The only exercise recommended is elongation of the contracted triceps surae muscle by passive stretching exercises performed manually or against the wall (Fig. 5–12).

In growing children over three or four years of age, the third-degree or severe flexible flat foot is treated by supporting the hindfoot and providing adequate room for the forepart of the foot. An attempt is made to shift weight-bearing laterally over the center of the foot to prevent foot strain. A common practice is to apply a wedged raise (1/8 to 3/16 inch) on the medial side of the heel and a Thomas heel to the shoe. A longitudinal arch support in the form of a 3/8-inch-thick flexible felt, leather, or rubber pad is glued to the insole; and, often, additional support is provided by extending the medial counter of the heel forward. The purpose is to tilt the hindfoot into inversion. This will not be accomplished, because the uprights of the heel of the shoe do not grip the heel snugly, and the hindfoot simply twists into eversion. Numerous

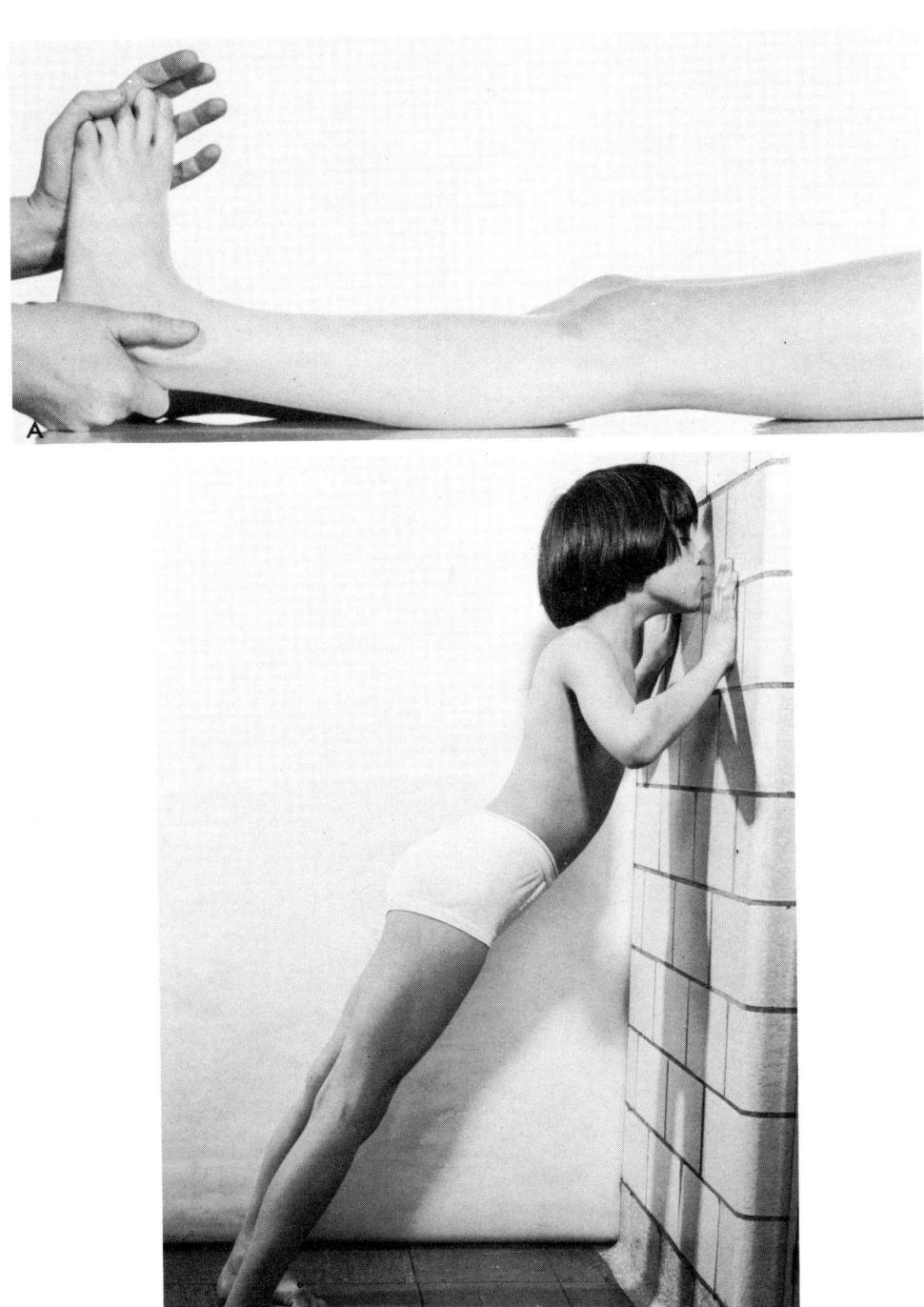

FIGURE 5–12. *Passive stretching of contracted triceps surae muscle.*

A. Manual stretching by the parents. Note the knee should be in extended position and the hindfoot slightly inverted. The child should not actively dorsiflex the ankle, as contraction of the anterior tibial muscle will relax the gastrocnemius-soleus muscles—its reciprocal antagonists. The maximally dorsiflexed position is maintained to the count of 10 and then relaxed. Exercises are performed 20 times each at three sessions a day. **B.** Passive stretching of triceps surae muscles against the wall is indicated in the older cooperative child. Note the feet are in inversion. The knees should not be hyperextended.

heel inserts (cups) are available commercially. Such devices satisfy the anxious parents and the shoe salesmen, but do little, if anything, to correct the deformity. In symptomatic flexible flat foot, however, they may relieve pain in a certain percentage of the cases.

Basta and Mital and their associates presented a clinical and roentgenographic study of 50 children with symptomatic flexible flat feet treated over a period of four years with varying combinations of shoes, custom-made arch supports, and pads. They concluded that conservative treatment of symptomatic flat feet in children can be successful in relieving subjective discomfort. They realized pain is a subjective patient response, but the success could be correlated with objective roentgenographic measurements. They recommended that children with symptomatic flexible flat foot should be fitted initially with laced high-top shoes containing a steel shank and firm counter. A custom-made navicular pad is added if the recommended shoe does not afford adequate symptomatic relief. Navicular "cookies" were found to be less effective than navicular pads.[6]

Bleck and Berzins performed a prospective study of 71 cases of flexible pes valgus with plantar-flexed talus followed up for periods of more than one year. The UCBL (University of California Biomechanics Laboratory) foot orthosis, shown in Figure 5–13, and Helfet heel seat improved the clinical and roentgenographic appearance of the feet in 79 per cent of the patients. These authors recommended the use of the Helfet heel seat when the plantar-flexion angle of the talus is 35 to 45 degrees, and the UCBL foot orthosis in those cases in which the plantar-flexion angle of the talus is greater than 45 degrees.[11]

Mereday, Dolan, and Lusskin reported the results of treatment of flexible pes planus by UCBL foot orthoses worn by 12 children over a two-year period. The study was documented by photographic and roentgenographic measurements, gait analysis, and a subjective questionnaire. It was

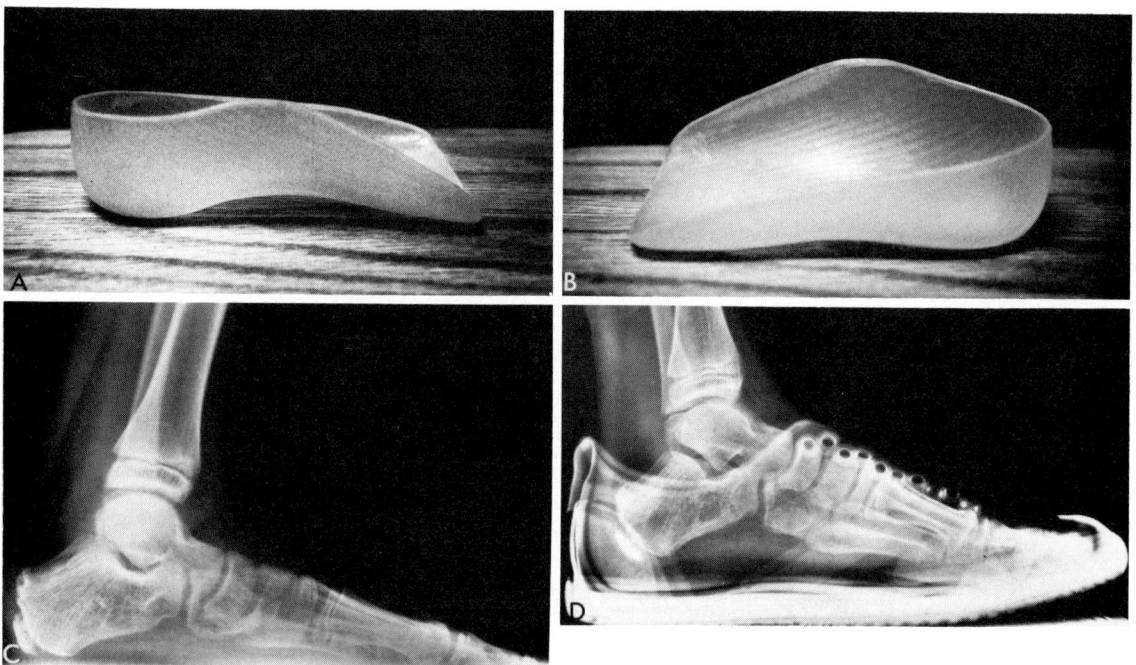

FIGURE 5–13. UCBL foot orthosis in treatment of severe flexible pes plano valgus.

A. Medial view of foot orthosis. **B.** Lateral view of foot orthosis. **C.** Standing lateral roentgenogram of left foot. Note the sag at the naviculocuneiform and talonavicular joints. **D.** Standing lateral roentgenogram with UCBL orthosis. The normal articular relations between the naviculocuneiform and talonavicular joints are restored, and the calcaneal pitch has improved to normal.

concluded (1) that protracted wearing of the UCBL foot orthosis relieved local pain in the anterior tibial muscles and diffuse pain in six children; (2) that there was some improvement in gait in eight patients, and that shoe wear was more even while the inserts were worn; and (3) that in the presence of relatively fixed foot deformity, the inserts failed to achieve lasting structural changes.[87]

In summary, factors to consider in treatment are (1) the age of the patient; (2) the severity of deformity; (3) the shoe wear; and (4) the symptoms. Mild and moderate degrees of flexible flat foot require no treatment in any age group. A well-fitted pair of good Oxford shoes is all that is needed. The symptomatic moderate flat foot in the older child is usually associated with contracture of the triceps surae; passive stretching exercises are performed to elongate the shortened calf muscles. A shoe prescription may be given for the symptomatic flat foot. It consists of a Thomas heel, a 1/8- to 3/16-inch medial heel wedge, an extended medial counter, and a 3/8-inch-high longitudinal arch support glued to the insole. The objective of such a shoe prescription is to relieve mild local discomfort of foot strain and not to correct flat foot. Older children with flat feet wear down the lateral part of the heels; raising the medial side of the shoe in such cases will increase the excessive wear of the lateral side of the heel. In these children the heel of the shoe is not altered; instead a Helfet plastic heel seat or, preferably, a UCBL foot orthosis is prescribed if the symptoms warrant it.

When a child presents with severe flexible flat foot one should rule out an underlying neuromuscular disorder such as benign congenital hypotonia, muscular dystrophy, Down's syndrome, Marfan's syndrome, osteogenesis imperfecta, or Ehlers-Danlos syndrome. These feet are symptomatic and cause rapid abnormal shoe wear. They should be supported by UCBL foot orthoses during the period of rapid skeletal growth of the foot (up to 8 to 10 years in girls and 10 to 12 years in boys). With the UCBL foot orthoses these children can wear any type of shoe and appear normal to their peers. The UCBL foot orthosis is also given to the juvenile or adolescent with severe flat foot to alleviate pain prior to consideration for surgery.

SURGICAL MANAGEMENT

Operative correction of pes planovalgus is indicated when the deformity is so marked that it causes rapid abnormal wear of the shoes as shown in Figure 5–14, or the discomfort in the foot persists despite proper conservative measures and prevents the patient from taking part in normal activities. Only a small percentage of patients with symptomatic flat foot fail to respond to conservative measures. Surgery should not be considered before the age of ten years.

Ideally surgical correction of flexible flat foot should provide a foot with a normal longitudinal arch that is free of pain and has normal range of motion and function. This is not always possible.

In the literature numerous operative procedures have been described for correction of flexible pes planovalgus. In general they can be divided into four groups: (1) soft-tissue procedures alone—ligamentous tightening, release of contracted soft tissue, and muscle-tendon transfer; (2) arthrodesis of tarsal joints; (3) osteotomy of tarsal bones with or without bone grafts (calcaneus, cuboid, or medial cuneiform); and (4) bone and joint operations combined with soft-tissue procedures (Table 5–2). Some of the operations have been discarded and are of historic interest only; they are therefore not considered in this text.

In the choice of operative procedure to correct flexible pes planovalgus the following factors should be considered: (1) the anatomic *site of the sag* in the longitudinal arch (Is it at the naviculocuneiform joint, at the talonavicular joint, or at both joints?); (2) the *plantar flexion angle of the talus* (Is it normal or is the talus tilted into an excessively equinus posture? Does the lateral roentgenogram of the foot indicate that the anatomic relationship between the talus and calcaneus and between the navicular and talar head can be restored to normal by full plantar flexion of the ankle and forefoot?); (3) the *degree of medial deviation of the talar axis* (What is the dorsoplantar talonavicular angle? Is the navicular displaced laterally in relation to the head of the talus?); (4) the *degree of hindfoot valgus deviation* (Is the anteroposterior talocalcaneal angle widened? Is there any valgus deformity of the ankle?) It is imperative to have standing antero-

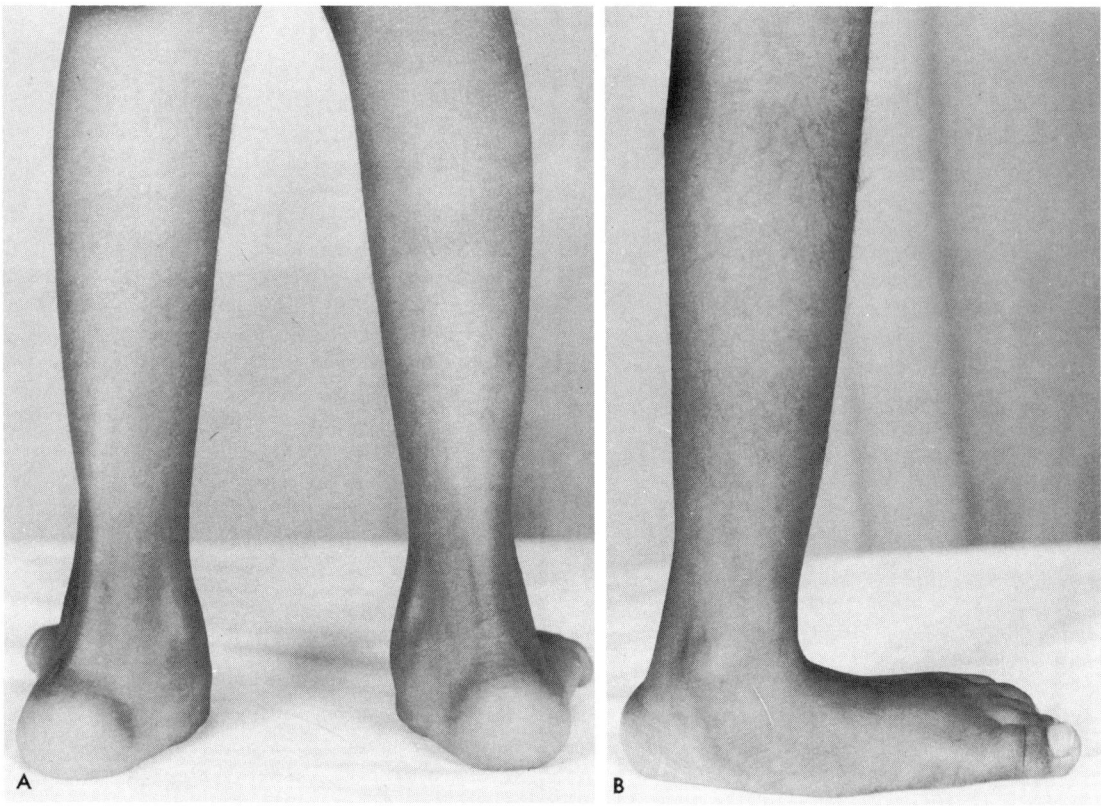

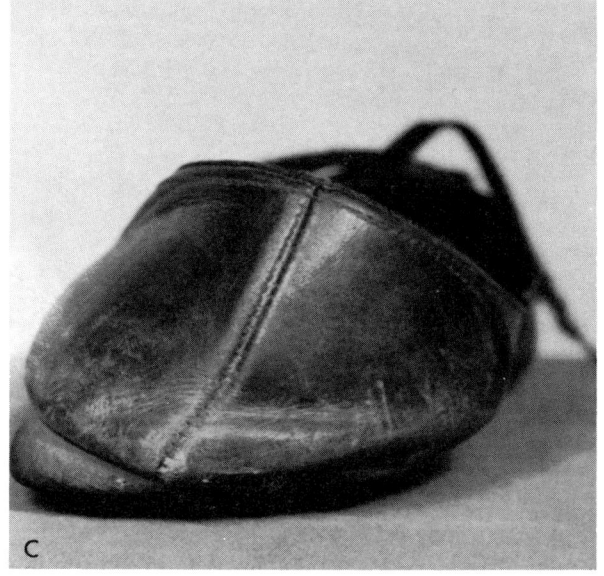

FIGURE 5–14. *Severe flexible flat foot in an eight-year-old girl.*

Surgical correction of deformity is indicated in such a case. **A.** Posterior view of both feet and legs. **B.** Medial view of left foot. **C.** Abnormal wear of left shoe.

posterior roentgenograms of the ankle and to note the relationship of the distal fibular physis to the level of the ankle. Is there abnormal lateral tilting of the dome contracture of the talus?); (5) the *calcaneal pitch* (Is it low or flat or at an equinus angle owing to contracture of the triceps surae muscle?); (6) the presence of *soft-tissue contracture* (Is it ligamentous or myostatic? Is there any muscle imbalance?); (7) the *age* of the patient; (8) the *rigidity* of flat foot (Can the foot be passively corrected to normal?

Are there arthritic changes in the tarsal joints?).

Treatment of Flexible Pes Planovalgus Due to Sag at Naviculocuneiform Joint

NAVICULOCUNEIFORM FUSION. Hoke, in 1931, introduced naviculocuneiform fusion for correction of flexible pes planus; he believed fusion gives a longer and more stable level on which the muscles act to maintain the longitudinal arch.[62] Butte, in 1937, reported unsatisfactory results in 50 per cent of the naviculocuneiform fusions for flat foot.[16] Crego and Ford, in 1952, criticized the operation as being insufficient to support the flattened longitudinal arch.[24] Jack, in 1953, reported the results of naviculocuneiform fusion in 46 feet in 25 patients, aged 11 to 14 years, with flexible flat foot with a break at the naviculocuneiform joint; 15 months to five years after operation, the results were excellent in 54 per cent, good in 28 per cent, and unsatisfactory in 18 per cent. Jack stressed that proper selection of patients was most important and that the procedure reconstructed the longitudinal arch only if roentgenographically verified collapse was restricted to the naviculocuneiform joint.[65] In 1967, 16 to 19 years after the surgery, Seymour reassessed 17 of the 25 patients on whom Jack had operated. The results were excellent in 31 per cent, good in 19 per cent, and unsatisfactory in 50 per cent. Seymour pointed out that it is unlikely that only naviculocuneiform ligaments are affected and solely responsible for the flattening of the medial longitudinal arch, and the stabilization of only one segment of the complex cannot be expected to prevent collapse of the entire arch. He also cautioned that the procedure will cause degenerative arthritis in the adjacent joints, which are subjected to additional load and stress following naviculocuneiform arthrodesis.[106] This author agrees with Seymour and does not recommend arthrodesis of the naviculocuneiform joint alone.

TENDON TRANSFERS AND LIGAMENTOUS TAUTENING PROCEDURES. In the literature a number of tendon transfers have been proposed to provide a dynamic force to elevate the apex of the medial longitudinal arch. Transfer of the anterior tibial tendon to the dorsum of the navicular bone (without arthrodesis of the tarsal joints) was first performed by Müller, modified by Legg, and popularized by Young.[76, 91, 126] Both peroneal tendons were transferred dorsally into the medial cuneiform by Ryerson.[99] Osmond-Clarke transferred the peroneus brevis to the head of the talus.

Transfer of the medial half of the Achilles tendon to the first metatarsal neck was described by Jones.[66] He emphasized the importance of the medial plantar fascia in maintaining the structural integrity of the longitudinal arch of the foot. He designed an operation by which the incompetent plantar fascia is reinforced by transferring the medial half of the Achilles tendon to the first metatarsal neck. A longitudinal incision is made on the medial side of the tendo Achillis. The subcutaneous tissue and paratenon are divided in line with the skin incision. The Achilles tendon is split sagittally into halves. The medial half with its fascial prolongations over the muscle belly is divided at its proximal end but is left attached at its insertion to the calcaneus. The plantar and medial aspects of the calcaneus are exposed by undermining and elevating subcutaneous tissues. Next, a second incision is made over the medial aspect of the first metatarsal neck. With an Ober tendon passer or Kocher forceps a subcutaneous tunnel is made from the metatarsal incision to the back of the heel. The free separated upper end of the medial strip of the Achilles tendon is pulled out and delivered into the second wound. A drill hole of appropriate diameter is made in the neck of the first metatarsal; the rolled-up fascial prolongation of the calcaneal tendon is passed through the hole and tautly sutured to itself, holding the longitudinal arch of the foot in the corrected position. After closure of the wounds, a below-knee cast is applied and worn for three months. During the last six weeks, a walking heel is added and weight-bearing is allowed. Jones reported satisfactory results in three patients, two, six, and seven years after surgery (Fig. 5–15).[66] This author has had no personal experience with this operation.

Phelps tautened the soft tissues on the medial aspect of the foot by division and shortening or by plication.[93] Schoolfield transferred the deltoid ligament proximally; he believed pes planovalgus is caused by insufficiency of the deltoid ligament,

Table 5–2. Surgical Procedures for Correction of Flexible Flat Foot

Operation	Objective	Indication	Comment
Operations on Soft Tissues			
Distal advancement of plantar calcaneonavicular ligament and posterior tibial tendon (Miller)	Tauten "sling" that supports medial longitudinal arch	Naviculocuneiform sag	Effective if combined with arthrodesis of naviculocuneiform joint
Transfer of anterior tibial tendon dorsally to the navicular bone (Lowman, Young)	Alter direction of pull of anterior tibial tendon from dorsiflexion of first metatarsal to dorsal elevation of navicular bone and apex of medial longitudinal arch	Naviculocuneiform sag	Effective if combined with stabilization of naviculocuneiform or talonavicular joint and distal advancement of posterior tibial tendon and plantar calcaneonavicular ligament
Transfer of medial half of Achilles tendon to first metatarsal neck (Jones)	Reinforce incompetent plantar fascia	Talonavicular and naviculocuneiform sag	No experience with this procedure
Proximal transfer of deltoid ligament (Schoolfield)	Maintain calcaneus in neutral position	Valgus hindfoot	Ineffective—will stretch out
Lengthening of Achilles tendon	Correct eversion pull on os calcis by contracted triceps surae	Taut triceps surae not responding to passive stretching exercises	Perform sliding lengthening. Section lateral half of heel cord insertion distally
Stabilization of Joints by Arthrodesis			
Naviculocuneiform fusion (Hoke)	Provide longer and more stable lever arm on which muscles act and maintain longitudinal arch	Naviculocuneiform sag	Effective if combined with distal transfer of plantar calcaneonavicular ligament and posterior tibial tendon. Caution—added stress on adjacent joints
Talonavicular fusion (Lowman)	Give stability of lever arm and correct plantar deviation of talus	Talonavicular sag	Lowman combined with transfer of anterior tibial tendon to navicular. Caution—causes stiffness of hindfoot. Grice or triple arthrodesis better

Table 5–2. *Surgical Procedures for Correction of Flexible Flat Foot (Continued)*

Operation	Objective	Indication	Comment
Extra-articular subtalar arthrodesis (Grice)	Stabilize subtalar joint in neutral position	Valgus malalignment at talocalcaneal and talonavicular joints	Does not correct midfoot valgus deformity. Transfer distally plantar calcaneonavicular and posterior tibial tendon if talonavicular and naviculocuneiform sag
Triple arthrodesis	Stabilize talocalcaneonavicular and calcaneocuboid joints	Valgus malalignment of all three components of longitudinal arch	Stiff hindfoot. Rule out ankle valgus deviation prior to surgery. Recommend lateral inlay graft technique of Williams/Menelaus
Osteotomies of Calcaneus			
Anterolateral part of calcaneus, beneath anterolateral facet of calcaneus and immediately posterior to calcaneocuboid joint (Chambers)	Provide bony buttress to maintain normal alignment of talocalcaneal joint	Plantar flexion and valgus malalignment of talocalcaneal joint	Preserves some subtalar motion. Causes incongruity of talocalcaneal joint—stiffness a postoperative problem. Not recommended by author
Horizontal osteotomy through base of posterior articular process of calcaneus with lateral wedge graft (Baker)	Invert os calcis without disturbing subtalar joint motion	Valgus malalignment of talocalcaneal joint	Good but technically difficult operation. Use iliac double cortical wedge graft. Do not break medial cortex of calcaneus!
Lateral open-up osteotomy of calcaneus with bone graft wedge (Dwyer)	Invert os calcis without disturbing subtalar joint motion	Valgus malalignment of talocalcaneal joint	Technically easier but not as effective as Baker operation. Not recommended in flexible pes planovalgus
Medial displacement osteotomy of calcaneus (Pridie, Koutsogiannis)	Restore normal weight-bearing on calcaneus	Valgus heel	Correct triceps surae contracture by heel cord lengthening. Medial displacement should be adequate
Elongation of lateral column of foot by osteotomy of os calcis and insertion of bone graft immediately behind calcaneocuboid joint (reverse Evans)	To elongate lateral column of foot	Valgus midfoot with lateral subluxation of navicular over head of talus and lateral tilting of calcaneocuboid joint	Effective in correcting midfoot valgus deformity

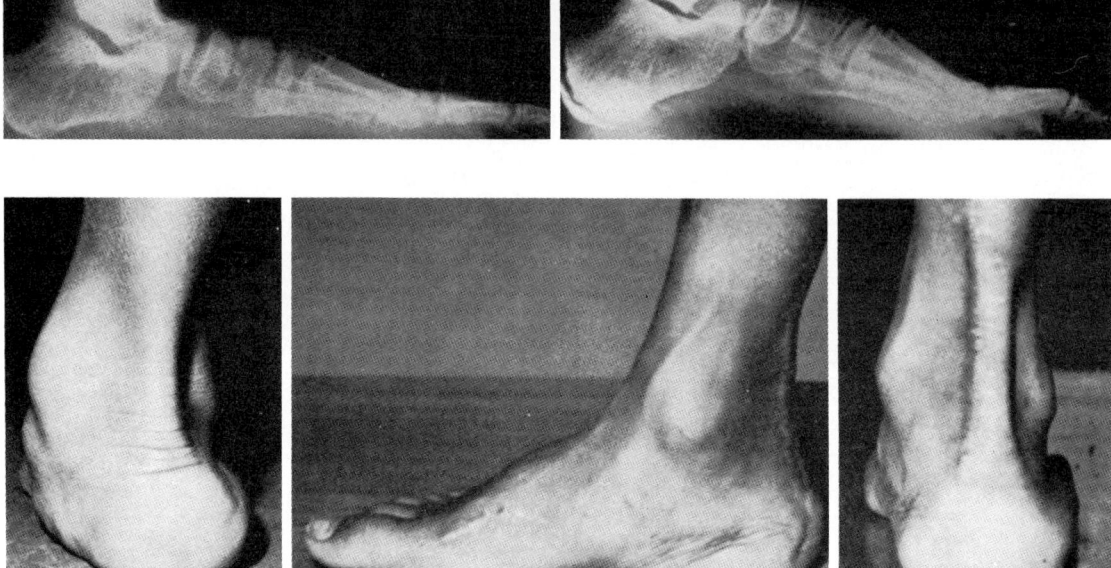

FIGURE 5–15. *Jones's operation for severe flatfoot.*

The medial half of the tendo Achillis is transferred to the first metatarsal neck to reinforce the incompetent plantar fascia. **A.** Roentgenogram of the foot before operation. **B.** Postoperative roentgenogram. **C.** Clinical appearance of the foot before surgery. **D** and **E.** Weight-bearing photographs of the foot three years after surgery. (From Jones, B. S.: Flat foot. A preliminary report of an operation for severe cases. J. Bone Joint Surg., 57-B:281, 1975. Reprinted by permission.)

which is unable to hold the calcaneus in erect attitude during weight-bearing. He therefore shortened the deltoid ligament by transferring it proximally with a periosteal flap. He claimed the advantage of the procedure was that mobility of the joints was preserved and not destroyed by arthrodesis.[103]

Ligamentous tightening and tendon advancement operations alone are not recommended by this author, as they generally do not stand the stresses of body weight and the deformity recurs.

COMBINATION OF NAVICULOCUNEIFORM FUSION AND SOFT-TISSUE TAUTENING WITH TENDON TRANSFER. In the properly selected patient, this combination of procedures is effective in correcting flat foot due to sag at the naviculocuneiform joint.

Miller described an operation in which the articulations between the navicular and medial cuneiform, and between the medial cuneiform and first metatarsal are fused in corrected position, and in which the plantar calcaneonavicular ligament and posterior tibial tendon are transferred distally, thus tightening the "sling" that supports the medial longitudinal arch and holding up the head of the talus in normal relationship with the anterior end of the calcaneus.[90] Fusion of the first metatarsal and medial cuneiform articulation is not recommended by this author because this joint is stable anatomically and does not sag.

The Durham operation differs from that of Miller in two aspects: first, the cuneiform–first metatarsal joint is not fused; second, a ligamentous-periosteal flap is raised from the medial and plantar aspect of the navicular and medial cuneiform with its base left attached distally at the base of the first metatarsal. After navicular cuneiform fusion the flap is pulled taut and attached to the sustentaculum tali, thereby reinforcing the plantar calcaneonavicular (spring) ligament and supporting the medial longitudinal arch.[17]

The Scottish-Rite operation, described by Lovell, differs from the Miller procedure in two ways: a dorsally based wedge osteotomy of the medial cuneiform is performed to elevate the longitudinal arch and the cuneiform–first metatarsal joint is left intact.[84]

Giannestras described an operation that is similar to that of Miller with the exceptions that the cuneiform–first metatarsal joint is not fused and that the tendons of the anterior tibial and posterior tibial muscles are transferred to the plantar surface of the navicular.[40] The Giannestras operation corrects the plantar sag of the naviculocuneiform joint and to a certain degree the medial sag of the talonavicular joint. This author finds it to be very effective. It is described in Plate 29. Giannestras strongly recommends that a suture be used to stabilize the medial cuneiform and navicular bones. He states that K-wires should not be used for internal fixation. This author, however, finds a small-fragment cancellous screw or two threaded K-wires are much more effective in transfixing the naviculocuneiform joint.

Treatment of Flexible Pes Planovalgus Due to Plantar Sag at Talonavicular Joint. In this type of flat foot the talus is tilted at an excessive equinus slant and the calcaneal pitch is low or flat owing to contracture of the triceps surae muscle. Often the talar axis is deviated medially and the dorsoplantar-talonavicular angle is markedly diminished (see Fig. 5–6). The navicular may be displaced laterally in relation to the head of the talus. The first step in treatment of this type of flat foot is correction of the contracture of the triceps surae muscle by passive stretching exercises and, if necessary, by a below-knee walking cast with an anteriorly placed heel. In the rigid equinus deformity that does not respond to a stretching cast, sliding lengthening of the heel cord is performed. The distal cut is made laterally. Excessive lengthening of the heel cord must be avoided.

Lowman advocated *fusion of the talonavicular joint* and transfer of the anterior tibial tendon dorsally to the navicular bone.[85] Fusion between the talus and navicular results in almost complete loss of motion of the talocalcaneonavicular joint. Because patients will have difficulty in walking on irregular terrain, this author does not recommend the Lowman operation.

Fogel and associates reported clinical, roentgenographic, and gait analysis of 11 patients in whom talonavicular fusion had been performed to relieve pain from isolated arthrosis. At a mean follow-up of 9.5 years (range 2.5 to 21 years) 3 of the 11 patients had roentgenographic evidence of arthrosis of adjacent tarsal joints that previously were unaffected. This late development of intertarsal arthrosis, however, did not cause symptoms. Isolated talonavicular arthrodesis did give relief of pain, and the patients were satisfied.[37] This author recommends talonavicular arthrodesis primarily for traumatic arthritis to provide relief of pain.

The patients who require surgical correction of flexible flat foot usually have disability and rapid abnormal wear of shoes because of valgus malalignment at the talocalcaneal and talonavicular joints. It is the pronated hindfoot that causes problems. *Extra-articular subtalar arthrodesis (Grice procedure)* corrects the hindfoot valgus deformity and restores the plantar flexion angle of the talus to normal; however, fusion eliminates motion of the subtalar joint. In paralytic pes planovalgus, stability provided by a talocalcaneal arthrodesis is desirable; for flexible pes planovalgus, however, the Grice extra-articular arthrodesis is not recommended by this author. The only indication is severe flexible pes planovalgus in syndromes with marked ligamentous hyperlaxity such as Marfan's syndrome. In such feet, valgus deformity is in the hindfoot as well as in the midfoot, and in the skeletally mature foot, triple arthrodesis is the most effective procedure (see section on triple arthrodesis). In the growing foot, a Grice extra-articular subtalar arthrodesis is recommended because it does not disturb the growth of the foot. The technique is described in Plate 15.

Dennyson and Fulford have described a technique of subtalar arthrodesis by means of metallic internal fixation and autogeneous cancellous bone grafting (Fig. 5–16). It is a modification of the Batchelor operation, but uses a metal screw instead of a bone peg to maintain the corrected position, and cancellous graft instead of cortical bone to stimulate union. The authors claim that it obviates technical problems of obtaining a satisfactory position of the hindfoot. Results of treatment of 48 feet with flexible pes planus by this method were satisfactory in 45 feet. Union occurred after an average

Text continued on page 588

Correction of Flexible Pes Planovalgus Due to Plantar Sag of Naviculocuneiform Joint and Medial Sag of Talonavicular Joint (Giannestras)

THE PROCEDURE

A. A slightly dorsally curved incision is made on the medial aspect of the foot; it begins immediately posterior to the medial malleolus, extends anteriorly to the navicular tubercle and ends at the middle of the midshaft of the first metatarsal. The subcutaneous tissue is divided in line with the skin incision; and the wound margins are undermined, elevated, and gently retracted. Avoid a short and inadequate incision.

B. The abductor hallucis muscle is detached and elevated from the medial and plantar surfaces of the medial cuneiform, navicular, plantar calcaneonavicular (spring), and laciniate ligaments. Care is taken not to injure its nerve supply.

C. Next, the posterior tibial tendon is identified. In the posterior part of the wound immediately behind the posterior tibial tendon are the flexor digitorum longus tendon and medial plantar branch of the tibial nerve; they are retracted posteriorly and plantarward. Over a blunt elevator the sheath of the posterior tibial tendon is split longitudinally from the medial malleolus to its insertion at the tuberosity of the navicular.

Plate 29. Correction of Flexible Pes Planovalgus Due to Plantar Sag of Naviculocuneiform Joint and Medial Sag of Talonavicular Joint (Giannestras)

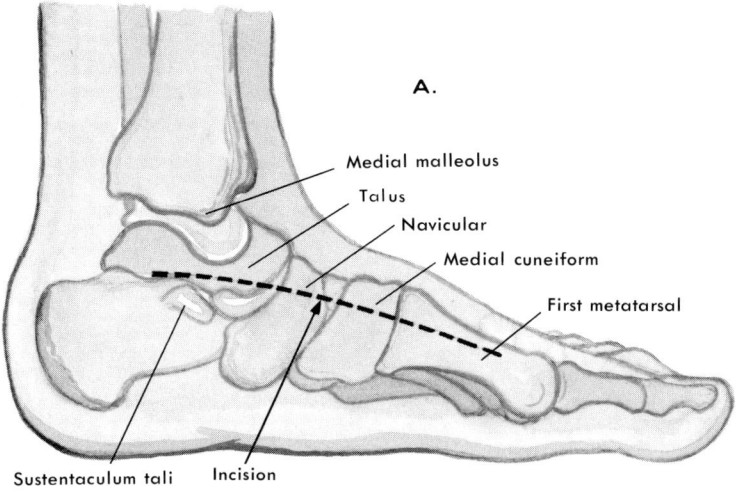

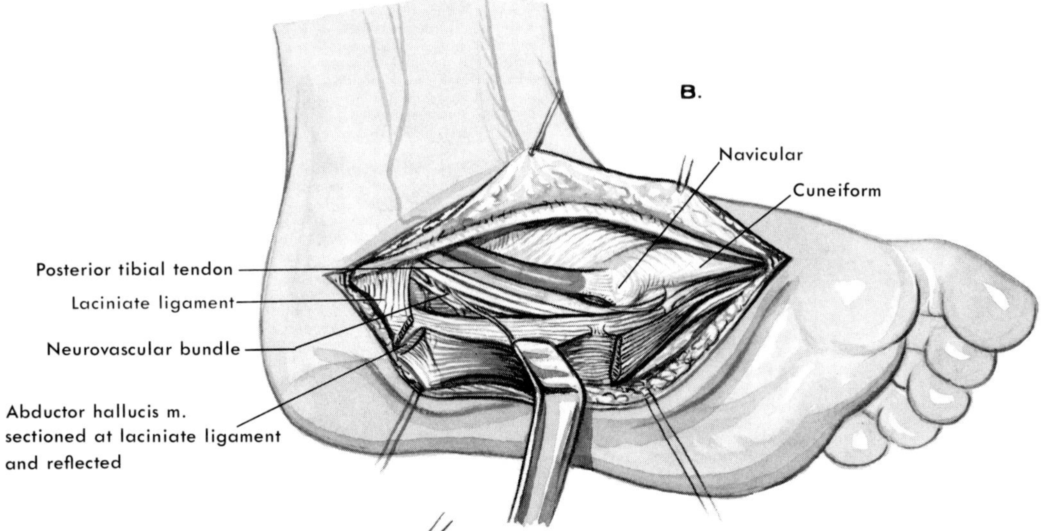

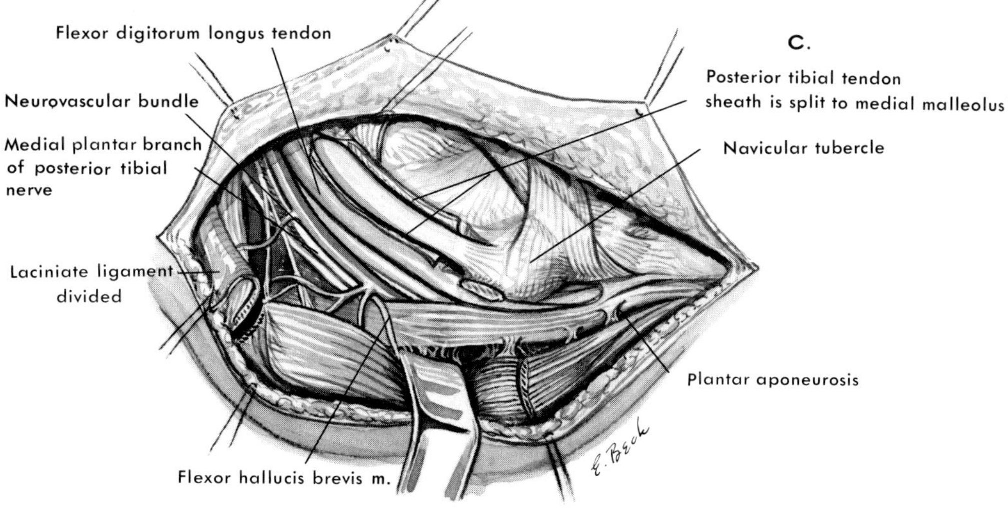

Correction of Flexible Pes Planovalgus Due to Plantar Sag of Naviculocuneiform Joint and Medial Sag of Talonavicular Joint (Giannestras) *(Continued)*

D. The posterior tibial tendon is sectioned from its insertion to the navicular tubercle and a 00 Mersilene "whip" suture is passed through the distal end of the tendon for traction and later reattachment. Caution! It is imperative to leave a moderate amount of stump of posterior tibial tendon covering the navicular tuberosity.

E. The anterior tibial tendon is identified in the dorsal and anterior part of the wound. The inferior extensor retinaculum is sectioned, and the sheath of the anterior tibial tendon is split longitudinally. The tendon is divided at its insertion to the base of the first metatarsal, and a 00 Mersilene suture is passed through its distal end.

F. The talonavicular, naviculocuneiform, and cuneiform–first metatarsal joints are identified; this should not be difficult, but, if in doubt, can be verified by making a roentgenogram with a Keith needle marking the first metatarsocuneiform joint. Next, on the medial aspect of the foot, 1.5 cm. apart, two parallel incisions are made down to underlying bone, dividing the capsule and ligamentous tissues; the two incisions extend from the distal end of the medial cuneiform to the neck of the talus adjacent to the sustentaculum tali. Do not divide the flexor digitorum longus tendon or the neurovascular bundle in the posterior part of the wound. The capsule of the first metatarsocuneiform joint is sectioned between the two parallel incisions, and with a sharp thin osteotome, an osteocartilaginous flap is elevated. The flap begins at the distal end of the medial cuneiform and extends proximally to include a thin cortical layer of the medial cuneiform and the navicular.

Plate 29. Correction of Flexible Pes Planovalgus Due to Plantar Sag of Naviculocuneiform Joint and Medial Sag of Talonavicular Joint (Giannestras)

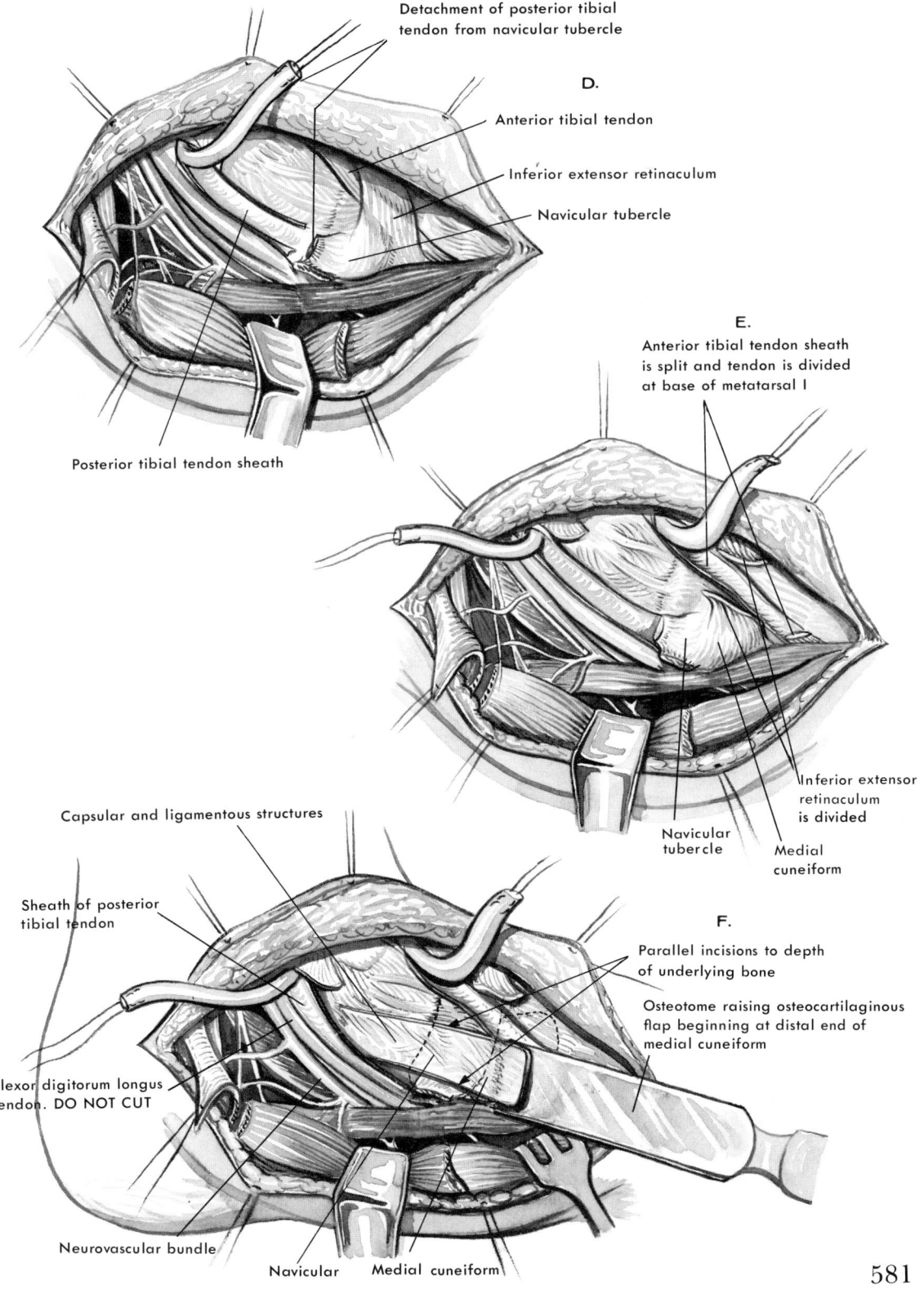

Correction of Flexible Pes Planovalgus Due to Plantar Sag of Naviculocuneiform Joint and Medial Sag of Talonavicular Joint (Giannestras) *(Continued)*

G. The osteocartilaginous flap and the capsular and ligamentous tissues are reflected. Care is taken not to tear the thin ligamentous structure between the navicular and cuneiform. The hyaline articular cartilage of the talonavicular joint should not be disturbed.

H. The plantar calcaneonavicular (or spring) ligament is identified and divided from its attachment to the navicular. It is dissected free and lifted back to its origin from the sustentaculum tali.

I. The ligamentous and capsular structures are gently dissected and elevated to expose the dorsal, medial, and plantar surfaces of the navicular and medial cuneiform bones.

Plate 29. Correction of Flexible Pes Planovalgus Due to Plantar Sag of Naviculocuneiform Joint and Medial Sag of Talonavicular Joint (Giannestras)

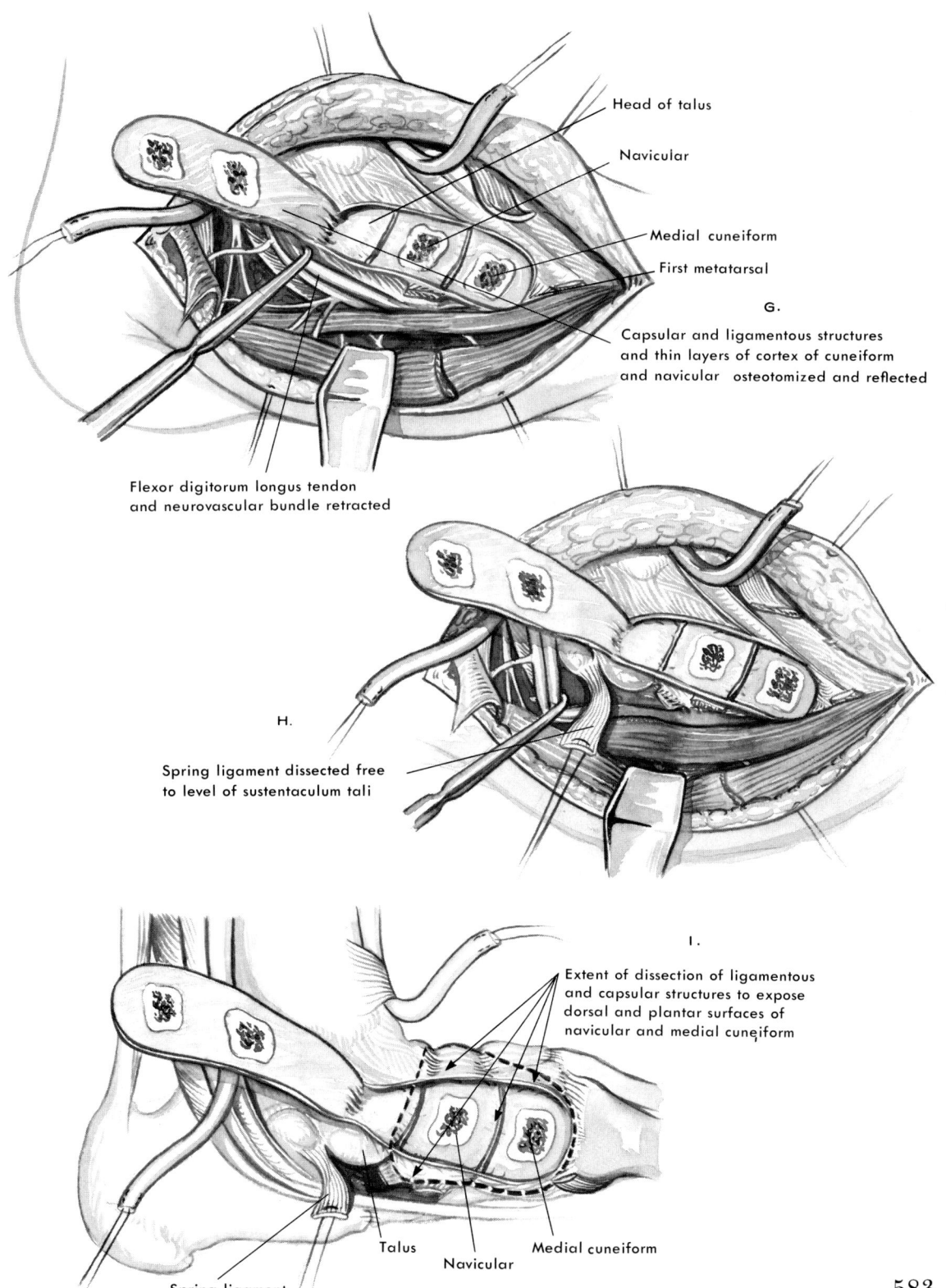

Correction of Flexible Pes Planovalgus Due to Plantar Sag of Naviculocuneiform Joint and Medial Sag of Talonavicular Joint (Giannestras) (Continued)

J. Next, the plantar aspect of the navicular is denuded of soft tissue, and the cortex is roughened with a sharp curet or rasp.

K. With a thin sharp osteotome, a wedge of bone is excised from the proximal surface of the medial cuneiform. The base of the wedge, directed plantarward, is about 2 to 3 mm. in width. The opposing distal articular cartilage of the navicular is excised, exposing the subjacent cortical bone.

L. Next, the adequacy of correction of the plantar sag of the naviculocuneiform joint is checked by pronation and plantar flexion of the forepart of the foot. There should be close apposition of the bone surfaces between the medial cuneiform and navicular. Then a drill hole 5/16 inch in diameter is made in the navicular, beginning on its plantar surface; it is directed dorsally and distally to exit at the center of the denuded distal articular surface of the navicular. A second drill hole, 5/16 inch in diameter, is made in the medial cuneiform; it begins on the plantar surface, extends dorsally and proximally, and exits on the proximal denuded joint surface immediately below the dorsal cortex. An adequate amount of cortex should be left in both bones so that the suture does not tear out of the cancellous bone.

M. Giannestras does not recommend the use of staples or Kirschner wires across the naviculocuneiform joint for internal fixation. A double No. 2 chromic suture is passed through the holes from the plantar surface of the navicular into the dorsal holes in the navicular and medial cuneiform, exiting on the plantar aspect of the cuneiform. The forefoot is held in plantar flexion and pronation, and the suture is tied. This author recommends the use of a small-fragment cancellous screw or two threaded K-wires for transfixing the naviculocuneiform joint.

Plate 29. Correction of Flexible Pes Planovalgus Due to Plantar Sag of Naviculocuneiform Joint and Medial Sag of Talonavicular Joint (Giannestras)

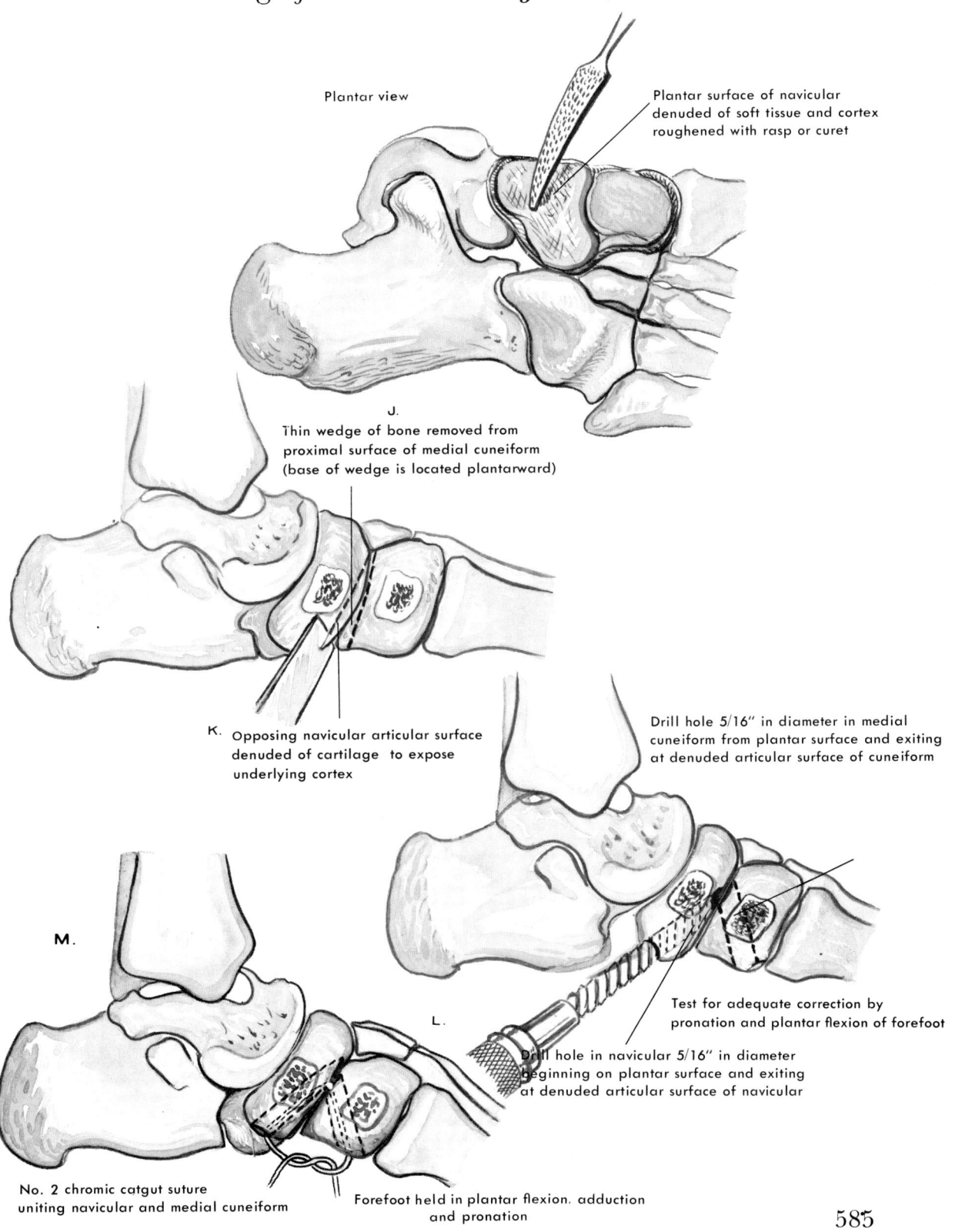

Correction of Flexible Pes Planovalgus Due to Plantar Sag of Naviculocuneiform Joint and Medial Sag of Talonavicular Joint (Giannestras) *(Continued)*

N. With the foot held in maximally corrected position—i.e., the forepart of the foot plantar-flexed and adducted—the osteocartilaginous flap is pulled distally with a Kocher clamp to cover the denuded surfaces of the navicular and cuneiform bones. The distal end is anchored securely to the base of the first metatarsal with 00 Mersilene suture. The flap should be taut, forming a bowstring on the medial and plantar aspect of the foot. With a fine small cutting needle, the dorsal and plantar margins of the flap are anchored to adjacent capsular structures with interrupted sutures. Any distal redundant portion of the flap is excised. The spring ligament is tautly resutured to the navicular. The security of fixation and degree of correction are checked with the foot released.

O. A drill hole 7/64 inch in diameter is made in the navicular from the dorsal to the plantar surface, approximately 1.5 to 2.0 cm. lateral to the medial edge of the navicular tubercle. The plantar surface of the navicular is denuded of all fibrous tissue and roughened with a sharp curet exposing raw cancellous bone.

P. The ends of the tibialis anterior and tibialis posterior tendons are sutured together with a 00 Mersilene suture, which is passed in a figure of eight fashion. The two ends of the suture are loose, one coming out of the end of the tibialis anterior and the other through the end of the tibialis posterior, similar to Bunnell's suture but without the pull-out wire. Then the two suture ends are threaded through a large slightly curved needle and passed through the plantar drill hole and up through the dorsal drill hole. The suture ends are then separated, and each one is threaded through a sharp cutting needle and passed separately through the overlying capsular and ligamentous soft tissues. Next, with a forceps the two tendons are pulled and held down snugly under the plantar aspect of the navicular and the sutures are tied. The tendons are against the plantar aspect of the navicular, but are not pulled up through the drill hole; only the sutures pass up through the drill hole. Additional sutures are applied through the two tendons to the overlying spring ligament.

The tourniquet is deflated and complete hemostasis obtained. It is best to insert a closed suction Hemovac unit. The subcutaneous tissues are closed with interrupted sutures and the skin with a subcuticular suture.

A below-knee cast is applied for immobilization. An overcorrected position should be avoided. The purpose of the cast is to retain the correction achieved surgically. Giannestras recommends that the cast be applied in two sections. The heel should be slightly varus, the plaster under the newly formed longitudinal arch well molded, and the forefoot in maximal pronation.[40]

Before the patient leaves the operating room, anteroposterior and lateral roentgenograms of the foot are made to determine the position of the talonavicular and naviculocuneiform joints.

POSTOPERATIVE CARE

Immobilization in the cast is maintained for eight weeks. The cast is changed as necessary. Roentgenograms of the foot are made to ascertain the fusion of the naviculocuneiform joint. If union is delayed or does not take place, a below-knee walking case is applied for another four weeks. Persistence of non-union is ignored, however, as it usually does not cause any symptoms.

Upon removal of the cast the foot may appear overcorrected; parents should be reassured that it will return to normal position after two to three weeks of walking. In the beginning three- or four-point crutch gait is used to protect the limb. Active exercises are performed to strengthen the triceps surae, toe extensor, tibialis posterior, and tibialis anterior muscles.

Initially the tendency is to walk on the lateral aspect of the foot. Proper heel-toe gait should be taught by the physical therapist. The child is fitted with simple Oxford shoes with a rigid shank. No arch supports of any type in the shoe are required.

Plate 29. Correction of Flexible Pes Planovalgus Due to Plantar Sag of Naviculocuneiform Joint and Medial Sag of Talonavicular Joint (Giannestras)

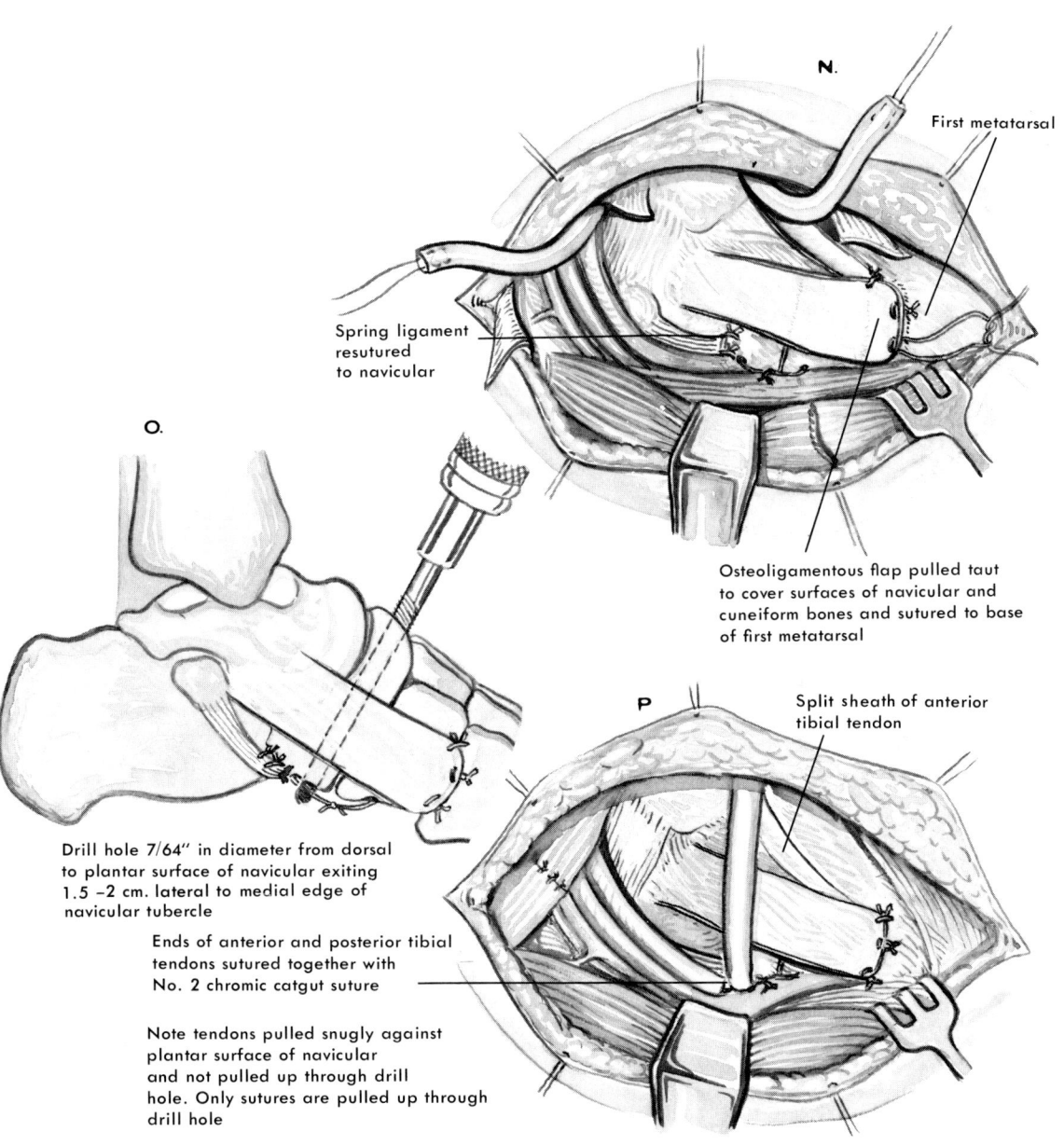

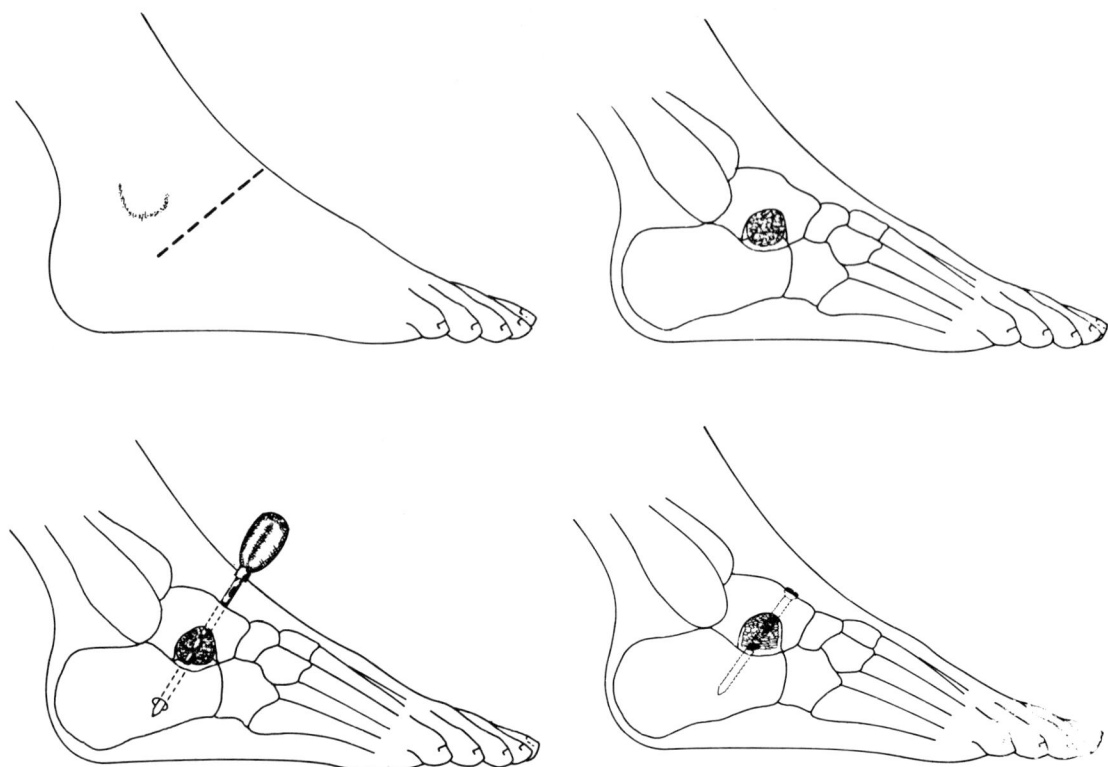

FIGURE 5–16. Subtalar arthrodesis by cancellous grafts and metallic internal fixation.

A. The incision. **B.** Area of cortical bone removed from sinus tarsi. **C.** Note the position of the bone awl. **D.** Internal fixation screw and packing of the sinus tarsi with cancellous bone chips. (From Dennyson, W. G., and Fulford, G. E. Subtalar arthrodesis by cancellous grafts and metallic internal fixation. J. Bone Joint Surg., *58-B*:507, 1976. Reprinted by permission.)

of seven and a half weeks in a below-knee weight-bearing plaster cast. An example is shown in Figure 5–17.[26]

In the experience of this author the technique described by Grice is very adequate, and he has found it unnecessary to use internal fixation by screw or transfixation by fibular bone graft.

In flexible pes planovalgus, relief of pain is the primary indication for *triple arthrodesis*. This author has performed it in adolescents with symptomatic flat feet caused by excessive ligamentous laxity associated with such generalized syndromes as Marfan's or Down's. Equinus deformity, if present, is corrected by elongating the tendo Achillis.

Arthrodesis by excision of articular cartilage and variable amounts of subjacent bone is not desirable in stabilization of the valgus foot. The base of the bone wedge to be removed must face medially. Following resection of bone, the foot becomes sloppy and shorter than its mate. It is much better to leave the joints undisturbed and to insert a lateral inlay graft to achieve stabilization. According to Williams and Menelaus, the operation was first elaborated by Littlejohn in 1930 (unpublished) and later popularized by Price.[125] The technique of the operation is described in Plate 30.

Williams and Menelaus reported the results of 88 triple arthrodeses by inlay grafting in 70 patients. The only significant complication was failure of fusion of the midtarsal joint; it occurred in 3 of 85 feet (3.5 per cent). In these three feet repeat inlay grafting of the midtarsal joint resulted in complete fusion. There were no failures of fusion of the subtalar joint.[125]

Osteotomies of Os Calcis to Correct Hindfoot Valgus Deformity

THE CHAMBERS PROCEDURE. The operation is illustrated in Figure 5–18 and is

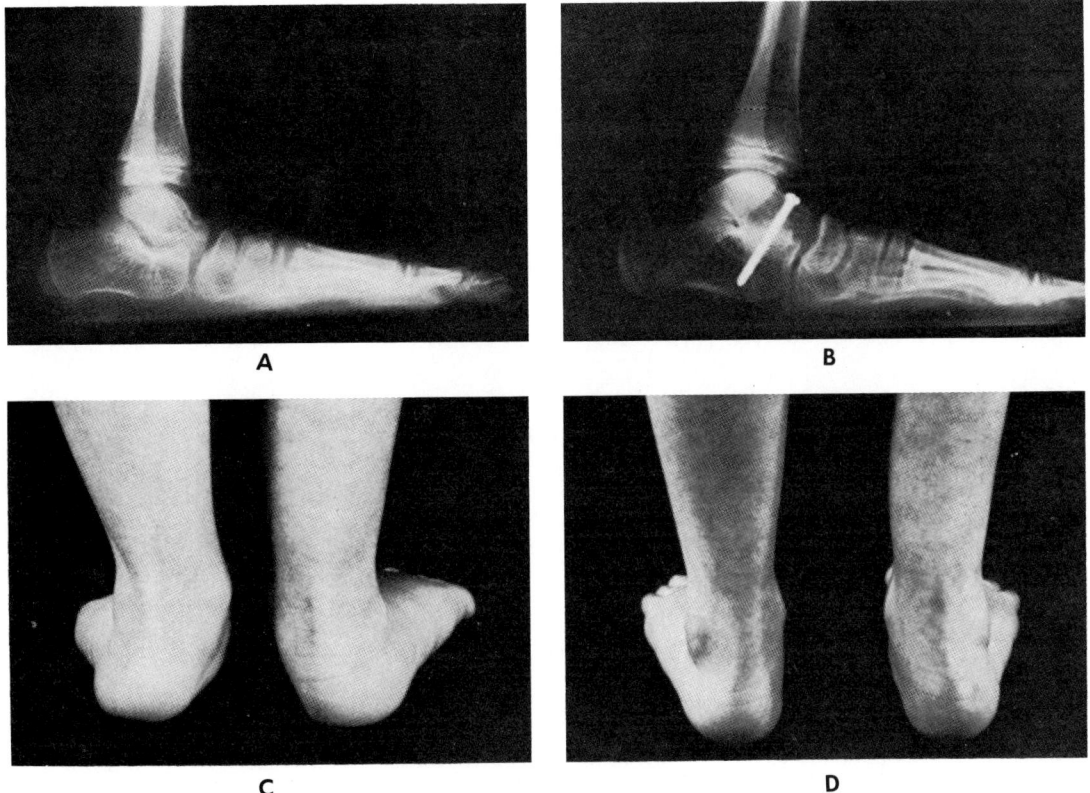

FIGURE 5–17. *Subtalar arthrodesis by cancellous grafts and internal fixation with a screw.*

A. Preoperative lateral roentgenogram of the foot. **B.** Lateral roentgenogram three years after operation. **C** and **D.** Preoperative and postoperative appearance of the foot. (From Dennyson, W. G., and Fulford, G. E.: Subtalar arthrodesis by cancellous grafts and metallic internal fixation. J. Bone Joint Surg., *58-B*:507, 1976. Reprinted by permission.)

performed as follows: first a lengthening of the tendo Achillis is carried out. Next the lateral part of the calcaneus is exposed through an oblique incision over the sinus tarsi, beginning 2 cm. inferior to the tip of the lateral malleolus and extending dorsally and distally to the talonavicular joint. The subcutaneous tissues are incised in line with the skin incision. Superficial fat is left intact. The deep fat in the sinus tarsi is excised. The talocalcaneal, calcaneocuboid, and talonavicular joints are identified. The capsule of the talonavicular joint is completely sectioned inferiorly, laterally, dorsally, and medially, to permit upward and backward shifting of the talus. With dorsal elevation of the head of the talus the calcaneus shifts medially and the sustentaculum tali rotates to lie underneath the talar head. The calcaneus becomes anteriorly displaced in relation to the talus. The soft-tissue release permits restoration of normal articular relations of the foot. Next, an osteotomy of the anterolateral part of the calcaneus is performed, beneath the anterolateral facet and immediately posterior to the calcaneocuboid joint. The osteotomized segment of the calcaneus is elevated dorsally and medially against the talus—cautiously, so as not to enter the subtalar joint. The position of the elevated calcaneal segment is maintained by a triangular autogenous bone graft. The wounds are closed, and an above-knee cast is applied and worn for four weeks, after which a below-knee walking cast is used for an additional eight weeks. By the end of this period there is usually solid bone healing and adequate remodeling of the anterior subtalar joint.[18]

Miller reported the results of the Cham-

Triple Arthrodesis by Inlay Grafting (Williams and Menelaus)

THE PROCEDURE

A. A curved longitudinal incision is made on the anterolateral aspect of the dorsum of the foot. It extends from immediately distal to the tip of the lateral malleolus to the second cuneiform. The subcutaneous tissue and deep fascia are divided in line with the skin incision.

B. The extensor digitorum brevis is elevated from its origin and reflected distally. The extensor digitorum longus tendons are retracted medially. The contents of the sinus tarsi and the capsules of the talonavicular, calcaneocuboid, and subtalar joints are excised.

C. Next, the foot is manipulated and securely held in the desired plantigrade position, with the valgus deviation corrected and a normal longitudinal arch. In the very flaccid foot it is best to stabilize the tarsus by drilling two stout Kirschner wires longitudinally, one across the talonavicular and the other across the calcaneocuboid joint. A square or oblong trough is cut across the midfoot—extending across the talonavicular, anterior subtalar, calcaneocuboid, and naviculocuboid joints.

D and E. A bone graft, slightly larger than the resected block, is taken from the upper third of the same tibia and is then hammered snugly into the trough in the tarsus.

With a gauge, the articular cartilage from the adjacent subtalar joint is removed and the defect is filled with the bone previously removed from the trough. The tourniquet is released, and after complete hemostasis the leg and foot wounds are closed in the usual fashion. Absorbable sutures are put in the skin. An above-knee cast is applied.

POSTOPERATIVE CARE

The foot and leg are immobilized in a plaster cast for a total period of three months. Then bone healing is assessed clinically and radiologically. The cortical bone graft may appear dense initially, but in time it will become revascularized.

Plate 30. Triple Arthrodesis by Inlay Grafting (Williams and Menelaus)

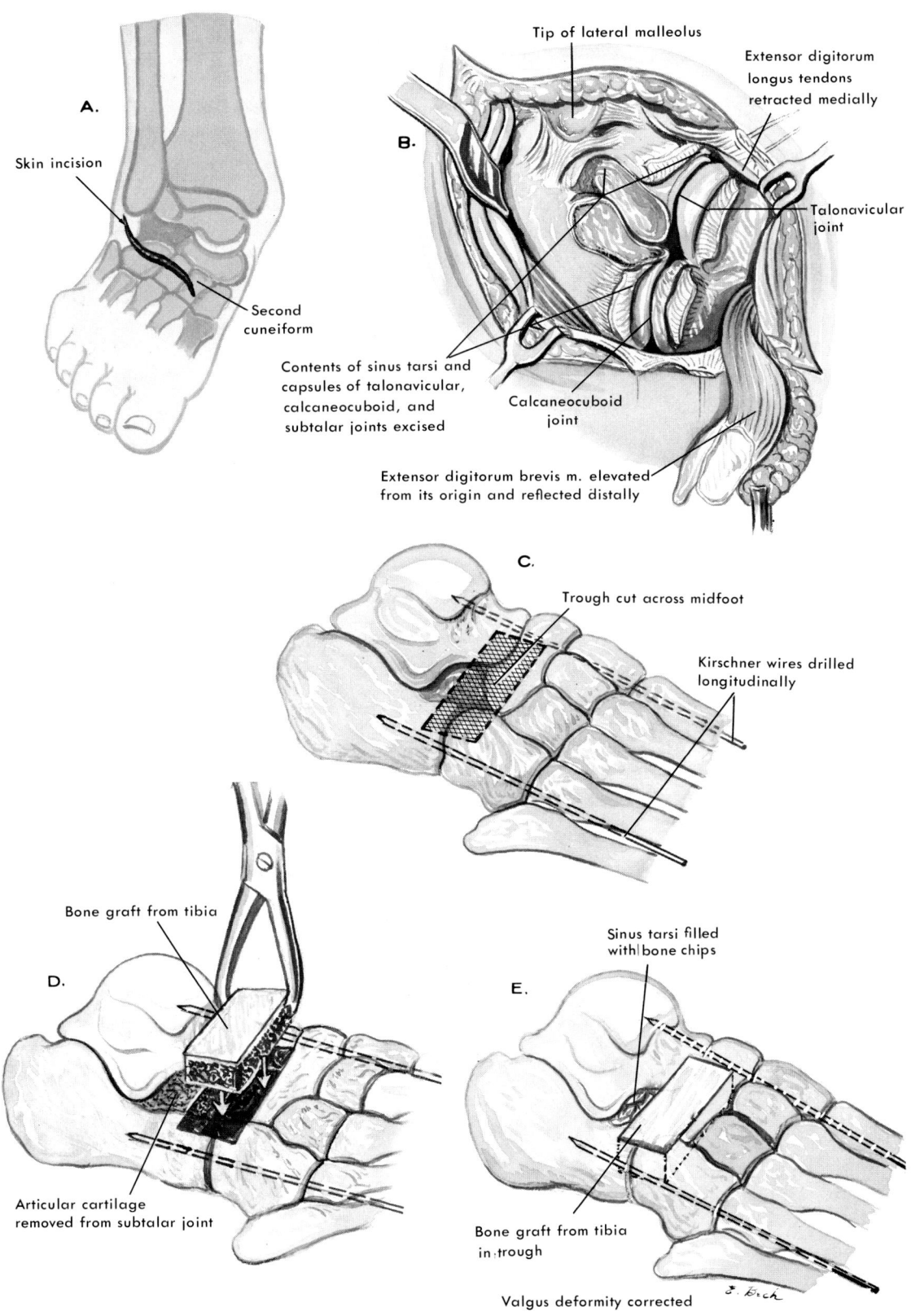

591

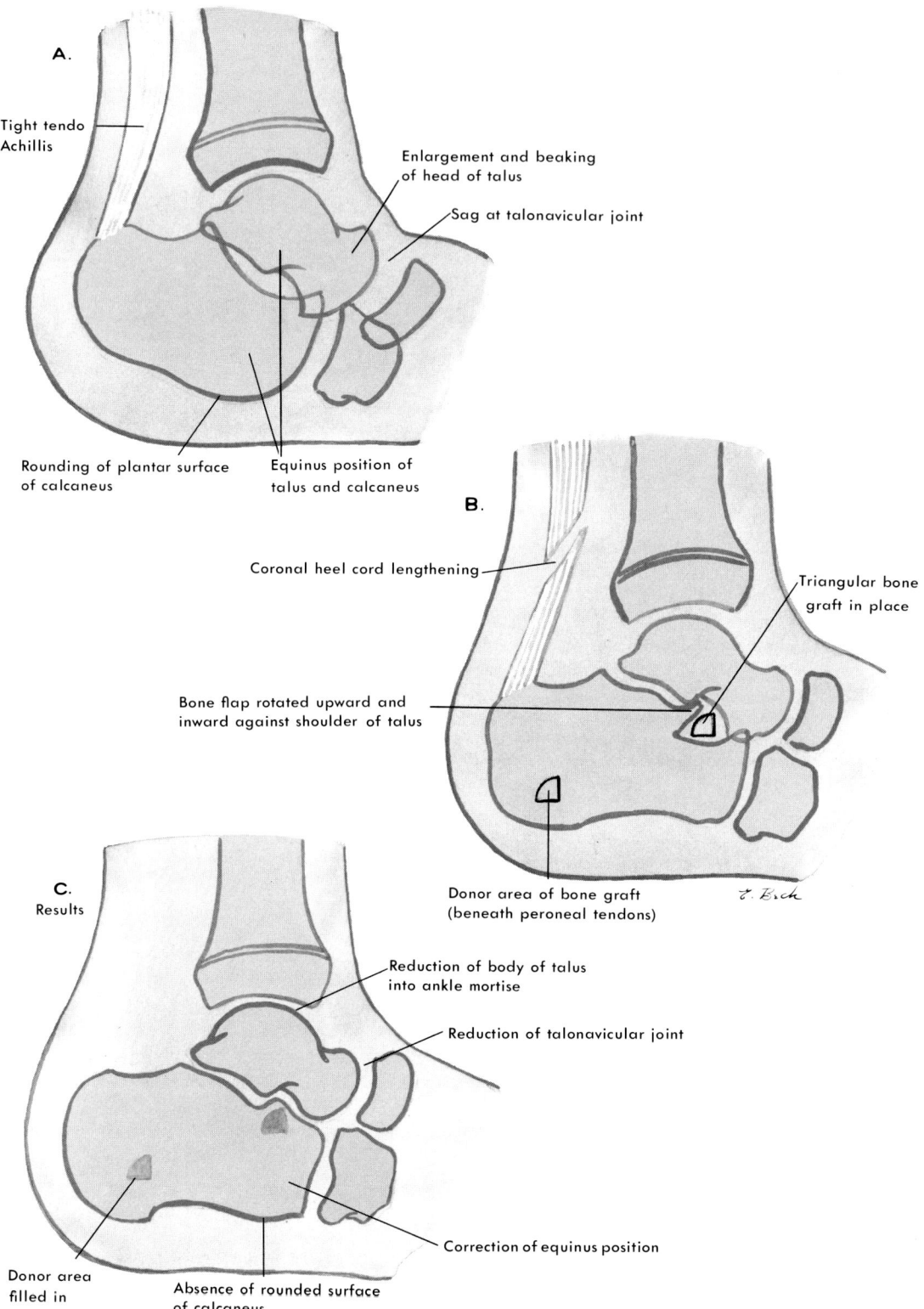

Figure 5–18. See legend on opposite page

bers osteotomy of the anterolateral aspect of the calcaneus in 81 hypermobile flat feet with an average follow-up of six and one half years (range—1 to 22 years). In 70 feet tendo Achillis lengthening was performed with the calcaneal osteotomy, and in 95 per cent of them an excellent or good clinical result was obtained. Roentgenograms disclosed normal foot alignment and normal articular cartilage spaces in only 72.8 per cent of the feet, however; in 22.2 per cent the talonavicular joint was narrowed, and in 5 per cent the subtalar joint was narrow. Postoperatively, in nine feet there was minimal loss of motion, in two feet moderate loss of motion, and in three feet marked restriction of joint motion. It seems the technique of complete release of the talonavicular joint disturbs circulation to the talus and damages articular cartilage. Miller states that should disabling pain develop later on, the feet are in good position for talonavicular or triple arthrodesis.[89] Because it causes incongruity and stiffness of the talocalcaneal joint, the Chambers procedure is not recommended by this author.

DWYER'S OSTEOTOMY. Dwyer's calcaneal osteotomy to correct valgus hindfoot may be either the lateral open-up or the medial close-up type. It is discussed in the section on cerebral palsy in Chapter 3. This author does not recommend this procedure for treatment of flexible pes planovalgus. The medial displacement osteotomy is simpler and as effective.

MEDIAL DISPLACEMENT OSTEOTOMY. Koutsogiannis described medial displacement osteotomy of the calcaneus; he credited Mr. Pridie with having been the first to perform the operation.[70] In flexible pes planovalgus the line along which body weight is transmitted through the talus passes medial to the calcaneus (Fig. 5–19B). The objective of the operation is to displace the posterior part of the calcaneus medially, thereby restoring normal weight-bearing (Fig. 5–19C). The patient is placed in prone position with the knee flexed 30 to 45 degrees by a sandbag under the lower leg. An incision is made on the lateral aspect of the body of the calcaneus, parallel and immediately posterior to the peroneal tendons. It extends proximally from the lateral margin of the tendo Achillis to the plantar aspect of the heel. Damage to the sural nerve should be avoided. The wound margins are undermined, elevated, and held apart by self-retaining retractors. Two Chandler elevator retractors are inserted, one on the superior and the other on the inferior surface of the os calcis, exposing its dorsal, lateral, and plantar surfaces. The periosteum is incised and elevated in line with the skin incision. With an electric oscillating saw or a wide osteotome the calcaneus is sectioned. If necessary, the segments are spread open with a laminectomy spreader to allow the periosteum on the medial aspect of the calcaneus to be divided; sometimes the taut plantar ligament is sectioned to achieve sufficient medial displacement. Next the posterior fragment of the calcaneus is displaced medially until its medial margin is in line with the sustentaculum tali. It is usually necessary to displace a third to a half of the width of the calcaneus. The calcaneal fragments are transfixed by one large threaded Steinmann pin, inserted obliquely from the posteroplantar aspect of the os calcis. The pin exits through the skin over the medial or intermediate cuneiform and should be subcutaneous or flush with the calcaneus posteriorly. The wound is closed in the usual fashion, and a well-padded above-knee cast is applied with the ankle in neutral position and the knee in 45 degrees of flexion.[70]

Four weeks after the operation the cast is changed. The threaded Steinmann pin and the sutures are removed. By then bony

---

FIGURE 5–18. *The Chambers procedure for flexible flat foot.*

A. Diagram illustrating preoperative abnormality. The talus and calcaneus are in equinus position owing to the taut triceps surae and the plantar sag at the talonavicular joint, with forward and downward displacement of the talus and posterolateral displacement of the calcaneus. **B.** Diagram of the operative correction showing the coronal lengthening of the heel cord and the osteotomy of the anterolateral part of the calcaneus beneath the anterolateral facet and immediately posterior to the calcaneocuboid joint. Note the triangular bone graft holding the osteotomized segment of the calcaneus dorsally and medially against the talus. **C.** Diagram showing remodeling of the calcaneal bone flap. It acts as a buttress to maintain normal alignment of the talocalcaneal joint. (Redrawn after Miller, G. R.: The operative treatment of hypermobile flatfeet in the young child. Clin. Orthop., *122*:95, 1977.)

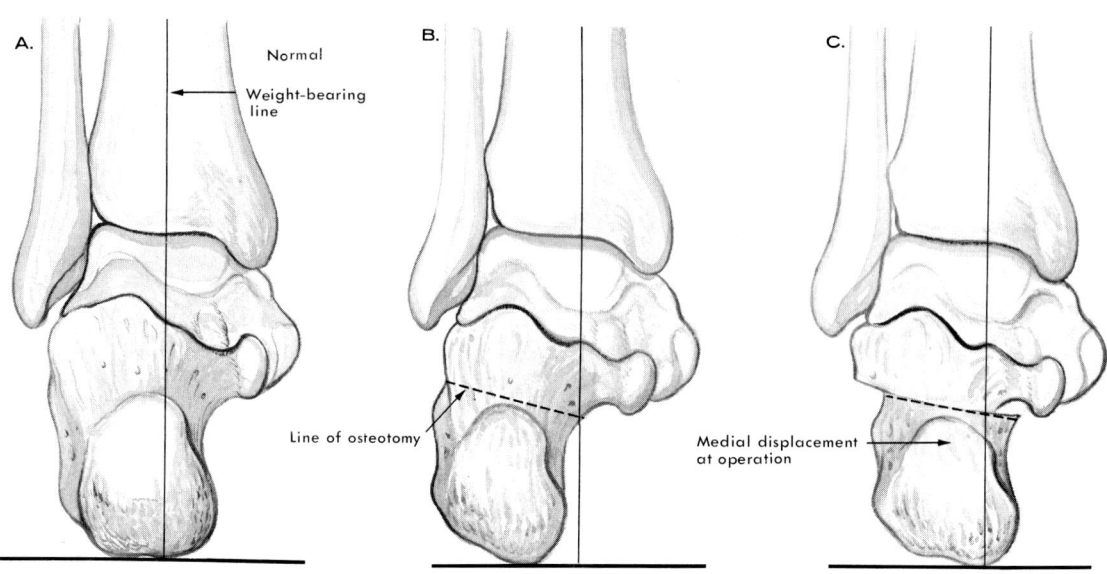

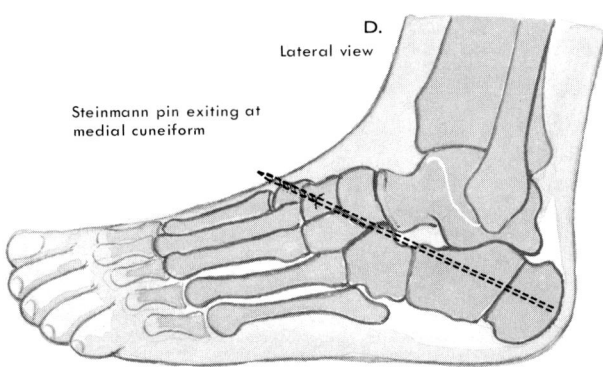

FIGURE 5–19. Medial displacement osteotomy of the calcaneus in severe pes planovalgus.

The weight-bearing line and relation of the talus to the calcaneus are visualized from the posterosuperior aspect. **A.** In normal foot. **B.** In pes planovalgus. Note that the weight transmitted through the talus passes medial to the calcaneus. The line of osteotomy of the calcaneus is shown. **C.** After medial displacement osteotomy of the calcaneus. The medial margin of the posterior calcaneal fragment is placed in line with the sustentaculum tali, and normal weight-bearing is restored. **D.** Threaded Steinmann pin transfixing the osteotomized calcaneus.

union usually has taken place. A below-knee walking cast is applied for an additional two weeks.

The operation was performed by Koutsogiannis in 34 feet in 19 patients. Two patients were over 17 years of age at the time of surgery; on exclusion of these two older patients, the mean age was 12 years. The follow-up ranged from six years to a few months. In 17 of the 19 patients, function was markedly improved. According to Koutsogiannis the two failures were probably due to a taut Achilles tendon or to inadequate medial displacement of the posterior calcaneal fragment.[70] This author highly recommends medial displacement osteotomy of the calcaneus to correct hindfoot valgus deformity in severe symptomatic flexible pes planovalgus.

EVANS OPERATIONS. Evans operation for

lengthening the lateral column of the foot for correction of calcaneovalgus deformity is performed as follows:

A 7-cm.-long incision is made over the lateral aspect of the calcaneus and cuboid bone, parallel with and immediately dorsal to the peroneal tendon. Subcutaneous tissue is divided in line with the skin incision. Avoid inadvertent division of the sural nerve. The calcaneocuboid joint is identified and the calcaneus is exposed. With a straight sharp osteotome the anterior end of the calcaneus is sectioned in front of the peroneal tubercle. The line of osteotomy is parallel with and 1.5 cm. behind the calcaneocuboid joint. The osteotomized segments are prised apart with a spreader. Broad straight osteotomes of various sizes (1.25 to 3.0 cm. or more) are inserted into the osteotomy site to determine the optimum width of the bone graft to be used. The foot is inspected clinically, and roentgenograms are made to ensure that the desired degree of correction is obtained. Next, a cortical bone graft is taken from the tibia. (This author prefers iliac bone with both cortices intact.) The graft is inserted between the calcaneal fragments. The spreader is removed, and the degree of correction is ascertained again by roentgenograms. The forepart of the foot should be adducted and the heel slightly inverted. The tourniquet is deflated, and after complete hemostasis, the wound is closed in the usual fashion. A below-knee cast is applied for immobilization.[32]

The cast is changed in four weeks. Roentgenograms are made to assess bone healing. A new below-knee cast with an anterior heel is applied, and weight-bearing is allowed. The total period of cast immobilization is two months for solid consolidation of the graft. (Mr. Evans recommended the plaster cast be retained for about four months; this author finds two months to be adequate.) No special corrective shoes or shoe inserts are needed when the plaster is removed.[32] This author recommends the reverse Evans procedure for midfoot valgus deformity with lateral subluxation of the navicular on the head of the talus and lateral tilting of the calcaneocuboid joint. If the calcaneocuboid joint is not tilted, he finds open-wedge osteotomy of the cuboid with iliac bone graft effective in correcting lateral subluxation of the navicular on the head of the talus. He combines it with tautening of the posterior tibial tendon and plantar calcaneonavicular ligament.

In summary, surgical treatment of pes planovalgus is rarely indicated and should not be performed in patients under the age of ten years. Contracture of the triceps surae muscle should be corrected in all cases; if it does not respond to passive stretching exercises or a below-knee walking cast with an anterior heel, a sliding lengthening of the heel cord is performed. The distal cut of the Achilles tendon should be lateral. When flexible pes planovalgus is due to sag at the naviculocuneiform joint, the recommended procedure is naviculocuneiform fusion and tautening of the posterior tibial tendon and plantar calcaneonavicular ligament. Proximal transfer of the anterior tibial tendon to the navicular will provide a dynamic force to elevate the medial longitudinal arch of the foot, and this author highly recommends the Giannestras modification. When the problem is severe hindfoot valgus deformity, medial displacement osteotomy of the calcaneus is the procedure of choice. This may be combined with naviculocuneiform fusion and tautening of the plantar calcaneonavicular ligament and distal transfer of the posterior tibial tendon. It is best to stage these two procedures. When the navicular is displaced laterally on the head of the talus and the medial column of the foot is elongated, elongation of the lateral column of the foot is recommended. If the calcaneocuboid joint is tilted laterally, the reverse Evans operation is performed with a wedge of bone graft placed in the anterior part of the calcaneus. If the calcaneocuboid joint orientation is normal, an open-up osteotomy of the cuboid bone is performed with the base of the wedge lateral; the plantar calcaneonavicular ligament and the posterior tibial tendon are tautened, but they should not be detached from the navicular or advanced distally. In severe flexible pes planovalgus due to excessive ligamentous laxity and in syndromes such as Down's or Marfan's, the inlay graft triple arthrodesis of Williams and Menelaus is recommended. When pes planovalgus is rigid and painful, a triple arthrodesis is performed with a subtalar bone block as in the Grice procedure and talonavicular and calcaneocuboid joint fusion with the wedges based plantarward.

References

1. Armstrong, G.: Evans elongation of lateral column of the foot for valgus deformity. J. Bone Joint Surg., *57-B*:530, 1975.
2. Asher, C.: Flat foot and valgus heel. *In* Postural Variations in Childhood. London, Butterworth & Co., Ltd., 1975, pp. 76:101.
3. Baker, L. D., and Hill, L. M.: Foot alignment in the cerebral palsy patient. J Bone Joint Surg., *46A*:1, 1964.
4. Basmajian, J. R., and Bentzon, J. W.: An electromyographic study of certain muscles of the leg and foot in the standing position. Surg. Gynec. Obstet., *98*:662, 1954.
5. Basmajian, J. R., and Stecko, G.: The role of muscles in arch support of the foot. An electromyographic study. J. Bone Joint Surg., *45-A*, 1184, 1963.
6. Basta, N. W., Mital, M. A., Bonadio, O., Johnson, A., Kang, S. Y., and O'Connor, J.: A comparative study of the role of shoe, arch supports, and navicular cookies in the management of symptomatic mobile flat feet in children. Int. Orthop., *1*:143, 1977.
7. Bettmann, E.: The treatment of flat-foot by means of exercise. J. Bone Joint Surg., *19*:821, 1937.
8. Bick, E. M.: Static deformities of the foot. *In* Source Book of Orthopaedics. Baltimore, Williams & Wilkins Co., 1948, pp. 449–458.
9. Bivings, L.: Heel printing in flat feet. Amer. J. Dis. Child., *46*:1050, 1933.
10. Bleck, E. E.: The shoeing of children: Sham or science? Develop. Med. Child Neurol., *13*:188, 1971.
11. Bleck, E. E., and Berzins, U. J.: Conservative management of pes valgus with plantar flexed talus flexible. Clin. Orthop., *122*:85, 1977.
12. Bohm, M., Der Foetal Fuss. Beiträge zur Entstehung des Pes planus, des Pes valgus und des Pes planovalgus. Z. Orthop. Chir., *57*:1932.
12a. Bordelon, R. L.: Correction of hypermobile flatfoot in children by molded insert. Foot Ankle, *1*:132, 1980.
13. Brahdy, B. M.: Flat-foot in children. Arch. Pediat., *44*:86, 1927.
14. Brown, L. T.: The end results of stabilizing operations on the foot. J. Bone Joint Surg., *6*:839, 1924.
15. Bruce, J. M., and Walmsley, R.: Some observations on the arches of the foot and flatfoot. Lancet, *2*:656, 1938.
16. Butte, F. L.: Navicular-cuneiform arthrodesis for flat-foot. J. Bone Joint Surg., *19*:496, 1937.
17. Caldwell, G. D.: Surgical correction of relaxed flatfoot by the Durham flatfootplasty. Clin. Orthop., *2*:221, 1953.
18. Chambers, E. F. S.: An operation for correction of flexible flat feet of adolescents. Western J. Surg., *54*:77, 1946.
19. Chandler, F. A.: Children's feet, normal and presenting common abnormalities. Amer. J. Dis. Child., *63*:1136, 1942.
20. Chigot, P. L., and Sananes, P.: Arthrodèse de Grice. Rev. Chir. Orthop., *51*:53, 1965.
21. Clark, W. A.: A rebalancing operation for pronated feet. J. Bone Joint Surg., *13*:867, 1931.
22. Compere, E. L.: Flat feet in children. Med. Clin. N. Amer. *30*:147, 1946.
23. Connolly, J., Regen, E., and Hillman, J. W.: Pigeon-toes and flatfeet. Pediat. Clin. N. Amer., *17*:291, 1970.
24. Crego, C. H., Jr., and Ford, L. T.: An end-result study of various operative procedures for correcting flat feet in children. J. Bone Joint Surg., *34-A*:183, 1952.
25. Debrunner, H. U.: Fussdeformitaten. Ther. Umsch., *29*:447, 1972.
26. Dennyson, W. G., and Fulford, G. E.: Subtalar arthrodesis by cancellous grafts and metallic internal fixation. J. Bone Joint Surg., *58-B*:507, 1976.
27. DeDoncker, E.: Le traitement du pied valgus souple. Acta Orthop. Belg., *28*:709, 1962.
28. Dickson, F. D., and Dively, R. L.: Functional Disorders of the Foot. Philadelphia, J. B. Lippincott Co., 1944.
29. Dommisse, G. F.: Flat foot. II. S. Afr. Med. J., *45*:726, July, 1971.
30. Dwyer, F. C.: Osteotomy of the calcaneum in the treatment of grossly everted feet with special reference to cerebral palsy. *In* Huitième Congrès de la Société Internationale de Chirurgie Orthopédique et de Traumatologie, New York, 4–9 September 1960. Brussels, Imprimerie des Sciences, 1961, pp. 892–897.
31. Dwyer, F. C.: The relationship of variations in the size and inclination of the calcaneus to the shape and function of the whole foot. Ann. Roy. Coll. Surg., *34*:120, 1964.
32. Evans, D. C.: Calcaneovalgus deformity. J. Bone Joint Surg., *57-B*:270, 1975.
33. Ewald, P.: Ueber den Knick-und Plattfuss. Z. Orthop. Chir., *25*:229, 1910.
34. Faggiana, F.: II piede piatto. Acta Orthop. Ital., *1*:141, 1955.
35. Ferciot, C. F.: The etiology of developmental flat foot. Clin. Orthop., *85*:7, 1972.
36. Ferguson, A. B.: Flat feet in childhood. Penn. Med. J., *57*:330, 1954.
37. Fogel, G. R., Katoh, Y., Rand, J. A., and Chao, E. Y. S.: Talonavicular arthrodesis for isolated arthrosis 9.5-year results and gait analysis. Foot Ankle, *3*:105, 1982.
38. Giannestras, N. J.: Static foot problems in the pre-adolescent and adolescent stages. *In* Foot Disorders. Medical and Surgical Management. Philadelphia, Lea & Febiger, 1967, pp. 119–155.
39. Giannestras, N. J.: Static deformities of the foot. Editorial comment. Clin. Orthop., *70*:2, 1970.
40. Giannestras, N. J.: Flexible valgus flatfoot resulting from naviculocuneiform and talonavicular sag. Surgical correction in the adolescent. *In* Bateman, J. E., (ed.): Foot Science. Philadelphia, W. B. Saunders Co., 1976, pp. 67–105.
41. Gleich, A.: Beitrag zur operativen Plattfussbehandlung. Arch. Klin. Chir., *46*:358, 1893.
42. Golding-Bird, C. H.: Pes valgus acquisitus. Pes pronatus acquisitus. Guy's Hosp. Rep., *41*:439, 1883.
43. Gomez, A. J.: Consideraciones Generales Acerca del Pie valgo Plano en el Nino. Conceptos Modernos de su Tratamiento Ortopedico y Quirurgico. Monograph. Caracas, Venezuela, 1965.
44. Gottlieb, A.: The acquired pes valgus in childhood. Arch. Pediat., *55*:166, 1938.
45. Gresham, J. L.: Correction of flat feet in children. Grice-Green subastragalar arthrodesis. Southern Med. J., *61*:177, 1968.
46. Grice, D. S.: An extra-articular arthrodesis of the subastragalar joint for correction of paralytic flat-feet in children. J. Bone Joint Surg., *34-a*:927, 1952.
47. Grice, D. S.: Further experience with extra-articular arthrodesis of the subtalar joint. J. Bone Joint Surg., *37-A*:246, 1955.
48. Grice, D. S.: The role of subtalar fusion in the treatment of valgus deformities of the foot. A.A.O.S. Instr. Course Lect., *16*:127, 1959.
49. Hackenbroch, M.: Der Plattfus. *In* Hohmann, G. (ed.): Handbuch der Orthopädie. Stuttgart, Georg Thieme Verlag, 1961, IV(II):998.
50. Haraldsson, S.: Operative treatment of pes planovalgus staticus juvenilis. Acta Orthop. Scand., *32*:492, 1962.
51. Haraldsson, S.: Pes plano-valgus staticus juvenilis and its operative treatment. Acta Orthop. Scand., *35*:234, 1965.
52. Harris, R. I., and Beath, T.: Hypermobile flat-foot with short tendo-Achillis. J. Bone Joint Surg., *30-A*:116, 1948.
53. Hatt, W. S., and Davis, L. A.: Analysis of the foot in infant, radiographic criteria and clinical aspects. Southern Med. J., *50*:720, 1954.
54. Hazlett, J. W.: Pes planus. Bull. Hosp. Spec. Surg., *3*:23, February, 1960.
55. Helfet, A. J.: A new way of treating flat feet in children. Lancet, *1*:262, 1956.
56. Henderson, W. H., and Campbell, J. W.: UCBL shoe insert: Casting and fabrication. The Biomechanics Laboratory. University of California at San Francisco and Berkeley. Technical Report 53, August, 1967.
57. Herzmark, M. H.: Floor pad for foot-exercising. J. Bone Joint Surg., *29*:1098, 1947.
58. Hicks, J. H.: The function of the plantar aponeurosis. J. Anat., *85*:414, 1951.
59. Hicks, J. H.: The mechanics of the foot. I. The joints. J. Anat., *87*:343, 1943.
60. Hicks, J. H.: The mechanics of the foot. II. The plantar aponeurosis and the arch. J. Anat., *88*:25, 1954.
61. Hohmann, G.: Zur operativen Plattfussbehandlung. Chirurg., *3*:593, 1931.
62. Hoke, M.: An operation for the correction of extremely relaxed flat feet. J. Bone Joint Surg., *13*:773, 1931.
63. Imhauser, G., and Schoberlein, J.: What does Schede flatfoot operation accomplish? Assessment based on fol-

low-up examinations after two decades. Z. Orthop., *112*:139, 1974.
64. Inman, V. T.: UCBL dual axis control system and UCBL shoe insert. Bull. Prosthet. Res., *10*:11, 1969.
65. Jack, E. A.: Naviculocuneiform fusion in the treatment of flat foot. J. Bone Joint Surg., *35-B*:279, 1953.
66. Jones, B. S.: Flat foot. A preliminary report of an operation for severe cases. J. Bone Joint Surg., *57-B*:279, 1975.
67. Jones, R. L.: The human foot. An experimental study of the mechanics and role of its muscles and ligaments in the support of the arch. Amer. J. Anat., *68*:1, 1941.
68. Kite, J. H.: The treatment of flatfeet in small children. Postgrad. Med., *15*:75, 1954.
69. Kleinberg, S.: Flat or weak feet in children. Arch. Pediat., *40*:1923.
70. Koutsogiannis, E.: Treatment of mobile flat foot by displacement osteotomy of a calcaneus. J. Bone Joint Surg., *53-B*:96, 1971.
71. Krause, W.: The operative treatment of juvenile flat and abducted feet. Ortopädische Klinik Kassel-Wilhelmshöhe, West Germany, 1971.
72. Lake, N. C.: Flat foot. In The Foot. 3rd Ed. Baltimore, Williams & Wilkins Co., 1948, pp. 165–198.
73. Lange, F.: Neue Plattfusseneinlagen aus Celluloid-Stahldraht. Munchen. Med. Wschr., 7, 1903.
74. Lanfranchi, R., and Zinghi, G. F.: L'Artrodesi estraarticolare della sotta-astragalica associata alla transposizione del tibiale posteriore nel trattamento del piede plato dell'adulto. Chir. Organi Mov., *57*:395, 1968.
75. Leavitt, D. G.: Subastragaloid arthrodesis for the os calcis type of flat foot. Amer. J. Surg., *59*:501, 1943.
76. Legg, A.T.: The treatment of congenital flatfoot by tendon transplantation. Amer. J. Orthop. Surg., *10*:584, 1912–13.
77. Lelièvre, J.: Le pied plat valgus statique. In Pathologie du Pied. 2nd Ed. Paris, Masson & Cie, 1961, pp. 387–399.
78. Lelièvre, J.: Current concepts and corrections in the valgus foot. Clin. Orthop., *70*:43, 1970.
79. Leonard, M. H., Gonzalez, S., Breck, L. W. Basom, C., Palafox, M., and Kosick, Z. W.: Lateral transfer of posterior tibial tendon in certain selected cases of pes planovalgus (Kidner operation). Clin. Orthop., *40*:139, 1965.
80. L'Episcopo, J. B., and Sabatelle, P. E.: The Hoke operation for flat feet. J. Bone Joint Surg., *21*:92, 1939.
81. Lewin, P.: Flat foot in infants and children. Amer. J. Dis. Child., *31*:704, 1926.
82. Lonergan, R. C.: Surgical treatment of flat feet: Indication and technic. Surg. Clin. N. Amer., *19*:21, 1934.
83. Lord, J. P.: Correction of extreme flatfoot. Value of osteotomy of os calcis (Gleich operation). J.A.M.A., *81*:1502, 1923.
84. Lovell, W. W., Price, C. T., and Meehan, P. L.: In Winter, R. B., and Lovell, W. W. (eds.): Pediatric Orthopedics. Philadelphia, J. B. Lippincott Co., 1978.
85. Lowman, C. L.: An operative method for correction of certain forms of flat foot. J.A.M.A., *81*:1500, 1923.
86. Lund, S. H.: Arthrodesis for flat foot. Acta Orthop. Scand., *33*:234, 1965.
87. Mereday, C., Dolan, C. M. E., and Lusskin, R.: Evaluation of the University of California Biomechanics Laboratory shoe insert in "flexible" pes planus. Clin. Orthop., *82*:45, 1972.
88. Mitch, H.: Reinforcement of the deltoid ligament for pronated foot. Surg. Gynec. Obstet., *74*:876, 1942.
89. Miller, G. R.: The operative treatment of hypermobile flatfeet in the young child. Clin. Orthop., *122*:95, 1977.
90. Miller, O. L.: A plastic flat foot operation. J. Bone Joint Surg., *9*:84, 1927.
91. Muller, E.: Ueber die Resultate der Ernst Muller'schen Plattfussoperation. Beitr. Klin. Chir., *75*:424, 1913.
92. Niederecker, K.: Der Plattfuss. Stuttgart, F. Enke, 1959.
92a. Ogilvy, C.: An operation for the permanent correction of weak feet in children. J. Orthop. Surg., *1*:343, 1919.
93. Ogston, A.: On flatfood and its cure by operation. Brit. Med. J., *9*:110, 1884.
93a. Osmond-Clarke, H.: Congenital vertical talus. J. Bone Joint Surg., *38-B*:334, 1956.
94. Penneau, K., Lutter, L. D., and Winter, R. B.: Pes planus: Radiographic changes with foot orthoses and shoes. Foot Ankle, *2*:299, 1982.
94a. Phillips, G. E.: A review of elongation of os calcis for flat feet. J. Bone Joint Surg., *65-B*:15, 1983.

95. Purvis, G. D.: Surgery of the relaxed flat foot. Clin. Orthop., *57*:221, 1968.
96. Rose, G. K.: Correction of the pronated foot. J. Bone Joint Surg., *40-B*:674, 1958.
97. Rose, G. K.: Correction of the pronated foot. J. Bone Joint Surg., *44-B*:642, 1962.
98. Rugtveit, A.: Extra-articular subtalar arthrodesis according to Green-Grice in flat feet. Acta Orthop. Scand., *34*:367, 1964.
99. Ryerson, E. W.: Tendon transplantation in flatfoot. Amer. J. Orthop. Surg., *7*:505, 1909.
100. Schede F.: Die Operation des Platfusses. Z. Orthop. Chir., *50*:528, 1929.
101. Schellenberg, K: Extra-artikulare subtalar arthrodese nach Grice. Arch. Orthop. Unfallchir., *56*:604, 1964.
102. Schmied, H. R.: Late results of translocation of the anterior tibial tendon around the navicular bone in plano-valgus feet. Z. Orthop., *104*:309, 1968.
103. Schoolfield, B. L.: An operation for the cure of flatfoot. Ann. Surg., *110*:437, 1939.
104. Schwartz, R. P., and Heath, A. L.: Conservative treatment of functional disorders of feet in adolescents and adults. J. Bone Joint Surg., *31-A*:501, 1969.
105. Seitz, D. G., and Carpenter, E. B.: Triple arthrodesis in children. A ten-year review. Southern Med. J.: *67*:1420, 1974.
106. Seymour, N: The late results of naviculo-cuneiform fusion. J. Bone Joint Surg., *49-B*:558, 1967.
107. Seymour, N., and Evans, D. K.: A modification of the Grice subtalar arthrodesis. J. Bone Joint Surg., *50-B*:372, 1968.
108. Sharrard, W. J. W.: Minor orthopedic disabilities in childhood. Practitioner, *180*:415, 1958.
109. Silver, C. M., Simon, S. D., Spindell, E., Litchman, H. M., and Scala, M.: Calcaneal osteotomy for valgus and varus deformities of the feet in cerebral palsy. J. Bone Joint Surg., *49*:232, 1967.
110. Smith, J. B., and Westin, G. W.: Follow-up notes on articles previously published, subtalar extra-articular arthrodesis. J. Bone Joint Surg., *50-A*:1027, 1968.
111. Smith, J. W.: Muscular control of the arches of the foot in standing, an electromyographic assessment. J. Anat., *88*:152, 1954.
112. Staheli, L. T.: Corrective shoes for children. Pediatr. Digest, *20*:22, 1978.
113. Staheli, L. T., and Griffin, L.: Corrective shoes for children: A survey of current practice. Pediatrics, *65*:13, 1980.
114. Steindler, A.: The pathomechanics of the static deformities of foot and ankle. In Kinesiology of the Human Body Under Normal and Pathological Conditions. 2nd Ed. Springfield, Ill., Charles C Thomas, 1970, p. 399.
115. Tanz, S. S.: The so-called tight heel cord. Clin. Orthop., *16*:184, 1960.
116. Thomson, J. E. M.: Treatment of congenital flat foot. J. Bone Joint Surg., *28*:787, 1946.
117. Trendelenburg, F.: Über Plattfussoperationen. Arch. Klin. Chir., *39*:751, 1889.
118. B. Vanden Brink, K. D.: Childhood foot and leg problems. Pediatr. Ann., *5*:61, 1976.
119. Voutey, H.: Traitment chirurgical du pied plat de l'enfant. Rev. Chir. Orthop., *58*:489, 1972.
120. Walsham, W. J., and Hughes, W. K.: Treatment of acquired flat foot. In The Deformities of the Human Foot. London, Balliere, Tindall & Cox, 1895, pp. 412–448.
121. Walsham, W. J., and Hughes, W. K.: Treatment of acquired flat foot. In The Deformities of the Human Foot. London, Balliere, Tindall & Cox, 1895, pp. 449–489.
122. Weissman, S. L., Torok, G., and Kharmosh, O.: L'arthrodèse extraarticulaire avec transplantation tendineuse concomitante dans le traitement du pied plat valgus paralytique du jeune enfant. Rev. Chir. Orthop., *43*:79, 1957.
123. Wetzenstein, H.: Prognosis of pes calcaneovalgus congenita. Acta Orthop. Scand., *41*:122, 1970.
124. Westin, G. W., and Hall, C. B.: Subtalar extra-articular arthrodesis. J. Bone Joint Surg., *39A*:501, 1957.
125. Williams, P. F., and Menelaus, M. B.: Triple arthrodesis by inlay grafting—a method suitable for the undeformed or valgus foot. J. Bone Joint Surg., *59-B*:333, 1977.
126. Young, C. S.: Operative treatment of pes planus. Surg. Gynec. Obstet., *68*:1099, 1939.
127. Zadek, I.: Transverse wedge arthrodesis for the relief of pain in rigid flatfoot. J. Bone Joint Surg., *17*:453, 1935.

6. Acquired Affections of Bones, Joints, and Soft Tissues

INFECTIONS AND INFLAMMATORY DISORDERS
   Osteomyelitis
   Tuberculosis
   Septic arthritis
   Rheumatoid arthritis
CIRCULATORY DISTURBANCES
   Osteochondrosis
      Köhler's disease of the tarsal navicular
      Freiberg's infraction of the metatarsal head
      Miscellaneous osteochondroses
      Osteochondritis dissecans of the talus
AFFECTIONS OF THE TOES
   Hallux rigidus
TUMORS OF THE FOOT
   Soft-tissue tumors
   Bone tumors
SKIN AND NAIL LESIONS
FRACTURES AND DISLOCATIONS OF THE FOOT AND ANKLE

Infections and Inflammatory Disorders of the Foot

PYOGENIC OSTEOMYELITIS

Osteomyelitis is an inflammation of bone and indicates a pyogenic infection unless the term *osteomyelitis* is otherwise modified. The disease most frequently occurs in infants and children, although it may occur at any age. It is about three times as common in the male as in the female.

In about 10 per cent of children with osteomyelitis the primary site of involvement is one of the bones of the foot.[19] The calcaneus is the most common (6 to 8 per cent), and in order of decreasing frequency, the metatarsals, cuboid, talus, phalanges, and cuneiforms.

The infection may be of hematogenous origin or caused by external inoculation of organisms, as in puncture wounds.

Pseudomonas osteomyelitis is a serious

complication of puncture wounds of the foot.[5, 14, 15, 20, 26, 27] The child may step on a nail, a thorn, a sharp piece of glass, or in the nursery, the heel of a newborn may be infected by a contaminated needle. Mixed infection with more than one organism may occur.

Clinically osteomyelitis of the bones of the foot is an indolent infection with a paucity of systemic manifestations such as pyrexia and leukocytosis. The most constant symptoms are pain and limp. Soon soft-tissue swelling and tenderness develop, and the affected phalanx or metatarsal will appear swollen and be chronically painful.

Early diagnosis is possible before changes become apparent in the roentgenogram.[34] Bone imaging with radionuclides such as technetium-99m diphosphate will detect the osteomyelitis very soon after the onset of symptoms. The earliest roentgenographic findings are loss and distortion of trabecular pattern. Bone resorption and periostitis develop in two to three weeks (Fig. 6–1). Sequestration appears later. Abscess cavities may have marginal sclerosis (Fig. 6–2).

An important aid in diagnosis is aspiration of the site of maximum tenderness. A 16- or 18-gauge lumbar puncture needle with a stylet inside is used; it is imperative to prepare the skin thoroughly for asepsis. If subperiosteal pus is not found, the needle is advanced to penetrate the cortex and the intertrabecular spaces. Often, in the first few days of the disease only serosanguineous fluid or blood will be obtained. The aspirated material is sent to the laboratory for culture and sensitivity studies. A smear and Gram stain are also done. Every attempt should be made to isolate the pathogenic organism.

Immediate treatment is vital. Once material has been obtained for culture, antibiotic therapy is started promptly. If Gram's stain discloses gram-negative bacteria, *Pseudomonas aeruginosa* is the probable organism. Carbenicillin alone or in combination with gentamicin is the antibiotic of choice in the case of *Pseudomonas* osteomyelitis. If the smear shows gram-positive cocci, aqueous penicillin or sodium methicillin is given intravenously in appropriate dosage. As soon as the pathogenic organism and its sensitivities are determined, the antibiotic is changed to the most effective one. Dosages of antibiotics used for therapy of bone and joint infections are given in Table 6–1.

The affected foot and leg are immobilized in a well-padded splint with the ankle in functional position. The patient is much more comfortable, and the rest is good treatment for osteomyelitis. The foot is in-

*Table 6–1. Dosages of Antibiotics Used for Therapy of Bone and Joint Infections**

Drug	Dosage (mg./kg./day)	Intervals of Doses (hours)	Route
Amikacin	15–20	q 8–12	I.V., I.M.
Amoxicillin	100	q 6	P.O.
Ampicillin	150	q 6	I.V., I.M., or P.O.
Carbenicillin	400–600	q 4–6	I.V.
Cefaclor	150	q 6	P.O.
Cefamandole	120	q 6	I.V., I.M.
Cefazolin	75	q 8	I.V.
Cephalexin	100	q 6	P.O.
Cephalothin	150	q 4–6	I.V.
Chloramphenicol	75	q 6	I.V., P.O.
Clindamycin	30	q 8	I.V., P.O.
Cloxacillin	100	q 6	P.O.
Dicloxacillin	75	q 6	P.O.
Gentamicin	6(children)—7.5(infants)	q 8	I.V., I.M.
Kanamycin	20–30	q 8	I.V., I.M.
Methicillin	200	q 6	I.V.
Oxacillin or nafcillin	150	q 6	I.V., P.O.
Penicillin	100 (150,000 units)	q 4–6	I.V., P.O.
Ticarcillin	200–300	q 4–6	I.V.
Vancomycin	40	q 6	I.V.

*From Jackson, M. A., and Nelson, J. D.: Etiology and medical management of acute suppurative bone and joint infections in pediatric patients. J. Pediat. Orthop., 2:319, 1982. Reprinted by permission.

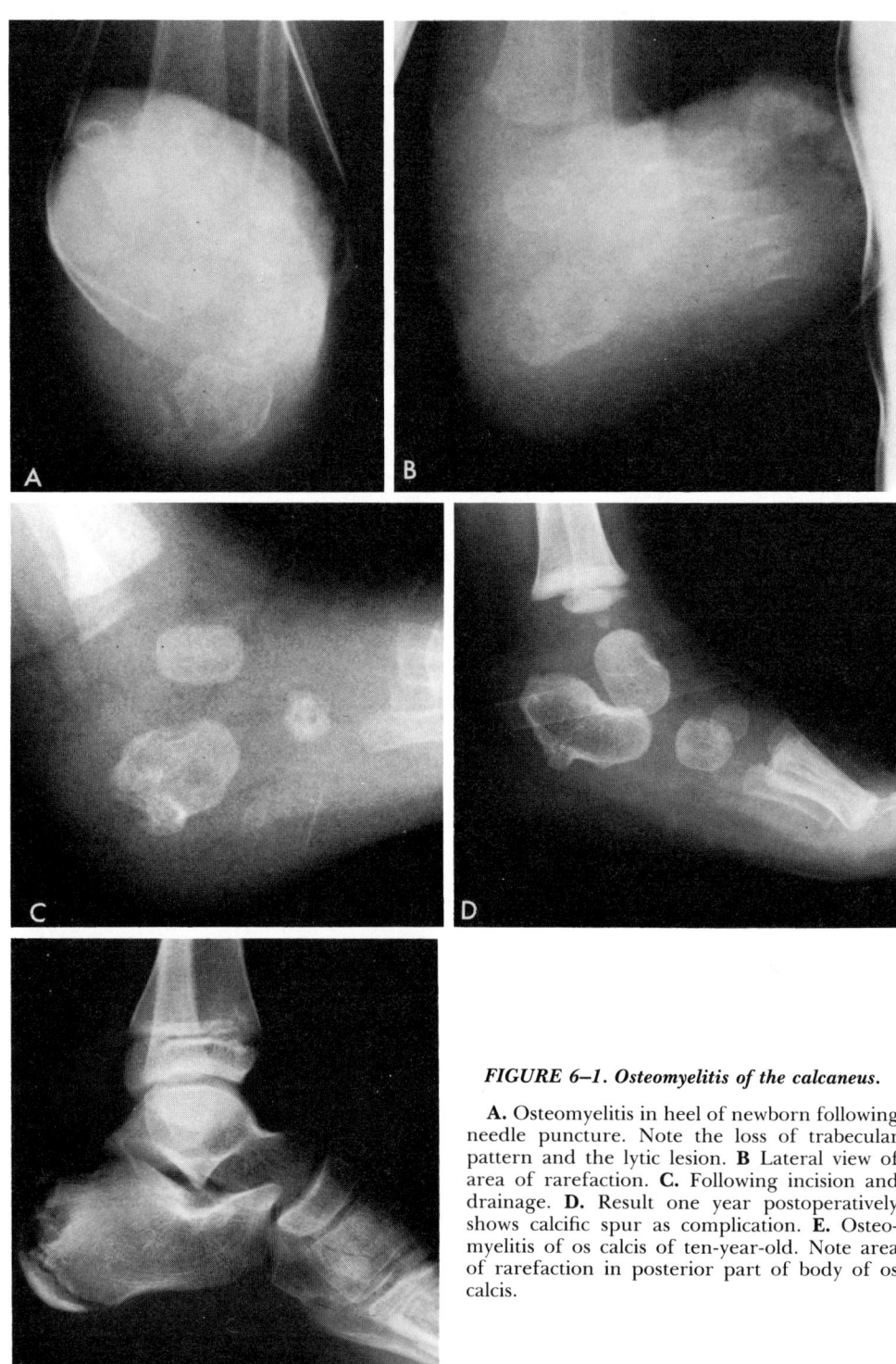

FIGURE 6–1. Osteomyelitis of the calcaneus.

A. Osteomyelitis in heel of newborn following needle puncture. Note the loss of trabecular pattern and the lytic lesion. **B** Lateral view of area of rarefaction. **C.** Following incision and drainage. **D.** Result one year postoperatively shows calcific spur as complication. **E.** Osteomyelitis of os calcis of ten-year-old. Note area of rarefaction in posterior part of body of os calcis.

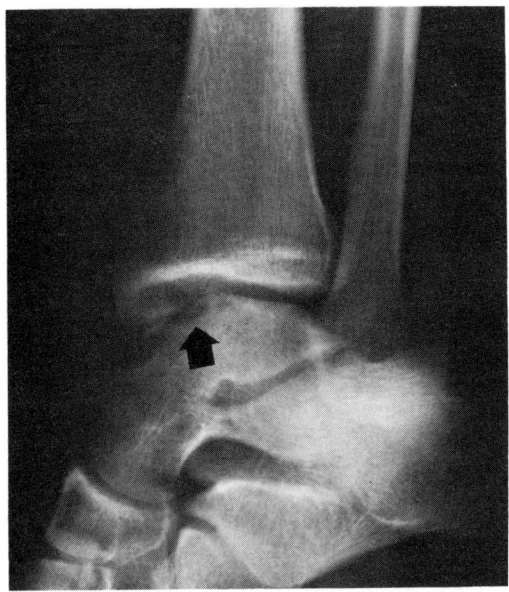

FIGURE 6–2. Osteomyelitis of the talus.

Note the area of radiolucency surrounded by marginal sclerosis *(arrow)*.

spected daily to assess the status of the local signs in response to antibiotic therapy and to see that the adjacent joints are not involved.

If pus is aspirated or if the systemic antibiotic therapy does not effect rapid improvement within 24 to 48 hours, surgical decompression in the form of incision and drainage is carried out.

In adults, partial or complete resection of the calcaneus has been advocated for osteomyelitis. The split-heel technique of Gaenslen is favored by most surgeons.[13] In children a more conservative surgical approach is preferable. Broudy, Scott, and Watts reported 16 cases of calcaneal osteomyelitis, 14 of which required surgical treatment; in 11 treatment with appropriate antibiotics, debridement, and curettage through medial and lateral incisions resulted in cure. A split-heel technique is used when extensive debridement of the calcaneus is required in cases of chronic osteomyelitis or those in which less extensive debridement has failed.[6] The growth of the apophysis of the calcaneus should be preserved when possible. In children, excision of the calcaneus for chronic osteomyelitis is not recommended.

The scar after the Gaenslen approach is deeply located and painless; the tissues on each side of the incision curl in and form thick cushions for weight-bearing. This author, however, objects to the cosmetic appearance of the hindfoot after the Gaenslen incision; he finds the surgical approach described by Banks and Laufman to be very satisfactory. The patient is placed in prone position. The skin incision is made along the posterior aspect of the heel in line with one of the skin creases; it extends as far as necessary on the medial and lateral aspects of the hindfoot to facilitate exposure. The skin flaps are undermined and elevated, the periosteum is incised in line with the skin incision, and the plantar soft tissues are stripped from their origin on the os calcis. The body of the calcaneus is exposed medially, laterally, and inferiorly (Fig. 6–3).[3]

Antoniou and Conner reported seven cases of osteomyelitis of the talus (five children and two adults). The characteristic finding was formation of an abscess in the body of the talus. In three of the five children the cavity was apparent on the initial roentgenograms. The pus from three of the abscesses contained coagulase-negative micrococci; from one abscess, the organism cultured was penicillin-resistant *Staphylococcus*, and the other abscess was sterile. The osteomyelitis responded to curettage and antibiotic therapy.[1]

Osteomyelitis of the Sesamoid Bones*

The sesamoid bones of the first metatarsophalangeal joint are occasionally the site of hematogenous osteomyelitis. These bones are named after the seeds of *Sesamum indicum* because of their configuration. Their cartilaginous anlagen develop at the third month of fetal life, and ossification begins at the age of eight years. Normally the sesamoid bones may ossify from one, two, or more centers of ossification. Bipartite or multipartite sesamoids are present in 7 to 10 per cent of feet, most commonly occurring in the medial sesamoid (90 per cent). Normal partition of the sesamoids is unilateral in about 75 per cent of cases; therefore, comparison roentgenograms of the other foot are not reliably helpful.[4]

The sesamoid bones of the hallux are

---

*See references 7, 14, 29, 33.

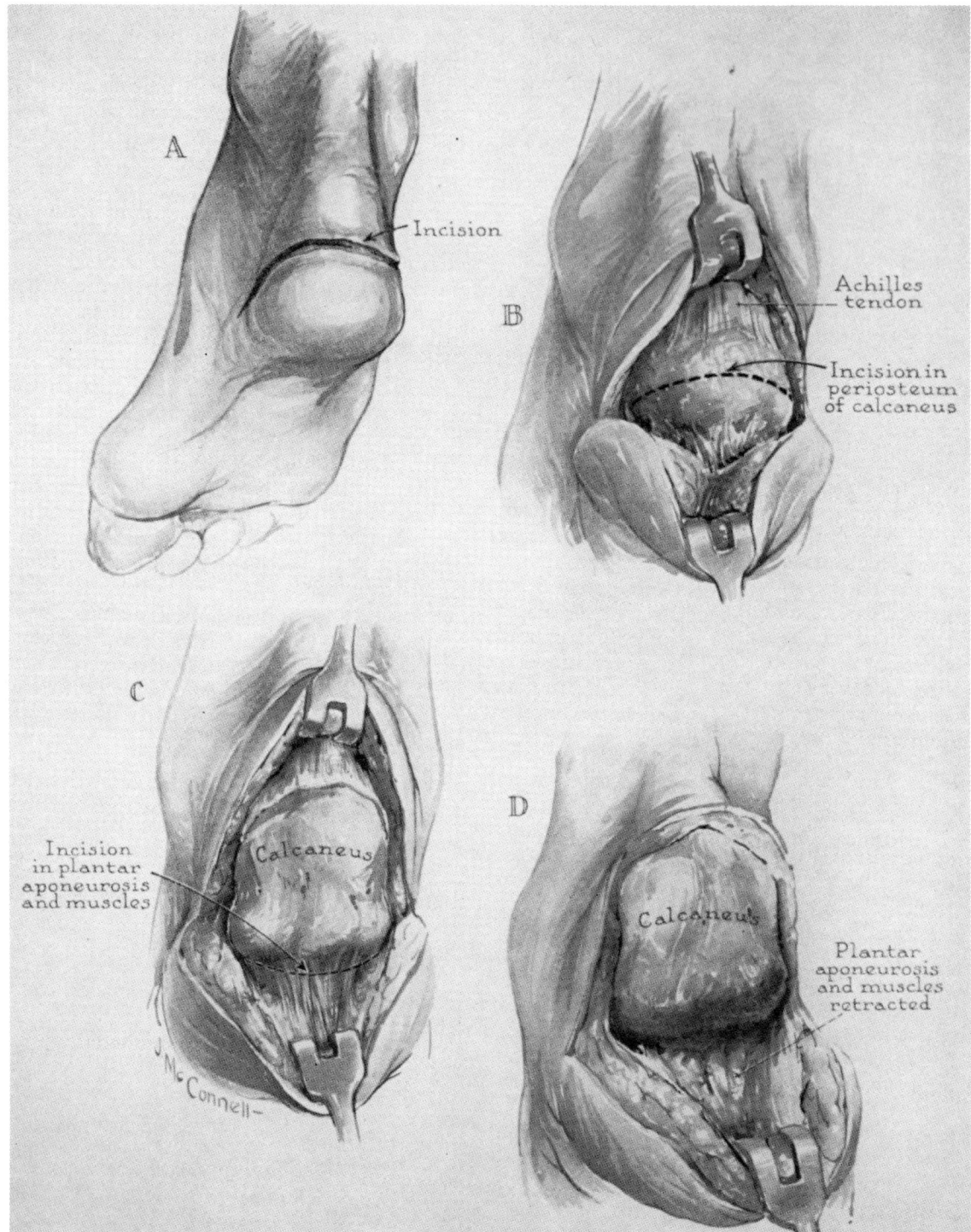

FIGURE 6–3. Surgical exposure of the calcaneus through a circumferential heel incision.

(From Banks, S. W., and Laufman, H.: An Atlas of Surgical Exposures of the Extremities. Philadelphia, W. B. Saunders Co., 1953, p. 379. Reprinted by permission.)

almost always located in the tendon of the flexor hallucis brevis; on their plantar aspect lies the thick fibrous pad of the ball of the foot, and dorsally they articulate with the articular surface of the first metatarsal head.

In the dorsoplantar projection of the roentgenogram of the foot, the medial (tibial) sesamoid lies within the outline of the first metatarsal head and is larger than the lateral (fibular) sesamoid, which extends beyond the lateral margin of the first metatarsal head. For better visualization of the sesamoid, axial views in the anteroposterior and lateral planes are necessary. Occasionally tomography may be helpful.

Osteomyelitis of the sesamoids usually occurs in children over eight years of age and in young adults. Occasionally it may be seen in adults. Often there is no history of recent acute injury. The presenting complaint is pain in the forepart of the foot. In the early stages of the disease there is little local or systemic evidence of infection. The diagnosis is frequently delayed or overlooked because the symptoms are thought to be due to foot strain or cellulitis. In the adult male the condition may be misdiagnosed as gout. On examination there are local tenderness of the affected sesamoid and swelling and redness in the region of the first metatarsophalangeal joint.

The initial roentgenograms are normal, but within 10 to 14 days the sesamoid appears to be irregular and fragmented (Fig. 6–4). This stage is followed by relatively increased density and sequestration and migration of the dead bone fragments.

Eventually an abscess develops on the medial and dorsal aspects of the head of the first metatarsal; the abscess does not extend into the thick plantar surface under the sesamoid bone. Periostitis of the first metatarsal shaft may develop.

Treatment consists of incision, drainage, and removal of the sesamoid bone, combined with chemotherapy. The prognosis is good, with permanent healing as a rule.

References

1. Antoniou, D., and Connor, A. N.: Osteomyelitis of the calcaneus and talus. J. Bone Joint Surg., 56-A:338, 1974.
2. Bailey, H.: Infections of the foot. J. Int. Coll. Surg., 27:475, 1957.
3. Banks, S. W., and Laufman, H.: Surgical Exposure of the Extremities. Philadelphia, W. B. Saunders Co., 1953, p. 378.
4. Bennet, K.: Septische Osteomyelitis als Ätiologie der sog. typischen Erkrankung der Sesambeine des Metatarsalknochens. Acta Chir. Scand., 76:103, 1935.
5. Brand, R. A., and Black, H.: Pseudomonas osteomyelitis following puncture wounds in children. J. Bone Joint Surg. 56-A:1637, 1974.
6. Broudy, A. S., Scott, R. D., and Watts, H. G.: The split-heel technique in the management of calcaneal osteomyelitis in children. Report of three cases. Clin. Orthop., 119:202, 1976.
7. Cowill, M.: Osteomyelitis of the metatarsal sesamoids. J. Bone Joint Surg., 51-B:464, 1969.
8. Cox, C. E.: Gentamicin. Med. Clin. N. Amer., 54:1305, 1970.
9. Dell, J. M., Jr.: Demonstrations of sinus tracts, fistulas and infected cavities by Lipiodol. Amer. J. Roentgen., 61:223, 1949.
10. Eid, A. M.: Treatment of chronic haematogenous osteomyelitis of the os calcis. Acta Orthop. Scand., 48:712, 1977.
11. Feigin, R. D., McAlister, W. H., San Joaquin, V. H., and Middlekamp, J. N.: Osteomyelitis of the calcaneus. Amer. J. Dis. Child., 119:61, 1970.
12. Frank, T. J. F.: Osteomyelitis of the sesamoid bone of the great toe. Roy. Melbourne Hosp. Clin. Rep., 14:80, 1943.
13. Gaenslen, F. J.: Split heel approach in osteomyelitis of the os calcis. J. Bone Joint Surg., 13:759, 1931.
14. Gordon, S. L., Evans, C., and Greer, R. B., III: Pseudomonas osteomyelitis of the metatarsal sesamoid of the great toe. Clin. Orthop., 99:188, 1974.
15. Hagler, D. J.: Pseudomonas osteomyelitis puncture wounds of the feet. Pediatrics, 48:672, 1971.
16. Horwitz, T.: Partial resection of the os calcis and primary closure in the treatment of resistant large ulcers of the heel, with or without osteomyelitis of the os calcis. Clin. Orthop., 84:149, 1972.
16a. Howie, D. W., Savage, J. P., Wilson, T. G., and Paterson, D.: The technetium phosphate bone scan in the diagnosis of osteomyelitis in childhood. J. Bone Joint Surg., 65-A:431, 1983.
17. Hubay, C. A.: Sesamoid bones of the hands and feet. Amer. J. Roentgen., 61:493, 1949.

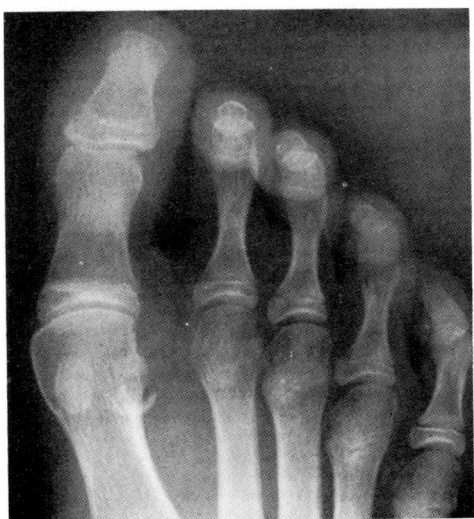

FIGURE 6–4. Osteomyelitis of the lateral sesamoid bone of the first metatarsophalangeal joint of the right foot.

The anteroposterior roentgenogram shows definite fragmentation of the lateral sesamoid bone with increased density of the proximal fragment. (From Torgerson, W. R., and Hammond, G.: Osteomyelitis of the sesamoid bones of the first metatarsophalangeal joint. J. Bone Joint Surg., 51-A:1421, 1969. Reprinted by permission.)

18. Jackson, A. W., Neviaser, R. J., and Adams, J. P.: Talectomy for osteomyelitis of the talus. In Bateman, J. E. (ed.): Foot Science. Philadelphia, W. B. Saunders Co., 1976, pp. 168–178.
18a. Jackson, M. A., and Nelson, J. D.: Etiology and medical management of acute suppurative bone and joint infections in pediatric patients. J. Pediat. Orthop., 2:313, 1982.
19. Jacobs, J. C.: Acute osteomyelitis. New York J. Med., 5:90, 1978.
20. Johanson, P. H.: Pseudomonas infections of the foot following puncture wounds. J.A.M.A., 204:170, 1968.
21. Kewenter, Y.: Die Sesambeine des 1. Metatarsophalangealgelenks des Menschen. Acta Orthop. Scand., Suppl. 2, 1936.
22. Lange, M.: Die typische Sesambeinerkrankung des 1. Metatarsal-knochens mit Ausgang in Vereiterung. Z. Orthop. Chir., 49:595, 1928.
23. Mansoor, I. A.: Typhoid osteomyelitis of the calcaneus due to direct inoculation. J. Bone Joint Surg., 49-A:732, 1967.
24. Martini, M., Martini-Benkeddache, Y., Bekhechi, T., and Daoud, A.: Treatment of chronic osteomyelitis of the calcaneus by resection of the calcaneus. A report of twenty cases. J. Bone Joint Surg., 56-A:542, 1974.
25. Maylahn, D. J.: Thorn-induced "tumors" of bone. J. Bone Joint Surg., 34-A:386, 1952.
26. Miller, E. H., and Semian, D. W.: Gram-negative osteomyelitis following puncture wound of the foot. J. Bone Joint Surg., 57-A:535, 1975.
27. Minnefor, A., Olson, M., and Carver, D.: Pseudomonas osteomyelitis following puncture wounds of the foot. Pediatrics, 47:598, 1971.
28. Pollock, S. F., and Morris, J. M.: Infectious disorders and noninfectious inflammatory diseases of the foot. In Inman, V. T. (ed.): DuVries' Surgery of the Foot. St. Louis, C. V. Mosby Co., 1973, pp. 299–317.
29. Rowe, M. M.: Osteomyelitis of metatarsal sesamoid. Brit. Med. J., 1:1071, 1963.
30. Schweitzer, G.: Acute hematogenous osteomyelitis of the os calcis. Med. J. Aust., 1:1179, 1967.
31. Smith, R.: Osteitis of the metatarsal sesamoid. Brit. J. Surg., 29:19, 1941.
32. Swischuk, L. E., Jorgenson, F., Jorgenson, A., and Capen, D.: Wooden splinter induced "pseudotumors" and "osteomyelitis-like lesions" of bone and soft tissue. Amer. J. Roentgen., 122:176, 1974.
33. Torgerson, W. R., and Hammond, G.: Osteomyelitis of the sesamoid bones of the first metatarsophalangeal joint. J. Bone Joint Surg., 51-A:1420, 1969.
34. Treves, S., Khettry, J., Broker, F. H., Wilkinson, H. R., and Watts, H.: Osteomyelitis: Early scintigraphic detection in children. Pediatrics, 57:173, 1976.
35. Waldvogel, F. A., Medoff, G., and Swartz, M. N.: Osteomyelitis: A review of clinical features, therapeutic considerations and unusual aspects (First of three parts.) New Eng. J. Med., 282:198–206, 260–266, and 316–322, 1970.
36. Weston, W. J.: Thorn and twig-induced pseudotumours of bone and soft tissues. Brit. J. Radiol., 36:323, 1963.
37. Wiltse, L. L., Bateman, J. G., and Kase, S.: Resection of the major portion of the calcaneus. Clin. Orthop., 13:271, 1959.
38. Zverev, A. F.: On the most rational surgical approach in children with chronic osteomyelitis of the calcaneus. Khirurgiia (Moskva), 42:117, 1966.

TUBERCULOSIS OF BONES AND JOINTS

In the foot and ankle tuberculosis infection may occur as tuberculous dactylitis (or spina ventosa) affecting the metatarsals and phalanges; as tuberculous osteomyelitis (of the calcaneus, talus, navicular, cuboid, or cuneiform bones); or as tuberculous arthritis involving the metatarsophalangeal, tarsometatarsal, and intertarsal joints.

Not too long ago tuberculosis was the most common disease affecting the skeleton; this is still true in certain parts of the world. In economically well-developed countries it is now rare and may be easily overlooked. Bergdahl, Fellander, and Robertson reported 18 cases of bone and joint tuberculosis in children in the Stockholm area over the period from 1961 to 1974. BCG infection was verified by culture and identification of bacterial type in seven, all after 1968 (the same origin is presumed in the remaining 11 cases). In Sweden all newborn children are vaccinated with BCG in the first few weeks of life. It is of interest to note that in 3 of the 18 cases the site of infection was the foot (one talus, one calcaneus, and one cuboid).[2]

Tuberculous dactylitis, or spina ventosa, occurs in children, usually under five years of age.[7] Occurring more frequently in the hand than in the foot, the infection may affect the metacarpals, metatarsals, or phalanges. It may involve several digits, which become swollen and fusiform or spindle-shaped. There is little if any pain, and disability is minimal. Shortening and contracture of the affected digit will result. Roentgenograms disclose expansion of the infected short tubular bone by cystlike rarefaction with some subperiosteal new bone formation. The condition should be distinguished from solitary enchondroma or multiple enchondromatosis, in which periosteal reaction is minimal or absent, unless complicated by a fracture; from fusiform enlargement of the fingers seen in pauciarticular arthritis, in which there is no cystlike rarefaction of bone; and from syphilitic dactylitis, in which there is marked subperiosteal new bone formation and the serologic test for syphilis is positive.

Treatment consists of chemotherapy with antituberculous drugs and splinting in functional position. The prognosis is good.

Tuberculous arthritis is often monarticular. The onset of the disease is insidious. The initial symptom may be a slight limp due to discomfort. The affected joint is stiff and boggy. Local heat is usually absent, and tenderness is minimal. Atrophy of the calf muscles soon develops. Temperature elevation is ordinarily not marked.

The roentgenograms will show regional bone atrophy and soft-tissue swelling. In the metatarsophalangeal joint the capsule will be distended. High-quality radiography is of vital importance. The normal trabecular structure of bone disappears, and soon areas of radiolucency develop in the epiphysis or metaphysis, indicating bone destruction. Reactive new bone formation is characteristically absent in the early stages; it is only in the late healing period that it develops. Sequestra may occasionally be present. If tuberculous arthritis remains untreated, the entire articular cartilage will eventually be eroded, and extensive destruction of subjacent bone will take place, resulting in gross deformity of the joint. Abscesses are usually not seen in the foot.

An elevated erythrocyte sedimentation rate and positive tubercular skin test are almost always present. Evidence of associated visceral tuberculosis (lungs, kidneys, lymph nodes) is the rule and is demonstrated by findings in the chest roentgenogram, in the intravenous pyelogram, or in the film of the abdomen.

Tuberculosis is a great deceiver because of its rarity. To make a diagnosis of tuberculosis one must consider it as a possibility in the differential diagnosis. Tuberculous arthritis of the ankle or metatarsophalangeal joint may be regarded as a chronic sprain, or that of the subtalar or midtarsal joints as cellulitis. The diagnosis is often long delayed.

Synovial fluid analysis is usually not feasible because of the difficulty of aspirating adequate amounts of joint fluid in the foot. The diagnosis is confirmed by histologic examination of synovial tissue obtained by biopsy, which should not be delayed if reasonable suspicion exists. Cultural studies and guinea pig inoculations are made; they will be positive for tuberculosis.

Treatment consists of administration of antituberculous drugs and resting the part by splinting it in functional position. Weight-bearing is not permitted. When the disease process is well advanced, synovectomy and curettage may be indicated.

References

1. Allred, S. W., and Minear, W. L.: Statistical study of tuberculosis of the bones and joints in children. Amer. Surg., *18*:58, 1952.
2. Bergdahl, S., Fellander, M., and Robertson, B.: BCG osteomyelitis. Experience in the Stockholm region over the years 1961–1974. J. Bone Joint Surg., *58-B*:212, 1976.
3. Bosworth, D. M.: Treatment of bone and joint tuberculosis in children. J. Bone Joint Surg., *41-A*:1255, 1959.
4. Campos, O. P.: Bone and joint tuberculosis and its treatment. J. Bone Joint Surg., *37-A*:937, 1955.
5. Crofton, J.: The chemotherapy of tuberculosis. Brit. Med. Bull., *16*:55, 1960.
6. Girdlestone, G. R., and Somerville, E. W.: Tuberculosis of Bone and Joint. London, Oxford University Press, 1952.
7. Hardy, J. B., and Hartman, J. R.: Tuberculous dactylitis in childhood. J. Pediat., *30*:146, 1947.
8. Kallesoe, O., and Jespersen, A.: Metastatic osteomyelitis following BCG vaccination. Acta Orthop. Scand., *49*:134, 1978.
9. Lelèvre, J.: Tuberculose du pied. In Pathologie du Pied. 2nd Ed. Paris, Masson & Cie, 1961, pp. 533–548.
10. Miltner, L. J., and Fang, H. C.: Prognosis and treatment of tuberculosis of the bones of the foot. J. Bone Joint Surg., *18*:287, 1936.
11. Phemister, D. B.: Changes in the articular surfaces in tuberculosis and pyogenic infection of joints. Amer. J. Roentgen., *12*:1, 1924.
12. Phemister, D. B.: Changes in the articular surfaces in tuberculous arthritis. J. Bone Joint Surg., 7:835, 1925.
13. Reeves, J. D.: Differential diagnosis in case 44122: Presentation of case. New Eng. J. Med., *258*:612, 1958.
14. Stuart, D.: Local osteo-articular tuberculosis complicating closed fractures. J. Bone Joint Surg., *58-B*:248, 1976.
15. Umansky, A. L., Schlesinger, P. T., and Greenberg, B. B.: Tuberculous dactylitis in the adult. Arch. Surg. (Chicago), *54*:67, 1947.
16. Walker, G. F.: Failure of early recognition of skeletal tuberculosis. Brit. Med. J., *1*:682, 1968.
17. Wilkinson, M. C.: Synovectomy and curettage in the treatment of tuberculosis of joints. J. Bone Joint Surg. *35-B*:209, 1953.
18. Wilkinson, M. C.: Chemotherapy of tuberculosis of bones and joints. J. Bone Joint Surg., *36-B*:23, 1954.

SUPPURATIVE OR SEPTIC ARTHRITIS

Acute suppurative, or septic, arthritis is an inflammation of the joint caused by pus-forming organisms. The ankle joint is infrequently involved, and the talocalcaneonavicular, midtarsal, and other smaller joints of the foot are rarely infected.

Staphylococcus aureus and *Streptococcus hemolyticus* are the common causative organisms in infection in the ankle joint, but in the foot *Pseudomonas aeruginosa* is not infrequently the culprit. The bacteria may gain entrance by the hematogenous route, by direct extension from an adjacent focus of osteomyelitis, or by direct inoculation into the joint by accidental puncture wounds.

In infection in the ankle, the onset of symptoms is usually acute. Pain in the ankle or foot is the most prominent complaint. The child walks with an antalgic limp; soon weight-bearing becomes very painful, and he may not be able to walk at all. The child is apprehensive, irritable, and feverish. His temperature may be as high as 39° or 40°C. In infection in the foot, the onset of symptoms may be insidious, and systemic manifestations may be minimal.

The ankle, subtalar, or other affected

joints of the foot are warm and swollen. The joint is held in the position of minimal pressure—the ankle in 15 to 20 degrees of plantar flexion, the talocalcaneonavicular joint in slight inversion. On palpation there is diffuse tenderness over the joint line. Active and passive motions of the affected joint are extremely painful.

Roentgenograms will show the capsule distended with fluid. Rarefaction of bone and narrowing of articular cartilage space will eventually develop as infection persists.

Diagnosis

The diagnosis is made by aspiration of the joint suspected of being infected. It should be performed under strict aseptic conditions. An 18-gauge lumbar puncture needle with a stylet inside is used. The route of aspiration of the ankle joint is anterior, lateral to the long extensor tendons (Fig. 6–5). One has to feel his way, so to speak, into the distended capsule. To avoid spreading infection into bone, he should take care not to penetrate the articular surface. The tip of the needle should always be double-checked to ensure that it is not broken. A stylet inside prevents such an accident and also serves to prevent thickened synovium and fibrin from plugging the needle.

When the joint contains little fluid or the fluid is very thick, one may introduce 1 ml. of sterile normal saline into the joint and reaspirate it. The joint fluid is then cultured, and smears are made with Gram stain to identify the causative organism under the microscope. Demonstration of the presence of bacteria by Gram stain not only strengthens the diagnosis but also aids in the selection of the antibiotic to be used. Sensitivity studies should always be performed.

In the early stages the joint fluid may be serosanguineous. Within a few days it becomes cloudy with an elevated cell count (usually between 15,000 and 20,000 cells per millimeter) and a high polymorphonuclear leukocyte differential count. The joint fluid sugar is reduced, averaging 50 mg per 100 ml. less than the blood sugar. The mucin, measured on the acid precipitation test, is poor or very poor.

In the differential diagnosis one should consider osteomyelitis, acute rheumatoid arthritis, and acute rheumatic fever. *Osteomyelitis*, particularly if associated with sympathetic effusion in the adjacent joint, presents a difficult problem in differential diagnosis, as most of its signs and symptoms resemble those of suppurative arthritis. In osteomyelitis the point of maximal tenderness is over the metaphysis, whereas in septic arthritis it is directly over the joint line. On gentle examination of the joint, motion is much less restricted and less painful in osteomyelitis than it is in septic arthritis. The limb as a whole is more swollen in osteomyelitis; in septic arthritis, it is the joint that is swollen. It is often necessary to aspirate the joint in order to make the diagnosis. One should exercise considerable caution not to contaminate a clean joint from an infected focus in the metaphysis. The joint fluid of sympathetic effusion in osteomyelitis will be straw-colored with only a few thousand leukocytes.

Rheumatoid arthritis may involve only one joint. Its onset, as a rule, however, is gradual, and usually the child is not acutely ill. The affected joint has a better range of motion, is not as tender, and is less swollen than in septic arthritis. The total leukocyte count in rheumatoid arthritis may be as high as that in septic arthritis, but the differential count will disclose many fewer polymorphonuclear cells. Mucin is poor in both conditions. Gram stain and culture, however, are negative in rheumatoid ar-

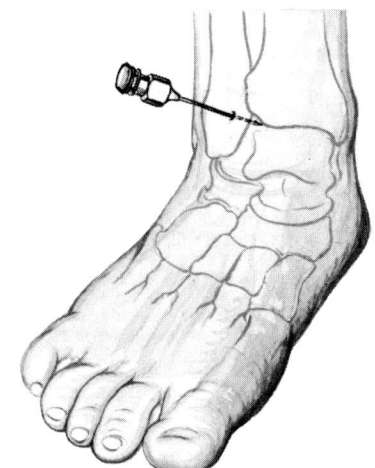

FIGURE 6–5. Route of aspiration of ankle joint.

The approach is anterior, lateral to the long extensor tendons.

thritis, and the glucose content is not diminished as much as in septic joint.

The hot, red, swollen, and painful joints and high temperature of *rheumatic fever* may be mistaken for suppurative arthritis. Fleeting migratory joint involvement and cardiac manifestations are the hallmarks of rheumatic fever. The response of acute rheumatic fever to an adequate dose of salicylates is dramatic, with relief of swelling and pain in the joints and return of temperature and pulse rate to normal. Salicylates, however, should not be given as a diagnostic test until sepsis has been ruled out, as their administration will only cloud the picture and cause delay in treatment of a pyogenic joint.

Treatment

Suppurative arthritis is a serious condition and must be treated immediately as an emergency. The purposes of treatment are sterilization of the joint; evacuation of the fibrin, debris, and bacterial products associated with infection; prevention of deformity; restoration of the joint motion to normal; and resumption of proper functional use.

As soon as suppurative arthritis of the ankle or joints of the foot is definitely suspected, the foot and ankle are immobilized in a posterior splint in functional position.

If diagnosis is made early, the septic joint fluid may still be serosanguineous. In such an instance the joint is thoroughly irrigated with normal saline solution, but antibiotics are not instilled into it.

Systemic antibiotics are immediately administered intravenously. The author prefers penicillin and methicillin (Staphcillin) unless the patient is allergic to them. The antibiotics may have to be changed, depending on the results of culture and sensitivity studies. Aqueous penicillin is given at a dosage of 1,000,000 to 3,000,000 units every four hours; methicillin dosage is 200 mg. per kilogram of body weight per day (up to a maximum daily dose of 8 to 10 gm.). This total daily amount is administered in six divided doses.

Treatment of septic arthritis is usually surgical drainage. On occasion, however, the infection is diagnosed early when the disease is of short duration and the organism is very sensitive to the antibiotic (as are meningococcus and streptococcus). In these cases response to conservative treatment may be dramatic, with immediate relief of local pain and tenderness, rapid increase in motion, return of elevated temperature to normal, and subsidence of local symptoms such as effusion and synovial thickening. The joint should then be reaspirated and irrigated, and cultures should be taken to check its sterility. The joints that respond to conservative management are protected in bivalved casts, and active and passive exercises are performed until full function is restored.

Surgical drainage of the affected joint is indicated when pus is obtained on initial diagnostic aspiration or when there is no dramatic response to conservative treatment. The ankle joint is incised and drained through the anterolateral approach, and the talocalcaneonavicular joint through a lateral incision. The wound is closed primarily with closed suction irrigation tubes connected to a Hemovac evacuator. A posterior splint is applied. Systemic antibiotics are continued for three weeks following surgical drainage.

Local care of the joint should be meticulous to ensure a normal joint. The foot and ankle are protected in a splint and with crutches until they attain anatomic and functional normality.

References

1. Argen, R. J., Wilson, C. H., and Wood, P.: Suppurative arthritis. Arch. Intern. Med. (Chicago), 117:661, 1966.
2. Baitch, A.: Recent observations of acute suppurative arthritis. Clin. Orthop., 22:157, 1962.
3. Borella, L., Goodbar, J. E., Summit, R. L., and Clark, G. M.: Septic arthritis in childhood. J. Pediat., 62:742, 1963.
4. Clawson, D. K., and Dunn, A. W.: Management of common bacterial infections of bones and joints. J. Bone Joint Surg., 49-A:164, 1967.
5. Compere, E. L., Metzger, W. I., and Mitra, R. N.: The treatment of pyogenic bone and joint infections by closed irrigation (circulation) with a non-toxic detergent and one or more antibiotics. J. Bone Joint Surg., 49-A:614, 1967.
6. Curtiss, P. H.: Changes produced in the synovial membrane and synovial fluid by disease. J. Bone Joint Surg., 46-A:873, 1964.
7. Curtiss, P. H., and Klein, L.: Destruction of articular cartilage in septic arthritis. J. Bone Joint Surg., 45-A:797, 1963.
8. Curtiss, P. H., and Klein, L.: Destruction of articular cartilage in septic arthritis. J. Bone Joint Surg., 47-A:1595, 1965.
9. Daniel, D., Boyer, J., Green, S., Amiel, D., and Akeson, W.: Cartilage destruction in experimentally produced Staphylococcus aureus joint infections: In vivo study. Surg. Forum, 24:479, 1973.

10. Drutz, D. J., Schaffner, W., Hillman, J. W., and Koenig, M. G.: The penetrations of penicillin and other antimicrobials into joint fluid. J. Bone Joint Surg., 49-A:1415, 1967.
11. Griffin, P. P.: Bone and joint infections in children. Pediat. Clin. N. Amer., 14:533, 1967.
12. Lloyd-Roberts, G. C.: Suppurative arthritis of infancy. J. Bone Joint Surg., 42-B:706, 1960.
13. Lloyd-Roberts, G. C.: Orthopaedics in Infancy and Childhood. London, Butterworth, 1971.
14. Nade, S., Robertson, F. W., and Taylor, T. K. F.: Antibiotics in the treatment of acute osteomyelitis and acute septic arthritis in children. Med. J. Aust., 2:703, 1974.
15. Nelson, J. D.: Antibiotic concentrations in septic joint effusions. New Eng. J. Med., 284:349, 1971.
16. Nelson, J. D., and Koontz, W. C.: Septic arthritis in infants and children: A review of 117 cases. Pediatrics, 38:966, 1966.
17. Parker, R. H., and Schmid, F. R.: Antibacterial activity of synovial fluid during therapy of septic arthritis. Arthritis Rheum., 14:96, 1971.
18. Paterson, D. C.: Acute suppurative arthritis in infancy and childhood. J. Bone Joint Surg., 52-B:474, 1970.
19. Phemister, D. B.: The effect of pressure on articular surfaces in pyogenic and tuberculous arthritides and its bearing upon treatment. Ann. Surg., 80:481, 1924.
20. Samilson, R. L., Bersani, F. A., and Watkins, M. B.: Acute suppurative arthritis in infants and children. Pediatrics, 21:798, 1958.
21. Schmid, F. R., and Parker, R. H.: Ongoing assessment of therapy in septic arthritis. Arthritis Rheum., 12:529, 1969.
22. Ward, J., Cohen, A. S., and Bauer, W.: The diagnosis and therapy of acute suppurative arthritis. Arthritis Rheum., 3:522, 1960.

JUVENILE RHEUMATOID ARTHRITIS

Rheumatoid arthritis in children is a generalized disease in which the arthritis is but one manifestation. It may affect the collagen and connective tissue of any organ system. The term *rheumatoid disease* is more appropriate. A discussion of the etiology, pathology, various clinical manifestations, and general management of rheumatoid arthritis is beyond the scope of this book but can be found in the cited references.[1-28]

The many variants of rheumatoid arthritis may be arbitrarily grouped into (1) pauciarticular arthritis, (2) polyarthritis with minimal systemic manifestations, and (3) severe rheumatoid disease with polyarthritis. The foot may be involved in any one of these forms of rheumatoid disease.

Pauciarticular arthritis is characterized by involvement of a few large joints with minimal or no systemic manifestations. The joints of the lower limb are involved more often than those of the upper limb, the knee, the ankle, and the subtalar joints being the three common sites (Fig. 6–6). In some children the toes are involved, with tumefaction of the entire digit.

The condition is more common in girls,

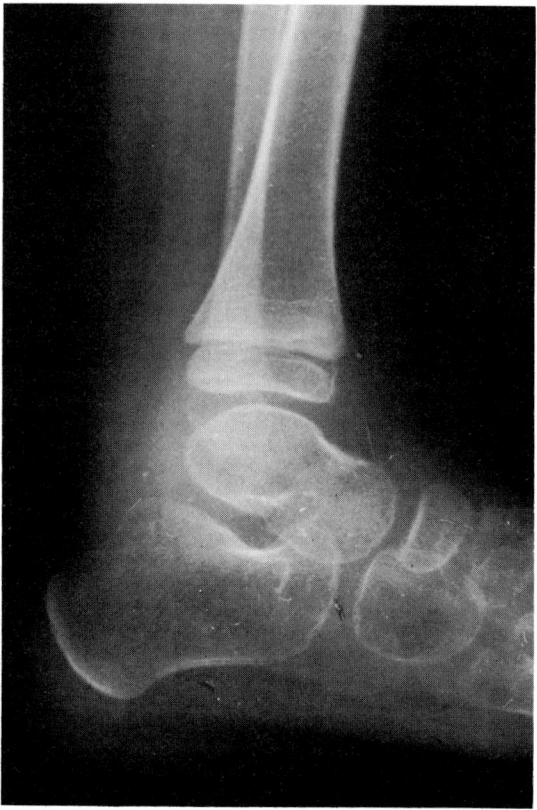

FIGURE 6–6. *Rheumatoid arthritis of left ankle.*

Roentgenogram shows soft-tissue swelling and capsular distention.

the female-to-male ratio being seven to three. The incidence is greatest between the ages of two and four years, with over 50 per cent of cases having their onset before the fourth year. The disease may, however, begin at any time between 4 months and 15 years of age.

In about 50 per cent of the patients, involvement is monarticular; in 25 per cent two joints are affected, and in 18 per cent three joints are involved. Occasionally four or five joints may be affected.

In rheumatoid polyarthritis and systemic rheumatoid disease with polyarthritis the foot and ankle are involved as often as the hand and wrist. The major disabling deformities are varus or valgus hindfoot, hallux valgus, hallux rigidus, and claw toes. Subluxation of the metatarsophalangeal joints is not infrequent in severe chronic cases. Less common and less disabling deformities are hammer toes, interphalangeal valgus deformity, and interphalangeal fusion. Treatment of rheumatoid disease requires multidisciplinary management; its general medical care is discussed in the cited references.[2, 4, 22–25]

Surgical correction of deformities of the foot in rheumatoid disease is rarely indicated in children. Orthopedic management is conservative. Local care of the joint is essential, as it determines the end result when the disease becomes quiescent. Basic principles of care include rest of the joint, relief of muscle spasm, prevention of deformity, and maintenance of motion, as effected by a combination of rest in a splint and exercises.

When the ankle or subtalar joints are involved, a bivalved cast or well-padded plastic splint is used initially, providing support, relieving muscle spasm, and preventing deformity. The limb is taken out of the splint several times a day, and active and passive exercises are performed. Forced wedging casts should not be employed to correct equinus angulation.

Motion is necessary for good nutrition of a joint. Exercises maintain and increase range of motion and strengthen the muscles, preventing muscular atrophy. Fatigue and pain should be avoided. The joint is moved through its maximal range short of the point at which there is discomfort. Range of motion is gradually increased with each succeeding movement. Active exercises are performed: first, lying on one side and with gravity eliminated, and then against gravity. Gentle passive stretching exercises are indicated when there is myostatic contracture of muscles.

Initially, the bivalved cast or splint is worn at all times, except for the exercise periods. As effusion subsides and synovial thickening decreases, the periods out of the cast are gradually increased. Use of the splint is eventually discontinued during the day, but it is continued at night until the disease is completely inactive.

Weight-bearing is not allowed during the acute inflammatory phase. With subsidence of the arthritis, walking with crutches is permitted, and the amount of weight-bearing and the periods of walking are gradually increased. When only one lower limb is involved, three-point crutch gait is utilized; but when both lower limbs are affected, four-point crutch gait is used. Crutch protection in a young child may not be feasible or practicable; in such an instance, weight-bearing is delayed until the acute inflammatory process has completely subsided. On occasion, a patellar tendon–bearing orthosis is used to protect the foot or the ankle (Fig. 6–7).

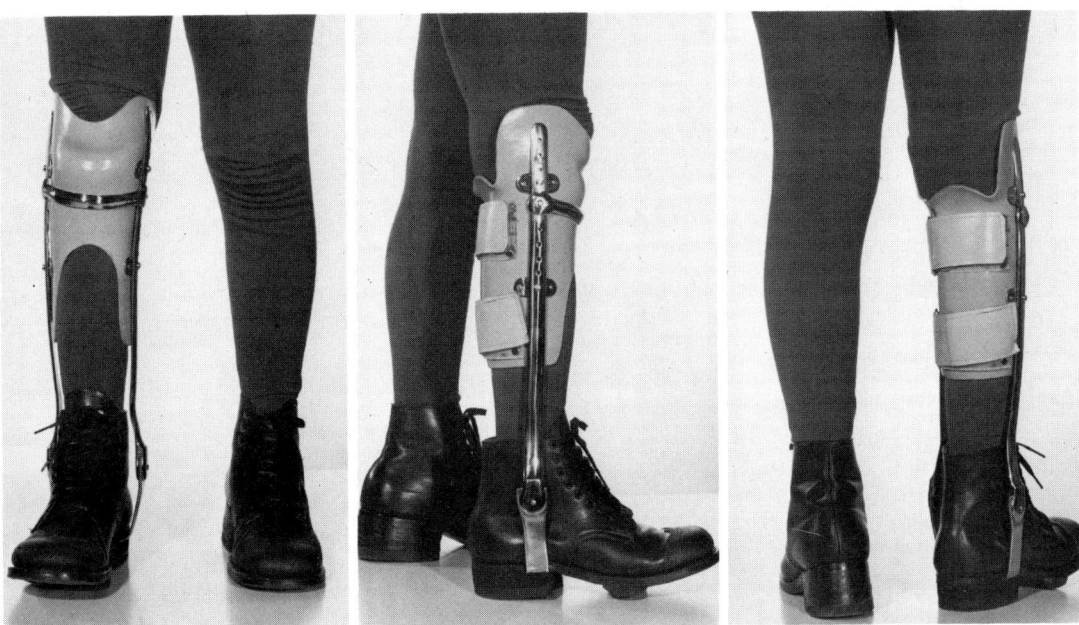

FIGURE 6–7. Patellar tendon–bearing orthosis for arthritis of ankle.

When care of joints during the acute inflammatory phase has been ineffective, deformities of the foot and ankle may be quite rigid, requiring surgical correction.

Synovectomy of the ankle and subtalar joint may be performed when 12 months of conservative management has failed to bring about subsidence of acute synovial inflammation. Partial rather than total synovectomy is safer in children. During the operation care should be taken not to damage the growth plates.

Surgical correction of the various deformities of the foot, such as hallux valgus, is described in other sections of this book.

References

1. Branemark, P. I., Ekholm, R., Goldie, I., and Lindstrom, J.: Synovectomy in rheumatoid arthritis. Acta Rheum. Scand., 13:161, 1967.
2. Brewer, E. J., Blattner, R. J., and Wing, H.: Treatment of rheumatoid arthritis in children. Pediat. Clin. N. Amer., 10:207, 1963.
3. Calabro, J. J.: A critical evaluation of the diagnostic features of the feet in rheumatoid arthritis. Arthritis Rheum., 5:19, 1962.
4. Calabro, J. J.: The natural evolution and nonoperative treatment of juvenile rheumatoid arthritis. A.A.O.S. Instr. Course Lect., 23:26, 1974.
5. Dixon, A. St. J., and Gheith, S. L.: Tangential x-ray of the forefoot in rheumatoid arthritis. Ann. Rheum. Dis., 32:92, 1973.
6. Eyring, E. J.: Braces and splints for patients with juvenile rheumatoid arthritis. A.A.O.S. Instr. Course Lect., 23:31, 1974.
7. Eyring, E. J., Longert, A., and Bass, J. C.: Synovectomy in juvenile rheumatoid arthritis. J. Bone Joint Surg., 53-A:638, 1971.
8. Fink, C. W., Baum, J., Paradies, L. H., and Carrell, B. C.: Synovectomy in juvenile rheumatoid arthritis. Ann. Rheum. Dis., 28:612, 1969.
9. Fitzgerald, J. A. W.: A review of the long-term results of arthrodesis of the first metatarso-phalangeal joint. J. Bone Joint Surg., 51-B:488, 1969.
10. Granberry, W. M., and Brewer, E. J., Jr.: Early surgery in juvenile rheumatoid arthritis. A.A.O.S. Instr. Course Lect., 23:32, 1974.
11. Griffin, P. P., Tachdjian, M. O., and Green, W. T.: Pauciarticular arthritis in children. J.A.M.A., 184:23, 1963.
12. Isaacson, A. S.: Operative procedures on patients with juvenile rheumatoid arthritis. A.A.O.S. Instr. Course Lect., 23:37, 1974.
13. Kalliomaki, J. L., and Vanha-Perttula, T.: Activity of four hydrolytic enzymes in serum and synovial fluid of patients with rheumatoid arthritis. Scand. J. Rheum., 1:21, 1972.
14. Kellgren, J. H., and Ball, J.: Tendon lesions in rheumatoid arthritis. Ann. Rheum. Dis., 9:48, 1950.
15. Key, J. A.: The reformation of synovial membrane in the knees of rabbits after synovectomy. J. Bone Joint Surg., 8:793, 1925.
16. Kirkup, J. R., Vidigal, E., and Jacoby, R. K.: The hallux and rheumatoid arthritis. Acta Orthop. Scand., 48:527, 1977.
17. Kuhns, J. G.: The care of the feet in chronic arthritis. J.A.M.A., 109:1108, 1937.
18. Lipscomb, P. R.: The role of the orthopaedist in the management of juvenile rheumatoid arthritis. A.A.O.S. Instr. Course Lect., 23:25, 1974.
19. MacSween, R. N. M., Dalakos, T. K., Jasani, M. K., and Buchanan, W. W.: Rheumatoid factor in serum and synovial fluid. Scand. J. Rheum., 1:177, 1972.
20. Martel, W.: Acute and chronic arthritis of the foot. Seminars Roentgen., 5:391, 1970.
21. Preston, R. L., and McEwen, C.: The Surgical Management of Rheumatoid Arthritis. Philadelphia, W. B. Saunders Co., 1968.
22. Schaller, J.: Juvenile rheumatoid arthritis. Postgrad. Med., 611:177, 1977.
23. Schaller, J., and Wedgewood, R. J.: Juvenile rheumatoid arthritis: A review. Pediatrics, 50:940, 1972.
24. Schaller, J., Kupfer, C., and Wedgewood, R. J.: Iridocyclitis in juvenile rhuematoid arthritis. Pediatrics, 44:92, 1969.
25. Spahr, R. C.: Juvenile rheumatoid arthritis: A review. Bull. Geisinger Med. Cent., 29:31, 1977.
26. Vidigal, E., Jacoby, R. K., Dixon, A. St. J., Ratcliff, A. H., and Kirkup, J.: The foot in chronic rheumatoid arthritis. Ann. Rheum. Dis., 34:292, 1975.
27. Williams, R. C.: Immunopathology of rheumatoid arthritis. Hosp. Pract., 13:53, 1978.
28. Wolcott, W. E.: Regeneration of the synovial membrane following typical synovectomy. J. Bone Joint Surg., 9:67, 1927.

Circulatory Disturbances

KÖHLER'S DISEASE OF THE TARSAL NAVICULAR

In 1908, Köhler described a self-limited disease of the tarsal navicular characterized by flattening, sclerosis, and irregular rarefaction in the roentgenogram.[11] The condition is uncommon, occurring more frequently in boys (about 75 to 80 per cent) than in girls. The age incidence is related to the sex of the patient, the average age of onset of symptoms being five years for boys and about four years for girls, the disease occurring at least a year earlier in the female. In about one third of the cases both feet are involved. Köhler's disease may occur simultaneously with Legg-Perthes disease.[6]

There is evidence that Köhler's disease has a mechanical basis. The tarsal navicular is located at the apex of the longitudinal arch of the foot and is subjected to constant strain during locomotion. The navicular, according to Karp, is the last bone of the foot to ossify, the average age of appearance of its ossific nucleus being between 18 and 24 months in girls and between 24 and 30 months in boys. Karp also noted that irregularities of ossification of the navicular bone are not uncommon.[9] Waugh, in a study of serial roentgenograms of the feet of 52 normal children (26 girls and 26 boys), made the same observation as Karp: that the ossification of the tarsal navicular occurs later in boys than in girls. He also reported that abnormalities of ossification are more frequent in boys and that they are more common in naviculars that ossify late. Waugh also states that abnormal ossification results from compression of the bony nucleus at a critical phase of the growth of the navicular bone whose appearance is delayed.[23] These same compressional forces occlude the vessels in the spongy osseous tissue and produce aseptic necrosis of bone. Histologic examination of the affected bone obtained by biopsy or excision of the involved navicular has disclosed areas of necrosis, resorption of dead bone, and formation of new bone.[10, 13, 21]

The child will walk with an antalgic limp, bearing his weight on the lateral side of the foot to relieve stress on its medial longitudinal arch. Other clinical manifestations consist of local pain and tenderness over the navicular bone, and not infrequently, reactive thickening and swelling over the affected area. The posterior tibial tendon may be inflamed near its insertion to the scaphoid. On testing, the midtarsal and subtalar joints have full range of motion, an important differential diagnostic point in distinguishing Köhler's disease from acute inflammatory arthritis, e.g., rheumatoid.

The roentgenographic picture is characteristic. Diagnosis rests on the demonstration of flattening of the tarsal navicular, narrowing in its anteroposterior diameter

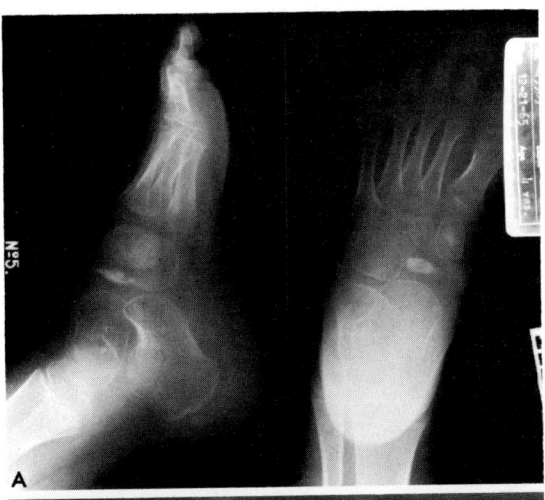

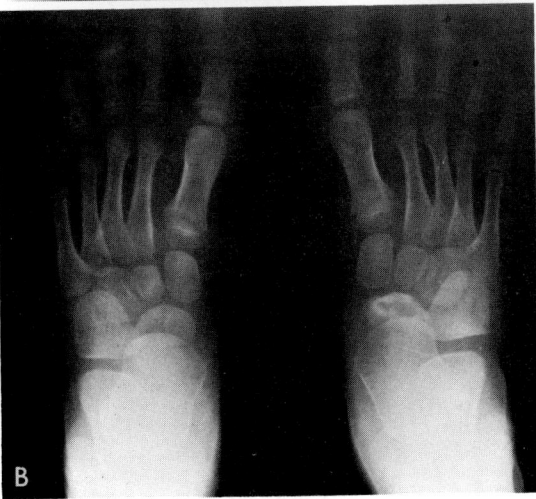

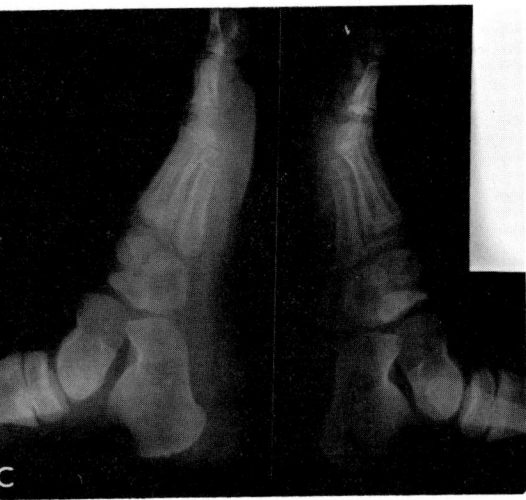

FIGURE 6–8. Köhler's disease of left tarsal navicular.

A. Note the sclerosis and flattening of the tarsal navicular. **B** and **C.** Anteroposterior and lateral roentgenograms of both feet two years later, showing healing of the left navicular.

(as seen in the lateral view), and irregular rarefaction and sclerosis of the affected bone (Fig. 6–8). Irregular ossification of the tarsal navicular is not infrequent in normal feet and should not be mistaken for Köhler's disease. Roentgenograms of both feet should be made to detect possible bilateral involvement, as, on occasion, equally severe changes may be noted in a totally asymptomatic foot.

Treatment varies with the severity of the condition. When there is moderate pain, it is best to protect the foot in a below-knee walking cast with the foot in 10 to 15 degrees varus and 20 degrees equinus position for a period of six to eight weeks. During the initial three weeks, it is best to prevent weight-bearing by the use of crutches. Following removal of the plaster cast, strain on the foot is relieved by a soft longitudinal arch support with a ⅛-inch inner heel wedge and a Thomas heel. Strenous physical activity, such as running, long walks, and active sports, should be avoided. When a foot is asymptomatic or when pain is minimal, a longitudinal arch support is the only necessary treatment. Keeping the child from bearing weight on the foot has no effect on the course of the disease.

In Köhler's disease, the prognosis is very good. The navicular reconstitutes itself in a minimum of six months, but usually between one and one half and three years. Waugh reports normal naviculars in 12 patients who have been followed for ten years or more. Most affected navicular bones become normal before the foot has completed its growth, and there is no residual deformity or disability.

References

1. Axhausen, G.: Die Ätiologie der Köhler'schen Erkrankung der Metatarsalkoptchen. Bruns Beitr. Klin. Chir., 126:451, 1922.
2. Axhausen, G.: Die Köhler'sche Erkrankung der Metatarsophalangealgelenke. Med. Klin., 19:561, 1923.
3. Bader, L.: Patologia e clinica del morbo di Koehler, II. Gorizia, Tipografia Paternelli, 1940.
4. Brailsford, J. F.: Osteochondritis of the adult tarsal navicular. J. Bone Joint Surg., 21:111, 1939.
5. Camerer, J. W.: Zur Ätiologie der Köhlerschen Erkrankung des Os naviculare pedis. Deutsch. Med. Wschr., 61:713, 1935.
6. Froelich, R.: Des apophysites de croissance. Paris Méd., 37:430, 1920.
7. Haboush, E. J.: Bilateral disease of the internal cuneiform bone with an associated disease of the right scaphoid bone (Köhler's). J.A.M.A., 100:41, 1933.
8. Hermodsson, I.: Zur Ätiologie der Köhlerschen Krankheit des Os naviculare tarsi. Acta Radiol., 17:68, 1936.
9. Karp, M.: Köhler's disease of the tarsal scaphoid. J. Bone Joint Surg., 19:84, 1937.
10. Kidner, F. C., and Muro, F.: Köhler's disease of the tarsal scaphoid or os naviculare pedis retardatum. J.A.M.A., 83:1, 650, 1924.
11. Köhler, A.: Über eine haüfige bisher anscheinend unbekannte Erkrankung einzelner kindlicher Knochen. München. Med. Wschr., 55:1923, 1908.
12. Köhler, A.: Eine typische Erkrankung des 2. Metatarsophalangealgelenkes. München. Med. Wschr., 67:1289, 1920.
13. Lecène, P., and Mouchet, A.: La scaphoidite tarsienne. Rev. Orthop., 3:série 11:105, 1928.
14. Lelièvre, J.: Scaphoidite tarsienne de l'enfant (maladie de Koehler-Mouchet). In Pathologie du Pied. 2nd Ed. Paris, Masson & Cie, 1961, pp. 409–410.
15. Martinie-Dubousquet, J.: Scaphoïdite tarsienne (premiére maladie de Köhler). Sem. Hôp. Paris–Ann. Chir., 32:177, 1956.
16. Nagura, S., and Kosuge, S.: Die Entstehung und das Wesen der Köhler'schen Krankheit des Navikulare. Zbl. Chir., 66:1186, 1939.
17. O'Donoghue, A. F., Donohue, E. S., and Zimmerman, W. W.: Bilateral osteochondritis of the tarsal navicular and first cuneiform. J. Bone Joint Surg., 30-A:780, 1948.
18. Scaglietti, O., Stringa, G., and Mizzau, M.: Plus-variant of the astragalus and subnormal scaphoid space, two important findings in Koehler's scaphoid necrosis. Acta Orthop. Scand., 32:500, 1962.
19. Schultze, E. O. P.: Das Alb. Köhlersche Knochenbild des Os naviculare pedis bei Kindern. Arch. Klin. Chir., 100:431, 1913.
20. Smets, W.: La maladie de Köhler du scaphoïde tarsien. J. Chir. (Brux.), 33:389, 1936.
21. Speed, K.: Köhler's disease of the tarsal scaphoid bone. Trans. Amer. Surg. Assoc., 45:179, 1927.
22. Wagner, A.: Isolated aseptic necrosis in the epiphysis of the first metatarsal bone. Acta Radiol., 11:80, 1930.
23. Waugh, W.: The ossification and vascularization of the tarsal navicular and their relation to Köhler's disease. J. Bone Joint Surg., 40-B:765, 1958.
24. Zeitlin, A.: Some reflections on the etiology of Köhler's disease. Radiology, 24:360, 1935.

FREIBERG'S INFRACTION

Freiberg, in 1914, described a form of anterior metatarsalgia in which the second metatarsal head has a "crushed in" appearance, terming the condition *infraction of the second metatarsal bone*.[10] In the European literature, this entity is also known as Köhler's No. 2 disease, distinguishing it from Köhler's No. 1 disease of the tarsal navicular. Priority should be given to Freiberg, however, as he was the first to report the condition.

The disease is seen in adolescents, usually after 13 years of age. It is more prevalent in the female, with about 75 per cent of the cases occurring in girls. Though the second metatarsal head is the most common site of involvement, other metatarsals may be affected. It may be bilateral.

The exact cause of the condition is not definitely known. It is generally regarded as caused by vascular insufficiency and re-

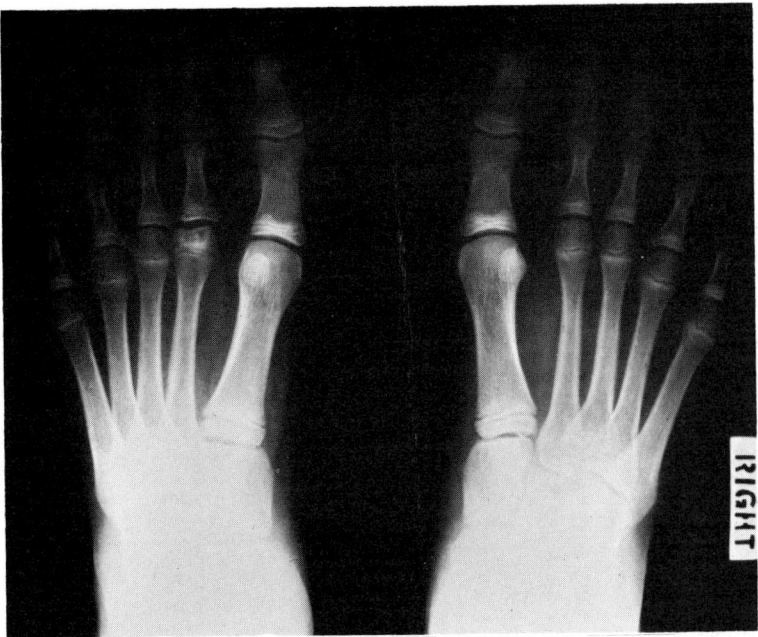

FIGURE 6–9. *Freiberg's infraction of the second metatarsal of the left foot.*
Note the flattening and irregularity of the epiphyses.

lated to aseptic necrosis of other bones. Histologic examination of the affected metatarsal heads has shown areas of necrosis.[1] Smillie thought the process to be traumatic in nature, postulating stress rather than a single injury.[25] Braddock, in his experimental studies of the strength of the second metatarsal and proximal phalanx in various age groups, found that the second metatarsal epiphysis was vulnerable; he believed Freiberg's infraction to be caused by a fracture somewhat modified by its proximity to the epiphyseal plate and articular cartilage.[3]

Clinical manifestations consist of pain under the second or any other affected metatarsal head, local swelling, and limitation of motion of the metatarsophalangeal joint. Roentgenograms of the metatarsal head demonstrate flattening and irregularity (Fig. 6–9).

Treatment is conservative in the adolescent. In the acute painful stage, the foot is protected in a below-knee walking cast until the symptoms subside, usually in three to four weeks. Then the pressure from the metatarsal head is relieved with a metatarsal pad. In adult life, if symptoms occur and persist, surgical measures consisting of resection of the head with a portion of the adjacent shaft are often indicated. To prevent recession of the corresponding toe, it is surgically syndactylized with its adjacent normal toe (Fig. 6–10).[15] The silicone elastomer (Silastic) implant prosthesis to replace the head of the metatarsal after resection is not recommended by this author.

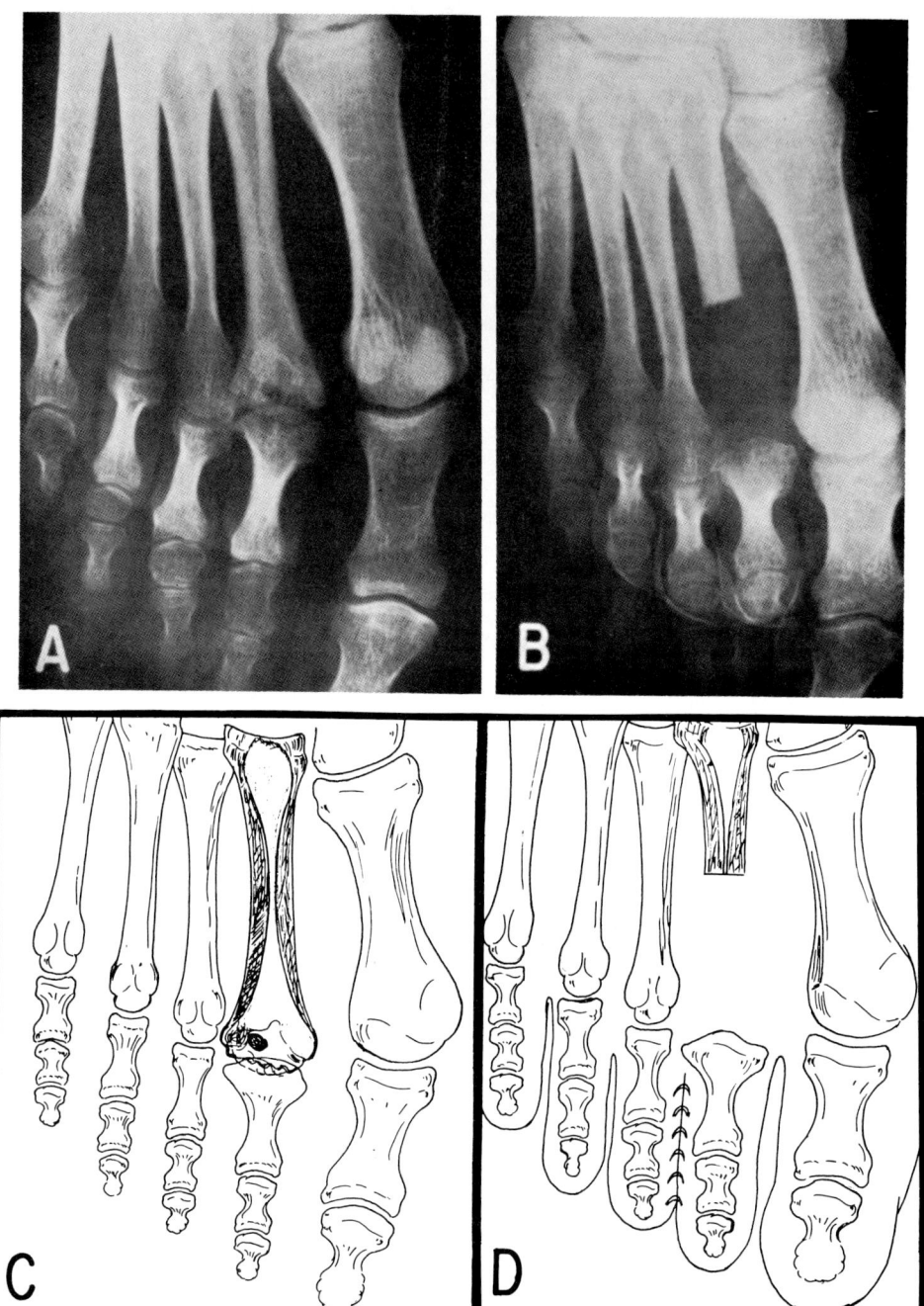

FIGURE 6–10. Freiberg's infraction of the second metatarsal.

A. Preoperative roentgenogram of the foot. **B.** Postoperative roentgenogram of the foot. A resection of the flattened head and distal shaft was performed, and the second toe was syndactylized to the third toe. **C** and **D.** Line drawings of the roentgenograms. (From Kelikian, H.: Hallux Valgus, Allied Deformities of the Forefoot and Metatarsalgia. Philadelphia, W. B. Saunders Co., 1965, p. 377. Reprinted by permission.)

References

1. Axhausen, G.: Die Koehlersche Erkrankung der Metatarsophalangealgelenke. Med. Klin. Wschr., 48:318, 1922.
2. Bordelon, R. L.: Silicone implant for Freiberg's disease. Southern Med. J., 70:1002, 1977.
3. Braddock, G. T. F.: Experimental epiphysial injury and Freiberg's disease. J. Bone Joint Surg., 41:154, 1959.
4. Brandes, M., and Ruschenburg, E.: Eine operative Behandlung der (II.) Köhlerschen Krankheit und Köpfchen des Os metatarsale. Z. Orthop., 69:353, 1939.
5. Cristallo, V.: Riparazione chirurgica della osteocondrosi di Freiberg Köhler. Minerva Ortop., 17:684, 1966.
6. Derivaux, J.: L'importance de l'ostéonécrose dans la maladie de Köhler II. Ann. Anat. Path., 17:394, 1947.
7. Dini, P.: Localizzazioni rare dell' osteocondrite del metatarsi. Arch. Putti, 15:280, 1961.
8. Doub, H. P.: Aseptic necrosis of the epiphyses and short bones: roentgen studies. J.A.M.A., 127:311, 1945.
9. Fasiani, G. M.: Contributo allo studio della malattia di Köhler del secondo metataseo. Arch. Ital. Chir., 13:741, 1925.
10. Freiberg, A. H.: Infraction of the second metatarsal bone; a typical injury. Surg. Gynec. Obstet., 19:191, 1914.
11. Freiberg, A. H.: The so-called infraction of the second metatarsal bone. J. Bone Joint Surg., 8:257, 1926.
12. Gauthier, G.: Maladie de Freiberg ou deuxiéme maladie de Koehler. Proposition d'un traitement de reconstitution au state evolué de l'affection (34 cas traités). Rev. Chir. Orthop., 60:Suppl.:337, 1974.
13. Hoskinson, J.: Freiberg's disease: A review of the long-term results. Proc. Roy. Soc. Med., 67:106, 1974.
14. Jewett, E. L.: A case of Freiberg's disease treated by a walking cast. J. Bone Joint Surg., 21:778, 1939.
15. Kelikian, H.: Hallux Valgus, Allied Deformities of the Forefoot and Metatarsalgia. Philadelphia, W. B. Saunders Co., 1965, p. 372.
16. Köhler, A.: Eine typische Ekraukung des 2. Metatarsophalageagelenkes. München. Med. Wschr., 67:1289, 1920; Typical disease of the second metatarsophalangeal joint. Amer. J. Roentgen., 10:705, 1923.
17. Konig, E., and Rauch, H.: Zur Histologie und Ätiologie der Köhler'schen Metatarsalerkrankung. Arch. Klin. Chir., 128:369, 1924.
18. Lelièvre, J.: Epiphysite des têtes métatarsiennes (maladie de Freiberg). In Pathologie du Pied. 2nd Ed. Paris, Masson & Cie, 1961, pp. 411–413.
19. Lewin, P.: Juvenile deforming metatarsophalangeal osteochondritis. J.A.M.A., 81:189, 1923.
20. Margo, M. K.: Surgical treatment of conditions of the fore part of the foot. J. Bone Joint Surg., 49-A:1667, 1967.
21. Moutier, G.: L'épiphysite métatarsienne. Rev. Orthop., 12:235, 1925.
22. Painter, C. F.: Infraction of the second metatarsal head. Boston Med. Surg. J., 184:533, 1921.
23. Panner, H. J.: A peculiar characteristic metatarsal disease. Acta Radiol., 1:319, 1921–1922.
24. Skillern, P. G., Jr.: Eggshell fracture of head of metatarsal. Ann. Surg., 61:371, 1915.
25. Smillie, I. S.: Freiberg's infarction (Koehler's second disease). J. Bone Joint Surg., 37:580, 1955.
26. Swanson, A. B.: Flexible Implant Resection Arthroplasty in the Hand and Extremities. St. Louis, C. V. Mosby Co., 1973, pp. 1–32; 296–305.
27. Wagner, A.: Isolated aseptic necrosis in the epiphysis of the first metatarsal bone. Acta Radiol., 11:80, 1930.

MISCELLANEOUS OSTEOCHONDROSES

Other rare sites in which osteochondrosis may occur include:
Distal tibial epiphysis.[10, 20]
Medial cuneiform.[1–3, 5, 9, 11]
Intermediate cuneiform.[12, 17]
Proximal epiphysis of first metatarsal.[7]
Epiphysis of fifth metatarsal.[8, 14–16, 22, 23]
First metatarsal sesamoid.[13, 18]
Epiphyses of phalanges.[19, 21, 24]

References

1. Barclay, M.: A case of duplication of the internal cuneiform bone of the foot. J. Anat., 67:175, 1932.
2. Barlow, T. E.: Os cuneiforme I bipartitum. Amer. J. Physic. Anthrop., 29:95, 1942.
3. Böker, H., and Müller, W.: Das Os cuneiforme I bipartitum, eine fortschreitende Umkonstruktion des Quergewölbes im menschlichen Fuss. Anat. Anz., 83:193, 1936.
4. Brown, I. D., and Shaw, D. G.: Multiple osteochondroses of the feet in West Indian family. J. Bone Joint Surg., 55-B:864, 1973.
5. Buchman, J.: Osteochondritis of the internal cuneiform. J. Bone Joint Surg., 15:225, 1933.
6. Burman, M. S.: Epiphysitis of the proximal or pseudometatarsal epiphyses of the foot. J. Bone Joint Surg., 15:538, 1933.
7. Burman, M. S., and Pomeranz, M.: Epiphysitis of the proximal epiphysis of the first metatarsal and of the first phalanx of the big toe; coincidental presence of proximal or pseudometatarsal epiphysis. J. Bone Joint Surg., 14:177, 1932.
8. De Cuveland, E.: Die Apophyse des Metatarsale V und Os vesalianum. Fortschr. Röntgenstr., 82:251, 1955.
9. Haboush, E. J.: Bilateral disease of the internal cuneiform bone with an associated disease of the right scaphoid bone (Köhler's). J.A.M.A., 100:41, 1933.
10. Hassler, W. L., Heyman, C. H., and Bennett, G. W.: Osteochondrosis of the distal tibial epiphysis: A report of two cases. J. Bone Joint Surg., 42-A:1261, 1960.
11. Heidsieck, E.: Os cuneiforme I bipartitum. Röntgenpraxis, 8:712, 1936.
12. Hicks, B. T. G.: Osteochondritis of the tarsal second cuneiform bone. Brit. J. Radiol., 26:214, 1953.
13. Ilfeld, F. W., and Rosen, V.: Osteochondritis of the first metatarsal sesamoid. Clin. Orthop., 85:38, 1972.
14. Iselin, H.: Die Wenzel-Brubersche fibulare Epiphyse der Tuberositas metatarsi quinti im Roentgenbild. Deutsch. Z. Chir., 92:561, 1910.
15. Iselin, H.: Wachstumsbeschwerden zur Zeit der knoechernen Entwicklung der Tuberositas metatarsi quinti. Deutsch. Z. Chir., 118:529, 1912.
16. Kirschner, A.: Die Epiphyse am proximalen Ende des Os metatarsi V, aus den anatomischen Heften. Arch. Klin. Chir., 80:719, 1908.
17. Meilstrup, D. B.: Osteochondritis of the internal cuneiforms. Amer. J. Roentgen., 58:329, 1947.
18. Renander, A.: Two cases of typical osteochondropathy of the medial sesamoid bone of the first metatarsal. Acta Radiol., 3:521, 1924.
19. Shaw, E. W.: Avascular necrosis of the phalanges of the hands (Thiemann's disease). J.A.M.A., 156:711, 1954.
20. Siffert, R. S., and Arkin, A. M.: Post-traumatic aseptic necrosis of the distal tibial epiphysis. J. Bone Joint Surg., 32-A:691, 1950.
21. Staples, O. S.: Osteochondritis of the epiphyses of the terminal phalanx of the fingers. J. Bone Joint Surg., 25:917, 1943.
22. Steller, K.: Epiphyseonekrosen des Kopfchens von Metatarsale V. Röntgenpraxis, 15:156, 1943.
23. Tessore, A., Carly, M., and Tos, L.: Epiphysitis of the bases of the 5th metatarsus (Iselin's disease). Arch. Putti Chir. Organi Mov., 26:235, 1971.
24. Thieman, H.: Juvenile Epiphysenstorungen. Fortschr. Röntgenstr., 14:79, 1909.

OSTEOCHONDRITIS DISSECANS

Osteochondritis dissecans is a condition in which a segment of articular cartilage with its underlying subchondral bone gradually separates from the surrounding osteocartilaginous tissue. The separation of the fragment may be partial or complete; in the latter case, it becomes detached and lodges in the contiguous joint as a loose body. The term *dissecans* is derived from the prefix *dis*, meaning "from," and *secare*, "to cut out." It is important to differentiate the word *dissecans* from *dessicans*, the latter being derived from *dessicare*, "to dry up."

The disease was first described in 1870 by Sir James Paget, who called it "quiet necrosis."[48] The name *osteochondritis dissecans* was given, in 1887, by König, who believed that necrosis of part of the articular bone surface was caused by trauma and that this was followed by "dissecting inflammation," which eventually caused the fragment to separate.[32]

Osteochondritis dissecans has been described as a disease of the young adult. Green and Banks, in 1953, pointed out that it is not uncommon in children. It has not been reported as occurring under the age of four years. Males are affected three to four times as often as females.[23]

The knee joint is most commonly affected, although other joints, such as the elbow, ankle, and hip, may also be involved. Characteristically, there is a particular site on the articular surface of each joint that is affected, examples being the lateral surface of the medial femoral condyle in the knee, the capitellum in the elbow, the superior surface of the talus in the ankle, and the superior area of the capital femoral epiphysis in the hip.

Etiology

The exact cause of osteochondritis dissecans remains a matter of conjecture; no theory is fully accepted. Heredity, constitutional predisposition, trauma, and ischemia are etiologic factors to be considered.

Heredity and Constitutional Predisposition. There are many examples of familial incidence mentioned in the literature.[50] Wagoner and Cohn described osteochondritis dissecans of the knee in a boy, his father, a paternal uncle, and his two brothers.[74] Stougaard, in 1964, reported a family in which ten members of the second and third generations were involved.[69] Neilson, in a survey of osteochondritis dissecans of the humeral capitellum, found the incidence to be 4.1 per cent of 1,000 men who were otherwise normal; the incidence in male relatives of affected men, however, was 14.6 per cent.[41] Petrie reported a family study in which 34 patients with osteochondritis dissecans and 86 of their first-degree relatives were examined clinically and radiologically. Only one relative was found to have osteochondritis dissecans. Association with other forms of osteochondritis, endocrinological abnormalities, and dwarfism could not be demonstrated. Petrie concluded that the common form of osteochondritis dissecans is not familial; this is in contradiction to previous reports that osteochondritis dissecans can appear in a familial form.[50]

Multiple joint involvement in the same patient is not uncommon, indicating a constitutional factor in its etiology.[74] White reported multiple osteochondritis dissecans in association with dwarfism in three patients, suggesting an underlying endocrine imbalance as a possible factor in its pathogenesis.[75]

Trauma. Injury plays a principal role in the causation of osteochondritis dissecans.[3, 22, 63] In studying the reaction of articular cartilage to mechanical trauma, a number of investigators have been able to produce lesions experimentally that are similar to those of osteochondritis dissecans. Rehbein did so by repeated and forced hyperextension of the knee and by exerting force on the femoral condyles through the patella.[54] Langenskiöld postulated that cartilage fractures in childhood may be the cause of osteochondritis dissecans. He based his conclusions on experimental work in four- to seven-day-old rabbits. A segment of hyaline cartilage from the articular surface of the distal femur was excised but left attached to the bone by a strand of synovial tissue in the intercondylar notch. The cartilaginous fragment was then replaced in its crater. When the rabbits were sacrificed one to four months postoperatively, an osseous nucleus similar to the osteochondral fragment of osteochondritis dissecans was found in most of the cartilage fragments.[33] Tallqvist repeated these experiments and confirmed the findings of Langenskiöld.[70]

Buchner and Rieger, however, in their experiments in cadavers, found that a force of 614 kg. was necessary to fracture an area of the femoral condyle by pressure of the patella against it and that a force of 184 kg. was required to detach a piece of bone at the insertion of the cruciate ligament.[11] In children and adolescents, force of such severity is not very likely.

Fairbank believed that injury from a relatively long tibial spine is the cause of osteochondritis dissecans in its usual location on the medial femoral condyle. His theory was that during medial rotation of the leg, the tibial spine impinges against the medial femoral condyle and causes a fracture through the subchondral bone, with no discontinuity of overlying joint cartilage. Nonunion of the fracture results from continued normal use of the knee, and eventually the fragment with the articular cartilage separates from the rest of the bone.[22] The roentgenographic findings of flattening of the femoral condyle, especially of the lateral one, supports the tibial spine theory, as this would allow a normal tibial spine to impinge upon the medial condyle.

Smillie maintains that likelihood of contact between the tibial spine and the femoral condyle is increased by some additional factors, such as genu recurvatum, instability of the knee (resulting from lesions of the menisci, rupture of the anterior cruciate ligament, or recurrent subluxation of the patella), and decreased joint space due to removal of the meniscus or to osteoarthritis.[62, 63] There are a number of objections to the "tibial spine" theory, as it does not account for the presence of lesions in other joints or at other areas in the knee, and anatomically, it is difficult to visualize repeated impingement of the tibial spine on the intercondylar notch during locomotion.

A direct relationship between injury and the development of osteochondritis dissecans is supported by reports of osteochondral fractures that failed to unite and that progressed to lesions that were roentgenographically and histologically indistinguishable from osteochondritis dissecans. These have been described in the patella, in the lateral femoral condyle, and the talus.[37, 59, 62, 63, 73]

Linden and Telhag performed histologic and autoradiographic studies of the cartilage and bone in osteochondritis dissecans in 14 adults. They demonstrated a fissure at a varying distance from the cartilage surface, which could also be seen in radiographs. From both sides the fissure tended to be filled out with fibrous cartilage, a sign of a reparative process, but blocked by a poor blood supply to the fragment.[36] The limited uptake of tetracycline and strontium-85, demonstrated by Linden and Nilson in 1976, is an indication of a poor blood supply.[35] The articular cartilage of the lesion was normal in all respects, and no thymidine-labeled chondrocytes were found; i.e., there was no DNA synthesis and consequently no cell division. The thickness of the cartilage was normal in all preparations.[36]

Unstable osteochondral fractures fail to unite.[1] The histologic appearance of these ununited fragments is very similar to that of osteochondritis dissecans—i.e., viable hyaline articular cartilage lying over acellular necrotic bone. Linden and Telhag proposed that osteochondritis dissecans in adults represents a form of subchondral fracture with intact articular cartilage. With delay or restriction of the healing process, the mobility of the fragment causes fissures in the cartilage.[36]

Ischemia. It has been proposed that an interruption in the blood supply to an area of subchondral bone is the cause of osteochondritis dissecans and that blockage of vessels may be produced by emboli of bacteria, fat, or clumps of erythrocytes.[2] These embolic ischemic theories are refuted by the findings of Rogers and Gladstone, which show that the blood supply of the lower end of the femur is rich with numerous anastomoses in the cancellous bone and that the subarticular areas of the distal femur are not supplied by end-arteries.[58]

Smillie distinguishes two varieties of osteochondritis dissecans, a juvenile type and an adult type. In the form found in children and adolescents, there is a basic disturbance of epiphyseal development, with small accessory islets of bone being separated from the main osseous nucleus of the epiphyses. Minimal trauma may cause avascular necrosis to these bone islets because their circulation is inadequate. Smillie believes that the adult form is mainly due to trauma.[65]

Osteochondritis dissecans of the talus is uncommon. Berndt and Harty reviewed the literature in 1959 and found 2 cases of loose bodies in the ankle joint, 30 cases of flake fractures, and 151 cases of osteochondritis dissecans (8 with bilateral involvement), giving a total of 191 lesions.[6] Of the publications they examined, only three reported more than four cases; namely, Ray and Couglin—13, DeGinder—19, and Rodèn and associates—55.[19, 53, 57] Since then Bourrel and co-workers have reported 9 cases in 1972; Kerr, 9 cases in 1973; and Scharling, 19 cases in 1978.[8, 31, 60] Males are affected twice as commonly as females.

The site of the lesion is in either the upper medial or the upper lateral angle of the dome of the talus; occasionally it may appear in both medial and lateral angles of the same talus. It is not seen in the middle third of the trochlea. In the 19 cases reported by Scharling the lesion were medial in 13, lateral in 5, and both medial and lateral in 1.[60]

In the literature a definite distinction is

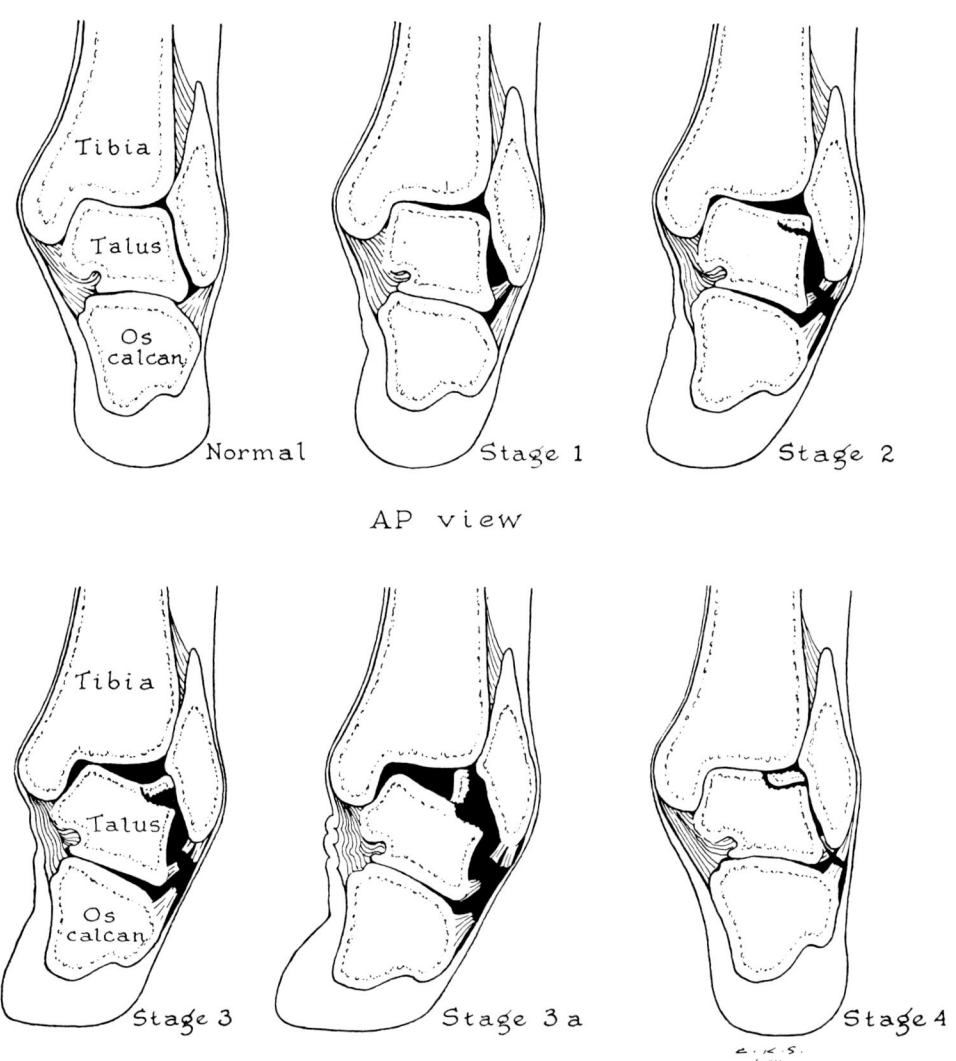

FIGURE 6–11. *Diagram showing mechanism of fracture of lateral border of the dome of the talus (see text).*

(From Berndt, A. L., and Harty, M.: Transchondral fractures (osteochondritis dissecans) of the talus. J. Bone Joint Surg., 41-A:988, 1959. Reprinted by permission.)

made between the lateral and medial lesions. It is generally accepted that lesions of the lateral angle of the talus are of traumatic origin, whereas in the medially localized changes, injury is not a causative factor. Eskesen proposed that osteochondritis dissecans localized to the lateral angle of the dome of the talus is a transchondral fracture.[21] Rasmussen published a report of one case of osteochondritis dissecans localized laterally in the talus that definitely followed an injury.[52] Rodèn and associates, Berndt and Harty, and O'Donoghue support the theory of the traumatic genesis of lateral angle lesions of the talus.[6, 44, 57] The role of injury in the etiology of medial lesions is not clear, however; Myhre does not feel that trauma is a causative factor.[39]

In the series of Scharling, in five of the six cases with changes in the upper lateral angle of the talus, symptoms had started following trauma; the sixth patient had a history of severe injury seven and a half years earlier, but the symptoms had not developed until five years afterward. Of the medially localized lesions, only 5 of 14 had a history of trauma.[60]

Berndt and Harty have studied the mechanism of transchondral fractures of the dome of the talus. In the lateral lesions, as the foot is inverted, the lateral border of the dome of the talus is compressed against the fibula. At first, *stage one*, the fibular collateral ligament is intact. Further inversion of the foot ruptures the lateral ligament and causes avulsion of the chip. In *stage two*, the fragment is completely detached and may remain in place or may be displaced by inversion (Fig. 6–11). Transchondral fracture of the medial border of the talar dome occurs when, with the foot in plantar flexion and inversion, lateral rotation of the tibia exerts compression on a small area of the medial upper border of the dome of the talus. In stage one the collateral ligaments remain intact. Greater force pushes the posteroinferior lip of the tibia so that it rides medially across the superiorly turned margin of the talus, gouging out an osteochondral chip. In *stage two* the fragment is partially detached; in *stage three* it is completely detached, and in *stage four* it is displaced within the joint (Fig. 6–12).[6]

Clinical Picture

The usual complaint is pain in the ankle joint on weight-bearing; the pain is usually intermittent and aggravated by strenuous physical activity such as running and sports. Antalgic limp is frequent. There may be episodes of "locking" in the ankle joint or a sensation of "missing" a step. At times, the condition is asymptomatic.

Physical findings depend upon the stage in the course of the disease and whether or not the fragment has become detached. The important finding is localized tenderness over the lesional area, detected by markedly plantar-flexing the ankle joint and palpating the medial and lateral corners of the dome of the talus. Pressure can be exerted on the dome of the talus by rotating the leg inward and outward while the foot remains on the floor in plantar flexion and inversion, then in dorsiflexion and eversion. When the fragment is displaced in the joint there will be effusion and synovial thickening of the ankle, clicking, and restriction of range of motion. Atrophy of the calf is common.

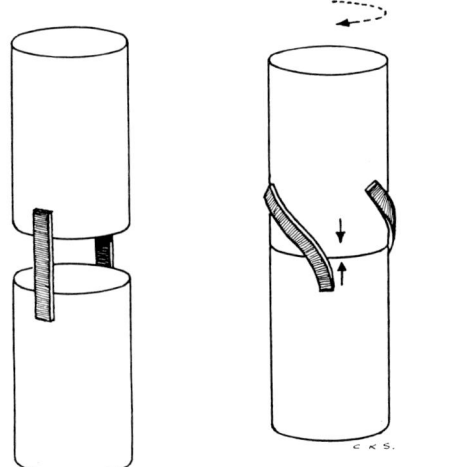

FIGURE 6–12. Diagram showing mechanism of transchondral fracture of the medial border of the dome of the talus (see text).

(From Berndt, A. L., and Harty, M.: Transchondral fractures (osteochondritis dissecans) of the talus. J. Bone Joint Surg., *41-A*:988, 1959. Reprinted by permission.)

Roentgenographic Findings

The roentgenographic picture is diagnostic. A fragment of subchondral bone is de-

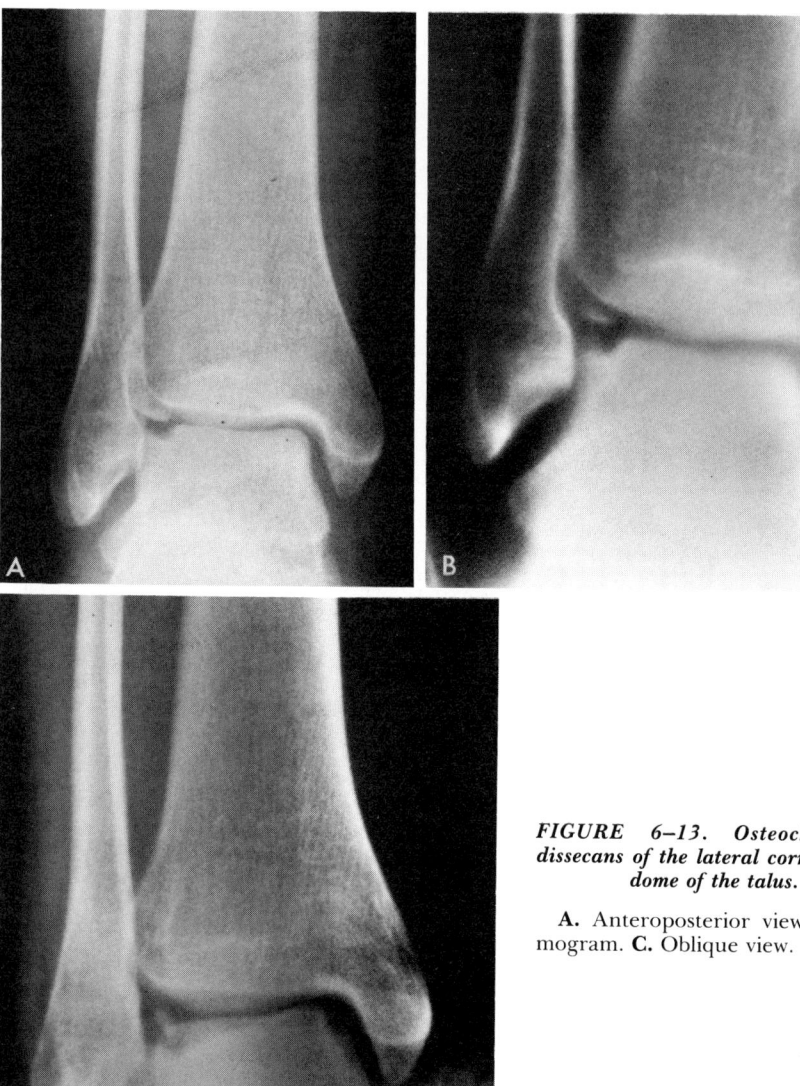

FIGURE 6–13. *Osteochondritis dissecans of the lateral corner of the dome of the talus.*

A. Anteroposterior view. **B.** Tomogram. **C.** Oblique view.

marcated by a radiolucent saucer-shaped line (Figs. 6–13 and 6–14). The lesional bone may appear denser than the surrounding parent bone. As the fragment separates from the dome, the continuity of subchondral bone is distorted, and a "crater" or depression is seen at the site from which it came. The detached loose body in the joint, which receives nutrition from the synovial fluid, will continue to grow.

Special views may be necessary to visualize the lesion. Oblique-lateral views of the ankle are essential. In some cases additional information can be obtained by lateral and anteroposterior tomography.

Treatment

In children, treatment is usually conservative unless the fragment has become detached. Osteochondritic lesions in children will heal without surgical intervention, provided the joint is protected from the stresses of weight-bearing.[23, 72, 76]

To do this, when the affected joint is the ankle, the author uses a below-knee cast or patellar tendon–bearing orthosis for two to three months. Then weight-bearing is gradually resumed over the ensuing three months. Healing will be apparent in the roentgenogram in about one year; it is not,

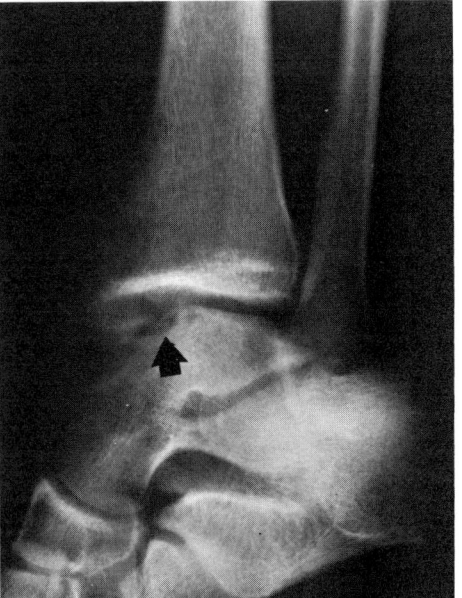

FIGURE 6–14. Osteochondritis dissecans of the medial corner of the dome of the talus.

however, necessary to use the orthosis that long. Absence of local tenderness on palpation is an important guideline.

When the diagnosis is made late, and the bone fragment has become partially detached and produces symptoms, conservative management for a period of three to four months is indicated. If there is no roentgenographic and clinical evidence of improvement, or if the fragment becomes completely detached, surgical measures should be taken. The lesion is not likely to heal after the age of 16 to 18 years.[76]

The type of operation depends upon the anatomic site affected and the size of the lesion. The author prefers simple excision of the partially detached fragment, and trimming and smoothing of the irregular crater bed with a sharp scalpel. The technique of surgical exposure of the lateral and medial angles of the dome of the talus is described and illustrated in Plate 31.

Bennett and Bauer have shown experimentally that such defects of the articular surface will heal. When articular cartilage and subchondral bone were removed from the articular surface of the distal femur in young adult dogs, the defect filled in with bone and a surface layer of fibrocartilage. This fibrocartilage and bone seemed to have developed from the vascular fibrous tissue that arose from the connective tissue of the marrow spaces of subchondral bone.[4]

Smillie advocates restoration of the articular surface by causing the osteochondritic fragment to unite with the underlying live cancellous bone. If the fragment is only partially detached, he recommends simple drilling of the lesional area; and if complete separation has occurred, he replaces the fragment in its bed. Added bone is placed underneath and the crater is drilled, if necessary. The fragment is held securely in place by Kirschner wire fixation. The Smillie procedure may be considered when the area affected is very extensive and involves a weight-bearing area of a knee or a hip.[62, 63]

The objection to the Smillie method is that it is technically difficult to reposition the displaced fragment perfectly so that it is flush with the rest of the articular surface. If the fragment is placed too deeply, a defect in the articular surface will still persist, whereas if the fragment projects, it creates an irregularity and incongruity of the joint, damaging a normal articular area of the coresponding opposing bone. This technique also requires a second operation for removal of the pins.

Arthroscopy of the ankle, which allows direct visualization of the lesion, has opened new vistas in the management of osteochondritis dissecans. One can resect and curet the osteochondritic lesion, shave the articular cartilage, and remove loose bodies if necessary.[12a, 29a, 48a]

Exposure of the Angles of the Dome of the Talus for Excision of Osteochondritis Dissecans

LATERAL PART OF THE DOME OF THE TALUS

A. A curvilinear incision is made in front of the ankle, beginning at its medial margin and extending laterally; in front of the fibula it descends distally for a distance of 5 cm. The subcutaneous tissue and deep fascia are divided in line with the skin incision. The wound margins are elevated and retracted.

B. The long extensors are retracted medially and the peroneal tendons laterally. The capsule of the ankle joint is divided by a transverse incision.

C. Next, the talofibular ligament is identified and sectioned near its attachment to the talus. The ligament is tagged with a 00 Mersilene whip suture for later attachment.   **D.** The hindfoot is inverted and plantar-flexed, exposing the lateral half of the dome of the talus. It is not necessary to osteotomize the distal fibula to expose the lateral compartment of the ankle joint. After excision of the osteochondritic fragment and drilling of its base, the talofibular ligament is repaired. The wound is closed, and a below-knee cast is applied for six weeks.

Plate 31. Exposure of the Angles of the Dome of the Talus for Excision of Osteochondritis Dissecans.

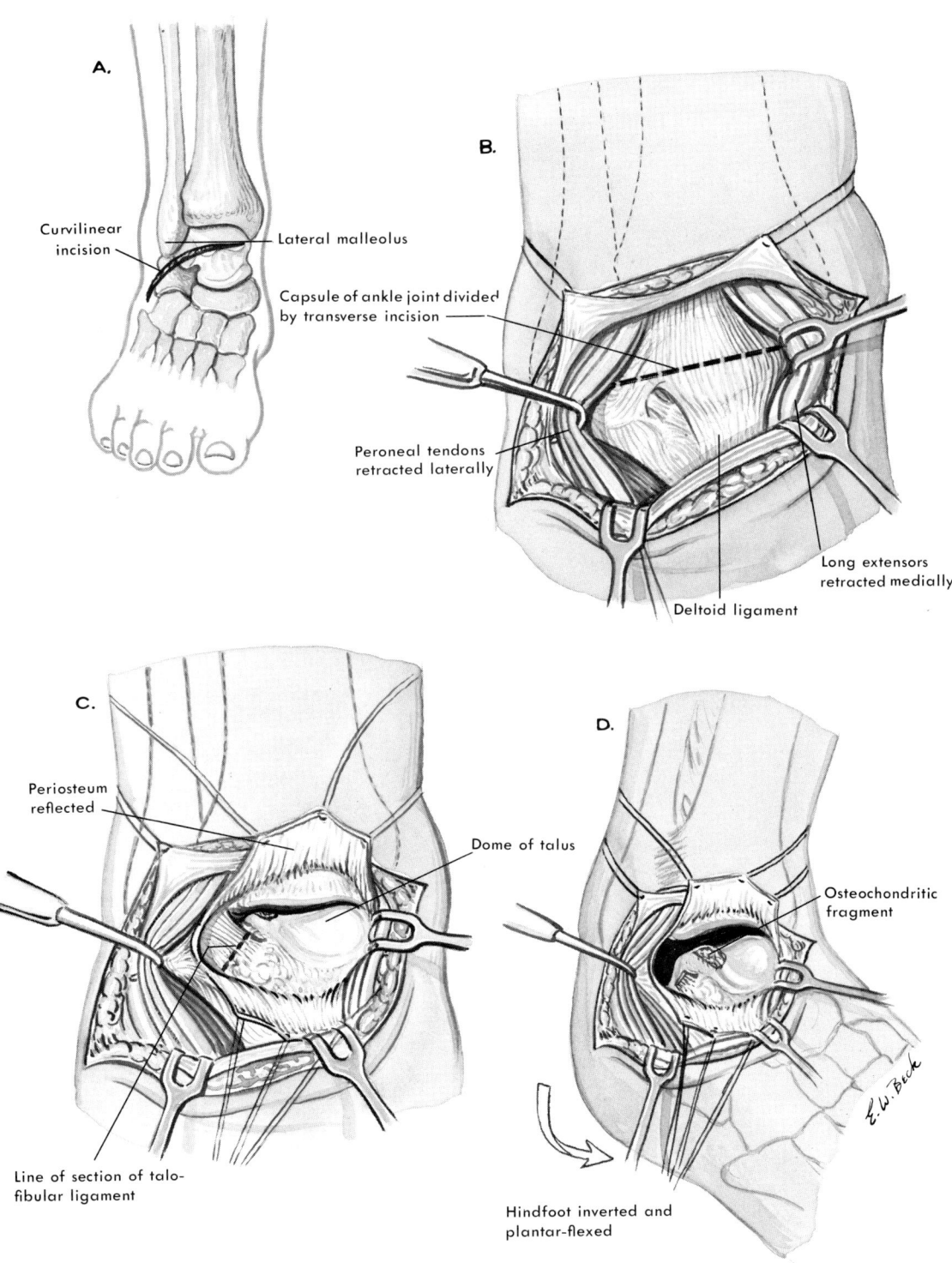

Exposure of the Angles of the Dome of the Talus for Excision of Osteochondritis Dissecans *(Continued)*

MEDIAL CORNER OF THE DOME OF THE TALUS

To expose the medial corner of the dome of the talus an osteotomy of the medial malleolus is required.

E. A medial incision about 7 to 9 cm. long is made centered over the medial malleolus. The subcutaneous tissue and deep fascia are divided in line with the skin incision.

F. The level of the ankle joint and the tip of the medial malleolus are identified. If the *distal tibial physis* is still open it should *not* be *injured*. The capsule of the ankle joint is opened by a transverse incision. The line of osteotomy of the medial malleolus is in line with the ankle joint.

G. The distal part of the medial malleolus is exposed subperiosteally. If the distal physis of the tibia is open, a transverse incision is made; if closed, a longitudinal incision.

H. Then a transverse osteotomy of the medial malleolus is performed at the level of the ankle joint. By rotating the medial malleolus downward 90 degrees and forcefully abducting the foot, the ankle joint and superior surface of the talus are visualized.

I. After excision of the osteochondritic fragment the medial malleolus is anatomically reduced and internally fixed with two or three *smooth* pins when the distal tibial physis is open, or with a single metal screw in the skeletally mature ankle. The capsule of the ankle joint and the wound are closed. A below-knee cast is applied for six weeks. The healing of the osteotomized malleolus is not a problem.

Plate 31. Exposure of the Angles of the Dome of the Talus for Excision of Osteochondritis Dissecans.

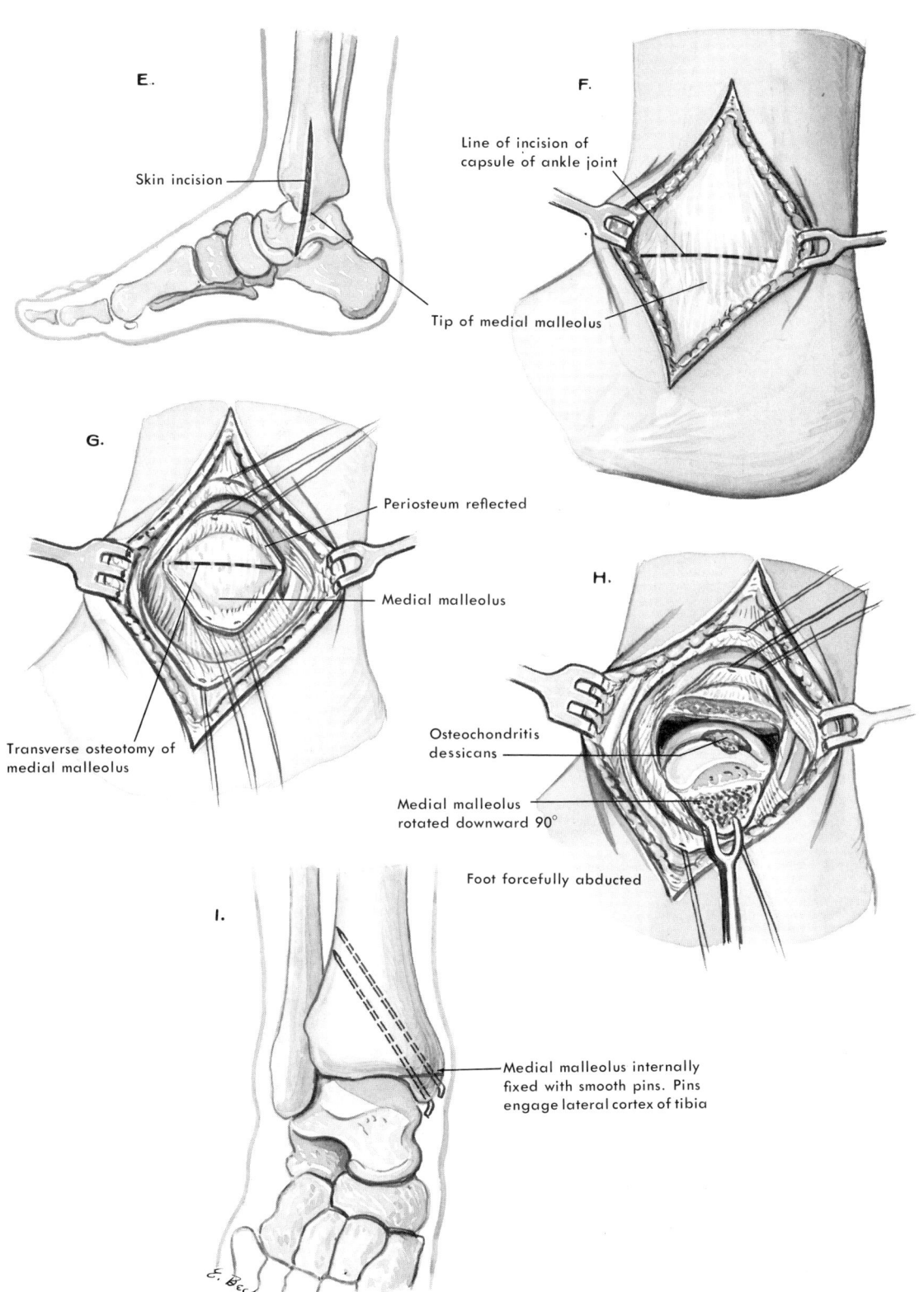

References (Osteochondritis Dissecans)

1. Aichroth, P.: Osteochondral fractures and their relationship to osteochondritis dissecans of the knee. J. Bone Joint Surg., 53-B:448, 1971.
2. Axhausen, G.: Die Ätiologie der Köhler'schen Erkrankung der Metatarsalköpfchen. Bruns Beitr. Klin. Chir., 126:451, 1922.
3. Bandi, W.: Über die Ätiologie der Osteochondritis dissecans. Helv. Chir. Acta, 18:221, 1954.
4. Bennett, G. A., and Bauer, W.: A study of the repair of articular cartilage and the reaction of normal joints of adult dogs to surgically created defects of articular cartilage, "joint mice," and patellar displacement. Amer. J. Path., 8:499, 1932.
5. Bernau, A.: Spätformen der Osteochondrosis dissecans. Z. Orthop., 115:468, 1977.
6. Berndt, A. L., and Harty, M.: Transchondral fractures (osteochondritis dissecans) of the talus. J. Bone Joint Surg., 41-A:988, 1959.
7. Besson, J., and Wellinger, C.: L'ostéochondrite de l'astragale. A propos de 12 observations. Rev. Rhum., 34:552, 1967.
8. Bourrel, P., Maistre, B., Palinacci, J. C., Gourul, J. C., and Jardin, M.: Ostéochondrite de l'astragale. A propos de 9 observations. Rev. Chir. Orthop., 58:609, 1972.
9. Breitlander: Osteochondritis dissecans tali. Arch. Klin. Chir., 148:149, 1927.
10. Brickey, P. A., and Grow, J. B.: Osteochondritis dissecans. Report of cases involving elbow, ankle and metatarsophalangeal joints. Amer. J. Surg., 48:463, 1940.
11. Buchner, L., and Rieger, H.: Konnen freie Gelenkkorper durch Trauma entstehen. Arch. Klin. Chir., 116:460, 1921.
12. Calandruccio, R. A., and Gilmer, W. S., Jr.: Proliferation, regeneration, and repair of articular cartilage of immature animals. J. Bone Joint Surg., 4-A:431, 1962.
12a. Chen, Y-C.: Clinical and cadaver studies on the ankle joint arthroscopy. J. Jap. Orthop. Assoc., 50:631, 1976.
13. Chiroff, R. T., and Cooke, C. P.: Osteochondritis dissecans: A histologic and microradiographic analysis of surgically excised lesions. J. Trauma, 15:689, 1975.
14. Cobey, M. C.: Osteochondritis dissecans of the astragalus (following ankle sprains). Milit. Surg., 93:184, 1943.
15. Convery, F. R., Akeson, W. H., and Keown, G. H.: The repair of large osteochondral defects. An experimental study in horses. Clin. Orthop., 82:253, 1972.
16. Crane, A. R., and Scasano, J. J.: Synovial cysts (ganglia) of bone. J. Bone Joint Surg., 49-A:355, 1967.
17. Dashefsky, J. H.: Post-traumatic subarticular cyst of bone. J. Bone Joint Surg., 58-A:154, 1971.
18. Davis, M. W.: Bilateral talar osteochondritis dissecans with lax ankle ligaments. J. Bone Joint Surg., 52-A:168, 1970.
19. DeGinder, W. L.: Osteochondritis dissecans of the talus. Radiology, 65:590, 1955.
20. Devas, M.: Stress avulsions and osteochondritis. In Stress Fractures. Edinburgh, London, and New York, Churchill Livingstone, 1975, pp. 190–211.
20a. Drez, D., Guhl, J. F., and Gollehon, D. L.: Ankle arthroscopy: Technique and indications. Foot Ankle, 2:138, 1981.
21. Eskesen, B.: En sjaelden intraarticulaer talus-fractur. Nord. Med., 16:3436, 1942.
22. Fairbank, H. A. T.: Osteo-chondritis dissecans. Brit. J. Surg., 21:67, 1933.
23. Green, W. T., and Banks, H. H.: Osteochondritis dissecans in children. J. Bone Joint Surg., 35-A:26, 1953.
24. Guilleminet, M., and Barbier, J. M.: Osteochondritis dissecans of the hip. J. Bone Joint Surg., 39-B:268, 1957.
25. Hanley, W. B., McKusick, V. A., and Barranco, F. T.: Osteochondritis dissecans with associated malformations in two brothers. A review of familial aspects. J. Bone Joint Surg., 49-A:925, 1967.
26. Harbin, M., and Zollinger, R.: Osteochondritis of the growth centres. Surg. Gynec. Obstet., 51:145, 1930.
27. Harms: Osteochondritis dissecans at the trochlea tali? Zbl. Chir., 54:1017, 1927.
28. Hay, B. M.: Two cases of osteochondritis dissecans affecting several joints. J. Bone Joint Surg., 32-B:361, 1950.
29. Hutchinson, R. G.: Osteochondritis dissecans: Records of some unusual cases. Brit. J. Radiol., 16:147, 1943.
29a. Johnson, L. L.: Diagnostic and Surgical Arthroscopy. 2nd Ed. St. Louis, The C. V. Mosby Co., 1981, pp. 412–419.
30. Kappis, M.: Weitese Beitrage zur traumatisch-mechanischen Entstehung der "spontanen" Knospelablosungen. Deutsch. Z. Chir., 171:13, 1922.
31. Kerr, T. S.: Osteochondritis dissecans of the talus. Proc. Roy. Soc. Med., Section of Orthopedics, 66:517, 1973.
32. König, F.: Über freie Korper in den Gelenken. Deutsch. Z. Chir., 27:90, 1887.
33. Langenskiöld, A.: Can osteochondritis dissecans arise as a sequel of cartilage fracture in early childhood? Acta Chir. Scand., 109:206, 1955.
34. Linden, C. B.: Longterm follow-up of osteochondritis dissecans in the femur condyles. In Osteochondritis dissecans. Dissertation, University of Lund, 1976.
35. Linden, C. B., and Nilsson, B. E.: Strontium-85 uptake in knee joints with osteochondritis dissecans. Acta Orthop. Scand., 47:668, 1976.
36. Linden, C. B., and Telhag, H.: Osteochondritis dissecans: A histologic and autoradiographic study in man. Acta Orthop. Scand., 18:682, 1977.
37. Marks, K. L.: Flake fracture of the talus progressing to osteochondritis dissecans. J. Bone Joint Surg., 34-B:90, 1952.
38. Mensor, M. C., and Melody, G. F.: Osteochondritis dissecans of the ankle joint. The use of tomography as a diagnostic aid. J. Bone Joint Surg., 23:903, 1941.
39. Myhre, H.: On osteochondritis dissecans trochleae tali. Acta Radiol., 20:272, 1939.
40. Nagura, H.: The so-called osteochondritis dissecans of König. Clin. Orthop., 18:100, 1960.
41. Neilson, N. A.: Osteochondritis dissecans capituli humeri. Acta Orthop. Scand., 4:307, 1933.
42. Novotny, H.: Preventive and conservative treatment of osteochondritis dissecans. Acta Orthop. Scand., 21:40, 1951.
43. Novotny, H.: Osteochondritis in two brothers. The pre- and developed state. Acta Radiol., 37:493, 1952.
44. O'Donoghue, D. H.: Chondral and osteochondral fractures. J. Trauma, 6:469, 1966.
45. Ogden, J. A., and Griswold, D. M.: Solitary cyst of the talus. J. Bone Joint Surg., 54-A:1309, 1972.
46. Paaby, H.: Solitary cysts of the talus. Acta Orthop. Scand., 44:560, 1973.
47. Paatsama, S., Rokkanen, P., and Jussila, J.: Etiological factors in osteochondritis dissecans. Acta Orthop. Scand., 46:906, 1975.
48. Paget, J.: On the production of some of the loose bodies in joints. St. Bart. Hosp. Res., 6:1, 1870.
48a. Parisien, J. S., and Shereff, M. J.: The role of arthroscopy in the diagnosis and treatment of disorders of the ankle. Foot Ankle, 2:144, 1981.
49. Pavlansky, R.: Treatment of osteochondritis dissecans by use of a cortical bone graft. Rev. Chir. Orthop., 59:681, 1973.
50. Petrie, P. W. R.: Etiology of osteochondritis dissecans. Failure to establish a familial background. J. Bone Joint Surg., 59-B:366, 1977.
51. Pick, M. P.: Familial osteochondritis dissecans. J. Bone Joint Surg., 37-B:142, 1955.
52. Rasmussen, K. B.: Osteochondritis dissecans—et bidrag til sporgsmalet om aetiologien. Nord. Med., 28:2088, 1945.
53. Ray, R. B., and Coughlin, E. J., Jr.: Osteochondritis dissecans of the talus. J. Bone Joint Surg., 29:697, 1947.
54. Rehbein, F.: Die Entstehung der Osteochondritis dissecans. Arch. Klin. Chir., 265:69, 1950.
55. Ribbing, S.: Zur Ätiologie der Osteochondritis dissecans. Acta Radiol. (Stockholm), 25:Suppl.:732, 1944.
56. Ribbing, S.: The hereditary multiple epiphyseal disturbance and its consequences for the aetiogenesis of local malacias—particularly osteochondrosis dissecans. Acta Orthop. Scand., 24:286, 1955.
57. Rodèn, S., Tillegard, P., and Unander-Scharin, L.: Osteochondritis dissecans and similar lesions of the talus. Acta Orthop. Scand., 23:51, 1953.
58. Rogers, W. M., and Gladstone, H.: Vascular foramina and arterial supply of the distal end of the femur. J. Bone Joint Surg., 32-A:867, 1950.
59. Rosenberg, N. J.: Osteochondral fractures of the lateral femoral condyle. J. Bone Joint Surg., 46-A:1013, 1964.
60. Scharling, M.: Osteochondritis dissecans of the talus. Acta Orthop. Scand., 49:89, 1978.
61. Shipp, F. L.: Osteochondritis dissecans. Surg. Clin. N. Amer., 32:713, 1952.

62. Smillie, I. S.: Injuries of the Knee Joint. 2nd Ed. Edinburgh, E. & S. Livingstone, Ltd., 1951, p. 255.
63. Smillie, I. S.: Osteochondritis Dissecans. Edinburgh and London, E. & S. Livingstone, Ltd.; Baltimore, Williams & Wilkins Co., 1960.
64. Sontag, L. W., and Pyle, S. L.: Variations in the calcification pattern in epiphyses. Their nature and significance. Amer. J. Roentgen., 45:50, 1941.
65. Spranger, M.: Tierexperimentelle und histologische Untersuchungen zur Einordnung der Osteochondrosis dissecans. Z. Orthop., 115:466, 1977.
66. Stadil, F., and Paaby, H.: Synoviale knoglecyster. Nord. Med., 83:109, 1970.
67. Stougaard, J.: Osteochondritis dissecans. Igeskr. Laeg., 122:1391, 1960.
68. Stougaard, J.: The hereditary factor in osteochondritis dissecans. J. Bone Joint Surg., 43-B:256, 1961.
69. Stougaard, J.: Familial occurrence of osteochondritis dissecans. J. Bone Joint Surg., 46-B:542, 1964.
70. Tallqvist, G.: The reaction to mechanical trauma in growing articular cartilage. Acta Orthop. Scand., Suppl. 53, 1962.
71. Tobin, W. J.: Familial osteochondritis dissecans with associated tibia vara. J. Bone Joint Surg., 39-A:1091, 1957.
72. Van Demark, R. E.: Osteochondritis dissecans with spontaneous healing. J. Bone Joint Surg., 34-A:143, 1952.
73. Vaughan, C. E., and Stapleton, J. G.: Osteochondritis dissecans of the ankle. Radiology, 49:72, 1947.
74. Wagoner, G., and Cohn, B. N. E.: Osteochondritis dissecans. A résumé of the theories of etiology and the consideration of heredity as an etiologic factor. Arch. Surg. (Chicago), 23:1, 1931.
75. White, J.: Osteochondritis dissecans in association with dwarfism. J. Bone Joint Surg., 39-B:261, 1957.
76. Wiberg, G.: Spontanheilung von Osteochondritis dissecans im Kniegelenk. Acta Chir. Scand., 85:421, 1941.
77. Wolff, A. O.: Osteochondritis dissecans i talo-cruralleddet. Hospitalstidende, 70:36, 1926.
78. Zellweger, H., and Ebnother, M.: A familiar skeletal disorder with multilocular aseptic bone necrosis, and with osteochondritis dissecans in particular. Helv. Paediat. Acta, 6:95, 1951.

Affections of the Toes

HALLUX RIGIDUS

Pain and stiffness in the metatarsophalangeal joint of the great toe are quite common in adults but occur in children only very occasionally. The condition is referred to by a variety of terms—as *hallux rigidus* by Cotterill, as *hallux flexus* by Davies-Colley, as *hallux dolorosus* by Walsham and Hughes, and as *metatarsus primus elevatus* by Lambrinudi.[5, 6, 17, 23]

Etiology

In adolescent patients, hallux rigidus is often a familial affliction. Bonney and Macnab report that 50 per cent of patients whose symptoms began prior to the age of 20 had a positive family history.[2]

More preponderant in females in adolescence, the condition shows equal sex incidence in the adult.

Hallux rigidus may be caused either by intrinsic disorders of the metatarsophalangeal joint or by extrinsic mechanical abnormalities acting on the joint.

Elevation of First Metatarsal. Lambrinudi observed that hallux rigidus is associated with dorsal hyperextension of the first metatarsal.[17] In about two thirds of the cases of Jack and of Bonney and Macnab, metatarsus primus elevatus was found in hallux rigidus.[2, 12] Kessel and Bonney reported two adult patients with acquired metatarsus primus elevatus (resulting from an osteotomy of the first metatarsal done for hallux valgus in one and following triple arthrodesis in the other) who developed typical hallux rigidus later. Thus evidence was presented that in some patients, hyperextension of the first metatarsal is the primary deformity and hallux rigidus is secondary.[15] One must, however, add that cases have been observed in which metatarsus primus elevatus developed because of marked flexor spasm following the operative production of a stiff and painful first metatarsophalangeal joint. The question of which is the cause and which the effect in adolescent hallux rigidus has not, as yet, been answered. Bingold and Collins believe that in the majority of cases metatarsus primus elevatus is secondary to flexor spasm of the first metatarsophalangeal joint.[1]

Relative Length of First and Second Metatarsals. Nilsonne observed that most of his adolescent patients with hallux rigidus had long narrow feet with a first metatarsal that was longer than the second.[20] This finding was also noted by Bonney and Macnab in 22 of the 53 feet examined, the discrepancy in length being 0.5 cm. or more.[2] The common association of a long great toe with hallux rigidus was also noted by McMurray.[18] It seems the pathomechanical factor is the increased pressure transmitted from the hallux to the first metatarsal head.

Stress on First Metatarsophalangeal Joint. A number of other conditions predispose to excessive pressure on the base of the proximal phalanx of the great toe. In hallux rigidus, the feet are frequently pronated and the center of gravity of body weight is shifted toward the first metatarsal head. Bingold and Collins proposed that the cause of hallux rigidus is an abnormal gait developed either to protect an injured or inflamed metatarsophalangeal joint from the pressure of weight-bearing or to stabilize a hypermobile first metatarsal. As a result, excessive pressure is transmitted from the flexor hallucis brevis tendon and the two sesamoids to the base of the first phalanx and the great toe. They found evidence of this abnormal gait in the peculiarities of wear seen in old shoes and observed a high degree of correlation between unilateral hallux rigidus and the patient's foot dominance.[1]

Local Inflammation of the Joint. In some cases, there is a definite history of injury precipitating these symptoms, and traumatic arthritis may be a factor. In other patients, hallux rigidus may be a local manifestation of generalized rheumatoid arthritis.

Osteochondritis Dissecans of First Metatarsal Head. This may be an occasional cause of hallux rigidus (Fig. 6–15). Increased density and fragmentation of the epiphysis of the proximal phalanx of the great toe was considered by Glissan to represent aseptic necrosis of bone, a condition similar to Legg-Perthes disease of the femoral head.[8] Pathologic studies by Bingold and Collins have, however, demonstrated that the increased density of the epiphysis of the proximal phalanx is caused by close packing of live trabeculae, and that fragmentation of the epiphysis represents irregular ossification, not aseptic necrosis.[1] Similar changes are observed in normal feet of adolescents; they are of no etiologic significance in hallux rigidus.

Clinical Features

The presenting complaint is pain in and around the metatarsophalangeal joint of the great toe. Usually the symptoms are of gradual onset, developing in adolescence. Occasionally pain occurs suddenly, precipitated

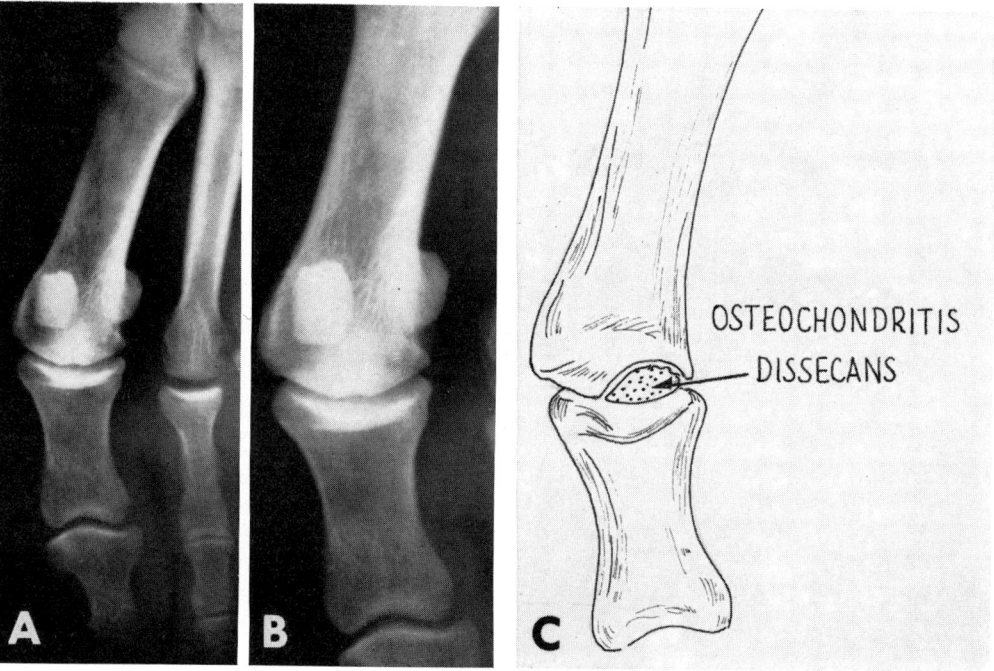

FIGURE 6–15. *Osteochondritis dissecans of the first metatarsal head.*

This condition is an occasional cause of hallux rigidus. (From Kelikian, H.: Hallux Valgus, Allied Deformities of the Forefoot and Metatarsalgia. Philadelphia, W. B. Saunders Co., 1965, p. 273. Reprinted by permission.)

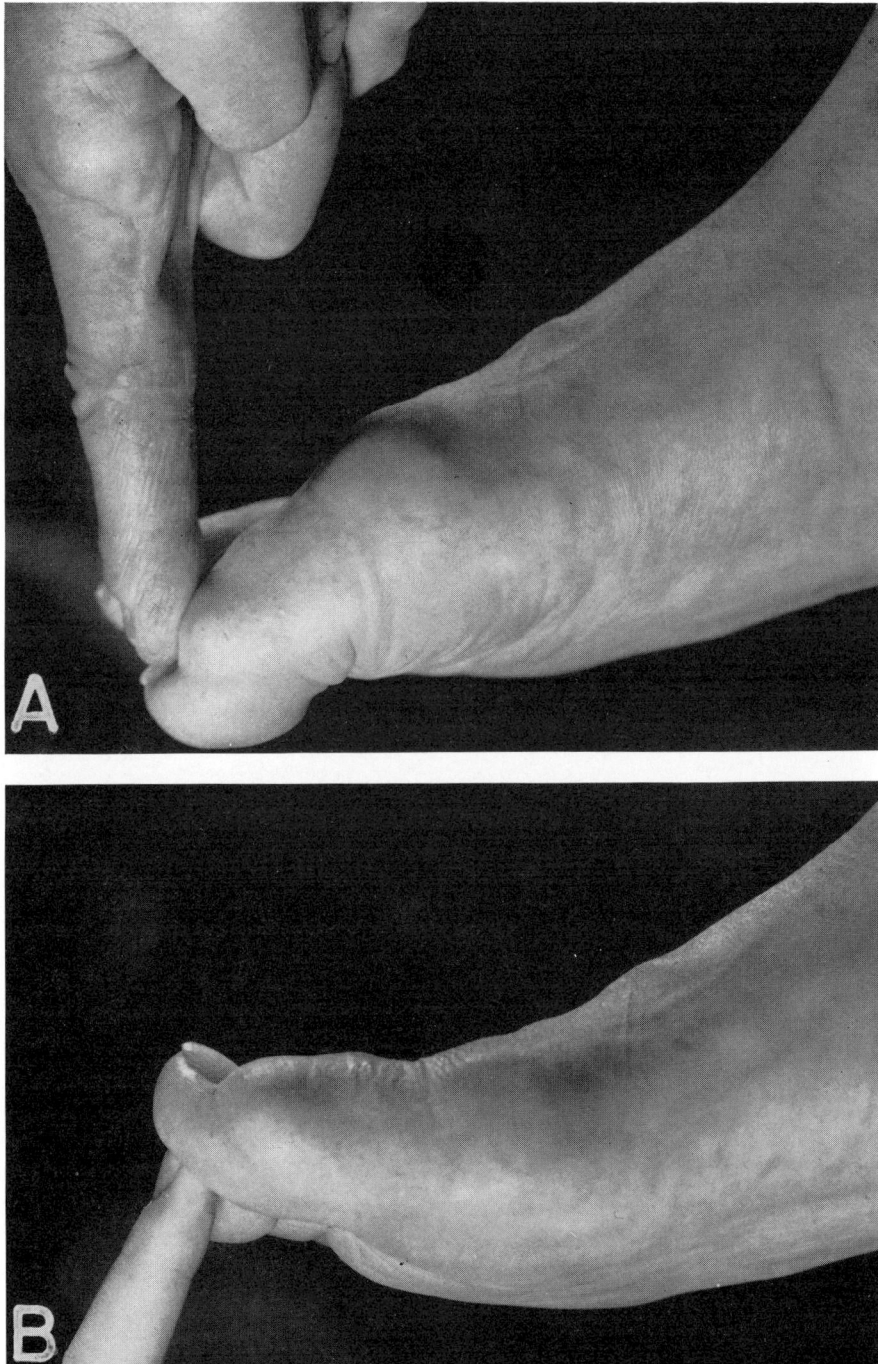

FIGURE 6–16. Hallux rigidus.

The metatarsophalangeal joint is enlarged, and dorsiflexion of the great toe is markedly limited. (From Kelikian, H.: Hallux Valgus, Allied Deformities of the Forefoot and Metatarsalgia. Philadelphia, W. B. Saunders Co., 1965, p. 268. Reprinted by permission.)

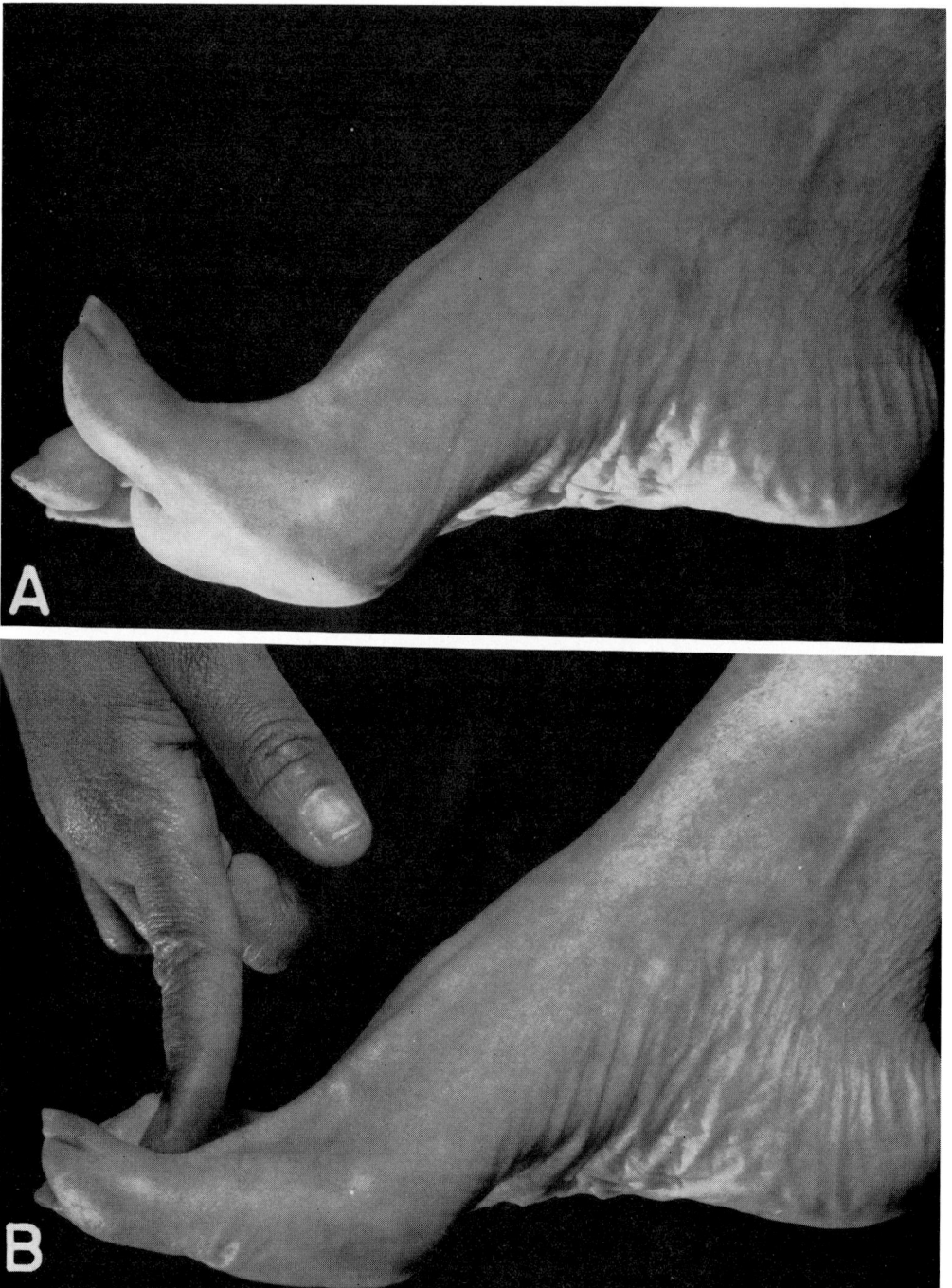

FIGURE 6–17. Hallux extensus.

A rare variety of hallux rigidus in which the first metatarsal is plantar-flexed and the great toe is held in hyperextension at the metatarsophalangeal joint. Note the hallux cannot be pushed plantarward. (From Kelikian, H.: Hallux Valgus, Allied Deformities of the Forefoot and Metatarsalgia. Philadelphia, W. B. Saunders Co., 1965, p. 269. Reprinted by permission.)

by acute trauma. It is aggravated by walking or rising on the toes and is relieved by rest.

Abnormal patterns of wear in the shoes are suggestive of hallux rigidus. The shoes are often too narrow and short, and show excessive wear on the outer side of the heel, the posterior half of the sole, and under the terminal phalanx of the great toe. The uppers are bulged outward over the outer side of the heel and the posterior half of the sole. Their toe spring is shortened, and there are furrows over the medial side of the toe cap caused by the hypermobile interphalangeal joint of the great toe. In gait the foot is inverted on push-off.

The feet of these patients are long and narrow and are usually pronated. The base of the first metatarsal is pushed plantarward, and its head is tilted dorsally. The first metatarsophalangeal joint is enlarged, and the great toe is held in a varying degree of flexion (hallux flexus). There is a callosity underneath the base of the proximal phalanx of the great toe, but the skin on the plantar aspect of the first metatarsal head is smooth (lacking its normal thickness). On palpation the metatarsophalangeal joint of the great toe is found to be tender and thickened. In severe cases one may palpate osteophytes at the articular margins. Active extension of the metatarsophalangeal joint is markedly restricted, but in the early stages of the disease, flexion is within normal range. Passive dorsiflexion of the great toe is limited and very painful (Fig. 6–16). Passive motions of the joint may be accompanied by crepitus. A taut flexor hallucis brevis may be palpated on the plantar aspect. The interphalangeal joint of the great toe is hypermobile in adolescents; in adults, its motion may be restricted and somewhat painful.

There is a rare variety of hallux rigidus referred to as hallux extensus in which the first metatarsal is plantar-flexed and the great toe is fixed in hyperextension at the metatarsophalangeal joint (Fig. 6–17).

Roentgenographic Features

Early in the course of the disease, the x-rays may be normal or show thickening of the soft tissues around the affected joint. The standing lateral roentgenogram of the foot shows the first metatarsal hyperextended with its head tilting dorsally. Later on, the articular cartilage space becomes narrowed and the metatarsal head flattened. Soon osteophytes form at the joint margins (Fig. 6–18).

In hallux rigidus due to rheumatoid arthritis there will be local osteoporosis and erosion at the articular margins. Gout is very rare in the adolescent, but in the adult a punched-out erosion due to a tophus on the articular surface is characteristic.

Treatment

Initially conservative treatment should always be tried. The sole of the shoe between the shank and toe portions medially under the first metatarsal head is stiffened. A slightly larger shoe with its leather softened dorsally over the first metatarsophalangeal joint will give symptomatic relief. Passive manipulative exercises are performed several times a day to increase the range of dorsiflexion of the great toe. In most cases, with conservative management, the symptoms will regress if the joint is protected for a few weeks or months. If the symptoms persist and disability remains moderately severe, operative correction of the deformity is required.

In these resistant cases, Kessel and Bonney (following an earlier suggestion of Bonney and Macnab) perform an extension osteotomy at the base of the proximal phalanx of the great toe, converting the normal range of plantar flexion at the metatarsophalangeal joint to a functional range of dorsiflexion and plantar flexion (Fig. 6–19).[2, 15]

The operative technique is as follows:

A curved dorsal incision about 4 cm. long is made, centering over the base of the proximal phalanx. The subcutaneous tissue is divided. The extensor hallucis longus tendon and digital nerves are retracted to one side to expose the proximal phalanx and metatarsophalangeal joint of the great toe. With small osteotomes, a wedge of bone with a dorsal base of predetermined width is resected from the phalanx as far proximally as possible. The cortex and periosteum on the plantar aspect are left intact.

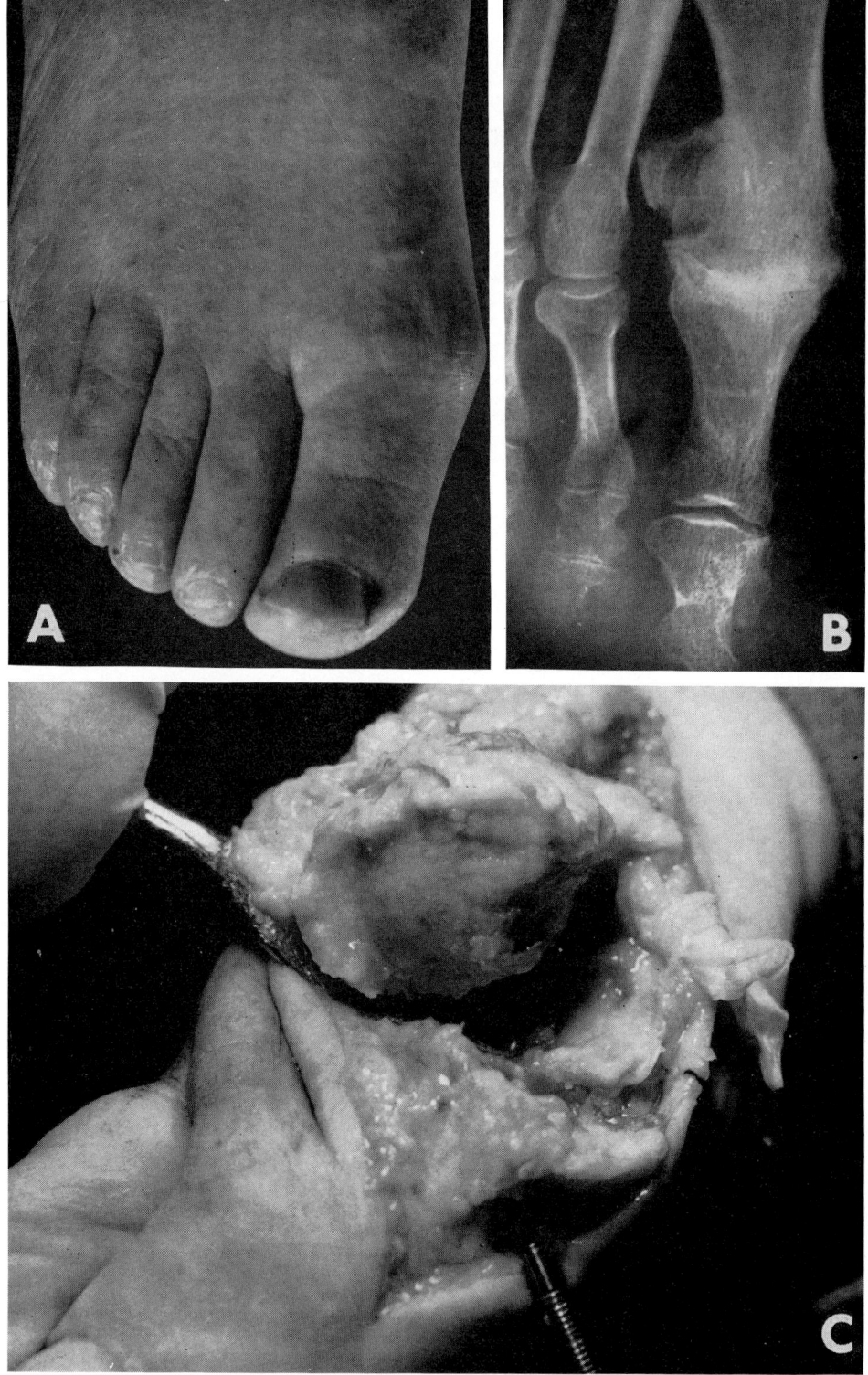

FIGURE 6–18. Hallux rigidus.

A. Photograph of the forefoot, showing enlargement of the first metatarsophalangeal joint. **B.** Roentgenograms. Note the degenerative changes—the articular cartilage space is obliterated and osteophytes have formed at the joint margins. **C.** Findings at operation. The hyaline articular cartilage is eroded, the synovium is thickened, and there is marked proliferation of new bone. (From Kelikian, H.: Hallux Valgus, Allied Deformities of the Forefoot and Metatarsalgia. Philadelphia, W. B. Saunders Co., 1965, p. 271. Reprinted by permission.)

Affections of the Toes   633

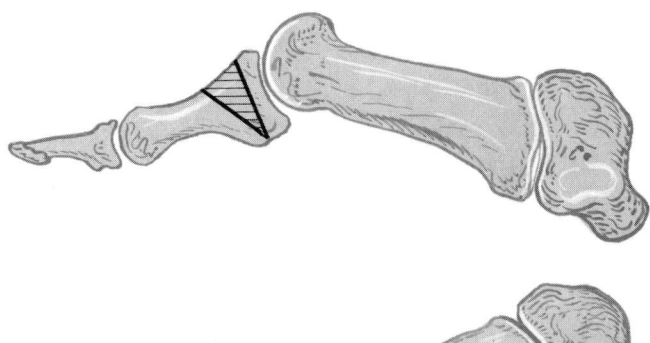
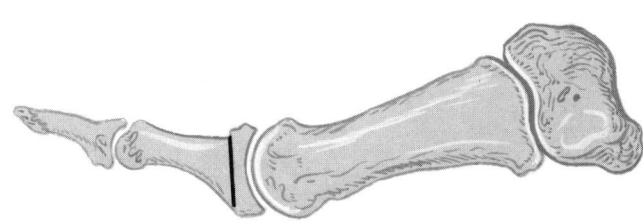

FIGURE 6–19. *Kessel and Bonney osteotomy.*

It is best to use drill holes to mark and control the extent of osteotomy. The phalanx is angulated dorsally to close the gap. One or two Kirschner wires are placed obliquely to keep the osteotomized fragments firmly together. The wound is closed, and a below-knee walking cast with a sturdy toe plate is applied. The great toe should be held in extension by appropriate padding underneath. In four to six weeks the osteotomy will heal.

Kessel and Bonney report satisfactory results following their procedure, with a mean improvement of dorsiflexion from 5 degrees before operation to 44 degrees afterward (Fig. 6–19).[15]

Watermann, in 1927, recommended a cuneiform osteotomy of the head of the first metatarsal with the base of the wedge directed dorsally and including the hypertrophic spurs (cf. Fig. 6–20).[24] Kelikian recommends the Watermann osteotomy in growing children in order to avoid injury to the growth plate of the proximal phalanx.[14]

A plantar capsulotomy of the first metatarsophalangeal joint is performed if the capsule is contracted and limits extension. One may have to release the flexor hallucis brevis from the proximal phalanx.

Whether extension osteotomy of the base of the proximal phalanx or the first metatarsal head will prevent the development of hallux rigidus in adult life has not been determined, as long-term follow-ups are not available. If metatarsus primus elevatus is the primary cause of hallux rigidus, the symptoms being due to restriction of dor-

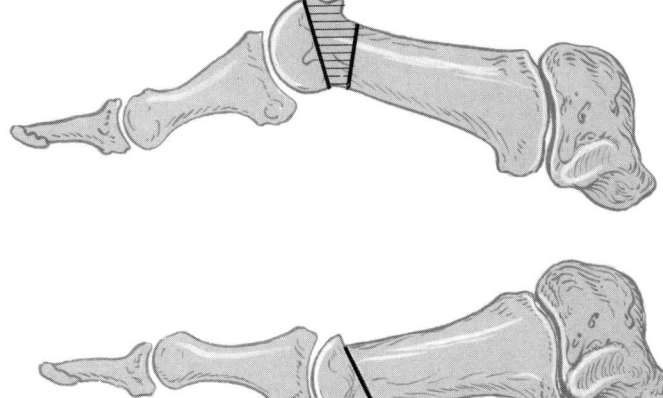

FIGURE 6–20. *Watermann's cuneiform osteotomy of the first metatarsal bone.*

Base of the wedge is directed dorsally and includes the hypertrophic spurs.

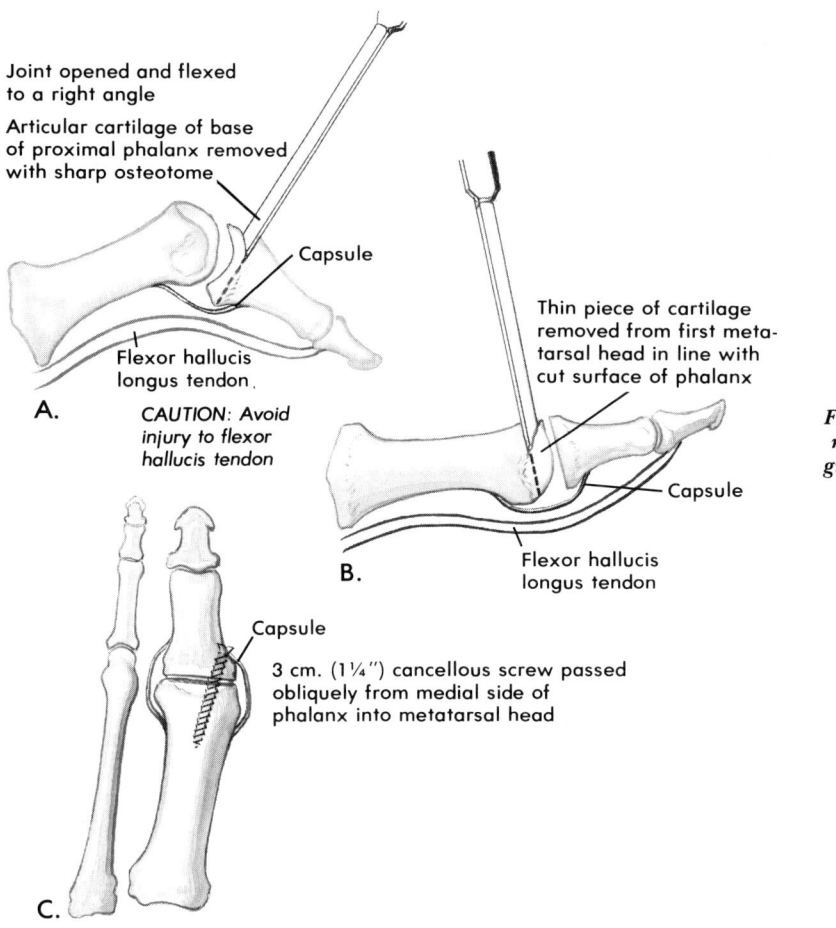

FIGURE 6–21. Arthrodesis of metatarsophalangeal joint of great toe and internal fixation with screw.

siflexion of the first metatarsophalangeal joint, extension osteotomy of the base of the first phalanx is worth a trial.

Depression of the first metatarsal head by a wedge osteotomy (with its base on the plantar aspect) was recommended by Jack.[12] This may prevent the development of hallux rigidus; however, experience with this procedure is limited.

In the adult in whom hallux rigidus is symptomatic and disabling, resection of the proximal half of the first phalanx of the great toe is recommended. If the sesamoid bones are involved in the arthritic process, they are also excised.

When hallux valgus is accompanied by metatarsalgia, Kelikian recommends fusion of the metatarsophalangeal joint of the great toe; in such an instance, the distal third of the second metatarsal is resected and its digit is syndactylized with the first or third toe. The optimum position of arthrodesis is 20 to 30 degrees valgus and 10 to 15 degrees of dorsiflexion in the male, 15 to 20 degrees of dorsiflexion in the female.

The operation is performed through a dorsomedial longitudinal incision. The joint cartilage is excised, and the denuded bony surfaces of the first metatarsal head and base of the proximal phalanx are snugly held in the desired position and internally fixed with a screw. The drill is directed proximally through the base of the proximal phalanx into the metatarsal, emerging on the side of the metatarsal. The screw head is countersunk and lies against the flare of the base of the proximal phalanx (Fig. 6–21). The foot is immobilized in a below-knee walking cast for six weeks.

Other methods are compression arthrodesis (used by Harrison and Harvey) or cone fusion (used by Wilson).[11, 25] Long-term results of metatarsophalangeal joint fusion of the great toe reported by Fitzgerald are excellent.[7]

References

1. Bingold, A. C., and Collins, D. H.: Hallux rigidus. J. Bone Joint Surg., *32-B*:214, 1950.
2. Bonney, G., and Macnab, I.: Hallux valgus and hallux rigidus. A critical survey of operative results. J. Bone Joint Surg., *34-B*:366, 1952.
3. Breitenfelder, G.: Hallux rigidus Jugendlicher. Verh. Deutsch. Orthop. Ges., *80*:313, 1951.
4. Cochrane, W. A.: An operation for hallux rigidus. Brit. Med. J., *1*:1095, 1927.
5. Cotterill, J. M.: On the condition of stiff great toe in adolescents. Edinburgh, Trans. Med. Chir. Soc., 1886-87, p. 277.
6. Davies-Colley, N.: On contraction of the metatarsophalangeal joint of the great toe (hallux flexus). Trans. Clin. Soc. London, *20*:165, 1887.
7. Fitzgerald, J. A. W.: Review of long-term results in arthrodesis of the first metatarsophalangeal joint. J. Bone Joint Surg., *51-B*:488, 1969.
8. Glissan, D. J.: Hallux valgus and hallux rigidus. Med. J. Aust., *2*:585, 1946.
9. Goodfellow, J.: Aetiology of hallux rigidus. Proc. Roy. Soc. Med., *59*:821, 1966.
10. Judas, G. J.: An etiology of hallux rigidus. J. Foot Surg., *10*:113, 1971.
11. Harrison, M. H. M., and Harvey, F. J.: Arthrodesis of the first metatarsophalangeal joint for hallux valgus and rigidus. J. Bone Joint Surg., *45-A*:471, 1963.
12. Jack, E. A.: The aetiology of hallux rigidus. Brit. J. Surg., *27*:492, 1940.
13. Jansen, M.: Hallux valgus, rigidus and malleus. J. Orthop. Surg., *3*:27, 1921.
14. Kelikian, H.: Hallux Valgus, Allied Deformities of the Forefoot, and Metatarsalgia. Philadelphia, W. B. Saunders Co., 1965, p. 273.
15. Kessel, L., and Bonney, G.: Hallux rigidus in the adolescent. J. Bone Joint Surg., *40-B*:668, 1958.
16. Kingreen, O.: Zur Aetiologie des Hallux flexus. Zbl. Chir., *60*:2116, 1933.
17. Lambrinudi, C.: Metartarsus primus elevatus. Proc. Roy. Soc. Med. (Section of Orthopaedics), *31*:1273, 1938.
18. McMurray, T. P.: The treatment of hallux valgus and rigidus. Brit. Med. J., *2*:218, 1936.
19. Moynihan, F. J.: Arthrodesis of the metatarsophalangeal joint of the great toe. J. Bone Joint. Surg., *49-B*:544, 1967.
20. Nilsonne, H.: Hallux rigidus and its treatment. Acta Orthop. Scand., *1*:295, 1930.
21. Severin, E.: Removal of the base of the proximal phalanx in hallux rigidus. Acta Orthop. Scand., *17*:77, 1947.
22. Steinhauser, W.: Osteochondrose der basalen Epiphyse der Grundphalanx, Grosszehe und Hallux rigidus. Beitr. Ges. Orthop., *6*:177, 1959.
23. Walsham, W. J., and Hughes, W. K.: The Deformities of the Human Foot. London, Baillière, Tindall & Cox, 1895, pp. 512–514.
24. Watermann, H.: Die Arthritis deformans Grosszehengrundgelenkes. Z. Orthop. Chir., *48*:346, 1927.
25. Watson-Jones, R.: Treatment of hallux rigidus. Brit. Med. J., *1*:1165, 1927.
26. Wilson, J. N.: Oblique displacement osteotomy of hallux valgus. J. Bone Joint Surg., *45-B*:552, 1963.

Tumors of the Foot

Tumors of the foot are uncommon in children. If they do occur, they may originate in either the soft tissues or bone, and may be either benign or malignant. Metastatic tumors distal to the knee are extremely rare.

The usual presenting complaints are a swelling or mass, difficulty in fitting shoes, and local pain or a limp. To detect minimal findings, it is essential to examine both feet, comparing the suspected pathologic limb with the contralateral normal limb. The exact site of the problem should be determined, whether it is in the soft tissues (subcutaneous tissue, fascia, muscle, tendon, or nerve), the joint, or the bone. Is the consistency of the swelling cystic, firm, or bony? Is the mass fixed to subjacent bone or is it freely movable? Are its boundaries well delineated or ill-defined and does it infiltrate adjacent tissues? Can it be transilluminated? What is the color of the overlying skin? Are the superficial veins dilated? Is there increased local heat? Does the mass pulsate? Upon tourniquet ischemia, does it decrease in size? The regional lymph nodes of the entire lower limb are also palpated for enlargement and tenderness. Roentgenograms of the foot are made to determine bony and soft-tissue alterations. The more common tumors causing problems in the foot are briefly described here.

SOFT-TISSUE TUMORS

Lipoma

Lipoma, one of the more common tumors in the foot, is seen in infants as well as in older children. It is usually located in the subcutaneous tissue of the instep of the foot, or deep to the plantar fascia (Figs. 6–22 and 6–23). Occasionally it may be found on the dorsum of the foot involving tendon sheaths or digital nerves. The mass is soft, generally lobulated, and surrounded by a definite capsule. The histologic picture varies, depending upon the amount of fibrous and myxomatous tissue associated with the fat.

On palpation, the mass has a soft flabby feeling, suggesting fluctuation. Its boundaries are usually not distinct. In the roentgenograms, the lipoma casts a soft-tissue shadow of "fatty density."

Treatment consists of surgical excision of

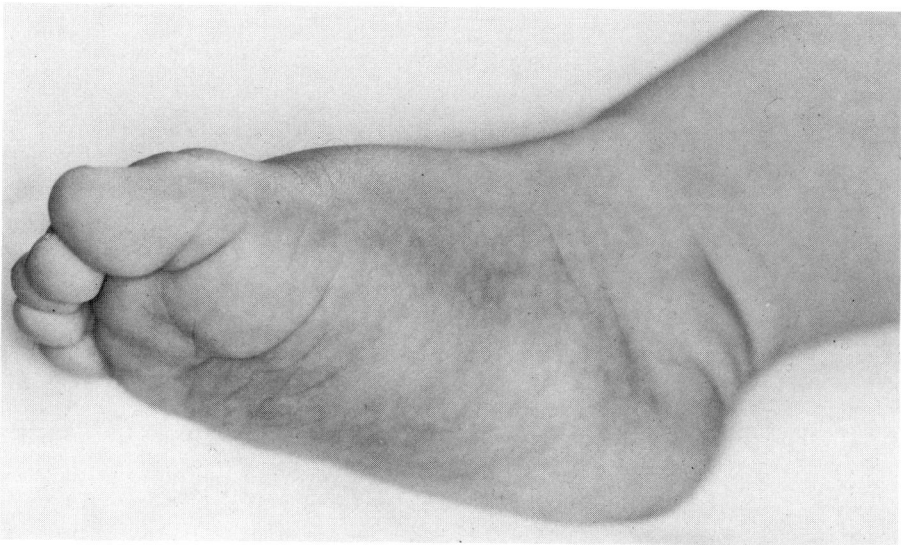

FIGURE 6–22. Lipoma of the right foot.

The mass was encapsulated and located deep to the plantar fascia.

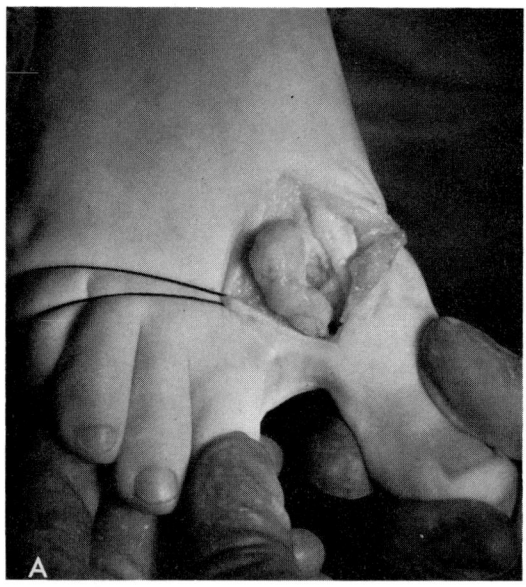
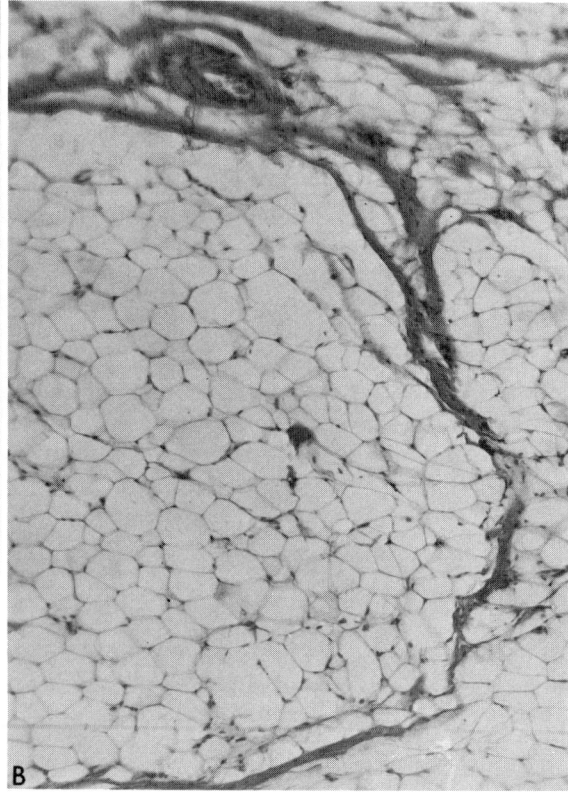

FIGURE 6–23. Lipoma on dorsum of the foot between the first and second metatarsal heads.

A. Appearance at surgery. **B.** Photomicrograph showing the fat cells ($\times$ 100).

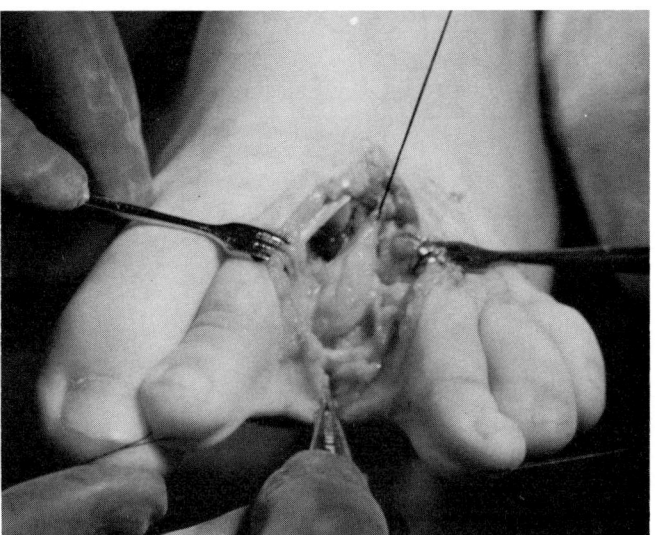

FIGURE 6–24. Ganglion between the second and third toes.

Gross appearance of the cyst at operation.

the tumor. If the lesion is not completely removed, it may recur. It is best to perform the procedure with tourniquet ischemia with the child under general anesthesia.

Ganglion

The usual locations of this common tumorous lesion are on the dorsum of the foot in the midtarsal area, in between the toes, and in the region of the ankle adjacent to the lateral or medial malleolus (Figs. 6–24 and 6–25). The thin-walled cyst contains clear colorless gelatinous fluid and seems to arise from tendon sheaths or from within the connective tissue of the subjacent joint capsule. Surgical excision of ganglia is usually indicated if they interfere with the normal fit of the shoe or if they are painful on weight-bearing (Fig. 6–26). Rupture of the cyst by external force or aspiration of its contents and injection of hydrocortisone are, as a rule, inadequate, and the ganglion eventually recurs. The best treatment is complete excision, which should be performed in the operating room under general anesthesia and tourniquet ischemia. The ligamentous tissue at the base of the stalk of the ganglion should be removed or scarified to prevent recurrence.

Hemangioma

Angiomata may be of congenital origin, presenting at birth, or they may develop in childhood or adolescence. The cavernous type is more common. In the foot, hemangioma may involve the skin and subcutaneous tissue, or it may involve the muscle and tendon (Figs. 6–27, 6–28, and 6–29). The tarsal bones may be invaded. The instep and plantar aspect of the foot are favored locations. Occasionally the lesion affecting the foot may be part of diffuse hemangiomatosis affecting the entire lower limb (Fig. 6–30).

The presenting complaint is of a compressible mass, which may be irritated by the shoe. When one obstructs the venous return, the mass enlarges. Occasionally the lesion may be painful when it invades nervous tissue or when it is located in bone and expansion is taking place. When hemangioma involves the skin, its external appearance is characteristic and diagnosis is not difficult.

Treatment consists of meticulous and complete excision of the lesion. Large tumors may require surgical resection in two or three stages. Tourniquet ischemia controls hemorrhage, but it is disadvantageous because part of the lesion may be overlooked. Because the tissues often heal poorly, careful handling and hemostasis of the wound are required. Roentgen therapy should not be employed in the treatment of hemangioma in children, but cryotherapy may occasionally be indicated.

Aneurysm in the foot and ankle may result from blunt trauma, which weakens the vessel walls, or from penetrating wounds. During triple arthrodesis, aneurysm of the posterior tibial vessels may be

Text continued on page 642

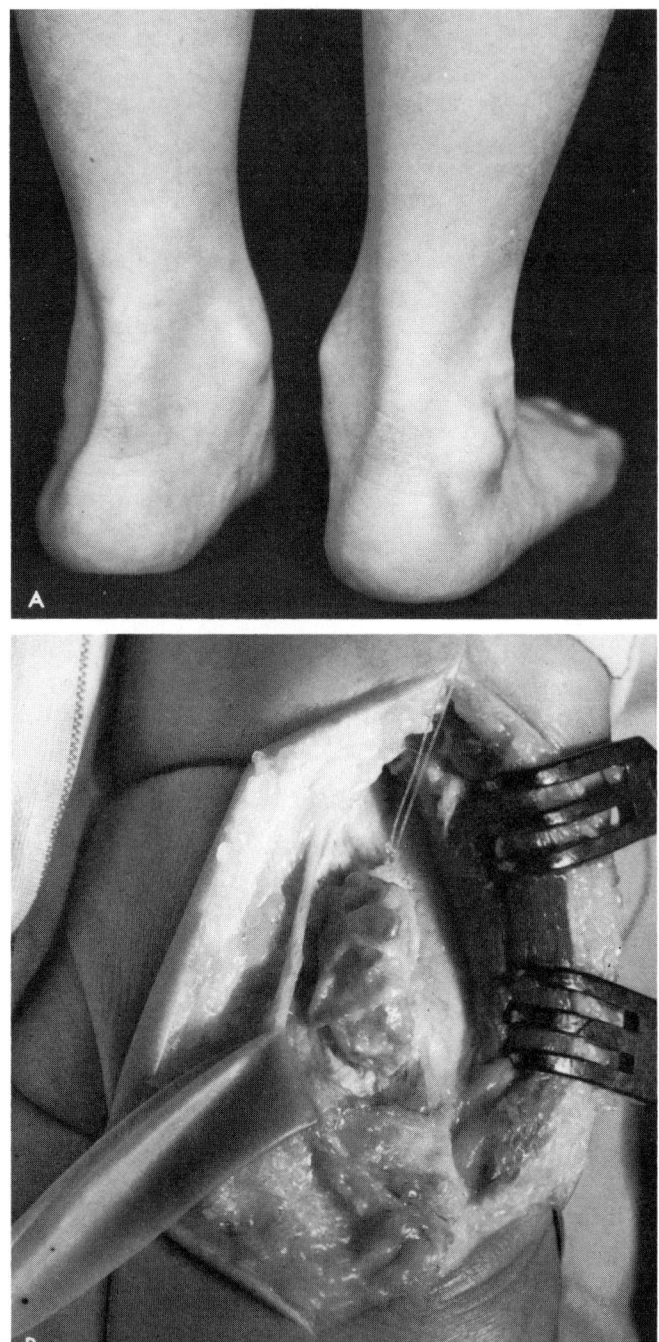

FIGURE 6–25. Ganglion in the region of the right ankle behind the lateral malleolus.

A. Photograph shows the mass behind the lateral malleolus. **B.** Gross appearance of the cyst at surgery.

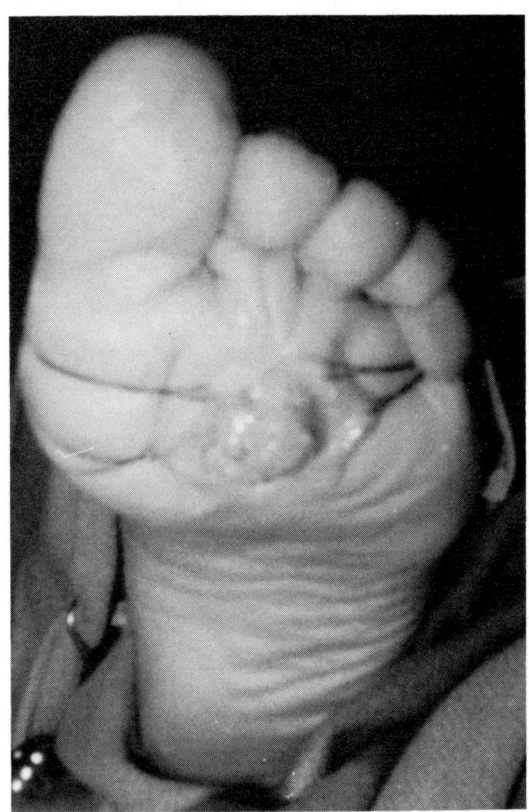

FIGURE 6–26. Ganglion on the sole of the foot, presenting as a painful mass.

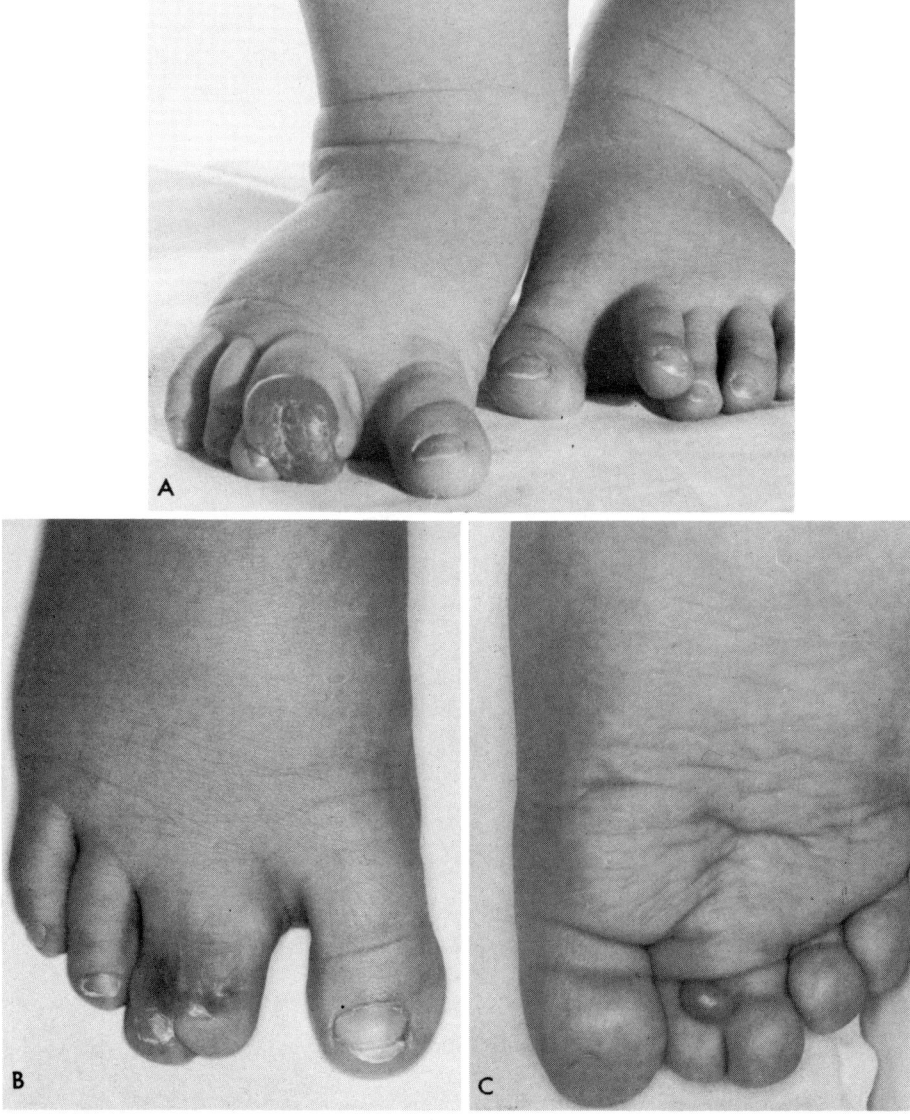

FIGURE 6–27. Hemangioma involving skin and subcutaneous tissue of the second and third toes.

A. Preoperative appearance. **B** and **C.** The lesion recurred one year following surgical removal. Again it was totally excised and the second and third toes were surgically syndactylized. Five-year follow-up showed no recurrence of the tumor.

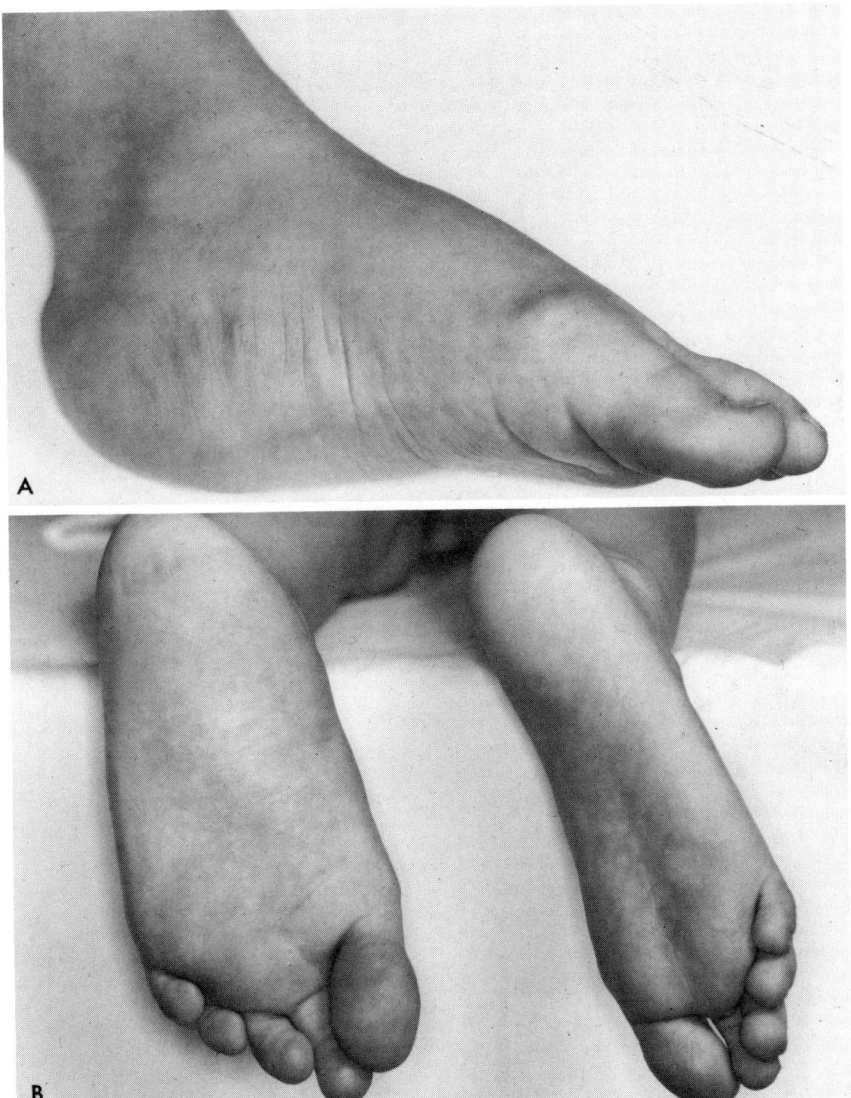

FIGURE 6–28. Cavernous hemangioma involving the subcutaneous tissue of the instep and the short plantar muscles.
A and **B.** Clinical appearance.

Illustration continued on following page

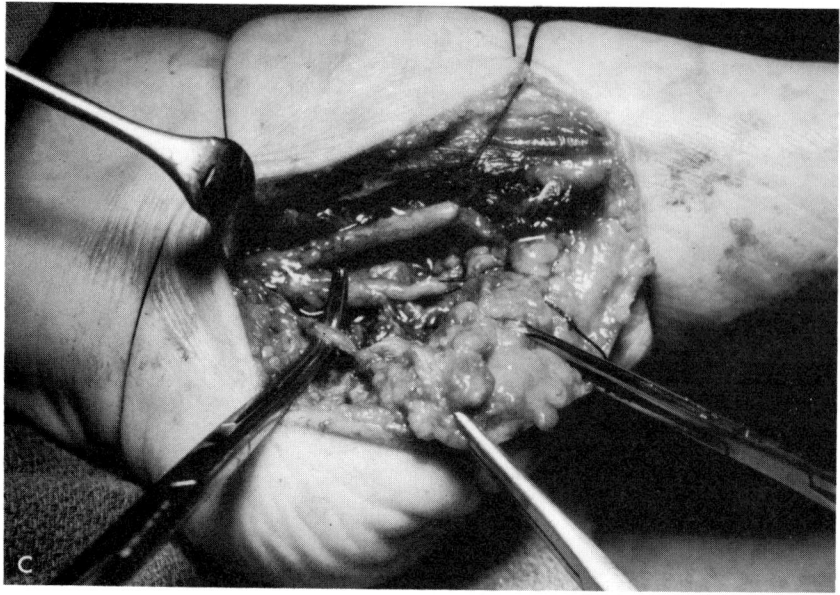

FIGURE 6–28 Continued. Cavernous hemangioma involving the subcutaneous tissue of the instep and the short plantar muscles.

C. Gross appearance at surgery.

caused by injury with an osteotome (Fig. 6–31).

Lymphangiectasis

In this condition the foot and often the entire lower limb are edematous and enlarged owing to replacement of normal subcutaneous tissue by dilated lymphatics (Fig. 6–32). In later life, fibrous changes take place in the lesion. When the abnormality is familial, it is known as "Milroy's disease." The condition should not be mistaken for a tumor; in doubtful cases, lymphangiography will establish the diagnosis.

Treatment consists of application of elastic bandages or stockings at night to shrink the dilated lymphatics. Excision of abnormal tissue is difficult but possible. The resulting defects are covered by salvaged skin and skin grafts.

Recurrent Digital Fibroma in Childhood

Digital fibrous tumors in infancy and childhood are rare.* They are limited to the fingers and toes and have a marked tendency to recur. There is no sex predilection. The lesions are multiple in about 50 per cent of cases. The tumors are either present at birth or, with few exceptions, develop in the first few months of infancy.

The tumors appear as small nodules on the lateral surfaces of the distal parts of the fingers and toes; occasionally they may be on the dorsal aspect of a digit. In multicentric cases the opposing surfaces of the toes are affected. The color of the overlying skin is normal or slightly red. The mass is firm in consistency, nontender, and fixed to the skin and underlying deep tissues. The tumor may grow either slowly or rapidly, reaching enormous size and encircling the digit. It is grayish-white in color, fibrous, and not encapsulated.

On histologic examination of the lesion the epidermis is normal. The tumor is located in the dermis and consists of interlacing bands of fibrous connective tissue with abundant collagen. The size of nuclei varies; mitosis is infrequent.

Two forms of fibroblasts can be visualized on electron microscopy: in Type I the nucleus is large and lobulated with scanty endoplasmic reticulum; and in Type II the nucleus is small and flattened with a greater amount of endoplasmic reticulum. Some

Text continued on page 648

---

*See references 1, 2, 4, 7, 8, 29, 32, 41.

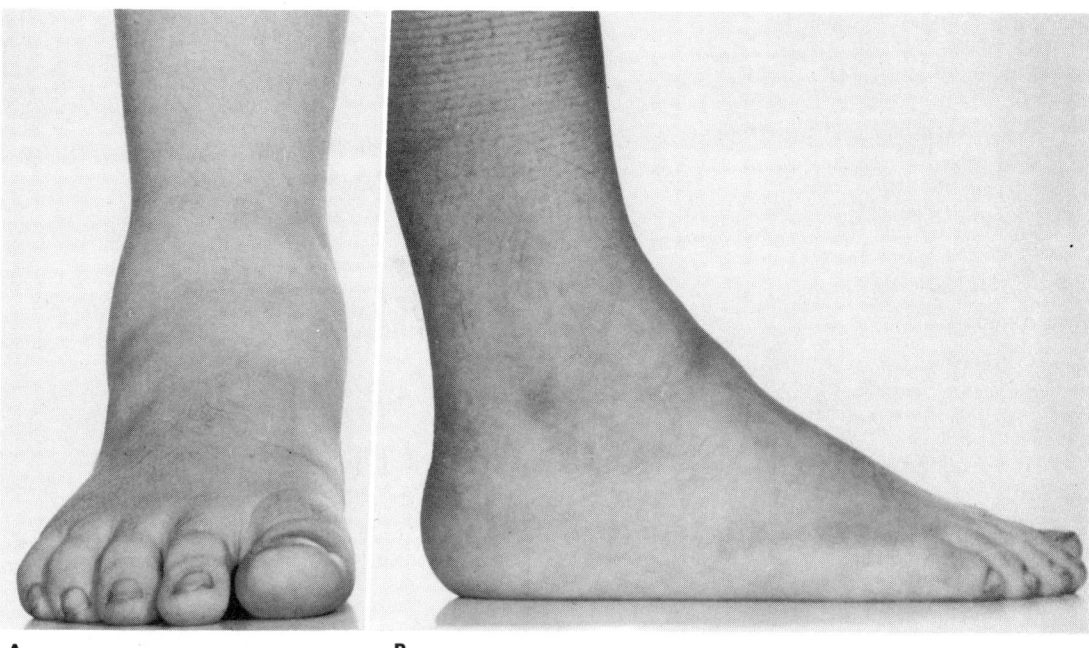
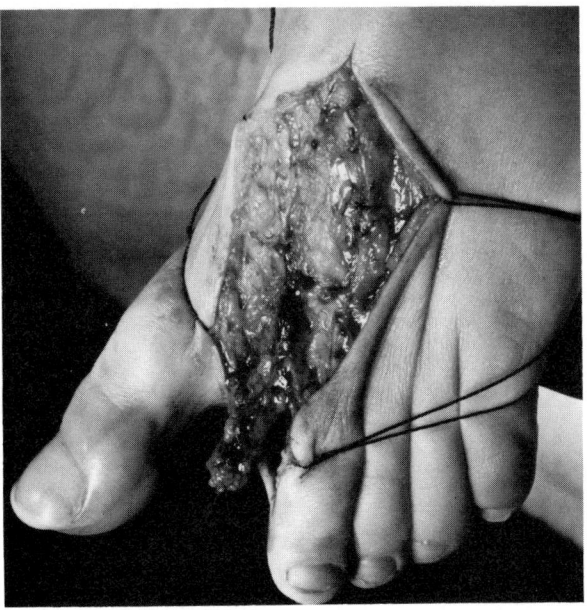

FIGURE 6–29. Cavernous hemangioma involving tendon sheaths on the dorsum of the foot.

A and **B.** Preoperative appearance. The condition was misdiagnosed, and the patient was treated for rheumatoid arthritis of the ankle and subtalar joints. Note the soft-tissue swelling. **C.** Gross appearance at surgery.

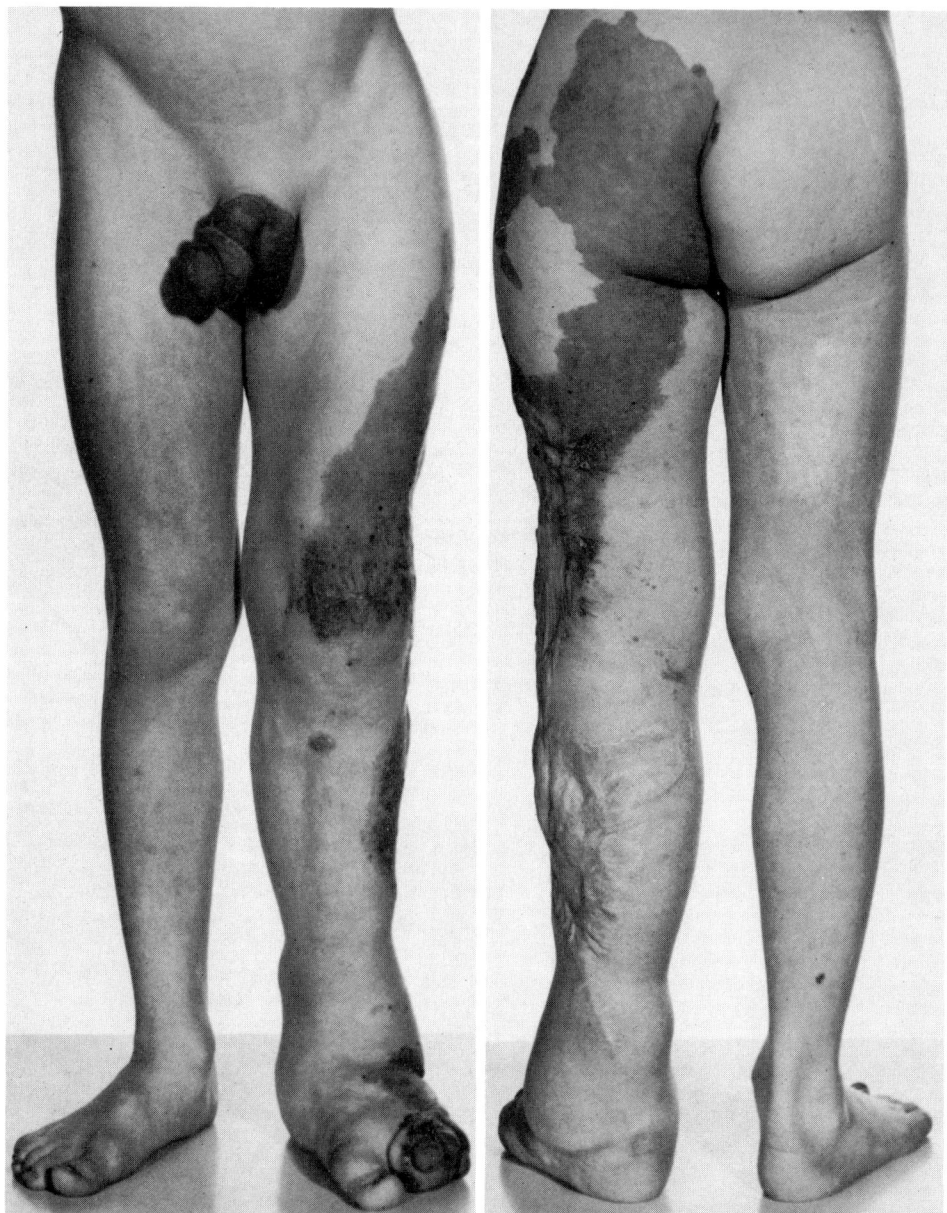

FIGURE 6–30. Massive hemangiomatosis involving the entire left lower limb.

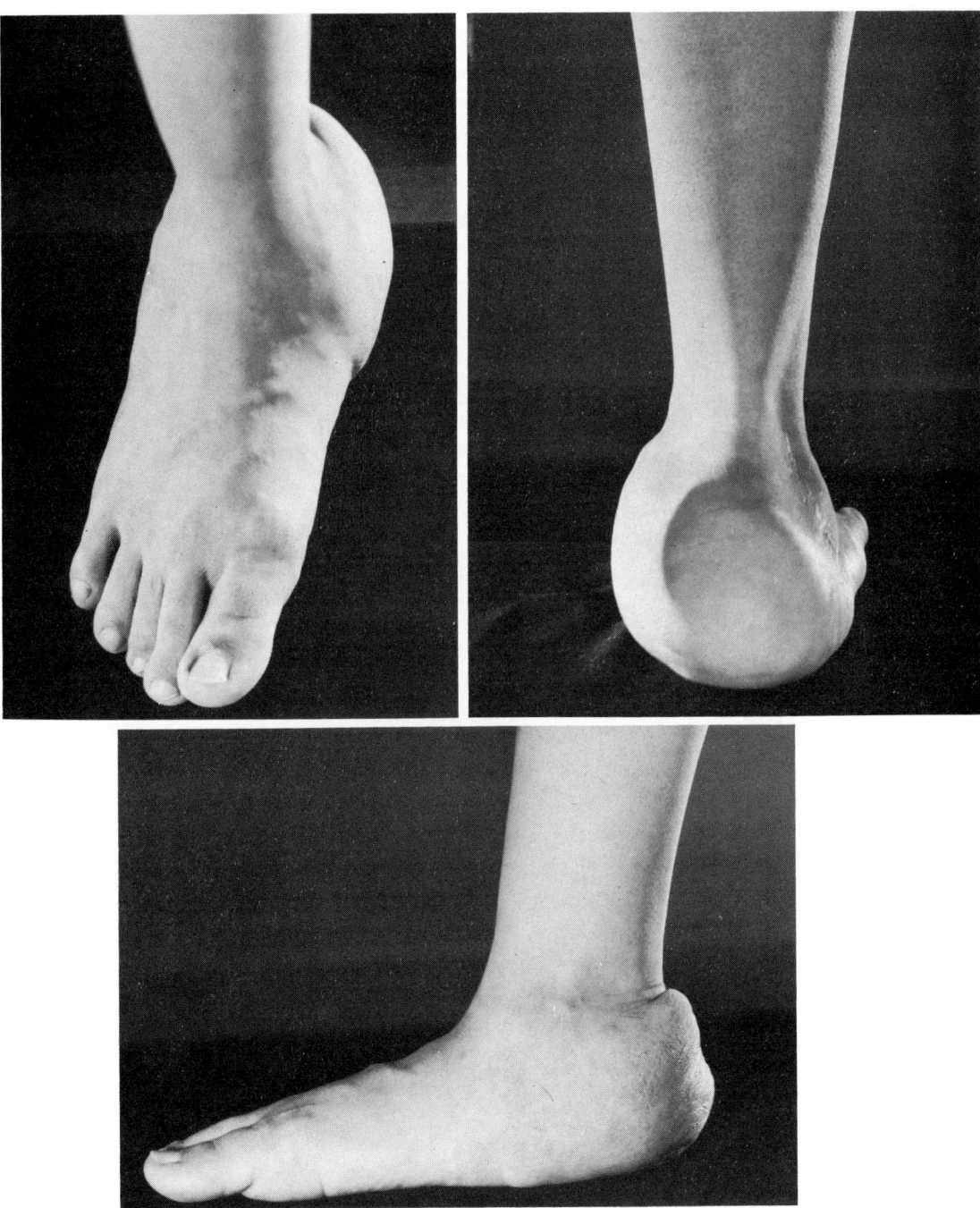

FIGURE 6–31. Aneurysm of the posterior tibial artery caused by injury during triple arthrodesis.

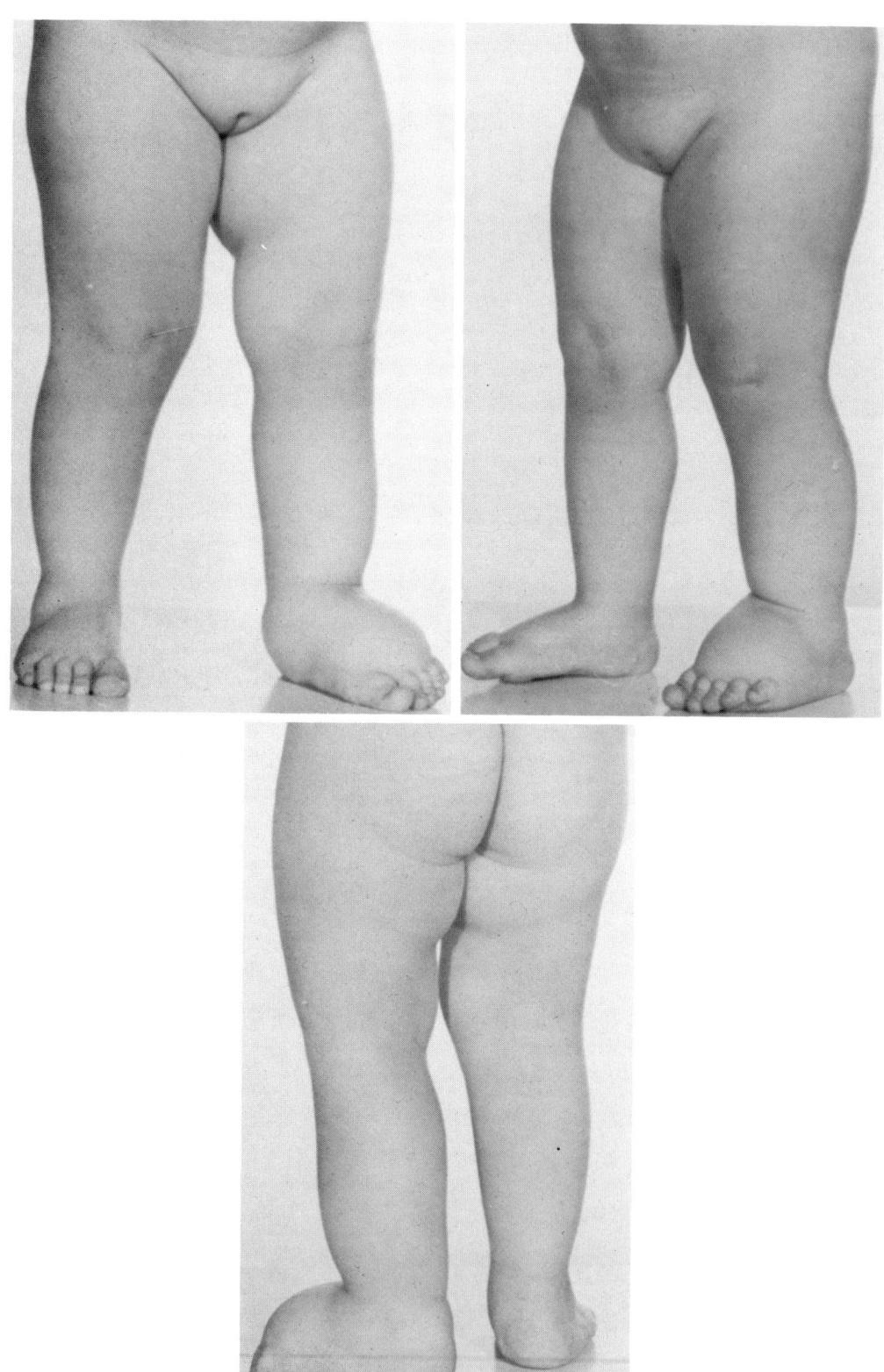

FIGURE 6–32. Lymphangiectasis of the left foot and leg.

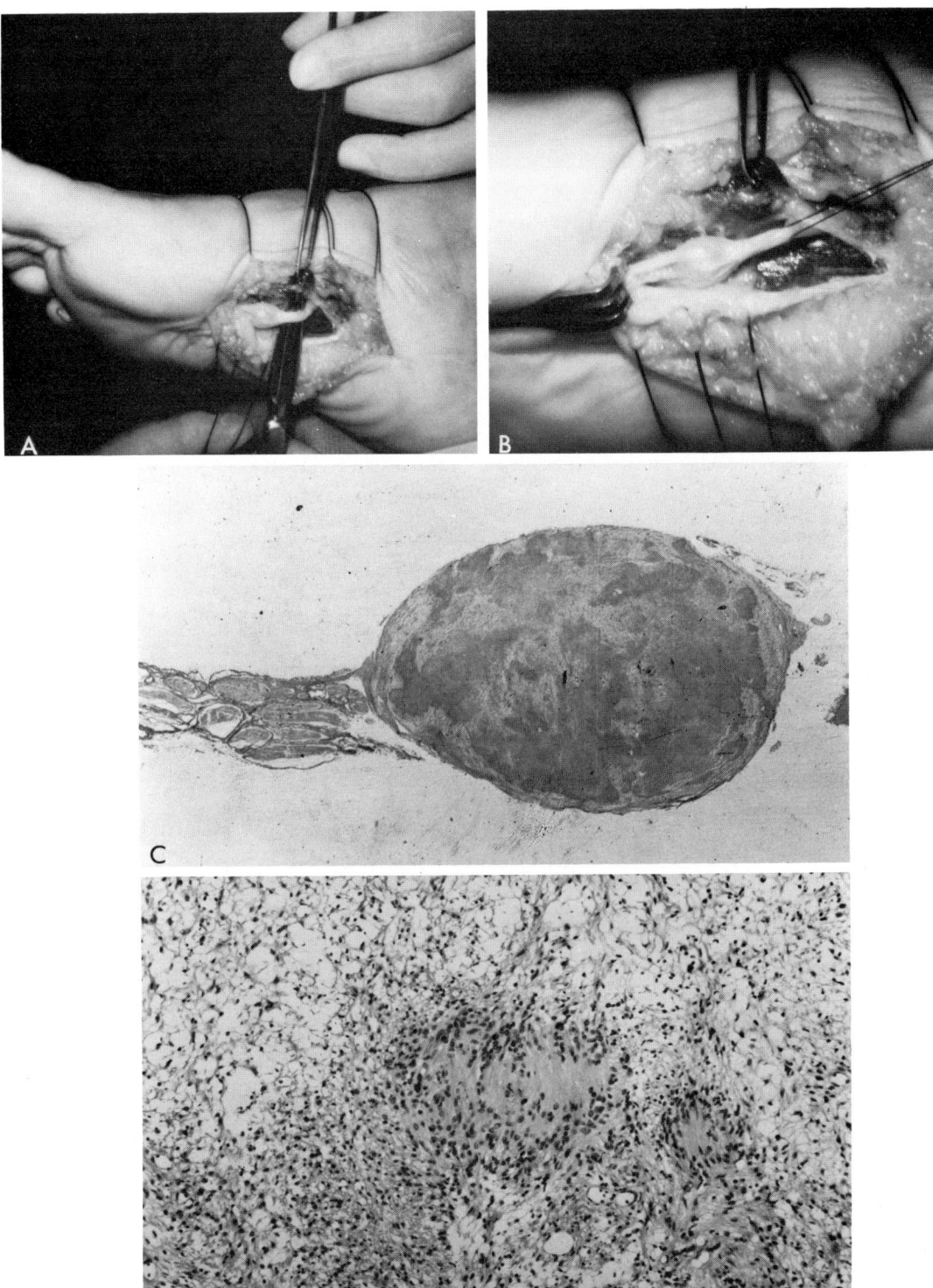

FIGURE 6–33. Solitary benign encapsulated neurilemoma of the medial plantar nerve.

A. Gross appearance in the wound. **B.** Close-up view showing the fusiform encapsulated mass. **C.** Photomicrograph of tumor (× 10). **D.** Photomicrograph showing palisading of long slender cells mixed with areas of loose reticulum cells with small nuclei (× 100). Note areas of cystic degeneration.

authors have demonstrated the presence of cytoplasmic inclusion bodies; others were unable to find them despite a thorough search.[4]

A virus is believed to be the cause of the tumor, but its presence has not been demonstrated by tissue culture.

The natural history of the tumor is local recurrence after excision, followed by slow spontaneous regression. There is no recorded case of metastasis and no reported case of persistence into adult life. Therefore, a conservative approach in management is recommended. Treatment consists of local excision with skin grafting, if necessary. The surgeon is strongly urged to refrain from amputation and impairment of the function of the part. In certain cases,

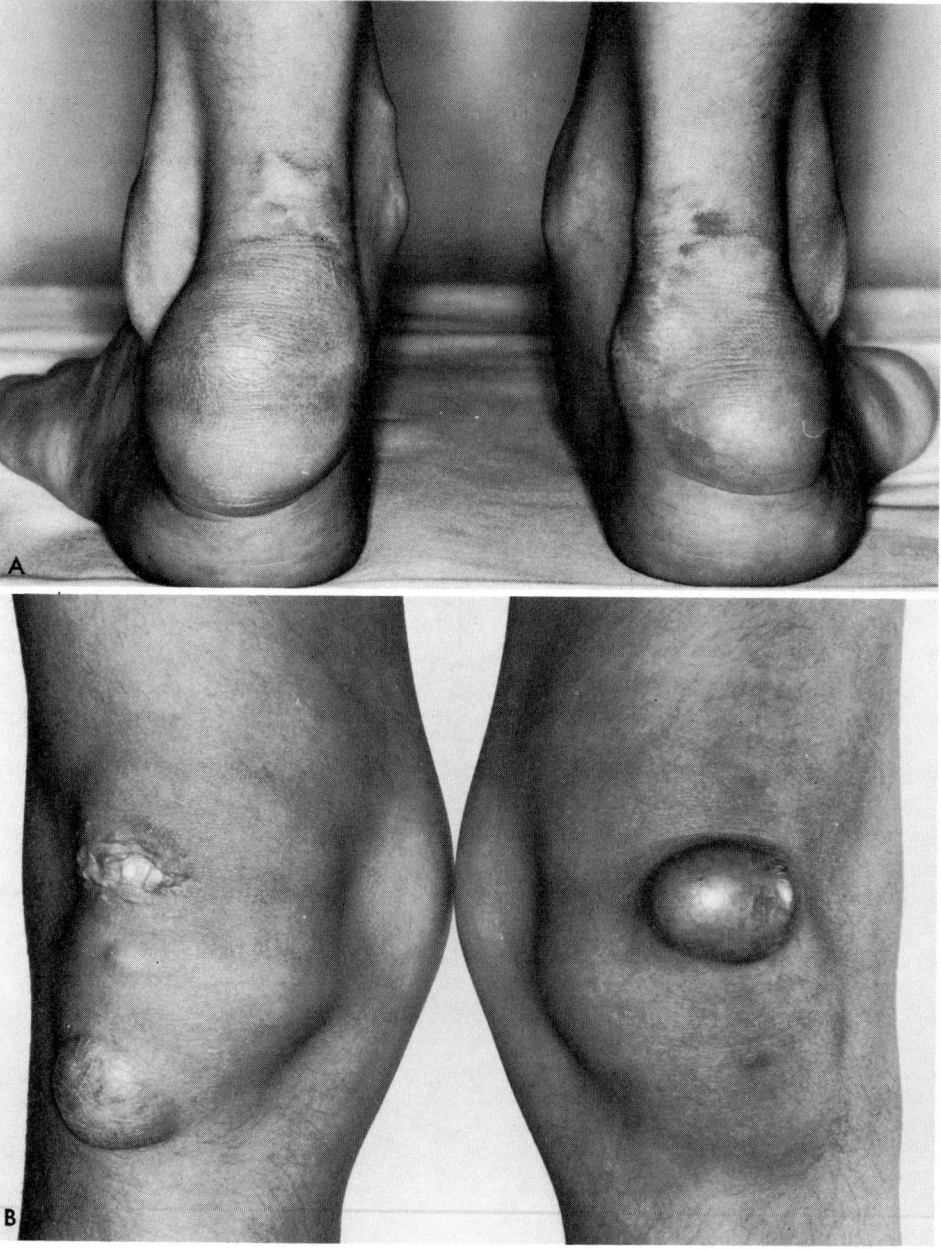

FIGURE 6–34. *Multiple xanthomatosis involving both heels and the extensor surfaces of knees.*

this calls for the establishment of a high level of confidence between parent and surgeon.

Nerve Sheath Tumors

The *benign encapsulated neurilemoma* is the most common type. In the past there has been some controversy as to its origin, but tissue culture studies favor development from the Schwann cells.[27] The tumor presents as a round or fusiform white mass within the sheath of the medial or lateral plantar nerve or in the smaller digital branches (Fig. 6–33). On palpation the tumor is firm in consistency, although occasionally it may be cystic. When located in weight-bearing areas of the foot it is painful and tender on pressure. It is usually solitary, but may be multiple.

On surgical exploration the tumor is usually well encapsulated. When the capsule is opened by a longitudinal incision it can be easily enucleated. Histologically the lesion is classified by Thorsrud into three types: in *Type I* there are a loose reticulum of cells with small nuclei and radiating fibrils with areas of cystic degeneration (Antoni B areas); in *Type II* the lesion predominantly consists of long slender cells with the nuclei arranged in a palisade fashion (Antoni A areas); *Type III* is a combination of Type I and Type II.[41]

Treatment is surgical excision; the encapsulated tumors are easy to shell out without damaging continuity of the nerve. The lesion is benign and the prognosis excellent.

Malignant neurilemomas are extremely rare in children; often they are associated with von Recklinghausen's disease.

Miscellaneous Tumors

Solitary fibroma is rare but may occur at any site in the foot and ankle; treatment is by surgical excision. Fibromatosis of plantar fascia does occur in adolescents, causing pain and disability; it is treated by excision of the plantar fascia.

Other soft-tissue tumors that may affect the foot are multiple xanthomatosis, tumoral calcinosis, and pigmented villonodular synovitis (Figs. 6–34 to 6–36). Glomus tumor is rarely found in children. Foreign body granuloma may present as a mass in the feet (Fig. 6–37).

Text continued on page 655

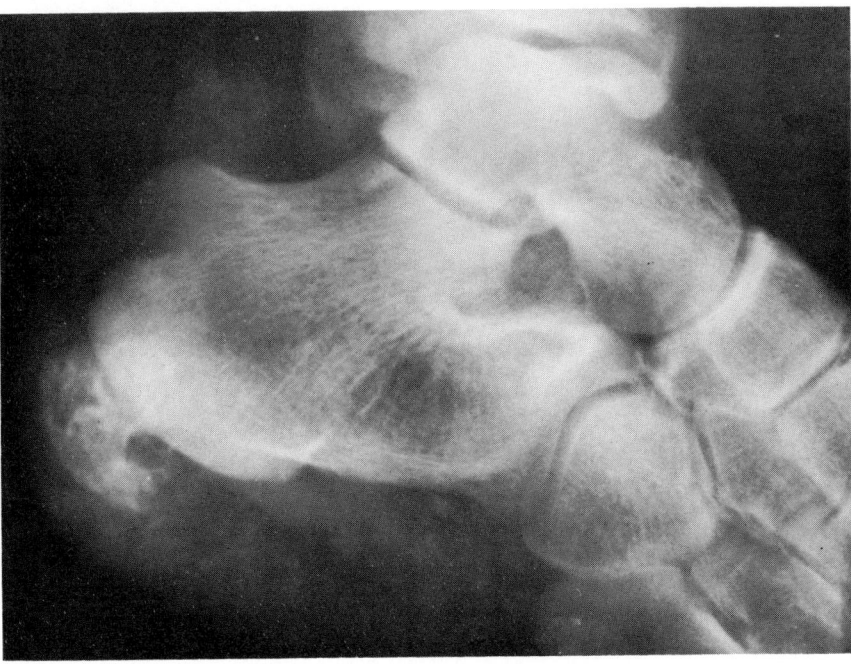

FIGURE 6–35. Tumoral calcinosis presenting as firm calcified mass in the posterior aspect of the heel.

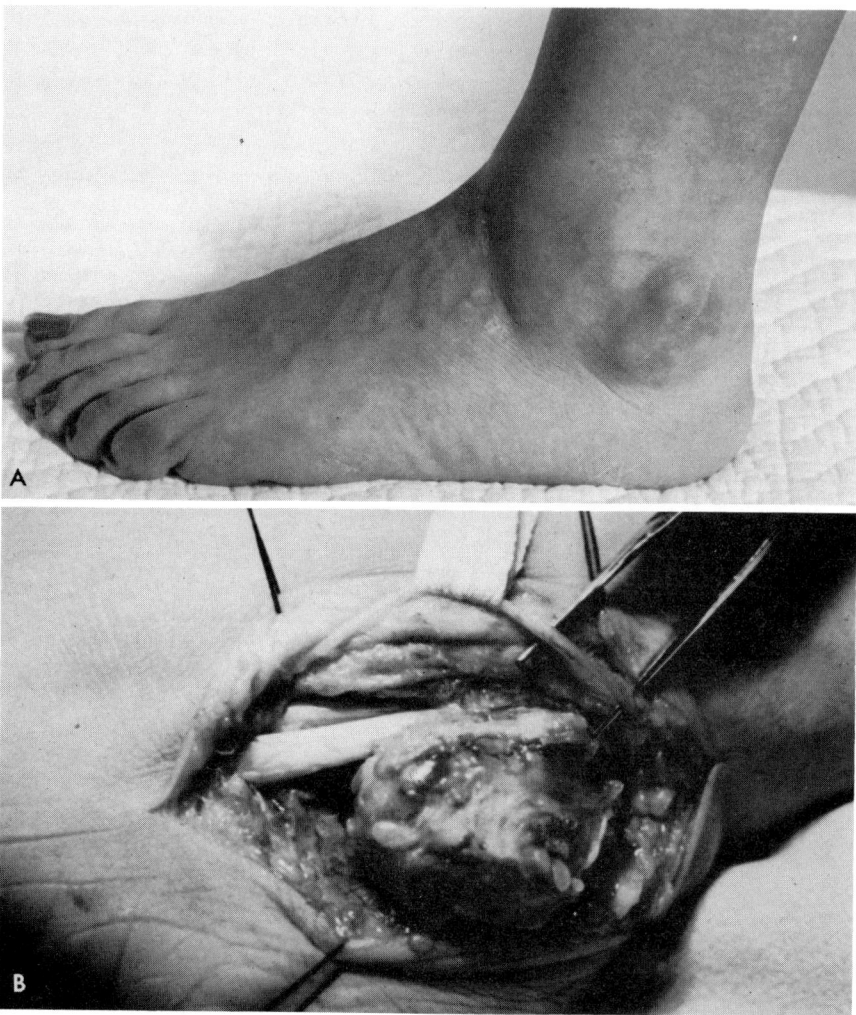

FIGURE 6–36. Pigmented villonodular synovitis of subtalar joint.
A. Photograph showing soft-tissue mass below the lateral malleolus. **B.** Gross appearance at surgery.

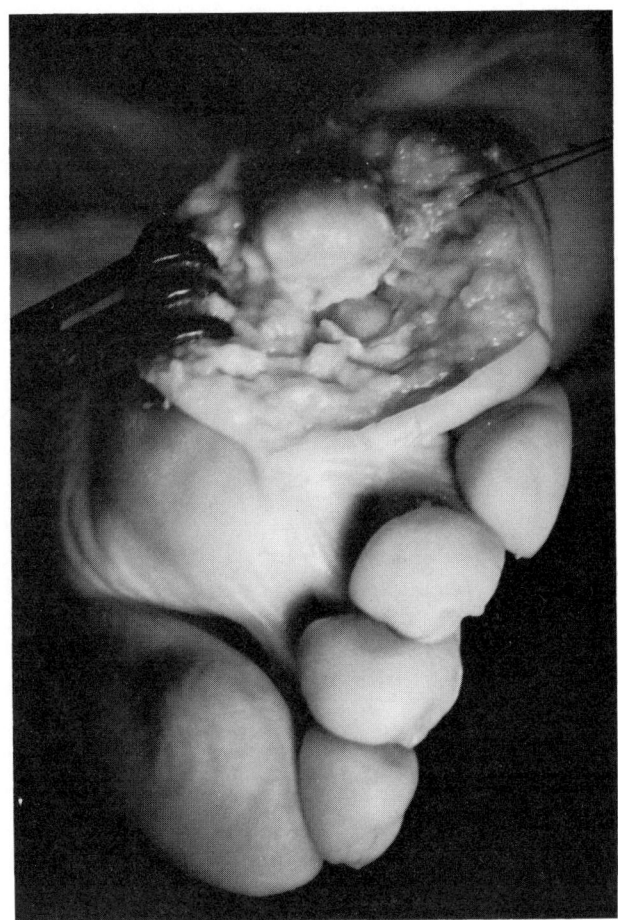

FIGURE 6–37. Foreign body granuloma in sole of foot—caused by a piece of broken glass.

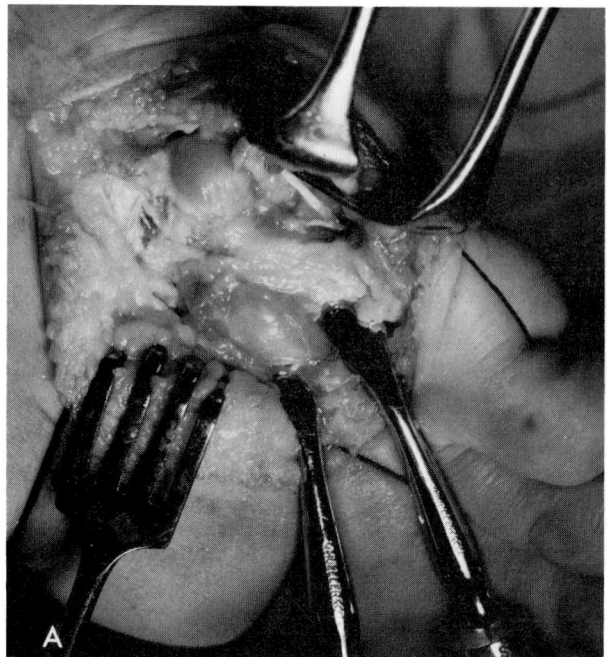

FIGURE 6–38. Synovioma in the plantar aspect of the foot.

A. Gross appearance at surgery. **B.** Photomicrograph (× 130).

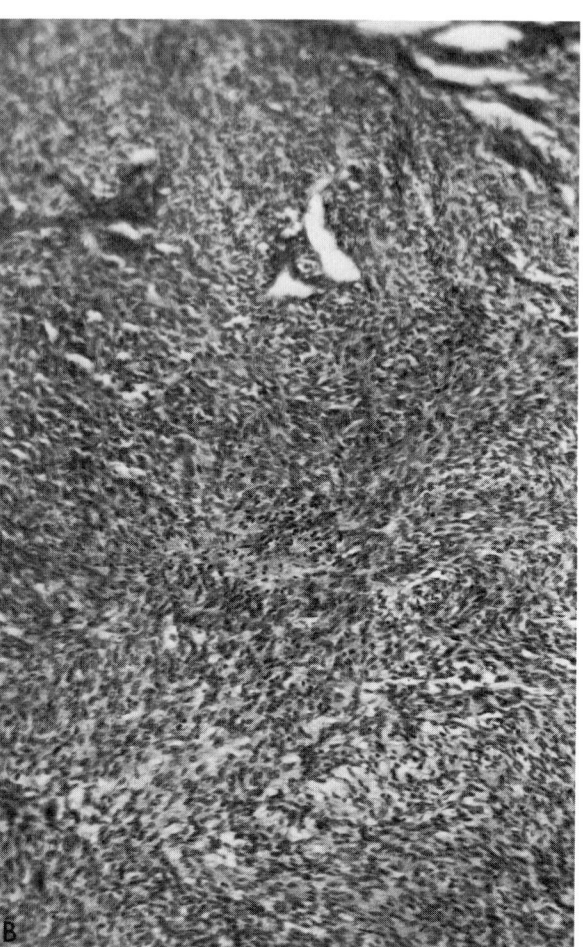

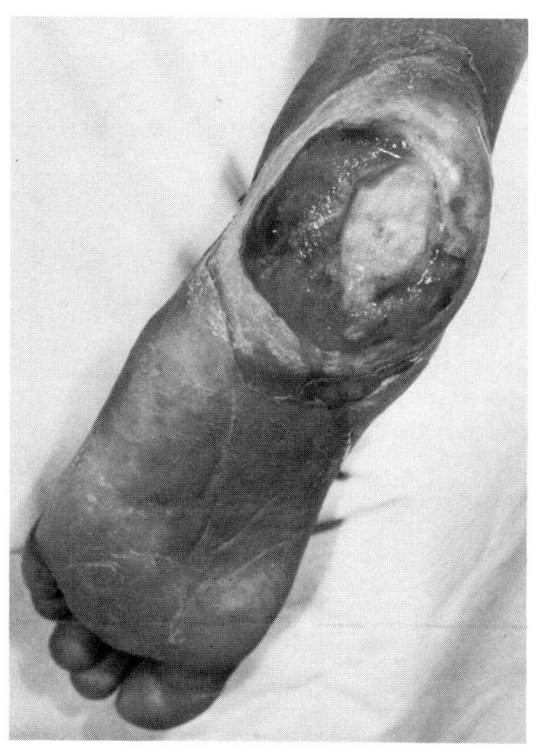

FIGURE 6–39. Fibrosarcoma of the heel.

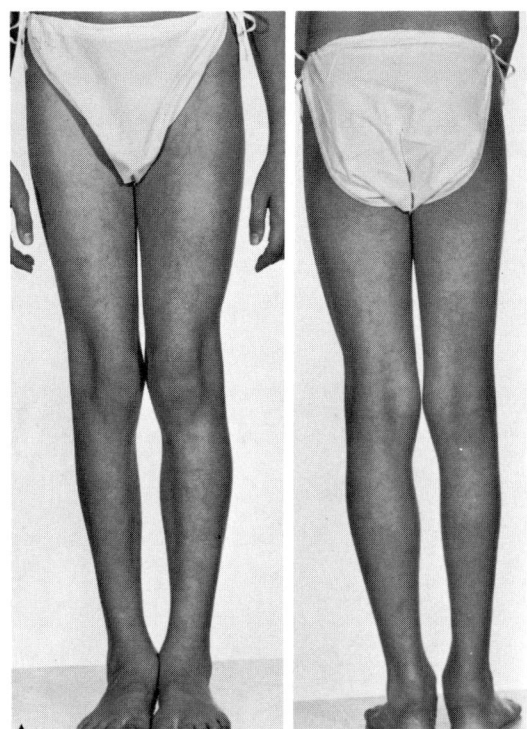

FIGURE 6–40. Osteoid osteoma of the talus.

A 12-year-old girl presented with a right antalgic limp of one year's duration. **A.** Photographs of the patient show disuse atrophy of the right leg. **B** and **C.** Roentgenograms of ankle. Note the radiolucent lesion in the superomedial area of the talus. Clinically, there was excruciating local tenderness on palpation.

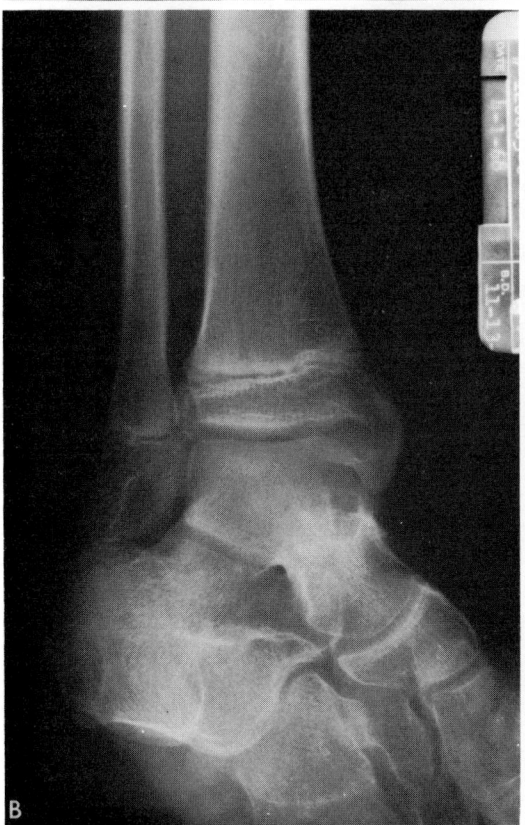
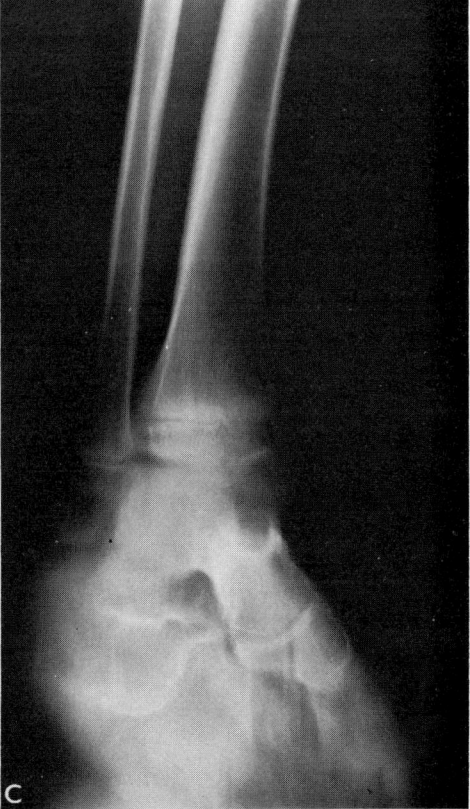

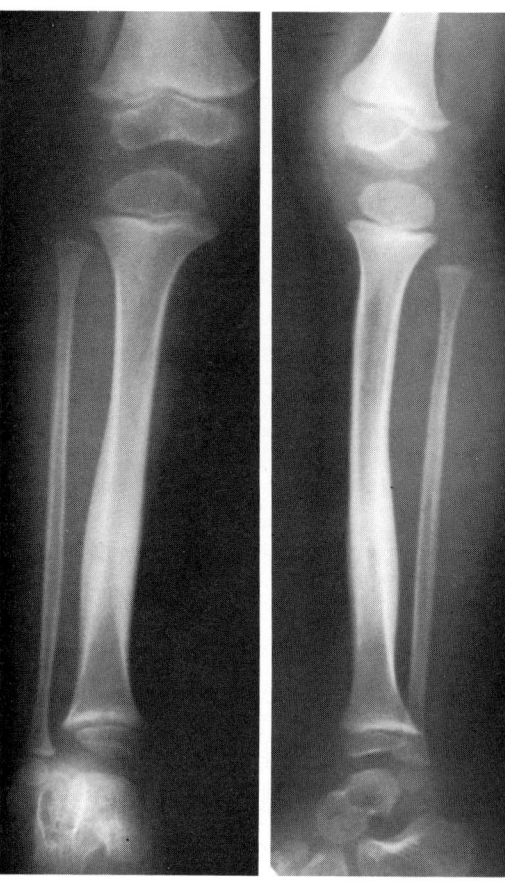

FIGURE 6–41. Osteoid osteoma of the tibia.

Roentgenograms show the extensive cortical hyperostosis, which is obscuring the intracortical nidus at the junction of the middle and distal thirds of the diaphysis.

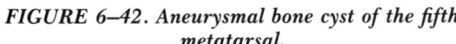

FIGURE 6–42. Aneurysmal bone cyst of the fifth metatarsal.

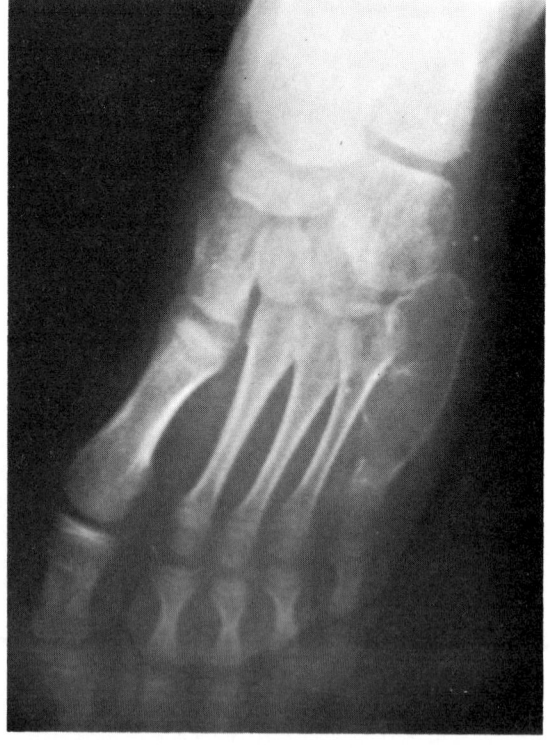

Synovioma is very rare in childhood and adolescence but can occur (Fig. 6–38). Fibrosarcoma is extremely rare (Fig. 6–39).

TUMORS OF BONE

Tumors of bone occasionally occur in the foot, involving the tarsal and metatarsal bones. Osteoid osteoma (shown in Figures 6–40 and 6–41), enchondroma, aneurysmal bone cyst (shown in Figure 6–42), unicameral bone cyst (shown in Figures 6–43 and 6–44), and multiple hereditary exostoses are some of the lesions encountered; the reader is referred to the excellent textbooks of Dahlin, Jaffe, and Lichtenstein.[9, 19, 22]

A bony tumor characteristically found in the foot is subungual exostosis. It presents as a bony growth from the dorsal surface of the distal part of the terminal phalanx of a toe, usually the great toe. A history of previous injury may be obtained in some cases; its cause, however, is unknown. The

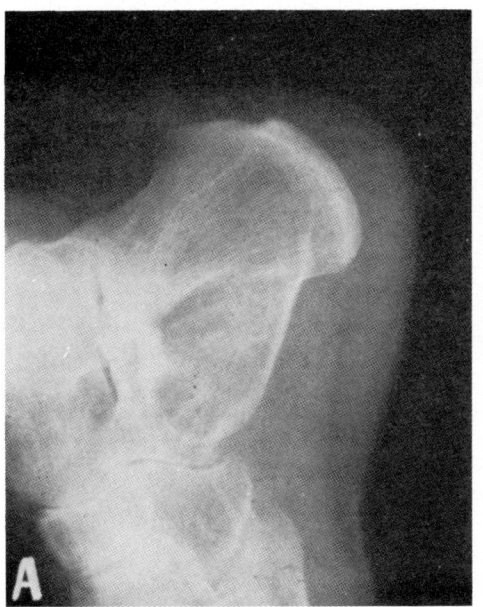
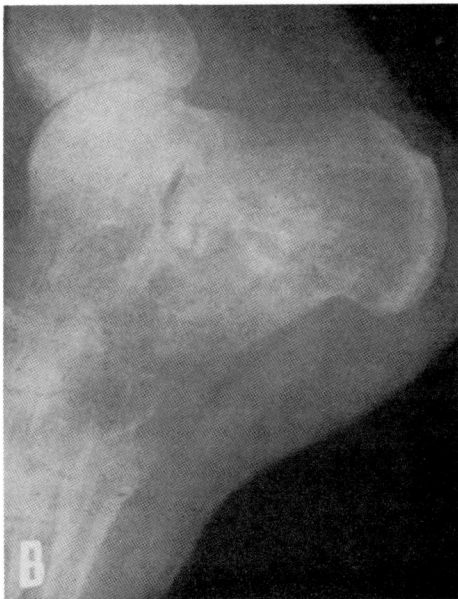
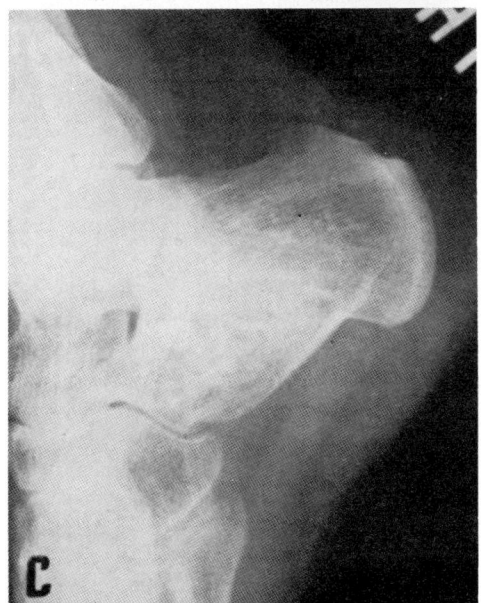

FIGURE 6–43. Roentgenograms of hindfoot showing solitary unicameral bone cyst in the calcaneus.

A. Preoperative. Note the radiolucency of the cyst. **B.** After curettage and implantation of bone chips. **C.** Five years after operation. (From Garceau, G. J., and Gregory, C. F.: Solitary unicameral bone cyst. J. Bone Joint Surg., *36-A*:267, 1954. Reprinted by permission.)

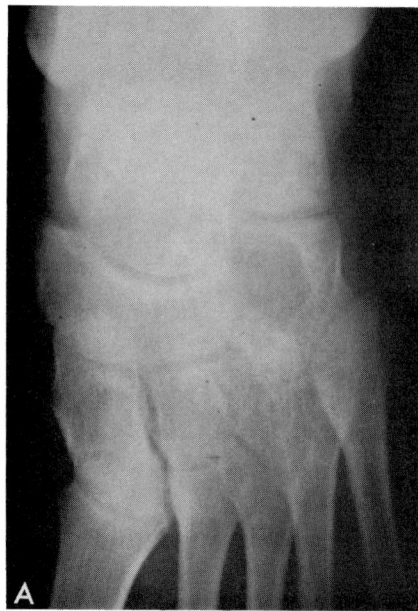
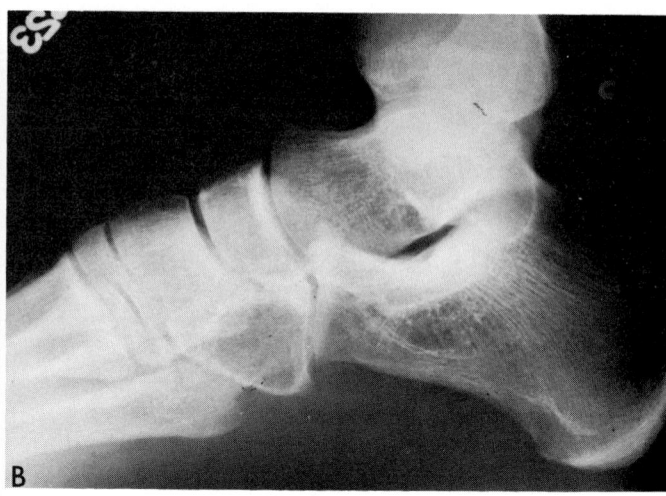

FIGURE 6–44. *Roentgenograms of the foot showing a radiolucent lesion in the cuboid.*

On biopsy, histologic findings were consistent with solitary bone cyst. **A.** Anteroposterior view. **B.** Lateral view.

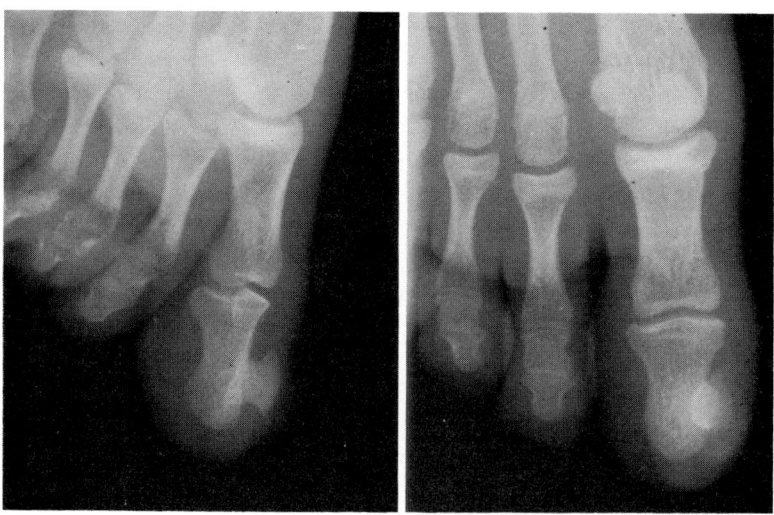

FIGURE 6–45. *Subungual exostosis of the distal phalanx of the great toe.*

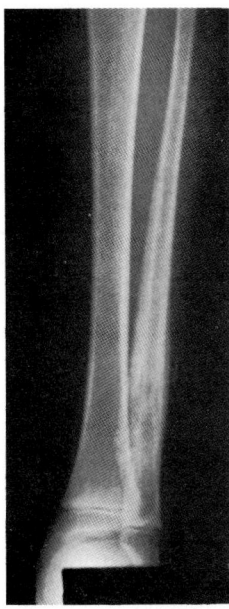

FIGURE 6–46. Osteogenic sarcoma in distal fibula of a five-and-a-half-year-old girl.

The child complained of local pain of about one month's duration. Initial roentgenogram of left leg shows a destructive lesion of the distal metaphysis of the fibula with periosteal new bone formation and soft-tissue swelling. Skeletal survey, chest roentgenograms, intravenous pyelogram, and bone marrow examination were normal. Histologic examination of biopsy tissue disclosed the tumor to be osteogenic sarcoma. A total of 5,000 r irradiation to the area was administered during a period of four weeks: 1,000 r was given before biopsy. The fibula was resected in toto, and a below-knee amputation was performed 3½ inches distal to the joint line. The child had immediate prosthetic fitting and was walking the day following the operation. Monthly follow-up roentgenograms of chest and skeletal survey were normal until ten months later, when metastatic lesions developed in left lower and right lower lobes.

condition is usually encountered in adolescents or young adults and is preponderant in females. The tumor projects upward and forward between the tip of the nail and the terminal pulp. The nail is deformed, becomes elevated, and eventually undergoes degenerative changes. The tumor is very painful, especially when pressure is applied over the nail. Diagnosis is made by demonstration of the exostosis in the roentgenogram (Fig. 6–45). It is treated by excision through a transverse incision at the distal end of the nail.

Malignant tumors of the bone in the region of the foot and ankle are very rare in childhood (Fig. 6–46).

References

1. Ahlqvist, J., Pohjanpelto, P., Hjelt, L., and Hurme, K.: Recurring digital fibrous tumor of childhood. 1. Clinical and morphological aspects of a case. Acta Path. Microbiol. Scand., 70:291, 1967.
2. Battifora, H., and Hines, J. R.: Recurrent digital fibromas of childhood. Cancer, 27:1530, 1971.
3. Bergstrand, H.: Über eine eigenartige wahrscheinlich bisher nicht beschriebene osteoblastische Krankheit in den longen Knochen der Hand und der Fusses. Acta Radiol., 11:597, 1930.
4. Bloem, J. J., Vuzevski, V. D., and Huffstadt, A. J. C.: Recurring digital fibroma of infancy. J. Bone Joint Surg., 56-B:746, 1974.
5. Boyle, W. J.: Cystic angiomatosis of bone. A report of three cases and review of the literature. J. Bone Joint Surg., 54-B:626, 1972.
6. Brown, R. C., and Ghormley, R. K.: Solitary eccentric (cortical) abscess in bone. Surgery, 14:541, 1943.
7. Burry, A. F., Kerr, J. F. R., and Pope, J. H.: Recurring digital fibrous tumour of childhood: An electron microscopic and virological study. Pathology, 2:287, 1970.
8. Cutler, E. C., and Gross, R. E.: The surgical treatment of tumors of peripheral nerves. Ann. Surg., 104:436, 1936.
9. Dahlin, D. C.: Bone Tumors. 3rd Ed. Springfield, Ill., Charles C Thomas, 1978.
10. Enneking, W. F.: Clinical Musculoskeletal Pathology. Gainesville, Fla., Storter Printing, 1977.
11. Glynn, J. J., and Lichtenstein, L.: Osteoid-osteoma with multicentric nidus. A report of two cases. J. Bone Joint Surg., 55-A:855, 1973.
12. Golding, J. S. R.: The natural history of osteoid osteoma. J. Bone Joint Surg., 36-B:218, 1954.
12a. Gould, N.: Articular osteoid osteoma of the talus: A case report. Foot Ankle, 1:284, 1981.
13. Grunnet, N., Genner, J., Mogensen, B., and Myhre-Jensen, O.: Recurring digital fibrous tumour of childhood. Acta Path. Microbiol. Scand., Section A, 81:167, 1973.
14. Heiple, K., Perrin, E., and Aikawa, M.: Congenital generalized fibromatosis. A case limited to osseous lesions. J. Bone Joint Surg., 54-A:663, 1972.
15. Huvos, A. G.: Bone Tumors: Diagnosis, Treatment, Prognosis. Philadelphia, W. B. Saunders Co., 1979.
16. Kauffman, S. L., and Stout, A. P.: Histiocytic tumors (fibrous xanthoma and histiocytoma) in children. Cancer, 14:469, 1961.
17. Keller, R. B., and Baez-Giangreco, A.: Juvenile aponeurotic fibroma. Report of three cases and review of the literature. Clin. Orthop., 106:198, 1975.
18. Jaffe, H. L.: Osteoid osteoma. A benign osteoblastic tumor composed of osteoid and atypical bone. Arch. Surg. (Chicago), 31:709, 1935.
19. Jaffe, H. L.: Tumors and Tumorous Conditions of the Bones and Joints. Philadelphia, Lea & Febiger, 1958.
20. Jaffe, H. L., and Lichtenstein, L.: Osteoid-osteoma: Further experience with this benign tumour of bone. J. Bone Joint Surg., 22:645, 1940.
21. Jensen, A. R., Martin, L. W., and Longino, L. A.: Digital neurofibrosarcoma in infancy. J. Pediat., 51:566, 1957.
22. Lichtenstein, L.: Bone Tumors. 5th Ed. St. Louis, C. V. Mosby Co., 1977.
23. Lichtenstein, L., and Goldman, R. L.: Cartilage tumors in soft tissues, particularly in the hand and foot. Cancer, 17:1203, 1964.
24. Lichtenstein, L., and Goldman, R. L.: The cartilage analogue of fibromatosis. A reinterpretation of the condition called "juvenile aponeurotic fibroma." Cancer, 17:810, 1964.
25. Lindbom, A., Lindvall, N., Soderberg, G., and Spjut, H.: Angiography in osteoid osteoma. Acta Radiol., 54:327, 1960.
26. Moberg, E.: The natural course of osteoid osteoma. J. Bone Joint Surg., 33-A:166, 1951.
27. Murray, M. R., and Stout, A. P.: Schwann cell versus fibroblast as the origin of the specific nerve sheath tumor. Amer. J. Path., 16:41, 1940.
28. Norman, A., and Dorfman, H. D.: Osteoid-osteoma inducing pronounced overgrowth and deformity of bone. Clin. Orthop., 110:233, 1975.
29. Pohjanpelto, P., Ahlqvist, J., Hurme, K., and Hjelt, L.: Recurring digital fibrous tumor of childhood. 2. Isolation

of a cell transforming agent. Acta Path. Microbiol. Scand., 70:297, 1967.
30. Posch, J. L.: Tumors of the hand. J. Bone Joint Surg., 38-A:517, 1956.
31. Quick, D., and Cutler, M.: Neurogenic sarcoma. Ann. Surg., 86:810, 1927.
32. Reye, R. D. K.: Recurring digital fibrous tumors of childhood. Arch. Path. (Chicago), 80:228, 1965.
33. Schaffzin, E. A., Chung, S. M. K., and Kaye, R.: Congenital generalized fibromatosis with complete spontaneous regression. A case report. J. Bone Joint Surg., 54-A:657, 1973.
34. Schajowicz, F., Aiello, C. L., Francone, M. V., and Giannini, R. E.: Cystic angiomatosis (hamartous haemolymphangiomatoisis) of bone. A clinicopathological study of three cases. J. Bone Joint Surg., 60-B:100, 1978.
35. Shapiro, L.: Infantile digital fibromatosis and aponeurotic fibroma. Arch. Derm. (Chicago), 99:37, 1969.
36. Sim, F. J., Dahlin, D. C., and Beabout, J. W.: Osteoid-osteoma: Diagnostic problems. J. Bone Joint Surg., 57-A:154, 1975.
37. Soren, A.: Pathogenesis and treatment of ganglion. Clin. Orthop., 48:173, 1966.
38. Spjut, H. J., Dorfman, H. D., Fechner, R. E., and Ackerman, L. V.: Tumors of Bone and Cartilage. Washington, D.C., Armed Forces Institute of Pathology, 1971.
39. Stout, A. P.: Juvenile fibromatoses. Cancer, 7:953, 1954.
40. Stout, A. P., and Lattes, R.: Tumors of the Soft Tissues. Washington, D.C., Armed Forces Institute of Pathology, 1967.
41. Thorsrud, G.: Neurinoma. Acta Chir. Scand., Suppl. 252:3–38, 1960.

Skin and Nail Lesions

The skin of the foot responds to the stress of body weight and to external pressure from the shoes. The *epidermis,* the outermost layer of the skin, is an epithelial tissue derived from ectoderm; the *dermis,* the subjacent deeper layer, is of mesodermal origin and consists of dense connective tissue. In the sole of the foot, the epidermis is very thick. In the embryo, the nails first appear in the third lunar month as invasions of epidermis into the subjacent dermis over the distal ends of the toes. This epidermal plate forms the matrix of the nail from which the epidermal cells proliferate and gradually become transformed into hard keratinous nail tissue that is pushed distally over the nail bed. The matrix of the nail, extending from its root to the crescentic whitish lunula, is the only site where longitudinal growth of the nail takes place, normal growth being about 1 mm. per week. If the matrix of the nail is destroyed, longitudinal growth of the nail will be arrested, and instead of a hard smooth nail appendage, the nail bed will be covered with irregular, corrugated, horny tissue.

The skin and nails are affected by a great variety of lesions; only the commoner ones are briefly discussed here. More extensive details are given in general textbooks of dermatology and the cited references.

HARD CORN (Clavus Durus)

A hard corn is a localized cornification of the skin resulting from shoe pressure on a bony prominence. It is most commonly seen over the dorsolateral aspect of the proximal interphalangeal joint of the fifth toe and over the tip of a flexed toe close to its nail. In the central area of the corn there is a deeply penetrating nucleus of hyperkeratosis that is partly degenerated. Beneath this hyperkeratotic central nucleus, there may be a sac containing fluid; irritation and inflammation of this sac and consequent pressure on the nerve endings in the papillary layer of the dermis are the cause of pain.

The immediate cause of the corn must be corrected to eliminate the possibility of recurrence; it may be a badly fitted shoe, deformed toes, or excessive use of the feet. The keratinized skin is softened with preparations containing salicylic acid; the horny layer and central nucleus will then eventually separate and fall away. Occasionally surgical excision of deep-rooted corns is required; this should be done under strict aseptic conditions to prevent infection.

SOFT CORN (Clavus Mollis)

Soft corns are rare in children. They usually occur between the toes, the most frequent sites being the fourth and fifth toes, where they are caused by bony pressure from a small exostosis on the lateral aspect of the base of the proximal phalanx of the fourth toe. They are soft, of whitish appearance, and have a depressed central area (Fig. 6–47).

The condition is painful and disabling. Treatment consists of excision of the interdigital clavus, resection of the exostosis or the proximal half of the proximal phalanx

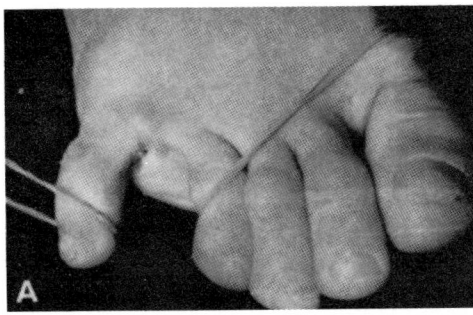 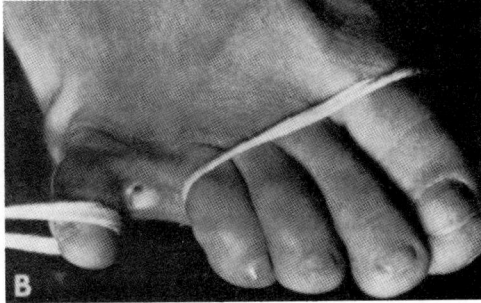

FIGURE 6–47. Two cases of interdigital soft corn.

(From Kelikian, H.: Hallux Valgus, Allied Deformities of the Forefoot and Metatarsalgia. Philadelphia, W. B. Saunders Co., 1965, p. 290. Reprinted by permission.)

of the fourth toe, or surgical syndactylism of the fourth and fifth toes.

PLANTAR WART (Verruca Plantaris)

These are very common in children and may be found on any part of the plantar aspect of the foot, on either weight-bearing or non-weight-bearing surfaces. Frequent sites are the heel, under the metatarsal heads, and the big toe. They may be single or may be surrounded by a whole crop of daughter warts, their size ranging from a few millimeters to two or three centimeters. A multitude of tiny warts may conglomerate into a large "mosaic wart." Plantar warts are infectious and may be transferred from one child to another by direct contact or indirectly by agents such as bath mats. Epidemics have been known to occur in schools.

Anatomically, a plantar wart is a papillomatous growth, but instead of projecting beyond the skin surface (like warts elsewhere), they are buried under the stratum corneum of the skin, with only the ends of the papillae showing through. They are extremely vascular and bleed profusely when trimmed. Plantar warts have a dark, punctate surface and are clearly demarcated from the surrounding skin. On direct pressure and lateral compression of the skin, the lesion is markedly tender.

Treatment

In children, a conservative approach is advised. Small lesions can be ignored, but if they are especially painful, the area is padded to relieve pressure of body weight on the wart. Larger or persistent lesions are destroyed by a caustic or keratolytic agent. Lapidus recommends applying 50 per cent salicylic acid ointment, covering the entire area of the wart with 40 per cent salicylic acid plaster (manufactured by Duke Laboratories, Inc.), and strapping it with adhesive tape. In three or four days, the dressing is removed and the foot is re-examined. The keratolytic medication may not be tolerated by some children and may produce irritation and aggravate the pain, in which case the dressing is removed and the foot is soaked in pHisoHex solution and zinc oxide ointment is applied. Most patients do tolerate the salicylic acid ointment. At weekly intervals the macerated skin is debrided, bleeding vessels are cauterized with silver nitrate stick, and again salicylic acid ointment and plaster are applied. Intractable plantar warts, particularly the mosaic warts, may require several weeks of treatment before being cured. Parents should be advised of the stubborn nature of the condition.[1]

Electrocoagulation of the plantar wart under local infiltration anesthesia may result in an intractable ulcer; it should be performed in only a few selected cases. Excision of the lesion may result in a disabling postoperative scar and is not recommended. Irradiation is contraindicated, as it may cause chronic indolent ulceration.

Reference

1. Lapidus, P. W.: Orthopedic skin lesions of the soles and the toes. Clin. Orthop., *45*:87, 1966.

INGROWING TOENAIL

Ingrowing toenail most commonly involves the great toe. It is caused by external pressure from tight shoes or hose on an improperly trimmed nail that has been cut too short so that its corners dig into the pulp. The edges of the nail become thickened and press into the neighboring soft tissues, which respond by hypertrophy. Soon the overgrown soft tissues obliterate the medial or lateral nail groove. This mechanical irritation is followed by infection of the skin fold. Pus then spreads around the edge of the nail and between the nail and the matrix, the great toe becoming red, swollen, locally tender, and painful.

Conservative treatment is indicated in mild and early cases. A pledget of cotton or gauze soaked in an antiseptic (such as aqueous Zephiran) is tucked beneath the corner of the nail so that it does not dig into the skin. This is done once or twice a day; then the nail is allowed to grow until its edges project beyond the skin folds. Local hot soaks may be used three or four times a day or continuously, depending upon the severity of infection. The toenails should subsequently be cut with square corners and the child should be fitted with proper shoes and socks to prevent recurrence.

Surgery is indicated in long-standing cases or when conservative measures have failed, the simplest method being excision of a wedge of nail bed together with the margin of skin fold. In very severe or recurrent cases, permanent ablation of the nail by excision of the nail bed is indicated.

Fractures and Dislocations

FRACTURES OF THE ANKLE

The ossific nucleus of the distal tibial epiphysis appears between six and ten months of life. The medial malleolus ossifies as a downward prolongation from the main nucleus, appearing at the age of seven years in girls and eight years in boys (Fig. 6–48). Occasionally the medial malleolus develops from a separate center of ossification; this should not be mistaken for a fracture. By 14 or 15 years of age, the entire lower end of the tibia (including the medial malleolus) is completely ossified; it unites with the diaphysis at about the eighteenth year. The lower epiphysis contributes to 45 per cent of the growth of the tibia.

The distal epiphysis of the fibula begins to ossify during the second year of life, usually between the ages of 18 and 20 months. Occasionally its ossification may be delayed until the end of the third year. Union with the diaphysis occurs around the twentieth year.

Fractures involving the lower tibial epiphyseal plate constitute 11 per cent of all physeal injuries. They are more common in boys, who account for about 80 per cent of the cases. The common age of incidence ranges from 11 to 15 years, the median ages being 14 years in males and 12 years in females.

Fractures involving the distal fibular physis may occur alone or in association with those of the distal tibial physis. They usually take place in the age range of 8 to 15 years.

Classification and Mechanism of Injury

The ankle is a true mortise joint that moves in only one plane—into plantar flexion and dorsiflexion—and is stable and distinctly limited in all other planes. This shape of the ankle joint renders the distal tibial epiphysis particularly vulnerable to crushing injuries.

All the ligaments of the ankle are attached to the distal epiphyses of the tibia and fibula. Ligamentous injuries are rare in children because the ligaments are stronger than the growth plate, and tension on them will cause fracture separation of the physis.

The tibia and fibula are bound together by the interosseous membrane. In adduction-inversion injuries, fracture through both physes may take place and the distal epiphyses of the tibia and fibula will move

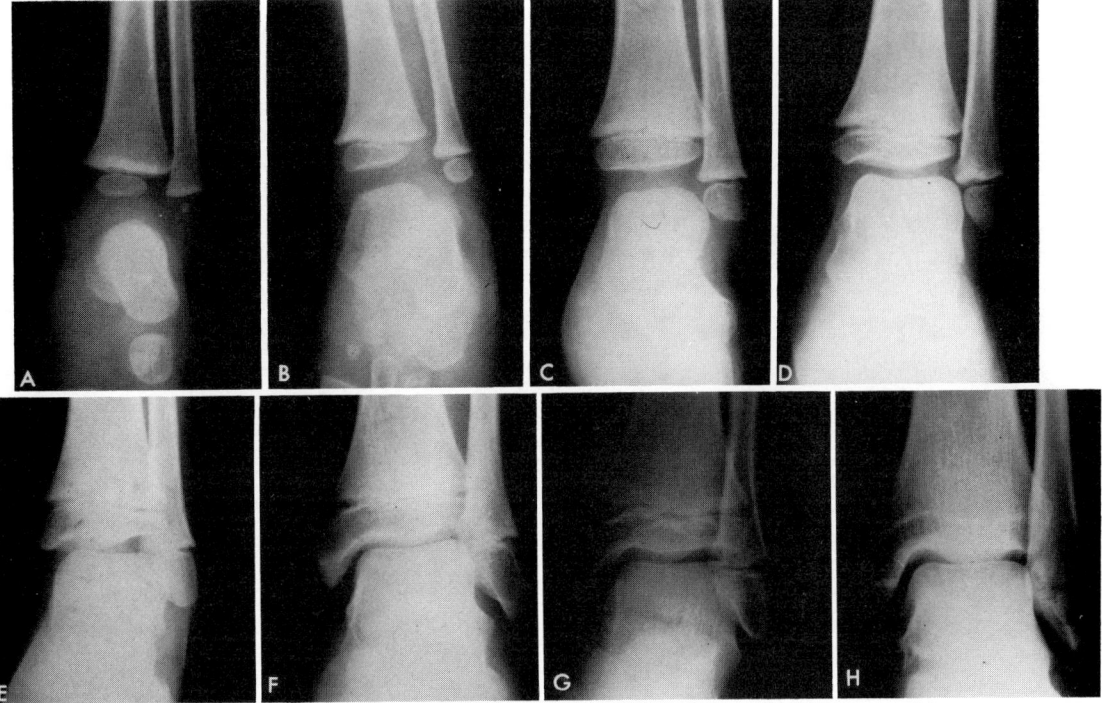

FIGURE 6–48. Ossification of distal epiphyses of tibia and fibula.

A. One year of age. **B.** Two years. **C.** Four years. **D.** Six years. **E.** Seven years. **F.** Ten years. **G.** Twelve years. **H.** Adult.

as a unit, as shown in Figure 6–49; or only the distal fibular physis may separate, and the talus will shift medially to impinge on the medial malleolus and the medial corner of the weight-bearing articular surface of the tibia, resulting in the intra-articular fracture (Fig. 6–49B). The lower fibular physis lies farther distal than that of the tibia. When the distal tibial epiphysis moves laterally it impinges on the metaphysis of the fibula and causes a fracture of the fibula at a higher level. Occasionally the interosseous membrane will rupture (Fig. 6–49C).

ANATOMIC CLASSIFICATIONS

Poland believed it difficult to classify injuries of the ankle on a mechanistic basis. He proposed an anatomic subdivision of the fractures involving the physis into the following types: *Type A*, pure and complete separation; *Type B*, partial separation with fracture of the diaphysis; *Type C*, partial separation with fracture of the epiphysis; and *Type D*, complete separation with fracture of the epiphysis (Fig. 6–50).[53]

Aitken designated three types of fractures involving the epiphyseal cartilage plate as: *Type I*, an avulsion type of fracture due to shearing or twisting force in which the fracture line passes through the zone of degenerating cartilage cells and emerges through a portion of the metaphyseal bone. Displacement in this type of fracture may be marked, but ultimate deformity due to displacement or growth disturbance is rare. *Type II*, a compression type of fracture caused by a combination of crushing and shearing force, commonly involves the distal tibial epiphysis, but rarely the distal femoral epiphysis. The line of fracture originates in the joint and may emerge between the bony epiphysis and the zone of the degenerative cartilage cells of the physis; or the fracture line may cross the physis and emerge between it and the diaphysis. In the former, growth will not be disturbed, but in the latter, a premature arrest of growth and deformity will follow. *Type III* is a compression type of injury in which the physis has been crushed between the bony epiphysis and the diaphysis. In this type, the fracture

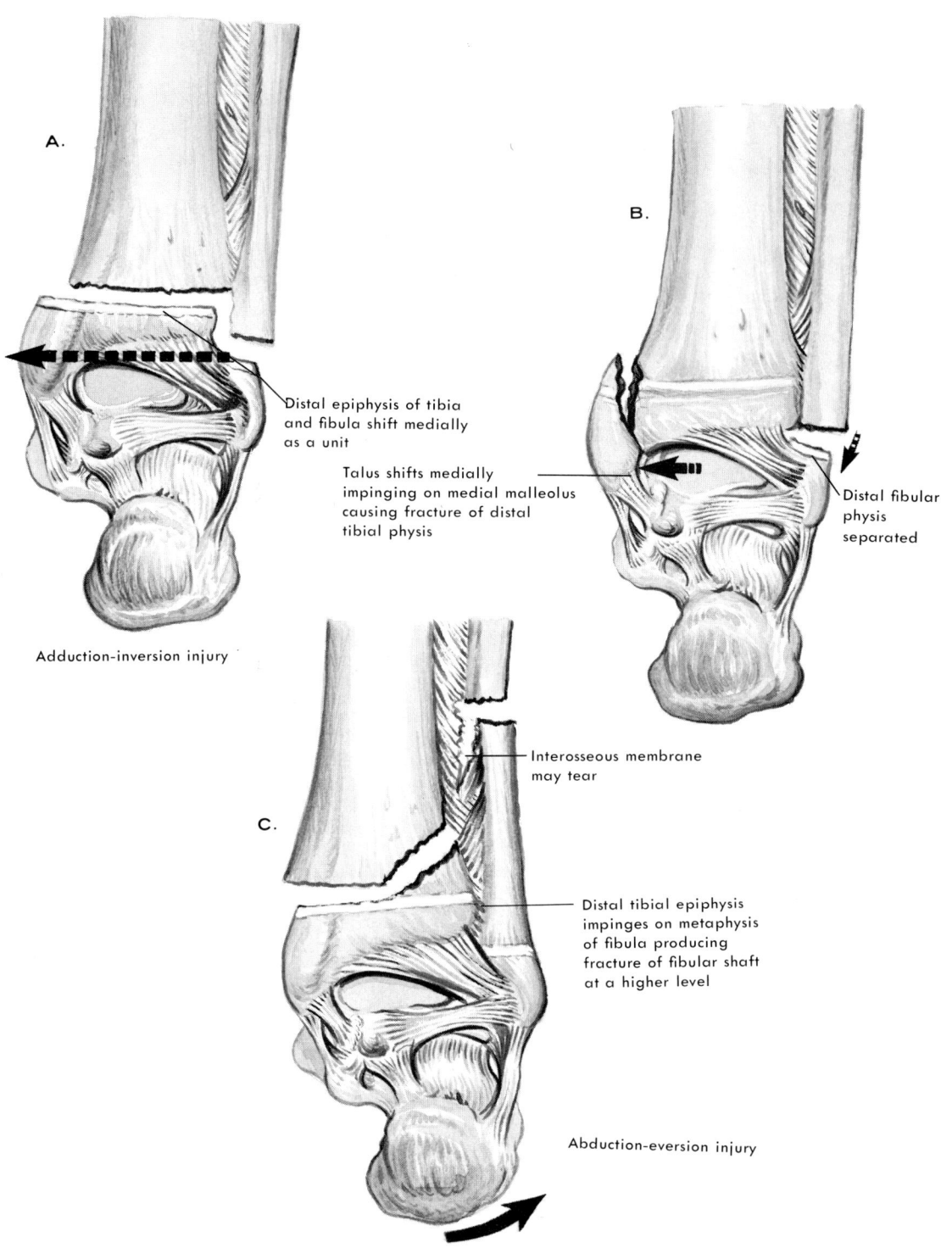

FIGURE 6–49. *Diagram of the ankle showing that all the ligaments of the ankle are attached to the distal epiphyses of the tibia and fibula.*

The lower physis of the fibula lies more distal than that of the tibia. The fibula and tibia are bound together by the interosseous membrane. **A** and **B.** On adduction-inversion injury, the distal epiphyses of the tibia and fibula may shift medially as a unit or the distal fibular physis may separate and the talus shift medially, impinging on the medial malleolus or the medial corner of the weight-bearing articular surface of the tibia and causing a Salter-Harris Type III or IV fracture of the distal tibial epiphysis. **C.** On abduction-eversion injuries the distal epiphysis of the tibia impinges on the metaphysis of the fibula, producing a fracture of the fibular shaft at a higher level; occasionally the interosseous membrane may tear.

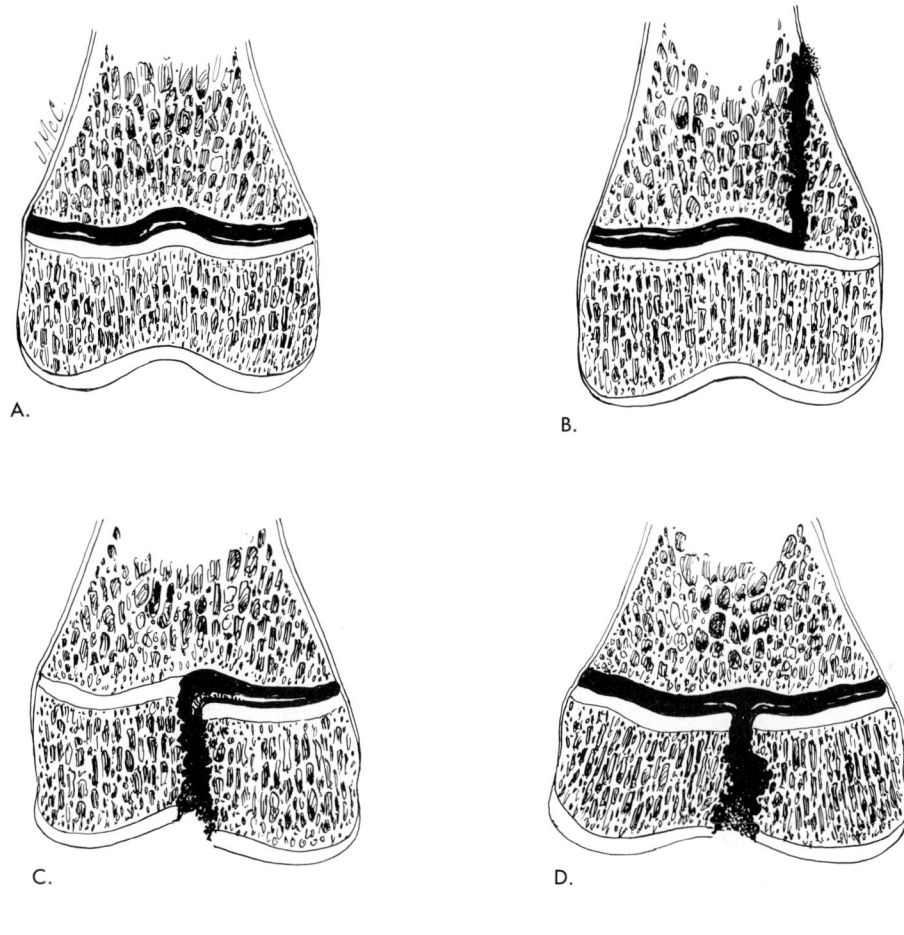

Partial   Complete

FIGURE 6–50. Poland's classification of epiphyseal separation.

A. Pure and complete separation. **B.** Partial separation with fracture of the diaphysis. **C.** Partial separation with fracture of the epiphysis. **D.** Complete separation with fracture of the epiphysis. (Redrawn after Poland, J.: Traumatic separation of the epiphysis. London, Smith, Elder & Co., 1898, p. 80.)

line may be so small as to be overlooked or may be considered of no clinical importance.[1]

Salter and Harris presented the following thorough and practical classification of physeal injuries, based on the mechanism of injury, the relationship of the fracture line to the germinal layer of the physis, and the prognosis concerning disturbance of growth.

Type I. This is produced by a shearing or avulsion force and is commonly encountered in infants whose physes are relatively thick. It may also occur in pathologic fractures such as those seen in rickets, scurvy, or osteomyelitis. The epiphysis separates from the metaphysis without any bony fragment, and the plane of cleavage is through the zone of the hypertrophic cells, with the germinal cells of the physis remaining with the epiphysis (Fig. 6–51A). Displacement of fragments is checked by the intact thick periosteal attachments. Reduction is usually unnecessary. Growth is not disturbed, unless there is associated aseptic necrosis and premature closure of the physis due to interruption of its blood supply as, for example, in acute traumatic separation of the capital femoral epiphysis.

Type II. A shearing or avulsion force causes this fracture, which is the commonest type of physeal injury. It frequently occurs

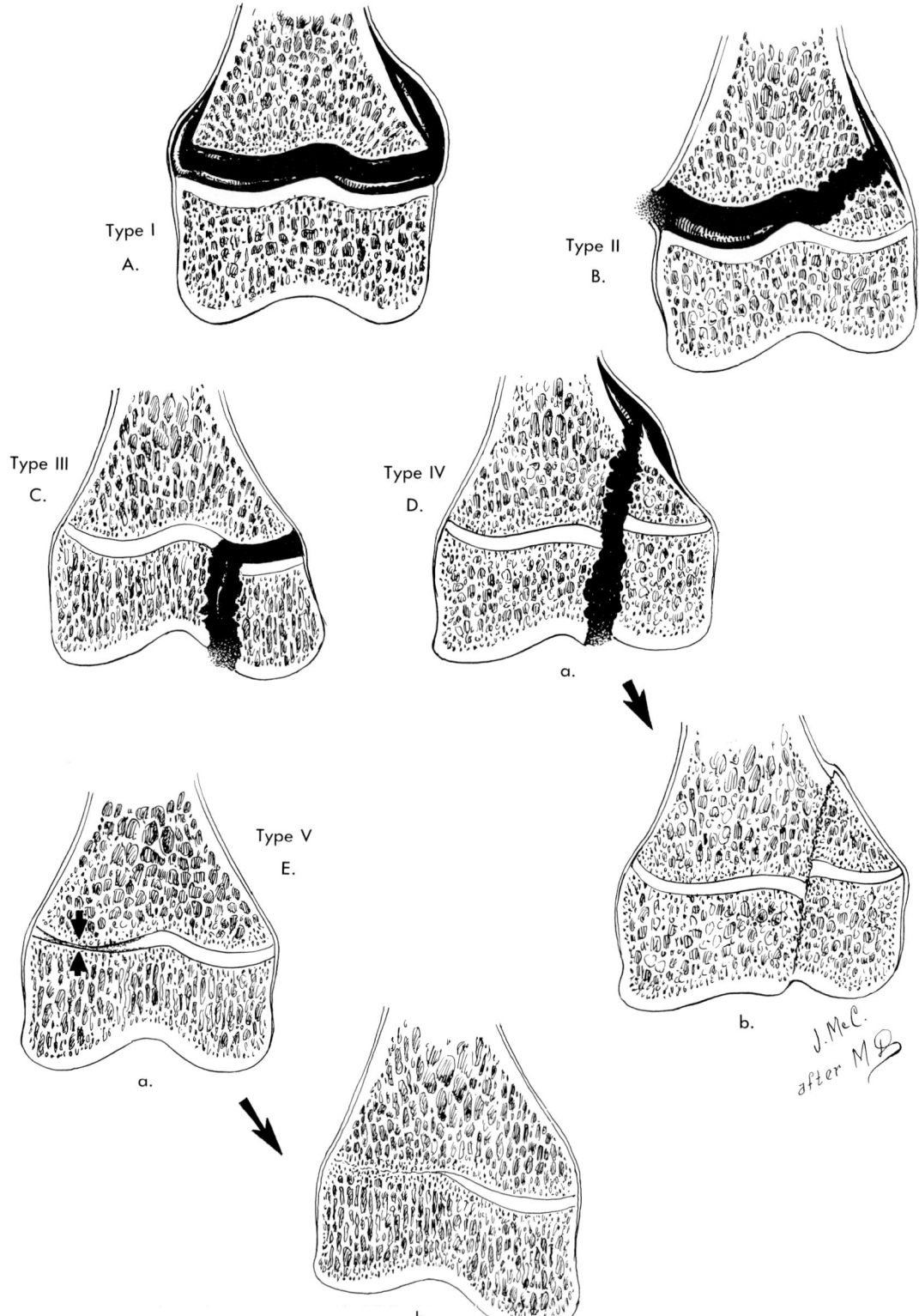

FIGURE 6–51. *Classification of epiphyseal plate injuries according to Salter and Harris.*

(Redrawn after Salter, R. B., and Harris, W. R.: Injuries involving the epiphyseal plate. J. Bone Joint Surg., 45-A:587, 1963.)

in children over ten years of age. The line of separation extends along the hypertrophic zone of the physis for a variable distance and then out through a portion of the metaphyseal bone (Fig. 6–51B). In the roentgenogram, a triangular metaphyseal fragment is readily visible, which is referred to as Thurston Holland's sign. The periosteum is intact on the concave side of the angulation (i.e., the side with the metaphyseal fragment), whereas on the convex side the periosteum is stripped and torn from the diaphysis but still remains attached to the epiphysis. This is accounted for by the thickness, the great vascularity, and the loose connection of the periosteum with the diaphysis, and the intimate connection of the periosteum with the perichondrium of the epiphysis. In Type II physeal injury, reduction is ordinarily achieved and maintained with relative ease. The intact periosteal hinge on the concave side and the metaphyseal bone fragment prevent overreduction. Growth is not disturbed, as the germinal layer of chondrocytes remains attached to the epiphysis and circulation to the epiphysis is not interrupted.

Type III. This rare injury is caused by an intra-articular shearing force, which usually occurs in the proximal or distal tibial epiphysis. There is an intra-articular fracture of the epiphysis in which the plane of cleavage extends from the joint surface to the weak zone of hypertrophic cells of the physis and then parallel with the growth plate to its periphery (Fig. 6–51C). Restoration of the congruous articular surface is essential in its treatment; in markedly displaced fractures, open surgery is often necessary to obtain accurate anatomic reduction. Prognosis for future growth is good, provided there is no impairment of circulation to the separated fragment of the epiphysis.

Type IV. This injury is most commonly seen at the lower end of the humerus in fractures of the lateral condyle. The fracture line begins at the articular surface and extends through the epiphysis, across the full thickness of the physis, and then through a segment of the metaphysis. There is a complete vertical split that involves the important germinal layer of the physis (Fig. 6–51D). The fracture fragments may be undisplaced or separated to a varying extent. It is imperative to achieve perfect anatomic reduction in order to restore a smooth articular surface and also to prevent osseous bridging across the physis with consequent local premature growth arrest. Only fine smooth Kirschner wires should be used for internal fixation; they should traverse the plate perpendicularly and be removed after four to six weeks.

Type V. This rare injury usually occurs in the knee or ankle—articulations that normally move in only one plane into flexion and extension. On the application of marked abduction or adduction strain, a severe compression force is transmitted through the epiphysis to a segment of the physis, crushing the germinal layer of the chondrocytes (Fig. 6–51E). Displacement of the epiphysis is minimal in this type of physeal injury. Often the seriousness of the condition is not suspected and the injury is misdiagnosed as a simple sprain. In treatment, the part is supported in a cast, and weight-bearing is avoided for at least three weeks. The prognosis in Type V epiphyseal plate injury is poor, since premature arrest of growth almost always occurs.[60]

MECHANISTIC CLASSIFICATIONS

Ankle fractures are usually caused by indirect violence; the fixed foot is forced into either abduction, adduction, lateral or medial rotation, eversion or inversion, or plantar flexion or dorsiflexion. Pronation and supination are the positions of the foot attained by rotational movement around the axis of the talocalcaneonavicular joint. Medial and lateral rotational movements of the talus take place around the sagittal axis of the weight-bearing articular surface of the tibia. These forces are transmitted by the deltoid and lateral collateral ligaments to the epiphyses of the distal tibia and fibula, exerting tension at the physes. Ankle fractures may also be caused by direct violence, as in an automobile accident or a fall. In direct crush injuries, the fractures may be open.

In 1932, Bishop modified the Ashhurst-Bromer classification of ankle fractures and subdivided ankle injuries in children on a mechanical basis.[7] Carothers and Crenshaw considered the direction of the injuring force and, in 1955, further modified the

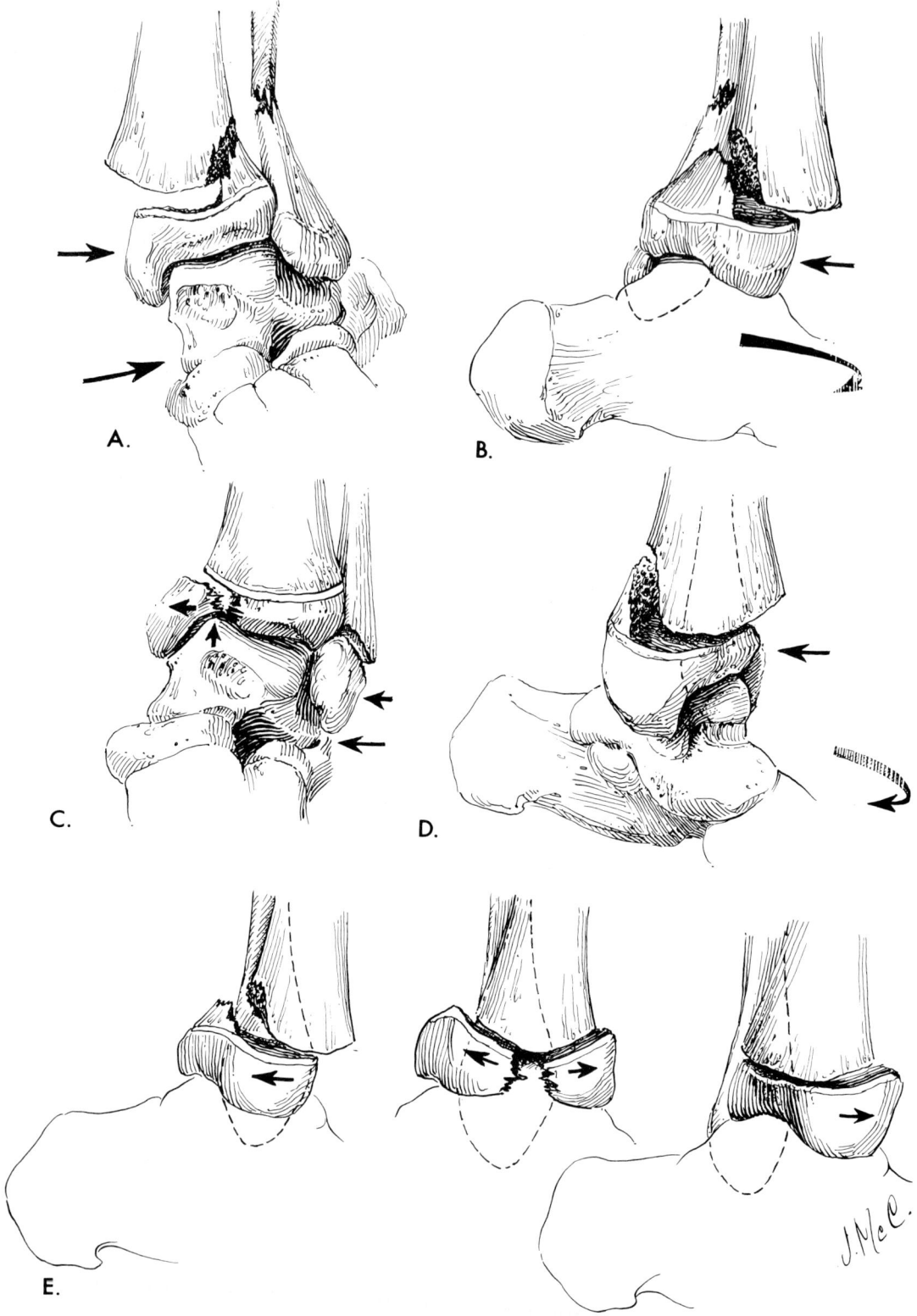

FIGURE 6–52. *Classification of fractures involving distal physis of tibia according to Carothers and Crenshaw.*

A. Abduction injury. **B.** External rotation injury. **C.** Adduction injury. **D.** Plantar flexion injury. **E.** Axial compression injury and injury caused by direct violence.

classification, listing (1) abduction injuries; (2) external rotation injuries; (3) adduction injuries; (4) plantar flexion injuries; and (5) axial compression injuries and injuries caused by direct violence (Fig. 6–52).[15]

Lauge-Hansen showed that in the study of the mechanism of ankle fractures in the adult three factors should be considered: the axial load, the position of the foot at the moment of trauma, and the direction of the abnormal force.[40–44] In children, an additional factor determining the pattern of fracture is the state of maturity of the physis.

Dias and Tachdjian devised a classification of physeal injuries of the ankle in children that utilizes Lauge-Hansen's categories of foot position and direction of abnormal force in correlation with the Salter-Harris classification. Four mechanisms are proposed; in each, the first term refers to the position of the foot at the time of injury and the second, to the direction of injuring force on the ankle joint. Grades of injury are described in a progressively increasing order of severity (Table 6–2).[24] The fracture patterns and displacement of fragments are quite characteristic for each mechanism. In classifying an ankle fracture, one should study the roentgenograms carefully to determine the type of Salter-Harris physeal injury, the direction of the fracture line, and the direction of displacement of the epiphyseal-metaphyseal fracture fragment in relation to localized swelling and tenderness.

Supination-Inversion Injury. In this type of ankle fracture an inversion force is exerted on a foot that is fixed in supination.

In *grade 1* supination-inversion injury, traction by the lateral ligaments of the ankle will produce a Salter-Harris Type I or II fracture separation of the distal fibular physis (Fig. 6–53A and B, and Fig. 6–54). Occasionally the calcaneofibular and talofibular ligaments may rupture, as shown in Figure 6–53C, or a fracture of the distal tip of the lateral malleolus may take place (Figs. 6–53D and 6–55). In almost all cases the displacement of the distal fibular epiphysis is medial and minimal. Injury to the distal fibular physis usually goes undiagnosed because the displacement of the epiphysis is slight. After twisting the ankle, the patient walks with an antalgic limp and complains of pain. There is local tenderness and swelling. In the routine anteroposterior and lateral roentgenograms of the ankle, this physeal injury is usually not visualized; oblique views are required to depict the minimal displacement (Fig. 6–56).

In *grade 2* supination-inversion injury, following fracture of the distal fibular epiphysis, the inversion force will medially displace the talus against the medial malleolus. The medial border of the upper surface of the talus impinges on the medial half of the lower end of the tibia and exerts a crushing force at this point. The intra-articular shearing force causes either a Type IV Salter-Harris physeal injury (in which the epiphysis, physis, and a portion of the metaphysis are completely split and there is upward and medial displacement of the medial fragment, as shown in Figures 6–57A and 6–58) or a Type III Salter-Harris physeal injury (in which the fracture extends from the articular surface to the zone of the hypertrophic cartilage cells of the physis and then along the plate to its medial border, as seen in Figures 6–57B and 6–59 to 6–63). Occasionally the inversion-adduction force will displace the entire distal tibial epiphysis medially with a medial metaphyseal tibial fragment attached to it (Type II physeal injury, shown in Figure 6–57C) or without a metaphyseal fragment (Type I physeal injury). The displacement of the fracture fragments is usually medial, occasionally posteromedial.

Supination–Plantar Flexion Fracture. With the foot fixed in full supination, a plantar flexion force exerted on the ankle causes this type of injury.

The common pattern (grade 1) is a Salter-Harris Type II physeal injury of the distal tibial epiphysis with posterior displacement of the epiphyseal-metaphyseal fracture fragment. The metaphyseal fragment is posterior. The fracture is best visualized in the lateral projection. There is no associated fibular fracture (Figs. 6–64 and 6–65).

Supination–Lateral Rotation Fracture. This type of fracture occurs when, with the foot in full supination, a lateral rotation force is exerted on the ankle joint. The fracture caused by this mechanism may fall into one of two grades. In the *grade 1* injury a Salter-Harris Type II fracture of the distal tibial epiphysis occurs with a long spiral

Text continued on page 677

Table 6–2. Classification of Physical Injuries of the Ankle in Children (Modified From Lauge-Hansen)

Type	Grade	Position of Foot	Injuring Force	Pattern of Fracture	Comment
Supination–inversion	1	Supinated	Inversion	Usually Salter-Harris I or II fracture separation of distal fibular physis. Occasionally rupture of lateral ligament or fracture of tip of lateral malleolus	Displacement minimal and almost always medial
	2	Supinated	Inversion	Usually Salter-Harris III or IV of medial part of tibial epiphysis. Rarely Salter-Harris I or II with medial displacement of entire tibial epiphysis	Caution! Asymmetric growth arrest causes varus ankle
Supination–plantar flexion	1	Supinated	Plantar flexion	Commonly Salter-Harris II of tibial epiphysis. Rarely Salter-Harris I of tibial physis. No associated fracture of fibula. Metaphyseal fragment and displacement posterior. Fracture line best seen in lateral x-ray	Prognosis good. Caution! Do not damage growth plate by forced manipulation. Posterior displacement will remodel
Supination–lateral rotation	1	Supinated	Lateral rotation	Salter-Harris II of distal tibial epiphysis with long spiral fracture of distal tibia starting laterally at distal tibial growth plate	Distinguishing feature is direction of fracture line starting laterally and running medially and proximally
	2	Supinated	Lateral rotation	Grade 1 plus spiral fracture of distal fibular shaft	—

Type		Position	Mechanism	Description	Notes
Pronation–eversion–lateral rotation	1	Pronated	Eversion–lateral rotation	Salter-Harris II of distal tibial epiphysis. Metaphyseal fragment lateral or posterolateral. Displacement lateral or posterolateral. Fibular fracture short, oblique, 4 to 7 cm. from tip of lateral malleolus	—
Miscellaneous Adolescent Tillaux	—	? Neutral?	Lateral rotation	Salter-Harris III of lateral part of distal tibial epiphysis. Should not be any metaphyseal fragment. Displacement anterolateral	Medial part of distal tibial physis closed
Triplane three-fragment	—	?	Lateral rotation	Fracture in three planes—coronal, sagittal, and transverse. Combination of Salter-Harris II and III. Fracture produces three fragments	Medial part of distal tibial physis open
Triplane two-fragment	—	?	Lateral rotation	Fracture in three planes—coronal, sagittal, and transverse. Combination of Salter-Harris II and III. Fracture creates two fragments	Medial part of distal tibial physis usually closed
Comminuted fracture of distal end of tibia	—	?	Crushing injuries. Direct violence	Comminuted fracture involving distal tibial epiphysis. Physis often damaged. Fibular fracture at various levels	Poor prognosis

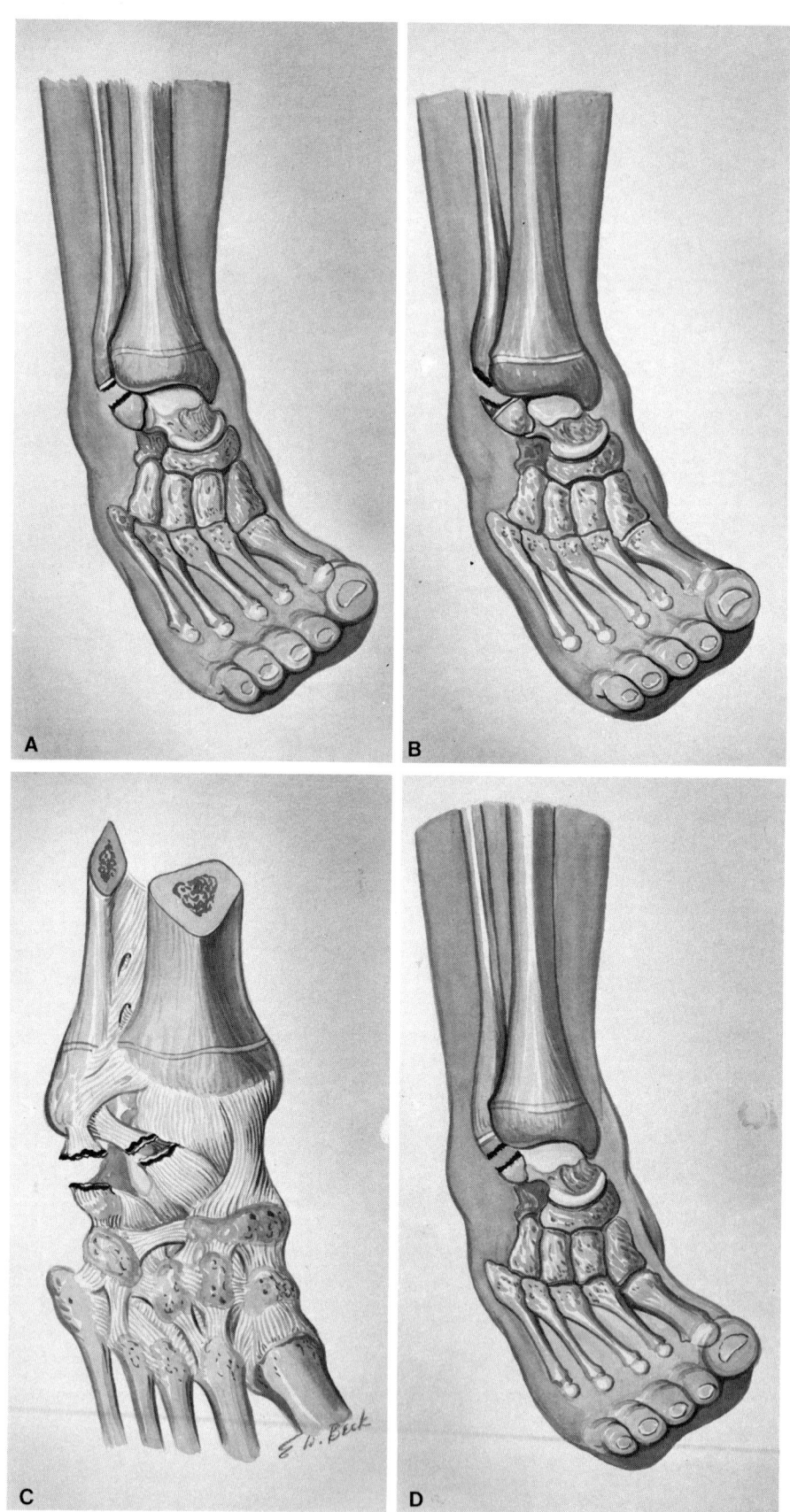

Figure 6–53 See legend on opposite page

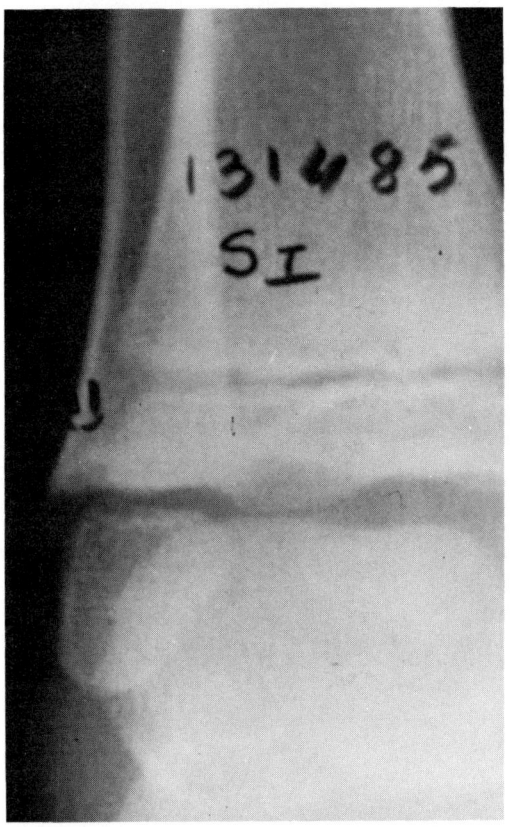

FIGURE 6–54. *Fracture-separation of distal fibular epiphysis with minimal displacement (supination-inversion grade 1 physeal injury of the ankle).*

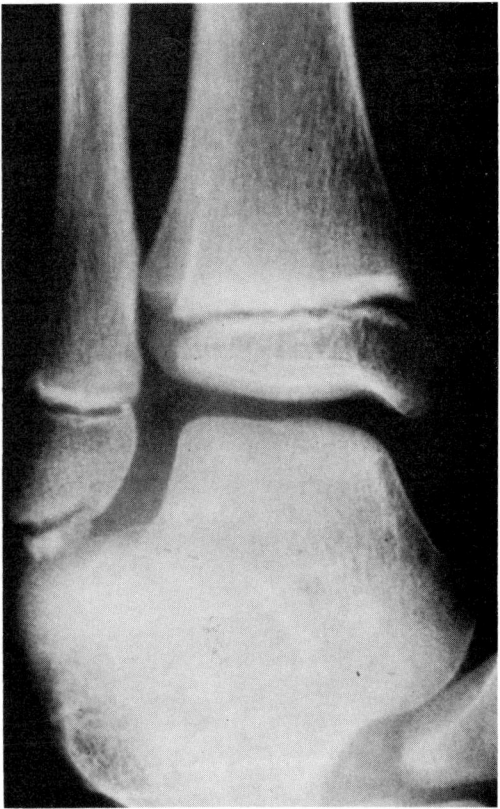

FIGURE 6–55. *Fracture of distal tip of lower fibular epiphysis (supination-inversion grade 1 injury of the ankle).*

FIGURE 6–53. *Supination-inversion physeal injury of the ankle in children—grade 1.*

An inversion force exerted with the foot fixed in supinated position will produce: **A** and **B**. Salter-Harris Type I or II physeal injury of the distal fibular physis. **C**. Occasionally rupture of the calcaneofibular or talofibular ligaments may result. **D**. The distal tip of the lateral malleolus may be fractured. Note that the displacement of the distal fibular epiphysis is medial and not marked.

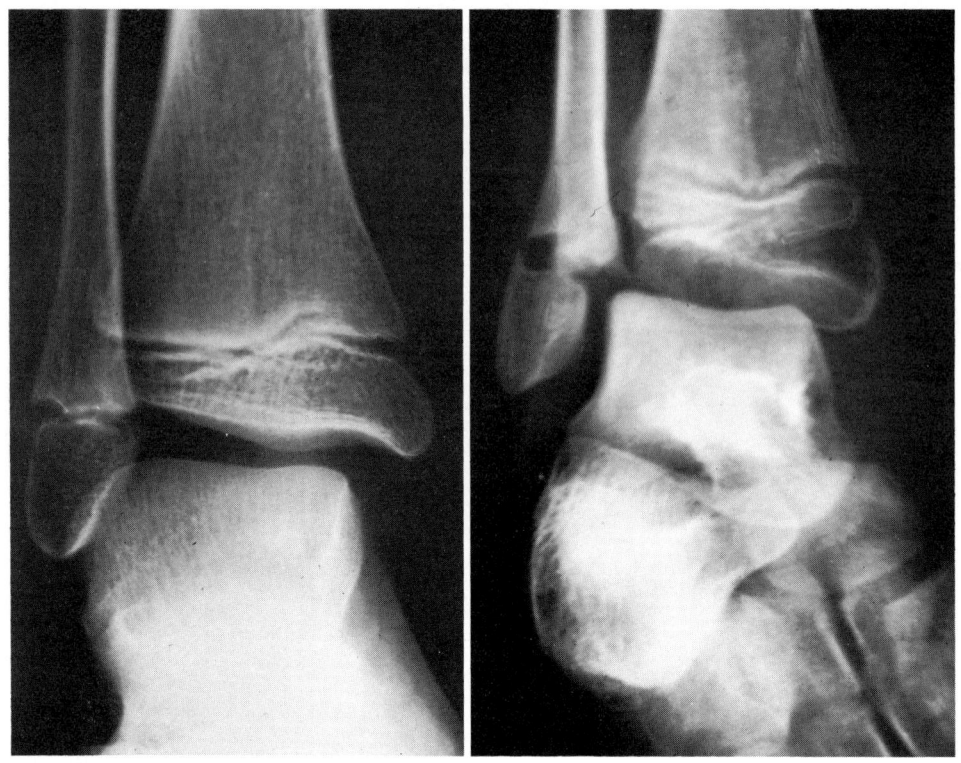

FIGURE 6–56. Anteroposterior and lateral roentgenograms of the ankle showing fracture-separation of the distal fibular epiphysis.

The importance of taking oblique views is obvious.

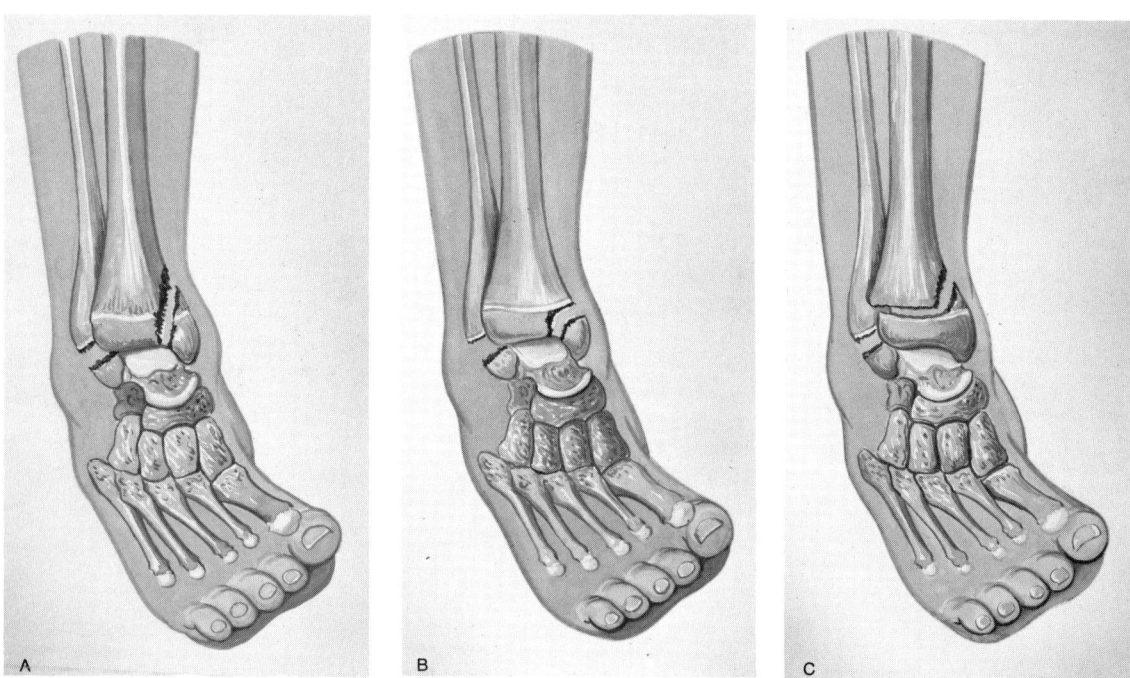

FIGURE 6–57. Supination-inversion fracture of the ankle—grade 2.

After separation of the distal fibular epiphysis the inversion-adduction force against the medial malleolus will produce: **A.** Type IV Salter-Harris physeal injury. **B.** Type III Salter-Harris physeal injury. **C.** Occasionally, a Type II Salter-Harris physeal injury.

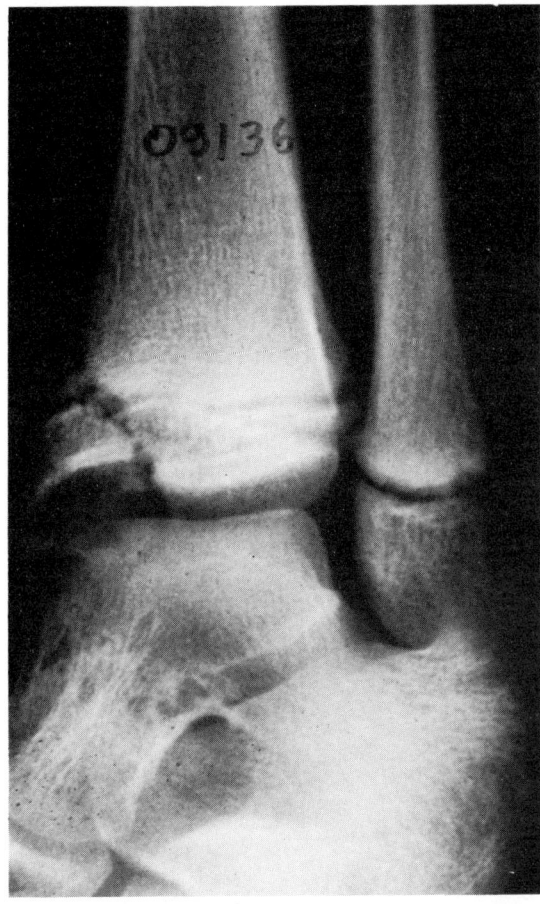

FIGURE 6–58. Oblique roentgenogram of the ankle showing Type III Salter-Harris physeal injury of the distal tibial epiphysis and Type I physeal injury of the distal fibular epiphysis (grade 2 supination-inversion ankle fracture).

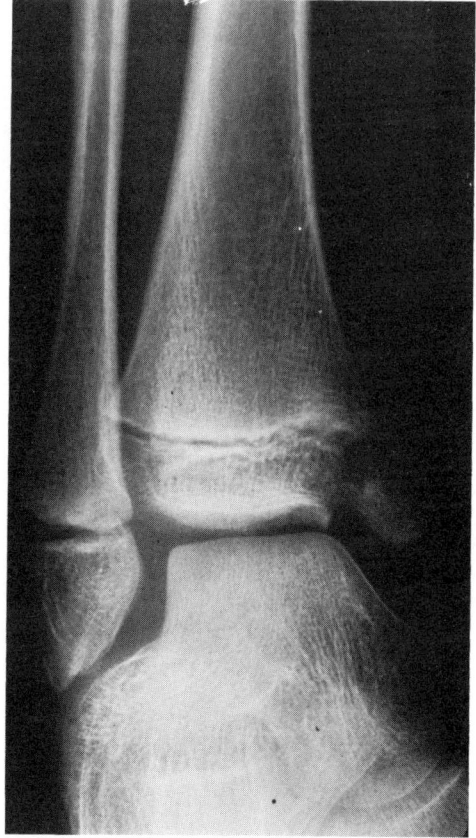

FIGURE 6–59. Oblique roentgenogram of the ankle showing grade 2 supination-inversion fracture of the ankle.

Note the Type III Salter-Harris physeal injury of the distal tibial epiphysis and Type I Salter-Harris injury of the distal fibular epiphysis.

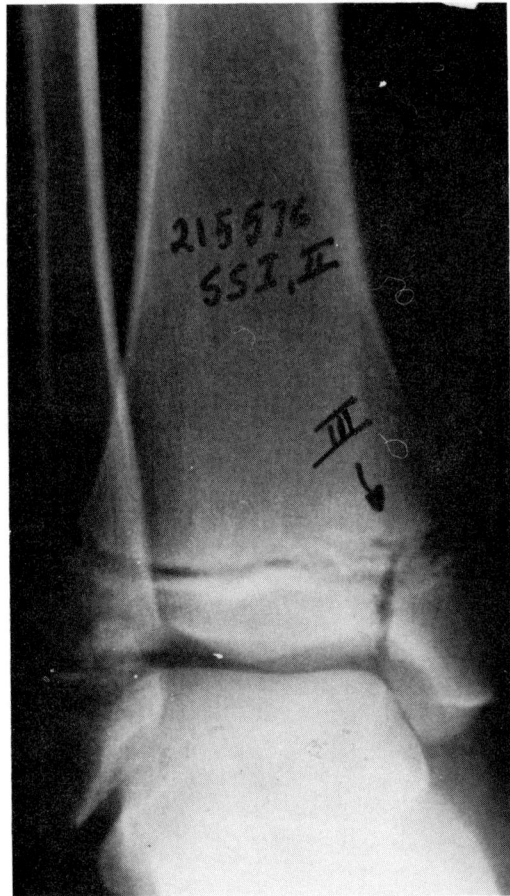

FIGURE 6–60. Supination-inversion grade 2 fracture of the ankle with Salter-Harris Type I injury of the distal fibula and Type III injury of the medial part of the distal tibial epiphysis.

The displacement is less than 2 mm.

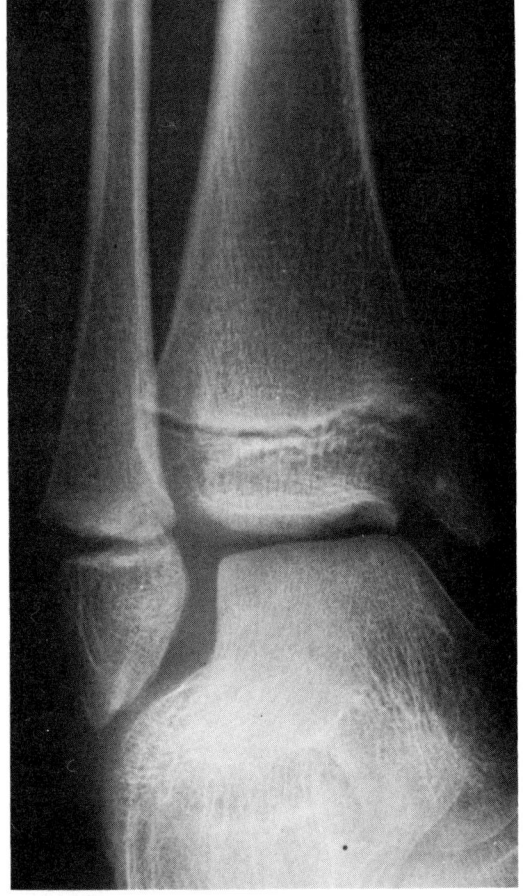

FIGURE 6–61. Supination-inversion grade 2 fracture of the ankle.

Note the Salter-Harris Type I injury of the distal fibula and the marked displacement of the Salter-Harris Type III injury of the medial part of the distal tibia. Open reduction and anatomic alignment are mandatory.

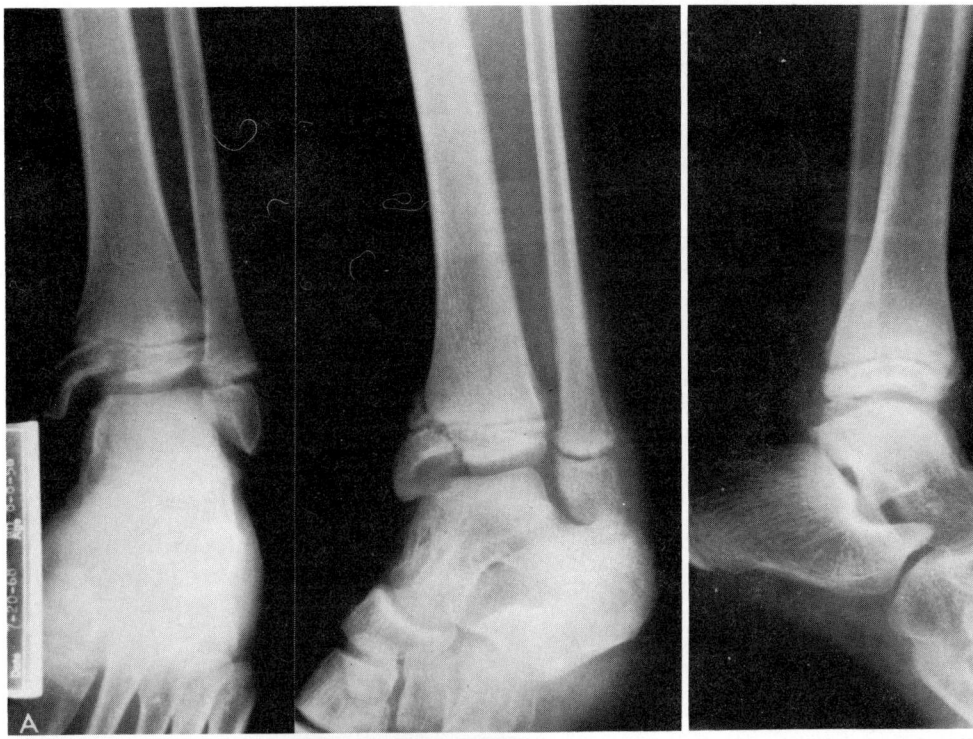

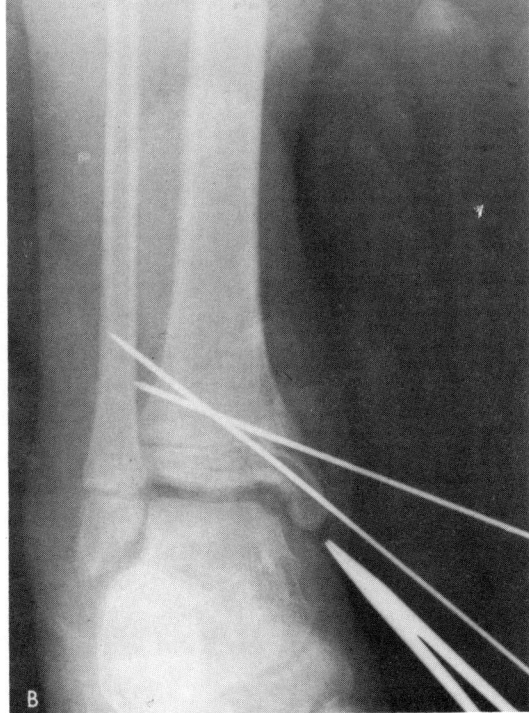

FIGURE 6–62. Supination-inversion grade 2 fracture of the ankle—Salter-Harris Type III physeal injury of the distal tibial epiphysis and Salter-Harris Type I injury of the distal fibular epiphysis.

A. Anteroposterior, oblique, and lateral roentgenograms. Note the superior and medial displacement of the tibial fracture fragment. Anatomic reduction is vital. **B.** Roentgenogram made in the operating room. Open reduction and internal fixation with two smooth Kirschner wires was carried out.

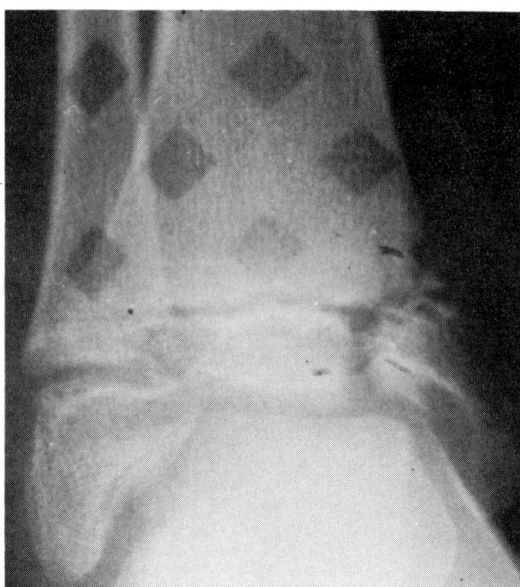

FIGURE 6–63. Supination-inversion grade 2 fracture of the ankle.

Note the Salter-Harris Type IV physeal injury of the medial part of the distal tibial epiphysis. The prognosis is poor because of the asymmetric growth arrest. This fracture should be treated by open reduction and internal fixation. There is also a Salter-Harris Type I fracture of the distal fibular physis.

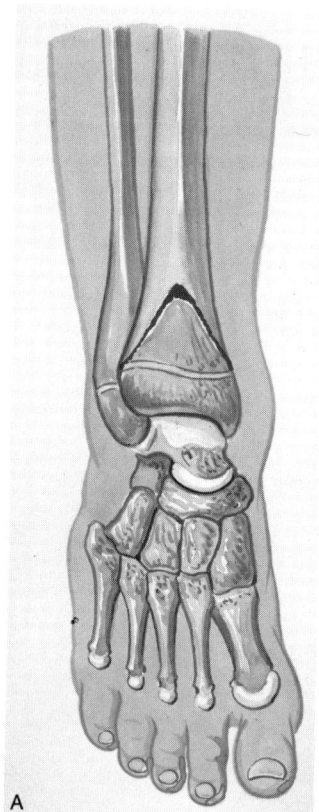
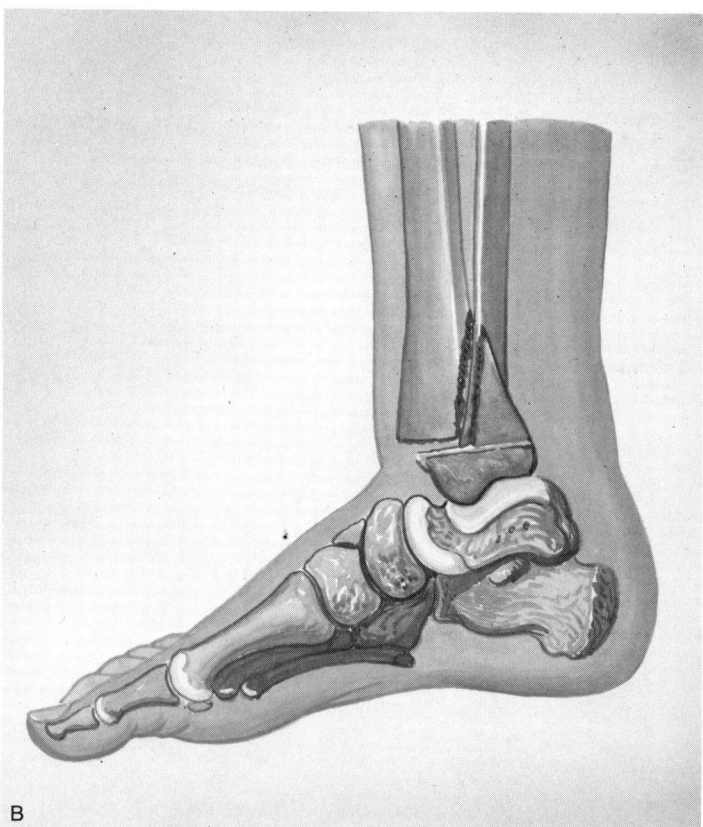

FIGURE 6–64. Grade 1 supination–plantar flexion fracture of the ankle.

Note the Salter-Harris Type II physeal injury of the distal tibial epiphysis. There is no associated fracture of the fibula. The metaphyseal fragment is posterior and the fracture fragment is displaced posteriorly. The fracture line is best visualized in the lateral projection.

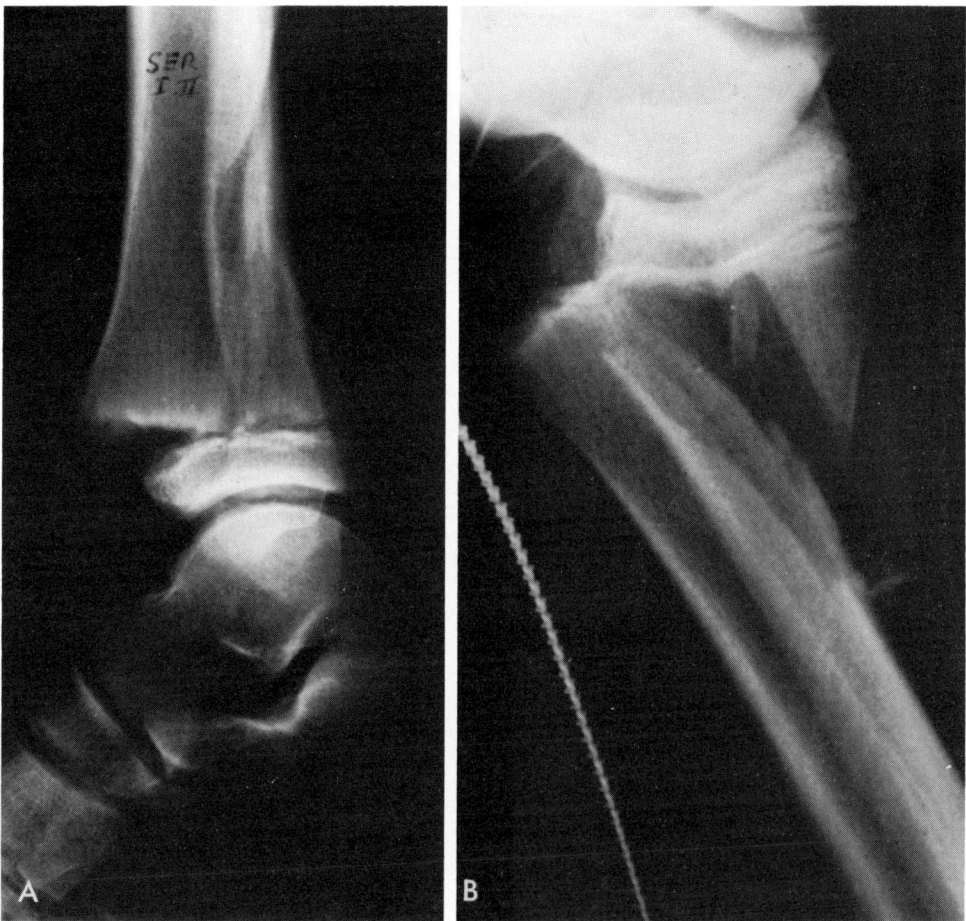

FIGURE 6–65. *Supination–plantar flexion injury of the ankle with Salter-Harris Type II fracture of the distal tibial physis.*

A. The posterior metaphyseal fragment is partially displaced backward. **B.** It is markedly displaced backward.

fracture of the distal tibia beginning at the lateral (fibular) end of the distal tibial physis and extending proximally and medially. The metaphyseal-diaphyseal segment is posteriorly located, and the displacement of the fracture segment is posterior. The fibula is intact (Figs. 6–66 and 6–67). In the lateral projection the grade 1 supination–lateral rotation fracture is very similar to supination–plantar flexion fracture; on careful analysis of the anteroposterior view, however, the characteristic feature of supination–lateral rotation type is that the fracture line starts laterally and runs medially and proximally. In *grade 2* supination–lateral rotation fracture of the ankle, continuation of the lateral rotation force produces in addition a spiral fracture of the fibula; the fracture line of the fibula begins medially and runs superiorly and posteriorly. There is no injury to the distal fibular physis (Fig. 6–68).

Pronation–Eversion–Lateral Rotation Fracture. In this type of injury an eversion and lateral rotation force is applied on the distal tibial epiphysis while the foot is pronated. The metaphyseal fragment is characteristically located *laterally* and posteriorly. The displacement of the fracture fragment is posterior and lateral. There is a short oblique fracture of the lower fibular shaft, located approximately 4 to 7 cm. proximal to the tip of the lateral malleolus (Figs. 6–69 and 6–70).

Text continued on page 682

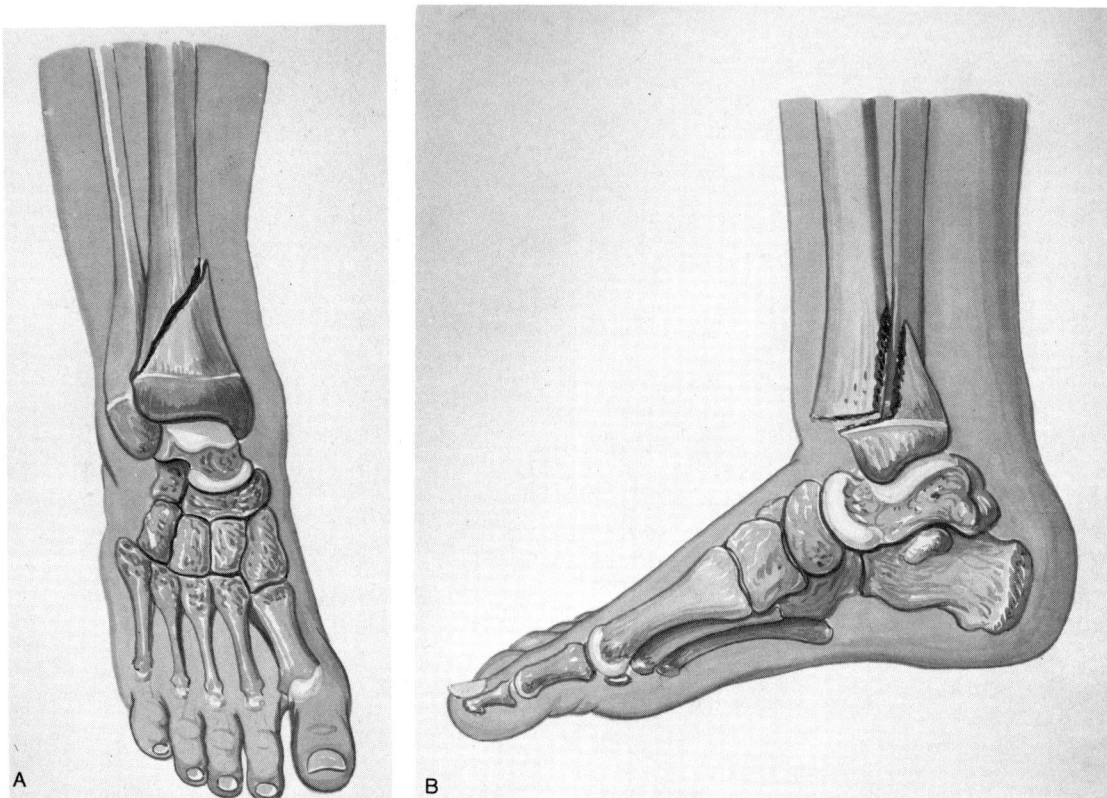

FIGURE 6–66. Supination–lateral rotation fracture of the ankle, grade 1.

A. Anteroposterior view. **B.** Lateral view. Note the Salter-Harris Type II physeal injury of the distal tibial epiphysis. The metaphyseal-diaphyseal segment is posteriorly located. Displacement of the fracture fragment is posterior. The fibula is intact. The fracture line starts laterally at the physis and extends proximally and medially. This is a characteristic feature of supination–lateral rotation fracture of the ankle, distinguishing it from supination–plantar flexion fracture.

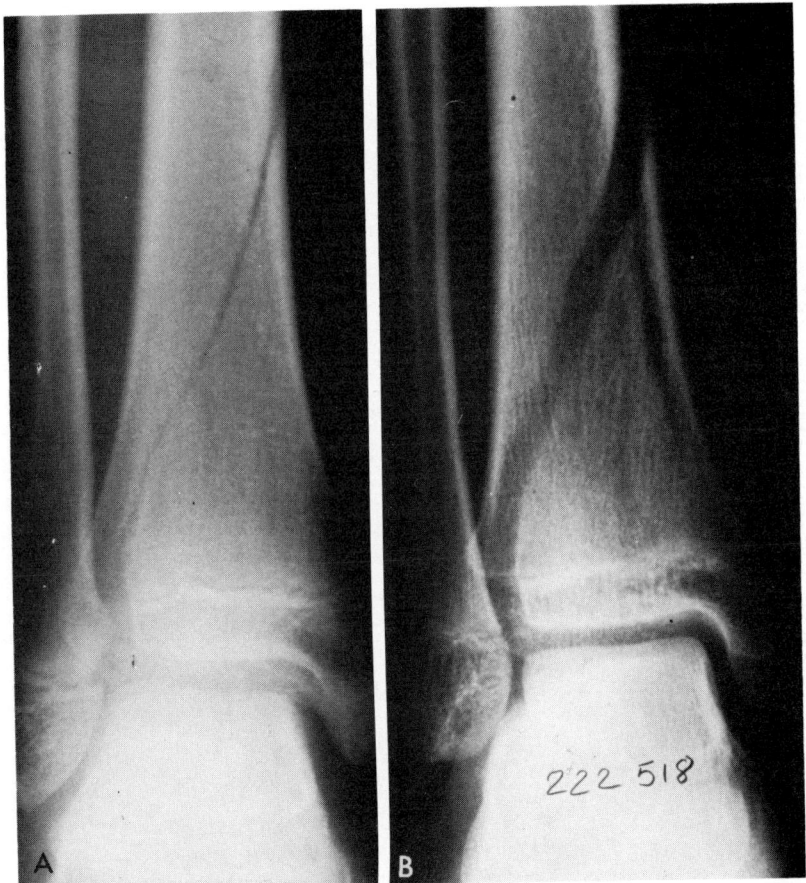

FIGURE 6–67. Roentgenograms of the ankle showing grade 1 supination–lateral rotation fracture of the ankle.

In this Salter-Harris Type II fracture of the distal tibial epiphysis, the fracture line starts laterally at the physis and extends proximally and medially. The fibula is intact. **A.** The fracture is minimally displaced. **B.** The displacement is marked.

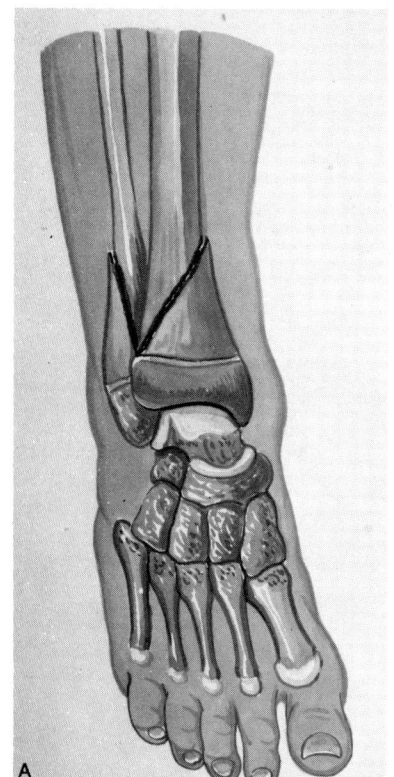 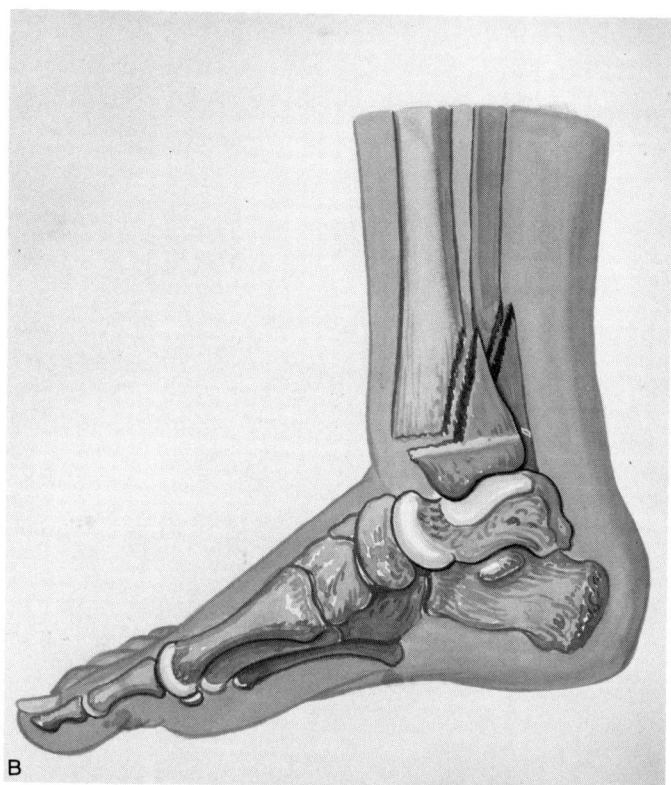

FIGURE 6–68. Diagrams illustrating grade 2 supination–lateral rotation fracture of the ankle.

In addition to the Salter-Harris Type II physeal injury of the distal tibial epiphysis there is a spiral fracture of the lower fibular shaft that starts medially and runs superiorly and laterally. Displacement is lateral or posterolateral. **A.** Anteroposterior view. **B.** Lateral view.

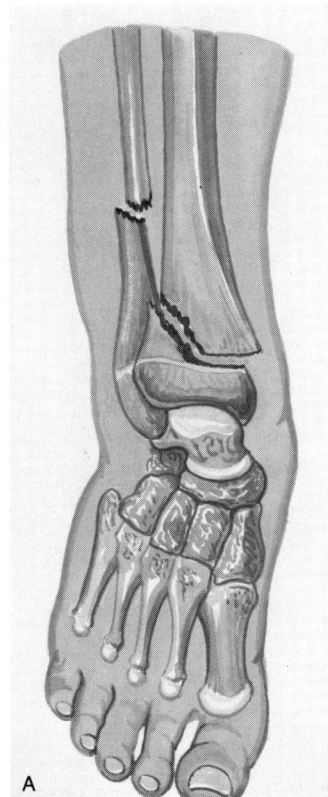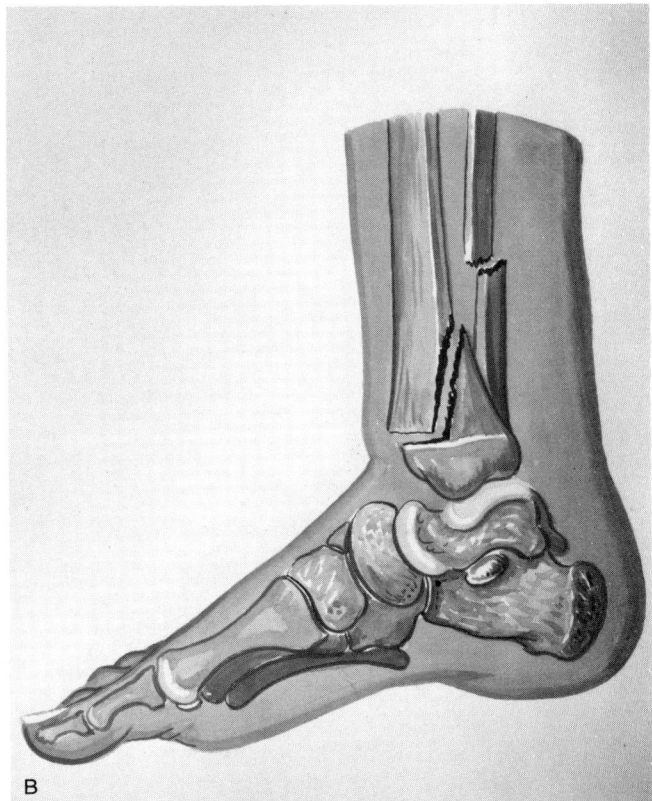

FIGURE 6–69. Diagrams illustrating grade 1 pronation–eversion–lateral rotation fracture of the ankle.

Note the Salter-Harris Type II physeal injury of the distal tibial epiphysis; the metaphyseal segment is located laterally and posteriorly. The displacement of the fracture fragment is posterolateral. Also note the fracture of the lower diaphysis of the fibula, running a short oblique course and located 4 to 7 cm. proximal to the tip of the lateral malleolus.

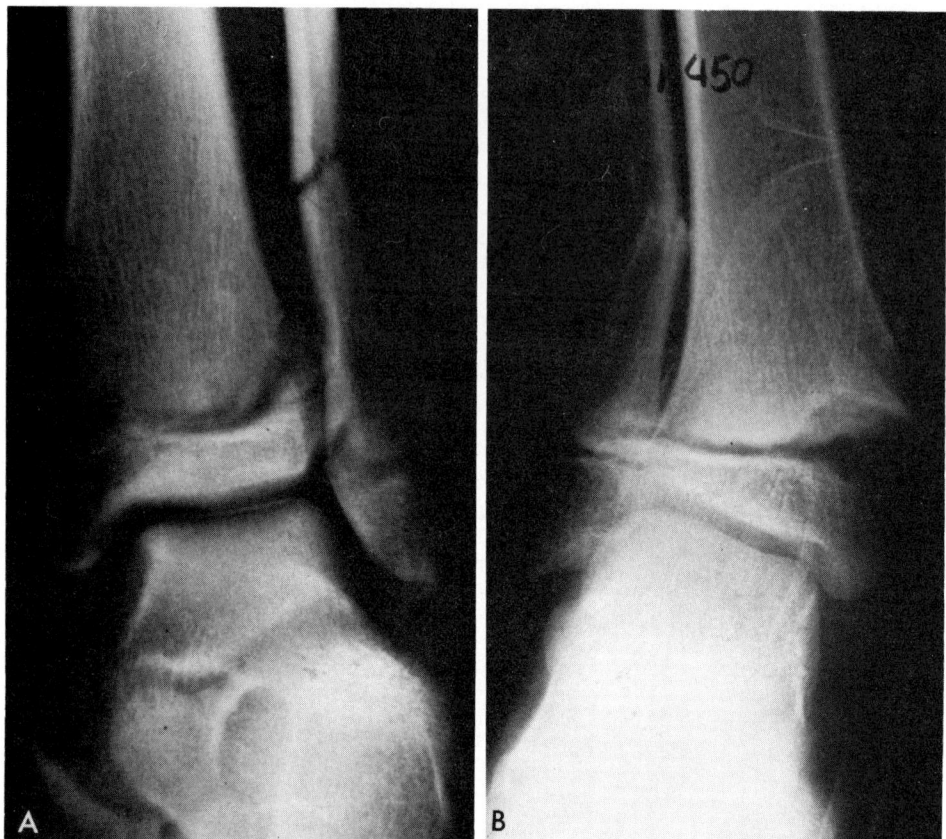

FIGURE 6–70. *Roentgenograms of the ankle showing pronation–eversion–lateral rotation fracture of the ankle.*

A. The laterally and posteriorly placed metaphyseal fragment is clearly seen. **B.** The metaphyseal fragment is very small.

MISCELLANEOUS FRACTURES

Fracture of Tillaux in the Adolescent. Fracture of the lateral portion of the distal end of the tibia in the adult was first described by Sir Astley Cooper; in the literature, however, it is referred to as the fracture of Tillaux.[20, 34]

The distal physis of the tibia closes first on its medial half at the age of 13 or 14 years; the lateral part closes at 14½ to 16 years. Thus there is a period of 18 months during which the lateral part of the distal tibial growth plate is open while the medial half is closed. The lower metaphysis of the fibula is connected with the anterolateral part of the tibial epiphysis by the anterior talofibular ligament. A lateral rotatory force may fracture the tibial epiphysis at the junction of the open and closed portions of the physis. The fracture line is vertical, extending from the articular surface proximally and then laterally to exit on the lateral cortex of the tibia. The more skeletally mature the child, the more lateral is the vertical fracture line. The physeal injury is Salter-Harris Type III of the lateral part of the distal tibial epiphysis (Figs. 6–71 and 6–72). The anterolateral and posterolateral tibiofibular ligaments are intact, and the fractured fragment rotates anterolaterally; the displacement is usually minimal, but occasionally it may be marked.[21, 34]

On clinical examination there is local tenderness and swelling over the anterolateral part of the distal tibial epiphysis. When displacement of the fragment is minimal, the vertical and horizontal fracture lines may be difficult to visualize in the anteroposterior and lateral roentgenograms of the ankle. Oblique views are essential, and computed tomography will clearly depict the fracture.

In the triplane fracture of the distal end of the tibia the fracture occurs in three planes—sagittal, transverse, and coronal—giving the roentgenographic appearance of a combination of Salter-Harris Types II and III physeal injuries (Fig. 6–73). In the lateral projection there is a vertical fracture line that separates the posterior metaphyseal triangular fragment from the distal tibial diaphysis. This fracture line becomes indistinct as one traces it distally into the epiphysis; i.e., the fracture line does not cross the epiphysis but runs along the physis for a varying distance, depending upon the stage of fusion of the growth plate in its different parts. The size of the posterior metaphyseal segment also varies, its vertical height measuring from 1 to 6 cm. above the physis and its width (measured along the physis from the fracture line to the posterior tibial cortex) between one tenth and one half that of the metaphysis.

In the anteroposterior projection there is a vertical fracture line in the bony epiphysis that extends proximally from the articular surface of the ankle to the physis and then courses along the growth plate (Salter-Harris Type III). This vertical fracture line in the sagittal plane is usually at or close to the center of the width of the physis or occasionally medial to the center. The degree of displacement of the fracture fragments on the anteroposterior roentgenogram varies; in the series of 15 cases of Cooperman and associates it measured more than 2 mm. in four, 2 mm. in seven, and less than 2 mm. in four.[21]

There is disagreement in the literature as to whether the triplane fracture gives rise to three or two major fragments. According to both Lynn and Rang, it produces three major fragments: (1) a rectangular fragment representing the anterolateral quadrant of the distal tibial epiphysis, (2) a posterior triangular metaphyseal segment along with the medial and posterior portion of the epiphysis, and (3) the distal tibial metaphysis (Fig. 6–74 A and B). The triplane fracture separates fragments 2 and 3 in the coronal plane, and fragments 1 and 2 in the sagittal plane, and courses through the physis in the transverse plane.[47, 56]

Cooperman, Spiegel, and Laros studied the three-dimensional configuration of the triplane fracture by tomography in five

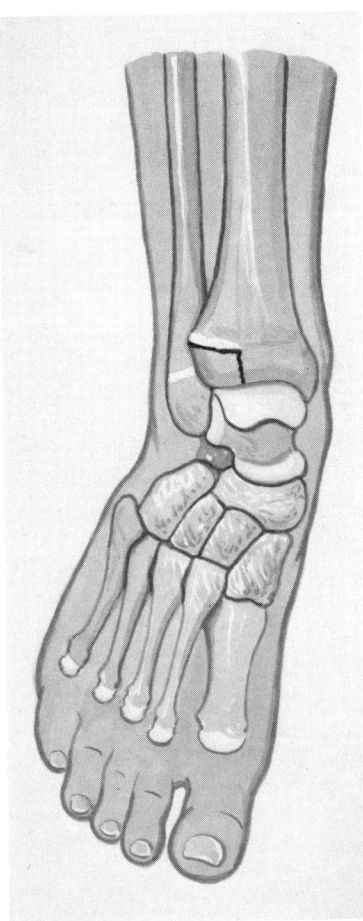

FIGURE 6–71. *Diagram showing fracture of Tillaux in the adolescent.*

Note the Salter-Harris Type III fracture of the lateral part of the distal tibial physis. The medial part of the physis is closed. There is no metaphyseal fragment.

Triplane Fracture of the Distal End of the Tibia. This unusual fracture was first reported by Marmor, in 1970.[49] Lynn, in 1972, described two additional cases and gave it the name *triplane fracture*.[47] Torg and Ruggiero reported a similar fracture in 1975.[65] Cooperman, Spiegel, and Laros, in 1978, reported 15 cases of triplane fracture of the distal end of the tibia, representing 6 per cent of 237 consecutive physeal injuries of the ankle.[21]

The fracture usually occurs in adolescents near skeletal maturity, the average age being 13½ years and the age range 10 to 16 years. It seems a maturing or partially fused physis is particularly susceptible to this injury.

Text continued on page 687

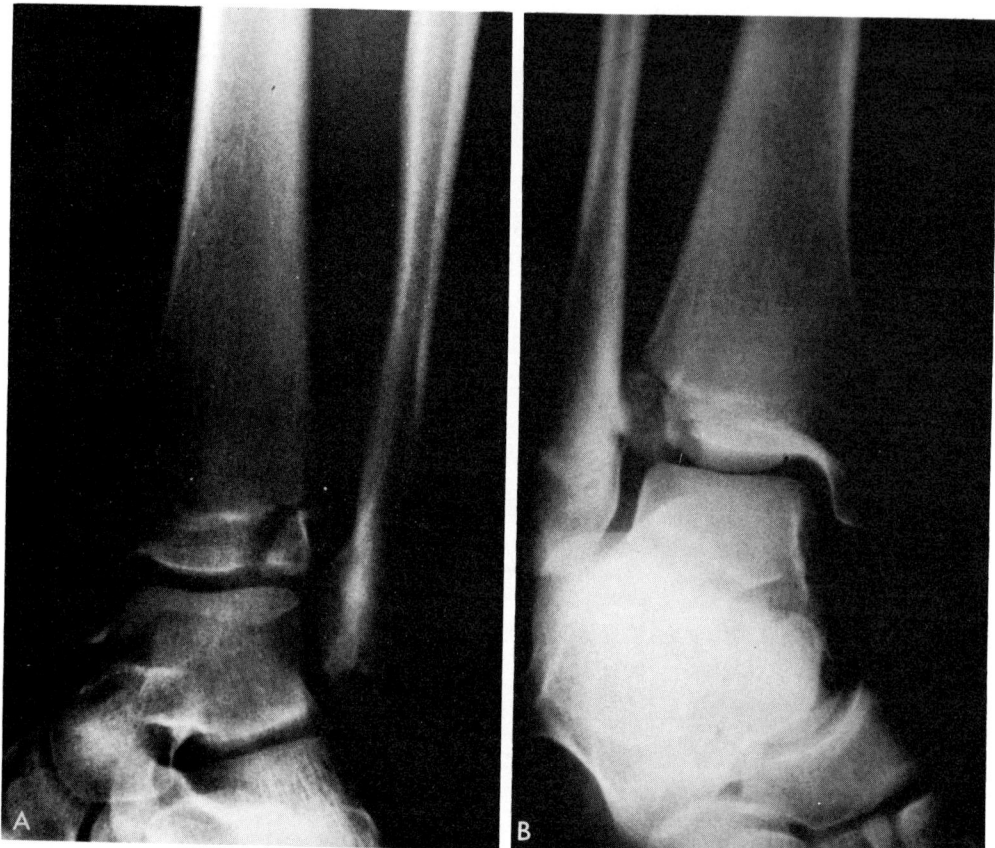

FIGURE 6–72. Fracture of Tillaux in the adolescent.

A. The growth plate of the medial part of the distal tibia is closed. The fracture is a Salter-Harris Type III physeal injury of the lateral part of the distal tibia. The displacement is anterolateral. **B.** Fracture of Tillaux in the more skeletally mature adolescent. The lateral part of the physis of the distal tibia is almost completely closed.

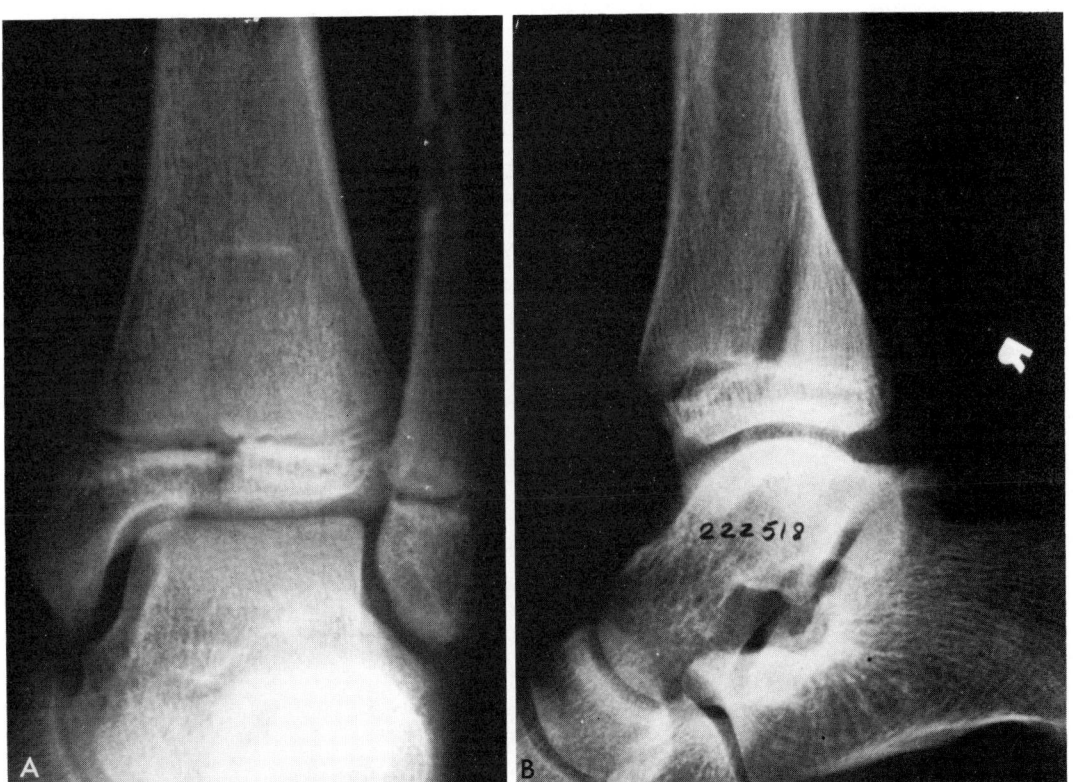

FIGURE 6–73. Triplane fracture of the ankle—three fragments.

The medial and lateral parts of the distal tibial physis are open. **A.** Anteroposterior view showing the Salter-Harris Type III physeal injury. **B.** Lateral projection showing Salter-Harris Type II injury.

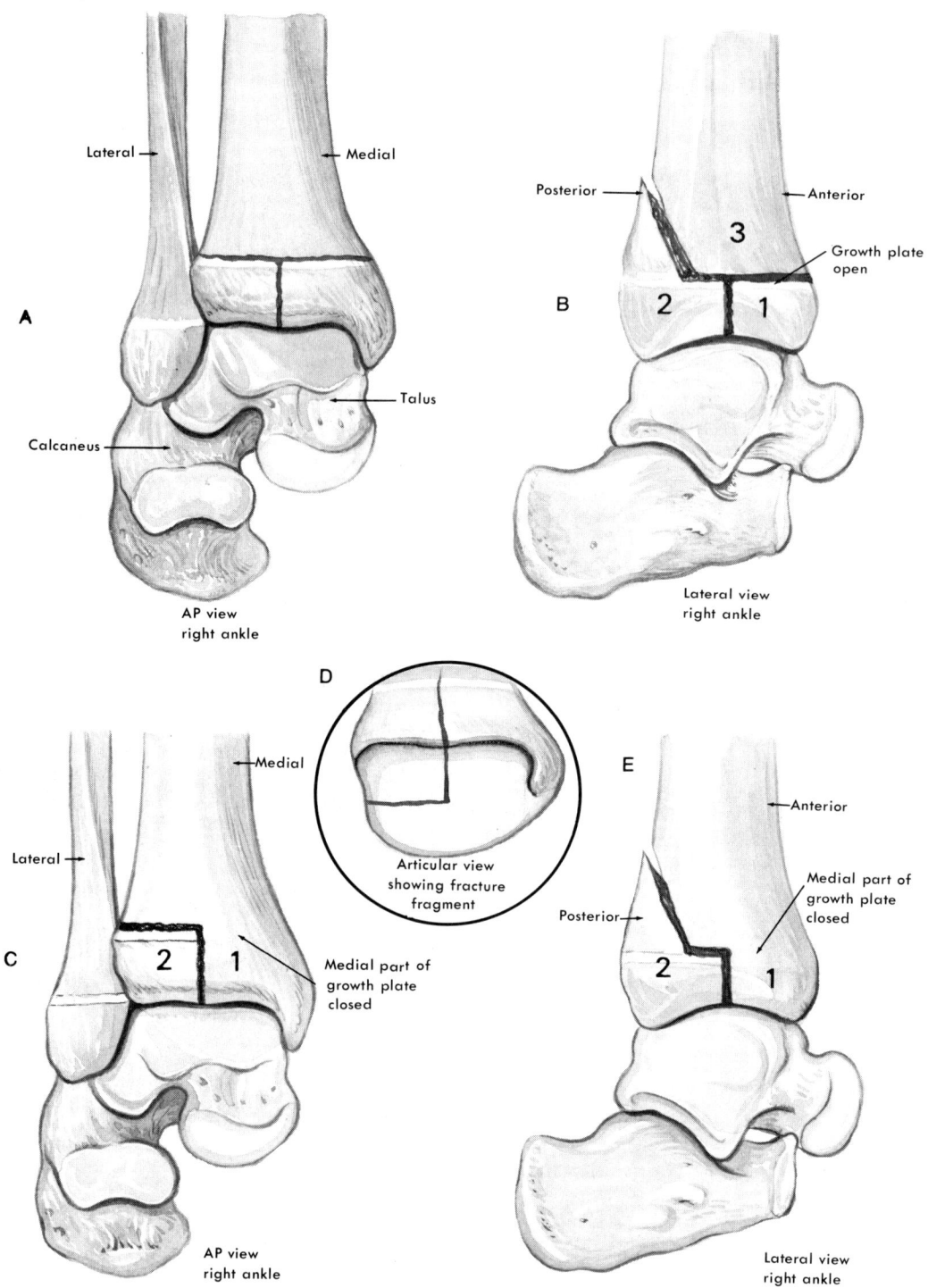

FIGURE 6–74. *Diagram illustrating triplane fracture.*

A and **B.** *Three-fragment type.* The medial part of the distal tibial physis is open. The fragments are: (1) a rectangular one representing the anterolateral quadrant of the distal tibial epiphysis; (2) a posterior triangular metaphyseal segment along with the medial and posterior portion of the tibial metaphysis; and (3) the distal tibial metaphysis. The fracture through the physis is in the transverse plane; fragments 1 and 2 are separated in the sagittal plane, and fragments 2 and 3 in the coronal plane. **C** to **E.** *Two-fragment type.* The medial part of the distal tibial physis is closed. (1) The anteromedial fragment consists of the major part of the tibial diaphysis and the attached medial malleolus; (2) the posterolateral fragment consists of the remainder of the distal tibial epiphysis—the posterior tibial metaphyseal fragment and the fibula connected with strong interosseous ligaments.

cases. In all of them the triplane fracture produced *two* and not three fragments; the anteromedial fragment consisted of the major part of the tibial shaft, the attached medial malleolus, and the anteromedial part of the distal tibial epiphysis; the posterolateral fragment consisted of the remainder of the distal tibial epiphysis; the posterior tibial metaphyseal fragment, and the fibula connected with strong interosseous ligaments (Figs. 6–74 C to E and 6–75).[21] In a triplane fracture studied by computed tomography, the two-fragment configuration of the fracture was also noted (Fig. 6–75H).

The pattern of fracture varies not only with the direction and degree of severity of the axial lateral rotation load and the position of the foot but also with the degree of skeletal maturity of the distal tibial physis. This author has found that the triplane fracture may produce a three-fragment fracture when the medial part of the distal

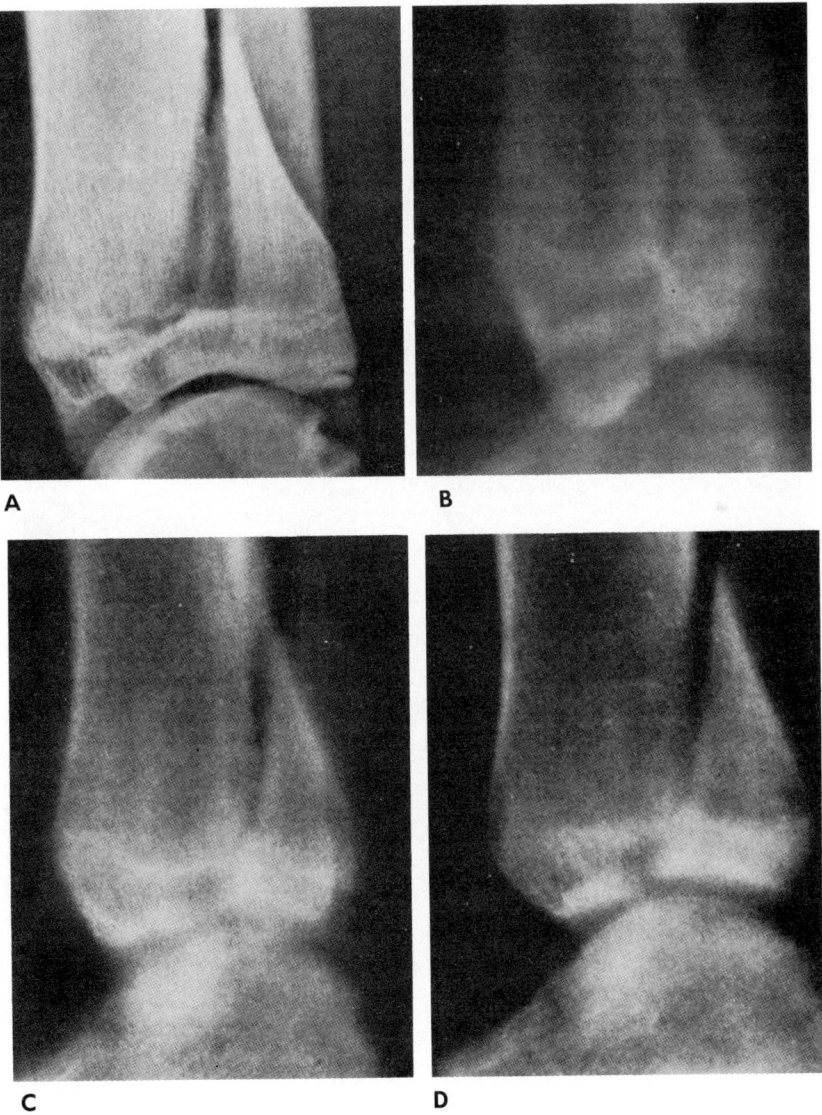

FIGURE 6–75. *Triplane fracture in a girl 12 years and nine months old.*

A. The routine lateral x-ray shows a coronal fracture with the medial malleolus and tibial diaphysis displaced forward as a unit. **B** to **E.** Lateral tomograms. In **B** the cut is at 9.0 cm. and shows the fracture line in the coronal plane along the posterior border of the medial malleolus; in **C** (8.5 cm. cut) and **D** (8.0 cm. cut), the continuity of the medial malleolus and tibial shaft is obvious. Note the articular step-off in **D**.

Illustration continued on following page

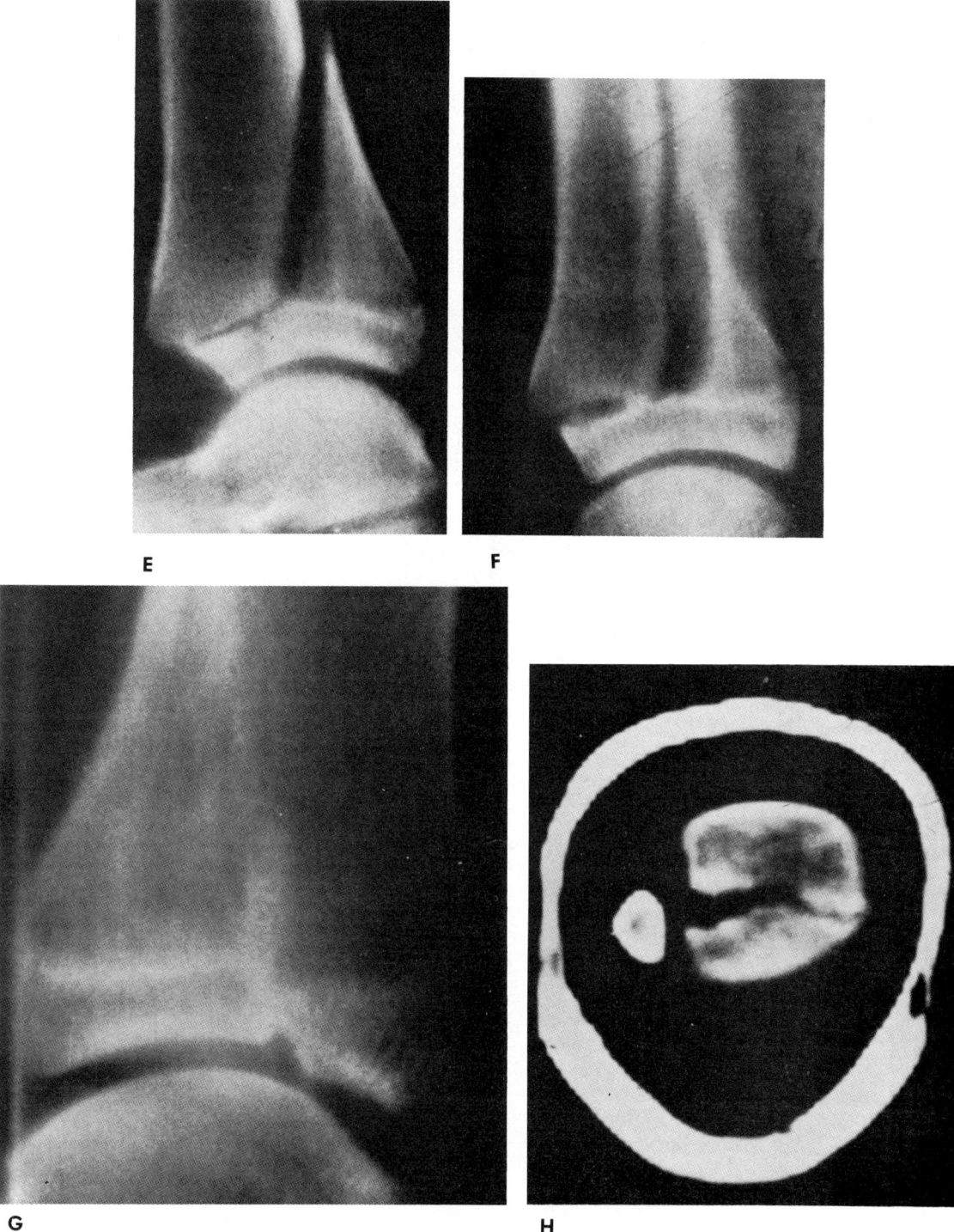

FIGURE 6–75 Continued. Triplane fracture in a girl 12 years and nine months old.

E and **F**. Tomographic cuts at 7.0 and 6.0 cm. show that the posterior epiphysis and metaphyseal fragment are continuous with the lateral epiphysis as a unit. **G.** A lateral tomogram, six months post fracture; note the persistence of articular incongruity. **H.** Computed tomography, one month post injury, at a level 4 mm. superior to the epiphysis. Note the fracture line in the tibia; the fragments are not displaced medially but are widely separated laterally. (From Cooperman, D. R., Spiegel, P. G., and Laros, G. S.: Tibial fracture involving the ankle in children—the so-called triplane fracture. J. Bone Joint Surg., 60-A:1042–1043, 1978. Reprinted by permission.)

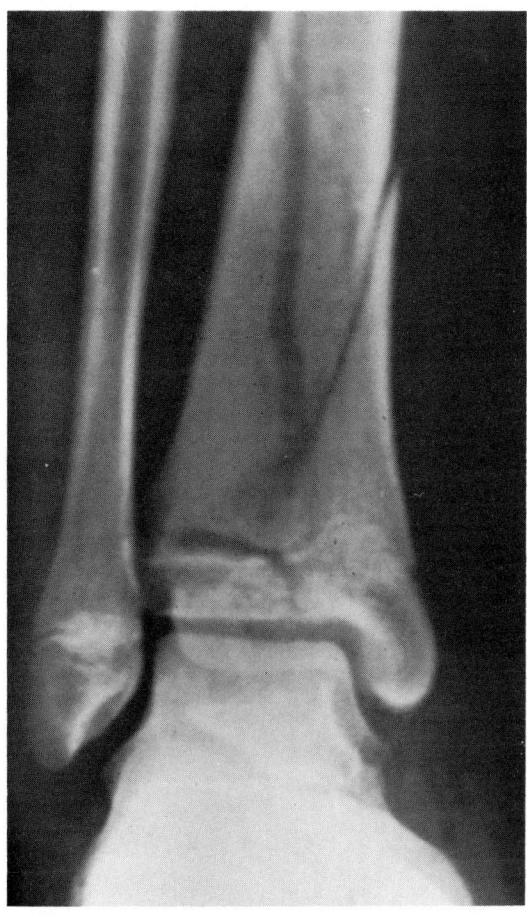

FIGURE 6–76. Comminuted fracture of the distal end of the tibia, involving the ankle joint.

tibial physis is open and will result in a two-fragment fracture when the medial part of the distal tibial physis is closed.

Comminuted fracture of the distal end of the tibia is usually caused by axial compression injury or direct violence. The distal tibial epiphysis is shattered, involving the joint (Fig. 6–76). The crushing often damages the physis, and the prognosis is poor.

Treatment

Principles of management of fractures involving the physis are well delineated by Salter and Harris.[60]

All reductions, whether closed or open, should be performed with the utmost gentleness in order to avoid damage to the delicate cartilage of the physis. Forceful manipulations are condemned. During open reduction, direct pressure on the physis by blunt instruments should be avoided.

Epiphyseal separations should be reduced immediately; each day of delay will make it progressively more difficult. In fact, after ten days, physeal injuries of Types I and II cannot be reduced without exerting undue force and damaging the cartilaginous growth plate. When such a fracture is seen late (i.e., after seven to ten days), it is better to accept malunion than to cause growth arrest by forceful manipulation or open surgery. In Type III or IV physeal injuries, congruity of articular surfaces is essential; in such cases, delayed reduction is performed, if indicated.

As stated earlier, reduction of Type I and Type II fractures involving the physis can be readily obtained and maintained. In Type III physeal injuries, open reduction may be indicated to restore a congruous articular surface, particularly in weight-bearing joints. Open reduction is required in almost all cases of Type IV fractures of the epiphyseal plate. Care must be taken not to compromise circulation of the epiphysis. Only smooth Kirschner wires must be used for internal fixation, and under no circumstances should screws or threaded wires be inserted across the physis. The internal fixation device is removed when the fracture has healed.

Type III and Type IV physeal injuries require accurate anatomic reduction. In Type I and Type II fractures of the physis, perfect reduction is desirable but not mandatory; bone remodeling will correct moderate residual deformities. In general, one can accept a greater degree of deformity in multiplane joints (such as the shoulder) than in single plane joints (such as the knee and ankle).

Types I, II, and III injuries consolidate very rapidly, usually in about half the time required for a fracture through the metaphysis of the same bone. Type IV injuries require the same period for union as metaphyseal fractures.

Fractures involving the physis should be closely followed for possible development of growth disturbance. Parents should be warned of potential complications, but without causing much anxiety. As already indicated, the factors that determine the prognosis are the type of epiphyseal plate injury, the age of the child at the time of fracture, the integrity of the blood supply to the epiphysis, the method of reduction, and whether the fracture is open or closed.

Treatment varies according to the type of fracture. Post-traumatic reactive swelling is prevented by the immediate application of a well-padded compression dressing and a posterior splint. The routine roentgenograms should include anteroposterior, lateral, and oblique views. In difficult cases, such as triplane fracture, plain tomography or computed tomography may be indicated. Closed reduction should be performed as soon as possible; each day of delay will make reduction much more difficult. Time is of the essence.

The reverse of the mechanism of injury will reduce the fracture. The golden rule is *be gentle*. A major manipulation, especially in an uncooperative child, is best performed under general anesthesia. Relaxation of muscles and absence of pain will make the manipulation easy and least traumatic. The knee is flexed 90 degrees and the foot is plantar-flexed to relax the triceps surae muscle. An assistant applies countertraction by pulling up on the leg. With one hand, the surgeon grasps the foot by the heel while steadying the anterior aspect of the lower fourth of the tibia with the palm of his other hand. First, distal traction is applied in the line of deformity and then in the direction opposite to the injuring force to reduce the fracture.

In *supination-inversion injuries,* first longitudinal distal traction is applied medially, and then the hindfoot is everted (Fig. 6–77).

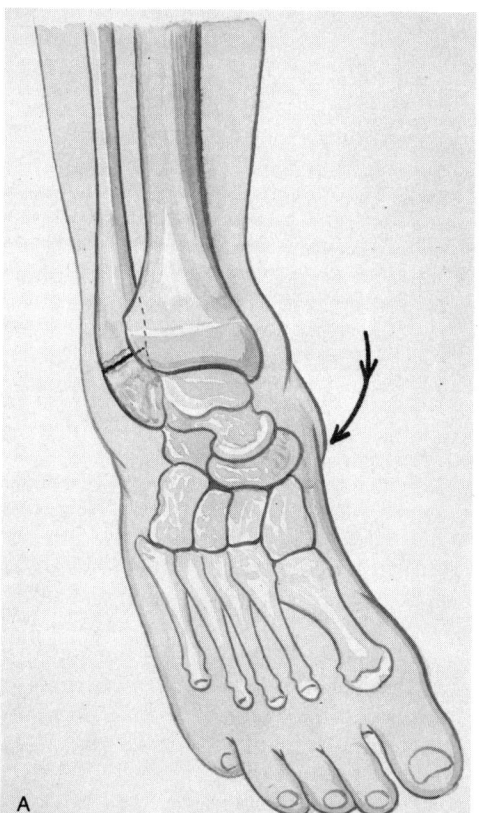
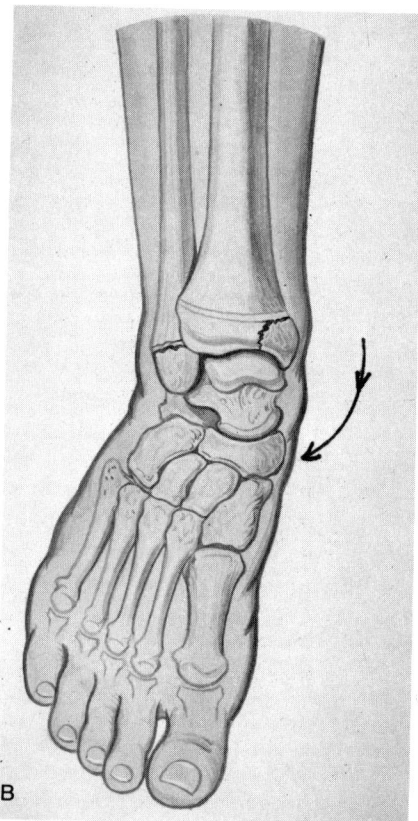

FIGURE 6–77. *Method of reduction of supination-inversion injury.*

A. Apply longitudinal traction distally in the line of deformity, i.e., in inversion. **B.** Then *evert* the hindfoot and apply cast with the foot in slight pronation and the ankle in neutral dorsiflexion. In Salter-Harris Type III physeal injuries anatomic reduction is imperative. Open reduction is required if separation of fracture fragments of the tibial epiphysis is greater than 2 mm.

The foot is immobilized in slight pronation with the ankle in neutral dorsiflexion. In Salter-Harris Type I or II fractures of the distal physis of the fibula the cast is worn for three to four weeks. The prognosis is excellent. The rare fracture of the tip of the lateral malleolus and rupture of the lateral collateral ligament is treated by a below-knee walking cast for three weeks. In *grade 2* supination-inversion injuries there is Salter-Harris Type III or IV physeal fracture of the distal tibial epiphysis. Anatomic reduction is mandatory. Separation of fracture fragments should be less than 2 mm. If one is unable to reduce and maintain anatomic reduction by closed method, open surgical reduction is performed. Smooth Kirschner wires or a cancellous screw is used for internal fixation (see Fig. 6–62). After closed or open reduction an above-knee cast is applied with the knee in 45 degrees of flexion. The palms of the hands are used to mold the plaster carefully over the malleoli and the heel of the foot. The cast is extended above the flexed knee to relax the pull of the tendo Achillis and to prevent weight-bearing. Immobilization is continued for six to eight weeks, and then gradual weight-bearing is allowed. Restraint from weight-bearing for longer periods is of no value in preventing deformity once the physis has been injured. The risk of growth arrest of the medial part of the distal tibial physis is great. With asymmetric growth, varus deformity of the ankle and shortening of the leg will gradually develop.

In *supination–plantar flexion fracture*, first longitudinal traction is applied in plantar flexion, and then, while the downward traction is maintained, the ankle is gently dorsiflexed (Fig. 6–78). The limb is immobilized for four to six weeks in an above-knee cast with the ankle in 5 to 10 degrees of dorsiflexion. The common physeal injury is a Salter-Harris Type II fracture of the distal tibial epiphysis with a posterior metaphyseal fragment and posterior displacement. Moderate residual deformity tends to disappear spontaneously with subsequent growth and remodeling. Posterior displacement corrects itself readily, as it is in the plane of ankle motion. The danger in management of su-

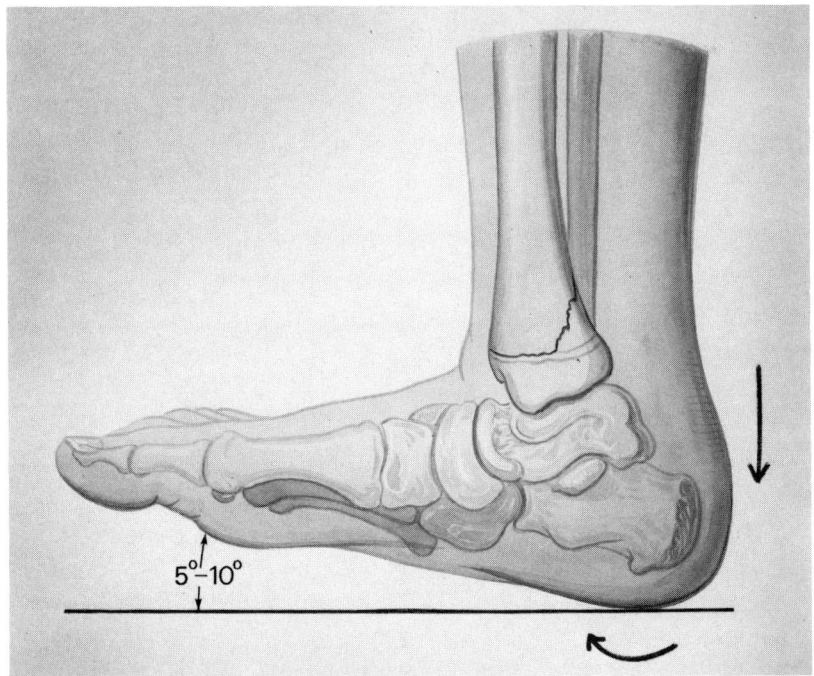

FIGURE 6–78. Method of reduction of supination–plantar flexion fracture of the ankle.

First, longitudinal traction is applied distally and in plantar flexion; then, the ankle is gently dorsiflexed. The limb is immobilized in an above-knee cast with ankle in 5 to 10 degrees of dorsiflexion and the foot in slight pronation.

pination–plantar flexion injury of the ankle is iatrogenic trauma by repeated forceful manipulation. If after two attempts accurate reduction cannot be achieved, it is wise to accept the deformed position.

Supination–lateral rotation fractures of the ankle, both grade 1 and grade 2, are reduced by longitudinal axial traction and medial rotation of the foot (Fig. 6–79). An above-knee cast is applied with the foot and ankle in slight inversion. The period of immobilization is eight weeks. The prognosis is excellent for complete healing with no deformity or disability.

Pronation–eversion–lateral rotation fracture of the ankle is reduced first by longitudinal axial traction in the line of deformity (i.e., in lateral rotation and with the hindfoot everted), and distal traction is maintained on the hindfoot, which is then *inverted and medially rotated* (Fig. 6–80). An above-knee cast is applied with the foot and ankle in inversion and medial rotation. The physeal injury is a Salter-Harris Type II fracture of the distal tibial epiphysis with the metaphyseal fragment located on the lateral or posterolateral side. The displacement is lateral, producing a valgus lateral rotation deformity of the ankle. A valgus tilt of the ankle up to 15 degrees can be accepted. In the report of Crenshaw, roentgenograms made soon after the reduction showed a valgus tilt of the ankle in 6 of the 20 abduction fractures, and by the time of skeletal maturity, this tilt had disappeared spontaneously in every instance. The most severe tilt measured 12 degrees (in a 13½-year-old patient) and the least severe was 4 degrees (in a 10-year-old child). One patient with a lateral rotation fracture had a valgus tilt at the ankle of 10 degrees immediately following treatment, but the deformity disappeared completely during later growth.[22]

If a valgus tilt of more than 15 degrees is present at the ankle, a well-padded below-knee cast is applied, and after three or four

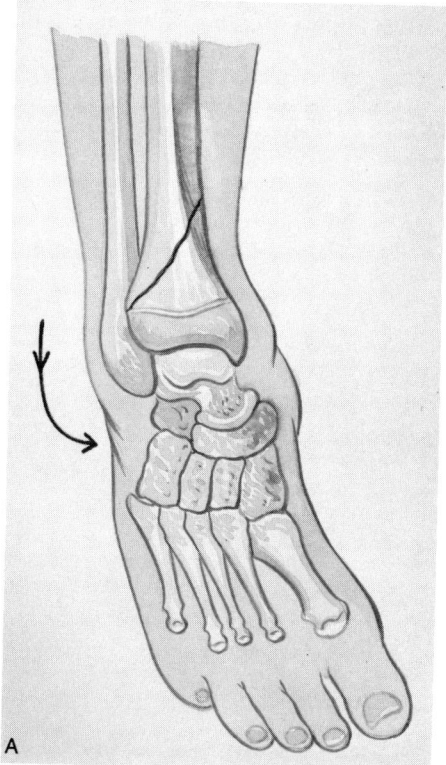 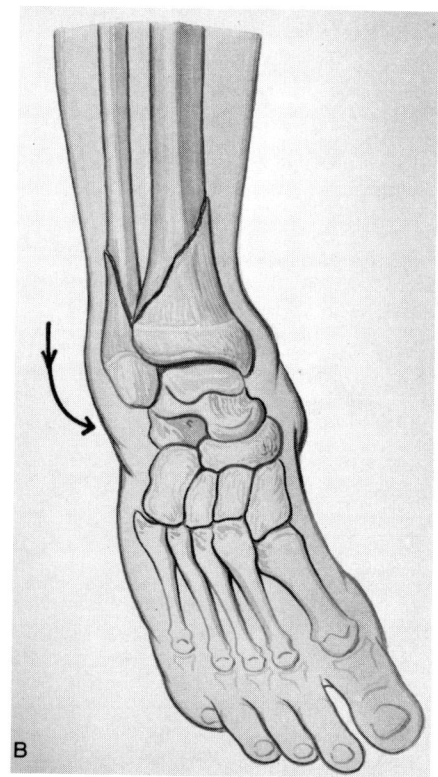

FIGURE 6–79. *Method of reduction of supination–lateral rotation fracture of the ankle.*

A. Grade 1. **B.** Grade 2. Longitudinal axial traction is applied, and while distal traction is maintained, the foot is medially rotated. An above-knee cast is applied with the foot in slight inversion. The period of immobilization in the cast is eight weeks.

injury is Salter-Harris Type III, involving the lateral part of the distal tibial epiphysis. Anatomic reduction is mandatory. If the fracture fragments are displaced more than 2 mm., open reduction and internal fixation with a cancellous screw or smooth Kirschner wires is required through an anterolateral approach. With accurate reduction the prognosis is excellent. Deformity due to asymmetric growth from physeal injury does not follow this fracture. Joint incongruity can be prevented by anatomic reduction. The only significant problem of Tillaux fracture in the adolescent is tendon adhesions.

The undisplaced or minimally displaced (less than 2 mm.) *triplane fracture* is reduced by medial rotation of the hindpart of the

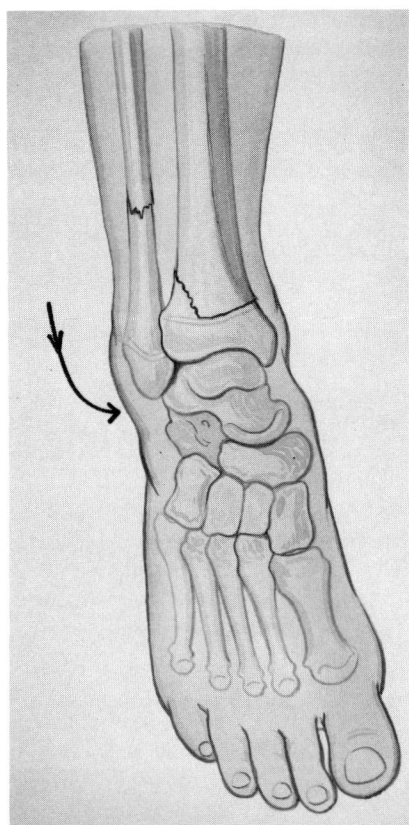

FIGURE 6–80. Method of reduction of pronation–eversion–lateral rotation fracture of the ankle.

First, apply longitudinal traction in the line of deformity—in lateral rotation and with the hindfoot everted, and then, while maintaining distal traction, *invert* and medially rotate the hindfoot.

days, gentle closed reduction is reattempted under general anesthesia; by then the reactive swelling will have subsided under the compression from the cast and the elevation of the leg. If reduction fails and more than 15 degrees of lateral angulation of the ankle mortise persists, open reduction should not be performed. The fracture is allowed to heal, and if, after two or three years, the deformity still persists, a supramalleolar osteotomy is performed to correct the valgus deformity at the ankle.

The *adolescent fracture of Tillaux* is reduced by applying longitudinal axial traction and, while traction is maintained, medially rotating the hindfoot on the leg. The limb is immobilized in an above-knee cast for six to eight weeks (Fig. 6–81). The physeal

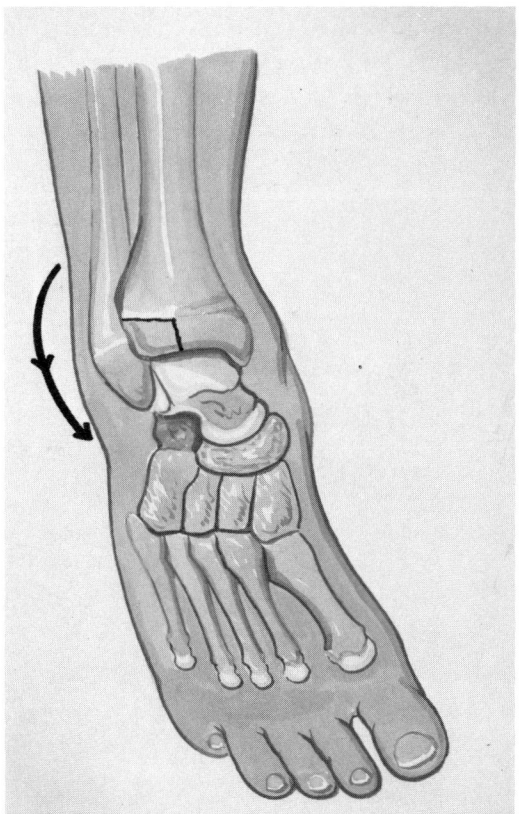

FIGURE 6–81. Method of reduction of adolescent Tillaux fracture.

While longitudinal axial traction is applied, the hindfoot is medially rotated. Caution! This is a Salter-Harris Type III fracture of the lateral part of the distal tibial epiphysis. If the fragments are separated by 2 mm. or more, open reduction and internal fixation are required.

foot on the tibia. The limb is immobilized in an above-knee non-weight-bearing cast for four weeks, then by a below-knee non-weight-bearing cast for an additional two to four weeks. In the cast the hindpart of the foot should be in medial rotation.

If on the routine anteroposterior and lateral roentgenograms the fracture is displaced more than 2 mm. and the fibula is intact, closed reduction under general anesthesia is ordinarily required. Medial rotation of the heel on the leg will usually be successful in reducing the fracture. Tomograms are made, if necessary, to delineate the accuracy of anatomic reduction. An associated greenstick or displaced fracture of the fibula may prevent reduction of the triplane fracture of the distal end of the tibia; the strong ligmentous attachments to the fibula and the lateral part of the tibia will maintain its angular deformity and the resultant shortening of the attached tibial fragment. Reduction of the triplane fracture cannot be accomplished until the fibular fracture is reduced.

If closed reduction is unsuccessful, open reduction and internal fixation with pins or cancellous screws is performed. In the reported cases of Marmor, Lynn, and Torg and Ruggiero, the triplane fracture of the distal end of the tibia was found to be unstable, requiring open reduction and internal fixation.[47, 49, 65] In the series of Cooperman and co-workers, however, only 2 of the 15 triplane fractures were treated by open surgical reduction.[21] First, the posterior fragment is reduced through a posteromedial approach and fixed internally with two cancellous screws. If in the anteroposterior roentgenogram the vertical fracture line through the sagittal plane is 2 mm. or more in width, an anterior approach is used to visualize the fracture; it is anatomically reduced and fixed securely with a transverse

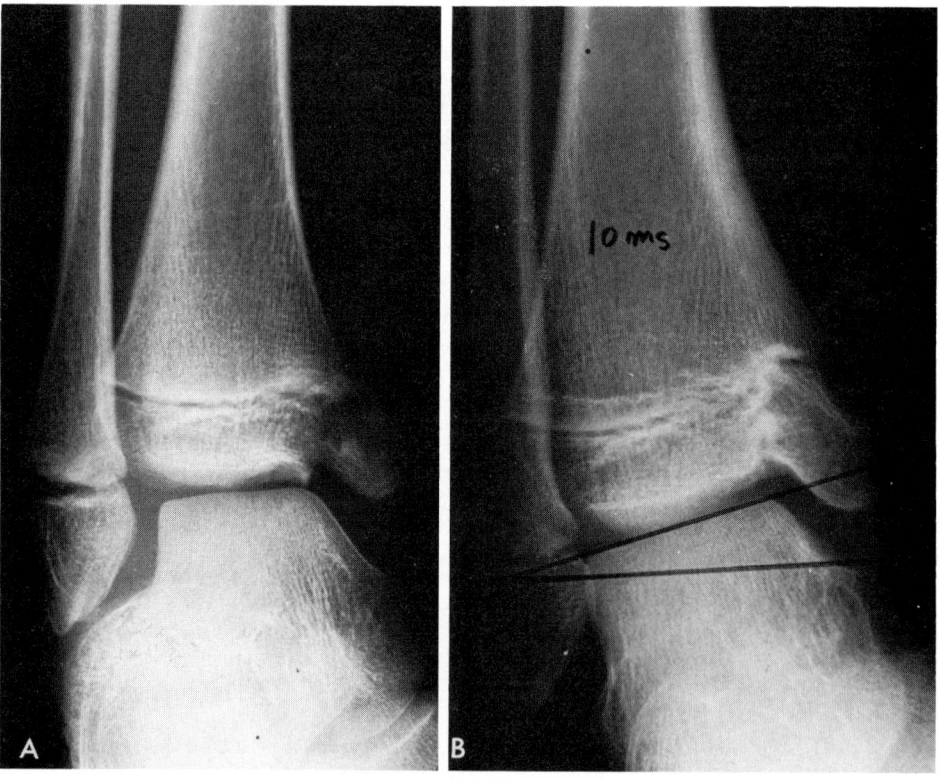

FIGURE 6–82. *Supination-inversion grade 2 fracture of the ankle.*

A. Note the Salter-Harris Type I fracture separation of the distal fibular physis and the Type IV fracture of the medial part of the distal tibial physis. **B.** Ten months later, there is varus ankle deformity secondary to asymmetric growth arrest of the medial part of the distal tibial physis and continued growth of the lateral part of the distal tibial physis and the lower fibular physis.

cancellous screw inserted immediately above the medial malleolus. Injury to the growth plate or penetration of the articular surface by the screw should be avoided. The limb is immobilized in an above-knee cast for six to eight weeks.

Complications

Premature Closure of Physis. Asymmetric and symmetric growth arrest results from crushing of the germinal layer of the physis. It may be complete, causing leg length inequality, or partial and asymmetric, causing angular deformity.

In grade 2 supination-inversion injury of the ankle with Salter-Harris Type IV or V fracture the medial part of the tibial physis will fuse, whereas the lateral portion of the tibial physis and the distal fibular physis will remain open and continue to grow, causing progressive varus deformity of the ankle (Figs. 6–82 and 6–83). The younger the patient, the greater will be the deformity.

The extent of fusion of the growth plate is determined by anteroposterior and lateral tomography of the ankle joint. If less than 40 per cent of the growth plate is fused, the bone bridge is resected and replaced with adipose tissue from the gluteal region (Figs. 6–84 and 6–85). The excision of the bony bridge should be complete; it is performed with a dental drill and image intensifier control. Langenskiöld has demonstrated that interposition of fatty tissue will prevent regeneration of bone and fusion across the physis.[39]

If the size of the bony bridge across it is greater than 50 per cent of the width of the physis, the varus deformity at the ankle joint may be corrected by either "close-up" or "open-up" supramalleolar osteotomy of the tibia. The age of the patient and the amount of shortening will determine the operative procedure chosen. If surgery is postponed until ossification of the physis is complete in children and young adolescents (under 12 years of age for girls and under 14 years for boys), structural changes due to walking in inversion may take place in the ankle mortise. Also, resultant shortening of the leg and overgrowth of the fibula may be of considerable magnitude. Thus, it is best to perform an open-up osteotomy without disturbing the lateral portion of the distal tibial physis. With growth, the varus deformity will recur, and a second osteotomy will be required for correction; this should be explained to the parents.

The technique of open-up supramalleolar wedge osteotomy is as follows: A 3-cm. linear incision is made over the lateral aspect of the distal diaphysis of the fibula. The peroneal tendons are retracted posteriorly, the periosteum is divided, and the fibula is osteotomized obliquely at a level 2 cm. proximal to its distal physis. Then a 5-cm. linear incision is made over the medial aspect of the tibia, beginning at the distal tibial physis and extending proximally. The subcutaneous tissue is divided, exposing the periosteum. The level of osteotomy is 1 cm. proximal to the distal tibial physis. A smooth Kirschner wire is drilled into the tibia, and an anteroposterior roentgenogram is made to ascertain its site. Next, with starters and

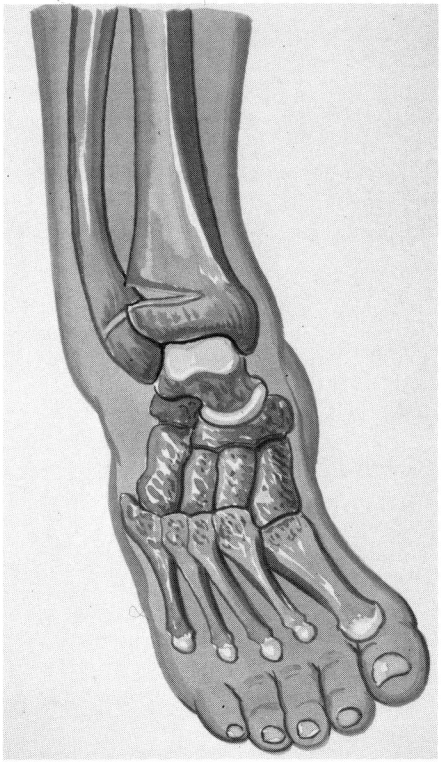

FIGURE 6–83. Diagram showing ankle varus deformity secondary to grade 2 supination-inversion fracture of the ankle.

Note the closure of the medial part of the distal tibial physis; the lateral part of the distal tibial physis and the fibular physis are open and continue to grow.

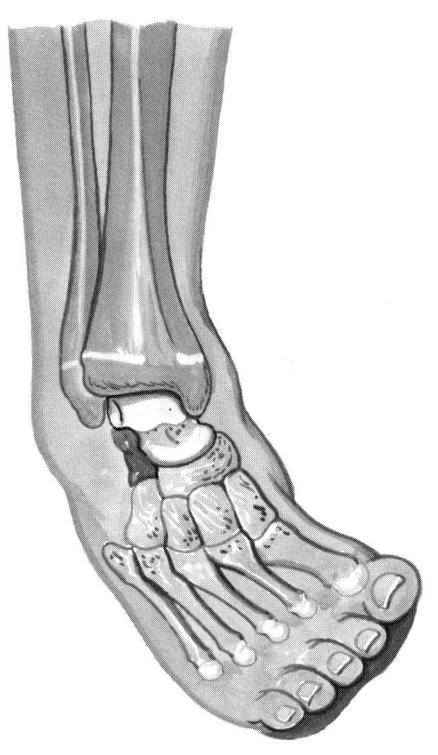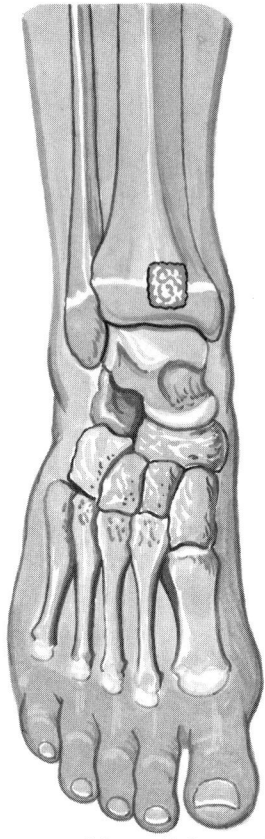

FIGURE 6–84. Diagram showing treatment of asymmetrical growth arrest of the medial part of the distal tibial physis.

The bony bridge across the growth plate is resected and replaced with adipose tissue from the gluteal region. Interposition of fatty tissue will prevent regeneration of bone.

a drill, holes are made through the medial four fifths of the tibia, which is divided transversely with sharp osteotomes, leaving the lateral cortex intact. An alternative method is the use of an oscillating electric saw. The distal fragment of the tibia and the foot are angulated laterally, opening up the osteotomy site. Wedges of iliac bone of appropriate width are obtained and inserted into the gap on the medial side of the tibia (a laminectomy spreader may be used to keep the tibial bone fragments apart while the iliac bone grafts are being inserted). Roentgenograms are made to determine the degree of correction obtained. The osteotomy is fixed internally with either two wide staples or criss-cross Kirschner wires. Caution is exercised to avoid overstretching of the tibial vessels and ischemia of the foot. The tourniquet is released, and after complete hemostasis and return of normal circulation in the limb, the wound is closed and an above-knee plaster cast is applied. The osteotomy will heal and the bone graft will be incorporated in about two to three months.

In the author's experience, in the young child supramalleolar open-up wedge osteotomy has been a satisfactory procedure. It is important to correct overgrowth of the fibula by wedge resection of the lower fibular diaphysis or by epiphysiodesis of the distal fibula at the appropriate age.

The author does not recommend "close-up" supramalleolar osteotomy to correct varus deformity of the ankle joint because it will aggravate the leg length discrepancy.

In an older patient (girls over 12 years and boys over 14 years) epiphysiodesis of the distal fibula and of the lateral half of the distal tibial physis is performed to prevent the development of varus deformity of the ankle. If significant ankle varus deformity has already occurred, the procedure is combined with an open-up wedge osteotomy of the medial aspect of the distal tibia.

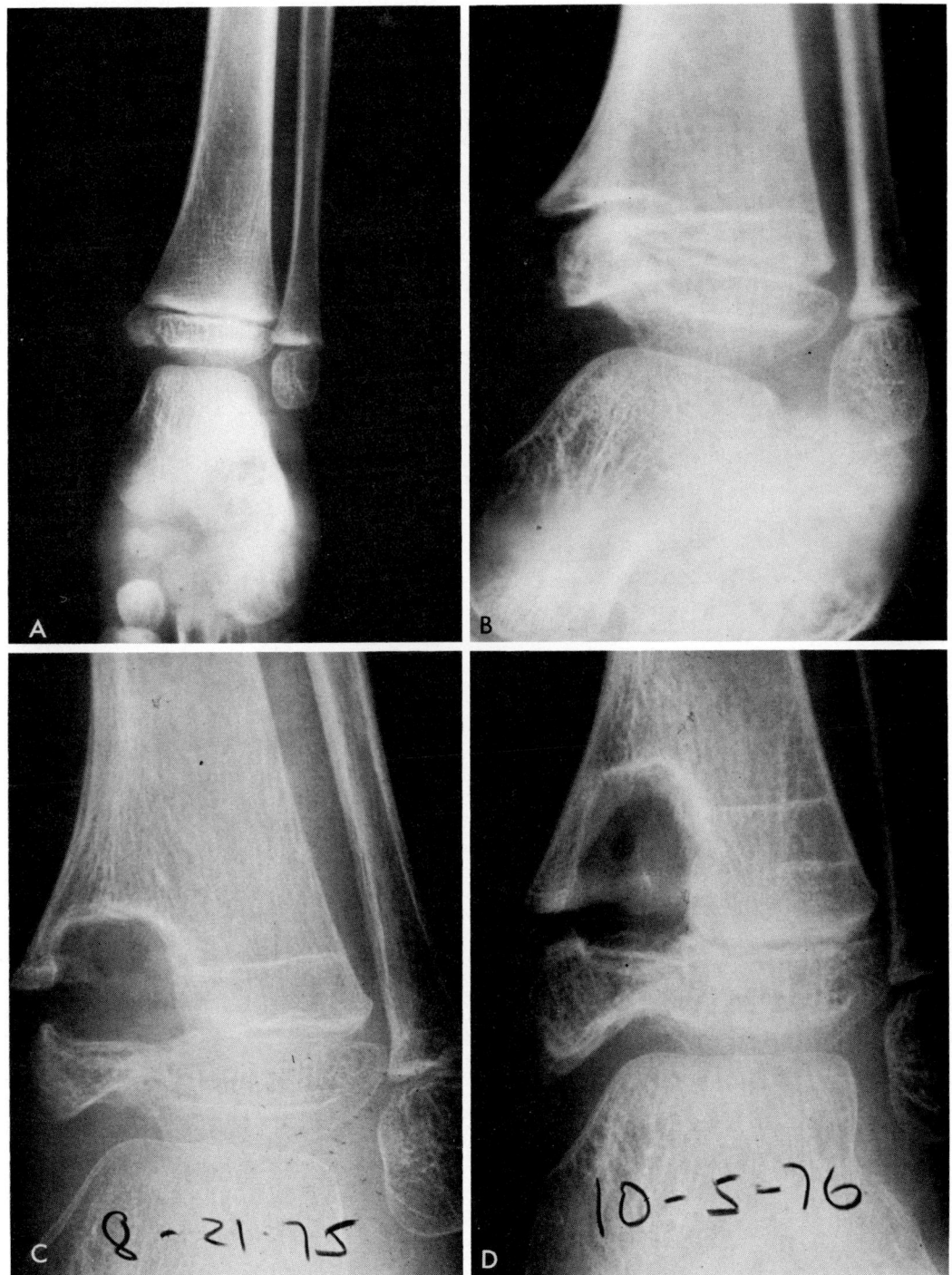

FIGURE 6–85. Roentgenograms of the ankle showing varus deformity due to asymmetrical growth arrest of medial part of the distal tibial physis.

The deformity was treated by excision of the bony bridge across the physis and its replacement in the defect with adipose tissue from the gluteal region to prevent regeneration of bone. Note in the follow-up roentgenograms the continued growth of the medial part of the tibial physis and correction of varus deformity.

Premature growth arrest of the entire distal tibial epiphysis will result in shortening of the tibia. In the older patient, this is inconsequential clinically because of the proximity to termination of skeletal growth, whereas in the younger child, leg length discrepancy may be so marked that an epiphyseal arrest of the contralateral leg will be indicated. An epiphysiodesis of the distal fibula on the affected side is performed to prevent its overgrowth.

Lateral Rotation Deformity. This complication is caused by inadequate reduction. It occurred in 3 of the 15 cases of triplane fracture of Cooperman, Spiegel, and Laros, who, by computed tomography, demonstrated the fracture gap to be wider laterally than medially. This was verified by lateral tomography, which showed the persistent posterior position of the fibula and its attached tibial fragment. In another case Cooperman and his associates studied the mechanism of reduction by premanipula-

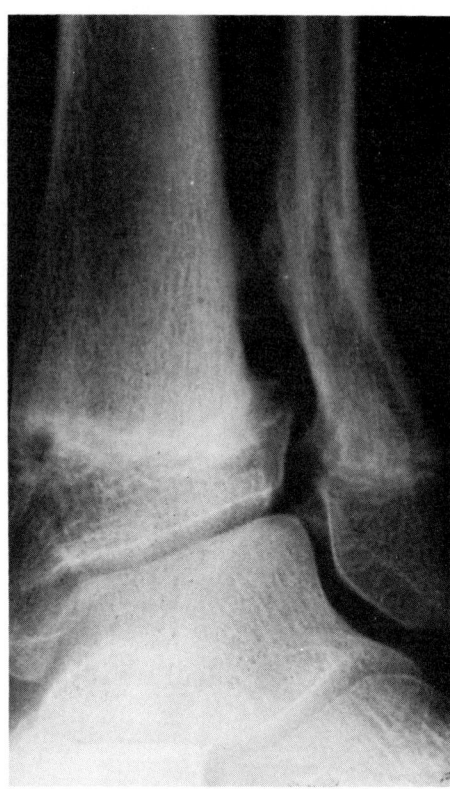

FIGURE 6–87. *Anteroposterior roentgenogram showing valgus ankle due to poor reduction of pronation–eversion–lateral rotation fracture of the ankle.*

A valgus tilt of greater than 15 degrees will usually not be remodeled.

tion and postmanipulation tomography; medial rotation of the foot in relation to the tibia closed the fracture gap.[21]

Valgus Deformity. Ankle valgus deformity usually results from inadequate reduction of pronation–eversion–lateral rotation fracture of the ankle (Figs. 6–86 and 6–87). A valgus tilt of the ankle greater than 15 to 20 degrees will not correct itself by remodeling with skeletal growth and cannot be accepted. It should be corrected surgically. If sufficient growth potential of the distal tibial epiphysis is present, the deformity may be corrected by epipheal arrest of the medial side of the distal tibia. Stapling of the medial side of the physis may be performed if it is difficult to calculate the exact skeletal age of the child. Growth arrest will cause further shortening of the limb.

If skeletal growth is complete, osteotomy of the distal tibia and fibula is performed to correct the deformity. A simple close-up

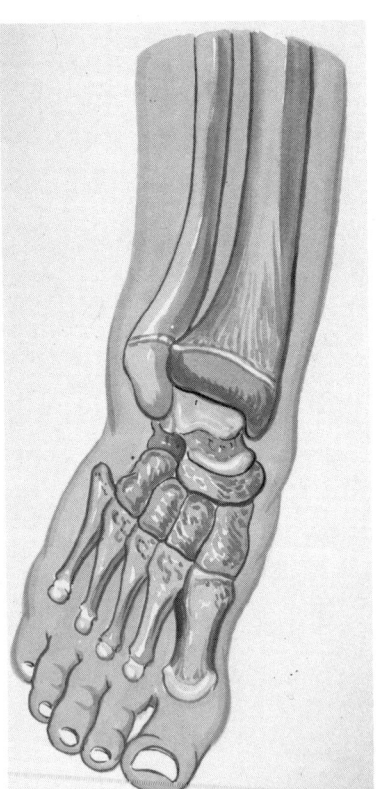

FIGURE 6–86. *Valgus deformity of the ankle results from inadequate reduction of pronation–eversion–lateral rotation fracture of the ankle.*

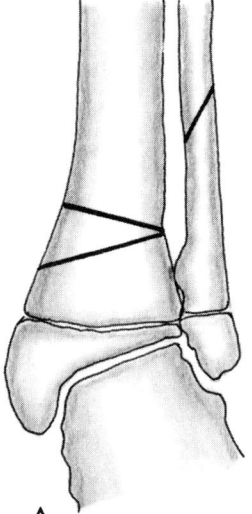
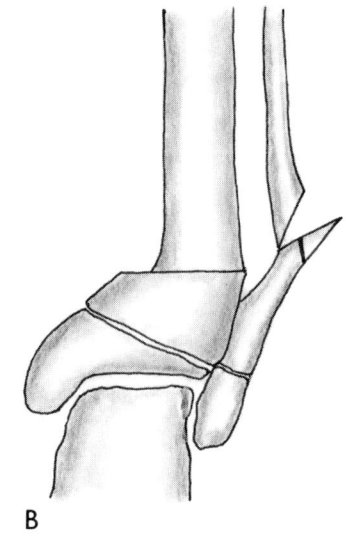

FIGURE 6–88. Close-up wedge osteotomy to correct valgus ankle.

This procedure will shorten the limb and cause an unsightly prominence of the medial malleolus.

wedge osteotomy of the distal tibia will cause unsightly prominence of the medial malleolus and shortening of the limbs (Fig. 6–88). Wiltse has designed a technique of tibial osteotomy in which a triangular segment of bone from the tibia is resected with its apex pointing proximally and the fibula is cut obliquely (from distal-lateral to proximal-medial). The distal fragments of tibia and fibula are rotated medially and shifted laterally, thereby producing normal alignment of the ankle without an unsightly appearance of the medial malleolus (see Fig. 3–55, page 438). The limb will be shortened less than by a simple closing wedge osteotomy. Osteosynthesis is achieved by staples in a three- or four-hole plate, as shown in Figure 3–55.[67]

Joint Incongruity. A potentially serious complication, joint incongruity may cause early degenerative arthritis. Separation of fracture fragments greater than 2 mm. should not be accepted.

Johnson and Fahl reported three additional complications, each of which occurred once following significant displacement of Salter-Harris Type II abduction fractures. In the first case, circulation in the distal part of the foot was decreased, but it quickly returned following reduction of the fracture. With the second (abduction injury), the anterior tibial tendon and periosteum were interposed between the epiphysis and the tibia. Open reduction was necessary to remove the tendon and periosteum before accurate repositioning of the epiphysis could be carried out. In the third case, adhesions developed about the extensor hallucis longus tendon. Following operative lysis of these adhesions, full function was restored.[28]

References

1. Aitken, A. P.: The end results of the fractured distal tibial epiphysis. J. Bone Joint Surg., *18*:685, 1936.
2. Apley, A. G.: The ankle. *In* A System of Orthopaedics and Fractures. 4th Ed. London, Butterworth, 1973, pp. 503–511.
3. Ashhurst, A. P. C., and Bromer, R. S.: Classification and mechanism of fractures of the leg bones involving the ankle. Arch. Surg. (Chicago), *4*:51, 1922.
4. Bartl, R.: Die traumatische Epiphysenlösung am distalen Ende des Schienbeines und des Wadenbeines. Hefte Unfallheilk., *54*:228, 1957.
5. Bergenfeldt, E.: Beiträge zur Kenntnis der traumatischen Epiphysenlösungen an den langen Röhrenknochen der Extremitäten. Eine Klinisch-Röntgenologische Studie. Acta Chir. Scand., Suppl. 28, 1933.
6. Berridge, F. R., and Bonnin, J. G.: The radiographic examination of the ankle joint including arthrography. Surg. Gynec. Obstet., *79*:383, 1944.
7. Bishop, P. A.: Fractures and epiphyseal separation fractures of the ankle. A classification of 332 cases according to the mechanism of their production. Amer. J. Roentgen., *28*:49, 1932.
8. Blount, W. P.: Injuries of the leg and ankle. *In* Fractures in Children. Huntington, N.Y., R. E. Krieger Publishing Co., 1977, pp. 183–193.
9. Bonnin, J. G.: Injuries to the Ankle. London, William Heinemann Medical Books Ltd., 1950.
10. Brashear, H. R.: Epiphyseal fractures of the lower extremity. Southern Med. J., *51*:845, 1958.
11. Bright, R. W.: Surgical correction of partial epiphyseal plate closure in dogs by bone bridge resection and use of silicone rubber implants. J. Bone Joint Surg., *54-A*:1133, 1972.
12. Bright, R. W., Burstein, A. H., and Elmore, S.: Epiphyseal plate cartilage. A biomechanical and histological analysis of failure modes. J. Bone Joint Surg., *56-A*:688, 1974.
13. Brook, G. J., and Greer, R. B.: Traumatic rotational displacement of the distal tibial growth plate. J. Bone Joint Surg., *52-A*:1666, 1970.

14. Cameron, H. U.: A radiologic sign of lateral subluxation of the distal tibial epiphyses. J. Trauma, 15:1030, 1975.
15. Carothers, C. O., and Crenshaw, A. H.: Clinical significance of a classification of epiphyseal injuries at the ankle. Amer. J. Surg., 89:879, 1955.
16. Cassidy, R. H.: Epiphyseal injuries of the lower extremities. Surg. Clin. N. Amer., 38:125, 1958.
17. Chigot, P. L., and Estève, P.: Traumatologie Infantile. 2nd Ed. Paris, Expansion Scientifique Française, 1967, pp. 299–311.
18. Chigot, P. L., and Thuilleux, G.: Traitement des fractures-décollement épiphysaire de la malléole interne, dites de MacFarland. Chirurgie, 98:229, 1972.
19. Chironi, P.: Considerazioni sulla frattura isolata del margine esterno dell'epifisi tibiale inferiore. Minerva Ortop., 6:123, 1955.
20. Cooper, A.: A Treatise on Dislocations and Fractures of the Joints. London, Longman, Hurst, Orme and Brown; E. Cox and Sons, 1822, pp. 238–240.
21. Cooperman, D. R., Spiegel, P. G., and Laros, G. S.: Tibial fractures involving the ankle in children. The so-called triplane epiphyseal fracture. J. Bone Joint Surg., 60-A:1040, 1978.
22. Crenshaw, A. H.: Injuries to the distal tibial epiphysis. Clin. Orthop., 41:98, 1965.
23. Dias, L. S., and Foerster, T. P.: Traumatic lesions of the ankle joint. The supination-external rotation mechanism. Clin. Orthop., 100:219, 1974.
24. Dias, L. S., and Tachdjian, M. O.: Physeal injuries of the ankle in children. Classification. Clin. Orthop., 136:230, 1978.
25. Dias, L. S., Guise, E. R., and Foerster, T.: Classification of ankle fracture. A mechanistic approach. Scientific Exhibit, A.A.O.S., October, 1974. Detroit, Henry Ford Hospital, 1974.
26. Frain, P.: Les décollements épiphysaires de l'extrémité inférieure du tibia. J. Chir. (Paris), 91:113, 1966.
27. Gill, G., and Abbott, L. C.: Varus deformity of ankle following injury to the distal epiphyseal cartilage of the tibia in growing children. Surg. Gynec. Obstet., 72:659, 1941.
28. Johnson, E. W., and Fahl, J. C.: Fractures involving the distal tibial epiphysis of the tibia and fibula in children. Amer. J. Surg., 93:778, 1957.
29. Judet, J., and Judet, R.: Fractures et Orthopaedie de l'Enfant. Paris, Librairie Maloine, 1974.
30. Judet, R., Judet, J., and LaGrange, J.: Les Fractures des Membres chez l'Enfant. Paris, Librairie Maloine, 1958, pp. 235–238.
31. Kaplan, L.: Epiphyseal injuries in children. Surg. Clin. N. Amer., 17:1637, 1937.
32. Kleiger, B.: The mechanism of ankle injuries. J. Bone Joint Surg., 38-A:59, 1956.
33. Kleiger, B., and Barton, J.: Epiphyseal ankle fractures. Bull. Hosp. Joint Dis., 25:240, 1964.
34. Kleiger, B., and Mankin, H. J.: Fracture of the lateral portion of the distal tibial epiphysis. J. Bone Joint Surg., 46-A:25, 1964.
35. Kristensen, T. B.: Treatment of malleolar fractures according to Lauge-Hansen's method. Preliminary results. Acta Chir. Scand., 97:362, 1949.
36. Kristensen, T. B.: Fractures of the ankle. VI. Follow-up studies. Arch. Surg. (Chicago), 73:112, 1956.
37. Kump, W. L.: Vertical fractures of the distal tibial epiphysis. Amer. J. Roentgen., 97:676, 1966.
38. Langenskiöld, A.: Traumatic premature closure of the distal tibial epiphyseal plate. Acta Orthop. Scand., 38:520, 1967.
39. Langenskiöld, A.: An operation for partial closure of an epiphyseal plate in children and its experimental basis. J. Bone Joint Surg., 57-B:325, 1975.
40. Lauge-Hansen, N.: Fracture of the ankle: I. Analytic historic survey as the basis of new experimental, roentgenologic and clinical investigations. Arch. Surg. (Chicago), 56:259, 1948.
41. Lauge-Hansen, N.: Fractures of the ankle: II. Combined experimental surgical and experimental-roentgenologic investigations. Arch. Surg. (Chicago), 60:957, 1950.
42. Lauge-Hansen, N.: Fractures of the ankle. IV. Clinical use of genetic roentgen diagnosis and genetic reduction. Arch. Surg. (Chicago), 64:488, 1952.
43. Lauge-Hansen, N.: Fractures of the ankle. V. Pronation-dorsiflexion fracture. Arch. Surg. (Chicago), 67:813, 1953.
44. Lauge-Hansen, N.: Fractures of the ankle. III. Genetic roentgenologic diagnosis of fractures of the ankle. Amer. J. Roentgen., 71:456, 1954.
45. Laurin, C., and Mathieu, J.: Sagittal mobility of the normal ankle. Clin. Orthop., 108:99, 1975.
46. Lovell, E. S.: An unusual rotatory injury of the ankle. J. Bone Joint Surg., 50-A:163, 1968.
47. Lynn, M. D.: The triplane distal tibial epiphyseal fracture. Clin. Orthop., 86:187, 1972.
48. McFarland, B.: Traumatic arrest of epiphyseal growth of the distal end of the tibia. Brit. J. Surg., 19:78, 1931.
49. Marmor, L.: An unusual fracture of the tibial epiphysis. Clin. Orthop., 73:132, 1970.
50. Maylahn, D. J., Zemel, N. P., and Fahey, J. J.: Fractures involving the epiphyseal cartilage plate of the distal tibia. Personal communication, 1976.
51. Nevelos, A. B., and Colton, C. L.: Rotational displacement of the lower tibial epiphysis due to trauma. J. Bone Joint Surg., 59-B:331, 1977.
52. Paleari, G. L.: Sul meccanismo di produzione dei distacchi antero-esterni dell'epifisi distale della tibia. Arch. Ortop., 73:1146, 1960.
53. Poland, J.: Traumatic Separation of the Epiphyses. London, Smith, Elder & Co., 1898.
54. Pollen, A. G.: Ankle and foot. In Fractures and Dislocations in Children. Baltimore, Williams & Wilkins Co., 1973, Chapter 10, pp. 198–215.
55. Quigley, T. B.: Analysis and treatment of ankle injuries produced by rotatory, abduction, and adduction forces. A.A.O.S. Instr. Course Lect., 19:172, 1970.
56. Rang, M.: Children's Fractures. Toronto, Philadelphia, J. B. Lippincott Co., 1974, pp. 198–209.
57. Robertson, D. E.: Post traumatic osteochondroses of the lower tibial epiphysis. J. Bone Joint Surg., 46-B:212, 1964.
58. Robichon, J., Pegington, J., Mooje, V. B., and Des Jardins, J. P.: Functional anatomy of the ankle joint and its relationship to ankle injuries. Canad. J. Surg., 15:145, 1972.
59. Salter, R. B.: Injuries of the ankle in children. Orthop. Clin. N. Amer., 5:147, 1974.
60. Salter, R. B., and Harris, W. R.: Injuries involving the epiphyseal plate. J. Bone Joint Surg., 45-A:587, 1963.
61. Sammarco, G. J., Burstein, A. H., and Frankel, V. H.: Biomechanics of the ankle: A kinetic study. Orthop. Clin. N. Amer., 4:75, 1973.
62. Schweitzer, G.: Injuries to the distal tibial epiphysis. S. Afr. Med. J., 43:1258, 1969.
63. Siffert, R. S., and Arkin, A. M.: Post-traumatic aseptic necrosis of the distal tibial epiphysis. J. Bone Joint Surg., 32-A:691, 1950.
64. Spiegel, P. G., Cooperman, D. R., and Laros, G. S.: Epiphyseal fractures of the distal ends of the tibia and fibula. J. Bone Joint Surg., 60-A:1046, 1960.
65. Torg, J. S., and Ruggiero, R.: Comminuted epiphyseal fracture of the distal tibia. Clin. Orthop., 110:215, 1971.
66. Wilson, F. C.: Fractures and dislocations of the ankle. In Rockwood, C. A. (ed.): Fractures. Philadelphia, J. B. Lippincott Co., 1975. Chapter 18, pp. 1361–1399.
67. Wiltse, L. L.: Valgus deformity of the ankle as a sequel to acquired or congenital anomalies of the fibula. J. Bone Joint Surg., 54-A:595, 1972.

FRACTURES OF THE FOOT

The flexibility and resiliency of a child's foot make it relatively immune to injury. The forces of indirect violence are transmitted proximally, causing fractures of the tibia or fibula.

In children fractures of the foot are usually produced by direct violence in a crushing injury, such as is caused by a heavy object being dropped on the foot, by being run over by the wheels of an automobile, or by falling from a height and landing on the heels. The crushing force may not break the skin, but it will cause marked soft-tissue injury to the child's foot.

In treatment, the first step is to decrease the soft-tissue swelling by application of a Jones compression dressing and elevation of the foot and leg. Often it is wise to admit the child to the hospital for observation and treatment. During the first few days following trauma the neurovascular and muscular status and the skin are thoroughly assessed. Management of soft-tissue injury takes priority over that of the fracture. When the soft-tissue swelling has subsided and the vascular and skin status permits, the fracture is reduced and immobilized in a plaster of Paris cast. Fractures of the individual bones of the foot are briefly discussed next.

Fractures of the talus are rare in children.[6, 9, 11, 16, 18, 22, 23] They usually occur in the adolescent. In general they heal adequately without serious complications, such as aseptic necrosis. A vertical fracture through the *neck of the talus* is the most common injury. If not displaced or minimally displaced, it is treated by immobilization in a below-knee cast for four to six weeks. Weight-bearing is not permitted.

When the talar neck fracture is displaced, the head of the talus is usually displaced dorsally. The fracture is reduced by closed manipulation and immobilized with the foot in 30 degrees of plantar flexion in a non-weight-bearing below-knee cast for six to eight weeks. Malunion should be avoided. If closed reduction is unsuccessful, open reduction and internal fixation with two Kirschner wires is carried out. It is best to utilize a lateral approach and dissect minimally to prevent further injury to the medial artery to the body of the talus. The reduced but unstable fracture may be fixed by percutaneous pinning under an image intensifier.

Talar neck fracture may be associated with subtalar dislocation. The distal talar fragment and the foot are medially luxated, and the talar body is rotated posteromedially. If the distal fragment is displaced anteriorly, the risk of aseptic necrosis to the body of the talus is very great. The dislocation usually can be reduced by closed manipulation; occasionally, however, open reduction may be required.

Fractures of the *body of the talus* result from violent trauma, as in a fall from a height or an automobile accident. The fracture usually consists of compression of the dome of the talus with varying degrees of comminution and collapse. A conservative approach is recommended in such cases. A below-knee cast is applied for eight weeks and is followed by protection in a patellar tendon–bearing foot-ankle orthosis for one or two years. It is surprising how well the fracture is remodeled and how much functional range of ankle motion is achieved. Primary ankle fusion should not be performed; it is reserved as a salvage procedure for relief of pain, later on in adult life, if necessary.

Indirect violence, such as is sustained in a fall with the foot caught in the spokes of a bicycle, may cause a transverse oblique fracture through the body of the talus. Undisplaced fractures are treated by immobilization in a below-knee cast for two months. Displaced fractures require restoration of anatomic alignment, often by open reduction and internal fixation with Kirschner wires.

Fracture of the *lateral process of the talus* is usually caused by a twisting injury of the ankle; the process is avulsed by the pull of the anterior talofibular ligament.[11] Careful palpation reveals point tenderness immediately anterior to the lateral malleolus. Oblique roentgenograms of the ankle in 10 to 20 degrees of medial rotation will demonstrate the fractured fragment. Sometimes tomography is indicated. Persistent and disabling pain may require excision of the loose fragment.

Osteochondral fracture fragments of the dome of the talus, if displaced, are best removed by arthrotomy (see section on osteochondritis dissecans).

Fractures of the calcaneus are very infrequent in children and usually do not involve the subtalar joint. Treatment consists of application of a Robert Jones compression dressing and elevation of the foot and leg for several days. It is best to admit the child to the hospital. Then the limb is immobilized in a below-knee cast for three to four weeks.[8, 17, 22, 25] Open surgical reduction of displaced os calcis fractures is contraindicated. Malunions will undergo marked remodeling with restoration of normal structure. The occasional persistent varus deviation of the heel may be corrected by Dwyer's osteotomy of the calcaneus.

Lisfranc's *tarsometatarsal fracture-dislocations* are treated by closed manipulation; if adequate reduction cannot be achieved, open surgery is indicated.[16, 26]

Fractures of the navicular, cuboid, and cuneiforms are caused by crushing injury.[7] Primary treatment is directed toward control of soft-tissue swelling with a Robert Jones compression dressing and elevation of the foot. After soft-tissue swelling has subsided a below-knee walking cast is applied and worn for four weeks.

Metatarsal fractures are produced by direct compression force, and usually more than one metatarsal bone is involved.[12] Treatment consists of simple immobilization of the foot in a below-knee cast for four weeks. Markedly displaced fractures may require open reduction and internal fixation with Kirschner wires. Nonunions and malunions may result in shortened rays and metatarsalgia due to depression of the metatarsal heads.

Fractures of the proximal end of the fifth metatarsal are of two distinct types: a fracture through the tuberosity (known as Jones's fracture, since Sir Robert Jones first described it in 1902), and a fracture through the proximal part of the diaphysis within a distance of 1.5 cm. from the tuberosity.[5, 13, 24]

Fractures through the tuberosity of the fifth metatarsal are caused by forced inversion of the plantar-flexed foot. Treatment is symptomatic. An elastic bandage and partial weight-bearing with crutches are used for about three weeks. If symptoms are severe, for the greater comfort of the patient and convenience of the surgeon, a below-knee cast is applied. Roentgenographic osseous union takes place almost uniformly in less than two months.

The problem with fractures of the tuberosity of the fifth metatarsal is erroneous diagnosis. Dameron has clearly described the anatomic variations of the proximal portion of the fifth metatarsal, where the secondary center of ossification in the tuberosity may be mistaken for a fracture line. Study of the roentgenograms of one foot of 164 unselected children (56 girls and 108 boys) ranging in age from 7 to 16 years disclosed no roentgenographic evidence of this secondary ossification center before the age of 8 years. It became visible in the roentgenogram between 9 and 11 years in girls and between 11 and 14 years in boys. The apophysis was seen to be united to the shaft before the age of 12 in all the girls and before the age of 15 in all the boys.[5]

The secondary center of ossification appears as a fleck of bone located within the plantar and lateral parts of the cartilaginous flare and obliquely oriented with respect to the metatarsal shaft. At this stage of maturation it can closely resemble a fracture.

Other structures that may cause difficulty in diagnosis are the *os peroneum* (located in the peroneus longus tendon and present in 15 per cent of roentgenograms of the foot) and *os vesalianum* (which is thought to be either an ossicle in the peroneus brevis tendon or part of the tuberosity of the fifth metatarsal and present in 0.1 per cent of roentgenograms of the feet). Both ossicles have smooth, sclerotic opposing surfaces that are easily differentiated from the jagged margin of a recent fracture. A transverse radiolucent line in the proximal end of the fifth metatarsal is another anomaly that may cause confusion. This apophyseal line does not extend proximally to the cuboid–fifth metatarsal joint or medially into the articulation between the fourth and fifth metatarsals, and its line of orientation is oblique (almost parallel) to the long axis of the shaft. In contrast, a fracture is perpendicular to the fifth metatarsal shaft, and usually the fracture line extends into one or both articulations between the fourth and fifth metatarsals and between the fifth metatarsal and the cuboid bone.

Fractures through the proximal part of the fifth metatarsal usually take place 1.5 cm. distal to the tuberosity. They are notorious for slow healing. It is best to treat them by immobilization in a below-knee cast for six weeks. In case of delayed healing, Dameron recommends consideration of early bone grafting in professional athletes and symptomatic treatment in sedentary persons.[5]

References

1. Anderson, L. D.: Injuries of the forefoot. Clin. Orthop., *122*:18, 1977.
2. Blount, W. P.: Injuries of the foot. *In* Fractures in Children. Huntington, New York, E. Krieger Publishing Co., 1977, pp. 195–201.

3. Bovill, E. G., Jr., and Inman, V. T.: Fractures and fracture-dislocations of the foot and ankle. In Inman, V. T. (ed.): DuVries' Surgery of the Foot. St. Louis, C. V. Mosby Co., 1973, pp. 119–167.
4. Brown, D. C., and McFarland, G. B.: Dislocation of the medial cuneiform bone in tarsometatarsal fracture-dislocation. J. Bone Joint Surg., 57-A:858, 1975.
5. Dameron, T. B.: Fractures and anatomical variation of the proximal portion of the fifth metatarsal. J. Bone Joint Surg., 57-A:788, 1975.
6. Dunn, A. R., Jacobs, B., and Campbell, R. D.: Fractures of the talus. J. Trauma, 6:443, 1966.
7. Elghawabi, M. H.: Fractures of the cuneiform bones. Classification and treatment. Egypt. Orthop. J., 7:206, 1972.
8. Essex-Lopresti, P.: The mechanism, reduction, technique and results of fractures of the os calcis. Brit. J. Surg., 39:395, 1952.
9. Fahey, J. J., and Murphy, J. L.: Dislocations and fractures of the talus. Surg. Clin. N. Amer., 45:79, 1965.
10. Giannestras, N. J., and Sammarco, G. J.: Fractures and dislocations in the foot. In Rockwood, C. A., and Green, D. P. (eds.): Fractures. Philadelphia, J. B. Lippincott Co., 1975, Vol. 2, pp. 1400–1495.
11. Hawkins, L. G.: Fractures of the lateral process of the talus. J. Bone Joint Surg., 47-A:1170, 1965.
12. Jaffe, A. C., and Lasser, D. H.: Multiple metatarsal fractures in child abuse. Pediatrics, 60:642, 1977.
13. Jones, R.: Fracture of the base of the fifth metatarsal bone by indirect violence. Ann. Surg., 35:697, 1902.
14. Joplin, R. J.: Injuries of the foot. In Cave, E. F., Burke, J. F., and Boyd, R. J. (eds.): Trauma Management. Chicago, Year Book Medical Publishers, Inc., 1974, pp. 837–868.
15. Kenwright, J., and Taylor, R. G.: Major injuries of the talus. J. Bone Joint Surg., 52-B:36, 1970.
16. Main, B. J., and Jowett, R. L.: Injuries of the midtarsal joint. J. Bone Joint Surg., 57-B:89, 1975.
17. Matter, R., and Frymoyer, J.: Fracture of the calcaneus in young children. J. Bone Joint Surg., 55-A:1091, 1973.
18. Mukherjee, S. K., and Young, A. B.: Dome fracture of the talus. A report of ten cases. J. Bone Joint Surg., 55-B:319, 1973.
19. Ogden, J. A.: Skeletal Injury in the Child. Philadelphia, Lea & Febiger, 1982, pp. 621–641.
20. Pathi, K.: Fractures of the neck of the talus in children. J. Indian Med. Assoc., 63:157, 1974.
21. Pollen, A. G.: Ankle and foot. In Fractures and Dislocations in Children. Baltimore, The Williams & Wilkins Co., 1973, pp. 198–215.
22. Spak, I.: Fractures of the talus in children. Acta Chir. Scand., 107:533, 1954.
23. Stephens, N. A.: Fracture dislocation of the talus in childhood: A report of two cases. Brit. J. Surg., 42:600, 1956.
24. Stewart, I. M.: Jones fracture: Fracture of base of fifth metatarsal. Clin. Orthop., 16:190, 1960.
25. Thomas, H. M.: Calcaneal fracture in childhood. Brit. J. Surg., 56:664, 1969.
26. Wilson, D. W.: Injuries of the tarso-metatarsal joints. J. Bone Joint Surg., 54-B:677, 1972.

STRESS FRACTURES

Stress (or fatigue) fracture is a gradual localized dissolution of bone caused by prolonged repetitive muscular action on a bone in a limb that is not accustomed to it. The break takes place in a bone with normal elastic resistance and occurs in individuals who engage in physical activities such as jogging or cross-country skiing.

The fatigue type of stress fracture should be distinguished from the *insufficiency* fracture, which occurs in a bone with deficient elastic resistance.[85] The stress exerted on the bone is physiologic and not strenuous. Conditions predisposing to insufficiency fractures may be classified as *those due to developmental affections* (osteogenesis imperfecta, osteopetrosis [marble bone disease], arachnodactyly), *those due to vitamin deficiency and endocrine disorders* (rickets, scurvy, primary or secondary hyperparathyroidism, hyperpituitarism [Cushing's syndrome], cortisone treatment), *those due to disuse atrophy* (immobilization, paralytic diseases such as myelomeningocele, cerebral palsy, and arthrogryposis multiplex congenita), and *those due to inflammatory conditions* (rheumatoid arthritis).

The term *pathologic fracture* should be restricted to fractures that are caused by trivial trauma in bones that are weakened by pre-existing local lesions such as benign or malignant tumors, osteomyelitis, or postirradiation local osteoporosis.

Sites of Involvement

Historically "stress fracture" was synonymous with the "march fracture" of the metatarsals seen in military recruits.* During the past three decades, however, it has been recognized that stress fractures occur in many bones. Their sites are often predictable, depending upon the activity causing them. For example, stress fracture of the sesamoids of the first metatarsal is produced by prolonged standing; that of the metatarsal shafts by marching, prolonged standing, or ballet; of the tarsal navicular by long-distance running or stamping on the ground as in aerobic exercise; of the calcaneus by prolonged standing (especially on a recently immobilized limb); of the distal shaft of the fibula and proximal diaphysis of the tibia by long-distance running; of the patella by hurdling, of the femur (shaft and neck) by ballet, gymnastics, and long-distance running; of the ischial pubic rami of the pelvis by bowling, stooping, and gymnastics; of the pars interarticularis of the lumbar vertebrae by heavy lifting and ballet; of the ribs by golf, carrying heavy packs, and coughing; of the ulnar shaft by propelling a wheelchair, and of the coronoid proc-

---

*See references 5, 8, 16, 19, 23, 40, 70.

ess of the ulna and the distal humeral shaft by pitching a ball.*

In children the tibia and fibula are frequent sites of stress fractures; they differ from similar fractures in the adult because in children bone has a richer blood supply and greater biologic plasticity.

Pathogenesis

Stress fractures are produced by muscular activity on bone and not from direct impact upon a bone. For example, during running, contraction of the triceps surae muscle plantar-flexes the ankle, dorsiflexion of the foot is restricted, and the tibia and fibula are pulled together maximally at a point immediately above the lateral malleolus. This is a common site of stress fracture in runners, especially children.

Resorption of cortical bone is a normal process that takes place in childhood, adolescence, and early adult life. Osteoclastic activity produces many microscopic channels in the cortex. Eventually these resorption cavities are filled by mature Haversian systems, and the circumferential lamellar bone is gradually replaced by the structurally sounder osteomal bone of the adult.

Bone responds to excessive stress and strain by acceleration of the normal process of cortical resorption. The bony cortex is weakened by the formation of numerous resorption channels. In an attempt to splint the cortex, the endosteal and periosteal tissues respond by forming new bone adjacent to the areas of cortical resorption. If the buttressing process is adequate, the periosteal and endosteal new bone will mature, and the cortical resorption cavities will fill in and eventually become osteomal bone. If this buttressing process does not take place rapidly enough, and if continued excessive stress is applied to the bone, fracture will occur. Stress fracture begins as a small cortical crack.[122] With increase and continuation of stress, the crack progresses by initiation of subcortical infraction ahead of the main crack.

Clinical Findings

When the bones in the lower limb are affected, the child has an antalgic limp, usually of gradual but occasionally of sudden onset. There is no history of acute trauma, although it may be ascertained that the child has recently taken part in some vigorous activity to which he has previously been unaccustomed.

---

*See references: tarsal navicular, 111; calcaneus, 11, 26, 51, 62, 106, 120; fibular, 12, 13, 45, 58, 66, 69, 77, 94; proximal diaphysis of tibia, 3, 4, 14, 27, 41, 49, 54, 55, 56, 58, 59, 67, 71, 95, 97, 105, 107; patella, 28; femur (shaft and neck), 7, 31, 36, 74, 78, 91, 121; ischial ramus, 115; lumbar vertebra, 24, 39, 46, 102, 119; ribs, 93; coronoid process of ulna and distal humeral shaft, 37, 110, 112.

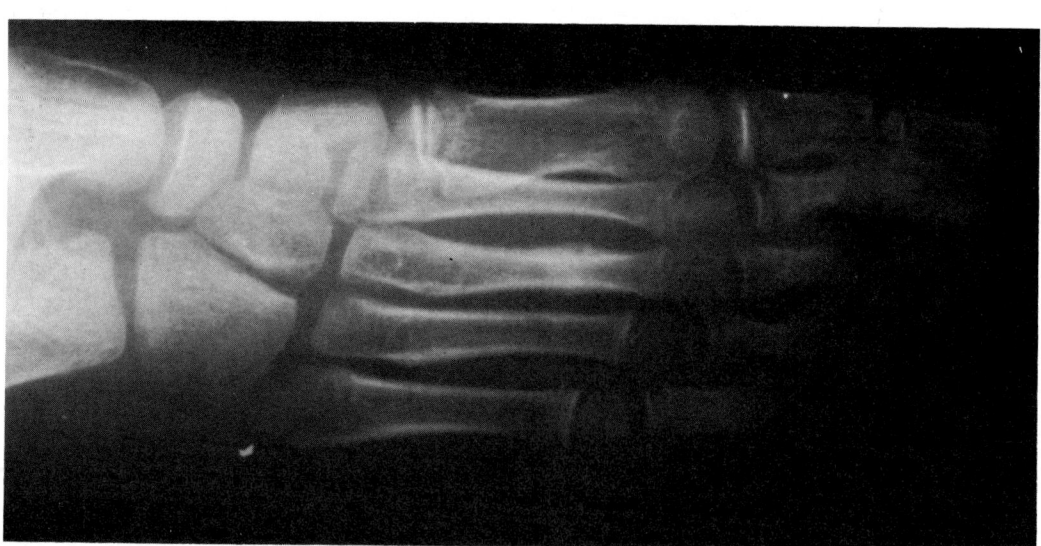

Figure 6–89. Stress fracture of the third metatarsal.

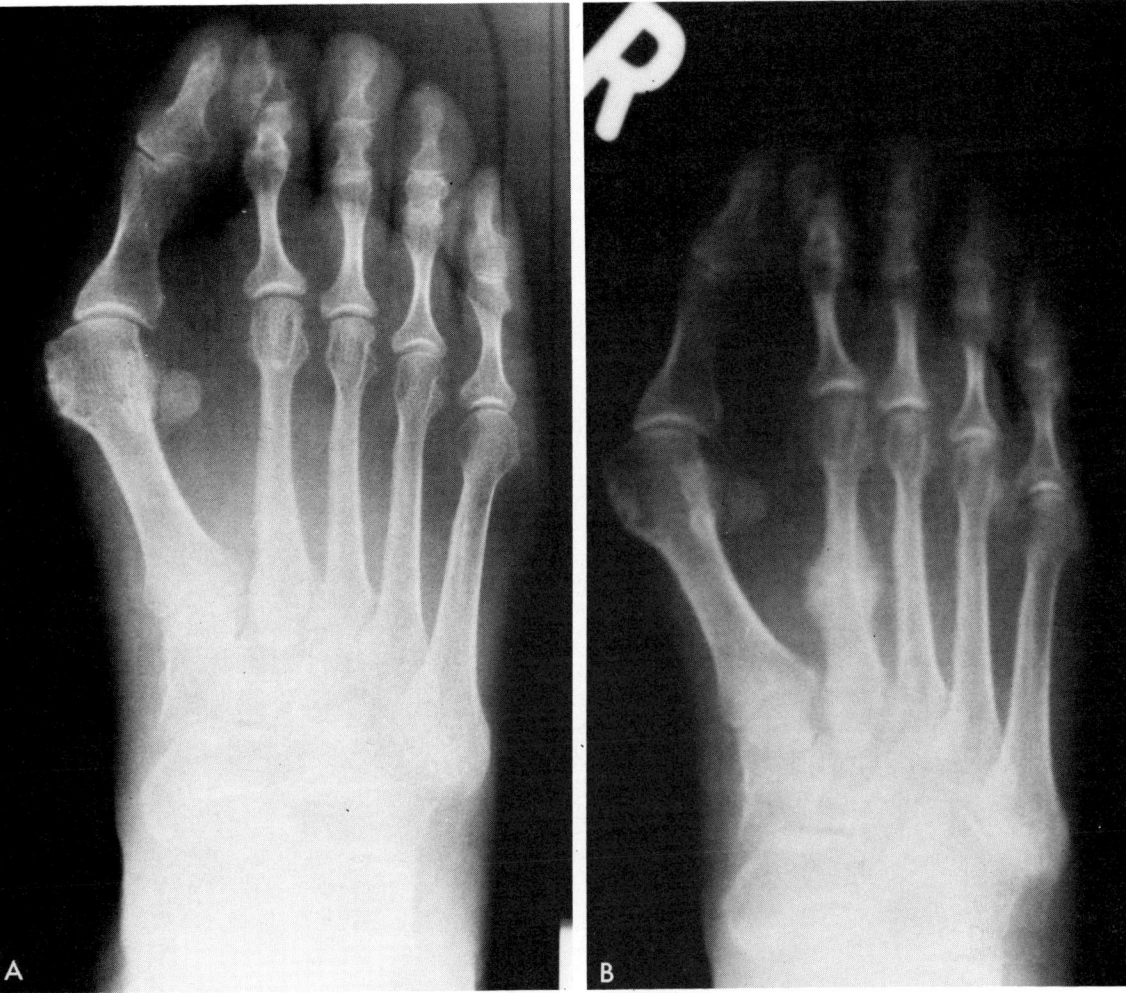

Figure 6–90. Stress fracture of the second metatarsal.

A. Initial roentgenogram. Note the periosteal thickening and the absence of a fracture line. **B.** Two weeks later anteroposterior roentgenogram of the foot shows rapid consolidation of subperiosteal callus and fracture line.

Local pain is frequently present; it is aggravated by activity and relieved by rest.

On palpation, there is a varying degree of local swelling and tenderness. The adjacent joints have full range of motion, but when the ischiopubic ramus or the femoral neck is involved, the hip joint is restricted in abduction and rotation (medial rotation with femoral neck fracture and lateral rotation with ischiopubic ramus fracture).

Roentgenographic Findings

Factors that determine the appearance of a fracture on the roentgenogram are the location of the fracture and the time between injury and the initial radiographic examination. In the early phase a stress fracture in a long bone will manifest itself as a radiolucent zone through the cortical surface without periosteal reaction or callus. With repeated injury and healing, solid or thick laminar periosteal reaction may be seen (Figs. 6–89 and 6–90). In a cancellous bone such as the calcaneus or in the metaphyseal region of a long bone, a stress fracture may appear as an area of focal sclerosis.

Two types of stress fractures have been described by Devas: a *compression type*, common in children, is seen in the calcaneus or the femoral neck, and a *distraction type* begins in one cortex and may be oblique (the most frequent), transverse, or longitudinal.[32] Oblique roentgenographic views and tomography (laminagraphy) will assist in delineating osseous detail.

In the *tibia* the site of stress fracture is nearly always in its proximal third, involving the posteromedial or posterolateral cortex; it rarely occurs on the anterior aspect of the tibia (Fig. 6–91).[107] There are a haze of internal callus across the diaphysis, subperiosteal new bone formation, and slight disruption of the cortex. An actual linear fracture across the shaft is not seen.

In the *fibula* the earliest roentgenographic

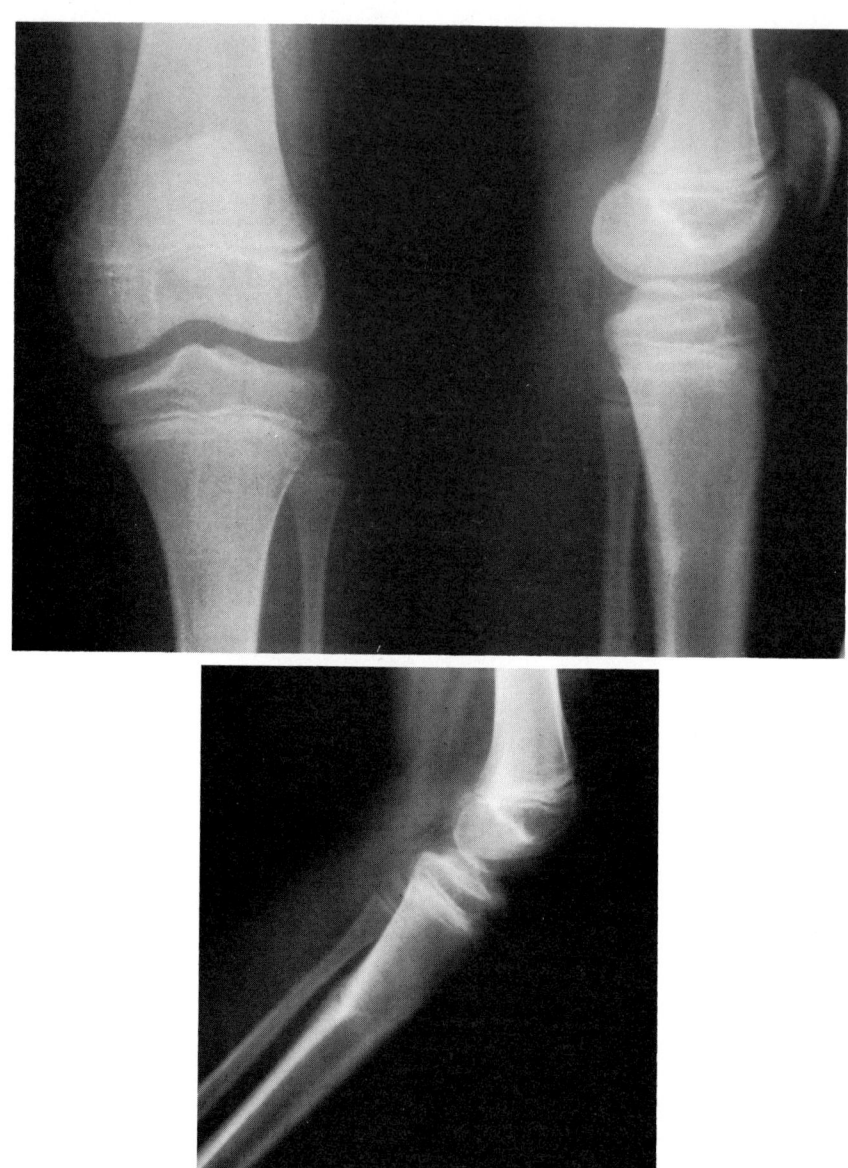

Figure 6–91. Stress fracture of the proximal tibial diaphysis.

Anteroposterior, oblique, and true lateral projections show slight disruption of the cortex on the posterolateral aspect, haze of internal callus, and subperiosteal new bone formation.

sign is the presence of thin layers of "egg shell" callus along the diaphysis. The fracture itself cannot be visualized because it is obscured by the exuberant callus that extends up and down the shaft.

Radioisotope scanning with technetium-99m will show increased isotope uptake due to osteoblastic new bone formation. The bone scan will be positive before plain roentgenograms show any changes.[43, 68, 84, 90, 117]

The diagnosis of stress fracture is made in the great majority of cases by clinical information, plain roentgenograms, and bone scan with technetium-99m. If in doubt, simple tomography is of great value. Occasionally one may have to resort to computed tomography (CT). CT scan will demonstrate lucent fracture lines in the cortex and periosteal reaction.[25, 76]

In the differential diagnosis, one should rule out osteoid osteoma, acute osteomyelitis, chronic sclerosing osteomyelitis, osteogenic sarcoma, Ewing's sarcoma, acute leukemia, and osteomalacia.[71]

In *osteoid osteoma,* a benign lesion, there is a history of pain at night that is relieved by aspirin. In stress fracture the pain occurs on strenuous physical activity and is relieved by rest. In the roentgenogram there is a lucent nidus surrounded by a dense area of sclerosis. The appearance of osteoid osteoma in the bone scan and CT scan is quite characteristic. *Osteogenic sarcoma* is usually a metaphyseal lesion with moth-eaten pattern of lysis in the medulla, tumor bone formation, and periosteal reaction that is aggressive, showing spiculation, thin lamination, coarse deposition, and sometimes Codman's triangle. In osteogenic sarcoma there is progressive destruction of bone. In time, it no longer resembles a healing fracture. The diagnosis of *acute osteomyelitis* is simple by thorough clinical examination. In *chronic sclerosing osteomyelitis* there is diffuse cortical sclerosis with no apparent radiolucency. There is absence of the linear sclerotic pattern of a healing fracture.

If stress fracture is suspected the limb is put to rest. Within 10 to 14 days roentgenograms are repeated; during this time there should be evidence of healing. Biopsy should not be performed unless there is clear-cut radiographic evidence that no healing is taking place and there is a suggestion of malignancy or infection.

Treatment

Treatment consists of rest of the affected part. The type of rest depends on the location of the fracture and whether the break involves one cortex or extends to be a complete fracture. In general, complete fractures are best treated in a plaster of Paris walking cast, whereas infractions are treated by abstinence from strenuous physical activity and use of crutches if necessary.

References

1. Adams, J.: Bone injuries in very young athletes. Clin. Orthop., *58*:129, 1968.
2. Bargren, J. H., Tilson, D. H., Jr., and Bridgeford, O. E.: Prevention of displaced fatigue fracture of the femur. J. Bone Joint Surg., *53-A*:1115, 1971.
3. Benedict, J. S.: Stress fractures of tibia; analysis of thirty-five cases. J. Int. Coll. Surg., *32*:174, 1959.
4. Berkebile, R. D.: Stress fracture of the tibia in children. Amer. J. Roentgen., *91*:588, 1964.
5. Bernstein, A., and Stone, J. R.: March fracture. A report of three hundred seven cases and a new method of treatment. J. Bone Joint Surg., *26*:743, 1944.
6. Bjelland, J. C., Pitt, M. J., and Capp, M. P.: Acute bowing fractures of the extremities: A frequently missed roentgen diagnosis. Medical Imaging, *3*:13, 1978.
7. Blickenstaff, L. D., and Morris, J. M.: Fatigue fractures of the femoral neck. J. Bone Joint Surg., *48-A*:1031, 1966.
8. Branch, H. E.: March fractures of the femur. J. Bone Joint Surg., *26*:387, 1944.
9. Bretagne, M. C., Mouton, J. N., Pierson, M., Prevot, J., Olive, D., and Treheux, A.: Periosteal appositions in paediatrics. (Author's transl.) J. Radiol. Electr., *58*:119, 1977.
10. Brubacker, C. E., and James, S. L.: Injuries to runners. Amer. J. Sports Med., *2*:189, 1974.
11. Buchanan, J., and Greer, R. B.: Stress fractures in the calcaneus of a child. A case report. Clin. Orthop., *135*:119, 1978.
12. Burrows, H. J.: Spontaneous fracture of the apparently normal fibula in its lowest third. Brit. J. Surg., *28*:82, 1940.
13. Burrows, H. J.: Fatigue fractures of the fibula. J. Bone Joint Surg., *30-B*:266, 1948.
14. Burrows, H. J.: Fatigue infraction of the middle of the tibia in ballet dancers. J. Bone Joint Surg., *38-B*:83, 1956.
15. Cail, W. S., Keats, T. E., and Sussman, M. D.: Plastic bowing fracture of the femur in a child. Amer. J. Roentgen., *130*:780, 1978.
16. Carlson, G. D., and Wertz, R. F.: March fracture, including others than those of the foot. Radiology, *43*:48, 1944.
17. Chamay, A.: Mechanical and morphological aspects of experimental overload and fatigue in bone. J. Biomech., *3*:263, 1970.
18. Chamay, A., and Tschants, P.: Mechanical influence in bone remodeling. Experimental research on Wolff's law. J. Biomech., *5*:173, 1972.
19. Childress, H. M.: March foot in a seven-year-old child. J. Bone Joint Surg., *28*:877, 1946.
20. Clement, D.: Tibial stress syndrome in athletes. Amer. J. Sports Med., *2*:81, 1974.
21. Collins, H. R., and Evarts, C. M.: Injuries to the adolescent athlete. Postgrad. Med., *49*:72, 1971.
22. Cullen, R. J., Jr., and Page, L. K.: Growing fractures in children. J.A.M.A., *60*:21, 1973.
23. Cwiklicki, Z.: Stress fracture of the third metatarsal bone in a child. Chir. Narzad. Ruchu. Ortop. Pol., *30*:333, 1965.

24. Cyron, B. M., Hutton, W. C., and Troup, J. D. G.: Spondylolytic fracture. J. Bone Joint Surg., 58-B:462, 1976.
25. Daffner, R. H.: Stress fractures. Current concepts. Skeletal Radiol., 2:221, 1978.
26. Darby, R. E.: Stress fractures of the os calcis. J.A.M.A., 200:1183, 1967.
27. Devas, M.: Stress fracture of the tibia in athletes or "shin soreness." J. Bone Joint Surg., 40-B:227, 1958.
28. Devas, M. B.: Stress fractures of the patella. J. Bone Joint Surg., 42-B:71, 1960.
29. Devas, M. B.: Compression stress fractures in man and the greyhound. J. Bone Joint Surg., 43-B:540, 1961.
30. Devas, M. B.: Stress fractures in children. J. Bone Joint Surg., 45-B:528, 1963.
31. Devas, M. B.: Stress fractures of the femoral neck. J. Bone Joint Surg., 47-B:728, 1965.
32. Devas, M. B.: Stress Fractures. Edinburgh, London, New York, Churchill Livingstone, Inc., 1975.
33. Devas, M. B., and Sweetnam, B.: Stress fractures of the fibula. J. Bone Joint Surg., 38-B:818, 1956.
34. Elton, R. C., and Abbott, H. G.: An unusual case of multiple stress fractures. Milit. Med., 130:1207, 1965.
35. Engh, C. A., Robinson, R. A., and Milgram, J.: Stress fractures in children. J. Trauma, 10:532, 1970.
36. Ernst, J.: Stress fractures of the femoral neck. J. Trauma, 4:71, 1964.
37. Evans, D. L.: Fatigue fracture of the ulna. J. Bone Joint Surg., 37-B:618, 1955.
38. Evans, F. G., and Riolo, M. L.: Relations between the fatigue life and histology of adult cortical bone. J. Bone Joint Surg., 52-A:1579, 1970.
39. Farfan, H. F., Osteria, V., and Lamy, C.: The mechanical etiology of spondylosis and spondylolisthesis. Clin. Orthop., 117:40, 1976.
40. Ford, L. T., and Gilula, L. A.: Stress fractures of the middle metatarsals following the Keller operation. J. Bone Joint Surg., 59-A:117, 1977.
41. Fructer, Z., and Enachesco, L.: Radiodiagnosis of tibial stress fractures in children. J. Radiol. Electr., 51:155, 1970.
42. Fuchs, G.: Diagnosis and therapy of spontaneous fractures in childhood and adolescence. Hefte Unfallheilkd., 102:76, 1970.
43. Geslein, G. E., Thrall, J. H., Espinosa, J. L., and Older, R. A.: Early detection of stress fractures using 99mTc-polyphosphate. Radiology, 121:683, 1976.
44. Gilbert, R. S., and Johnson, H. A.: Stress fracture in military recruits—a review of twelve years' experience. Milit. Med., 8:716, 1966.
45. Griffiths, A. L.: Fatigue fracture of the fibula in childhood. Arch. Dis. Child., 27:552, 1952.
46. Hadley, L. A.: Stress fracture with spondylolysis. Amer. J. Roentgen., 90:1258, 1963.
47. Haluzicky, M., and Szabad, F.: Fracture of long bones from fatigue in sportsmen. Acta Chir. Orthop. Traum. Cech., 42:72, 1975.
48. Hamilton, A. S., and Finklestein, H. E.: March fracture: Report of a case involving both fibulae. J. Bone Joint Surg., 26:146, 1944.
49. Hartley, J. B.: Fatigue fracture of the tibia. Brit. J. Surg., 30:9, 1942.
50. Hartley, J. B.: "Stress" or "fatigue" fractures. Brit. J. Radiol., 16:255, 1943.
51. Hullinger, C. W.: Insufficiency fracture of the calcaneus—similar to march fracture of the metatarsal. J. Bone Joint Surg., 26:751, 1944.
52. Ingersoll, C. F.: Ice skater's fracture. Amer. J. Roentgen., 50:469, 1943.
53. Jones, H. H., Priest, J. D., Hayes, W. C., Tichenor, C. C., and Nagel, D. A.: Humeral hypertrophy in response to exercise. J. Bone Joint Surg., 59-A:204, 1977.
54. Kelly, R. P., and Murphy, F. E.: Fatigue fractures of the tibia. Southern Med. J., 44:290, 1951.
55. Kimball, P. R., and Savastano, A. A.: Fatigue fractures of the proximal tibia. Clin. Orthop., 70:170, 1970.
56. Kochhar, V. S., and Srivastava, K. K.: Stress fracture of the tibia: Report of a case. Aust. N.Z. J. Surg., 43:266, 1973.
57. Kolisch, P. D.: Stress fractures in children. Letter. J.A.M.A., 237:2038, 1977.
58. Kozlowski, K., Pietron, K., and Puk, E.: Stress fracture of the tibia in children. Ann. Radiol. (Paris), 11:679, 1968.
59. Krause, G. R., and Thompson, J. R. G.: March fracture of tibia. Radiology, 41:580, 1943.
60. Kroenig, P. M., and Shelton, M. L.: Stress fractures. Amer. J. Roentgen., 89:1281, 1963.
61. Laferty, J. F., Winter, W. G., and Gambaro, S. A.: Fatigue characteristics of posterior elements of vertebrae. J. Bone Joint Surg., 59-A:54, 1977.
62. Leabhart, J. W.: Stress fractures of the calcaneus. J. Bone Joint Surg., 41-A:1285, 1959.
63. Leveton, A. L.: March (fatigue) fractures of the long bones of the lower extremity and pelvis. Amer. J. Surg., 71:222, 1946.
64. Levin, D. C., Blazina, M. E., and Levine, E.: Fatigue fractures of the shaft of the femur. Simulation of malignant tumor. Radiology, 89:883, 1967.
65. McBryde, A. M.: Stress fractures in athletes. Amer. J. Sports Med., 3:212, 1975.
66. McPhee, H. R., and Franklin, C. M.: March fracture of the fibula in athletes. J.A.M.A., 131:574, 1946.
67. Manoli, A.: Traumatic fibular bowing with tibial fracture. Orthopedics, 1:145, 1978.
68. Marta, J. B., Williams, H. J., and Smookler, R. A.: Gallium-67 uptake in a stress fracture. Letter. J. Nucl. Med., 23:271, 1982.
69. Martin, W., and Riddervold, H. D.: Acute plastic bowing fractures of the fibula. Radiology, 131:639, 1979.
70. Michetti, M. L.: March fracture following a McBride bunionectomy. A case report. J. Amer. Podiatr. Assoc., 60:286, 1970.
71. Milkman, L. A.: Pseudofractures (hunger osteopathy, late rickets, osteomalacia). Report of a case. Amer. J. Roentgen., 32:622, 1934.
72. Miller, B., Markheim, H. R., and Towbin, M. N.: Multiple stress fractures in rheumatoid arthritis. J. Bone Joint Surg., 49-A:1408, 1967.
73. Miller, E. H., Schneider, J. H., Bronson, J. L., and McLain, D.: A new consideration in athletic injuries. The classical ballet dancer. Clin. Orthop., 111:181, 1975.
74. Miller, F., and Wenger, D. R.: Femoral neck stress fracture in a hyperactive child. J. Bone Joint Surg., 61-A:435, 1979.
75. Morris, J. M., and Blickenstaff, L. D.: Fatigue Fractures. Clinical Study. Springfield, Ill., Charles C Thomas, 1967.
76. Murcia, M., Brennan, R. E., and Edeiken, J.: Computed tomography of stress fracture. Skeletal Radiol., 8:193, 1982.
77. Murray, D. S.: Fatigue fractures of the lower tibia and fibula in the same leg. J. Bone Joint Surg., 39-B:302, 1957.
78. Nand, S., and Shukla, R. K.: Fatigue fractures of the femoral neck. Int. Surg., 61:31, 1976.
79. North, K. A.: Multiple stress fractures simulating osteomalacia. Amer. J. Roentgen., 97:672, 1966.
80. O'Boyle, C. M.: Sports injuries in adolescents: Emergency care. Amer. J. Nurs., 75:1732, 1975.
81. Ollenquist, I. J.: Osteopathia itineraria tibiae. Acta Radiol., 18:526, 1937.
82. Orava, S., Jormakka, E., and Hulkko, A.: Stress fractures in young athletes. Arch. Orthop. Trauma. Surg., 98:271, 1981.
83. Orava, S., Puranen, J., and Ala-Ketola, L.: Stress fractures caused by physical exercise. Acta Orthop. Scand., 49:19, 1978.
84. Park, C. H., Kapadia, D., and O'Hara, A. E.: Three phase bone scan findings in stress fracture. Clin. Nucl. Med., 6:587, 1981.
85. Pentecost, R. L., Murray, R. A., and Brindley, H. H.: Fatigue, insufficiency, and pathologic fractures. J.A.M.A., 187:1001, 1964.
86. Percy, E. C., and Gamble, F. O.: An epiphyseal stress fracture of the foot and shin splints in an anomalous calf muscle in a runner. Brit. J. Sports Med., 14:110, 1980.
87. Perl, T., and Carsky, E. W.: Stress fractures in children. New York J. Med., 66:391, 1966.
88. Pilgaard, S., Poulsen, J. O., and Christensen, J. H.: Stress fractures. Acta Orthop. Scand., 47:167, 1976.
89. Podlaha, M., and Podlahov, A. J.: Creeping fatigue fractures in children. Cesk. Radiol., 22:57, 1968.
90. Prather, J. L., Nusynowitz, M. L., Snowdy, H. A., Hughes,

A. D., McCartney, W. H., and Bagg, R. J.: Scintigraphic findings in stress fractures. J. Bone Joint Surg., *59-A*:869, 1977.
91. Provost, R. A., and Morris, J. M.: Fatigue fracture of the femoral shaft. J. Bone Joint Surg., *51-A*:487, 1969.
92. Rappoport, A. S., Sosman, J. L., and Weissman, B. N.: Spontaneous fractures of the olecranon process in rheumatoid arthritis. Radiology, *119*:83, 1976.
93. Rasad, S.: Golfer's fractures of the ribs. Report of 3 cases. Amer J. Roentgen., *120*:901, 1974.
94. Richmond, D. A.: Fatigue fracture of the fibula: Report on two cases. Lancet, *1*:273, 1945.
95. Roberts, S. M., and Vogt, E. C.: Pseudofracture of the tibia. J. Bone Joint Surg., *21*:891, 1939.
96. Robin, P. A., and Thompson, S. B.: Fatigue fractures. J. Bone Joint Surg., *26*:557, 1944.
97. Samuel, E.: Fatigue (insufficiency) fracture of the tibia. S. Afr. Med. J., *29*:89, 1955.
98. Sandrock, A. R.: Another sports fatigue fracture. Stress fracture of the coracoid process of the scapula. Radiology, *117*:274, 1975.
99. Savoca, C. J.: Stress fractures. A classification of the earliest radiographic signs. Radiology, *100*:519, 1971.
100. Schneider, H. J., King, A. Y., Bronson, J. L., and Miller, E. H.: Stress injuries and developmental changes of lower extremities in ballet dancers. Radiology, *113*:627, 1974.
101. Schneider, R., and Kaye, J. J.: Insufficiency and stress fractures of the long bones occurring in patients with rheumatoid arthritis. Radiology, *116*:595, 1975.
102. Sherman, F. C., Wilkinson, R. H., and Hall, J. E.: Reactive sclerosis of a pedicle and spondylolysis in the lumbar spine. J. Bone Joint Surg., *59-A*:49, 1977.
103. Siffert, R. S., and Levy, R. N.: Athletic injuries in children. Pediat. Clin. N. Amer., *12*:1027, 1965.
104. Singer, M., and Maudsley, R. H.: Fatigue fractures of lower tibia: Report of five cases. J. Bone Joint Surg., *36-B*:647, 1954.
105. Stark, H. H., Jobe, F. W., Boyes, J. H., and Ashworth, C. R.: Fracture of the hook of the hamate in athletes. J. Bone Joint Surg., *59-A*:575, 1977.
106. Stein, R. E., and Stelling, F. H.: Stress fracture of the calcaneus in a child with cerebral palsy. J. Bone Joint Surg., *59*:131, 1977.
107. Subbarao, K.: Radiologic problem of the month. Stress fractures involving anterior tibial cortex. New York J. Med., *80*:1419, 1980.
108. Tondeur, G., and Bosman, J.: Spontaneous fractures in the child. Acta Orthop. Belg., *32*:825, 1966.
109. Torg, J. S., and Moyer, R. A.: Non-union of a stress fracture through the olecranon epiphyseal plate observed in an adolescent baseball pitcher. J. Bone Joint Surg., *59-A*:264, 1977.
110. Torg, J. S., Pollack, H., and Sweterlitsch, P.: The effect of competitive pitching on the shoulders and elbows of preadolescent baseball players. Pediatrics, *49*:267, 1972.
111. Towne, L. C., Blazina, M. E., and Cozen, L. N.: Fatigue fracture of the tarsal navicular. J. Bone Joint Surg., *52-A*:376, 1970.
112. Tullos, H. S., and Fain, R. H.; Little League shoulder: Rotational stress fracture of proximal epiphysis. J. Sports Med., *2*:152, 1974.
113. Volder, J. G.: A case of a stress fracture in a child. Arch. Chir. Nedrl., *24*:43, 1972.
114. Walter, N. E., and Wolf, M. D.: Stress fractures in young athletes. Amer. J. Sports Med., *5*:165, 1977.
115. Wang, C. C., Lowrey, C. W., and Severance, R. L.: Fatigue fracture of pelvis and lower extremity. New Eng. J. Med., *260*:958, 1959.
116. Weaver, J. B., and Francisco, C. B.: Pseudofractures: A manifestation of non-suppurative osteomyelitis. J. Bone Joint Surg., *22*:610, 1940.
117. Wilcox, J. R., Jr., Moniot, A. L., and Green, J. P.: Bone scanning in the evaluation of exercise-related stress injuries. Radiology, *123*:699, 1977.
118. Wilson, E. S., and Katz, F. N.: Stress fractures. Radiology, *92*:481, 1969.
119. Wiltse, L. L., Widell, E. H., Jr., and Jackson, D. W.: Fatigue fracture: The basic lesion in isthmic spondylolisthesis. J. Bone Joint Surg., *57-A*:17, 1975.
120. Winfield, A. C., and Dennis, J. M.: Stress fracture of the calcaneus. Radiology, 72:415, 1959.
121. Wolfgang, G. L.: Stress fracture of the femoral neck in a patient with open capital femoral epiphyses. A case report. J. Bone Joint Surg., *59-A*:680, 1977.
122. Wright, T. M., and Hayes, W. C.: The fracture mechanics of fatigue crack propagation in compact bone. J. Biomed. Mat. Res., *7*:637, 1976.

Index

Page numbers in *italic* type refer to illustrations; in **bold** type, to plates; and followed by (t), to tables. The abbreviation *vs.* indicates differential diagnosis.

Abduction. See also *Abduction bar, Abduction contracture,* and *Abduction injury.*
  definition of, 77
  forefoot, range of, 81, *82*
  hip, in cerebral palsy, 368, *369*
Abduction bar, contraindicated in congenital metatarsus varus, 297
Abduction contracture, hip, diagnosis of, 69, 74
Abduction injury, in ankle fracture, *666,* 667
Abductor digiti quinti (minimi) muscle, anatomic relations of, *11, 13, 21, 27–32, 36, 38*
  testing of, **114–115**
Abductor hallucis muscle (tendon), anatomic relations of, *11, 13, 17, 18, 28–32, 36, 38*
  in congenital hallux varus, 329
  in congenital metatarsus varus, 296, *296*
  testing of, **114–115**
  transfer of, in congenital metatarsus primus varus and hallux valgus, 310
Abscess, in osteomyelitis, 599, *601*
  of sesamoid bones, 603
Accessory bones (ossicles). See also *Accessory tarsal navicular.*
  as normal variations, 123–130, *123–129*
  congenital hallux varus with, 329
  in tarsal coalition, 268
Accessory muscles, *506,* 508, *508*
Accessory tarsal navicular, as normal variation, 123–125, *123–126*

Accessory tarsal navicular (*Continued*)
  flat foot from, 557(t)
  tarsal coalition and, 268
  vs. congenital convex pes valgus, 251
Achilles tendinitis, 509
Achilles tendon, anatomic relations of, *3, 4, 6, 17–20, 22*
  anterior advancement of (Murphy), 388, *389,* **392–393**
  congenital short, 508
  in cerebral palsy, 377, **378–380,** *381–384, 389,* **392–393,** 414, *414*
  in myelomeningocele, 428
  in talipes equinovarus, 152, 188–189(t), 213, 217, *220*
  in talipes equinus, 377, **378–380,** *381–384,* 383, 388, *389,* **392–393**
  lateral transfer of (Axer and Segal), 214
  pes calcaneus and, 414, *414,* 428
  sliding lengthening of (White), 377, **378–380,** *381–384*
  transfer of (Jones), in flexible pes planovalgus, 573, 574(t), *576*
  subcutaneous tenotomy of (Stromeyer), 383, *383*
  switch operation on (Stewart), 213
  Z-lengthening of, 383, *384*
  with Dwyer calcaneal osteotomy, 217, *220*
Action potentials, electrical testing of, 85
Adduction. See also *Adduction deformity* and *Adduction injury.*

Adduction (*Continued*)
  definition of, 77
  forefoot, range of, 81, *82*
Adduction deformity, hip, in cerebral palsy, 368, *369*
Adduction injury, in ankle fracture, *666*, 667
Adduction-inversion ankle fracture, 660, *662*
Adductor brevis muscle, in hip adduction deformity, 368, *369*
  neurosegmental innervation of, *421*
Adductor hallucis muscle, anatomic relations of, *30–32, 36, 38*
  testing of, **116–117**
  transfer of, in congenital metatarsus primus varus and hallux valgus, 310
Adductor longus muscle, function of, in gait, 57, *58*
  in hip adduction deformity, 368, *369*
  neurosegmental innervation of, *421*
Adductor magnus muscle, function of, in gait, 57, *58*
  in hip adduction deformity, 368, *369*
  neurosegmental innervation of, *421*
Adhesive strapping, in talipes equinovarus, application of, 180, *181*
  in myelomeningocele, 439
Adipose tissue, congenital hyperplasia of, macrodactylism in, 333
  interposition of, in calcaneonavicular coalition, 285, **290–291**
  in premature closure of physis after ankle fracture, 695, *696, 697*
  in progressive muscular dystrophy, 505
Adolescent(s), ankle fracture in, of Tillaux, 669(t), 682, *683, 684*
  treatment of, 693, *693*
  triplane, 669(t), 683, *685–688*
  congenital metatarsus primus varus in, 308
  fibromatosis of plantar fascia in, 649
  Freiberg's infraction of second metatarsal in, 612
  hallux rigidus in, 627
  subungual exostosis in, 657
Adrenal steroids, in hypertrophic interstitial neuritis, 506
Adult, hallux rigidus in, 634
Africoid talus, 128, *129*
Age, ambulation and, in myelomeningocele, 424
  choice of operation and, in talipes equinovarus, 187
  congenital contraction of triceps surae muscle correction and, 509
  congenital metatarsus primus varus and, 308
  congenital metatarsus varus treatment and, 301
  flexible pes planovalgus treatment and, 567, 572
  Freiberg's infraction of second metatarsal and, 612
  Friedreich's ataxia and, 500
  gait development and, 59, *64–71*
  hallux rigidus and, 627
  in myelomeningocele, talipes equinovarus correction and, 439
    valgus ankle correction and, 434
  in progressive muscular dystrophy, 505
  juvenile rheumatoid arthritis and, 608

Age (*Continued*)
  Köhler's disease of tarsal navicular and, 610
  of ossification, in ankle fractures, 660, *661*
  osteochondritis dissecans and, 616
  peroneal muscular atrophy and, 496
  premature closure of tibial physis after fracture and, 695
  preoperative assessment of cerebral palsy and, 365
  tarsal coalition symptoms and, 268
  tendon transfer and, in poliomyelitis, 454
  triple arthrodesis and, 483
Agonist, muscle function as, 353
Air arthrography, in os trigonum vs. fracture of talus, 126, *127*
Aitken classification of ankle fractures, 661
Ambulation, in Friedreich's ataxia, 501
  in myelomeningocele, 422, *423*
Amikacin, in osteomyelitis, 599(t)
Aminopterin-induced syndrome, talipes equinovarus in, 169
Amniocentesis, in antenatal diagnosis of myelomeningocele, 422
Amoxicillin, in osteomyelitis, 599(t)
Ampicillin, in osteomyelitis, 599(t)
Aneurysm, 637, *645*
Aneurysmal bone cyst, *654*, 655
Angle(s), declination, of talus, 145, *145, 146*
  roentgenographic measurement of, in talipes equinovarus, 170(t), 172, *172–174*
Angulation, valgus and varus, 75
Ankle, anatomic relations in, *10–13, 15–25*
  arthritis of, rheumatoid, *608*, 609, *609*
    suppurative, 605, *606*
  arthrodesis and, 471–492, 482(t), *483, 484, 486*
    Chuinard, **488–491**, 492
    in plantar flexor muscle paralysis, 471
    pantalar, 487
    triple, 477, **478–481**
  bones of, normal variations in, 123–130, *123–129*
    ossification in, 660, *661*
  congenital ball-and-socket joint in, 312–314, *312*
  flail, 446
    pantalar arthrodesis in, 487
  fractures of, 660–700
    classification of, 660, *662–664, 666, 668–669*(t), *670–689*
    complications of, *694–699*, 695
    mechanism of injury in, 660, *662–664, 666, 668–669*(t), *670–689*
    treatment of, 689, *690–693*
  ganglion of, 637, *638*
  hip and knee and, interdependence of, 356–358, *356–359*
  in myelomeningocele, deformity of, 424, 425(t), *426, 427*
    valgus, 429–438, *434, 435,* **436–437,** *438*
    flail, 446
  in poliomyelitis, 471–492, **478–481**, 482(t), *483, 484, 486,* **488–491**
  in talipes equinovarus, 156, *156–159,* 176, *177,* 188–189(t)
  in talipes equinus, in cerebral palsy, 370, *373*

Ankle (*Continued*)
  in talipes equinus, posture and, 358, *358, 359*
  ligaments of, nonoperative elongation of, 176, *177*
  motion of, as determinant of gait, 54, *54*
    innervation of reflexes and, *421*
    limitation of, bone blocks for, 492
    range of, 79–84, *80*
Ankle-foot orthosis, in cerebral palsy, after anterior tibial tendon transfer in pes varus, 402
  contraindicated, in talipes equinus, 376
  in tarsal coalition, 283
Ankle mortise, in talipes equinovarus, 146, *147, 158*
  obliquity of, *25*
Ankylosis, joint, pathologic gait in, 62
Annular constriction bands, congenital, talipes equinovarus and, 164, *165*
Antagonist, muscle function as, 356
Antalgic limp, 62
Antenatal diagnosis, of myelomeningocele, 422
Anterior horn cell, degeneration of, electromyography in, 118
  disease of, paralysis in, 353, 354–355(t)
  poliomyelitis as, 452
Anterior tibial artery, anatomic relations of, *2, 5, 7–9, 13*
Anterior tibial muscle (tendon), anatomic relations of, *2, 3, 5, 9–13, 16, 18–21, 34, 36, 37*
  function of, in gait, 58, *58*
  in cerebral palsy, 370, *375*, 389, **394–397**, 401, *401*
  in claw toes, 554
  in congenital convex pes valgus, *241*, 243, *246, 247*
  in flexible pes planovalgus, 573, 574(t), **578–587**
  in Friedreich's ataxia, 501
  in myelomeningocele, 425, *427*, **430–433**, 439
  in peroneal muscular atrophy, 496, *497*
  in pes calcaneus, *427*, 428, **430–433**
  in pes cavus, 510, 526, *527*
  in pes varus, 401, *401*
  in poliomyelitis, 456–457(t), 459, *464*, 465, *465*
  in talipes equinovalgus, 402
  in talipes equinovarus, 152, 210, 439
  in talipes equinus, 370, *375*, 389, **394–397**
  in tarsal coalition, *270*, 271
  innervation of, intrauterine posture and, 133, *133*
  neurosegmental, *421*
  paralysis of, deformities and, 456–457(t), 459, *464*, 465, *465*
  shortening of, 389, **394–397**
  transfer of, lateral, 210, 459
    posterior, *427*, 428, **430–433**
    split, 401, *401*
    to first metatarsal base, 526, *527*
    to navicular, 573, 574(t), **578–587**
Anterior tibial vein, anatomic relations of, *2, 5, 8*
Anterior transverse ligament, anatomic relations of, *3, 11, 17, 21*

Antibiotics, in osteomyelitis, 599, 599(t)
  in suppurative arthritis, 607
Apert's syndrome, tarsal coalition in, 262(t), *266*, 267
Arachnodactyly, insufficiency fractures in, 703
Arch, dorsal venous, anatomic relations of, *11, 12*
  longitudinal, anatomy and function of, 1
    in flexible pes planovalgus, 556, *558–560, 562–564, 566, 567*
Arch support(s), in flexible pes planovalgus, 568
  in Köhler's disease of tarsal navicular, 612
Arcuate artery, anatomic relations of, *12–14*
Arm, measurement of, in diagnosis of deformities, 74
Arsenic poisoning, vs. hypertrophic interstitial neuritis, 504
Artery (arteries). See also names of specific arteries.
  foot and ankle, anatomic relations of, *11–14, 17, 18, 21, 23, 24, 27–29, 31–33, 36*
  leg, anatomic relations of, *5–9*
  tarsal, development of, 40
Arthritis, flat foot in, 557(t)
  rheumatoid, 608–610. See also *Rheumatoid arthritis*.
  suppurative (septic), 605–608, *606*
  tuberculous, 604
Arthrodesis, ball-and-socket ankle joint following, 313
  Chuinard, 489, **490–493**. See also *Chuinard ankle arthrodesis*.
  extra-articular subtalar (Grice), 403, **404–407**. See also *Grice extra-articular subtalar arthrodesis*.
  in congenital metatarsus varus, 301
  in flexible pes planovalgus, 571, 574–575(t), *588, 589*, **590–591**
  in talipes equinovalgus, 403, **404–407**, *408, 409*
  in talipes equinovarus, 192, 224
  metatarsophalangeal joint, in hallux rigidus, 634, *634*
  proximal interphalangeal joint, in hammer toe, **348–349**, 350
  triple. See *Triple arthrodesis*.
Arthrography, air, in os trigonum vs. fracture of talus, 126, *127*
  in talipes equinovarus, 175
  in tarsal coalition, 280, *282*
Arthrogryposis multiplex congenita, congenital convex pes valgus with, 240
  insufficiency fractures in, 703
  talipes equinovarus in, 163, *164*
    open reduction of talocalcaneonavicular joint in, 192
Arthroscopy, ankle, in osteochondritis dissecans of talus, 621
Articulations. See *Joint(s)*.
Aseptic necrosis, Freiberg's infraction of second metatarsal and, 613
  open reduction of talocalcaneonavicular joint and, 209
Aspiration, bone, in osteomyelitis, 599
  joint, in suppurative arthritis, 606, *606*
Asymmetrical tonic neck reflex, in cerebral palsy, 360, *361*

Ataxia, cerebellar lesions and, 353, 354–355(t)
  gait in, 63
  hereditary spinocerebellar (Friedreich's), 501–503, 502(t)
    pes cavus in, 510
    vs. peroneal muscular atrophy, 498
Athetosis, extrapyramidal lesions and, 353, 354–355(t)
  pes cavus in, 510
  tension, vs. spasticity, 370
Atrophy, disuse, insufficiency fractures in, 703
  in diastematomyelia, 449
  in genu valgum, 68
  in osteochondritis dissecans of talus, 619
  in talipes equinovarus, 152, 162, 163(t)
  in tuberculous arthritis, 604
  paralysis and, in neuromuscular disease, 352, 354–355(t)
  peroneal muscular, 496–500. See also *Charcot-Marie-Tooth disease*.
  progressive muscular, electromyography in, 118
Automatic reflex, as test of motor strength, in cerebral palsy, 375
Autosomal trisomy, congenital convex pes valgus with, 240
Avulsion fracture, of ankle, 661
Axer and Segal Achilles tendon transfer, in talipes equinovarus, 214
Axial compression injury, in ankle fracture, *666*, 667
Axial rotation, in gait, 56–57, *65, 67, 70*

Baker horizontal calcaneal osteotomy, in flexible pes planovalgus, 575(t)
  in talipes equinovalgus, in spastic cerebral palsy, 412, *413*
Baker tongue-in-groove lengthening, of gastrocnemius aponeurosis, 383, *386*
Balance, in cerebral palsy, 360, *364, 368*
Ball-and-socket joint, ankle, congenital, 312–314
  following arthrodesis, 313
  tarsal coalition and, 262(t), *265*, 266
  talocalcaneonavicular joint as, 153
Bar, abduction, contraindicated in congenital metatarsus varus, 297
  intertarsal, 261. See also *Tarsal coalition* and names of specific coalitions.
Batchelor extra-articular subtalar arthrodesis, 410, *410, 411*
"Beak," navicular, in talipes varus, 483
"Beak" triple arthrodesis, 538, *539, 540*
Biceps femoris muscle, anatomic relations of, *4*
  function of, in gait, 58, *58*
  neurosegmental innervation of, *421*
Bifurcated ligament, anatomic relations of, *15, 22*
  in congenital convex pes valgus, 244, *245*
  in talipes equinovarus, 188–189(t)
Biopsy, in hypertrophic interstitial neuritis, 504
  in progressive muscular dystrophy, 505
  in tuberculous arthritis, 605

Blood supply, fibular periosteal, in Batchelor extra-articular subtalar arthrodesis, 411
  osteochondritis dissecans and, 617
  tarsal, development of, 40
Bone(s). See also names of specific bones.
  deformities of, in congenital talipes equinovarus, 145–149, *145–148*
  in pathologic gait, 62
  in pes calcaneus, in myelomeningocele, 429
  grafting of. See *Bone graft*.
  growth of, muscle action in, 356
  infection of, 598. See also *Osteomyelitis*.
  normal variations in, 123–130, *123–129*
  pathogenesis of stress fracture and, 704
  pathologic changes in, congenital convex pes valgus, 243, *244*
  procedures on, in talipes equinovarus, 214, *216*, **218–219**, *220*, **222–223**
  tuberculosis of, 604
  tumors of, **653–657**, 655–658
Bone block, in calcaneal dorsal wedge osteotomy, for pes calcaneocavus, 544
  to limit ankle motion, in poliomyelitis, 492
Bone cyst, aneurysmal, *654*, 655
  unicameral, 655, *655, 656*
Bone graft, autogenous cancellous, in subtalar arthrodesis, 577, *588, 589*
  in Batchelor extra-articular subtalar arthrodesis, 410, *410, 411*
  in Dwyer calcaneal osteotomy, in talipes equinovalgus, 412
  in talipes equinovarus, 217, **222–223**
  in Evans operation, in flexible pes planovalgus, 595
  in Grice extra-articular subtalar arthrodesis, 403, **406–407**, 408
  lateral inlay, in Williams and Menelaus triple arthrodesis, 575(t), 588, **590–591**
  lateral wedge, in Baker calcaneal osteotomy, 412, *413*
Bost-Schottstaedt-Larsen technique, for plantar soft-tissue release, 523
Bowleg. See *Genu varum*.
Brachial plexus palsy, neural level lesion in, 353, 354–355(t)
Brachymetatarsia, 314–317, *314–317*
Bridge, intertarsal, 261. See also *Tarsal coalition* and names of specific coalitions.
Bulbar palsy, progressive, spinal level lesion in, 353, 354–355(t)
Bunion, 308–311, *309, 311*
  dorsal. See *Dorsal bunion*.
Bursa, adventitious, accessory tarsal navicular bone and, *124*, 125
Butler operation, in congenital digitus minimus varus, 338, *342, 343*

Cadence, in gait, 50, 59
Calcaneal arteries, anatomic relations of, *21*
Calcaneal nerves, anatomic relations of, *21*
Calcaneal pitch, in flexible pes planovalgus, 561, *565*
  choice of operation and, 572

Calcaneocavus deformity. See *Pes calcaneocavus*.
Calcaneocuboid coalition, 262, 262(t)
Calcaneocuboid joint, fusion of, in pes cavus, 532
  in pantalar arthrodesis, 488
  in triple arthrodesis, 477
  pathologic change in, in congenital convex pes valgus, 244
  resection and fusion of (Evans), in talipes equinovarus, 192
Calcaneocuboid ligament, anatomic relations of, *22, 34*
Calcaneofibular ligament, anatomic relations of, *15, 22, 23, 34*
  in congenital convex pes valgus, 244, *245, 246*
  in talipes equinovarus, 152, 188–189(t)
Calcaneofibular tenodesis, in myelomeningocele, 435, **436–437**
Calcaneo–fifth metatarsal angle, measurement of, 173, *173*
Calcaneonavicular coalition, 261, 262(t), 268, *270, 271, 281*
  surgical treatment of, 284, **286–291**
Calcaneonavicular (spring) ligament, anatomic relations of, *19, 34, 36*
  in congenital convex pes valgus, 244, *245, 246*
  in talipes equinovarus, as obstacle to reduction, 152, *152*
  nonoperative elongation of, *178,* 180
  release of, 188–189(t)
  transfer of, in flexible pes planovalgus, 574(t), 576
Calcaneovalgus deformity. See *Talipes calcaneovalgus*.
Calcaneovarus deformity, muscle paralysis and, 456–457(t)
Calcaneus, anatomic relations of, 1, *3, 4, 10, 15–17, 19–23, 25, 26, 28–32, 34–36, 38*
  development and ossification of, 40, *40–43*
  fractures of, 701
  in flexible pes planovalgus, 557, *557, 559, 560, 562–565,* 575(t), 576, *588, 592, 594*
  in talipes equinovarus, deformity of, 148
    in open reduction of talocalcaneonavicular joint, 208
    malalignment of, 149, *150, 151, 153–156*
    manipulation of, nonoperative, *178, 179,* 180
  normal variations of, *123, 126,* 128, *128*
  osteomyelitis of, 598, *600, 602*
    tuberculous, 604
  osteotomy of, Baker horizontal, 412, *413*
    dorsal wedge, 540, *541*
    Dwyer, 217, *220,* **222–223**
    Dwyer lateral close-up wedge, in pes cavus, 539, **542–543**
    Dwyer lateral open-up, 412
    in flexible pes planovalgus, 575(t), 576, 588, *592, 594*
    in pes calcaneocavus, 540, *541, 544, 545,* **546–551**
    in talipes equinovalgus in cerebral palsy, 412, *413*
    in talipes equinovarus, 192, 217, *220,* **222–223**

Calcaneus (*Continued*)
  osteotomy of, posterior-superior displacement, 544, *544, 545,* **546–551**
  pathologic change in, in congenital convex pes valgus, 243, *244–247*
  resection of distal end of (Lichtblau), in talipes equinovarus, 192
  stress fracture of, 703
  unicameral bone cyst of, *655*
Calcaneus deformity. See *Talipes calcaneus*.
Calcaneus gait, 61, *62*
Calcaneus secundarius, as normal variation, *123,* 128
Calcinosis, tumoral, 649, *649*
Calf, atrophy of, in genu valgum, 68
  in osteochondritis dissecans of talus, 619
  in talipes equinovarus, 162, 163(t)
  in tuberculous arthritis, 604
  muscles of, anatomic relations of, *2–6, 8–10, 37, 38*
    in peroneal muscular atrophy, 497
    in talipes equinus, in spastic cerebral palsy, 371, *372*
Callus (callosity), ankle position in pantalar arthrodesis and, 487
  in brachymetatarsia, 316
  in congenital digitus minimus varus, 338
  in hallux rigidus, 631
  in hammer toe, 350
  in pes calcaneus, in myelomeningocele, 426
Campbell's bone block, ball-and-socket ankle joint following, 313
Capitular ligaments, transverse, anatomic relations of, *15, 34*
Capsule(s), joint, anatomic relations of, *19,* 22
  in congenital convex pes valgus, 244
  in talipes equinovarus, 160, 188–191
    as obstacle to reduction, 152
    nonoperative elongation of, 176, *177*
  release of, in congenital metatarsus varus, 301, **302–305**
    metatarsophalangeal, in congenital digitus minimus varus, 338, *339,* **340–341,** *342, 343*
    in congenital hallux varus, 329
Carbenicillin, in osteomyelitis, 599(t)
Carothers-Crenshaw classification of ankle fractures, 665, *666*
Carpal coalition, tarsal coalition and, 262, 262(t), *264, 265*
Cartilage, articular, in osteochondritis dissecans, 616
  injury to, in nonoperative treatment of talipes equinovarus, 187
  tarsal, embryonic formation of, *39, 40*
Cast(s), in congenital postural deformities, 136
  in Freiberg's infraction of second metatarsal, 613
  in Köhler's disease of tarsal navicular, 612
  in rheumatoid arthritis, 609
  in supination-inversion ankle fracture, 691
  in talipes equinovarus, application of, 183, *183*
    in myelomeningocele, 439
    retention in, in triple arthrodesis, 225
  in tendon transfers, 453
  manipulation and, in congenital metatarsus varus, 297, *298–300*

Cast(s) (*Continued*)
  stretching, contraindicated, in talipes equinus in cerebral palsy, 377
  in congenital contracture of triceps surae muscle, 509
Cavernous hemangioma, 637, *641–643*
Cavovarus deformity. See *Pes cavovarus*.
Cavus deformity. See *Pes cavus*.
Cefaclor, in osteomyelitis, 599(t)
Cefamandole, in osteomyelitis, 599(t)
Cefazolin, in osteomyelitis, 599(t)
Cephalexin, in osteomyelitis, 599(t)
Cephalothin, in osteomyelitis, 599(t)
Cerebellar ataxia, gait in, 63
Cerebellar level, lesion at paralysis in, 353, 354–355(t)
  pes cavus in, 510
Cerebral palsy, 358–418
  athetoid, paralysis at extrapyramidal level in, 353, 354–355(t)
  criteria for diagnosis of, 359
  flat foot in, 557(t)
  forefoot deformities in, 415
  insufficiency fractures in, 703
  paralytic pes valgus in, vs. congenital convex pes valgus, 251
  pes calcaneus in, 414, *414*
  pes cavus in, 510
  pes varus in, 398, *398–401*
  preoperative assessment in, 359, *360–364, 366–369*, 370(t)
  talipes equinovalgus in, 402, **404–407**, *408–410, 413*
  talipes equinus in, 370, *371–376*, **378–380**, *381–389*, **390–397**
  toe deformities in, 415
  triple arthrodesis in, 487
  types of, 360
Cerebrospinal fluid, in peroneal muscular atrophy, 498
Chambers procedure, in flexible pes planovalgus, 575(t), 588, *592*
Charcot-Marie-Tooth disease, 496–500, *497, 498*
  lesion at neural level in, 353, 354–355(t)
  pes cavus in, 502, 510
  tendon transfer in pes cavovarus in, 526
Chloramphenicol, in osteomyelitis, 599(t)
Chondrification, tarsal, embryonic, 39, *40*
Chondroectodermal dysplasia, polydactyly and, 325
Chopart's joint, anatomic relations at, *36*
Chuinard ankle arthrodesis, **488–491**, *492*
  in myelomeningocele, 446
  in plantar flexor muscle paralysis, 471
Cincinnati incision, *193*
Circulatory disorders, 610–627
Clavus durus, 658
Clavus mollis, 658, *659*
Clawfoot, pes cavus as, 510
Claw toes, 554, *554, 555*
  in Friedreich's ataxia, 501
  in myelomeningocele, 444, *445*
  in peroneal muscular atrophy, 497, *498*
  in pes cavus, 516, *516, 520*
  in rheumatoid arthritis, 608
Cleft foot, congenital, 317–322, *318–322*
Clindamycin, in osteomyelitis, 599(t)

Close-up, lateral wedge osteotomy of calcaneus (Dwyer), 539, **542–543**
Cloxacillin, in osteomyelitis, 599(t)
Clubfoot, postural congenital, 131, 132(t), 137
  vs. talipes equinovarus, 162, 163(t)
Coalition, tarsal, 261–294. See also *Tarsal coalition*.
Cock-up deformity, of toes, muscle paralysis and, 456–457(t), 459
Coleman's cavovarus test, in pes cavus, 520, *521, 522*
Community ambulators, in myelomeningocele, 422
Compression fracture, in nonoperative treatment of talipes equinovarus, 187, *187*
  of ankle, 661
  stress fracture as, 705
Computed tomography, in flexible pes planovalgus, 568
  in stress fracture, 707
Conduction velocity, nerve, in diagnosis, 119
  in hypertrophic interstitial neuritis, 504
  in peroneal muscular atrophy, 497
"Confusion," as test of motor strength, in cerebral palsy, 375
Congenital absence of muscles, 506
Congenital ball-and-socket ankle joint, 312–316
Congenital cavus foot, pes cavus as, 514
Congenital contracture, of triceps surae muscle, 508
Congenital convex pes planovalgus, vs. postural talipes calcaneovalgus, 134
Congenital convex pes valgus, 239–261
  clinical features of, 247, *248*
  differential diagnosis of, 250
  flat foot in, 557(t), *566*
  in myelomeningocele, 424, 425(t), *442–444*, 443
  pathologic anatomy of, 243, *244–247*
  roentgenographic findings in, 248, *249, 250*
  treatment of, 251, 251(t), *253*, **254–259**
Congenital curly (varus) toe, 344–350, *347*
Congenital deformities, 131–351. See also names of specific deformities.
  postural, 131–139, 132(t), *133–136, 138*
Congenital digitus minimus varus, 335–344, *339*, **340–341**, *342, 343*
Congenital flatfoot, due to vertical talus, 239. See also *Congenital convex pes valgus*.
Congenital hallux valgus interphalangeus, 344, *344–346*
Congenital hallux varus, 329, *330, 331*
Congenital metatarsus adductus, vs. congenital metatarsus varus, 294, 297
Congenital metatarsus primus varus, 308–311, *308, 309, 311*
Congenital metatarsus varus, 294–308, *295, 296, 298–300*, **302–307**
  differential diagnosis of, 294, 297
  vs. postural metatarsus adductus, 137, *138*, 297
Congenital short metatarsal, 314–317, *314–317*
Congenital split (cleft) foot, 317–322, *318–322*
Congenital talipes equinovarus, 139. See also *Talipes equinovarus*.

Congenital vertical talus, 239. See also *Congenital convex pes valgus.*
Congenital webbing, of toes, 335, *336*
Contracture(s), congenital, of triceps surae muscle, 508
　flat foot and, 557(t), 559
　in flexible pes planovalgus, choice of operation and, 572
　in progressive muscular dystrophy, 505
　in talipes equinovarus, as obstacles to reduction, 152
　　nonoperative elongation of, 176, *177–179*
　muscular fibrosis and, in pes cavus, 513
　myostatic. See *Myostatic contracture.*
　of hip, diagnosis of, 69, *73, 74*
　plantar, in pes cavus, release of, 522, **524–525**
　　in talipes equinovarus, nonoperative elongation of, *178*, 180
Convex pes valgus, congenital, 239. See also *Congenital convex pes valgus.*
Corn, hard, 658
　soft, 658, *659*
Cornuted navicular bone, 125, *125*
Cortex, bony, resorption of, stress fracture and, 704
　cerebral, disease of, paralysis in, 353, 354–355(t)
Corticospinal level, lesion at, paralysis in, 353, 354–355(t)
Cortisone treatment, insufficiency fractures from, 703
Counseling, genetic, in myelomeningocele, 419
　in talipes equinovarus, 140
Cowell technique, in calcaneonavicular coalition, 284, **290–291**
Coxa valga, angulation in, 75
Coxa vara, angulation in, 75
Craniocarpotarsal dysplasia, talipes equinovarus in, 164, *167*
Creatine phosphokinase, in progressive muscular dystrophy, 505
Crescentic osteotomy of calcaneus (Samilson), in pes calcaneocavus, 544, *544, 545*, **546–551**
Cruciate ligament, anatomic relations of, *3, 11, 12, 17, 21*
Crushing injury, in fractures, ankle, 660
　foot, 700
Crutch(es), contraindicated, in talipes equinus in cerebral palsy, 376
　in Köhler's disease of tarsal navicular, 612
　in rheumatoid arthritis, 609
　in suppurative arthritis, 607
　in tendon transfer training, 455
Cryotherapy, in hemangioma, 637
Cuboid bone, anatomic relations of, *1, 10, 14–16, 20, 22, 26, 34–36, 38*
　development and ossification of, 39, *42, 43*
　fractures of, 702
　malalignment of, in talipes equinovarus, 150,
　normal variations of, *123*, 130
　osteomyelitis of, 598
　　tuberculous, 604
　subluxation of, in open reduction of talocalcaneonavicular joint, 208, *208*

Cuboid bone (*Continued*)
　unicameral bone cyst of, *656*
Cuboideonavicular ligament, anatomic relations of, *22, 34*
Cubonavicular coalition, 262, 265
Cuneiform bone(s), anatomic relations of, *1, 10, 14–16, 19, 20, 26, 34, 36, 38*
　development and ossification of, 40, *42, 43*
　fractures of, 702
　medial, vertical opening-wedge osteotomy of, in pes cavus, 532
　normal variations of, *123*, 130
　osteochondrosis of, 615
　osteomyelitis of, 598
　　tuberculous, 604
Cuneiform osteotomy, in hallux valgus interphalangeus, 344, *345, 346*
　Watermann, in hallux rigidus, 633, *633*
Cuneonavicular ligament, anatomic relations of, *22, 34*
Curly (varus) toe, brachymetatarsia and, *315*, 317
　congenital, 344–350, *347*
Cushing's syndrome, insufficiency fractures in, 703
Cutaneous nerves, dorsal, anatomic relations of, *11, 13, 17, 21, 36*
Cyst, bone, aneurysmal, *654*, 655
　unicameral, 655, *655, 656*

Dactylitis, tuberculous, 604
Declination angle, of talus, 145, *145, 146*
Deep peroneal nerve, anatomic relations of, *2, 5, 8, 9, 11, 13, 18, 21, 36*
　in lateral transfer of anterior tibial tendon, 459
Deformities. See also names of specific deformities.
　as complication of ankle fracture, 694–698, 695
　congenital, 131–351
　diagnosis of, 68–75, *72–75*
　in myelomeningocele, 424, 425(t), *426, 427*
　in rheumatoid arthritis, 608
　preoperative assessment of, in cerebral palsy, 367
Degeneration, reaction of, electrical testing and, 85
　in neuromuscular disease, 352, 354–355(t)
Dehiscence, wound, open reduction of talocalcaneonavicular joint and, 192
Dejerine-Sottas interstitial neuritis, 503–505
　pes cavus in, 503, 510
　vs. peroneal muscular atrophy, 498
Deltoid ligament, anatomic relations of, *15, 19, 23*
　in congenital convex pes valgus, 244, *245, 246*
　in talipes equinovarus, 188, 188–189(t)
　transfer of (Schoolfield), in flexible pes planovalgus, 573
Denis Browne splint, contraindicated in congenital metatarsus varus, 297
　in congenital postural talipes calcaneovalgus, 136

Dennyson and Fulford subtalar arthrodesis, 577, *588*, *589*
Dermis, in skin lesions, 658
Diabetes, vs. hypertrophic interstitial neuritis, 504
Dias-Tachdjian classification of ankle fractures, 667, 668–669(t), *670–682*
Diastematomyelia, 449–451, *450*
　pes cavus in, 510
　talipes equinovarus in, 162, *164*
　vs. congenital contracture of triceps surae muscle, 509
Diastrophic dwarfism, congenital hallux varus in, 329
　talipes equinovarus in, 164, *166*
Dicloxacillin, in osteomyelitis, 599(t)
Digit(s), arteries of, anatomic relations of, dorsal, *11–14*, *36*
　　plantar, *27*, *29*, *33*
　nerves of, anatomic relations of, dorsal, *11–13*, *36*
　　plantar, *27–29*, *36*
　recurrent fibroma of, 642–649
　supernumerary, 323–328, *325–329*
　tuberculous dactylitis of, 604
Digitus minimus varus, congenital, 335–344, *339*, **340–341**, *342*, *343*
Dislocations, fractures and, 660–709
Distraction fracture, stress fracture as, 706
Disuse, atrophy from, insufficiency fractures in, 703
　muscle response to, 356
Dome osteotomy, in congenital metatarsus primus varus and hallux valgus, 310, *311*
Dorsal bunion, muscle paralysis and, 456–457(t), 458, *458*, *472*, *472*, *473*, *476*, *477*
　open-up osteotomy of base of first metatarsal in, **474–475**
　tendon transfer and, 453
Dorsal wedge osteotomy, in pes cavus, cuneiform-cuboid, 526, **530–531**
　metatarsal, 532, *533*, *538*
Dorsalis pedis artery, anatomic relations of, *12*, *14*
Dorsiflexion, ankle, range of, 80, *80*
　muscles of, paralysis of, deformities and, 458
Dorsiflexion-assist orthosis, in cerebral palsy, after split anterior tibial tendon transfer in pes varus, 402
　contraindicated in talipes equinus, 376
　in congenital contraction of triceps surae muscle, 509
Dorsoplantar talonavicular angle, in flexible pes planovalgus, *560*, 561, *562–564*
　choice of operation and, 571
Down's syndrome, flat foot in, 557(t), 571
Drop-foot gait in, 61
　paralytic, bone block operations in, 492
Drugs, antibiotic, in osteomyelitis, 599, 599(t)
　in suppurative arthritis, 607
　in tuberculosis, 604
Duchenne muscular dystrophy, 505. See also *Muscular dystrophy*.
Durham operation, in flexible pes planovalgus, 576
Dwarfism, diastrophic congenital hallux varus in, 329
　talipes equinovarus in, 164, *166*

Dwarfism (*Continued*)
　osteochondritis dissecans and, 616
Dwyer calcaneal osteotomy, dorsal wedge, in pes calcaneocavus, 540, *541*
　in flexible pes planovalgus, 575(t), 593
　in talipes equinovalgus in cerebral palsy, 412
　in talipes equinovarus, 217, *220*, **222–223**
　lateral close-up wedge, in pes cavus, 539, **542–543**
Dystonia musculorum deformans, pes cavus in, 510
Dystrophy, muscular. See *Muscular dystrophy*.

Ectrodactyly, congenital split (cleft) foot as, 317, *318–322*
Ehlers-Danlos syndrome, flat foot in, 557(t), 571
Elbow, range of motion of, 76, *76*
Electrocoagulation, of plantar wart, 659
Electrodiagnosis, 85–119
Electromyography, in diagnosis, 118
　in hypertrophic interstitial neuritis, 504
　in measurement of muscle action in gait, 57, *58*
　in myelomeningocele, 420
　in tendon transfer planning, 399, *399*, *400*
Ellis-van Creveld syndrome, polydactyly and, 325
Ely test, for hip flexion deformity, 367, *367*
Embryo, development of foot and leg in, 39, *40*, *42*
Enchondroma, 655
　vs. tuberculous dactylitis, 604
Endocrine abnormality, in osteochondritis dissecans, 616
　insufficiency fractures in, 703
Environment, intrauterine, in talipes equinovarus, 141
Epidermis, in skin lesions, 658
Epiphysis (epiphyses), development of, 41, *42*, *43*
　juvenile osteochondritis dissecans and, 617
　fusion of, in macrodactilism, 333
　of tibia and fibula, to prevent varus deformity after ankle fracture, 696
　ossification of, 41, *42*, *43*
　　distal, of tibia and fibula, in ankle fractures, 660, *661*
　osteochondrosis of, 615
　phalangeal, normal variations of, 130
　tibial, damage to, in nonoperative treatment of talipes equinovarus, 187, *187*
Equinocavus deformity, *513*, 514
Equinovalgus deformity. See *Talipes equinovalgus*.
Equinovarus deformity. See *Talipes equinovarus*.
Equinus deformity. See also *Talipes equinus*.
　forefoot, in Friedreich's ataxia, 502
　in pes cavus, 510, *512*, *513*, *515*
　　bony procedures for, 526, **530–531**, *533*, **534–537**, *538–540*
　in open reduction of talocalcaneonavicular joint, 209
　in peroneal muscular atrophy, 497, *497*
　in triple arthrodesis, 485

Erector spinae, function of, in gait, 57, *58*
Evans's procedure, in inflexible pes planovalgus, 575(t), 594
 in talipes equinovarus, 192, 214, *216*, **218–219**
Eversion, definition of, 77
 hindfoot, measurement of, 81, *81*
 muscles of, paralysis of, deformities and, 458
 talocalcaneonavicular joint in, in talipes equinovarus, 153
Ewing's sarcoma, vs. stress fracture, 707
Examination, 44–121
 deformity evaluation in, 68, *72–75*
 gait analysis in, 45, *49*, *51–58*, *60–62*, *64–71*
 muscle testing in, 82, 84(t), *86–89*(t), **90–117**
 of joints, range of motion in, 75, *76*, *78–84*
 physical, 44, *44*, *46*, *47*
 electrodiagnostic, 85
 neurologic, 84
 roentgenographic, 84. See also *Roentgenography*.
Exercise(s), in cerebral palsy, in talipes equinovalgus, 402
 in talipes equinus, 375
 in flexible pes planovalgus, 568, *569*
 in hallux rigidus, 631
 in hypertrophic interstitial neuritis, 504
 in suppurative arthritis, 607
 postoperative, after posterior tendon transfer, in pes calcaneus, 428, *429*
 in tendon transfer training in poliomyelitis, 454
 stretching, in congenital contracture of triceps surae muscle, 509
 in congenital metatarsus varus, 297, *298–300*
 passive, after nonoperative correction of talipes equinovarus, 184
 in congenital digitus minimus varus, 338
 in congenital postural talipes calcaneovalgus, 135
 in convalescent phase of poliomyelitis, 459
 in peroneal muscular atrophy, 498
 in pes cavus, 519
Exostosis, subungual, 655, *656*
Extension, definition of, 77
Extensor digiti quinti tendon, in congenital digitus minimus varus, 338
Extensor digitorum brevis muscle, anatomic relations of, *3*, *10–13*, *21*, *36*
 in peroneal muscular atrophy, 496, *497*
 innervation of, intrauterine posture and, 133, *133*
 interposition of, in resection of calcaneonavicular coalition, 285, **290–291**
 testing of, **98–99**
Extensor digitorum communis muscle, paralysis of, deformities and, 456–457(t), 458
Extensor digitorum longus muscle, anatomic relations of, *2*, *3*, *5*, *9–13*, *20*, *21*, *36*, *37*
 function of, in gait, 58, *58*
 in claw toes, 554
 in congenital convex pes valgus, *242*, *243*, *246*
 in myelomeningocele, in talipes equinovarus, 439

Extensor digitorum longus muscle (*Continued*)
 in myelomeningocele, level of lesion and, 425, *426*, *427*
 in peroneal muscular atrophy, 496, *497*
 innervation of, intrauterine posture and, 133, *133*
 neurosegmental, *421*
 paralysis of, deformities and, 459
 testing of, **96–97**
 transfer of, to metatarsal heads, in pes cavus, 523, **528–529**
Extensor hallucis brevis muscle, anatomic relations of, *11*, *13*, *21*, *30*
 in peroneal muscular atrophy, 496, *497*
 innervation of, intrauterine posture and, 133, *133*
 testing of, **98–99**
Extensor hallucis longus muscle (tendon), anatomic relations of, *2*, *3*, *5*, *9–13*, *16*, *18–21*, *36*, *37*
 function of, in gait, 58, *58*
 in congenital convex pes valgus, 244, *246*, *247*
 in peroneal muscular atrophy, 496, *497*
 innervation of, intrauterine posture and, 133, *133*
 neurosegmental, *421*
 paralysis of, deformities and, 456–457(t), 459
 rerouting of, in congenital hallux varus, 329
 testing of, **94–95**
 transfer of, in claw toes, 555
 in talipes equinus, 389, **394–397**
 to first metatarsal head, in pes cavus, 523, *527*, **528–529**
Extensor retinaculum, inferior, anatomic relations of, *3*, *11*, *12*, *17*, *21*
 superior, anatomic relations of, *3*, *11*, *17*, *21*
Extra-articular subtalar arthrodesis, in congenital metatarsus varus, 301
 in flexible pes planovalgus, 575(t), 577
 in paralysis in poliomyelitis, 488
 in talipes equinovalgus in cerebral palsy, Batchelor, 410, *410*, *411*
 Grice, 403, **404–407**, *408*, *409*
Extrapyramidal level, lesion at, in neuromuscular disease, 353, 354–355(t)
 pes cavus in, 510
Eyes, in hypertrophic interstitial neuritis, 505

Familial periodic paralysis, electrical stimulation in diagnosis of, 118
 lesion at myoneural level in, 353, 354–355(t)
Family, preoperative assessment in cerebral palsy and, 365
Faradic current, stimulation with, in diagnosis, 85
Fascia, plantar, fibromatosis of, 649
Fasciculations, in electromyographic testing, 118
 in paralysis in neuromuscular disease, 352, 354–355(t)
Fatigue (stress) fracture, 703–709, *704–706*
Fatty tissue. See *Adipose tissue*.
Femur, proximal focal deficiency of, tarsal coalition and, 262(t), 266

Femur (*Continued*)
  rotation of, in gait, 56, *65, 67, 70*
Fetus, developmental arrest in, in talipes equinovarus, 142–144, *143*, 144(t)
  myelomeningocele diagnosis in, 422
  posture in, sequential development of, 132, *133, 134*
  tarsal bones in, development and ossification of, 40, *42*
  relationships of, 240, *240*
Fibrillations, in electromyographic testing, 118
  in paralysis in neuromuscular disease, 352, 354–355(t)
Fibroma, recurrent digital, 642–649
  solitary, 649
Fibromatosis, of plantar fascia, 649
Fibrosarcoma, *652*, 655
Fibrosis, muscular, in pes calcaneus, 428
  in pes cavus, 513
Fibula, accessory bone of, *123*, 128
  anatomic relations of, *2, 3, 5, 7–16, 19–23, 25, 37, 38*
  bone graft from, in Batchelor procedure, 410, *410, 411*
  in Grice procedure, **406–407**, *408*
  epiphysiodesis of, to prevent deformity after ankle fracture, 696
  hypoplasia or absence of, congenital ball-and-socket ankle joint and, 313
  tarsal coalition and, 262(t), 266
  in talipes equinovarus, articular malalignment of, *147*, 149, *157, 158*
  injury to, as complication of nonoperative treatment, 187
  in valgus ankle in myelomeningocele, 429, *434, 435*, **436–437**
  ossification of, development and, *40*, 41, *42, 43*
  in fractures of ankle, 660, *661*
  stress fracture of, 703, 706
Fibular nerve, deep, anatomic relations of, *12*
Fibulotalar ligaments, anatomic relations of, *15, 22, 23*
Fick method, for measuring hip flexion deformity, 367
Fillauer bar, contraindicated in congenital metatarsus varus, 297
Fixation, muscles of, function of, 356
Flaccid paralysis, in peroneal muscular atrophy, 499
  muscle testing in, 82, 88–89(t)
Flail ankle, deformities and, in poliomyelitis, 456–457(t), 471
  in myelomeningocele, 446
Flail foot, in myelomeningocele, 424
  pantalar arthrodesis in, 487
Flat foot, classification of, 557(t)
  congenital, due to vertical talus, 239. See also *Congenital convex pes valgus*.
  flexible, 556. See also *Pes planovalgus*.
Flat-topped talus, in talipes equinovarus, 174, 187, *187*
Flexible pes planovalgus, 556–597
  clinical features of, 561, *566*, 567
  deformity in, 557, *557–560*
  roentgenographic features of, 557, *559, 560, 562–565*

Flexible pes planovalgus (*Continued*)
  treatment of, 567, *569, 570, 572,* 574–575(t), *576,* **578–587**, *588, 589,* **590–591**, *592, 594*
Flexion, definition of, 77
Flexion contracture, of hip, diagnosis of, 69, 73
  in cerebral palsy, 367, *366–369*
Flexion deformity, of hip, posture in, *357,* 358
  of knee, in cerebral palsy, 368
Flexor digiti quinti brevis, anatomic relations of, *31, 36, 38*
Flexor digitorum brevis muscle(s), anatomic relations of, *18–20, 28–32, 36, 38*
  in talipes equinus, in cerebral palsy, 371, *372*
  neurosegmental innervation of, *421*
  testing of, **112–113**
Flexor digitorum longus muscle (tendon), anatomic relations of, 1, *2–4, 6, 9, 16–19, 23, 24, 28–32, 34, 36, 38*
  function of, in gait, 57, *58*
  in claw toes, 554
  in myelomeningocele, 425, *427,* 439
  in talipes equinovarus, 151, 188–189(t), 439
  in talipes equinus, in cerebral palsy, 371, *372*
  level of lesion and, 425, *427*
  neurosegmental innervation of, *421*
  paralysis of, deformities and, 456–457(t), 458, 471
  testing of, **110–111**
  transfer of, in congenital curly toe, 346
Flexor hallucis brevis muscle, anatomic relations of, *3, 17–19, 28–32, 36, 38*
  in talipes equinus in cerebral palsy, 371, *372*
  neurosegmental innervation of, *421*
  testing of, **108–109**
Flexor hallucis longus muscle (tendon), anatomic relations of, 1, *3, 4, 6, 9, 17–19, 21, 23, 24, 28–32, 34, 36, 38*
  function of, in gait, 57, *58*
  in talipes equinovarus, 151, 188–189(t)
  in myelomeningocele, 439
  in talipes equinus in cerebral palsy, 371, *372*
  neurosegmental innervation of, *421*
  paralysis of, deformities and, 456–457(t), 471
  testing of, **106–107**
  transfer of, for dorsal bunion, **474–475**
Floor, reaction force of, in gait, 50, *51*
Foot, anatomic relations in, *2, 3, 5, 10–22, 26–38*
  arthrodesis of, alignment for, 482, *483*
  in paralysis in poliomyelitis, 471–492, **478–481**, 482(t), *483, 484, 486,* **488–491**
  bones of, normal variations in, 123–130, *123–129*
  deformities of, congenital postural, 131–139, 132(t), *133–136, 138*
  in myelomeningocele, 424, 425(t), *426, 427*
  flail, pantalar arthrodesis in, 487
  fractures of, 700–703
  interdependence of lower limb structures and, 356–358, *356–359*

Foot (*Continued*)
  motion of, as determinant of gait, 54, *54, 65, 67, 70*
    range of, *79–84*, 80
  normal growth of, 121, 121(t), *122*
  in talipes equinovarus, ridigity of, as complication of open reduction, 210
    shortening lateral column of, 214, *216*, **218–219**
  tumors of, 635. See also specific types of tumor.
Foot orthosis. See *University of California Biomechanics Laboratory foot orthosis.*
Force plate, in gait analysis, 50, *51, 68, 71*
Forefoot, anatomy of, 1
  deformity of, in cerebral palsy, 415
  in talipes equinovarus, 149
    as complication of open reduction of talocalcaneonavicular joint, 209, *210*
  range of motion in, 81, *82*
Foreign body granuloma, 649, *651*
Fowler opening-wedge osteotomy, in pes cavus, 526, *527*, 532
Fracture(s), 660–709
  ankle, 660, *661*
    classification of, 660, *662–664, 666,* 668–669(t), *670–689*
    complications of, *694–699,* 695
    mechanism of injury in, 660, *662–664, 666,* 668–669(t), *670–689*
    treatment of, 689, *689–693*
  cartilage, in osteochondritis dissecans, 616, *618–621*
  foot, 700
  in Freiberg's infraction of second metatarsal, 613
  in nonoperative treatment of talipes equinovarus, 187, *187*
  of Tillaux, 669(t), 682, *683, 684*
    treatment of, 693, *693*
  stress, 703, *704–706*
Fracture-dislocation, Lisfranc's tarsometatarsal, 702
Freeman-Sheldon syndrome, talipes equinovarus in, 164, *167*
Freiberg's infraction of second metatarsal, 612–615, *613, 614*
Friedreich's ataxia, 500–503, 502(t)
  gait in, 64, 500
  pes cavus in, 500, 510
  vs. peroneal muscular atrophy, 498
Function, neuromuscular system as unit of, 353–356
  of muscles for tendon transfer, principles of, 452
Functional metatarsus varus, vs. congenital metatarsus varus, 297

Gait, 46–68
  abnormal, hallux rigidus from, 628
  analysis of, 64, *64–71*
  axial rotation in, 56, *65, 67, 70*
  cycle of, 46, *49*
  determinants of, 51, *52–56*
  gravity in, 50, *51*

Gait (*Continued*)
  in congenital contracture of triceps surae muscle, 508
  in congenital convex pes valgus, 247
  in diastematomyelia, 449
  in Friedreich's ataxia, 502
  in hypertrophic interstitial neuritis, 503
  in peroneal muscular atrophy, 497
  in progressive muscular dystrophy, 64, 505
  in talipes equinus in cerebral palsy, 370, *372*
    training of, 376
      after heel cord lengthening, *382*
  mature, development of, 59
  muscle action in, 57, *58*
  pathologic, in diagnosis, 59, *60–62*
  tarsal coalition and, 269
Galvanic current, diagnostic stimulation with, 85
Ganglion, 637, *637–639*
Gastrocnemius muscle. See also *Triceps surae muscle.*
  anatomic relations of, *2–4, 6, 9, 37*
  atrophy of, in genu valgum, 68
  function of, in gait, 57, *58*
  in talipes equinus in cerebral palsy, 370, *371*
    lengthening of, 383, *385–388*
      neurectomy of motor nerves to, 388, **390–391**
  neurosegmental innervation of, *421*
  paralysis of, deformities and, 456–457(t), 458, 465, *470–473, 476–478*
    gait in, 61, *62*
  testing of, **104–105**
Genetics, in myelomeningocele, counseling in, 419
  in peroneal muscular atrophy, 496
  in pes cavus, 513
  in progressive muscular dystrophy, 505, 505(t)
  in talipes equinovarus, 139
Gentamicin, in osteomyelitis, 599(t)
Genu recurvatum, in talipes equinus, in cerebral palsy, 373
Genu valgum, foot alignment for arthrodesis and, 482
  in flexible pes planovalgus, 568
  measurement of, 68, *72*
Genu varum, foot alignment for arthrodesis and, 482
  measurement of, 68
Germ plasm, primary defect of, in talipes equinovarus, 144
Giannestras operation, in flexible pes planovalgus, 577, **578–587**
Gigantism, of toes, *332–334,* 333
Girdlestone-Taylor operation, for claw toes, 554
Glomus tumor, 649
Gluteus maximus muscle, function of, in gait, 57, *58*
  hip flexion deformity and, in talipes equinus, 377
  innervation of, intrauterine posture and, 133, *133*
    neurosegmental, *421*
  paralysis of, gait in, 61
Gluteus medius lurch, 60, *60*

Gluteus medius muscle of, in gait, 57, *58*
  neurosegmental innervation of, *421*
  paralysis of, in pathologic gait, 59, *60*
Gluteus minimus muscle, function of, in gait, 57, *58*
  neurosegmental innervation of, *421*
Goodwin and Swisher Y-plasty, in congenital digitus minimus varus, 338
Gout, hallux rigidus in, 631
Gracilis muscle, function of, in gait, 58, *58*
  in hip adduction deformity, 368, *369*
  neurosegmental innervation of, *421*
Graft, bone. See *Bone graft.*
Granuloma, foreign body, 649, *651*
Grasp reflex, in cerebral palsy, 360
Gravity, in gait, 50, *51*
Green-Baker fractional lengthening of gastrocnemius, 387, *388*
Green-Grice posterior tendon transfer, in myelomeningocele, 428, **430–433**
Grice extra-articular subtalar arthrodesis, ball-and-socket ankle joint following, 313
  in congenital metatarsus varus, 301
  in flexible pes planovalgus, 575(t), 577
  in poliomyelitis, 487
  in talipes equinovalgus in cerebral palsy, 403, **404–407**, *408, 409*
Growth, arrest of, in nonoperative treatment of talipes equinovarus, 187, *187*
  asymmetric, as complication of ankle fracture, *694–697*, 695
  bone, muscle action in, 356
  normal, of foot, 121–122, 121(t), *122*
Growth plate(s), anatomic relations of, *10, 15, 16, 20, 23*
  ankle fractures and, 661, 689

Hallux, normal variations of, 130
  range of motion of, 81, *83, 84*
Hallux dolorosus, 627. See also *Hallux rigidus.*
Hallux extensus, hallux rigidus as, *630*, 631
Hallux flexus, 627. See also *Hallux rigidus.*
Hallux rigidus, 627–635, *628–630, 632–634*
  in rheumatoid arthritis, 608
Hallux valgus, 308–311, *309, 311*
  hammer toe with, 350
  in cerebral palsy, 415
  in rheumatoid arthritis, 608
Hallux valgus interphalangeus, congenital, 344, *344–346*
Hallux varus, congenital, 329, *330, 331*
Hammer toe, **348–349**, 350–351
  in cerebral palsy, 415
  in rheumatoid arthritis, 608
Hamstring muscle(s), accessory, 508, *508*
  in cerebral palsy, in hip adduction deformity, 368, *369*
  in talipes equinus, 373
  innervation of, intrauterine posture and, 133, *133*
Hard corn, 658
Harris medial approach, in talocalcaneal coalition, *283*, 284
Heart, in Friedreich's ataxia, 501
  in progressive muscular dystrophy, 505

Heel, anatomic relations in, *16–35, 37, 38*
  in talipes equinovarus, clinical appearance of, 160, *161, 162,* 163(t)
  position of, in stance, 45, *48*
  Thomas, in flexible pes planovalgus, 568
  in Köhler's disease of tarsal navicular, 612
Heel cord. See *Achilles tendon.*
Helfet heel seat, in flexible pes planovalgus, 570
Hemangioma, 637–642, *640–644*
Hemangiomatosis, massive, 637, *644*
Hemiplegia, definition of, 82
  in cerebral palsy, 360, *374, 375*
  spastic, gait in, 371, *372*
    pes cavus in, 510
Hereditary spinocerebellar ataxia, 501–504, 502(t)
Heredity, in congenital convex pes valgus, 243
  in congenital talipes equinovarus, 139, 140(t)
  in flexible pes planovalgus, 556, 557(t)
  in Friedreich's ataxia, 500
  in hypertrophic interstitial neuritis, 503
  in myelomeningocele, 419
  in osteochondritis dissecans, 616
  in peroneal muscular atrophy, 496
  in pes cavus, 510, 513
  in polydactylism, 325
  in progressive muscular dystrophy, 505
  in tarsal coalition, 268
Heyman-Herndon-Strong soft-tissue release, in congenital metatarsus varus, 301, **302–305**
Hibbs method, for measuring pes cavus, 518, *518*
Hindfoot, anatomy of, 1
  deformity of, varus, in pes cavus, bony procedures for, 540, *541*, **542–543**, *544, 545*, **546–551**
    varus or valgus, in rheumatoid arthritis, 608
  inversion and eversion of, range of, 81, *81*
Hip, ankle and knee and, interdependence of, 356–358, *356–359*
  deformities of, diagnosis of, 69, *73, 74*
  flexion, posture in, *357*, 358
    intrauterine posture and, 131, 132(t)
  dislocation of, congenital, gait in, 63
    congenital convex pes valgus with, 240
    prevention of in cerebral palsy, 361
  in cerebral palsy, 361, 367, *366–369*, 377
  flexor release of, in talipes equinus, 377
  movement of, innervation of reflexes and, *421*
  pathologic change in, in talipes equinovarus, 156, *156*
  range of motion of, 77, *78*
Hoke naviculocuneiform fusion, in flexible pes planovalgus, 573, 574(t)
Home, preoperative assessment of in cerebral palsy, 365
Horizontal breach, in talipes equinovarus, 156, *157, 158*, 174
Horizontal osteotomy of calcaneus, Baker, in talipes equinovalgus, 412, *413*
Household ambulators, in myelomeningocele, 422
Hyperactivity, of intrinsic foot muscles, in pes cavus, 513

Hyperextension, definition of, 77
Hyperkinesis, toe walking in, vs. congenital contracture of triceps surae muscle, 509
Hyperlaxity, of ligaments, in flexible pes planovalgus, 556, 557(t), *558*
Hyperparathyroidism, insufficiency fractures in, 703
Hyperpituitarism, insufficiency fractures in, 703
Hypertrophic interstitial neuritis (Dejerine-Sottas), 503–505
　pes cavus in, 503, 510
　vs. peroneal muscular atrophy, 498
Hysteria, paralysis in, 353, 354–355(t)
　pes cavus in, 510

Iliopsoas (iliacus) muscle, function of, in gait, 58, *58*
　in hip flexion deformity, 366, 367
　innervation of, intrauterine posture and, 133
　　neurosegmental, *421*
Iliotibial tract, anatomic relations of, *2, 5*
Infant(s), ankle fractures in, 663
　gait pattern in, 59, *64, 65*
　talipes equinovarus in choice of operating procedures for, 187
　　foot and leg atrophy in, 152
　　roentgenography of tarsal bones in, 170
　tarsal coalition in, 268
Infection(s), 598–610, 599(t), *600–603, 606, 608, 609*
　in growing toenail, 660
　plantar wart as, 659
　viral, poliomyelitis as, 451
　wound, in open reduction of talocalcaneonavicular joint, 209
Inflammation, joint, in hallux rigidus, 628
Inflammation disorders, 598–610, 599(t), *600–603, 606, 608, 609.* See also *Infection(s).*
　insufficiency fractures in, 703
Ingrowing toenail, 660
Injury. See *Trauma.*
Innervation, muscle, evaluation of in cerebral palsy, 370, 370(t)
　segmental, 420, *421*
Insufficiency fracture, 703
Intelligence, of child, preoperative assessment in cerebral palsy and, 365
Intercapitular veins, anatomic relations of, *11, 12*
Intermetatarsal joints, mobilization of, in congenital metatarsus varus, 301, **302–305**
Intermuscular septum, anatomic relations of, *5, 8, 9*
Interosseous ligament(s), anatomic relations of, *15, 19, 22, 23, 36*
　as obstacle to reduction in talipes equinovarus, 152
　in flexible pes planovalgus, 557
Interosseous membrane, anatomic relations of, *2, 5, 7–9, 24*
　in mechanism of ankle fractures, 660, *662*
Interosseous muscles, anatomic relations of, *11, 13, 30, 32, 36–38*

Interosseous (*Continued*)
　in pes cavus, hyperactivity of, 513
　paralysis of, 511
Interphalangeal joints, in claw toes, 554, *554*
　in hammer toe, **348–349,** 350
　in rheumatoid arthritis, 608
Interstitial neuritis, hypertrophic (Dejerine-Sottas), 503–505
Intertarsal bridge (bar), 261. See also *Tarsal coalition* and names of specific conditions.
Intertarsal joints, tuberculous arthritis of, 604
Inversion, definition of, 77
　hindfoot, measurement of, 81, *81*
　muscles of, paralysis of, deformities and, 458
　talocalcaneonavicular joint in, in talipes equinovarus, 153
Irradiation, of plantar wart, 659
Ischemia, in osteochondritis dissecans, 617
　muscle response to, 356

Jack, toe-raising test of, 567, *567*
Japas V-osteotomy of tarsus, 532, **534–537**
Jeunes's infantile thoracic dystrophy, polydactylism and, 325
Joint(s). See also names of specific joints.
　anatomic relations in, *15, 19, 23, 25*
　deformity of, in pathologic gait, 62
　embryonic development of, 39
　in congenital convex pes valgus, 243, *244*
　in flexible pes planovalgus, 557, *557, 559, 560, 562–565*
　in talipes equinovarus, malalignment of, 149–151, *150–159*
　　roentgenography of, 170
　incongruity of, in ankle fracture, 699
　motion of, innervation of reflexes and, *421*
　range of, 75–82, *76, 78–84*
　rotation of, in gait, 50
　tuberculosis of, 604
Jones' fracture, of fifth metatarsal, 702
Jones tendon transfer, Achilles, in flexible pes planovalgus, 573, 574(t), *576*
　long toe extensor, **528–529**
Jump position, in cerebral palsy, 367, *368*
Juvenile rheumatoid arthritis, 608–610, *608, 609*

Kanamycin, in osteomyelitis, 599(t)
Kelikian operation, in congenital digitus minimus varus, **340–341**
Kelikian push-up test, in pes cavus, 520, *520*
Kessel and Bonney extension osteotomy, in hallux rigidus, 631, *633*
Kidner procedure, in accessory tarsal navicular, 125
Knee, ankle and hip and, interdependence of, 356–358, *356–359*
　deformities of, diagnosis of, 68, *72*
　in flexible pes planovalgus, 568
　in talipes equinus, 373
　extension contracture of, intrauterine posture and, 131
　in cerebral palsy, 368, 373

Knee (*Continued*)
  motion of, as determinant of gait, 51, *54, 55, 65, 67, 70*
  innervation of reflexes and, *421*
Knock-knee. See *Genu valgum.*
Köhler's disease No. 2, 612–615, *613, 614*
Köhler's disease of tarsal navicular, 610–612, *611*
  vs. congenital convex pes valgus, 250
Koutsogiannis medial displacement osteotomy, in flexible pes planovalgus, 575(t), 593, *594*

Laciniate ligament, anatomic relations of, *3, 6, 17, 24, 28–32*
Lambrinudi triple arthrodesis, 487
  ball-and-socket ankle joint following, 313
Larsen's syndrome, talipes equinovarus in, 164, *168*
Lateral displacement osteotomy of calcaneus, in pes cavovarus, 540
Lateral rotation deformity, as complication of ankle fracture, 698
Lateral rotation injury, in ankle fracture, *666, 667*
Lauge-Hansen classification of ankle fractures, 667, 668–669(t)
Lead poisoning, vs. hypertrophic interstitial neuritis, 504
Leg, congenital postural deformities of, 131–139, 132(t), *133–136, 138*
  length inequality of, deformities and, 69–75, *75*
  muscles of, anatomic relations of, *2–9, 37, 38*
  rotational deformity of, in talipes equinovarus, 156, *156, 158*
  shortening of, congenital, ball-and-socket ankle joint and, 313
  limp in, 62
Leukemia, vs. stress fracture, 707
Lichtblau procedures, in talipes equinovarus, 192, 216, **218–219**
Lichtblau test, in congenital metatarsus varus, 296, *296*
Ligament(s). See also names of specific ligaments.
  anatomic relations of, *15, 17, 19, 22–24, 29–32, 34, 36*
  ankle, in tarsal coalition, 269
  in congenital convex pes valgus, 244, *245, 246*
  in flexible pes planovalgus, hyperlaxity of, 556, 557(t), *558*
  tightening of, 571, 574(t)
  in fractures of ankle, 660, *662*
  in talipes equinovarus, bone deformities and, 150
    clinical characteristics of, 160
    nonoperative elongation of, 176, *177*
    pathologic change in, 152
Limbs, length inequality of, in deformities, 69–75, *75*
Limp, antalgic, 62
  in Köhler's disease of tarsal navicular, 611

Limp (*Continued*)
  in osteochondritis dissecans of talus, 619
  in osteomyelitis, 599
  in stress fracture, 704
  in suppurative arthritis, 605
  short-leg, 62
Lipoma, 635, *636*
Lisfranc's joint, anatomic relations at, *36*
  fracture-dislocation of, 702
  in metatarsal wedge resection in pes cavus, 532, *538*
Lobster claw, 317–322, *318–322*
Long arm 18 deletion syndrome, talipes equinovarus in, 169
Longitudinal arch, anatomy and function of, 1
  in flexible pes planovalgus, 556, *558–560, 562–564, 566, 567*
Longitudinal branch, in talipes equinovarus, 174
Lovell, Scottish-Rite operation of, in flexible pes planovalgus, 576
Lower motor neuron lesion, electrical stimulation in diagnosis of, 85
Lowman talonavicular fusion, in flexible pes planovalgus, 574(t), 577
Lumbrical muscles, anatomic relations of, *28–30, 36, 38*
  testing of, **116–117**
Lymphangiectasis, 642, *646*
Lymphatic tissue, congenital hyperplasia of, in macrodactylism, 333

Macrodactylism, *332–334*, 333
Malformations, congenital, vs. congenital postural deformities, 132, 132(t)
Malleolar arteries, anatomic relations of, *12, 14, 17, 21, 23*
Malleolus (malleoli), anatomic relations of, *2–5, 10–13, 16–24*
  development and ossification of, 41, *43*
  in talipes equinovarus, *147, 148, 150, 152*
  medial, accessory bone of, 126, *128*
Mallet toe, *350*, 351
  in cerebral palsy, 415
Manipulation, in congenital metatarsus varus, 297, *298–300*
  triple arthrodesis and, in talipes equinovarus, 225
March fracture, 703
Marfan's syndrome, flat foot in, 557(t), 571
Master knot of Henry, relations of, *17, 19, 30*
  in talipes equinovarus, 152
Maturation, delayed, vs. congenital contracture of triceps surae muscle, 509
  neurophysiologic, preoperative assessment in cerebral palsy and, 360
McFarland-Dwyer dorsal wedge osteotomy of calcaneus, in pes calcaneocavus, *541*, 544
McFarland operation, in congenital digitus minimus varus, 338, **340–341**
McKay technique, for open correction of talipes equinovarus, 192
  for tendon transfer in dorsal bunion, 472, *473, 476, 477*

Méary method, for measuring pes cavus, *518*, 519
Mechanical theory, of talipes equinovarus etiology, 141
Metatarsal arteries, anatomic relations of, dorsal, *12, 14*
    plantar, *31, 33*
Metatarsal bone(s), anatomic relations of, 1, *10, 14–17, 19–22, 26, 34, 35, 38*
    development and ossification of, 39, *40–43*
    fifth, aneurysmal bone cyst of, *654*, 655
    first, congenital short, 314–317, *314–317*
        elevation of, in hallux rigidus, 627
        osteotomy of, in congenital metatarsus primus varus and hallux valgus, 310, *311*
            open-up, for dorsal bunion, **474–475**
        short, hallux varus with, 329
    first and fifth, osteochondrosis of, 615
    fractures of, 702
    normal variations of, *123, 129*, 130
    osteomyelitis of, 598
    osteotomy of, at bases, in talipes equinovarus, 192, 227
        dorsal wedge, in pes cavus, 532, *533, 538*
    second, Freiberg's infraction of, 612–615, *613, 614*
    stress fracture of, 703, *704, 705*
    tendon transfers to, in pes cavus, 523, 527, **528–529**
    tuberculous dactylitis of, 604
Metatarsocuneiform joint(s), fusion of, in pes cavus, 532, *533*
Metatarsophalangeal joint(s), anatomic relations at, *36*
    arthritis of, rheumatoid, 608
        tuberculous, 604
    in claw toes, 554, *554*
    in hallux rigidus, 627, *629, 630, 632–634*
    sesamoid bones of, osteomyelitis of, 601, *603*
Metatarsus adductus, postural congenital, 131, 137, *138*
Metatarsus adductus varus, congenital ball-and-socket ankle joint and, 313
Metatarsus primus elevatus, 627–635, *628–630, 632–634*
    in rheumatoid arthritis, 608
Metatarsus primus varus, congenital, 308–311, *308, 309, 311*
Metatarsus varus, after open reduction of talocalcaneonavicular joint, 209, *210*
    brachymetatarsia and, *315*, 317
    congenital, 294–308, *295, 296, 298–300*, **309–307**
        vs. postural metatarsus adductus, 137, *138*
    hallux varus with, 329
    in cerebral palsy, 415
Methicillin, in osteomyelitis, 599, 599(t)
    in suppurative arthritis, 607
Microdactylism, 335
Midfoot (midtarsus), anatomy of, 1
    joints of, roentgenography of, in talipes equinovarus, 170
    range of motion in, 81, *82*
Milch method, for measuring hip flexion deformity, 367
Miller operation, in flexible pes planovalgus, 574(t), 576

Milroy's disease, 642
Minimal brain damage syndrome, hyperkinesia in, vs. congenital contracture of triceps surae muscle, 509
Mitchell posterior-superior displacement osteotomy, of calcaneus, 544, *550–551*
Möbius syndrome, talipes equinovarus in, 169, *169*
Moderator, muscle function as, 356
Monoplegia, definition of, 82
    in cerebral palsy, 360
Moro reflex, in cerebral palsy, 360
Mosaic wart, plantar, 659
Motion, innervation of reflexes and, *421*
    range of, in diagnosis, 75–82, *76, 78–84*
Motor power. See also *Muscle(s), strength of*.
    in gait, 57, *58*
    in neuromuscular disease, 352, 354–355(t)
    in peroneal muscular atrophy, 499
Mucin test, in suppurative arthritis, 606
Murphy anterior advancement of heel cord, in talipes equinus, 388, *389*, **392–393**
Muscle(s). See also names of specific muscles.
    accessory, *506, 508*, 508
    action of, in gait, 57–59, *58, 60–62*
        on bone, in pathogenesis of stress fracture, 704
        anatomic relations of, of foot, *2, 3, 5, 10–13, 16–21, 27–32, 36, 38*
        of leg, *2–9, 37, 38*
    choice of for tendon transfer, principles of, 452
    congenital absence of, 507
    contracture of, flat foot in, 557(t), 559
    electrical stimulation of, in diagnosis, 85
    examination of, 45, *47*
    imbalance of, in Friedreich's ataxia, 501
        in pes cavus pathogenesis, 510
    in congenital convex pes valgus, 244–247, *246, 247*
    in neuromuscular disease, 352, 354–355(t)
    in talipes equinovarus, 151
    innervation of, intrauterine posture and, 133, *133, 134*
    paralysis of, deformities caused by, 455, 456–457(t), *458, 464, 465, 470–478*
    spasm of, in diagnosis of deformities, 68
        in rheumatoid arthritis, 609
    strength of, testing of, 82–84, 86(t), 86–89(t), **90–117**
        in cerebral palsy, 370, 370(t), 375
        in lower leg, *79*, 80
        in myelomeningocele, 420
    transplantation of, definition of, 452
Muscular dystrophy, distal, vs. peroneal muscular atrophy, 498
    flat foot in, 557(t), 571
    gait in, 64, 505
    lesion at muscular level in, 353, 354–355(t)
    pes cavus in, 510
    progressive, 505–507, 505(t)
    vs. congenital contracture of triceps surae muscle, 509
Muscular level, lesion at, pes cavus from, 510
Myasthenia gravis, electrical stimulation in, diagnostic, 118
    lesion at myoneural level in, 353, 354–355(t)
Myelodysplasia, flat foot in, 557(t)

Myelography, in diastematomyelia, *450*, 451
  in hypertrophic interstitial neuritis, 504
Myelomeningocele, 418–449
  claw toes in, 444, *445*
  clinical features of, 419, *419–421*
  congenital convex pes valgus in, 240, *442–444*, 443
    vs. paralytic pes valgus, 251
  flail ankle in, 446
  incidence of, 418
  insufficiency fractures in, 703
  pes calcaneus in, 425, *426, 427, 429*, **430–433**
  pes cavus in, 444, 510
  pes equinus in, 441, *441*
  talipes equinovalgus in, Batchelor extra-articular subtalar arthrodesis in, 411
  talipes equinovarus in, 438, *438–440*
    open reduction of talocalcaneonavicular joint in, 192
    treatment principles in, 421, *423*, 425(t), *426, 427*
  valgus ankle in, 429, *434, 435*, **436–437**, *438*
Myoneural level, lesion at, in neuromuscular disease, 353, 354–355(t)
Myositis, electromyography in, 119
Myostatic contracture, Achilles tendon lengthening in, 377, **378–380**
  as response to injury, 356
  deformity and, in cerebral palsy, 367
  from neurectomy, 388
  in muscle weakness, 83
  peroneal, in flat foot, 557(t)
Myotonia congenita, electrical stimulation in diagnosis of, 118
Myotonia dystrophica, electrical stimulation in diagnosis of, 118

Nafcillin, in osteomyelitis, 595(t)
Nail(s), 658–660, *659*
Navicular bone, accessory, 123. See also *Accessory tarsal navicular*.
  anatomic relations of, 1, *10, 14–19, 20, 23, 26, 30, 34, 35, 38*
  "beak" of, in talipes varus, 483
  cornuted, 125, *125*
  development and ossification of, 39, *42, 43*
  fractures of, 702
  in congenital convex pes valgus, 243, *244*
  in flexible pes planovalgus, 557, *559, 560, 562–564*
  in talipes equinovarus, articular malalignment of, 149, *152, 153, 159*
    aseptic necrosis of, after open reduction of calcaneonavicular joint, 209
    displacement of, *147, 148, 148*
    nonoperative manipulation of, *179*, 180
  Köhler's disease of, 610–612, *611*
  normal variations of, os supranaviculare as, 130
  osteomyelitis of, tuberculous, 604
  stress fracture of, 703
Navicular pads, in flexible pes planovalgus, 570

Naviculocuneiform coalition, 262(t), 265
Naviculocuneiform joint, in flexible pes planovalgus, 557, *559, 560, 562–565*
  correction of sag at, 573, *576*, **578–587**
  fusion of, 573, 574(t)
Naviculocuneiform ligament, anatomic relations of, *19*
Naviculometatarsal angle, measurement of, 209, *210*
Necrosis, aseptic, after open reduction of talocalcaneonavicular joint, 209
Neoplasm. See *Tumors*.
Nerve(s). See also names of specific nerves.
  conduction velocity determination in, 119
  disorders of, pathologic gait in, 63
  electrical stimulation of, diagnostic, 85
  examination of, 84
  in diastematomyelia, 449
  in hypertrophic interstitial neuritis, 504
  in peroneal muscular atrophy, 496, 498
  in tendon transfer, 453
  injuries of, flat foot from, 557(t)
  plantar motor, section of, pes cavus, 526
Nerve sheath, tumors of, *647*, 649
Neural level, lesion at, in neuromuscular disease, 353, 354–355(t)
  pes cavus in, 510
Neurilemoma, benign encapsulated, *647*, 649
Neuritis, hypertrophic interstitial (Dejerine-Sottas), 503–505
  pes cavus in, 503, 510
  vs. peroneal muscular atrophy, 498
  peripheral, nerve conduction velocity studies in, 119
Neurofibromatosis, congenital convex pes valgus with, 240
  macrodactylism in, 333
Neuromuscular system, as functional unit, 353–356
  defect of, in talipes equinovarus etiology, 141
  development of function in, intrauterine posture and, 133, *133, 134*
  diseases of, 352. See also names of specific diseases.
    levels of paralysis in, 352, 354–355(t)
    muscle responses in, 356
  excitability tests of, 85–119
  interdependence of structures in, 356–358, *356–359*
Neutral Zero method, measurement of joint range of motion by, 75
Newborn, pes calcaneus in, in myelomeningocele, 428
  talipes equinovarus treatment in, 176
Nievergelt-Pearlman syndrome, tarsal coalition in, 262(t), *264, 265*, 266
Night splints, in cerebral palsy, after split anterior tibial tendon transfer, in pes varus, 402
  in talipes equinus, 376
  in hypertrophic interstitial neuritis, 504
  in peroneal muscular atrophy, 498
  in tendon transfer, in poliomyelitis, 455
Nonambulators, in myelomeningocele, 424
Nonfunctional ambulators, in myelomeningocele, 422

Ober's test, for abduction contracture of hip, 69, *74*
Obliquity, of ankle mortise, *25*
   of neck of talus, 145, *145, 146*
   pelvic, congenital, intrauterine posture and, 131
Obstetrical brachial plexus palsy, lesion at neural level in, 353, 354–355(t)
Obturator externus muscle, neurosegmental innervation of, *421*
Opening-wedge osteotomy (Fowler), of medial cuneiform, in pes cavus, 526, *527*, 532
Open-up osteotomy, in congenital metatarsus primus varus and hallux valgus, 310, *311*
   of base of first metatarsal, for dorsal bunion, **474–475**
Orthosis (orthoses), ankle-foot. See *Ankle-foot orthosis.*
   dorsiflexion-assist. See *Dorsiflexion-assist orthosis.*
   foot. See *University of California Biomechanics Laboratory foot orthosis.*
   in cerebral palsy, 365, 376, 402
   in hypertrophic interstitial neuritis, 504
   in pes varus, after split anterior tibial tendon transfer, 402
   in talipes equinovalgus, 402
   in talipes equinus, 376
   in tarsal coalition, 283
   patellar tendon–bearing, in osteochondritis dissecans of talus, 620
   in rheumatoid arthritis, 609, *609*
   postoperative, in tendon transfer training, 455
Os calcaneus secundarius, tarsal coalition and, 268, 272
Os calcis. See *Calcaneus.*
Os cuboideum secundarium, as normal variation, *123*, 130
Os fibulare, as normal variation, *123*, 128
Os intercuneiforme, as normal variation, *123*, 130
Os peroneum, tarsal coalition and, 268
   vs. fracture of fifth metatarsal, 702
Os supranaviculare, as normal variation, 130
Os sustentaculare, tarsal coalition and, 268
Os tibiale externum, 123. See also *Accessory tarsal navicular.*
Os trigonum, as normal variation, *123*, 125–126, *126, 127*
   tarsal coalition and, 268
Os vesalianum, as normal variation, *123*, *129*, 130
   vs. fracture of fifth metatarsal, 702
Ossicles, accessory. See *Accessory bones (ossicles)* and names of specific bones.
Ossification, 39–44, *40–43*
   age of, in fractures of ankle, 660, *661*
   tarsal coalition symptoms and, 269
   fifth metatarsal center of, vs. fracture, 702
   of fibula, valgus ankle and, in myelomeningocele, 429
   of navicular bone, Köhler's disease and, 610
   of tarsal bones, roentgenography and, in congenital convex pes valgus, 249, *249, 250*
      in talipes equinovarus, 170

Osteochondritis dissecans, 616–627, *618–621*, **622–625**
   etiology of, 616
   of first metatarsal head, in hallux rigidus, 628, *628*
   of talus, 618, *618–621*, **622–625**
   vs. accessory bone of fibula, 128
Osteochondroses, 615
Osteogenesis imperfecta, flat foot in, 557(t), 571
   insufficiency fracture in, 703
Osteogenic sarcoma, 657, *657*
   vs. stress fracture, 707
Osteoid osteoma, *653, 654*, 655
   vs. stress fracture, 707
Osteomalacia, vs. stress fracture, 707
Osteomyelitis, 598–604, 599(t), *600–603*
   ankle fracture in, 663
   pathologic fractures in, 703
   vs. stress fracture, 707
   vs. suppurative arthritis, 606
Osteopetrosis, insufficiency fracture in, 703
Osteophytes, in osteomyelitis of calcaneus, *600*
   of metatarsophalangeal joint, in hallux rigidus, 631, *632*
Osteoporosis, postirradiation, pathologic fractures in, 703
"Ostrich legs" appearance, in peroneal muscular atrophy, 497
Outflare (tarsal pronator) shoes, in talipes equinovarus, 185, *186*
Overcorrection, in talipes equinovarus, 208, 216, *216*
Oxacillin, in osteomyelitis, 599(t)

Pain, in congenital curly toe, 346
   in diagnosis of deformities, 68
   in flexible pes planovalgus, 561, 567
      as indication for arthrodesis, 577, 588
   in Freiberg's infraction of second metatarsal, 613
   in hallux rigidus, 628
   in hemangioma, 637
   in Köhler's disease of tarsal navicular, 611
   in osteochondritis dissecans of talus, 619
   in osteomyelitis, 599
   in stress fracture, 705
   in suppurative arthritis, 605
   in tarsal coalition, 270
      operative treatment for, 283, **286–291**
   muscle response to, 356
Palsy. See also *Paralysis.*
   cerebral, 358. See also *Cerebral palsy.*
   progressive bulbar, spinal level lesion in, 353, 354–355(t)
Pantalar arthrodesis, in poliomyelitis, 487
Paralysis, clubfoot in, Evans procedure in, 192
   vs. talipes equinovarus, 162
   definition of, 82
   familial periodic, electrical stimulation in diagnosis of, 118
   gait in, 59, *60–62*
   in cerebral palsy, distribution of, 360
   in diastematomyelia, 449
   in myelomeningocele, 424

Paralysis (*Continued*)
  in myelomeningocele, congenital convex pes valgus in, *442–444,* 443
    evaluation of, 420
  in peroneal muscular atrophy, 497
  in poliomyelitis, 452
    deformities caused by, 455, 456–457(t), *458, 464, 465, 470–478*
    insufficiency fractures in, 703
    levels of, in neuromuscular disease, 352, 354–355(t)
    muscle examination in, 82, 86–89(t)
    of intrinsic foot muscles, in pes cavus pathogenesis, 511
    pes cavovarus in, tendon transfer in, 526
    triple arthrodesis in, 540
    pes valgus in, vs. congenital convex pes valgus, 251
      roentgenography in, 249
Paraplegia, definition of, 82
  spastic, gait in, 63
    vs. congenital contracture of triceps surae muscle, 509
Parents, associations for, in myelomeningocele, 422
Paresis, definition of, 82. See also *Weakness.*
Patella, anatomic relations of, *2, 3, 5, 8*
  in talipes equinovarus, 156, *156, 158*
Patellar tendon–bearing orthosis, in osteochondritis dissecans of talus, 620
  in rheumatoid arthritis, 609, *609*
Pathologic fracture, 703
  type of injury in, 663
Pauciarticular arthritis, 608, *608*
  vs. tuberculous dactylitis, 604
Pectineus muscle, in hip adduction deformity, 368, *369*
  neurosegmental innervation of, *421*
Pelvis, as determinant of gait, lateral displacement of, 55, *56*
  rotation of, 51, *52, 56, 65, 67, 70*
  tilt of, 51, *53, 65, 67, 70*
  congenital obliquity of, intrauterine posture and, 131
Pelvofemoral angle, in hip flexion deformity, 367
Penicillin, in osteomyelitis, 599, 599(t)
  in suppurative arthritis, 607
Periodic paralysis, familial, electrical stimulation in diagnosis of, 118
Periosteum, blood supply to, in Batchelor extra-articular subtalar arthrodesis, 411
Peripheral nerves, in hypertrophic interstitial neuritis, 504
  in peroneal muscular atrophy, 496, 498
Peripheral neuritis, nerve conduction velocity in, 119
Peroneal artery, anatomic relations of, *6, 8, 9, 23*
Peroneal muscles (tendons). See also names of individual peroneal muscles.
  contracture of, flat foot in, 557(t)
  in cerebral palsy, 371, 373, *402*
  in congenital convex pes valgus, 246, *247*
  in flexible pes planovalgus, transfer of, 573
  in Friedreich's ataxia, 501
  in myelomeningocele, 425, *426, 427,* 439
  in peroneal muscular atrophy, 498, *498*

Peroneal muscles (tendons) (*Continued*)
  in talipes equinovalgus, 402
  in talipes equinovarus, 151, 439
  in talipes equinus, 371, *373*
  innervation of, intrauterine posture and, 133, *133*
  paralysis of, level of lesion and, 425, *426, 427*
Peroneal muscular atrophy, 496–500. See also *Charcot-Marie-Tooth disease.*
Peroneal nerves, anatomic relations of, *2, 5, 8, 9, 11, 13, 18, 21, 36*
Peroneal retinaculum, anatomic relations of, *6, 21*
  as obstacle to reduction in talipes equinovarus, 152
Peroneal spastic flatfoot, tarsal coalition and, 261, *269,* 271
  vs. congenital convex pes valgus, 251
Peroneal veins, anatomic relations of, *8*
Peroneus brevis muscle, anatomic relations of, *2–6, 9, 10, 21, 24, 34, 36, 37*
  function of in gait, 57, *58*
  in congenital convex pes valgus, 244
  in pes cavus pathogenesis, 510
  neurosegmental innervation of, *421*
  paralysis of, deformities and, 456–457(t), 458, *458*
  testing of, **100–101**
Peroneus longus muscle (tendon) anatomic relations of, 1, *2–6, 9, 19, 21, 23, 36, 37*
  function of in gait, 57, *58*
  in pes cavus pathogenesis, 510
  lengthening of, in pes cavovarus, 526
  neurosegmental innervation of, *421*
  paralysis of, deformities and, 456–457(t), 458, **458**
  testing of, **102–103**
  transfer of, anterior, to base of second metatarsal, **460–463**
    posterior, in pes calcaneus, *427, 428,* **430–433**
Peroneus tertius muscle, anatomic relations of, 3, *21, 36, 37*
  neurosegmental innervation of, *421*
  testing of, **100**
Pes calcaneocavus, *513,* 514
  calcaneal osteotomy for, dorsal wedge, 540, *541*
    posterior-superior displacement, 544, *544, 545,* **546–551**
  muscle paralysis and, 456–457(t), 470, *471*
  wedge resections for, in triple arthrodesis, 486, *487*
Pes calcaneus. See *Talipes calcaneus.*
Pes cavovarus, clinical features of, *513,* 514, 515–517
  Coleman's test for flexibility in, 520, *521, 522*
  in Friedreich's ataxia, 501
  in peroneal muscular atrophy, 497, *498*
  muscle paralysis and, 456–457(t), 459
  subtotal excision of talus in, 552
Pes cavus, 510–554
  clinical features of, *512, 513,* 514, *515–517*
  etiology of, 510
  in Friedreich's ataxia, 500, 510
  in hypertrophic interstitial neuritis, 503, 510

Pes cavus (Continued)
  in myelomeningocele, 444, 510
  roentgenographic findings in, 518, *518*
  treatment of, 519, *519–522*
    bony procedures in, 526, **530–531**, *533*, **534–537**, *538–541*, **542–543**, *544*, *545*, **546–551**
    soft-tissue procedures in, 522, **524–525**, **528–529**
    wedge resections for, in triple arthrodesis, 486, *487*
Pes equinocavus, *513*, 514
Pes planovalgus, flexible, 556. See also *Flexible pes planovalgus*.
  in progressive muscular dystrophy, 505
  muscle paralysis and, 511
  tarsal coalition and, *269*
Pes planus, classification of, 556, 557(t)
Pes valgus. See also *Talipes valgus*.
  after Evans procedure in talipes equinovarus, 216, *216*
  as complication of ankle fracture, 698, *698*, *699*
  congenital convex, 239. See also *Congenital convex pes valgus*.
  flexible, 556. See also *Flexible pes planovalgus*.
  in tarsal coalition, *269*, *270*
  talipes equinus and, in cerebral palsy, 373, *373*
  triceps surae contracture with, vs. congenital convex pes valgus, 250
  wedge resections for, in triple arthrodesis, 486
Pes varus. See *Talipes varus*.
Phalanx (phalanges), anatomic relations of, 1, *10*, *14–16*, *26*, *34*, *35*, *38*
  development and ossification of, 39, *42*, *43*
  normal variations of, 130
  osteochondrosis of, 615
  osteomyelitis of, 598
  range of motion of, 81, 83, 84
  tuberculous dactylitis of, 604
Phelps method, of physical therapy in cerebral palsy, 365
Phocomelia, tarsal coalition and, 262(t), 266
Physical therapy, in cerebral palsy, preoperative assessment and, 365
  in tendon transfer training in poliomyelitis, 454
Physis, injury to, in fractures, 660, *662–664*, *666*, 668–669(t), *670–689*
    premature closure as complication of, *694–697*, 695
Pigmented villonodular synovitis, 649, *650*
Plantar aponeurosis, anatomic relations of, *3*, *18*, *19*, *27–32*, *36*
  section of, in pes cavus, 522, **524–525**
Plantar arteries, anatomic relations of, *18*, *23*, *27*, *28*, *31–33*, *36*
Plantar fascia, fibromatosis of, 649
Plantar flexion, ankle, range of, *80*, 81
  paralysis of, muscles of, deformities and, 455
Plantar-flexion angle, of talus, in flexible pes planovalgus, 561
    choice of operation and, 571
Plantar flexion injury, in ankle fracture, 666, *667*

Plantar ligaments, anatomic relations of, *19*, *22*, *29–32*, *34*, *36*
Plantar muscles, cavernous hemangioma of, *641*, *642*
  short, section of in pes cavus, 255, **524–525**
Plantar nerve(s), anatomic relations of, *18*, *27–32*, *36*
  medial, benign encapsulated neurilemoma of, *647*
Plantar veins, anatomic relations of, *18*
Plantar wart, 659
Plantaris muscle, anatomic relations of, 3, 4, 9, 37
  neurosegmental innervation of, *421*
Plaster cast. See *Cast(s)*.
Plastizote shoe insert, in pes cavus, 519
Poisoning, lead or arsenic, vs. hypertrophic interstitial neuritis, 504
Poland's classification of ankle fractures, 661, *663*
Poliomyelitis, 451–497
  arthrodesis in, 471–492, **478–481**, *483*, *484*, *486*, **488–491**
  foot, ball-and-socket ankle joint following, 313
  denervation potentials in, 118
  flat foot in, 557(t)
  lesion at spinal level in, 353, 354–355(t)
  paralytic pes valgus in, vs. congenital convex pes valgus, 251
  pes cavus in, 510
  tendon transfer in, 452, 456–457(t), *458*, **460–463**, *464*, *465*, **466–469**, *470–473*, **474–475**, *476*, *477*
Pollex varus, congenital convex pes valgus with, 240
Polyarthritis, rheumatoid, 608
Polydactylism, 323–329, *323–328*
  congenital hallux varus with, 329, *330*, *331*
Polyneuritis, chronic, vs. peroneal muscular atrophy, 498
  pes cavus in, 510
Polypropylene splint, above-knee, in nonoperative correction of talipes equinovarus, 184
Popliteus muscle, anatomic relations of, 3, 4, 6, 9, 38
Positioning, for roentgenography, in talipes equinovarus, 171
Posterior-superior calcaneal displacement osteotomy, *544*, *545*, **546–551**
Posterior tibial artery, anatomic relations of, 6, 9, *18*, *23*, *24*, *27–33*
  aneurysm of, from triple arthrodesis, 637, *645*
Posterior tibial muscle (tendon), accessory tarsal navicular bone and, 125
  anatomic relations of, 1, *3*, 4, 6, 9, 11, *16–19*, *23*, *24*, *34*, *36*, *38*
  flat foot and, 557(t)
  function of, in gait, 57, *58*
  in cerebral palsy, 371, *374*, 398, *398–400*, 402
  in congenital convex pes valgus, 246, *246*
  in Köhler's disease of tarsal navicular, 611
  in myelomeningocele, 439
  in pes varus, 398, *398–400*
  in poliomyelitis, 456–457(t)

Posterior tibial muscle (tendon) (*Continued*)
  in talipes equinovalgus, 402
  in talipes equinovarus, 151, *152*, 160, 188–189(t), 439
    nonoperative elongation of, *17*, 180
    transfer of, 211
  in talipes equinus, 371, *374*
  in tarsal coalition, 271
  innervation of, intrauterine posture and, 133, *133*
    neurosegmental, *421*
  paralysis of, deformities and, 456–457(t)
  testing of, 92–93
  transfer of, anterior, through interosseous membrane, 398, **466–469**
    in flexible pes planovalgus, 574–575(t), 576
    in peroneal muscular atrophy, 499
Posterior tibial veins, anatomic relations of, *18*
Postoperative care, feasibility of, preoperative assessment of, in cerebral palsy, 365
Postural clubfoot, congenital, 131, 132(t), 137–138
  vs. talipes equinovarus, 162, 163(t)
Postural deformities, congenital, 131–139, 132(t), *133–136*, *138*
Postural metatarsus adductus, congenital, 131, 137, *138*
  vs. congenital metatarsus varus, 297
Postural talipes valgus, congenital, 131, 137
Postural talipes varus, congenital, 131, *136*, 137
Posture, calcaneus ankle deformity and, 358, *359*
  equinus ankle deformity and, 358, *358*, *359*
  examination of, 44
  hip flexion deformity and, *357*, 358
  in stance, requirements for, 356, *356*
  intrauterine, in congenital deformities, 131, *133*, *134*
Prehallux, as normal variation, 123–125, *123–126*. See also *Accessory tarsal navicular*.
Prewalker clubfoot shoe, contraindicated in congenital metatarsus varus, 297
  in talipes equinovarus, 184, *185*
Prime mover, muscle function as, 353
Progressive muscular atrophy, electromyography in, 118
  level of lesion in, 353, 354–355(t)
Progressive muscular dystrophy, 505–507, 505(t). See also *Muscular dystrophy*.
Pronation, definition of, 77
  range of motion in, 81, *83*
Pronation–eversion–lateral rotation ankle fracture, 668(t), 677, *681*, *682*
  treatment of, 692, *693*
Protective extension of arms reflex, 360, *362*
Pseudarthrosis, after Grice procedure, 409
Pseudohypertrophy, in progressive muscular dystrophy, 505
Pseudomonas aeruginosa, in osteomyelitis, 598
  in suppurative arthritis, 605
Psychomotor level, paralysis at, 353, 354–355(t)
Puncture wound, osteomyelitis as complication of, 598
Pyogenic osteomyelitis, 598–604, 599(t), *600–603*

Pyramidal level, lesion at, in neuromuscular disease, 353, 354–355(t)
  pes cavus in, 510
Pyruvate metabolism, hypertrophic interstitial neuritis, 504

Quadratus femoris muscle, congenital absence of, 507
Quadratus plantae muscle, anatomic relations of, *18*, *19*, *29–32*, *36*, *38*
  in congenital convex pes valgus, 246
  testing of, **110–111**
Quadriceps femoris muscle, congenital absence of, 507
  function of, in gait, 57, *58*
  innervation of, intrauterine posture and, 133, *133*
    neurosegmental, *421*
  in talipes equinus, in cerebral palsy, 373
  paralysis of, gait in, 61, *61*
Quadriplegia, definition of, 82
  in cerebral palsy, 360

Race, polydactylism and, 325
  talipes equinovarus incidence and, 139, 139(t)
Radiography. See *Roentgenography*.
Radionuclide bone imaging, in flexible pes planovalgus, 568
  in osteomyelitis, 599
  in stress fracture, 707
Range of motion, of joints, measurements of, 75–82, *76*, *78–84*
  of muscles for tendon transfer, principles of, 452
Reaction of degeneration, electrical testing and, 85
  in neuromuscular disease, 352, 354–355(t)
Rectus femoris muscle, in hip flexion deformity, *366*, 367, *367*
Recurrent tibial vein, anatomic relations of, *9*
Reduction (correction), loss of, in open reduction of talocalcaneonavicular joint, 208
Reflex(es), in cerebral palsy, 360, *361–364*
  automatic, as test of motor strength, 375
  in diastematomyelia, 449
  in Friedreich's ataxia, 501
  in hypertrophic interstitial neuritis, 503
  in myelomeningocele, 420, *421*
  in paralysis in neuromuscular disease, 352, 354–355(t)
  in peroneal muscular atrophy, 497
  innervation of, *421*
Reimann dynamic clubfoot splint, in talipes equinovarus, 184
Resorption, cortical, in stress fracture, 704
Retardation, in cerebral palsy, preoperative assessment in, 360
Rheumatic fever, vs. suppurative arthritis, 607
Rheumatoid arthritis, 608–610, *608*, *609*
  flat foot in, 557(t)
  hallux rigidus in, 631
  insufficiency fractures in, 703
  vs. Köhler's disease of tarsal navicular, 611
  vs. suppurative arthritis, 606

Rickets, ankle fracture in, 663
  insufficiency fractures in, 703
Rigidity, foot, after open reduction of talocalcaneonavicular joint, 210
Robert Jones strapping, application of, in talipes equinovarus, 180, *181*
Rocker-bottom deformity, in congenital convex pes valgus, *244*, 247, *247*, *566*
  in talipes equinovarus, 174, *175*
    as complication of manipulation, 182
Rocker-bottom flatfoot, congenital, 239. See also *Congenital convex pes valgus.*
Rocker-foot due to talonavicular dislocation, 239. See also *Congenital convex pes valgus.*
Roentgenography, for triple arthrodesis, 483
  in diagnosis, 84
  in diastematomyelia, 450, *450*
  in flexible pes planovalgus, 557–561, *559, 560, 562–565*
  in fractures, of ankle, 667, *671–677, 679, 682,* 690
    of Tillaux, 682, *684*
    stress, *704–706,* 705–707
    triplane, of tibia, 683, *685, 687, 688*
  in Freiberg's infraction of second metatarsal, 613, *613, 614*
  in hallux rigidus, 631, *632*
  in hypertrophic interstitial neuritis, 504
  in Köhler's disease of tarsal navicular, 611, *611*
  in osteochondritis dissecans of talus, 619, *620, 621*
  in osteomyelitis, 599, *600, 601, 603*
    of sesamoid bones, 603, *603*
  in pes cavus, 518, *518*
  in suppurative arthritis, 606
  in talipes equinovarus, 170–176, 170(t), *172–175*
    confirmation of reduction by, 182
  in tarsal coalition, *271–282,* 272–281
  in tuberculosis, 604
Rotation, angular, of joint, in gait, 50
  axial, in gait, 56, *65, 67, 70*
  medial and lateral, definition of, 77
Rotation deformity, in talipes equinovarus, 156, *156–159*
Rotation flap incision, 440, *440*
Rotator muscles, hip, neurosegmental innervation of, *421*
Roussy-Lévy syndrome, pes cavus in, 510
  vs. Friedreich's ataxia, 501
  vs. peroneal muscular atrophy, 498
Ryerson triple arthrodesis, 478, **480–483**

Sacrofemoral angle, in hip flexion deformity, 367
Salicylic acid, in skin lesions, 658
Salter-Harris classification of ankle fractures, 663, *664*
Samilson crescentic calcaneal osteotomy, 544, *544, 545,* **546–551**
Saphenous nerve(s), anatomic relations of, *8, 9, 11, 12, 17, 18, 36*
Saphenous vein(s), anatomic relations of, *8–12, 17, 18, 21, 24, 36*

Sarcoma, Ewing's, vs. stress fracture, 707
  osteogenic, 657, *657*
    vs. stress fracture, 707
Sartorious muscle, anatomic relations of, *3*
  function of, in gait, *58*
  neurosegmental innervation of, *421*
Schwann cell, tumors of, *647,* 649
Sciatic nerve, trauma of, pes cavus in, 510
Scoliosis, congenital, intrauterine posture and, 132, 132(t)
  diagnosis of, *44, 45,* 46
  in Friedreich's ataxia, 500
  in progressive muscular dystrophy, 505
Scottish-Rite operation (Lovell), in flexible pes planovalgus, 576
Scurvy, ankle fracture in, 663
  insufficiency fractures in, 703
Semimembranosus muscle, anatomic relations of, *3, 4*
  congenital absence of, 507
  function of, in gait, 58, *58*
  in hip adduction deformity, 368, *369*
  neurosegmental innervation of, *421*
Semitendinosus muscle, anatomic relations of, *3, 4*
  function of, in gait, 58, *58*
  in hip adduction deformity, 368, *369*
  neurosegmental innervation of, *421*
Sensory function, evaluation of, in myelomeningocele, 420, *420*
  in diastematomyelia, 450
  in Friedreich's ataxia, 501
  in hypertrophic interstitial neuritis, 503
  in neuromuscular disease, 353, 354–355(t)
  in peroneal muscular atrophy, 497
Septic (suppurative) arthritis, 605–608, *606*
Septum, intermuscular, anatomic relations of, *5, 8, 9*
Serpentine foot, 294. See also *Congenital metatarsus varus.*
Sesamoid bone(s), anatomic relations of, *19, 26, 35, 36*
  as normal variations, 130
  development and ossification of, 40
  excision of, in pes cavus, 545
  osteochondrosis of, 615
  osteomyelitis of, 601–603, *603*
  stress fracture of, 703
Sex, age of ossification and, in ankle fractures, 660
  congenital ball-and-socket ankle joint and, 313
  congenital metatarsus primus varus and, 308
  diastematomyelia and, 449
  Freiberg's infraction of second metatarsal and, 612
  hallux rigidus and, 627
  juvenile rheumatoid arthritis and, 608
  Köhler's disease of tarsal navicular and, 610
  myelomeningocele and, 419
  normal growth of foot and 121, 121(t), *122*
  osteochondritis dissecans and, 616
    of talus, 618
  osteomyelitis and, 598
  peroneal muscular atrophy and, 496
  polydactylism and, 325
  progressive muscular dystrophy and, 505, 505(t)

Sex (*Continued*)
  subungual exostosis and, 657
  talipes equinovarus and, 139
Shearing injury, in ankle fractures, 663
Shock absorbers, muscles as, in gait, 57, *58*
Shoe(s), abnormal wear of, in hallux rigidus, 631
  correction of congenital metatarsus varus and, 297
  examination of, diagnostic, 44
  in congenital metatarsus primus varus and hallux valgus, 310
  in flexible pes planovalgus, 568, *570*
  in pes cavus, 519, *519*
  in talipes equinovalgus, 402
  in talipes equinovarus, outflare (tarsal pronator), 185, *186*
    prewalker clubfoot, 184, *185*
  in talipes equinus, 377
Short-leg limp, 62
Siffert "beak" triple arthrodesis, in pes cavus, 538, *539, 540*
Silfverskiöld gastrocnemius recession, in talipes equinus, 383, *386*
Silfverskiöld test, in talipes equinus, 370, *371*
Sinus tarsi, anatomic relations of, *10, 20, 21*
Sitting balance, in cerebral palsy, 360, *364*
Skewfoot, 294, See also *Congenital metatarsus varus.*
Skin, 658–660, *659*
  in clinical appearance in talipes equinovarus, 160, *161, 162,* 163(t)
  in diastematomyelia, 449
  in hallux rigidus, 631
  in hemangioma, 637, *640*
  sensory innervation of, 420, *420*
Sliding lengthening, heel cord, in congenitally short triceps surae muscle, 509
  in talipes equinus, 377, **378–380,** *381, 382*
  posterior tibial muscle, in pes varus, 398, *398*
Smillie procedure, in osteochondritis dissecans of talus, 621
Soft corn, 658, *659*
Soft tissues, in congenital convex pes valgus, stretching of, 251
  in congenital metatarsus varus, 301, **302–305**
  in flexible pes planovalgus, 571, 574(t), 576, **578–587**
  in fractures of foot, 701
  in talipes equinovarus, 151–160, *152–159*
    nonoperative elongation of, 176, *177–179*
    surgical release of, in myelomeningocele, 439
      in open reduction of talocalcaneonavicular joint, **194–207**
    in triple arthrodesis, 224
  tumors of, 635–655, *636–652*
Sole, ganglion of, 637, *639*
Soleus muscle. See also *Triceps surae muscle.*
  accessory, *506,* 508
  vs. congenital contracture of triceps surae muscle, 509
  anatomic relations of, *3, 4, 6, 9, 10, 16, 37*
  function of, in gait, 57, *58*
  in talipes equinovarus, 151
  in talipes equinus, 370, *371*
    lengthening of, 383, *385*

Soleus muscle (*Continued*)
  neurosegmental innervation of, *421*
  paralysis of, deformities and, 456–457(t), 458, 465, *470–473, 476–478*
    gait in, 61, *62*
  testing of, **104–105**
Solitary fibroma, 649
Spasm, as muscle response to pain, 356
  flexor, in hallux rigidus, 627
  in diagnosis of deformities, 68
  in rheumatoid arthritis, 609
  peroneal tendon, tarsal coalition and, *269,* 271
Spastic cerebral palsy, 360. See also *Cerebral palsy.*
Spasticity, gait in, 63
  paralysis in, muscle testing in, 82, 86–87(t)
  vs. tension athetosis, in cerebral palsy, 370
Speech, in Friedreich's ataxia, 501
  in hypertrophic interstitial neuritis, 504
Spina ventosa, 604
Spinal ataxia, gait in, 63
Spinal cord, affections of, flat foot in, 557(t)
  in Freidreich's ataxia, 500
  lesion of, in pes cavus, 510
Spinal level, lesion at, paralysis in, 353, 354–355(t)
Spine, abnormalities of, talipes equinovarus and, 162, *164*
  cogenital postural deformities of, 132, 132(t)
  examination of, *44, 45,* 46
  fetal, for myelomeningocele, 422
  in diastematomyelia, 449, *450*
  in myelomeningocele, 418
Spinocerebellar tracts, heredofamilial disease of, pes cavus in, 510
Spinomuscular level, lesion at, paralysis in, 352, 354–355(t)
Splint(s), Denis Browne, contraindicated in congenital metatarsus varus, 297
  in congenital postural talipes calcaneovalgus, 136
  in congenital postural talipes varus, 137
  in rheumatoid arthritis, 609
  in suppurative arthritis, 607
  in talipes equinovarus, 184
  night. See *Night splints.*
Split foot, congenital, 317–322, *318–322*
Spring ligament. See *Calcaneonavicular (spring) ligament.*
Spurs, calcific, in hallux rigidus, 631, *633*
  in osteomyelitis of calcaneus, *600*
Stability, foot and ankle operations for, history of, 477, 483(t)
  in talipes equinovarus, 221
  in development of mature gait, 59
Stabilizers, muscles as, in gait, 57, *58*
Stance, as phase of gait, 46–50, *49*
  balance in, in cerebral palsy, 360, *368*
  examination of, 44, *48*
  heel position in, 45, *48*
  in progressive muscular dystrophy, 505
  posture in, requirements for, 356, *356*
Staphylococcus, in osteomyelitis, 601
Staphylococcus aureus, in suppurative arthritis, 605
Steindler stripping operation, in pes cavus, 523
Step length, in gait, *49,* 50

Step length (*Continued*)
  in mature gait, 59
Steppage gait, muscle paralysis in, 61
Steroids, adrenal, in hypertrophic interstitial neuritis, 504
Stewart Achilles tendon switch operation, in talipes equinovarus, 213
Stieda's process, ossification of talus and, 126
Strapping, adhesive, in talipes equinovarus, 439
    Robert Jones, application of, 180, *181*
Strayer gastrocnemius recession, in talipes equinus, 383, *387*
Streeter's dysplasia, talipes equinovarus in, 164, *165*
Strength, muscle. See *Muscle(s), strength of.*
Strength-duration curve, in neuromuscular excitability testing, 118
Streptococcus hemolyticus, in suppurative arthritis, 605
Stress fractures, 703–709, *704–706*
Stretching exercises. See *Exercise(s), stretching.*
Stride length, in gait, *49,* 50
Stromeyer subcutaneous tenotomy of Achilles tendon, 383, *383*
Strumpell test, of motor strength in cerebral palsy, 375
Subcutaneous section of plantar aponeurosis, in pes cavus, 522, **524–525**
Subluxation, dorsal, in open reduction of talocalcaneonavicular joint, 208, *208*
  of talocalcaneonavicular joint, in talipes equinovarus, 139
Subtalar joint(s), arthrodesis of, extra-articular, Batchelor, 410, *410, 411*
    Grice, 403, **404–407,** *408, 409*
    in poliomyelitis, 487
    in flexible pes planovalgus, 575(t), 577, *588, 589*
    in congenital convex pes valgus, 243, *244*
    in pantalar arthrodesis, 488
    in talipes equinovarus, 176, *177,* 188–189(t), 221
    in triple arthrodesis, 477
  motion in, ball-and-socket ankle joint and, 313
  nonoperative elongation of, 176, *177*
  pigmented villonodular synovitis of, *650*
  rheumatoid arthritis of, 609
  suppurative arthritis of, 605
  tarsal coalition symptoms and, 269, *269, 271*
Subungual exostosis, 655, *656*
Supination, definition of, 77
  range of motion in, 81, *83*
Supination-inversion ankle fracture, 667, 668(t), *670–676*
  treatment of, 690, *690*
  varus deformity as complication of, *694,* 695, *695, 697*
Supination–lateral rotation ankle fracture, 667, 668(t), *678–680*
  treatment of, 692, *692*
Supination–plantar flexion ankle fracture, 667, 668(t), *676, 677*
  treatment of, 691, *691*
Suppurative (septic) arthritis, 605–608, *606*
Supramalleolar osteotomy, for varus deformity after ankle fracture, 695, *696, 697*

Supramalleolar osteotomy (*Continued*)
  Wiltse, in valgus ankle in myelomeningocele, 438, *438*
Sural nerve, anatomic relations of, *8, 9, 21, 24*
Sustentaculum tali, anatomic relations of, *16–19, 23, 34*
  in congenital convex pes valgus, 243
  in flexible pes planovalgus, 557(t)
  in talipes equinovarus, 152
  in tarsal coalition, 262, *263, 275, 277, 278*
Swelling, in Köhler's disease of tarsal navicular, 611
  in osteomyelitis, 599
  in suppurative arthritis, 606
  popliteal, accessory hamstring muscle as, 508, *508*
Swing phase, of gait, *49, 50*
Switch operation (Stewart), on Achilles tendon, in talipes equinovarus, 213
Symmetrical tonic neck reflex, in cerebral palsy, 360, *363*
Symphalangism, in embryo, 40
  tarsal coalition and, 262, 262(t), *264, 265*
Synchondrosis, in tarsal coalition, 262
Syndactylism, 335, *335–337*
  surgical, in congenital curly toe, 346
  in congenital digitus minimus varus, 338
  tarsal coalition and, *226,* 267
Syndesmosis, in tarsal coalition, 262
Synergists, muscle function as, 356
Synkinesia, as test of motor strength, in cerebral palsy, 375
Synostosis, tarsal, 261. See also *Tarsal coalition* and names of specific synostoses.
Synovioma, 652, 655
Synovitis, pigmented villonodular, 649, *650*
Syphilis, dactylitis in, vs. tuberculous dactylitis, 604
  vs. hypertrophic interstitial neuritis, 504
Syringomyelia, paralysis at spinal level in, 353, 354–355(t)

Talectomy, in talipes calcaneus, 485
  in talipes equinovarus, 192, 225
  in myelomeningocele, 441
  subtotal, in pes cavovarus, 552
Talipes calcaneovalgus, congenital postural, 131, 134–137, *135*
  flat foot in, 557(t)
  in myelomeningocele, 425(t), *426*
  muscle paralysis and, in poliomyelitis, 456–457(t)
  vs. congenital convex pes valgus, 250
Talipes calcaneus, in cerebral palsy, 414, *414*
  in myelomeningocele, 424–429, 425(t), *426, 427, 429,* **430–433**
  muscle paralysis and, in poliomyelitis, 456–457(t)
  paralytic, bone block operations in, 492
  posture and, 358, *359*
  wedge resections for in triple arthrodesis, 485, *486*
Talipes cavus, congenital pes cavus as, 514
Talipes equinovalgus, in cerebral palsy, 402–414, **404–407,** *408–411, 413*
  muscle paralysis and, in poliomyelitis, 456–457(t), 459, *464*

Talipes equinovarus, 139–239
  brachymetatarsia and, 317
  congenital convex pes valgus with, 240
  diagnosis of, 160, *161, 162*, 163(t), *164–169*
  etiology of, 140, *143*, 144(t)
  heredity in, 139, 140(t)
  in cerebral palsy, 373, *374*
  in myelomeningocele, *419*, 424, 425(t), 438–441, *438–440*
  incidence of, 139, 139(t)
  muscle paralysis and, in poliomyelitis, 456–457(t), 465, *465*
  pathology of, 144, *145–148, 150–159*
  roentgenography in, 170, 170(t), *172–175*
  treatment of, nonoperative, 176, *177–179, 181, 183, 185, 186*
    complications of, 186, *187*
    operative, 186, *187*, 188–191(t), *193, 208, 210, 216, 220*
      Dwyer medial osteotomy of calcaneus in, **222–223**
      open reduction of talocaneonavicular joint in, **194–207**
      shortening lateral column of foot in, **218–219**
    strapping in, 180, *181*, 439
  vs. congenital metatarsus varus, 297
  vs. postural clubfoot, 162, 163(t)
Talipes equinus. See also *Equinus deformity, forefoot.*
  conservative management of, 375
  in cerebral palsy, 370–398, *371–376*
  in congenital contracture of triceps surae muscle, 509
  in myelomeningocele, 424, 425(t), 441, *441*
  muscle paralysis and, in poliomyelitis, 456–457(t), 459
  posture and, 358, *358, 359*
  surgical treatment of, 377, **378–380**, *381–387*, **390–397**
Talipes valgus. See also *Pes valgus.*
  flat foot in, 557(t)
  in myelomeningocele, 429–438, *434, 435,* **436–437,** *438*
  postural congenital, 131, 137
Talipes varus, congenital postural, 131, *136,* 137
  in cerebral palsy, 398–402, *398–401*
  in peroneal muscular atrophy, 496, *497*
  osteotomies and wedge resections for, in triple arthrodesis, 483, *484*
Talocalcaneal angle, in congenital convex pes valgus, 243, 249
  measurement of, in talipes equinovarus, 172, *172*
Talocalcaneal coalition, 261, *263, 267,* 268, *276–280*
  in embryo, 40, *40*
  medial, surgical treatment of, 284
Talocalcaneal index, in talipes equinovarus, 174
Talocalcaneal joint, in flexible pes planovalgus, 557, *557, 559, 560, 564, 565*
Talocalcaneal ligament(s), anatomic relations of, *15, 19, 22, 23*
  in congenital convex pes valgus, 244, *245*
Talocalcaneonavicular joint, closed reduction of, *179*, 182, 252

Talocalcaneonavicular joint (*Continued*)
  dorsolateral dislocation of, 239–261. See also *Congenital convex pes valgus.*
  in talipes equinovarus, 139, 144, *145, 147, 148*
    mechanics of, 153, *153–155*
    reduction of, closed, *179*, 182
      open, 187–227, 188–191(t), *193, 208, 210, 216, 220.* See also entry for *open reduction of, procedures for.*
    in myelomeningocele, 439
    roentgenography of, 170
  open reduction of, complications of, 192
    Dwyer open-up medial calcaneal osteotomy in, **222–223**
    procedures for, **194–207, 254–259**
    shortening lateral column of foot in, **218–219**
  soft-tissue procedures in, 192
  suppurative arthritis of, 607
Talo–first metatarsal angle, measurement of, 172, *172, 174*
Talonavicular coalition, 261, 262(t), 268, 271, 280
Talonavicular joint, in flexible pes planovalgus, 557, *559, 560, 562–565*
  in pantalar arthrodesis, 488
  in pes cavus, 532
  in triple arthrodesis, 477
Talonavicular ligament, anatomic relations of, 22
  in congenital convex pes valgus, 244, *245, 246*
Talotibial ligament, anatomic relations of, *19*
Talus, accessory bone of, os sustentaculi as, *123, 128*
  os trigonum as, *123,* 125, *126, 127*
  africoid, as normal variation, 128, *129*
  anatomic relations of, *1, 10, 15, 16, 19, 20, 22, 23, 25, 26, 35, 36, 38*
  "beaking" of, in tarsal coalition, 279, *280, 281*
  development and ossification of, 40, *40, 42, 43*
  excision of. See *Talectomy.*
  fractures of, 701
    vs. os trigonum, 126, *126, 127*
  in congenital convex pes valgus, 243, *244, 247*
  in flexible pes planovalgus, 557, *557, 559, 560, 562–565*
  in talipes equinovarus, articular malalignment of, 149, *150–152, 154, 155–159*
    aseptic necrosis of, in open reduction of talocalcaneonavicular joint, 209
    deformities of, 145–148, *145–148*
    nonoperative manipulation of, *178, 179,* 180
  osteochondritis dissecans of, 618, *618–621,* **622–625**
  osteoid osteoma of, *653*
  osteomyelitis of, 598, *601*
  tuberculous, 604
Talus secundarius, as normal variation, *123*
Tarsal coalition, 261–294
  classification of, 262, 262(t)
  clinical features of, 268, *269, 270*
  congenital ball-socket ankle joint and, 313

Tarsal coalition (*Continued*)
  etiology of, 267, *267*
  flat foot in, 557(t)
    peroneal spastic, vs. congenital convex pes valgus, 251
  heredity in, 268
  incidence of, 262, 262(t)
  roentgenographic findings in, *270–282*, 272
  treatment of, 282, *283*, **286–291**
Tarsal pronator shoes, contraindicated in congenital metatarsus varus, 297
  in talipes equinovarus, 185, *186*
Tarsometatarsal joints, Lisfranc's fracture-dislocation of, 702
  mobilization of, in congenital metatarsus varus, 301, **302–305**
  roentgenography of, in talipes equinovarus, 170
  tuberculous arthritis of, 604
Tarsometatarsal ligaments, anatomic relations of, *15, 19, 22, 34*
Tarsus, bones of, fetal relationships of, 240, *240*
  development of, embryonic, 39, *40, 42*
  reconstruction of, in talipes equinovarus, 192
  in triple arthrodesis, 225, **480–483**
Tenderness, in Köhler's disease of tarsal navicular, 611
  in osteochondritis dissecans of talus, 619
  in osteomyelitis, 599
  in suppurative arthritis, 606
Tendinitis, Achilles, 509
Tendo Achillis. See *Achilles tendon*.
Tendon(s). See also names of specific muscles.
  Achilles. See *Achilles tendon*.
  in congenital convex pes valgus, 244–247, *246, 247*
  in talipes equinovarus, 152, 160
  transfer of. See *Tendon transfer(s)*.
Tendon transfer(s), 452–572
  Achilles, Jones, 573, *576*
    lateral (Axer and Segal), 214
    Murphy, 388, *389*, **392–393**
  anterior and posterior tibial, to navicular (Giannestras), 577, **578–587**
  anterior tibial, lateral, 210, 459
    posterior, *427, 428*, **430–433**
    split, 401, *401*
    to first metatarsal base, 526, *527*
  flexor hallucis longus, for dorsal bunion, **474–475**
  in claw toes, 555
  in flexible pes planovalgus, 571, 574(t), *576*, **578–587**
  in pes varus in cerebral palsy, 398, *399, 400, 401*
  in poliomyelitis, 452, 456–457(t), *458*, **460–463**, *464, 465*, **466–469**, *470–473*, **474–475**, *476–478*
  in talipes equinovarus, 210
  long toe extensor, in pes cavus, 523, **528–529**
  peroneus longus, anterior, to base of second metatarsal, **460–463**
    posterior, in pes calcaneus, *427, 428*, **430–433**

Tendon transfer(s) (*Continued*)
  posterior tibial, in peroneal muscular atrophy, 499
    through interosseous membrane, 398, **466–469**
  postoperative care and training in, 454
  principles of, 452
Tenotomy, subcutaneous (Stromeyer), of Achilles tendon, 383, *383*
Tension athetosis, vs. spasticity, in cerebral palsy, 370
Tensor fasciae latae, function of, in gait, 57, *58*
  neurosegmental innervation of, *421*
Tetany, electrical stimulation in diagnosis of, 118
Tetraplegia, definition of, 82
Thomas heel, in flexible pes planovalgus, 568
  in Köhler's disease of tarsal navicular, 612
Thomas test, for hip flexion contracture, 69, *73*
  side-lying, in cerebral palsy, *366, 367*
Thomsen's disease, electrical stimulation in diagnosis of, 118
Thompson Z-plasty, in congenital digitus minimus varus, 338
Thurston Holland sign, in ankle fracture, 665
Tibia, anatomic relations of, *3–5, 7–17, 19, 20, 22–25, 37, 38*
  bone graft from, in Grice procedure, **406–407**, 408
  complications of ankle fracture and, *694–697*, 695
  fracture of, comminuted, 689, *689*
    of Tillaux, 669(t), 682, *683, 684*, 693, *693*
    stress, 703, 706, *706*
    triplane, 669(t), 683, *685–688*
  hypoplasia or absence of, polydactylism and, 325
  in talipes equinovarus, *147,* 149, *157, 158*
    damage to, in nonoperative treatment, 187, *187*
  osteotomy of, 192, 226
  ossification of, development and, 41, *42, 43*
  in fractures of ankle, 660, *661*
  osteochondrosis of, 615
  osteoid osteoma of, *654*
  rotation of, in gait, 56, *65, 67, 70*
  rotation osteotomy of, medial, 192
  torsion of, foot alignment for arthrodesis and, 482, *483*
Tibial nerve, anatomic relations of, *6, 8, 9, 18, 24*
  neurectomy of motor branches of, 388, *390–391*
Tibial spine, in osteochondritis dissecans, 617
Tibialis anterior muscle. See *Anterior tibial muscle (tendon)*.
Tibialis posterior muscle. See *Posterior tibial muscle (tendon)*.
Tibiocalcaneal angle, measurement of, 174
Tibiofibular ligaments, anatomic relations of, *15, 22, 23*
Tibiofibular supramalleolar osteotomy, in valgus ankle, 435, *438*
Tibionavicular ligament, in congenital convex pes valgus, 244, *245, 246*

Tibionavicular ligament (*Continued*)
  in talipes equinovarus, 152, *152, 177,* 180, 188–189(t)
Tibiotalar angle, measurement of, 174
Tibiotalar joint, roentgenography of in talipes equinovarus, 170
Ticarcillin, in osteomyelitis, 599(t)
Tillaux, ankle fracture of, 669(t), 682, *683, 684*
  treatment of, 693, *693*
Tilting reactions, in cerebral palsy, 360, *364*
Toe(s), absence of, tarsal coalition and, 262(t), 266
  acquired affections of, 627–635
  claw, 554, *554, 555*
  cock-up deformity of, muscle paralysis and, 456–457(t), 459
  convergent or divergent, 335, *338*
  fifth, congenital dorsal overriding of, 335, *339,* **340–341**, *342, 343*
  ganglion between, 637, *637*
  in cerebral palsy, 371, *372,* 415
  in congenital metatarsus primus varus and hallux valgus, 308, *308, 309, 311*
  in pes cavus, 516, *516,* 520
  macrodactylism of, *332–334,* 333
  muscles of, extensor, in peroneal muscular atrophy, 498, *498*
    flexor, in talipes equinus, 371, *372*
  normal variations of, 130
  range of motion of, 81, *83, 84*
Toeing-in, in flexible pes planovalgus, 558, *558,* 567
Toe-raising test, of Jack, 567, *567*
Toenail, ingrowing, 660
Tomography, computed, in flexible pes planovalgus, 568
  in stress fracture, 707
  in talipes equinovarus, 174
Tongue-in-groove lengthening (Baker), of gastrocnemius aponeurosis, 383, *386*
Torus fracture, in nonoperative treatment of talipes equinovarus, 187
Transplantation, definition of, 452
Transverse breach, in talipes equinovarus, 174, *175*
Transverse crural ligament, anatomic relations of, *3, 11, 17, 21*
Trauma, aneurysm from, 637, *645*
  flat foot from, 557(t)
  muscle response to, 356
  osteochondritis dissecans from, 616
  sciatic nerve, pes cavus in, 510
Trendelenburg test, 46, *47*
Triceps surae muscle. See also *Gastrocnemius muscle* and *Soleus muscle*
  action of, deformities and, in poliomyelitis, 458
  in gait, 57, *58*
  anatomic relations of, *16, 17, 19–21, 24*
  contracture of, congenital, 508
    flat foot in, 557(t), 559
    in flexible pes planovalgus, passive stretching of, 568, *569*
      toe-raising test for, 567
    pes valgus with, vs. congenital convex pes valgus, 250

Triceps surae muscle (*Continued*)
  in cerebral palsy, 227, 370, *371,* 378–380, *381–387,* 402, 414
  in claw toes, 554
  in congenital convex pes valgus, 244, *246, 247*
  in myelomeningocele, 425, *427,* 439
  in pes cavus, 512
  in progressive muscular dystrophy, 505
  in talipes equinovalgus, 402
  in talipes equinovarus, 160, 439
    nonoperative elongation of, 176, *177*
  in talipes equinus, 277, 370, *371,* 378–380, *381–387*
  innervation of, intrauterine posture and, 133, *133*
  lengthening of, 277, 378–380, *381–387*
    pes calcaneus from, 414
  paralysis of, deformities and, 456–457(t), 458, 465, *465*
    gait in, 61, *62*
    testing of, **104–105**
Triplane fracture, of ankle, 669(t), 683, *685–688*
  treatment of, 693
Triple arthrodesis, 477, **478–481**
  ball-and-socket ankle joint following, 313
  "beak", in pes cavus, 538, *539, 540*
  in cerebral palsy, 487
  in flexible pes planovalgus (Williams and Menelaus), 575(t), **590–591**
  in paralytic pes cavovarus, 540
  in peroneal muscular atrophy, 499
  in talipes equinovarus, 192, 224
  in tarsal coalition, 284
  posterior tibial artery aneurysm from, 637, *645*
Trisomy, autosomal, congenital convex pes valgus with, 240
Trunk, lower limb and, interdependence of, 356–358, *356–359*
Tuberculosis, 604–605
Tuberculous arthritis, 604
Tuberculous dactylitis, 604
Tumors, 635–658. See also specific types of tumor.
  bone, 653–657, *655*
  intraspinal, vs. hypertrophic interstitial neuritis, 504
  pathologic fractures in, 703
  soft-tissue, 635, *636–652*
  spinal cord, paralysis from spinal level lesion in, 353, *354–355*(t)
    pes cavus in, 510

UCBL foot orthosis. See *University of California Biomechanics Laboratory foot orthosis.*
Ulceration, in pes calcaneus, in myelomeningocele, 426
Ultrasound in antenatal diagnosis of myelomeningocele, 422
Unicameral bone cyst, 655, *655, 656*
University of California Biomechanics Laboratory foot orthosis, in flexible pes planovalgus, 570, *570*

University of California Biomechanics Laboratory foot orthosis (*Continued*)
  in talipes equinovalgus, 402
  in tarsal coalition, 282
Upper limb, motion of, in gait, 57

V-osteotomy (Japas), of tarsus, in pes cavus, 532, **534–537**
V- and Y-plasty, Wilson and DuVries, in congenital digitus minimus varus, 338
Valgus angulation, in diagnosis of deformities, 75
Valgus deformity. See *Pes valgus* and *Talipes valgus*.
Vancomycin, in osteomyelitis, 599(t)
Varus angulation, in diagnosis of deformities, 75
Varus deformity. See also *Talipes varus*.
  ankle, as complication of ankle fracture, *694*, 695, *695*, *697*
  forefoot, as complication of open reduction of talocalcaneonavicular joint, 209, *210*
  hindfoot, in pes cavus, bony procedures for, 540, *541*, **542–543**, *544*, *545*, **546–551**
  in Friedreich's ataxia, 502
  muscle paralysis and, in poliomyelitis, 456–457(t), 458, *458*
Vein(s). See names of specific veins.
Velocity, in gait, 50, 59
Venous arch, dorsal, anatomic relations of, *11*, *12*
Verruca plantaris, 659
Vertebra(e), in diastematomyelia, 449, *450*
  segmentation failure of, congenital ball-and-socket ankle joint and, 313
Vertical opening-wedge osteotomy (Fowler), in pes cavus, 526, *527*, 532
Vertical talus, congenital, 239. See also *Congenital convex pes valgus*.
Villonodular synovitis, pigmented, 649, *650*
Viral infection, poliomyelitis as, 451
Vitamin deficiency, insufficiency fractures in, 703
Vulpius technique, for gastrocnemius lengthening, 383, *385*

Walk cycle, 46, *49*. See also *Gait*.
Walking. See *Ambulation* and *Gait*.
Wart, plantar, 659

Watermann cuneiform osteotomy, in hallux rigidus, 633, *633*
Weakness, in peroneal muscular atrophy, 497
  isolated, of peroneus brevis muscle, in pes cavus, 511
Webbing, congenital, of toes, 335, *336*
Weight, ambulation and, in myelomeningocele, 424
  tarsal coalition symptoms and, 269
Weight-bearing, flexible pes planovalgus and, 557, *558–560*, *562–566*, 568
  in brachymetatarsia, 316
Werdnig-Hoffmann disease, spinal level lesion in, 353, 354–355(t)
White sliding heel cord lengthening, 377, **378–380**, *381*, *382*
Williams and Menelaus triple arthrodesis, 575(t), 588, **590–591**
Wilson and DuVries V- and Y-plasty, in congenital digitus minimus varus, 338
Wiltse tibial osteotomy, for valgus deformity, after ankle fracture, 699
  in myelomeningocele, 438, *438*
Wound, complications of in open reduction of talocalcaneonavicular joint, dehiscence as, 192
  infection as, 209
  puncture, osteomyelitis as complication of, 598
Wrist, radial and ulnar deviation of, definition of, 77

Xanthomatosis, multiple, *648*, 649

Y ligament, anatomic relations of, *15*, *22*
  in congenital convex pes valgus, 244, *245*
  in talipes equinovarus, 188–189(t)
Y-plasty, Goodwin and Swisher, in congenital digitus minimus varus, 338

Z-plasty, Achilles tendon, 383, *384*
  with Dwyer calcaneal, osteotomy, 217, *220*
  posterior tibial tendon, 211
  Thompson, in congenital digitus minimus varus, 338